The GALE ENCYCLOPEDIA *of* PUBLIC HEALTH

The GALE ENCYCLOPEDIA *of* PUBLIC HEALTH

VOLUME

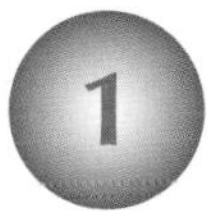

A–L

LAURIE J. FUNDUKIAN, EDITOR

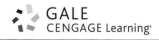

GALE
CENGAGE Learning

Detroit • New York • San Francisco • New Haven, Conn • Waterville, Maine • London

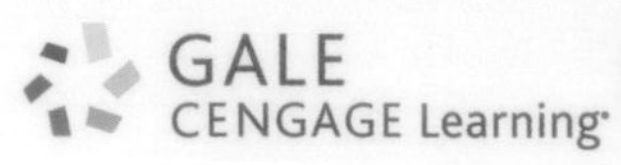

The Gale Encyclopedia of Public Health

Project Editor: Laurie J. Fundukian

Product Manager: Kate Hanley

Editorial Support Services: Andrea Lopeman

Indexing Services: Hawkeye Indexing

Rights Acquisition and Management: Sheila Spencer

Composition: Evi Abou-El-Seoud

Manufacturing: Wendy Blurton

Imaging: John Watkins

Product Design: Kristine Julien

LIBRARY OF CONGRESS CATALOGING-IN-PUBLICATION DATA

The Gale encyclopedia of public health / Laurie J. Fundukian, editor. –
First edition.
2 volumes ; cm
Summary: "Alphabetically arranged encyclopedia contains approximately 257 entries pertaining to important Public Health concerns. Topics include diseases and conditions, health and wellness efforts, nutrition, ethics and law related topics and statistics, sanitation issues, everyday environmental effects and more. Contains images, tables, and illustrations"– Provided by publisher.
Includes bibliographical references and index.
ISBN-13: 978-1-4144-9876-8 (set : hardback)
ISBN-10: 1-4144-9876-4 (set : hardback)
ISBN-13: 978-1-4144-9877-5 (v. 1 : hardback)
ISBN-10: 1-4144-9877-2 (v. 1 : hardback)
[etc.]
1. Public health–Encyclopedias. I. Fundukian, Laurie J.
RA423.G35 2013
362.103–dc23
2012051201

Gale
27500 Drake Rd.
Farmington Hills, MI, 48331-3535

ISBN-13: 978-1-4144-9876-8 (set) ISBN-10: 1-4144-9876-4 (set)
ISBN-13: 978-1-4144-9877-5 (vol. 1) ISBN-10: 1-4144-9877-2 (vol. 1)
ISBN-13: 978-1-4144-9878-2 (vol. 2) ISBN-10: 1-4144-7878-0 (vol. 2)

This title is also available as an e-book.
ISBN-13: 978-1-4144-9879-9 ISBN-10: 1-4144-9879-9
Contact your Gale, a part of Cengage Learning sales representative for ordering information.

Printed in China
1 2 3 4 5 6 7 17 16 15 14 13

CONTENTS

ALPHABETICAL LIST OF ENTRIES

F

G

H

I

J

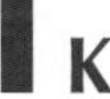

K

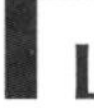

L

M

N

O

P

Public health administration
Public health engineers
Public Health Foundation
Public health nurses

Q

Q fever
Quarantine and isolation

R

Rabies
Radiation
Refugee health
Reproductive health
Ringworm
Risk factors and assessment
Road traffic safety
Rotavirus
Rubella
Rural health

S

Safe sex
Salmonella
Sanitation
Scarlet fever
Schistosomiasis
School health
Scurvy
Secondhand smoke
Senior health
Severe acute respiratory syndrome (SARS)
Sexual assault
Sexually transmitted diseases
Shigellosis
Shingles
Sick building syndrome
Sleep deprivation
Small pox
Smoking
Society for Public Health Educators (SOPHE)
Sociologists
Sodium
Staphylococcal infections
Stress
Stroke
Substance abuse and dependence
Suicide
Sun protection
Syphilis

T

Tetanus
Tobacco control
Trachoma
Travel health
Tuberculosis
Tularaemia
Typhoid fever
Typhus

U

United States Public Health Service

V

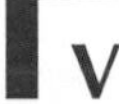

Vaccination
Variant Creutzfeldt-Jakob Disease
Veterinary medicine
Violence
Visual health
Vitamins

W

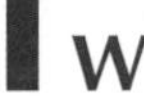

Water
West nile virus
Whooping cough
Women's health
Workplace safety
World Health Organization

Y

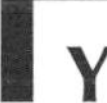

Yellow fever

Z

Zoonosis

PLEASE READ—IMPORTANT INFORMATION

The *Gale Encyclopedia of Public Health* is a health reference product designed to inform and educate readers about a wide variety of subjects pertaining to public health, such as diseases, related organizations, laws and industries, and practices and population. The Gale Group believes the product to be comprehensive, but not necessarily definitive. It is intended to supplement, not replace, consultation with a physician or other healthcare practitioners. While The Gale Group has made substantial efforts to provide information that is accurate, comprehensive, and up-to-date, The Gale Group makes no representations or warranties of any kind, including without limitation, warranties of merchantability or fitness for a particular purpose, nor does it guarantee the accuracy, comprehensiveness, or timeliness of the information contained in this product. Readers should be aware that the universe of medical knowledge is constantly growing and changing, and that differences of opinion exist among authorities. Readers are also advised to seek professional diagnosis and treatment for any medical condition, and to discuss information obtained from this book with their healthcare provider.

INTRODUCTION

The *Gale Encyclopedia of Public Health* is a source for readers who are looking to investigate health topics that effect the public. The encyclopedia minimizes medical jargon and uses language that any reader can understand, while still providing thorough coverage of each topic.

SCOPE

257 full-length articles are included in *The Gale Encyclopedia of Public Health*. Entries follow a standardized format that provides information at a glance. An example of such a format:

Diseases and conditions

- Definition
- Demographics
- Description
- Causes and symptoms
- Diagnosis
- Treatment
- Prognosis
- Prevention
- Effects on Public health
- Costs to Society

INCLUSION CRITERIA

A preliminary list of public health topics was compiled from a wide variety of sources, including professional medical guides and textbooks, as well as consumer guides and encyclopedias. An advisory board comprised of professionals in public health and medicine evaluated the topics and made suggestions for inclusion. The final selections were determined by Gale editors in conjunction with the advisory board.

ABOUT THE CONTRIBUTORS

The entries were written by experienced medical writers, including healthcare practitioners and educators, pharmacists, researchers, and other professionals. The essays were reviewed by advisors to ensure that they are appropriate, up-to-date, and accurate.

HOW TO USE THIS BOOK

The Gale Encyclopedia of Public Health has been designed with ready reference in mind:

- A timeline of historic events that were important within the scope and development of Public Health (which you'll find just before the entries begin)
- Straight **alphabetical arrangement** of topics allows users to locate information quickly.
- **Bold-faced terms** within entries direct the reader to related articles.
- Lists of **key terms** are provided where appropriate to define unfamiliar terms or concepts. A **glossary** of key terms is also included at the back of Volume 2.
- **Cross-references** placed throughout the *Encyclopedia* direct readers to primary entries from alternate names, drug brand names, and related topics.
- **Questions to Ask Your Doctor** sidebars provide sample questions that patients can ask their physicians.
- **Resources** at the end of every entry direct readers to additional sources of information on a topic.
- Valuable **contact information** for organizations and support groups is included with each entry and compiled in the back of Volume 2.
- A comprehensive **general index** at the back of Volume 2 allows users to easily find areas of interest.

GRAPHICS

The Gale Encyclopedia of Public Health is enhanced with approximately 200 full-color images, including photographs, tables, and custom illustrations.

INTRODUCTION

ADVISORY BOARD

Thank you to the following experts in health for providing invaluable assistance in the formulation of this encyclopedia. Advisors listed have also acted as contributing advisors—writing various articles related to their fields of expertise and experience.

Tamra J. Fairchild
MPH Health Educator and Public Information Officer
Wood County Health District
Genoa, Ohio

L. Fleming Fallon, Jr.
Distinguished Professor; MD, Dr. PH
Public Health
Bowling Green University
Bowling Green, OH

Brenda Wilmoth Lerner
Infectious disease specialist; R.N.
L&L Publishing, LLC
Montrose, AL

CONTRIBUTORS

Margaret Alic, Ph.D.
Science Writer
Eastsound, Washington

William Arthur Atkins
Science Writer
Atkins Research and Consulting
Pekin, Illinois

Rosalyn Carson-DeWitt, M.D.
Medical Writer
Durham, NC

Laura Jean Cataldo, RN, Ed.D.
Medical Writer
Myersville, MD

Rhonda Cloos, R.N.
Medical Writer
Austin, TX

Tish Davidson, A.M.
Medical Writer
Fremont, California

L. Fleming Fallon Jr., M.D., Dr. PH
Associate Professor of Public Health
Bowling Green State University
Bowling Green, OH

Karl Finley
Medical Writer
West Bloomfield, MI

Rebecca Frey, Ph.D.
Research and Administrative Associate
East Rock Institute
New Haven, Connecticut

Frances Hodgkins
Medical writer
Rockport, Maine

Sally J. Jacobs, Ed.D.
Medical Writer
Los Angeles, CA

Monique Laberge, PhD
Research Associate
Department of Biochemistry and Biophysics
University of Pennsylvania
Philadelphia, Pennsylvania

Leslie Mertz, PhD
Medical writer
Kalkaska, Michigan

David E. Newton
Medical Writer
Ashland, Oregon

Andrea Nienstedt, M.A.
Medical Writer
Lake Orion, Michigan

Melinda Granger Oberleitner, RN, DNS
Acting Department Head and Associate Professor
Department of Nursing
University of Louisiana at Lafayette
Lafayette, Louisiana

Teresa Odle
Medical Writer
Albuquerque, New Mexico

Judith Sims, M.S.
Medical Writer
Logan, UT

Carol Turkington
Medical Writer
Lancaster, PA

Samuel Uretsky, PharmD
Pharmacist and medical writer
Wantagh, New York

Ken Wells
Freelance Writer
Laguna Hills, California

CHRONOLOGY

Sample milestone world events involving public health throughout history.

1348: The Black Plague or Black Death, also known as the Bubonic Plague, reappeared in Europe after nearly a 1,000 year absence.

1700: Bernardino Ramazzini (1633–1714) published the first comprehensive occupational health treatise, which was the birth of occupational health.

1700–1800: In the United States, governmental agencies were created to address mounting health problems, sanitation and the protection of water supply, concerns that arose with the industrial revolution.

1761: World's first formal veterinary school was founded in Lyon, France.

1763: Smallpox infected blankets were distributed in the "New World" to Native Americans starting an epidemic that killed thousands.

1779: The first recognized Dengue epidemics occurred at about the same time in Asia, Africa, and North America in the 1780s.

1796: Edward Jenner (1749–1843) published his first paper on the potential for inoculation, which led to the development of the small pox vaccine.

1793: Yellow Fever appeared in the U.S. in the late 17th century. In 1793, Philadelphia was the scene of one of the worst outbreaks.

1799: The Lying-in Hospital of the City of New York is chartered, the first to provide obstetrical care for women in New York City.

1804: The first city water treatment plant was built in Scotland, initiating the idea that all people should have access to clean, safe drinking water.

1842: Social reformer Edwin Chadwick published his landmark report, "Report on the Inquiry into Sanitary Conditions of the Laboring Population of Great Britain", outlining the major public health challenges facing England at the time, leading to the beginnings of reform.

1831–1832: Cholera first came to Sunderland, England. Several epidemics appeared overtime throughout England, eventually killing more people than the Black Plague.

1840: The first dental college, the Baltimore College of Dental Surgery, was established.

1849: Swedish physician Magnus Huss (1807–1890) first coined the term alcoholism to systematically classify the damage that was attributable to the excessive consumption of alcohol.

1863: New York City conducted the first sanitation survey. New York's Association for the Improvement of the Condition of the Poor finds "dark, contracted, ill constructed, badly ventilated and disgustingly filthy" housing.

1869: Dr. Robert Dalton creates the world's first hospital ambulance, a horse-drawn carriage serving Bellevue Hospital in New York.

1872: The American Public Health Association was founded by American physician Stephen Smith, a pioneer in the U.S. public health movement.

1873: The nation's first nursing school based on Florence Nightingale's principles opens at Bellevue in New York City. Nursing students work on the hospital wards 12 hours a day, six days a week. By 1910, there are more than 1,000 nursing schools in the country.

1879: The National Board of Health was established.

1881: The first anthrax vaccine was perfected by Louis Pasteur.

1890: Naturopathy is recognized as a formal system of healthcare.

1891: Bisphenol A was first synthesized by Russian chemist Alexksandr Dianin.

1919: Methamphetamine was first synthesized in Japan.

1921: The Bureau of Indian Affairs Health Division was created.

1928: Scottish physician Alexander Fleming (1881–1955) inadvertently discovered Penicillin while studying moulds.

1938: Fair Labor Standards Act (FLSA) passed as part of President Roosevelt's New Deal, providing regulations for employers to improve conditions of workers.

1946: Centers for Disease Control and Prevention (CDC) was established in 1946 in Atlanta as the Communicable Disease Center.

1947: American cardiac surgeon Claude Schaeffer Beck (1894–1971) was the first to use a defibrillator on a human when he successfully applied it to a 14-year-old male during surgery.

1948: The World Health Organization (WHO) was established by the United Nations.

1949: National Institute of Mental Health is founded.

1950: Mass TB immunization with the bacille Calmette-Guerin (BCG) vaccine is under way to protect children from tuberculosis.

1960: G. D. Searle & Company receives FDA approval to sell Enovid as a birth control pill. The development of the first highly effective contraceptive transforms women's lives around the world and opens the door to the sexual revolution.

1962: President John F. Kennedy signed into law the Migrant Health Act, which provided for the establishment of health clinics across the nation designed to deal specifically with migrant health issues.

1962: Child abuse is formally acknowledged in the United States.

1963: Measles vaccine was developed.

1965: The Johnson Administration created Medicare and Medicaid.

1965: The first report on diabetes mellitus is issued.

1968: Noroviruses are named after the original strain that caused an outbreak of gastroenteritis in a Norwalk, Ohio school.

1969: Federal Coal Mine Health and Safety Act of 1969 is passed.

1970: Environmental Protection Agency (EPA) was established under the Nixon Administration.

1970: The Occupational Safety and Health Act of 1970 was passed, which requires employers to create a workplace free of known hazards.

1972: The Special Supplemental Nutrition Program for Women, Infants, and Children, commonly referred to as WIC, a federally funded nutrition-intervention program administered by the food and Nutrition Service of the U.S. Department of Agriculture, was founded.

1973: The American Psychiatric Association removed homosexuality from their list of mental disorders.

1973: Roe v. Wade is decided by the U.S. Supreme Court. The court rules that laws prohibiting abortions violate a constitutional right to privacy. Texas attorney Sarah Weddington argues the case on behalf of "Jane Roe."

1975: First cases of Lyme disease discovered in Lyme, Connecticut, where the disease got its name.

1977: The U.S. Consumer Product Safety Commission announces a ban on lead paint on toys and furniture, nearly 60 years after studies show that lead is dangerous to children and decades of opposition from the lead industry.

1980: The American Psychological Association adds Post Traumatic Stress Syndrome (PTSD) to its DSM-III (Diagnostic and Statistical Manual of Mental Disorders) classification system.

1981: A mysterious epidemic was identified as Acquired Immune Deficiency Syndrome (AIDS). It was found to be caused by the Human immunodeficiency virus (HIV).

1987: The F.D.A. approves Prozac, which becomes the most prescribed antidepressant drug worldwide.

1988: Congress passed the Medical Waste Tracking Act of 1988.

1990: The Nutrition Labeling Education Act was signed into law. The act required food manufacturers to disclose the fat (saturated and unsaturated), cholesterol, sodium, sugar, fiber, protein and carbohydrate content in their products.

1994: U.S. Congress passed the Violence Against Women Act, which established the Rape Prevention and Education(RPE) program at the CDC. It expired in 2012, but president Congress voted to renew it and president Obama signed the extension in March 2013.

2002: The Public Health Security and Bioterrorism Preparedness and Response Act of 2002 provided grants to improve hospitals' preparedness to respond to bioterrorism and other public health emergencies.

2003: Severe acute respiratory syndrome, or SARS, is a contagious and potentially fatal disease that first appeared in the form of a multi-country outbreak.

2005: The continued spread of a highly pathogenic avian influenza virus across eastern Asia and other countries raised concerns about a potential human pandemic.

Hurricane Katrina, one of the most destructive natural disasters in U.S. history, slams the Gulf Coast. Subsequent flooding from the failure of the New Orleans levee system adds to the crisis. Hospitals around the country respond by sending workers and supplies to the devasted areas.

2006: Two vaccines are introduced to protect against H.P.V. viruses that can cause cervical cancer and genital warts. H.P.V. is the most common sexually transmitted virus in the United States.

2009: President Barack Obama signs the Family Smoking Prevention and Tobacco Control Act, which gives the F.D.A. the power to regulate nicotine and ban tobacco advertising aimed at children.

2010: President Barack Obama signs the Affordable Health Care for America Act, with the intent of enabling millions of Americans to obtain health insurance.

2011: According to the WHO's 2011 Malaria Report, the global incidence of malaria dropped 17 percent since 2000 and by more than 50 percent in several endemic countries. Malaria-specific mortality rates fell by 26 percent worldwide. Much of this success is due to increased access to and use of insecticide-treated mosquito nets.

2012: On January 13th, India marks one year without any new polio cases diagnosed. This set the stage for India's removal from the list of polio endemic countries in February, leaving only Afghanistan, Nigeria and Pakistan as nations where transmission of the poliovirus has never been stopped

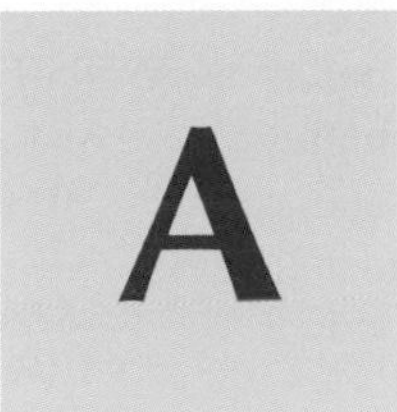

AARP

Definition

AARP is a nonprofit organization that advocates and provides services for retired people over the age of 50. Its name is derived from its previous official title, American Association of Retired Persons.

Purpose

The purpose of AARP is to help older and retired persons to choose lifestyle options that will maximize the benefits of their own lives and improve the society in which they live. The organization also lobbies from a nonpartisan standpoint for the types of public policy that will enhance the lives of senior citizens in the United States.

Description

AARP was founded in 1958 by retired principal Ethel Percy Andrus as an extension of an earlier organization she had also founded in 1947, the National Retired Teachers Association (NRTA). Andrus had established the NRTA because, at the time, there was essentially no way in which retired teachers could obtain health insurance. All existing insurance providers felt that offering health insurance programs to older citizens, including retired teachers, was too much of a risk. Andrus was finally able to find a company, the Continental Casualty Company, that would take on this risk, and she created NRTA to provide an organization through which health insurance could be provided. Before long, Andrus found that many retired Americans from professions other than teaching were also in need of health insurance, and she created a new company with a broader potential clientle, the American Association of Retired Persons, which took the acronym AARP. In 1999, the organization took this acronym as its official name.

AARP consists of two separate and distinct divisions, AARP Services, Inc., and AARP Foundation. AARP Services offers a host of services especially designed for older and retired individuals, such as health, life, auto, motorcycle, home, mobile home, property and casualty, and lifetime income insurance; health products; discounts on shopping, home and auto products, dining and entertainment opportunities, and health and wellness products; financial services, ranging from financial counseling to credit card programs; and travel programs, including hotel, car rental, air travel, and cruises and tours options. Through its website, AARP also provides information on virtually every topic in which senior citizens might be interested, including health, work and benefits, money issues, home and family, food, travel, entertainment, and politics.

In contract to AARP Services, the AARP Foundation is a nonprofit entity that works to improve the lives of seniors through direct assistance, legal advocacy, and awareness raising among decision makers. The Foundation currently has defined four areas of special interest and concern for senior citizens: hunger, income, housing, and isolation. For example, the Foundation works with other national, state, and local non-profit groups to develop ways of getting food to elderly individuals who are unable for financial or other reasons to maintain a healthy level of **nutrition**. These programs might include organizing food drives for the elderly, having high-school students participate in food drives or free meals programs, and lobbying local, state, and national legislators to develop programs for feeding the elderly.

True to its history, AARP has an important health component in its ongoing programs. One primary part of that component is a Medicare supplement health insurance (Medigap) program to which about seven million members belong. It is probably the largest and most profitable of all AARP programs, and it provides the additional coverage, beyond regular Medicare coverage, that most people need today. In addition to this profit-making element, AARP provides a vast amount of health information in its print publications and on its website on topics such as **influenza** and **shingles** immunizations, dry eye disorder, osteoporosis, hormone replacement therapy, statins, herbal supplements, **antibiotics**, and detailed information on many individual drugs.

AARP has long taken strong stands on important national health issues and, in particular, has long argued in support of the existing Social Security/Medicare/Medicaid program and has fought strongly against efforts to dismantle or weaken these programs. It was a strong supporter of President Barack Obama's 2010 Affordable Care Act. Although it does not take partisan stands on national, state, or local elections, it does critically analyze health care proposals made by political candidates and parties at all levels.

AARP publishes two print journals, the bimonthly *AARP The Magazine* (formerly *Modern Maturity*) and the monthly *AARP Bulletin*, both sent at no cost to members (making them by far the largest subscriber magazines in the United States). The organization also produces both radio and television programs, including Prime Time Radio, Prime Time Focus, Movies for Grownups, and My Generation.

Demographics

As of late 2012, the organization claims to have about 38 million members, making it one of the largest membership organizations in the United States, if not the world. Membership is available to anyone over the age of 50, whether he or she is retired or not.

Resources

BOOKS

Flower, Lynda, and Lynn Nonnemaker. *Improvements to Medicare's Preventive Services under Health Reform.* Washington, DC: AARP Public Policy Institute, 2010.

Lynch, Frederick R. *One Nation under AARP: The Fight over Medicare, Social Security, and America's Future.* Berkeley, CA: University of California Press, 2011.

PERIODICALS

Cagna, Robert. "AARP." *Journal of Consumer Health on the Internet* 14, 1. (2010): 51–56.

Correa, Frances. "Report Accuses AARP of Abusing Nonprofit Status." *Internal Medicine News* 44, 7. (2011): 70.

Paisner, Susan R. "RIPTA and AARP: Partnering to Keep Senior *sic* Mobile." *Passenger Transport* 70, 11. (2012): 11.

Wesbury, S., Jr. "An Unquestionable Role. AARP Can Fend off Congressional Critics by Leading Healthy-living Campaign." *Modern Healthcare* 41, 16. (2011): 24.

WEBSITES

"AARP Loses Members Over Health Care Stance." USA Today. http://usatoday30.usatoday.com/news/washington/2009-08-17-aarp-health-overhaul_N.htm. Accessed on October 30, 2012.

"AARP Topics Page." The New York Times. http://topics.nytimes.com/topics/reference/timestopics/organizations/a/aarp/index.html. Accessed on October 30, 2012.

"AARP Topics Page." USA Today. http://content.usatoday.com/topics/topic/Organizations/Non-profits,+Activist+Groups/AARP. Accessed on October 30, 2012.

Herger, Wally, and Dave Reichert. "Behind the Veil: The AARP America Doesn' Know." http://waysandmeans.house.gov/uploadedfiles/aarp_report_final_pdf_3_29_11.pdf. Accessed on October 30, 2012.

ORGANIZATIONS

AARP, 601 E St., N.W., Washington, DC USA 20049, (888) 687–2277, member@aarp.org, http://www.aarp.org/.

David E. Newton, Ed.D.

Abortion

Definition

Abortion is the intentional termination of a pregnancy before the fetus can live independently. An abortion may be elective or therapeutic. It can be performed either medically by administration of drugs that cause the uterus to contract and expel the fetus, or surgically, in which the fetus is removed mechanically in a surgical procedure. The choice of method usually depends on the stage of the pregnancy.

Purpose

An abortion is performed to end a pregnancy. An abortion is termed "induced" to differentiate it from a spontaneous abortion (often called a "miscarriage") in which the products of conception are lost naturally. An abortion is elective if a woman chooses to end her pregnancy for reasons other than maternal or fetal health. Some reasons a woman might choose to have an elective abortion are:

- continuation of the pregnancy may cause emotional or financial hardship
- the woman is not ready to become a parent
- the pregnancy was unintended and unwanted
- the woman is pressured into aborting by her partner, parents, or others
- the pregnancy was the result of rape or incest

KEY TERMS

Cervix—Narrow, lower end of the uterus forming the opening to the vagina.

Curette—A spoon-shaped instrument used to remove tissue from the inner lining of the uterus.

Ectopic pregnancy—Pregnancy in which a fertilized egg begins to develop outside the uterus. An ectopic pregnancy can be life-threatening to the woman and must be terminated.

Endocarditis—An infection of the inner membrane lining of the heart.

Fibroid tumors—Non-cancerous (benign) growths in the uterus. Fibroid tumors, which occur in 30–40% of women over age 40, do not need to be removed unless they are causing symptoms that interfere with a woman's normal activities.

Systemic lupus erythematosus (SLE)—A chronic, inflammatory, autoimmune disorder in which the individual's immune system attacks, injures, and destroys the body's own organs and tissues. It may affect many organ systems, including the skin, joints, lungs, heart, and kidneys.

Prostaglandins—Fatty acids produced by the body that are responsible for inflammation features, such as swelling, pain, stiffness, redness, and warmth as well as being involved in smooth muscle contractions.

Rh negative—Lacking the Rh factor, which is a genetically determined antigen on red blood cells that produce immune responses.

Rh disease—Illness caused when an Rh-negative woman is pregnant with an Rh-positive fetus, and her body produces antibodies against the fetus's blood.

Rh immune globulin (RhoGAM)—A vaccine given to a woman after an abortion, miscarriage, or prenatal tests in order to prevent sensitization to Rh disease. Sensitization to the disease occurs when the blood of a woman who is Rh positive is exposed to the blood of a previous fetus, which was Rh negative.

A therapeutic abortion is performed in order to preserve the health or save the life of a pregnant woman. A healthcare provider also may recommend a therapeutic abortion if the fetus is diagnosed with significant abnormalities, if it is not expected to live, or if it has died *in utero*.

A therapeutic abortion may be indicated if a woman has a pregnancy-related health condition that endangers her life. Some examples of such conditions include:

- severe, life-threatening hypertension (high blood pressure)
- cardiac disease
- severe depression or other psychiatric condition
- serious kidney or liver disease
- certain types of infection
- malignancy (cancer)
- ectopic pregnancy
- multifetal pregnancy (called a "multifetal pregnancy reduction," or MFPR) that may result from fertility treatments.

Demographics

Abortion has been a legal procedure in the United States since 1973. According to research published in a 2011 issue of *Contraception*, 49% of pregnancies among American women are unintended, and about 43% of those end in abortion. In 2008 (the latest data available as of 2012), the **Centers for Disease Control and Prevention (CDC)** received reports of 825,564 legal, induced abortions, or 16.0 abortions per 1,000 women aged 15–44. This represents an abortion ratio of 234 abortions per 1,000 live births. A separate study published in a 2011 issue of *Perspectives on Sexual and Reproductive Health* suggests that the number of abortions in 2008 was closer to 1.21 million, or 19.4–19.6 abortions per 1,000 women aged 15–44.

Abortions occur in women of all races and ethnic groups. According to a study published in a 2011 issue of *Obstetrics & Gynecology*, 36% of women who had abortions from 2000–2008 were non-Hispanic white, 30% were non-Hispanic black, 25% were Hispanic, and 9% were women of other races. The study did note an increase in abortions among poor women, who as a group accounted for 42.4% of abortions in 2008—a 17.5% increase from 2000 to 2008.

Description

Abortions are safest when performed within the first six to 10 weeks after the last menstrual period (a calculation used by healthcare providers to determine the stage of pregnancy) and experience few complications. Abortions performed between 13 and 24 weeks (during the second trimester) have a higher rate of complications. Abortions after 24 weeks, sometimes called "partial birth abortions," are extremely rare and are usually limited to situations where the life of the mother is in danger.

Most women have abortions at clinics or outpatient facilities if the procedure is performed early in pregnancy and the woman is in relatively good health. Women with **heart disease**, previous endocarditis, **asthma**, systemic lupus erythematosus, uterine fibroid tumors, blood-clotting disorders, poorly controlled epilepsy, or some psychological disorders typically require hospitalization so they may receive special monitoring and medications during the procedure. Late-term abortions are usually performed in hospitals.

Fewer complications occur among women who have an abortion during the first trimester. Second-trimester abortions are not uncommon, however, because the results of genetic testing often are not available until 16 weeks gestation. In addition, women, especially teens, might not recognize the pregnancy or come to terms with it emotionally soon enough to have a first-trimester abortion. Teens make up the largest group having second-trimester abortions.

As a general rule, the earlier the abortion, the less expensive it is. Second-trimester abortions carry more risk, in addition to more services, anesthesia, and sometimes a hospital stay, and are therefore more expensive than early abortions. Therapeutic abortions make up only a small percentage of all abortions; most abortions are elective.

Medical abortions

Medical abortions are those resulting from taking prescription drugs that end the pregnancy. Both mifepristone (Mifeprex, RU-486) and methotrexate (Rheumatrex, Folex PFS), sometimes in combination with misoprostol (Cytotec), are used for medical abortions. Other drugs may be used to enhance contractions, reduce bleeding, prevent infection (various **antibiotics**), or control **pain**.

Mifepristone works by blocking the action of progesterone, a hormone needed for pregnancy to continue. Approved by the Food and Drug Administration (FDA) in September 2000 as an alternative to surgical abortion, mifepristone can be taken for early abortions (up to 49 days gestation). On the first visit to the doctor, a woman takes a mifepristone pill, and if necessary, followed two days later by misoprostol, which causes the uterus to contract. Approximately 92–95% of women experience an abortion after the mifepristone-and-misoprostol regimen. A third follow-up visit to the doctor is necessary to confirm through observation or ultrasound that the procedure is complete. In the event that it is not, a surgical abortion is performed. Surgical abortion is then recommended because the fetus may be damaged. Side effects include nausea, vaginal bleeding, and heavy cramping. The bleeding is typically heavier than a normal period and may last up to 16 days.

Some women should not use mifepristone. For instance, it is not recommended for women with ectopic pregnancy or those who have been taking long-term steroidal therapy, have bleeding abnormalities, or are on blood-thinners such as Coumadin.

Methotrexate works differently than mifepristone. Methotrexate targets rapidly dividing fetal cells, thus preventing the fetus from developing further. It most often is used in conjunction with misoprostol, a prostaglandin that stimulates contractions of the uterus. Methotrexate may be taken up to 49 days after the first day of the last menstrual period. On the first visit to the doctor, the woman receives an injection of methotrexate, followed a week later, if necessary, by administration of misoprostol tablets vaginally to stimulate contractions of the uterus. Within two weeks, the woman will expel the contents of her uterus, ending the pregnancy. A follow-up visit to the doctor is necessary to ensure that the abortion is complete.

With this procedure, a woman will feel cramping and may feel nauseated from the misoprostol. This combination of drugs is approximately 92–96% effective in ending pregnancy, with about half experiencing the abortion soon after taking the misoprostol.

Methotrexate is not recommended for women with liver or kidney disease, inflammatory bowel disease, clotting disorders, documented immunodeficiency, or certain blood disorders.

Induction is a procedure used in second-term abortions; an abortion occurs by means of inducing labor via the administration of medications. The fetus is delivered within eight to 72 hours. Side effects of this procedure include nausea, vomiting, and diarrhea from the prostaglandin, and pain from uterine contractions. Anesthesia of the sort used in childbirth can be given to reduce pain. Many women are able to go home a few hours after the procedure.

Surgical abortions

The majority of surgical abortions performed in the United States are elective. Multiple surgical options exist, depending on the stage of the pregnancy. These include manual vacuum aspiration (MVA) and dilation and suction curettage (D&C).

MVA, also known as "menstrual extraction," "mini-suction,"or "early abortion," is typically used for abortions of up to 10 weeks gestation. In this procedure, the cervix is dilated, then the contents of the uterus are suctioned out through a thin plastic tube that is inserted through the cervix. The procedure generally lasts about 15 minutes, and the woman goes home after a few hours of observation. MVA has a very low rate of complications, although the amount of fetal material is so small at this stage of development, it is possible to miss extracting it. This results in an incomplete abortion, which means the pregnancy continues.

A D&C, also known as "suction dilation," "vacuum curettage," or "suction curettage," is often used for induced abortions occurring between 10 and 14 weeks. This procedure involves stretching of the cervix with a series of dilators or specific medications. The contents of the uterus are then removed with a tube attached to a suction machine, and walls of the uterus are cleaned using a narrow loop called a "curette." A D&C takes about 15 minutes, and the woman usually goes home after a few hours of observation. The procedure is 97–99% effective. The amount of discomfort a woman feels varies considerably. The local anesthesia given to numb the cervix does not mask uterine cramping.

Some second-trimester abortions occurring between 14 and 20 weeks are performed as a dilatation and evacuation (D&E). The procedures are similar to those used in a D&C, but a larger suction tube must be used, since more material is removed. This increases the amount of cervical dilation necessary and increases the risk and discomfort and complications from the procedure. A combination of suction and manual extraction using medical instruments is used to remove the contents of the uterus.

OTHER SURGICAL OPTIONS. After 20 weeks, abortions usually must be performed in a hospital. These are rare, usually performed to save the life of the mother. Surgical options include:

- Dilatation and extraction (D&X)—the cervix is prepared by means similar to those used in a dilatation and evacuation; however, the fetus is removed mostly intact, although the head must be collapsed to fit through the cervix. This procedure is sometimes called a "partial-birth abortion."
- Hysterotomy—a surgical incision is made into the uterus, and the contents of the uterus removed through the incision. This procedure is rarely done, and generally used only if induction methods fail to deliver the fetus.

AFTERCARE. Regardless of the method used to perform the abortion, a woman will be observed for a period of time to make sure her blood pressure is stable and that bleeding is controlled. The doctor may prescribe antibiotics to reduce the chance of infection. Women who are Rh negative should be given an injection of human Rh immune globulin (RhoGAM) after the procedure unless the father of the fetus also is Rh negative. This prevents blood-incompatibility complications in future pregnancies.

Bleeding will continue for about five days in a surgical abortion and longer in a medical abortion. To decrease the risk of infection, a woman should avoid intercourse, tampons, and douches for two weeks after the abortion. A follow-up visit two to four weeks after the abortion is a necessary part of the woman's aftercare. Contraception will be offered to women who wish to avoid future pregnancies, because menstrual periods normally resume within a few weeks.

Depending on the circumstances surrounding the abortion, some women find post-abortion counseling or grief counseling helpful.

Risks

Complications from abortions are rare, but risks increase with the duration of the pregnancy; the earlier an abortion is performed, the safer it is. Women who experience any of the following should call the clinic or doctor who performed the abortion immediately:

- severe pain
- fever over 100.4°F (38.2°C)
- heavy bleeding that soaks through more than one sanitary pad per hour
- foul-smelling discharge from the vagina
- continuing symptoms of pregnancy.

Results

The expected result is that the pregnancy is ended without complication and without altering future fertility. According to research cited by the Guttmacher Institute, abortions performed during first trimester pose virtually no long-term risk of various health problems, including **infertility**, ectopic pregnancy, spontaneous abortion (miscarriage), birth defect, or deliveries that are pre-term or of low birth weight. The risk of maternal death does, however, increase as pregnancies progress: For abortions performed at or before eight weeks gestation, the death rate is one per 1,000,000 abortions, but it increases to one per 29,000 at 16–20 weeks gestation, and to one per 11,000 for pregnancies of 21 weeks or more.

Effects on Public Health

Abortion laws vary substantially from country to country, ranging from easily available abortion on demand to complete illegality for any reason. Illegal abortions are likely to be performed in an unsafe manner, often by untrained or poorly trained individuals and in unclean environments where contamination often results in infection and maternal death. Unsafe abortion substantially increases the risk of complications, including compromised fertility and maternal death. The **World Health Organization (WHO)** has stated that unsafe abortion is a major public health problem in many developing countries.

QUESTIONS TO ASK YOUR DOCTOR

- What abortion options are available to me based on my stage of pregnancy?
- What are the short- and long-term complications of the procedure?
- What type of pain relief/anesthesia is available to me?
- Who can be in the procedure room with me?
- What will the abortion cost? What do the fees include? What, if anything, will my insurance pay toward the abortion?
- Is pre-abortion counseling offered?
- How is follow-up or emergency care provided?
- Does the doctor who will perform the abortion have admitting privileges at a hospital in case of a problem?

Costs to Society

According to the **WHO**, approximately 21.6 million unsafe abortions took place worldwide in 2008, almost all in developing countries. The WHO also reports that 13% of all maternal deaths are due to unsafe abortions. This often results in poorer care for the children these mothers have left behind.

Efforts and Solutions

In June 2012, the WHO issued updated recommendations for policy makers, program managers, and health providers in the second edition of its publication "Safe Abortion: Technical and Policy Guidance for Health Systems." The publication provides "the latest evidence-based guidance on clinical care," information on establishing and strengthening services, and an outline for a "human-rights-based approach" to laws and policies on safe, comprehensive abortion care. The guidelines are designed to help stem the number of unsafe abortions and associated maternal deaths.

For all women contemplating an abortion, pre-abortion counseling is important in helping them to resolve any questions about having the procedure. Some states require a waiting period (most often of 24 hours) following counseling before the abortion may be obtained. Some states require parental consent or notification if the patient is under the age of 18. A woman's physician will be able to provide counseling recommendations or referrals.

Resources

PERIODICALS

Finer, Lawrence B., and Mia R. Zolner. "Unintended Pregnancy in the United States: Incidence and Disparities, 2006" *Contraception* 84, no. 5 (2011): 478–485.

Jones, Rachel K., and Kathryn Kooistra. "Abortion Incidence and Access to Services In the United States, 2008." *Perspectives on Sexual and Reproductive Health* 43, no. 1 (2011): 41–50.

Jones, Rachel K., and Megan L. Kavanaugh. "Changes in Abortion Rates Between 2000 and 2008 and Lifetime Incidence of Abortion." *Obstetrics & Gynecology* 117, no. 6 (2011): 1358–1366.

Pazol, Karen, et al. "Abortion Surveillance—United States, 2008." *Morbidity and Mortality Weekly Report* 60, no. SS15 (2011): 1–41. http://www.cdc.gov/mmwr/preview/mmwrhtml/ss6015a1.htm?s_cid=ss6015a1_w(accessed September 21, 2012).

WEBSITES

"Are You in the Know?" Guttmacher Institute. http://www.guttmacher.org/in-the-know/index.html(accessed September 21, 2012).

"Facts on Induced Abortion in the United States. Guttmacher Institute." http://www.guttmacher.org/pubs/fb_induced_abortion.html(accessed September 21, 2012).

MedlinePlus. "Abortion." U.S. National Library of Medicine. http://www.nlm.nih.gov/medlineplus/abortion.html (accessed September 21, 2012).

"Preventing Unsafe Abortion." World Health Organization. http://www.who.int/reproductivehealth/topics/unsafe_abortion/magnitude/en/index.html(accessed September 21, 2012).

"Safe abortion: technical and policy guidance for health systems. Second Edition." World Health Organization, Department of Reproductive Health and Research.http://extranet.who.int/iris/bitstream/10665/70914/1/9789241548434_eng.pdf(accessed September 21, 2012).

ORGANIZATIONS

Guttmacher Institute, 125 Maiden Lane, New York, NY 10038, (212) 248-1111, (800) 355-0244, http://www.guttmacher.org

National Abortion Federation, 1660 L Street, NW, Suite 450, Washington, DC 20036, (202) 667-5881, naf@prochoice.org, http://www.prochoice.org

Planned Parenthood Federation of America, 434 West 33rd Street, New York, NY 10001, (212) 541-7800, http://www.plannedparenthood.org

World Health Organization, Avenue Appia 20, 1211 Geneva 27, Switzerland, +22 41 791 21 11, info@who.int, http://www.who.int.

Debra Gordon
Stephanie Dionne Sherk
Tish Davidson, AM
Brenda Lerner
Leslie Mertz, Ph.D.

Acrylamide

Definition

Acrylamide (chemical formula: C_3H_5NO) is a white crystalline solid that can be reactive though it is stable at room temperature and is dissolvable in a number of solvents including **water**. Acrylamide is a hazardous and potentially toxic chemical used to make polyacrylamide materials that have common industrial applications like water treatment; the manufacturing of cosmetics, paper, plastics, permanent press fabrics, and grout; and laboratory use with gel electrophoresis, though polyacrylamides contain small amounts of acrylamide and show a much lower toxicity. Acrylamide is found in cigarette smoke and in certain foods. The main producers of acrylamide are Japan, the United Sates, and Europe.

Description

Acrylamide has been used in industry since the 1950s, and in 2002, researchers in Sweden first discovered that acrylamide could be found in food. Acrylamide is most commonly found in plant-based foods, particularly foods that are high in starch. Naturally-occurring sugars and the amino acid, asparagine, combine to create acrylamide when certain foods are heated to high temperatures (above 120 degrees Celsius or 248 degrees Fahrenheit). These temperatures are generally achieved through cooking methods like frying, baking, and roasting. Boiling, microwaving, and steaming are less likely to produce acrylamide. Acrylamide is one of many Maillard reaction products (MRPs)—chemicals that are produced during the Maillard reaction. According to **Environmental Health** Perspectives, the Maillard reaction is "the chemical process that causes food to brown as it cooks—sugars including glucose, fructose, and lactose react with free amino acids in foods."

Acrylamide is most rapidly absorbed through the respiratory and gastrointestinal systems and then distributed almost uniformly throughout the body, in relation to the body's total water, though acrylamide tends to be more highly concentrated in testes, red blood cells, and plasma. Acrylamide is primarily released through the kidneys. Acrylamide is known to create DNA mutations and to be a human neurotoxicant. Researchers that fed rodents high oral doses of acrylamide showed that acrylamide is a carcinogen for rodents and since comparable human evidence is difficult to obtain, the International Agency for Research on **Cancer** (IARC), a division of the **World Health Organization (WHO)**, classified acrylamide as a probable human carcinogen.

A 2008 Danish study lead by Henrik Frandsen suggested a potential link between levels of acrylamide in diet and an elevated risk for breast cancer in postmenopausal women; however, these results were contested on the grounds that they were most significant for smokers, which may have received more acrylamide from **smoking** than diet. As of 2010, further studies were being conducted to determine the variations in how acrylamide is processed in both humans and animals—taking into account factors like age, metabolic rate, and accumulated levels of acrylamide.

KEY TERMS

Electrophoresis—A process used in molecular biology, biochemistry, and clinical chemistry to separate and identify specific proteins as well as DNA and RNA fragments. Polyacrylamide, a compound containing acrylamide, is used in this process.

Carcinogen—A substance that causes or increases the risk of cancer in human or animals.

Toxicity—The quality of being or the degree to which a substance is poisonous.

Neurotoxicant—A substance that is man-made or introduced to an environment by man and is poisonous to the human nervous system. Toxicants are similar to toxins except that they are artificially produced or introduced, where toxins are naturally-occurring.

Neuropathy—Damage to a nerve or group of nerves, resulting in lost or diminished ability to move, feel, or function.

Risks

The acrylamide found in food exceeds the levels that are deemed acceptable in **drinking water** by the **Environmental Protection Agency (EPA)** or levels that would be found in paper or cosmetics. Exposure from cigarette smoking and **secondhand smoke** may be significant.

Precautions

Research published in both the Journal of Agricultural and Food Chemistry in 2004 and in Molecular **Nutrition** and Food Research in 2008 suggests that blanching foods like potatoes prior to cooking, shortening cooking time, and drying food with hot air after cooking reduces the amount of acrylamide in some foods. The National Cancer Institute and Food and Drug Administration (FDA) maintain that there is insufficient evidence to justify eliminating any specific food from a normal diet. According to the FDA, the healthiest course is to maintain a balanced diet; this type of diet is "consistent with the Dietary Guidelines for Americans, that emphasizes fruits, vegetables, whole grains, and fat-free or low-fat milk and milk products, includes lean meats, poultry, fish, beans, eggs, and nuts; and is low in saturated fats, trans fats, cholesterol, salt (**sodium**) and added sugars."

Causes and Symptoms

Causes

Direct skin contact with or inhalation of acrylamide should be avoided as this type of chronic exposure can cause neurological damage. This type of contact is most likely to occur during industrial uses of acrylamide and regulations exist to help minimize this exposure. It is also possible for drinking water that has been treated with polyacrylamides to retain traces of acrylamide if not properly removed during water treatment.

Symptoms

Symptoms of neuropathy resulting from chronic acrylamide exposure include tingling feelings, fatigue, weakness, and minimized sensitivity and reflexes. Chronic skin exposure may result in skin irritation. The levels of acrylamide required to produce neurological or dermatological reactions would be consistent with chronic industrial levels of exposure.

Treatment

Neuropathy from acrylamide exposure usually ceases within one year of discontinued exposure to acrylamide, though some serious cases of exposure may leave permanent nerve damage.

Effects on Public Health

The biggest public health concern is the potential of acrylamide in food to cause cancer. However, as of 2012, the evidence attempting to link quantities of acrylamide in food to cancer was inconclusive, though research to examine this potential link is ongoing.

Efforts and Solutions

Beginning in 2002, the FDA developed a method to measure acrylamide in food. The agency analyzed over 2600 food samples, began research to study the effects of acrylamide and published this research in peer–reviewed journals. It also began to study ways to potentially reduce levels of acrylamide in food. As of 2012, the **EPA** regulated levels of acrylamide present in drinking water and the FDA regulated levels of acrylamide in many materials that commonly come in contact with food products, though not in the food itself.

Resources

BOOKS

Considine, Glenn D., ed. "Acrylamide." *Van Nostrand's Encyclopedia of Chemistry.* 15. Hoboken, NJ: Wiley-Interscience, 2005.

Larsen, Laura, ed. "Acrylamide From High–Temperature Cooking." *Environmental Health Sourcebook.* 493-497. Detroit, MI: Omnigraphics, Inc, 2010.

Schmidt, Robert F. and William D. Willis, eds. "Acrylamide." *Encyclopedia of Pain.* 7. New York, NY: Springer-Verlag, 2007.

Wexler, Philip, Bruce D. Anderson, et al, eds. "Acrylamide." *Encyclopedia of Toxicology.* 42-44. Oxford, United Kingdom: Elsevier, 2005.

PERIODICALS

Christensen, Jane, Henrik Frandsen, et al. "Pre–diagnostic acrylamide exposure and survival after breast cancer among postmenopausal Danish women." *Toxicology* 296, nos. 1-3 (2012).

Potera, Carol. "Diet & Nutrition: Acrylamide Study Suggests Breast Cancer Link." *Environmental Health Perspectives* 116, no. 4 (2008).

Spivey, Angela. "A Matter of Degrees: Advancing Our Understanding of Acrylamide." *Environmental Health Perspectives* 188, no. 4 (2010).

WEBSITES

FDA.gov. "Acrylamide." http://www.fda.gov/food/foodsafety/foodcontaminantsadulteration/chemicalcontaminants/acrylamide/ucm053569.html Accessed June 10, 2012.

Cancer.Gov. "Acrylamide in Food and Cancer Risk" http://www.cancer.gov/cancertopics/factsheet/Risk/acrylamide-in-food Accessed June 10, 2012.

WHO.int. "Frequently asked questions—acrylamide in food." http://www.who.int/foodsafety/publications/chem/acrylamide_faqs/en/index3.html Accessed June 10, 2012.

Andrea Nienstedt, MA

Addiction

Definition

Addiction is a disease of the brain that causes dependence upon or a persistent, compulsive need to use a habit-forming substance or an irresistible urge to engage in an activity, despite harmful consequences. Addictions are characterized by the increasing need for more of the substance or activity to obtain the same effect. Abstinence from the addiction may cause unpleasant or even life-threatening withdrawal symptoms.

Demographics

Addiction to substances and activities is very widespread in the United States and Canada and around the world. Substance abuse and addiction costs Americans more than $484 billion annually in healthcare costs, lost earnings, accidents, and crime. Every year, Americans suffer approximately 40 million debilitating illnesses or injuries as a result of tobacco, alcohol, and other addictive drug use. Likewise about one in ten Canadians age 15 and older is addicted to alcohol or drugs. Men are more than twice as likely as women to be addicted to a substance. However gender differences are much less pronounced among adolescents: teenage girls are almost as likely as boys to abuse a substance. Approximately 20% of people with addictions have other mental disorders as well.

Nicotine dependence is the most common type of addiction. It is estimated that worldwide tobacco use results in five million deaths annually. Cigarette **smoking** is the leading preventable cause of death in the United States, with 443,000 deaths annually, which is about one out of every five deaths. An additional 38,000 deaths annually are caused by exposure to **secondhand smoke**. According to the **Centers for Disease Control and Prevention (CDC)** as of 2012, about 19.3% of American adults smoked cigarettes, which equals aproximately 45.3 million people. In addition, the **CDC** reports about 19.5% of American high school students and 5.2% of middle school students smoked cigarettes. In recent years, there has also been an increase in the number of children under the age of 18 who used smokeless (chewing) tobacco.

Alcoholism is the most common addiction to a psychoactive substance. Alcohol addiction affects both sexes and all races and nationalities. In the United States 17.6 million people—about one in 12 adults—abuse or are addicted to alcohol. Alcohol addiction rates are highest among young adults aged 18–29 and lowest among those 65 and older.

An estimated four million Americans over the age of 12 use prescription **pain** relievers, sedatives, or stimulants for nonmedical reasons during any given month. In 2008, 15.4% of twelfth-graders reported using prescription drugs nonmedically. These included amphetamines, sedatives/barbiturates, tranquilizers, and opiates other than heroin.

Addictions most often first appear in adolescence. The CDC's most recent data show that 8.7% of young people, age 12 and older reported having used an illicit drug in the previous month. In this same age group, 6.6% report having used marijuana in the past month, and 2.8% report nonmedical use of psychotherapeutic medication. Young people aged 15–24 are more likely to report addictions than those in other age groups. However, the use of illegal drugs among American teenagers declined by 24% between 2001 and 2007. Cigarette smoking and alcohol use among American youth also declined significantly over the first decade of the twenty-first century.

Statistics on addictive activities are more difficult to obtain because these behaviors are less clearly defined than substance addiction. However, a Harvard University study found that an estimated 15.4 million Americans suffered from a gambling addiction. More than half (7.9 million) were adolescents.

Description

Addiction most commonly refers to the compulsive use or abuse of or physical or psychological dependence on addictive substances, including:

- tobacco
- alcohol
- cocaine, including crack cocaine
- amphetamines, including methamphetamine or "crank," an extremely addictive substance
- heroin
- prescription medications

Prescription painkillers, such as the opiates Vicodin and OxyContin, have emerged as drugs of special concern because of their widespread use by high school students.

In recent years, the term "addiction" has been used to describe a wide and complex range of behaviors. These so-called process addictions are compulsive behaviors involving activities such as:

- gambling
- eating
- working
- exercising
- shopping or otherwise spending money
- sex
- internet use, especially online gaming

Most addictions are associated with mood modification. Initially, at least, they make the addict feel better. Addicts often describe a release of tension or feelings of euphoria when using the substance or engaging in the activity. Most addictions are progressive syndromes—without treatment their severity increases over time. Furthermore, many addicts are addicted to more than one substance or activity. Addictions are characterized by frequent relapse—a return to the abused substance or activity following recovery.

Some substances are more addictive than others, either because they produce a rapid and intense change in mood or because they produce painful withdrawal symptoms when stopped suddenly. Drugs that are smoked or injected, giving an immediate short-lived "high," tend to be more addictive than substances that are otherwise ingested.

The American Psychiatric Association's *Diagnostic and Statistical Manual of Mental Disorders* (*DSM-IV-TR*) classifies **substance abuse and dependence** as psychological disorders that are major clinical syndromes (called "Axis 1"). Over time, repeated drug use changes brain structure and function in fundamental and long-lasting ways. Evidence suggests that these long-lasting brain changes are responsible for the distortions of cognitive and emotional functioning that characterize addicts, particularly the compulsion to use drugs. This explains why many addicts cannot stop using drugs by force of will alone.

Risk factors

Risk factors for addiction include:

- inherited factors
- adolescence
- addictive behavior in the home or among family members or peers
- early substance use
- early aggressive behavior
- academic failure
- lack of parental supervision
- poor social skills
- other mental disorders or illnesses
- substance abuse
- substance availability
- poverty

Causes and symptoms

For much of the twentieth century, addiction was viewed as a moral failing; however, today addiction is widely viewed as a disease. The disease model of alcohol and drug addiction was first introduced in the late 1940s by E.M. Jellinek and was adopted by the American Medical Association in 1956. According to the disease model, the compulsion to use alcohol and/or drugs is genetically and physiologically based and, although the disease can be arrested, it is progressive, chronic, and fatal if unchecked. However, some experts argue that addiction is better understood as a learned behavior and that the negative behavior can be unlearned and replaced by learning new positive behaviors. The causes of addiction remain the subject of ongoing research and debate.

The initial positive consequences of substance use or a potentially addictive activity can "hook" a susceptible person and turn into an addiction. Addiction comes about through an array of changes in the brain and the strengthening of new memory connections. The anterior cingulated cortex in the frontal lobe of the brain is the area responsible for the long-term craving in addicts that triggers relapse.

Many experts believe that addictive substances and activities affect neurotransmitters in the brain. The primary pathway involved in the development and persistence of addiction is the brain reward or mesolimbic pathway, which operates via a neurotransmitter called dopamine. Dopamine pathways may interact with those of other neurotransmitters, including opioid pathways. These neuronal pathways have been identified as underlying both substance and process addictions.

Whatever the brain chemistry involved in addiction, it usually results from the interaction of several factors:

- Social learning. This may be the most important single factor in addiction and includes patterns of substance use and activities in the addict's family or subculture, peer pressure, and advertising or media influence.
- Availability. There are marked increases in addiction rates when tobacco, alcohol, or drugs are inexpensive or readily available.
- Individual development. Before the 1980s, addiction was blamed on an "addictive personality," which was described as escapist, impulsive, dependent, devious, manipulative, and self-centered. Although individual development may play a role in addiction, many doctors now believe that these character traits develop in addicts as a result of the addiction rather than causing the addiction.
- Genetic factors. It is estimated that genetic factors account for 40–60% of an individual's vulnerability to addiction. Twin studies have shown that addiction has a strong inherited component. Some forms of addiction seem to run in families, and some people appear to be more vulnerable to addiction because of their body chemistry.

The continued use of an addictive substance or engagement in an addictive activity causes the addict's body to adjust and develop tolerance. Increasing amounts of the substance or more frequent engagement in the activity are needed to produce the same effect. In some cases, addicts routinely use amounts of a substance that would be lethal in someone who had not developed a tolerance.

The inability to hold a steady job and disruptions of social and familial relationships are common outcomes of all types of addiction. Over time, the physical symptoms of an addiction increase, and withdrawal symptoms can become more severe. These symptoms vary with the individual and with the substance or activity.

According to the *DSM-IV-TR*, alcohol abuse progresses through a series of stages from social drinking to chronic alcoholism. Danger signs that indicate the probable onset of addiction to alcohol include:

- a frequent desire to drink
- increasing alcohol consumption
- memory lapses (blackouts)
- morning drinking
- hiding alcohol from family and coworkers
- drinking in secret

Alcoholic psychoses are symptoms of late-stage alcohol addiction and include:

- alcohol withdrawal delirium (delirium tremens)
- hallucinations
- Korsakoff's psychosis, an irreversible brain disorder involving severe memory loss

Symptoms of withdrawal from alcohol and some drugs may include:

- flu-like aches and pains
- digestive upset
- seizures
- hallucinatory sensations, such as the feeling of bugs crawling over one's skin
- damage to organs, including the brain and liver
- dementia

Diagnosis

Examination

Addictions are usually readily diagnosed by their symptoms and by lifestyle factors. Alcoholism is usually diagnosed when drinking impairs a person's life, personal relationships, work, and/or health. A physician, psychologist, or social worker usually makes a diagnosis of addiction based on the following criteria:

- a pattern of frequent and compulsive substance use or engagement in an activity
- preoccupation with acquiring and using an abused substance
- tolerance or escalation of the substance use or activity
- loss of willpower
- harmful consequences
- unmanageable lifestyle
- withdrawal symptoms

The examination may include probing for underlying conditions such as depression, emotional upset, anxiety, or **stress**. A physician may also look for signs of malnutrition or other medical problems resulting from substance abuse.

Tests

Blood and urine tests may be ordered to check for substance use or for liver or other organ damage resulting from substance abuse.

Procedures

Imaging tests may be ordered to check for organ damage resulting from substance abuse.

Treatment

Addictions are notoriously difficult to treat. Treatment often requires a combination of medical, psychological, and social approaches.

KEY TERMS

Addictive personality—The concept that addiction is the result of pre-existing character defects.

Dopamine—A neurotransmitter in the brain.

Methamphetamine (Meth, Methadrine, "Speed")—A highly addictive medication that is used to treat attention deficit disorder and obesity, but is widely abused as a stimulant.

Neurotransmitter—A chemical that transmits impulses across a synapse between nerves.

Process addiction—Addiction to certain mood-altering behaviors, such as eating, gambling, sexual activity, overwork, and shopping.

Relapse—A recurrence of symptoms after a period of improvement or recovery.

Tolerance—The requirement for higher doses of a substance or more frequent engagement in an activity to achieve the same effect.

Withdrawal—The unpleasant, sometimes life-threatening physiological changes that occur due to the discontinuation of some drugs after prolonged regular use.

Traditional

Although addiction treatment may be provided by practicing clinicians, such as psychiatrists, psychologists, and social workers, it is more often provided by specialized addiction treatment programs and clinics. These programs usually rely upon confrontational tactics and re-education, often employing former or recovering addicts to treat newly admitted addicts. Residential settings can be effective in helping addicted individuals to stay away from the many cues—including people and places—that form the setting for their addiction. Substance addicts may need hospital treatment to manage withdrawal symptoms.

Individual or group psychotherapy is often helpful for treating addictions after the substance use or addictive activity has ceased. Many of the negative behaviors and personality problems associated with addictions disappear when the substance use or activity ceases. Family therapy can be helpful for addressing and changing "enabling behaviors" by family members who help maintain the addiction by providing money, food, shelter, and/or emotional support.

The effectiveness of addiction treatment based on behavioral and other psychotherapeutic methods is well-documented. Specific therapies to treat addiction include:

- cognitive-behavioral approaches to prevent relapse by helping addicts recognize, avoid, and cope with situations that encourage their addictions
- motivation-enhancing strategies that utilize positive reinforcement and incentives
- motivational interviewing that uses strategies to promote behavior changes
- solution-oriented and other brief therapy techniques
- harm-reduction approaches

Drugs

Research continues into pharmacological treatments for easing withdrawal and treating various addictions. Some promising drugs boost the levels of neurotransmitters in the brain. Medications that are used to treat addiction include:

- nicotine-replacement therapies including gum, patches, and inhalers
- bupropion (Zyban), an antidepressent, for tobacco addiction
- varenicline, which blocks the pleasant effects of nicotine on the brain
- disulfiram (Antabuse) and acamprosate (Campral) for treating alcoholism
- naltrexone (Depade, ReVia) for preventing relapse in alcohol and opioid addicts
- methadone, which blocks the euphoric effect of opiates
- buprenorphine (Subutex) or buprenorphine and naloxone (Suboxone) to prevent withdrawal symptoms and to treat addiction to opioids including heroin and narcotic painkillers
- sedatives for reducing anxiety and withdrawal symptoms
- antidepressants for treating underlying problems in addicts who have been "self-medicating"

Alternative

Over the past several decades, alternatives to the complete abstinence model have arisen. Controlled-use programs allow addicted individuals to reduce their use without committing to complete abstinence. This alternative is highly controversial, and the prevailing belief is that recovery is only possible by committing to complete lifelong abstinence from all substance use.

Home remedies

Many people turn to self-help groups such as Alcoholics Anonymous (AA) and Narcotics Anonymous (NA) to treat their addictions. The approach of one addict helping another to stay "clean," with or without additional professional help, is widely accepted in the United States and around the world.

The most frequently recommended social outpatient treatment is the 12-step program. The number of visits to 12-step self-help groups exceeds the number of visits to all mental health professionals combined. There are 12-step groups for all major substance and process addictions.

The 12 steps consist of:

- Admit powerlessness over the addiction
- Believe that a power greater than oneself can restore sanity
- Make a decision to turn your will and your life over to the care of your higher power
- Make a searching and fearless moral inventory of self
- Admit to your higher power, yourself, and another human being the exact nature of your wrongs
- Become willing to have your higher power remove all these defects from your character
- Humbly ask your higher power to remove your shortcomings
- Make a list of all persons harmed by your wrongs and become willing to make amends to them all
- Make direct amends to such people, whenever possible, except when to do so would injure them or others
- Continue to take personal inventory and promptly admit any future wrongdoings

- Seek to improve contact with the higher power of your understanding through meditation and prayer
- Carry the message of spiritual awakening to others and practice these principles in all your affairs

Prognosis

The prognosis for recovery from any addiction depends on the substance or process, the individual's circumstances, and the underlying personality structure. Patterns of relapse tend to be very similar regardless of the specific addiction. Two-thirds of all relapses occur within the first 90 days following treatment. Substance abusers often make repeated attempts to quit before they are successful. Physical addictions alter a person's brain chemistry in ways that make it difficult to be exposed to the addictive substance again without relapsing, and cravings may persist for years. Between 40 and 60% of drug addicts relapse following treatment. Multi-drug users have the worst prognosis for recovery.

Substance abuse can damage organs, including the brain and liver, and can lead to serious and even fatal illness, as well as mental disorders such as dementia. Drug addiction puts the addict at risk for:

- cardiovascular disease
- stroke
- cancer
- HIV/AIDS
- hepatitis B and C
- lung disease
- obesity
- other mental disorders

Prevention

Preventive approaches are most effective when targeted at young teenagers between the ages of 11 and 13. It is during these years that most young people are likely to first experiment with drugs and alcohol. Hence, reducing experimentation during this critical period holds promise for reducing the number of adults with addictions. Effective **prevention** programs focus on the concerns of young people with regard to the effects of tobacco, alcohol, and drugs. Training older adolescents to help younger adolescents resist peer pressure has shown considerable effectiveness in preventing experimentation.

Preventative measures against addiction include:

- fostering self-control and positive relationships
- promoting parental monitoring and support
- promoting anti-addiction policies
- educational programs for the public
- building strong communities

The most effective form of prevention appears to be a stable family that models responsible attitudes toward mood-altering substances and behaviors.

Effects on Public Health

The effects of addiction are complex and far-reaching. Addiction affects not only the addict but also the friends and family members of the addict. Through loss in productivity, healthcare costs, motor vehicle accidents, enforcement, and crime, addiction also places a heavy financial burden on society. According to the most recent data available from the National Institute on Drug Abuse (NIDA), illegal drug abuse and addiction costs the United States $181 billion per year, alcohol abuse and addiction costs $185 billion per year, and tobacco abuse and addiction costs $193 billion per year, bringing the total cost of drug and alcohol addictions to $559 billion per year in the United States. These numbers do not take into account similar costs that result from other forms of addiction.

The presence of alcohol or other drugs can increase the likelihood of **violence** and other crimes. The U.S. Department of Justice (DOJ) reports that 75% of spousal abuse incidents involve an offender who has been drinking alcohol, and that approximately one out of every four violent crimes and fatal motor vehicle accidents involves alochol.

Resources

BOOKS

American Psychiatric Association. *Diagnostic and Statistical Manual of Mental Disorders (DSM-IV-TR)*, 4th ed., text rev. Arlington, VA: American Psychiatric Association, 2007.

Califano, Joseph A., Jr. *High Society: How Substance Abuse Ravages America and What to Do About It.* New York: Public Affairs Press, 2007.

DiClemente, Carlo C. *Addiction and Change: How Addictions Develop and Addicted People Recover.* New York: Guilford Press, 2006.

Erickson, Carlton K. *The Science of Addiction: From Neurobiology to Treatment.* New York: W. W. Norton, 2007.

Fleming, John C. *Preventing Addiction.* Garland, TX: CrossHouse Publishing, 2006.

Hoffman, John, and Susan Froemke. *Addiction: Why Can't They Just Stop?* Emmaus, PA: Rodale Books, 2007.

National Center on Addiction and Substance Abuse (CASA) at Columbia University. *Women Under the Influence.* Baltimore: Johns Hopkins University Press, 2006.

PERIODICALS

Adler, Jerry. "Rehab Reality Check: As the Traditional Treatment Centers Do Battle With Glitzy Newcomers, Everyone is Debating What Works." *Newsweek* (February 19, 2007): 44.

Grant, Jon E., Judson A. Brewer, and Marc N. Potenza. "The Neurobiology of Substance and Behavioral Addictions." *CNS Spectrums* 11 (2006): 924–930.

Johnson, Brian, et al. "Reducing the Risk of Addiction to Prescribed Medications." *Psychiatric Times* (April 15, 2007): 35.

Kienast, T., and A. Heinz. "Dopamine and the Diseased Brain." *CNS & Neurological Disorders—Drug Targets* 5 (2006): 109–131.

Kushlick, Danny. "Stopping the Conveyor Belt to Addiction: Addressing the Underlying Issues of Addiction Will Help Us to Tackle It." *New Statesman* (May 21, 2007): S4–S5.

Lemonick, Michael D. "The Science of Addiction." *Time* (July 16, 2007): 42.

Lobo, Daniela S. S., and James L. Kennedy. "The Genetics of Gambling and Behavioral Addictions." *CNS Spectrums* 11 (2006): 931–939.

Pallanti, Stefano. "From Impulse-Control Disorders Toward Behavioral Addictions." *CNS Spectrums* 11 (2006): 921–922.

Rutledge, Barbara. "Disulfiram, Vaccine May Curb Cocaine Addiction." *Clinical Psychiatry News* (May 2007): 38.

Throop, John. "Cyber-Addictions." *Marriage Partnership* (Summer 2007): 7.

WEBSITES

Centers for Disease Control and Prevention "Illegal Drug Use." http://www.cdc.gov/nchs/fastats/druguse.htm Accessed November 11, 2012.

Centers for Disease Control and Prevention "Smoking & Tobacco Use." http://www.cdc.gov/tobacco/index.htm Accessed November 11, 2012.

Department of Justice "Bureau of Justice Statistics." http://bjs.ojp.usdoj.gov/ Accessed November 11, 2012.

National Institute on Alcohol Abuse and Alcoholism"Drinking Statistics." http://www.niaaa.nih.gov/alcohol-health/overview-alcohol-consumption/drinking-statistics Accessed November 11, 2012.

"Drugs, Brains, and Behavior—The Science of Addiction." *National Institute on Drug Abuse.* http://www.nida.nih.gov/scienceofaddiction. Accessed November 11, 2012.

ORGANIZATIONS

Al-Anon/Alateen, 1600 Corporate Landing Parkway, Virginia Beach, VA 23454-5617, (757) 563-1600, Fax: (757) 563-1655, wso@al-anon.org, http://www.al-anon.alateen.org

Alcoholics Anonymous, PO Box 459, New York, NY 10163, (212) 870-3400, http://www.aa.org

American Psychiatric Association, 1000 Wilson Blvd., Ste. 1825, Arlington, VA 22209-3901, (703) 907-7300, apa@psych.org, http://www.psych.org

Center for Internet Addiction Recovery, P.O. Box 72, Bradford, PA 16701, (814) 451-2405, Fax: (814) 368-9560, http://www.netaddiction.com

Centre for Addiction and Mental Health, 33 Russell St., Toronto, Ontario, Canada M5S 2S1, (416) 535-8501, (800) 463-6273, http://www.camh.net

European Cities Against Drugs, Hantverkargatan 3D, City Hall, S-105-35, Stockholm, Sweden, 46-8-5082-9362, Fax: 46-8-5082-9436, ecad@ecad.net, http://www.ecad.net

National Center on Addiction and Substance Abuse at Columbia University, 633 Third Avenue, 19th Floor, New York, NY 10017-6706, (212) 841-5200, http://www.casacolumbia.org

National Clearinghouse for Alcohol and Drug Information, P.O. Box 2345, Rockville, MD 20847-2345, (877) SAMHSA-7, Fax: (240) 221-4292, http://ncadi.samhsa.gov

National Institute on Alcohol Abuse and Alcoholism (NIAAA), 5635 Fishers Lane, MSC 9304, Bethesda, MD 20892-9304, (301) 443-3860, http://www.niaaa.nih.gov

National Institute on Drug Abuse (NIDA), 6001 Executive Boulevard, Room 5213, Bethesda, MD 20892-9561, (301) 443-1124, information@nida.nih.gov, http://www.drugabuse.gov/NIDAHome.html.

Barbara S. Sternberg, PHD
Emily Jane Willingham, PHD
Bill Asenjo, MS, CRC
Ken R. Wells
Margaret Alic, PHD
Andrea Nienstedt, MA

Aging

Definition

Aging is the accumulation of physical, psychological, and social changes for a person over a lifetime. Starting at what is commonly called "middle age," operations of the human body begin to be more vulnerable to daily wear and tear, and there is a general decline in physical and possibly mental functioning. However, other facets may increase as one ages, such as knowledge and wisdom. The length of life is often into the 70s for men and 80s for women. The upward limit of the life span for humans, however, can be as high as 120 or more years. During the latter half of life, an individual is more prone to having problems with the various functions of the body and to developing any number of chronic or fatal diseases. The cardiovascular, digestive, excretory, nervous, reproductive, and urinary systems are particularly affected. The most common diseases of aging include Alzheimer's disease, arthritis, **cancer**, **diabetes**, depression, and **heart disease**.

Description

Human beings reach a peak of growth and development around the time of their mid-20s. Aging is the normal transition time after that flurry of activity. Although there are quite a few age-related changes that tax the body, disability is not necessarily a part of aging. Health and lifestyle factors, together with the genetic makeup of the

10 leading causes of death: United States, 2007

Rank	Cause of death	Number	Percent of total deaths	Death rate
...	All causes	1,755,567	100.0	4,633.6
1	Diseases of heart	496,095	28.3	1,309.4
2	Malignant neoplasms	389,730	22.2	1,028.6
3	Cerebrovascular diseases	115,961	6.6	306.1
4	Chronic lower respiratory diseases	109,562	6.2	289.2
5	Alzheimer's disease	73,797	4.2	194.8
6	Diabetes mellitus	51,528	2.9	136.0
7	Influenza and pneumonia	45,941	2.6	121.3
8	Nephritis, nephrotic syndrome and nephrosis	38,484	2.2	101.6
9	Accidents (unintentional injuries)	38,292	2.2	101.1
10	Septicemia	26,362	1.5	69.6
...	All other causes	369,815	21.1	976.1

SOURCE: Heron, M. "Deaths: Leading Causes for 2007." *National Vital Statistics Reports*, vol. 59, no. 8. Hyattsville, MD: National Center for Health statistics, 2011.

(Table by PreMediaGlobal. © 2013 Cengage Learning)

individual, help to determine the response to these changes. Body functions that are most often affected by age include:

- A decline in hearing, which decreases especially in relation to the highest pitched tones.
- The proportion of fat to muscle, which may increase by as much as 30%. Typically, the total padding of body fat directly under the skin thins out and accumulates around the stomach. The ability to excrete fats is impaired, and therefore the storage of fats increases, including cholesterol and fat-soluble nutrients.
- The amount of water in the body decreases, which therefore decreases the absorption of water-soluble nutrients. Also, there is less saliva and other lubricating fluids.
- The liver and the kidneys cannot function as efficiently, thus affecting the elimination of wastes.
- A decrease in the ease of digestion, with a decrease in stomach acid production.
- A loss of muscle strength and coordination, with an accompanying loss of mobility, agility, and flexibility.
- A decline in sexual hormones and sexual functioning.
- A decrease in the sensations of taste and smell.
- A reduction in the cardiovascular and respiratory systems, leading to decreased oxygen and nutrients throughout the body.
- A decreased functioning of the nervous system so that nerve impulses are not transmitted as efficiently, reflexes are not as sharp, and memory and learning are diminished.
- A decrease in bone strength and density.
- A gradual decline in hormone levels. The thyroid and sexual hormones are particularly affected.
- A decline in visual abilities. Age-related changes may lead to diseases such as macular degeneration.
- A compromised ability to produce vitamin D from sunlight.
- A reduction in protein formation, leading to shrinkage in muscle mass and decreased bone formation, possibly leading to osteoporosis

Demographics

The number of deaths per year per 1,000 people is called the "crude death rate" (CDR). As of the period from 2005 to 2010, the United Nations estimates that the CDR for the world is 8.5 per 1,000 people. Roughly 100,000 people die each day around the world from age-related problems. According to the **World Health Organization**, the 10 leading causes of death (in order of highest frequency) in the world are:

- ischaemic heart disease
- cerebrovascular disease
- lower respiratory infections
- human immunodeficiency virus/acquired immune deficiency syndrome (HIV/AIDS)
- chronic obstructive pulmonary disease
- diarrheal diseases
- tuberculosis
- trachea/bronchus/lung cancers
- malaria
- road traffic accidents

Effects on Public Health

Between 2000 and 2050, the percentage of older people in the United States is projected to increase by 135%. During this same period, the percentage of people who are 85 years or over is projected to increase by 350%. Thus, the aging of the U.S. **population** will have a dramatic effect on the public health care system. There is already a shortage of health care workers, especially nurses, in the United States. This situation will most likely require that medical professionals focus more on chronic diseases such as Alzheimer's disease and heart disease rather than acute illnesses.

Costs to Society

According to the Daily Finance article "The Price of Aging: Will It Break National Budgets?," Growing old is costlier than ever, and in many countries, the rising expense of caring for graying populations threatens to

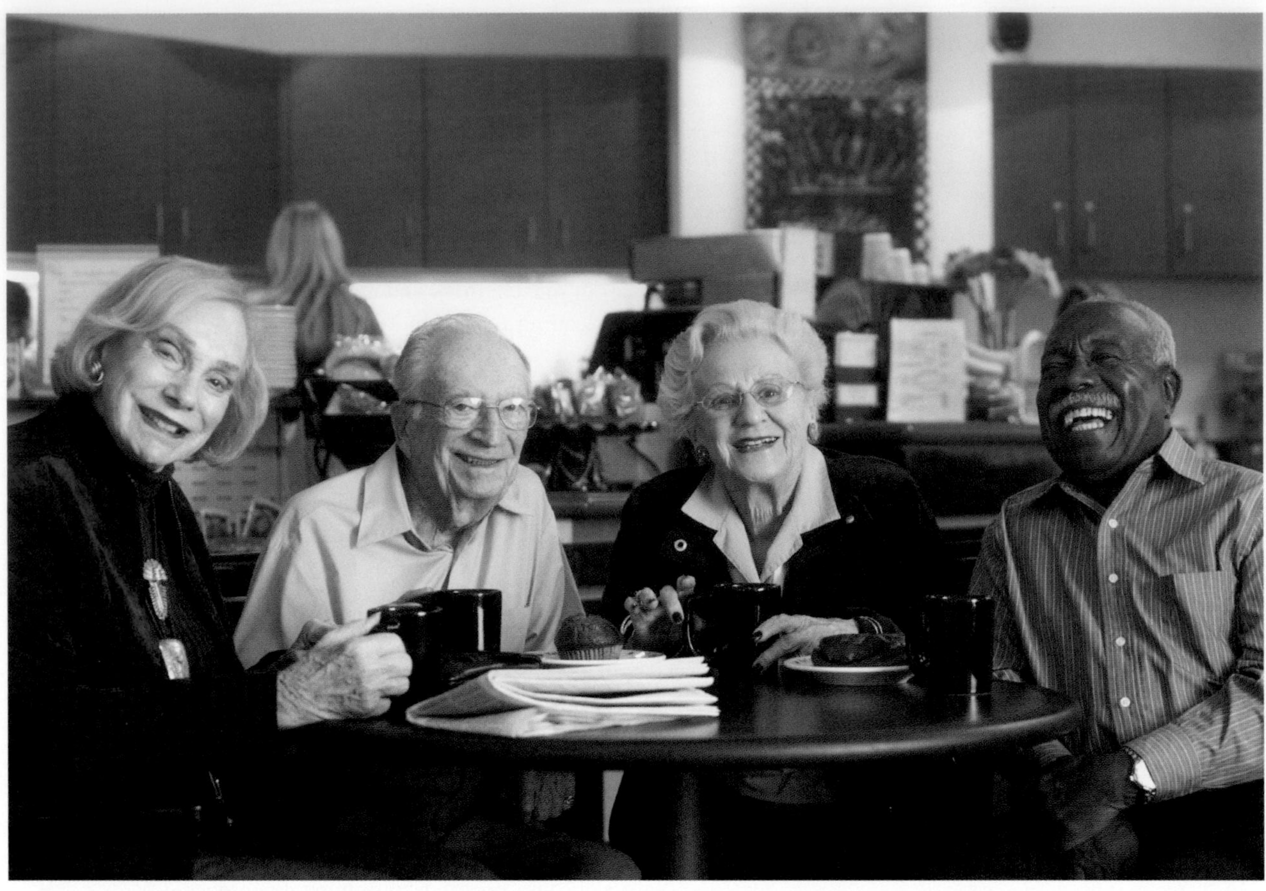

A group of seniors enjoying tea and social interaction, both of which are part of a healthy retirement. *(© istockPhoto.com/ Catherine Yeulet)*

inflate national debts to unsustainable levels. The article states, "If current policies remain in place, age-related expenses could launch Japan's national debt into an unsustainable 750% of its gross domestic product [GDP] by 2050, according to the [Standard & Poor's] report. The credit-rating agency estimates those costs could soar to nearly 600% of GDP in the Netherlands and 415% of GDP in the U.S. by that time. Currently, national age-related expenses average less than 40% of countries' GDPs."

Causes and symptoms

Several theories have been proposed as to the causes of aging. Many symptoms are quite apparent as one ages, while others are more subtle.

Causes

There are several theories as to why the aging body loses functioning. It may be that several factors work together or that one particular factor is at work more than are others in a given individual. Some of these theories as to what causes aging are:

- Programmed senescence, or aging clock, theory. The aging of the cells of each individual is programmed into the genes, and there is a preset number of possible rejuvenations in the life of a given cell. When cells die at a rate faster than they are replaced, organs do not function properly, and they are soon unable to maintain the functions necessary for life.
- Genetic theory. Human cells maintain their own seed of destruction at the level of the chromosomes.
- Connective tissue, or cross-linking theory. Changes in the make-up of the connective tissue alter the stability of body structures, causing a loss of elasticity and functioning, and leading to symptoms of aging.
- Free-radical theory. As the most commonly held theory of aging, it is based on the fact that ongoing chemical reactions of the cells produce free radicals. In the presence of oxygen, these free radicals cause the cells of the body to break down. As time goes on, more cells

die or lose the ability to function, and the body soon ceases to function as a whole.

- Immunological theory. There are changes in the immune system as it begins to wear out, and the body is more prone to infections and tissue damage, which may finally cause death. Also, as the system breaks down, the body is more apt to have autoimmune reactions, in which the body's own cells are mistaken for foreign material and are destroyed or damaged by the immune system.

Symptoms

The most apparent sign of aging is changes to the skin. Aging skin becomes thinner, is more apt to wrinkle, and becomes less elastic. It also takes longer to heal after being injured. These changes occur when the fat layer beneath the skin becomes diminished. Without such a fat layer, the skin begins to sag and wrinkle, and lines and furrows begin to form. Dementia is another sign that often results as one ages. This involves a gradual diminishing of mental capacity to perform tasks that involve memory, physical coordination, and general functioning. The most common form of dementia is Alzheimer's disease. Its symptoms include memory loss, emotional and behavioral disturbances, and cognitive and communication difficulties. Other signs of aging include graying hair, balding, **hearing loss**, and diminished eyesight, such as difficulty in reading small print.

Diagnosis

Many problems can arise due to age related changes in the body. Although there is no single test to be given, a thorough physical examination and a basic blood screening and blood chemistry panel can point to areas in need of further attention. When older people become ill, the first signs of disease are often nonspecific. Further exams should be conducted if any of the following occurs:

- diminished or lack of desire for food
- increasing confusion
- failure to thrive
- urinary incontinence
- dizziness
- weight loss
- falling

Prevention

Preventive health practices such as healthy diet, daily exercise, **stress** management, and control of lifestyle habits, such as not smoking tobacco products and drinking alcoholic beverages, can lengthen the life span and improve the quality of life as people age. Exercise can improve the appetite, the health of the bones, the emotional and mental outlook, and the digestion and circulation.

Drinking plenty of fluids aids in maintaining healthy skin, good digestion, and proper elimination of wastes. Up to eight glasses of **water** should be consumed daily, along with plenty of herbal teas, diluted fruit and vegetable juices, and fresh fruits and vegetables with high water content.

Because of a decrease in the sense of taste, older people often increase their intake of salt, which can contribute to high blood pressure and nutrient loss. Use of sugar is also increased. Seaweeds and small amounts of honey can be used as replacements.

Alcohol, nicotine, and caffeine all have potential damaging effects and should be limited or completely eliminated from consumption.

A diet high in fiber and low in fat is recommended. Complex carbohydrates such as whole grains should replace processed foods. If chewing becomes a problem, there should be an increased intake of protein drinks, freshly juiced fruits and vegetables, and creamed cereals.

Treatment

For the most part, doctors prescribe medications to control the symptoms and diseases of aging. In the United States, about two-thirds of people 65 years or older take medications for various complaints. More women than men use these medications. The most common drugs used by the elderly are painkillers, diuretics or water pills, sedatives, cardiac drugs, **antibiotics**, and mental health drugs.

Estrogen replacement therapy (ERT) is commonly prescribed to postmenopausal women for symptoms of aging. It is often used in conjunction with progesterone. ERT functions to help keep bones strong, reduce risk of heart disease, restore vaginal lubrication, and improve skin elasticity. Evidence suggests that it may also help maintain mental functions.

Alternative Treatment

Various alternative treatments can also be used for aging. These include nutritional supplements, hormone supplements, and herbs.

NUTRITIONAL SUPPLEMENTS. Consumption of a high quality multivitamin is recommended. Common nutritional deficiencies connected with aging include B **vitamins**, vitamins A and C, folic acid, calcium, magnesium, zinc, iron, chromium, and trace minerals. Since stomach acids may be decreased, it is suggested that the use of a powdered multivitamin formula in gelatin capsules be used, as this form is the easiest to digest. Such formulas may also contain enzymes for further help with digestion.

Antioxidants can help to neutralize damage by the free radical actions thought to contribute to problems of aging. They are also helpful in preventing and treating cancer and in treating cataracts and glaucoma. Supplements that serve as antioxidants include:

- Vitamin E, 400–1,000 international units (IUs) daily. It protects cell membranes against damage; and it shows promise in prevention against heart disease, and Alzheimer's and Parkinson's diseases.
- Selenium, 50 milligrams (mg) taken twice daily. Research suggests that selenium may play a role in reducing the risk of cancer.
- Beta-carotene, 25,000–40,000 IUs daily. It may help in treating cancer, colds and flu, arthritis, and immune support.
- Vitamin C, 1,000–2,000 mg per day. It may cause diarrhea in large doses. If this occurs, however, all that is needed is a decrease in the dosage.

Other supplements that are helpful in treating age-related problems including:

- B_{12}/B-complex vitamins; studies show that B_{12} may help reduce mental symptoms, such as confusion, memory loss, and depression.
- Coenzyme Q10 may be helpful in treating heart disease, as up to three-quarters cardiac patients have been found to be lacking in this heart enzyme.

HORMONES. Hormone supplements may be taken to prevent or to treat various age-related problems. However, caution should be taken before beginning treatment, and the patient should consult his or her health care professional.

Dehydroepiandrosterone (DHEA) improves brain functioning and serves as a building block for many other important hormones in the body. It may be helpful in restoring declining hormone levels and in building up muscle mass, strengthening the bones, and maintaining a healthy heart.

Melatonin may be helpful for insomnia. It has also been used to help fight viruses and bacterial infections, reduce the risk of heart disease, improve sexual functioning, and protect against cancer.

Human growth hormone (hGH) has been shown to regulate blood sugar levels and to stimulate bone, cartilage, and muscle growth while reducing fat.

HERBS. Garlic (*Allium sativa*) is helpful in preventing heart disease, as well as improving the tone and texture of skin. Garlic stimulates liver and digestive system functions, and also helps in dealing with heart disease and high blood pressure.

Siberian ginseng (*Eleutherococcus senticosus*) supports the adrenal glands and immune functions. It is believed to be helpful in treating problems related to stress. Siberian ginseng also increases mental and physical performance and may be useful in treating memory loss, chronic fatigue, and immune dysfunction.

Proanthocyanidins—sometimes shortened to PCOs for procyanicolic oligomers or OPCs for oligomeric proanthocyanidins—are part of the bioflavonoid family of organic compounds. With the chemical term "pycnogenol," they are derived from grape seeds and skin, and from pine tree bark, and may help in the **prevention** of cancer and poor vision.

In Ayurvedic medicine, aging is described as a process of increased *vata* (a principle within traditional Hindu medicine), in which there is a tendency to become thinner, drier, more nervous, more restless, and more fearful, while having a loss of appetite as well as sleep. Bananas, almonds, avocados, and coconuts are some of the foods used in correcting such conditions. One of the main herbs used for such conditions is gotu kola (*Centella asiatica*), which is used to revitalize the nervous system and brain cells and to fortify the immune system. Gotu kola is also used to treat memory loss, anxiety, and insomnia.

In Chinese medicine, most symptoms of aging are regarded as symptoms of a yin deficiency. Moistening foods such as millet, barley soup, tofu, mung beans, wheat germ, spirulina, potatoes, black sesame seeds, walnuts, and flax seeds are recommended. Jing tonics may also be used. These include deer antler, dodder seeds, processed rehmannia, longevity soup, mussels, and chicken.

KEY TERMS

Antioxidants—Substances that reduce the damage of the highly reactive free radicals that are the byproducts of the cells.

Alzheimer's disease—A condition causing a decline in brain function that interferes with the ability to reason and to perform daily activities.

Senescence—The state or process of aging.

Vata—One of the three main constitutional types found under Ayurvedic principles. Keeping one's particular constitution in balance is considered important in maintaining health.

QUESTIONS TO ASK YOUR DOCTOR

- Am I up to date on my vaccinations?
- Are my medications still appropriate?
- Is memory loss a normal part of aging?
- How much exercise do I need daily?
- What are my best options for preventative care?
- Are vitamin and mineral supplements necessary for me at my age?
- How much alcohol consumption is safe for me?
- Where can I learn more about senior nutrition?
- Where can I find useful and reliable information on the aging process?

Prognosis

Although the aging process is inevitable, people can take important steps to reduce the risk of disease and maintain a high quality of life.

Results

Aging is unavoidable, but major physical impairment is not. People can lead a healthy, disability-free life well through their later years. A well-established support system of family, friends, and health care providers, together with focus on good **nutrition** and lifestyle habits and good stress management, can prevent disease and lessen the impact of chronic conditions. Maintaining an active lifestyle with high cognitive and physical functions will help to slow the aging process.

Precautions

As one grows older, it is imperative that precautions are taken to maintain one's health and vitality. The diet of older people should be balanced and well planned out. Check with a dietitian or a family doctor for the proper diet best suited for older people. Good nutrition is very important for healthy aging; and to prevent diseases associated with aging. A regular, routine checkup with a family doctor is also imperative. During such checkups, make sure all medicines and supplements are reviewed for appropriateness.

Risks

Risks during aging come into play based on genetics and lifestyle. Some of the biggest risks for women as they age are: osteoporosis (because women tend to have more bone loss than men), breast cancer (with an increased incidence of it after the age of 65 years), chronic obstructive pulmonary disease (women are twice as likely as men to be diagnosed with it), and urinary incontinence (over 30% of women between the ages of 35 and 55 years develop the condition). In men, prostate problems are common after the age of 50 years, and they become even more common after the age of 60. Some doctors recommend regular blood tests to check the prostate specific antigen (PSA) level. The PSA level tends to be high in men with an enlarged prostate gland or prostate cancer.

Resources

BOOKS

Bales, Connie Watkins, and Christine Seel Richie, editors. *Handbook of Clinical Nutrition and Aging.* Totowa, NJ: Humana Press, 2009.

Cress, Cathy Jo, editor. *Handbook of Geriatric Care Management.* Sudbury, MA: Jones & Bartlett Learning, 2012.

Dangour, Alan, Emily Grundy, and Asrtrid Fletcher, editors. *Aging Well: Nutrition, Health, and Social Interventions.* Boca Raton, FL: CRC Press, 2007.

Preedy, Victor R., Ronald Ross Watson, and Colin R. Martin, editors. *Handbook of Behavior, Food and Nutrition.* New York: Springer, 2011.

Roth, Ruth A. *Nutrition & Diet Therapy.* Clifton Park, NY: Delmar Cengage Learning, 2011.

Touhy, Theris A., and Kathleen Jett. *Ebersole & Hess' Toward Healthy Aging: Human Needs & Nursing Response.* St. Louis: Elsevier/Mosby, 2012.

Watson, Ronald R. *Handbook of Nutrition in the Aged.* Boca Raton, FL: CRC Press, 2009.

WEBSITES

Beattie, Leanne. *Nutrition and the Elderly.* SparkPeople.com. (January 18, 2011). http://www.sparkpeople.com/resource/nutrition_articles.asp?id=869 (accessed February 18, 2012).

50+: Live Better, Longer. WebMD. http://www.webmd.com/healthy-aging/default.htm (accessed July 25, 2012).

Haas, Elson M. *Nutritional Program for Anti-Aging.* Healthy .net. http://www.healthy.net/scr/article.aspx?ID=1272 (accessed July 25, 2012).

Haas, Elson M. *Nutritional Programs for the Elderly.* Healthy. net. http://www.healthy.net/hwlibrarybooks/haas/lifestage/elderly.htm (accessed July 25, 2012).

Healthy Aging: Over 50. Mayo Clinic. http://www.mayoclinic .com/health/healthy-aging/MY00374/ (accessed July 25, 2012).

The Joy of Eating Well and Aging Well. HelpGuide.org. http://helpguide.org/life/senior_nutrition.htm (accessed February 18, 2012).

ORGANIZATIONS

Academy of Nutrition and Dietetics, 120 South Riverside Plaza, Ste. 2000, Chicago, IL U.S.A. 60606-6995, 1 (312) 899-0040, (800) 877-1600, http://eatright.org

Administration on Aging, One Massachusetts Ave., N.W., Washington, D.C. U.S.A. 20001, 1 (202) 619-0724,

Fax: 1 (202) 357-3555, aoainfo@aoa.hhs.gov, http://www.aoa.gov/

Food and Nutrition Information Center, U.S. Department of Agriculture, 10301 Baltimore Ave., Rm. 105 (National Agricultural Library), Beltsville, MD U.S.A. 20705, 1 (301) 504-5414, Fax: 1 (301) 504-6409, http://fnic.nal.usda.gov

National Institute on Aging, Bldg. 31, Rm. 5C27; 31 Center Dr., Bethesda, MD U.S.A. 20892, (800) 222-2225, niaic@nia.nih.gov, http://www.nia.nih.gov/.

Patience Paradox
William A. Atkins, BB, BS, MBA

AIDS

Definition

AIDS, or acquired immune deficiency syndrome, is the end stage of an **infectious disease** caused by the human immunodeficiency virus, or HIV. There are two variants of the HIV virus, HIV-1 and HIV-2, both of which ultimately cause AIDS. The virus damages the immune system, leaving the patient vulnerable to certain cancerous tumors and increasingly severe opportunistic infections. HIV can be transmitted whenever a body fluid containing the virus—semen, saliva, blood, or breast milk—comes into contact with a mucous membrane or the bloodstream itself. A person can get AIDS through sexual intercourse, anal or oral sex, childbirth, breastfeeding, blood transfusion, tattoos or body piercing, or sharing hypodermic needles.

Demographics

As of 2009, about 0.6% of the world's **population** was infected with HIV, or about 35 million people. Ninety-five percent of these cases are in Africa or southeastern Asia. About 25 million people have died of AIDS since 1981, making the disease one of the deadliest pandemics in history. In the United States, the CDC's recently revised estimates indicate that about 945,000 people have been diagnosed with AIDS since 1981, and about 1.2 million are currently living with HIV infection. About a quarter of these people are unaware that they are infected with the virus. The **CDC** estimates that there are 56,300 new cases of HIV infection in the United States each year.

The CDC gives the following statistics for specific groups within the United States:

- Males account for 74% of persons with HIV infection in the United States, although worldwide, the figure for males is 50%.
- In terms of race or ethnicity, 47% of persons with HIV infection are African American, 34% are Caucasian, 17% are Hispanic, and 2% are Native American or Asian American.
- In terms of method of transmission, 50% of infected persons are men who had sex with men; 33% had high-risk heterosexual sex; 13% are injection drug users; and the remainder are people who engaged in more than one high-risk behavior.
- In terms of age group, one percent of infected persons are under 13 years of age; 15% are between the ages of 13 and 24; 26% are between the ages of 25 and 34; 32% are between the ages of 35 and 44; 20% are between the ages of 45 and 54; 8% are 55 or older.

A worrisome new trend as of 2009 is the return and increase of high-risk behaviors among men who have sex with men in Canada and the United States. This trend appears to have been triggered by the spread of **methamphetamine addiction** from the West Coast to the Eastern Seaboard since the early 2000s.

AIDS in women

Women exposed to HIV infection through heterosexual contact are the most rapidly growing risk group in the United States. The gender demographics of HIV infection within the United States are changing, with women accounting for more new cases in 2009 than was the case in 1999. The percentage of AIDS cases diagnosed in American women has risen from 7% in 1985 to about 26% in 2006, the last year for which data are available. According to the CDC, in 2006 approximately 278,400 women in the United States were living with HIV/AIDS. The rate was highest among black women, who had 23 times as many cases as Caucasian women and 4 times as many cases as Hispanic women. About 75% of these women contracted HIV through high-risk heterosexual activity; almost all of the remainder acquired the infection through needle sharing.

The prevalence of women with HIV in the United States is low, however, compared to the rate in many countries in the developing world. Worldwide, about half the people living with HIV are women. According to the United Nations, in 2005 about 59% of women living in sub-Saharan Africa are infected with HIV. The vast majority of them were infected through having unprotected sex with an infected male partner. One theory that has been proposed to explain the higher rate of AIDS in women in Africa is the prevalence of **schistosomiasis** in the region. Schistosomiasis is a parasitic disease caused by a trematode (a type of flatworm) that affects as many as 50% of women in some parts of Africa; while it is

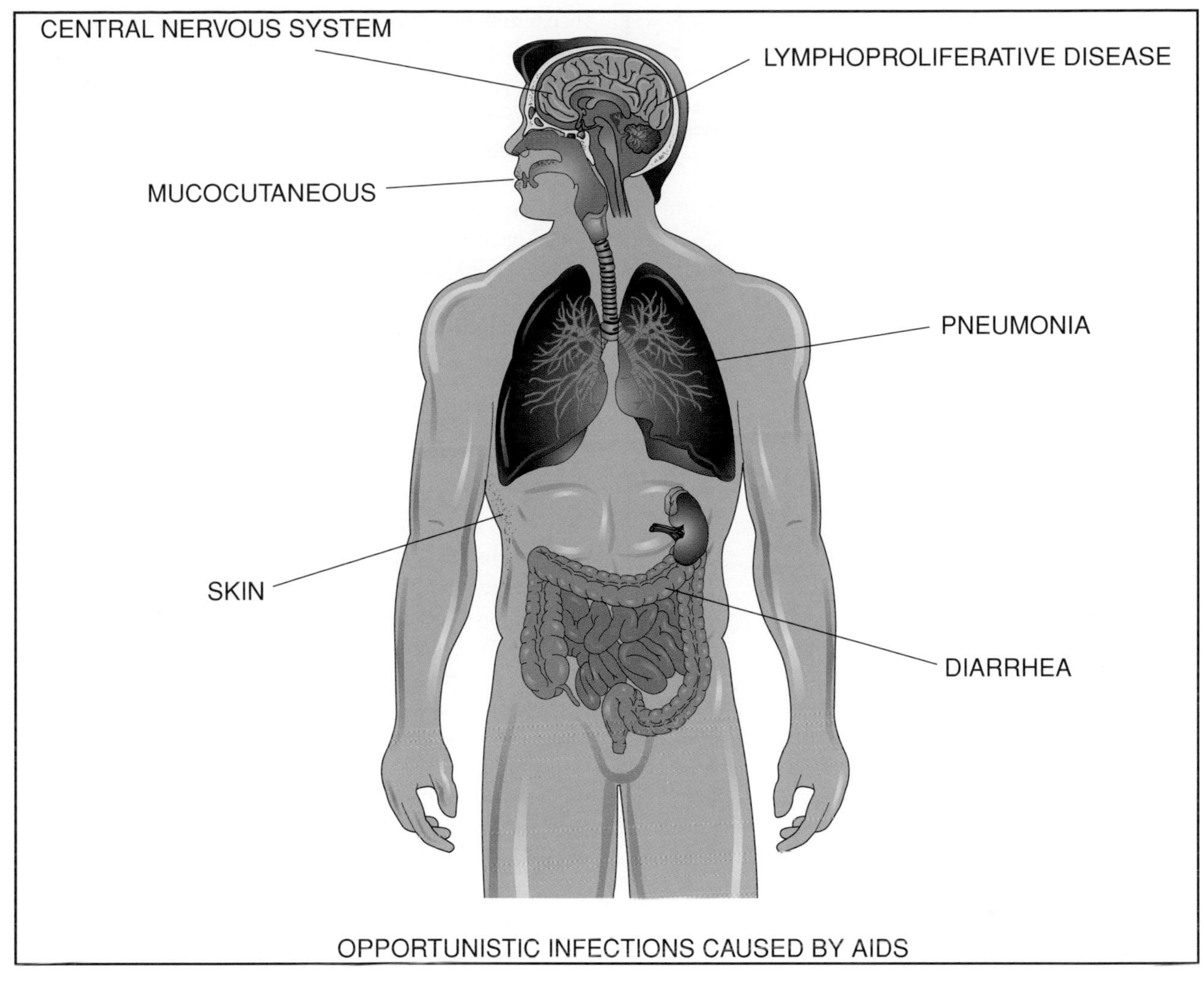

(Illustration by Electronic Illustrators Group. © 2013 Cengage Learning)

rarely fatal, schistosomiasis damages the tissues lining the vagina, making them more vulnerable to the AIDS virus.

AIDS in children

Since AIDS can be transmitted from an infected mother to a fetus during pregnancy or to an infant during the birth process or through breastfeeding, all infants born to HIV-positive mothers are considered a high-risk group. However, prenatal drug treatment of HIV-positive mothers in developed countries has reduced the number of children born infected with HIV. In the developing world, drug treatment is either not available or not affordable. According to the United Nations Children's Fund (UNICEF) worldwide 2.3 million children under age 13 were living with HIV in 2006. The previous year, about 380,000 children died of AIDS and more than half a million children were newly infected. UNICEF estimates that at least 15 million children have lost at least one parent to AIDS.

AIDS is the leading causes of death in children under age five in many parts of Africa and Southeast Asia. One reason for this tragedy is that only 1% of sexually active women in these regions get tested for HIV infection, and these women can become pregnant before they develop symptoms of the disease. The interval between exposure to HIV and the development of AIDS is shorter in children than in adults. Infants infected with HIV have a high chance of developing AIDS within one year and dying before age three. In the remainder, AIDS progresses more slowly; the average child patient survives to about seven years of age. Some survive into early adolescence.

AIDS in older adults

The demographics of HIV infection among the elderly have changed since the early days of the AIDS

Risk of acquiring HIV infection by entry site

Entry site	Risk virus reaches entry site	Risk virus enters	Risk inoculated
Conjunctiva	Moderate	Moderate	Very low
Oral mucosa	Moderate	Moderate	Low
Nasal mucosa	Low	Low	Very low
Lower respiratory	Very low	Very low	Very low
Anus	Very high	Very high	Very high
Skin, intact	Very low	Very low	Very low
Skin, broken	Low	High	High
Sexual:			
Vagina	Low	Low	Moderate
Penis	High	Low	Low
Ulcers (STD)	High	High	Very high
Blood:			
Products	High	High	High
Shared needles	High	High	Very high
Accidental needle	Low	High	Low
Traumatic wound	Moderate	High	High
Perinatal	High	High	High

(Illustration by Electronic Illustrators Group. © 2013 Cengage Learning)

epidemic. In the mid-1980s, most cases of AIDS among older adults in the United States were the result of transfusions with contaminated blood. The introduction of effective screening tests for blood products has virtually eliminated this path of HIV transmission, however; as of 2009, almost all cases of AIDS in seniors are the result of sexual activity. In the United States, about 10% of all cases of AIDS occur in people over 50, and 3% in people over 60. About 35% of seniors who develop AIDS are homosexual or bisexual men; others are heterosexual men living in urban areas who engage in high-risk sex with prostitutes. In addition, the number of older adults with HIV/AIDS is rising; the CDC estimates that by 2015, half of all persons living with HIV/AIDS in North America will be over the age of 50.

One reason that sexually active seniors are particularly at risk for HIV infection is that they are rarely concerned about contraception. Adults over 50 are five times more likely than younger people to have unprotected sex because they think of condoms as a method of birth control rather than a means of preventing disease transmission. In addition, older women have thinner and more fragile tissues lining the walls of the vagina; these tissues are more likely to be bruised or damaged during unprotected intercourse, making it easier for the virus to enter the underlying tissues. Several studies done in 2006 and 2007 reported that older women are less likely than their younger counterparts to take precautions against HIV infection, in part because they are less sexually active than older men, and partly because they do not perceive themselves as being at risk for HIV infection.

According to the *Merck Manual of Geriatrics*, "Practically no **prevention** information on AIDS is targeted at elderly persons, although most elderly persons are sexually active." According to statistics compiled by the **Centers for Disease Control and Prevention**, about 2100 men between the ages of 55 and 59 are diagnosed with HIV infection each year, and 800 over the age of 65. Since the epidemic began in 1981, 15,000 adults over age 65 have been diagnosed with HIV in the United States.

Description

Background

AIDS is now considered a **pandemic** because it has spread to every country in the world. According to the **World Health Organization (WHO)**, 34 million people around the world were living with HIV infection in 2009; 2.1 million people died in 2008 from the disease, 330,000 of them children. Scientists think that the virus that causes AIDS originated somewhere in the African rainforest as an infection of chimpanzees and Old World monkeys. At some point in the twentieth century the virus jumped the species barrier from monkeys into humans, most likely somewhere in western Africa. The earliest known case of HIV infection was found in a blood sample collected from a man in Kinshasa in the Congo in 1959. AIDS was first defined as an epidemic human disease in June 1981 by the **Centers for Disease Control and Prevention (CDC)**. The virus that causes AIDS was identified by two teams of French and American scientists in 1983–1984.

The first cases of AIDS in the United States were not diagnosed until 1981, when the CDC reported a cluster of five cases of an opportunistic lung infection among homosexual men in Los Angeles. In the first 15 years of the epidemic, there were no effective treatments for HIV infection (there is still no cure). In 1996, a team of researchers in California introduced a form of treatment known as highly active antiretroviral therapy or HAART. While drug therapy is not a cure for AIDS, it can slow the progress of the disease and improve the patient's quality of life.

Course

HIV infection progresses in stages as the virus gradually weakens the body's immune system. It takes an average of 11 years for HIV infection to progress to AIDS, although the disease progresses faster in children and the elderly. AIDS is diagnosed when the count of certain white blood cells in the patient's blood drops to a critical level or the patient develops life-threatening tumors or opportunistic infections.

In the early stage of HIV infection, the patient may have no symptoms at all or a mild flu-like illness with fever and headache within a few days or weeks of getting infected. These symptoms usually go away without treatment and the person feels normal, even though they are a carrier and can transmit the infection to others. The infected person may continue to feel well for a period ranging from a few months to several years.

Risk factors

AIDS can be transmitted in several ways. The risk factors for HIV transmission vary according to the method of transmission.

- Sexual contact. People at greatest risk are those who do not practice safer sex by always using a condom, those who have multiple sexual partners, those who participate in anal intercourse, and those who have sex with a partner who has HIV infection and/or other sexually transmitted diseases (STDs). In the United States and Europe, most cases of sexually transmitted HIV infection result from homosexual contact, whereas in Africa, the disease is spread primarily through sexual intercourse among heterosexuals. Most people with AIDS in the United States are between 25 and 44 years of age.
- Transmission in pregnancy. High-risk mothers include women sexually active with bisexual men, intravenous drug users, and women living in neighborhoods with a high rate of HIV infection among heterosexuals. The chances of transmitting the disease to the child are higher in women in advanced stages of the disease. Breast feeding increases the risk of HIV transmission as HIV passes into breast milk. The rate of pediatric HIV transmission in the United States had decreased substantially because of HIV testing and improved drug treatment for infected mothers, so fewer than 1% of AIDS cases now occur in children under age 15. In the developing world, mother to infant transmission remains epidemic. In 2006, AIDS was the single most common cause of death in children under age 5 in South Africa, while worldwide children account for about 10% of all AIDS cases.
- Exposure to contaminated blood. Risk of HIV transmission among intravenous drug users increases with the frequency and duration of intravenous use, frequency of needle sharing, number of people sharing a needle, and the rate of HIV infection in the local population. In 2006, about 19% of men with AIDS and 25% of women with AIDS contracted the disease through sharing needles during intravenous drug injection. With the introduction of new blood product screening in the mid-1980s, HIV transmission through blood transfusions became rare in the developed world. However, contaminated blood is still a significant source of infection in the developing world.
- Transmission via improperly sterilized tattooing or body piercing needles.
- Needle sticks or body fluid splashes among health care professionals. Transmission through theses sources accounts for fewer than 0.3% of all HIV infections in the United States. This rate reflects the emphasis on universal safety precautions (e.g., use of gloves, face shields, proper disposal of needles) among health care professionals and first responders.

Some older adults are at higher risk than others of HIV infection. In order to determine whether HIV testing should be a personal priority, an adult 55 years of age or older should use the following checklist of high-risk behaviors for 1978 and later:

- Shared needles for injecting drugs or steroids
- If a male, had unprotected sex with other males
- Had unprotected sex with someone known or suspected to be infected with HIV
- Had a blood transfusion between 1978 and 1985
- Had another sexually transmitted disease
- Had unprotected sex with anyone with any of the five previous risk factors

Causes and symptoms

Causes

The cause of AIDS is infection with human immunodeficiency virus or HIV. HIV is a retrovirus that reproduces by inserting its own genetic material into a type of white blood cell called a CD4 lymphocyte. When the virus copies break out of the infected white blood cell, they attack other CD4 cells and the cycle repeats. The virus has a short life cycle, needing as little as 1.5 days to enter a cell, replicate, and release new copies of itself to infect other cells. Eventually so many of the white blood cells have been destroyed that the body's immune system is weakened and the person can no longer fight off opportunistic infections. The patient may also develop certain cancers associated with a weakened immune system.

Symptoms

STAGES. The symptoms of HIV infection vary according to the progress of the infection. As mentioned above, about 30% of patients develop an acute syndrome resembling flu within a month of exposure to HIV. The patient typically

KEY TERMS

Acquired immune deficiency syndrome (AIDS)—HIV infection that has led to certain opportunistic infections, cancers, or a CD4+ T-lymphocyte (helper cell) blood cell count lower than 200/mL.

Acute retroviral syndrome (ARS)—A syndrome that develops in about 30% of HIV patients within a few weeks of infection. ARS is characterized by nausea, vomiting, fever, headache, general tiredness, and muscle cramps.

AIDS dementia complex—A type of brain dysfunction caused by HIV infection that causes difficulty thinking, confusion, and loss of muscular coordination.

Carrier—A person who bears or carries a disease agent in or on their body and can transmit the disease to others, but is immune to the disease or has no symptoms of it.

CD4—A type of protein molecule in human blood. The HIV virus infects cells with CD4 surface proteins and, as a result, depletes the number of T cells, B cells, natural killer cells, and monocytes in the patient's blood.

Dietitian—A health care professional who specializes in individual or group nutritional planning, public education in nutrition, or research in food science. To be licensed as a registered dietitian (RD) in the United States, a person must complete a bachelor's degree in a nutrition-related field and pass a state licensing examination. Dietitians are also called nutritionists.

Highly active antiretroviral therapy (HAART)—An individualized combination of three or more antiretroviral drugs used to treat patients with HIV infection. It is sometimes called a drug cocktail.

Kaposi's sarcoma—A cancer of the connective tissue that produces painless purplish red (in people with light skin) or brown (in people with dark skin) blotches on the skin. It is a major diagnostic marker of AIDS.

Lipodystrophy—The medical term for redistribution of body fat in response to HAART, insulin injections in diabetics, or rare hereditary disorders.

Lymphoma—A cancerous tumor in the lymphatic system that is associated with a poor prognosis in AIDS patients.

Malabsorption syndrome—A condition characterized by indigestion, bloating, diarrhea, loss of appetite, and weakness, caused by poor absorption of nutrients from food as a result of HIV infection itself, giardiasis or other opportunistic infections of

has a fever, headache, swollen lymph nodes, and fatigue. This illness is called acute retroviral syndrome or ARS. The symptoms then disappear; however, the infected person is highly contagious in this early phase and can readily pass on the virus to others. The patient may or may not have developed antibodies to HIV (a process known as seroconversion) at this point; thus a test for HIV infection in this early period may not yield positive results even though the patient is in fact infected.

In the second phase, the virus may be silent, but more commonly it produces complications. Patients in this stage of infection may have the following symptoms:

- Swelling of the lymph nodes that lasts three months or longer
- Fevers and night sweats
- Loss of energy
- Weight loss
- Frequent yeast infections of the vagina or mouth and throat. Yeast infections of the mouth are sometimes called thrush
- Skin rashes or flaky skin that does not go away
- Short-term memory loss. This symptom helps to explain why HIV infection in seniors is often misdiagnosed as early-stage Alzheimer's

In full-blown AIDS, the person develops one or more of the following opportunistic infections. Death usually results from one of these infections or from an AIDS-related **cancer**.

- Lung infections: these include a type of pneumonia caused by an organism known as *Pneumocystis jirovecii*, a yeast-like fungus; and tuberculosis.
- Mouth infections: these include oral candidiasis, or thrush.
- Infections of the digestive tract: these include parasitic as well as bacterial infections, and are often marked by severe diarrhea.
- Infections of the central nervous system: these include meningitis and toxoplasmosis. AIDS dementia complex (ADC), which is often misdiagnosed as Alzheimer's disease, is caused by destruction of brain tissue by

KEY TERMS (continued)

the digestive tract, or certain surgical procedures involving the stomach or intestines.

Non-nucleoside reverse transcriptase inhibitors—The newest class of antiretroviral drugs that work by inhibiting the reverse transcriptase enzyme necessary for HIV replication.

Nucleoside analogues—The first group of effective anti-retroviral medications. They work by interfering with the AIDS virus' synthesis of DNA.

Opportunistic infection—An infection caused by an organism that does not cause disease in a person with a healthy immune system.

Pandemic—An infectious disease that spreads across a large region or even worldwide.

Post-exposure prophylaxis (PEP)—A four-week course of antiretroviral drugs given to people immediately following exposure to HIV infection from rape, unprotected sex, needlestick injuries, or sharing needles.

Protease inhibitors—The second major category of drug used to treat AIDS that works by suppressing the replication of the HIV virus.

Retrovirus—A virus that uses its RNA to produce DNA and add that DNA to the genetic material of infected cells.

Seroconversion—The development of detectable specific antibodies in a patient's blood serum as a result of infection or immunization.

T-lymphocyte—A type of white blood cell, also known as a T-helper cell, a T_h cell, an effector T cell, or a CD4+ T cell, whose numbers in a blood sample can be used to monitor the progression of HIV infection.

Viral load—A measure of the severity of HIV infection, calculated by estimating the number of copies of the virus in a milliliter of blood.

Wasting syndrome—A combination of weight loss and change in composition of body tissues that occurs in patients with HIV infection. Typically, the patient's body loses lean muscle tissue and replaces it with fat as well as losing weight overall.

Western blot—A procedure that uses electrical current passed through a gel containing a sample of tissue extract in order to break down the proteins in the sample and detect the presence of antibodies for a specific disease. The Western blot method is used in HIV testing to confirm the results of an initial screening test.

Window period—The period of time between a person's getting infected with HIV and the point at which antibodies against the virus can be detected in a blood sample.

toxins secreted by HIV. AIDS dementia complex affects between 10 and 20% of AIDS patients in the United States and is often the first symptom of full-blown AIDS. Like Alzheimer's, ADC is characterized by memory loss, inability to concentrate, loss of motor ability, poor balance, and mood changes.

AIDS-related cancers include Kaposi's sarcoma, a skin cancer occasionally found in older men who do not have HIV infection; and cervical cancers in women. AIDS patients are also at increased risk of developing Hodgkin's disease, Burkitt's lymphoma, and cancers of the anus or rectum.

Diagnosis

The diagnosis of HIV infection and AIDS is complicated by the fact that many people are afraid to be tested for the disease. They may fear that a positive test will lead to the loss of housing, jobs, relationships, or the chance to complete their education. Because many infected persons put off getting tested and telling their partners, the disease continues to spread. In 2006, the CDC recommended routine HIV screening for all adults, adolescents, and pregnant women within health care settings, not just those considered to be high-risk. As of 2009, the CDC recommends that people engaging in high-risk behaviors be tested for HIV infection every year.

Examination

The patient's history is often the most important single diagnostic clue to HIV infection, particularly if he or she admits to unsafe sexual practices or intravenous drug use. If the doctor suspects HIV infection on the basis of the flu-like symptoms of acute retroviral syndrome, or if the patient requests HIV testing, the doctor will usually order appropriate blood or oral fluid tests.

AIDS-related dementia is the first symptom to appear in 4–15% of patients with AIDS in the United States. In those cases the doctor will include a neurologic examination and a mental status examination as part of the office physical. The patient may be referred to a psychiatrist for further evaluation if he or she appears to be suicidal or homicidal.

Tests

LABORATORY TESTS. Testing for HIV is a two-step process. The first test is a screening test, which usually involves taking a sample of the patient's blood. There are also newer screening tests that can use a sample of the person's urine or saliva. These rapid screening tests look for antibodies to the HIV virus and give results in about 20 minutes. If the person tests positive for HIV infection, a second test, called a Western blot test, is performed. This test uses a technique for separating out proteins in a blood sample to identify antibodies against HIV.

In 1996 the Food and Drug Administration (FDA) approved a test kit that people can use at home called the Home Access HIV-1 Test. The person pricks their finger on a special blotting card and mails it back to the company. The sample is identified only by a code number, which allows the person to remain completely anonymous. The test costs about $45 and results are available in seven days.

An important point to keep in mind is that it may take the body several weeks to three months after a person is infected to produce enough antibodies to HIV to be detected by a blood test. This period of time is called the window period. A person who tests negative for HIV infection after high-risk behaviors should wait three months and have another blood test to make sure they are not infected.

The doctor may also order a complete blood count and a stool test if the patient is suspected of having intestinal **parasites**.

IMAGING TESTS. The doctor may order a chest x-ray if opportunistic infections of the lung are suspected, or a magnetic resonance imaging (MRI) study of the brain if the patient has signs of AIDS dementia complex (ADC).

Diagnosis in children

The CDC recommends HIV testing as a part of standard prenatal care for all pregnant women. When a pregnant woman tests positive for HIV, testing of her infant ideally begins within 48 hours of birth. Testing is repeated at between one and two months of age and again at age 3–6 months. Testing of infants uses a different technique to detect the presence of HIV virus. Infants can be diagnosed by direct culture of the HIV virus, PCR testing, and p24 antigen testing. By one month of age, results are highly accurate. Diagnostic blood testing in children older than 18 months is similar to adult testing, with ELISA screening confirmed by Western blot.

In terms of symptoms, children are less likely than adults to have an early acute syndrome. They are, however, likely to have delayed growth, a history of frequent illness, recurrent ear infections, a low white blood cell count, failure to gain weight, and unexplained fevers. Children with AIDS are more likely to develop bacterial infections, inflammation of the lungs, and AIDS-related brain disorders than are HIV-positive adults.

Procedures

If the patient appears to have an opportunistic infection of the nervous system, the doctor may order a lumbar puncture in order to test a sample of spinal fluid. In some cases the doctor may take a sample of nerve, skin, or muscle tissue for a biopsy.

Treatment

Because there is no cure for AIDS, all forms of HIV/AIDS therapy are focused on improving the quality and length of life for people who are infected by slowing or halting the replication of the virus and treating or preventing infections and cancers that often develop in people with AIDS.

Traditional

Drugs

Medications are the mainstay of AIDS treatment. Drug treatment guidelines for HIV/AIDS change frequently as new drugs are approved and new drug regimens developed. Two principles currently guide doctors in developing drug regimens for AIDS patients: using combinations of drugs rather than one medication alone; and basing treatment decisions on the results of the patient's viral load tests. Current information on United States Food and Drug Administration-(FDA) approved drugs by class can be found at the United States **Department of Health and Human Services** Aids Info Website at http://www.aidsinfo.nih.gov/DrugsNew/Default.aspx?MenuItem=Drugs. Individuals interested in participating in a trial of new HIV/AIDS drugs under development can find a list of clinical trials currently accepting volunteers at http://www.clinicaltrial.gov. There is no cost to volunteers to participate and some medical care and testing is provided.

POST-EXPOSURE PROPHYLAXIS (PEP). Post-exposure prophylaxis (PEP) is a four- to eight-week course of antiretroviral drugs given to persons immediately after exposure (through rape, unprotected sex, or needlestick injuries) to HIV to prevent them from being infected by the virus. To be effective, PEP must be started within

48 hours of exposure. It has some unpleasant side effects, including severe nausea and headaches.

TREATMENT OF OPPORTUNISTIC INFECTIONS AND MALIGNANCIES. Most AIDS patients require complex long-term treatment with medications for infectious diseases. This treatment is often complicated further by the development of resistance in the disease organisms. AIDS-related malignancies in the central nervous system are usually treated with **radiation** therapy. Cancers elsewhere in the body are treated with chemotherapy.

PROPHYLACTIC TREATMENT FOR OPPORTUNISTIC INFECTIONS. Prophylactic treatment is treatment that is given to prevent disease. AIDS patients with a history of *Pneumocystis* pneumonia, with CD4+ counts below 200 cells/mm^3 or 14% of lymphocytes, weight loss, or thrush should be given prophylactic medications. Drugs that may be given include **antibiotics** such as trimethoprim-sulfamethoxazole (Bactrim) or pentamidine (Pentam-300, Pentacarinat) and anti-fungals such as amphotericin B (AmBisome), flucytosine (Ancobon), and clotrimazole (Lotrim AF, Mycelex, Femizole-7). All these drugs can have undesirable side effects.

ANTIVIRAL TREATMENTS. When a person tests positive for HIV infection, the doctor will measure the amount of virus in the patient's blood. This level is called the viral load. The viral load helps the doctor to decide when to start drug treatment for HIV. The current method of treatment is called highly active antiretroviral therapy or HAART. Introduced in 1996, HAART consists of combinations of three or more different drugs from two or more of the seven classes of antiretroviral drugs presently available. HAART is not a cure for AIDS, but it reduces the viral load, improves the patient's overall quality of life, and extends **life expectancy** by four to 12 years.

Antiviral drugs suppress HIV replication, as distinct from treating its effects on the body. These drugs fall into several classes:

- Nucleotide reverse transcriptase inhibitors (also called nucleoside analogues). These drugs work by interfering with the action of HIV reverse transcriptase inside infected cells, thus ending the virus's replication process. These drugs include zidovudine (Retrovir), lamivudine (Epivir), and abacavir (Ziagen) and many others. They are often used in used in multi-drug combinations.
- Non-nucleoside reverse transcriptase inhibitors. This class of drugs binds to an enzyme that is necessary for the HIV virus to reproduce. Examples of drugs in this class are viramune, delavirdine (Rescriptor), and efavirenz (Sustiva) and others.
- Protease inhibitors. Protease inhibitors work by disabling protease, an enzyme necessary for HIV reproduction. Protease inhibitors include saquinavir (Invirase), ritonavir (Norvire), indinavir (Crixivan), nelfinavir (Viracept), amprenavir (Agenerase), kaletra, and many others.
- Integrase inhibitors. Integrase inhibitors prevent the virus from inserting its own genetic material into the DNA of the infected cell. This stops the virus from replicating. Integrase was the only FDA-approved drug in this class as of early 2009. Several investigational drugs in this category were in clinical trials at that time.
- Fusion inhibitors and entry inhibitors. Fusion inhibitors block specific proteins on the surface of the virus or the CD4+ cell. These proteins help the virus gain entry into the cell. The only FDA-approved fusion inhibitor as of early 2009 was enfuvirtide (Fuzeon). Entry inhibitors block HIV from entering cells. The only FDA-approved fusion inhibitor as of early 2009 was maraviroc (Selzentry). Several drugs in this class are, in pre-approval clinical trials.

HAART has several drawbacks. First, it is a very expensive form of treatment. In addition, many of the drugs used in HAART have troublesome side effects; as a result, some AIDS patients simply stop taking their medications. Last, some patients develop resistance to the antiretroviral drugs and no longer respond to treatment. The doctor can sometimes switch one of the drugs in the patient's combination to another drug within the same class.

Another problem with HAART is the complicated dosing schedules of the different drugs prescribed for an individual patient. To encourage adherence to treatment schedules (which must be at least 98 percent complete to protect the patient from developing a strain of the virus resistant to HAART), some pharmaceutical companies have developed fixed-dose combinations—medications in which several antiretroviral drugs that are known to work well together are combined in a single pill.

STIMULATION OF BLOOD CELL PRODUCTION. Because many patients with AIDS have abnormally low levels of both red and white blood cells, they may be given medications to stimulate blood cell production. Epoetin alfa (erythropoietin) may be given to anemic patients. Patients with low white blood cell counts may be given filgrastim or sargramostim.

Alternative

AIDS patients turn to **alternative medicine** when conventional treatments are ineffective and to supplement conventional treatment, reduce disease symptoms, counteract drug effects, and improve quality of life. Because alternative medicines may interact with conventional medicines, it is important for patients with HIV infection to inform their doctors of all treatments being used.

CAM treatments that have been recommended for AIDS patients include multivitamin therapy, acupuncture, yoga, massage therapy, and the use of relaxation techniques to improve mood and relieve depression. Some studies indicate that naturopathic treatments slow the progression of HIV infection even though they cannot cure it. Interestingly, a study published in 2007 reported that seniors with AIDS are just as likely to use complementary therapies since the introduction of HAART as they were before 1996. The study also reported that men who used CAM were more likely to be college-educated, to have contracted HIV through intravenous drug use rather than through sex with other men, and to be African American rather than Caucasian.

The National Center for Complementary and Alternative Medicine (NCCAM) announced plans in 2007 to conduct a three-year study of CAM therapies used by adults diagnosed with HIV. According to the center, between 47 and 74% of HIV-positive persons in the United States have used some type of CAM approach—most often to relieve the side effects of HAART as well as to improve overall well-being. The study is scheduled to run from 2009 through 2011.

Prognosis

There was no cure for AIDS as of 2010. Without treatment, HIV infection progresses to AIDS in an average of 11 years. After diagnosis with AIDS, the patient has a life expectancy of 9.2 months without treatment. A person diagnosed with HIV infection who begins treatment with HAART has a life expectancy of about 20 years as of 2010. Unfortunately, about half of patients who begin treatment with HAART fail to benefit from it as much as they had hoped and discontinue it.

About 37% of patients with AIDS eventually develop AIDS dementia complex, with another 30% showing milder symptoms of dementia. Women with AIDS are at slightly higher risk than men of developing ADC.

Older adults generally have a worse prognosis than younger adults diagnosed with AIDS. The earlier stages of HIV infection progress more rapidly to AIDS in seniors, the initial CD4+ T cell counts are lower, and the survival period is shorter. Whereas 80 percent of younger adults survive for a year after being diagnosed with AIDS, only 40% of seniors survive that long.

The reasons for the poorer prognosis in older adults were not fully understood as of 2010. Various explanations include delayed diagnosis due to the fact that the early symptoms of HIV infection are easily confused with those of other diseases commonly found in older persons; inadequate treatment; the high rate of other diseases and disorders in the elderly that can further weaken the immune system; a lower rate of compliance with treatment regimens; and age-related changes in the immune system itself. It is thought that the immune system in older adults is less efficient in replacing T helper cells and so is more easily overwhelmed by HIV infection.

Prevention

There is no vaccine against HIV infection; moreover, it is unlikely that an effective vaccine will be developed in the foreseeable future because the retrovirus that causes AIDS mutates so rapidly. Although various vaccines against HIV have been tested by the National Institutes of Health since 1996, none have so far been approved for use outside clinical trials.

Researchers are, however, actively working on producing preventative and therapeutic vaccines for HIV. Preventative vaccines immunize an individual against a disease, so that he or she does not become infected. A therapeutic vaccine, also called a treatment vaccine, does not keep someone from getting a disease the way a preventative vaccine does. Instead, therapeutic vaccines are used to boost the body's immune system in order to help control infection. The potential exists to prolong life indefinitely using these and other drug therapies to boost the immune system, keep the virus from replicating, and ward off opportunistic infections and malignancies.

People can lower their risk of HIV infection by taking the following precautions recommended by the CDC:

- Limit sexual activity to a single partner who is known to be uninfected and is faithful
- Use a condom when having sex with anyone whose HIV status is unknown
- Do not share needles or inject illegal drugs
- Do not exchange sex for drugs
- Health care workers should follow guidelines for protecting against needle sticks and other accidental exposures to body fluids that may be contaminated with HIV
- Get tested for HIV infection after engaging in high-risk activities; if the test results are positive, inform all current sexual partners

Diet and nutritional concerns

Diet and **nutrition** are a major part of managing HIV infection and AIDS. While there is no standard "HIV diet" or "AIDS diet" because patients' symptoms, medication regimens, and corresponding nutritional needs vary so widely, there are general practices followed by registered dietitians who work with doctors and other health care professionals to care for these patients.

The function of nutritional education and dietary management in patients with HIV infection and AIDS is to maintain the patient's energy level and ability to carry out normal activities of daily life; lower the risk of opportunistic infections of the digestive system; and minimize the side effects of HAART on the patient's ability to eat and enjoy food.

Dietetics consultation and follow-up

Patients with HIV infection should consult a registered dietitian (RD) as soon as possible after diagnosis, because good nutrition is essential to maintaining a normal level of activity and self-care as well as supporting the patient's immune system. RDs use several screening questionnaires to evaluate patients for potential nutritional problems. On the patient's first visit, he or she is given a quick nutrition screen or QNS to fill out. The QNS identifies such problems as unintentional weight loss, nausea, difficulty swallowing, and diarrhea. The dietitian then measures the patient's height, weight, skinfold thickness, and the circumference of the muscles on the patient's midarm. These last two measurements are needed in order to monitor changes in body fat distribution and muscle wasting that often accompany HIV infection.

The next step in the initial assessment is the patient's completion of a food intake record (FIR). The patient is asked to record everything he or she eats or drinks in a 24-hour period, including snacks and alcoholic beverages. If possible, the patient will fill out two FIRs, one for a working day and one for a weekend day or holiday. The FIR allows the dietitian to evaluate the patient's usual eating habits, portion sizes, food preferences, and average calorie intake. It also establishes a baseline for the individual patient, so that loss of appetite later on or other nutritional problems can be detected as quickly as possible.

Follow-up visits to the dietitian are scheduled according to the degree of the patient's nutritional risk. The American Dietetic Association and the Los Angeles County Commission on HIV Health Services use the following timelines for HIV patients at nutritional risk:

- Low risk: The patient's weight is stable, with a balanced and adequate food intake; normal blood levels of cholesterol, triglycerides, and glucose; no evidence of kidney or liver disorders; regular physical exercise; and low levels of psychosocial stress. Low-risk patients are evaluated by the RD as needed, but at least once a year.
- Moderate risk: The patient is obese or suffers from changing patterns of body fat distribution; has high blood cholesterol levels or high blood pressure; has developed an eating disorder, nausea, vomiting, or diarrhea; has been recently diagnosed with type 2 diabetes or food allergies; is in recovery from substance abuse; or is under psychosocial stress. Moderate-risk patients should be seen by the RD within a month.
- High risk: The patient is pregnant; suffers from poorly controlled diabetes; has lost 10% of body weight over the previous 4–6 months; has lost 5% of body weight in the previous 4 weeks; has dental problems, involvement of the central nervous system, severe nausea or vomiting, severe pain on swallowing, or chronic diarrhea; has one or more opportunistic infections; or is under severe psychosocial stress. These patients should be seen by an RD within one week.

In addition to assessment of the patient's nutritional needs, RDs also evaluate his or her living situation and other issues that may affect receiving adequate nutrition.

Specific issues in nutritional care of HIV patients

NAUSEA, VOMITING, AND DIARRHEA. Nausea and vomiting are common symptoms of HIV infection as well as side effects of HAART. They can lead to long-term damage to the esophagus and dental problems as well as weight loss and inability to take needed medications. About 30% of patients develop nausea and vomiting within one to four weeks following infection as part of a condition called acute retroviral syndrome or ARS, which resembles **influenza** or mononucleosis. Most patients, however, develop nausea, vomiting, and diarrhea later on in the course of the disease as side effects of HAART or from opportunistic infections of the gastrointestinal system. Patients with HIV infection are highly susceptible to such diseases as giardiasis, cryptosporidiosis, **listeriosis**, *Campylobacter* infections, and *Salmonella* infections.

Treatment of nausea, vomiting, and diarrhea in patients with HIV infections may require a number of diagnostic tests and imaging studies as well as evaluation of the patient's medications in order to determine the cause(s) of the symptoms.

LIPODYSTROPHY. Lipodystrophy is the medical term for the redistribution of body fat that sometimes occurs in patients with HIV infection as a result of HAART, genetic factors, the length of time a person has been HIV-positive, and the severity of the disease. It is not completely understood why antiretroviral drugs and other factors have this effect. The patient may notice new deposits of fat at the back of the neck (sometimes called "buffalo humps") and around the abdomen. Conversely, fat may be lost under the skin of the face, resulting in sunken cheeks, or lost under the skin of the buttocks, arms, or legs. Lipodystrophy is not necessarily associated with weight loss.

Lipodystrophy may be accompanied by other changes in the patient's metabolism, particularly insulin resistance and higher levels of blood cholesterol and triglycerides. One recommendation nutritionists often give to patients with lipodystrophy and metabolic changes is to follow the Mediterranean diet, which is high in fiber-rich whole grains and vegetables and low in saturated fats. Another recommendation is to maintain a schedule of regular physical exercise (particularly weight training), which has been shown to lower insulin resistance and decrease abdominal fat deposits.

WASTING. Wasting refers to rapid unintentional weight loss (usually defined as 5% of body weight over a period of six months) combined with changes in the composition of body tissue. Specifically, the patient is losing lean muscle tissue and replacing it with fat. The patient's outward appearance may not be a reliable guide to wasting, particularly if he or she also has lipodystrophy. Weight loss associated with wasting may result from nausea and vomiting related to opportunistic infections of the digestive tract as well as from reactions to medication.

Nutrition is the first line of defense against wasting. To help the patient maintain weight, nutritionists recommend raising the daily calorie intake from 17–20 calories per pound of body weight (a guideline used for patients whose weight has been stable) to 25 calories per pound. Patients with wasting syndrome may require as much as 3500 calories per day to maintain their weight. Nutrient ratios should be 15–20% protein, 50–60% carbohydrates, and 25% fats to protect the body's muscle tissue. Patients who need more calories or protein may benefit from adding such supplements as Ensure or Instant Breakfast to their daily diet. In addition, weight training or other forms of regular exercise help to maintain muscle tissue.

Other treatments for wasting include the use of appetite stimulants to increase food intake and hormonal treatments to build lean muscle tissue, particularly in male patients.

MEDICATION INTERACTIONS. Most medications used in HAART have the potential to cause nausea and vomiting. Some antiretroviral medications should be taken with food to minimize these side effects. Digestive disturbances are the single most common reason given by patients for discontinuing antiretroviral therapy. In some cases, switching to a different combination of drugs helps to relieve nausea, vomiting, or diarrhea.

FOOD SAFETY ISSUES. **Food safety** is an important concern for patients with HIV infection because their immune systems have difficulty fighting off food or water-borne disease organisms. While most people can get food **poisoning** or parasitic infections of the digestive tract if they drink contaminated **water** or do not prepare food properly, patients with HIV infection can get severely ill as a result of these diseases. Food-borne illnesses are also much more difficult to treat in persons with AIDS or HIV infection, and may lead to malabsorption syndrome, a condition in which the body cannot absorb and make use of needed nutrients in food.

The CDC and NIH have brochures with detailed instructions for patients about safety issues in purchasing and preparing foods, particularly when traveling abroad. Basic safeguards include the following:

- Wash hands repeatedly in warm soapy water before and after preparing or eating food; instant hand sanitizers should be used when away from home
- Cook all meats, fish, and poultry to the well-done stage; do not eat sushi, raw oysters, or raw meat in any form
- Do not use unpasteurized milk or dairy products
- Do not eat raw, soft-boiled, or "wet" scrambled eggs, or Caesar salad made with raw egg in the dressing; hard-boiled or hard-scrambled eggs are safe
- Rinse all fruits and vegetables carefully in clean, safe water, and clean all cutting boards and knives that touch chicken and meat with soap and hot water before using these utensils with other food items
- Keep all refrigerated foods below 40°F; check expiration dates on food packaging
- Completely reheat leftovers before eating, and do not eat leftovers that have been stored in the refrigerator for longer than 3 days
- Do not drink water that comes directly from lakes, streams, rivers, or springs, and ask for drinks without ice in restaurants

Caregiver concerns

A caregiver for an older adult with AIDS should be concerned with the following:

- Complete compliance with the senior's HAART regimen. Failure to take the medications exactly as directed can lead to resistant forms of HIV and eventual treatment failure. A handout for patients on how to take antiretroviral medications is available on the American Academy of Family Physicians website at http://www.aafp.org/afp/20030815/689ph.html
- Nausea, vomiting, and weight loss, or signs of lipodystrophy or wasting syndrome; the doctor may recommend a consultation with a professional dietitian
- Signs of dementia; AIDS-related dementia in seniors is often misdiagnosed as Alzheimer's disease

- Signs of drug interactions between the senior's antiretroviral therapy and medications he or she may be taking for other diseases
- Signs of upper respiratory infections, particularly pneumonia or thrush
- Skin disorders, including changes in the skin that may indicate cancer

Resources

BOOKS

Beers, Mark H., M. D., and Thomas V. Jones, MD. *Merck Manual of Geriatrics*, 3rd ed., Chapter 134, "Human Immunodeficiency Virus Infection." Whitehouse Station, NJ: Merck, 2005.

Currie-McGhee, Leanne K. *AIDS*. Detroit, MI: Lucent Books, 2009.

Gallant, Joel. *100 Questions and Answers about HIV and AIDS*. Sudbury, MA: Jones and Bartlett Publishers, 2009.

Klausner, Jeffrey D., and Edward W. Hook, III, eds. *Current Diagnosis and Treatment of Sexually Transmitted Diseases*. New York: McGraw-Hill Medical, 2007.

Lee, Sharon Dian. *HIV and Aging*. New York: Informa Healthcare USA, 2008.

Weeks, Benjamin, and I. Edward Alcamo. *AIDS: The Biological Basis*, 5th ed. Sudbury, MA: Jones and Bartlett, Publishers, 2010.

PERIODICALS

Akers, A., L. Bernstein, S. Henderson, et al. "Factors Associated with Lack of Interest in HIV Testing in Older At-Risk Women." *Journal of Women's Health (Larchmont)* 16 (July-August 2007): 842-858.

Branson, B. M. "State of the Art for Diagnosis of HIV Infection." *Clinical Infectious Diseases* 45 (December 15, 2007): S221-225.

Fitzpatrick, A. L., L. J. Standish, J. Berger, J. G. Kim, C. Calabrese, and N. Polissar. "Survival in HIV-1-positive Adults Practicing Psychological or Spiritual Activities for One Year." *Alternative Therapy Health Medicine* (September/October 2007): 18-20, 22-24.

Foley, J., et al. "Emerging Issues in the Neuropsychology of HIV Infection." *Current HIV/AIDS Reports* 5 (November 2008): 204–11.

Hammer, S. M., et al. "Antiretroviral Treatment of Adult HIV Infection: 2008 Recommendations of the International AIDS Society-USA Panel." *Journal of the American Medical Association* 300 (August 6, 2008): 555-70.

Johnson, C. J., et al. "Adherence to Antiretroviral Medication in Older Adults Living with HIV/AIDS: A Comparison of Alternative Models." *AIDS Care* 21 (May 2009): 541-51.

Letendre, S. L., et al. "Neurologic Complications of HIV Disease and Their Treatment." *Topics in HIV Medicine* 17 (April-May 2009): 46-56.

Llibre, J. M., et al. "The Changing Face of HIV/AIDS in Treated Patients." *Current HIV Research* 7 (July 2009); 365–77.

Mangili, A., D. H. Murman, A. M. Zampini, and C. A. Wanke. "Nutrition and HIV Infection: Review of Weight Loss and Wasting in the Era of Highly Active Antiretroviral Therapy from the Nutrition for Healthy Living Cohort." *Clinical Infectious Diseases* 42 (March 15, 2006): 836-842.

Robinson-Papp, J., et al. "HIV-related Neurocognitive Impairment in the HAART Era." *Current HIV/AIDS Reports* 6 (August 2009): 146-152.

Shushan, S., et al. "Laryngeal Cancer in Acquired Immunodeficiency Syndrome." *International Journal of STD and AIDS* 20 (August 2009): 582-84.

Vidrine, D. J. "Cigarette Smoking and HIV/AIDS: Health Implicats, Smoker Characteristics and Cessation Strategies." *AIDS Education and Prevention* 21 (June 2009): 3-13.

OTHER

Centers for Disease Control and Prevention (CDC). *CDC Revised Recommendations for HIV Testing (2006)*. http://www.cdc.gov/hiv/topics/testing/resources/factsheets/pdf/healthcare.pdf

Centers for Disease Control and Prevention (CDC). *Fact Sheet: Estimates of New HIV Infections in the United States*. http://www.cdc.gov/hiv/topics/surveillance/resources/factsheets/incidence.htm

Centers for Disease Control and Prevention (CDC). *HIV/AIDS*. http://www.cdc.gov/hiv

Dubin, Jeff. "HIV, Early Recognition and Rapid Testing." *eMedicine*, April 7, 2009. http://emedicine.medscape.com/article/783434-overview

Food and Drug Administration (FDA). *Eating Defensively: Food Safety Advice for Persons with AIDS*. http://www.fda.gov/ForConsumers/ByAudience/ForPatientAdvocates/HIVandAIDSActivities/ucm135844.htm

Mayo Clinic. *HIV/AIDS*. http://www.mayoclinic.com/health/hiv-aids/DS00005

National Institute of Allergy and Infectious Diseases (NIAID). *HIV/AIDS*. http://www3.niaid.nih.gov/healthscience/healthtopics/HIVAIDS/default.htm

Public Broadcasting System (PBS) Frontline. *The Age of AIDS*. http://www.pbs.org/wgbh/pages/frontline/aids

ORGANIZATIONS

Centers for Disease Control and Prevention (CDC), 1600 Clifton Road, Atlanta, GA 30333, 800-232-4636, cdcinfo@cdc.gov, http://www.cdc.gov

Food and Drug Administration (FDA), 10903 New Hampshire Ave., Silver Spring, MD 20993, 888-INFO-FDA, http://www.fda.gov/

Gay Men's Health Crisis (GMHC), Tisch Building, 119 West 24th Street, New York, NY 10011, 212-367-1000, http://www.gmhc.org/

Infectious Diseases Society of America (IDSA), 1300 Wilson Blvd, Suite 300, Arlington, VA 22209, 703-299-0200, Fax: 703-299-0204, http://www.idsociety.org/

National Institute of Allergy and Infectious Diseases (NIAID), 6610 Rockledge Drive, MSC 6612, Bethesda,

MD 20892-6612, 301-496-5717, 866-284-4107, Fax: 301-402-3573, http://www3.niaid.nih.gov

International AIDS Society (IAS), Ave. Louis Casaï 71, P. O. Box 28, Geneva, Switzerland CH - 1216 Cointrin, +41-(0) 22-7 100 800, Fax: +41-(0)22-7 100 899, info@iasociety.org, http://www.iasociety.org/

World Health Organization (WHO), Avenue Appia 20, 1211 Geneva 27, Switzerland, + 41 22 791 21 11, Fax: + 41 22 791 31 11, info@who.int, http://www.who.int/en/.

Genevieve Pham-Kanter
Tish Davidson, A.M.
Rebecca J. Frey, Ph.D.

Air pollution

Definition

Air pollution is a general term that covers a broad range of contaminants in the atmosphere. Pollution can occur from natural causes or from human activities. Discussions about the effects of air pollution have focused mainly on human health, but attention is being directed to environmental quality and amenity as well. Air pollutants are found as gases or particles, and on a restricted scale, they can be found inside buildings as indoor air pollutants. Urban air pollution has long been an important concern for civic administrators, but increasingly, air pollution has become an international problem.

Origins

Air pollution began in prehistoric times when humans first used fire. Discoveries within prehistoric caves show evidence of soot on the ceilings caused by inadequate ventilation from open fires. In addition, outdoor air pollution was present when early humans began to forge metals. In fact, core samples taken by scientists from glaciers in Greenland confirm pollution from metal production by the ancient Chinese, Greeks, and Romans.

Since historic times, air pollution has been a matter of concern in large urban areas. Indeed, there were complaints about smoke in ancient Rome. The use of

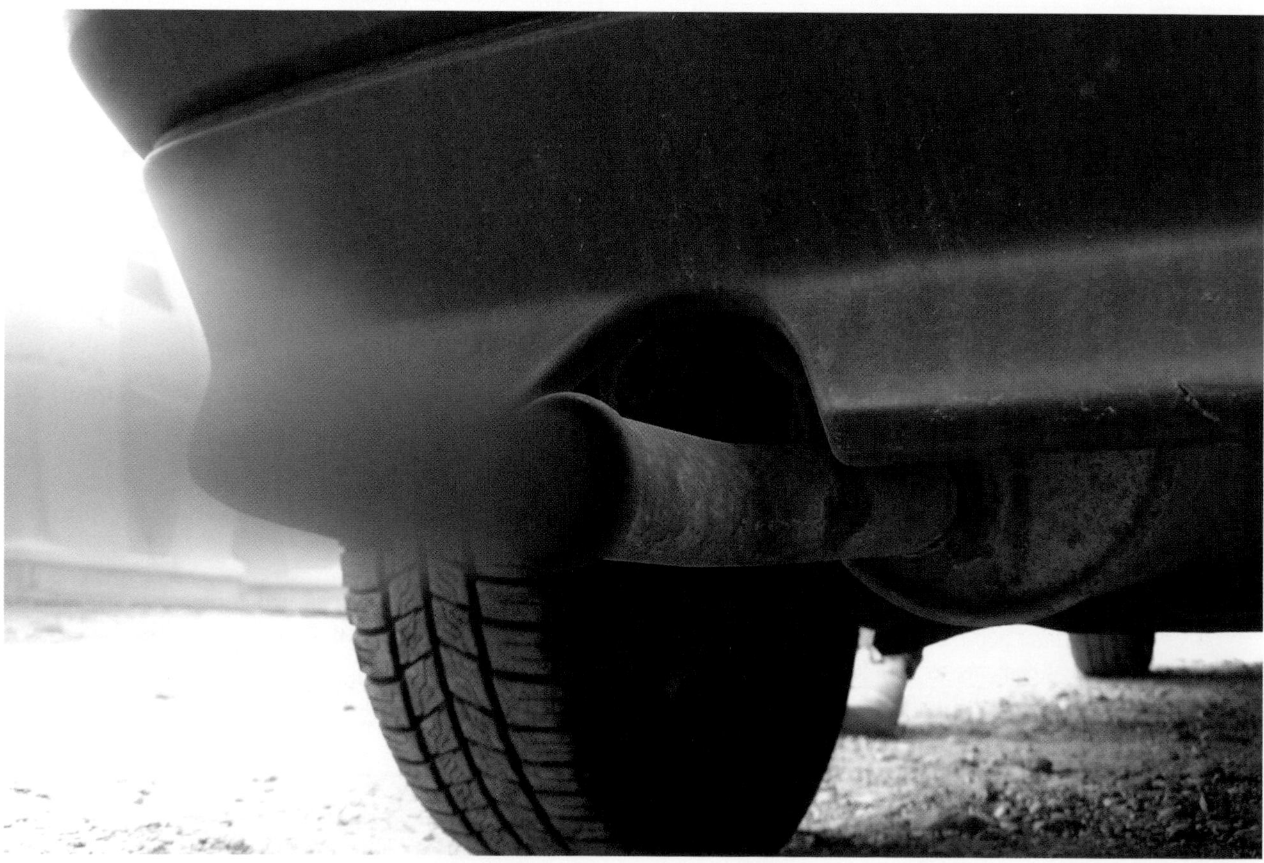

Exhaust fumes from a car. *(©iStockimages.com/matteo69)*

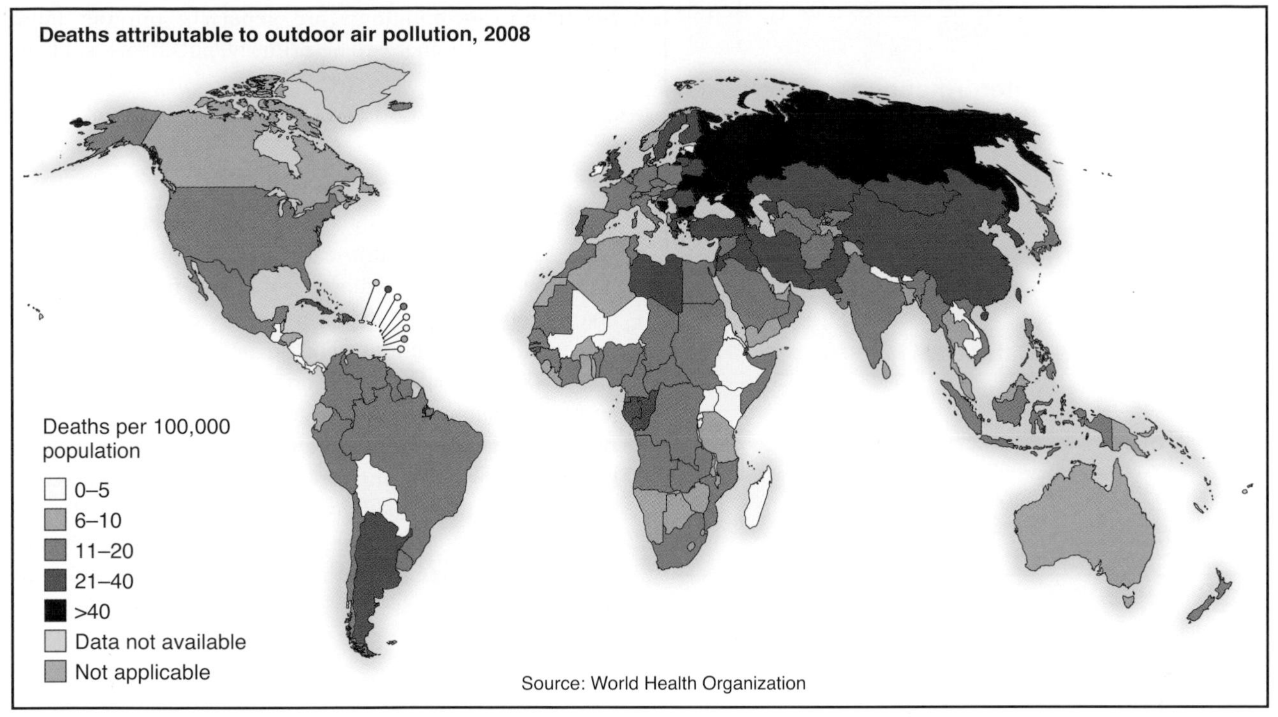

(Illustration by Electronic Illustrators Group. © 2013 Cengage Learning)

coal throughout the centuries caused cities to produce dense smoke. Along with smoke, large concentrations of sulfur dioxide (SO_2) were produced. The mixture of smoke and sulfur dioxide typified the foggy streets of nineteenth-century, industrialized London, England. Such situations are far less common in the cities of North America and Europe today. However, until recently, they were evident in other cities, such as Ankara, Turkey, and Shanghai, China, that rely heavily on the use of coal.

Description

The most common sources of air pollution are the combustion processes. The most obvious pollutant is smoke. However, the widespread use of fossil fuels have made sulfur (S) and nitrogen oxides (NO_x) pollutants of great concern. With increasing use of petroleum-based fuels, a range of organic compounds have become widespread in the atmosphere.

Risk factors

Coal is still burnt in large quantities to produce electricity or to refine metals, but these processes are frequently undertaken outside cities. Within urban areas, fuel use has shifted toward liquid and gaseous hydrocarbons (petrol and natural gas). These fuels typically have a lower concentration of sulfur, so the presence of sulfur dioxide has declined in many urban areas. However, the widespread use of liquid fuels in automobiles has meant increased production of carbon monoxide (CO), nitrogen oxides, and volatile organic compounds (VOCs).

Primary pollutants such as sulfur dioxide or smoke are the direct emission products of the combustion process. Many key pollutants in the urban atmospheres are secondary pollutants, produced by processes initiated through photochemical reactions. The photochemical smog in Los Angeles, California, is now characteristic of urban atmospheres dominated by secondary pollutants.

Although motorized vehicles, such as automobiles, are the main source of air pollution in contemporary cities, there are other equally significant sources. Stationary sources are still important and the oil-burning furnaces that have replaced the older coal-burning ones are responsible for a range of gaseous emissions and fly ash. Incineration is also an important source of complex combustion products, especially where incineration burns a wide range of refuse. These emissions can include chlorinated hydrocarbons such as dioxin. When plastics, which often contain chlorine (Cl), are incinerated, the result is hydrochloric acid (HCl) in the waste gas stream. Metals, especially where they are volatile at high temperatures, can migrate to smaller, respirable particles. The accumulation of toxic metals, such as cadmium (Cd),

Air Pollution Stages

Index value	Interpretations
0	No concentration
100	National ambient air quality standard
200	Alert
300	Warning
400	Emergency
500	Significant harm

PSI Range	Category
0 to 50	Good
50 to 100	Moderate
100 to 200	Unhealthful
200 to 300	Very unhealthful
300 to 500	Hazardous

(Illustration by Electronic Illustrators Group. © 2013 Cengage Learning)

on fly ash gives rise to concern about harmful effects from incinerator emissions. Many questions have been raised about the completeness of the destruction process in specialized incinerators designed to destroy toxic compounds such as polychlorinated biphenyls (PCBs). Even under optimum conditions where the furnace operation has been properly maintained, great care needs to be taken to control leaks and losses during transfer operations (fugitive emissions).

The enormous range of compounds used in modern manufacturing processes have also meant that there has been an ever-widening range of emissions from both the industrial processes and the combustion of their wastes. Although the amounts of these exotic compounds are often rather small, they add to the complex range of compounds found in the urban atmosphere. The deliberate loss of effluents through discharge from pipes and chimneys is not the only source that needs attention. Fugitive emissions of volatile substances that leak from valves and seals require careful control.

Control procedures

Air pollution control procedures are increasingly an important part of civic administration, although their goals are far from easy to achieve. It is also troubling that, although many urban concentrations of primary pollutants (for example, smoke and sulfur dioxide) are on the decline in developed countries, such is not the case in developing countries. Here the desire for rapid industrial growth has often lowered urban air quality. Secondary air pollutants are generally proving more difficult to eliminate than primary pollutants such as smoke.

Demographics

Air pollution was the cause of a major disease outbreak in London, England, in 1952. According to the U.K. Ministry of Health, early in December, severe air pollution caused by airborne pollutants from the use of coal was made worse by exceptionally cold temperatures and windless conditions. The air pollution event caused about 4,000 people to die, primarily from the airborne particles being inhaled. The air pollution quickly disappeared when the weather changed. However, over the following few months, another estimated 8,000 people may have died as the result of the pollution event. In all, about 100,000 people were sickened by the air pollution. The historic incident is often referred to as the Great Smog of '52.

Financial news company 24/7 Wall St. conducted a study in 2010 based on numerous studies on air quality over the previous few years and data from government and private sources. Its study examined data on the following pollutants: sulfur dioxide, nitrogen dioxide, and particulates. It concluded that the cities with the world's worst air pollution were: (1) tied for first place, Beijing, China, and New Delhi, India; (2) Santiago, Chile; (3) Mexico City, Mexico; (4) Ulaanbaatar, Mongolia; (5) Cairo, Egypt; (6) Chongqing, China; (7) Guangzhou, China; (8) Hong Kong, and (9) Kabul, Afghanistan. The DailyFinance.com article *The 10 Cities with the World's Worst Air*, which reported the findings, stated: "Beijing's air quality has become so bad that the city has recently been engulfed in a hazardous haze.... As a result, schools have been forced to cancel outdoor activities, and health experts have asked that children, the elderly and people with respiratory ailments stay indoors. The city recorded the world's highest level of sulfur dioxide concentrations for 2000 to 2005 and has the third-highest level of nitrogen dioxide behind only Sao Paulo and Mexico City."

Common diseases and disorders

Urban air pollutants have a wide range of effects, with health problems being the most enduring concern. In atmospheres filled with smoke and sulfur dioxide, various bronchial diseases were intensified. In atmospheres where the air pollutants are not so obvious, the effects may be more difficult to identify and address. For example, in photochemical smog, eye irritation from the secondary pollutant peroxyacetyl nitrate (PAN) is one on the most characteristic direct effects of the smog. High concentrations of carbon monoxide in cities where automobiles operate at high density force the human heart to work harder to make up for the oxygen displaced from the blood's hemoglobin by carbon monoxide. This extra **stress** appears to reveal itself by increased incidence of complaints among people with heart problems. Many suspect that contemporary air pollutants are involved in the increases in **asthma**, but the links between asthma and air pollution are complex and related to a whole range of factors. Lead (Pb), from automotive exhausts, is thought by many to be a factor in lowering the intelligence quotients (IQs) of urban children.

Air pollution also affects materials in the urban environment. Soiling has long been regarded as a problem, originally the result of the smoke from wood or coal fires, but in modern times increasingly the result of fine black soot from diesel exhausts. The acid gases, particularly sulfur dioxide, erode building materials. This effect is most noticeable with calcareous stones, which are the predominant building material of many important historic structures. Metals also suffer from atmospheric acidity. In modern photochemical smog, natural rubbers crack and deteriorate rapidly.

Health problems relating to indoor air pollution have existed since ancient times. Anthracosis, or **black lung disease**, has been found in mummified lung tissue. The late 1990s and early 2000s witnessed a shift from the concern about outdoor air pollution to worry about indoor air quality.

The production of energy from combustion and the release of solvents is so pervasive in the contemporary world that it causes air pollution problems on a regional and global nature. Acid rain, which is widely observed throughout the world, is produced when emissions of sulfur oxides (SO_x) and nitrogen oxides react with **water** and oxygen in the air to form acids. Precipitation and fog deposit these acids in water bodies, on the ground, on structures, and on plants, which can all be damaged by these acidic compounds. Carbon dioxide (CO_2) emitted in the combustion process is increasing the concentration of carbon dioxide in the atmosphere and enhancing the greenhouse effect, which is the increased temperature of Earth as a result of greenhouse gases, absorbing and trapping heat in the lower atmosphere (troposphere). The warming of Earth is referred to as climate change. Power plants are responsible for about one-half of the energy-producing fossil fuel emissions, whereas vehicles contribute approximately one-third of these emissions.

Moreover, gases leak indoors from the polluted outdoor environment, but more often the serious pollutants arise from processes that take place indoors.

KEY TERMS

Fly ash—Fine particles of ash produced from the combustion of solid fuel.

Fossil fuels—Any type of fuel, such as coal, natural gas, peat, and petroleum, derived from the decomposed remains of prehistoric plants and animals.

Hydrocarbons—Any organic chemical compound containing hydrogen (H) and carbon (C).

Greenhouse effect—The overall warming of Earth's atmosphere as the result of atmospheric pollution by gases.

Greenhouse gases—Any gas (such as carbon dioxide and ozone) that absorbs radiation and contributes to the warming of Earth's atmosphere by reflecting radiation from the surface of Earth.

Polychlorinated biphenyls—Any compound derived from biphenyl and containing chlorine (Cl), which is considered an hazardous environmental pollutant; with the abbreviation PCBs.

Concern with indoor air quality focuses on the nitrogen oxides generated by sources such as gas stoves. Similarly, formaldehyde (CH_2O) from insulating foams causes illnesses and adds to concerns about human exposure to a substance that may induce **cancer** over time. In the early twenty-first century, it was clear that radon (Rn) leaks from the ground expose some people to high levels of this radioactive gas within their own homes. Cancers may also result from the emanation of solvents from consumer products, glues, paints, and mineral fibers (such as asbestos). More generally, these compounds and a range of biological materials, animal hair, skin and pollen spores, and dusts can cause allergic reactions in some people. At one end of the spectrum these simply cause annoyance, but in extreme cases, such as found with the bacterium *Legionella*, a large number of deaths can occur.

There are also important issues surrounding the effects of indoor air pollutants on materials. Many industries, especially the electronics industry, must take great care over the purity of indoor air where a speck of dust can destroy a microchip or low concentrations of air pollutants change the composition of surface films in component design. Museums must care for objects over long periods of time, so precautions must be taken to protect delicate dyes from the effects of photochemical smog; and paper and books from sulfur dioxide; and metals from sulfide gases.

QUESTIONS TO ASK YOUR DOCTOR

- What can I do to reduce indoor air pollution?
- Will indoor air pollution compromise my health?
- Am I susceptible to indoor air pollution? Outdoor air pollution?
- How can air pollution harm me?
- What are the risks associated air pollution?

Public health role and response

In many countries, including the United States, steps are being taken to minimize and even prevent air pollution from damaging the environment. Scientists are studying the damaging effects on animals and plants, while politicians are writing laws to control pollution emissions. At the same time, teachers are teaching their students about the effects of air pollution. In the United States, the **Environmental Protection Agency (EPA)** is required by the Clean Air Act (CAA) of 1990 to set standards for air quality termed the national ambient air quality standards (NAAQS). The NAAQS are established for pollutants that are deemed harmful to public health and the environment.

Solvents such as carbon tetrachloride (CCl_4) and aerosol propellants such as chlorofluorocarbons (CFCs) are detectable all over the globe and are responsible for such problems as ozone layer depletion. Because of their effects, these compounds have been targeted under the CAA for phaseout to prevent further breakdown of the ozone layer. Although air quality in the United States improved between 1980 and 2010, many problems remain to be addressed with regards to the public health and the environment.

Effects on public health

The effects on the public health with respect to air pollution are considerable. In fact, as of 2012, the **World Health Organization (WHO)** estimated that approximately 800,000 people around the world die each year from the effects of air pollution. Further, respiratory diseases in children are exacerbated due to air pollution.

Efforts and solutions

According to the *Scientific American* article "5 Steps to Clean Up Air Pollution," the American Lung Association and many other public health and environmental organization recommend the following five ways to curb air pollution in the United States:

- Clean up coal-fired power plants
- Strengthen ozone air standards voluntarily
- Clean up oceangoing vessels
- Improve the pollution-monitoring network
- Enforce the law

Resources

BOOKS

Feinstein, Stephen. *Solving the Air Pollution Problem: What You Can Do*. Berkeley Heights, NJ: Enslow Publishers, 2011.

Franchetti, Matthew John, and Defne Apul. *Carbon Footprint Analysis: Concepts, Methods, Implementation, and Case Studies*. Boca Raton, FL: CRC Press, 2013.

Gold, Susan Dudley. *Clean Air and Clean Water Acts*. New York: Marshall Cavendish Benchmark, 2012.

Phalen, Robert F., and Robert N. Phalen. *Introduction to Air Pollution Science: A Public Health Perspective*. Burlington, MA: Jones & Bartlett Learning, 2013.

Tiwary, Abhishek, and Jeremy Colls. *Air Pollution: Measurement, Modelling and Mitigation*. London: Routledge, 2010.

Wentz, Dave, and Myron Wentz. *The Healthy Home: Simple Truths to Protect Your Family from Hidden Household Dangers*. New York: Vanguard Press, 2011.

WEBSITES

Environmental Protection Agency. "Air Pollutants." http://www.epa.gov/oar/airpollutants.html (accessed September 10, 2012).

Environmental Protection Agency. "Air Quality and Public Health." http://www.epa.gov/oia/air/pollution.htm (accessed September 10, 2012).

Environmental Protection Agency. "National Ambient Air Quality Standards (NAAQS)." http://www.epa.gov/air/criteria.html (accessed September 10, 2012).

McIntyre, Douglas. "The 10 Cities with the World's Worst Air." DailyFinance.com. http://www.dailyfinance.com/2010/11/29/10-cities-with-worlds-worst-air/ (accessed September 10, 2012).

Nolen, Janice. "5 Steps to Clean Up Air Pollution." Scientific American. http://www.scientificamerican.com/article.cfm?id=5-steps-to-clean-up (accessed September 10, 2012).

ORGANIZATIONS

American Lung Association, 1301 Pennsylvania Ave. NW, Ste. 800, Washington, DC 20004, (202) 785-3355, Fax: (202) 452-1805, info@lung.org, http://www.lung.org

American Medical Association, 515 N State St., Chicago, IL 60654, (800) 621-8335, http://www.ama-assn.org

Environmental Protection Agency, 1200 Pennsylvania Ave. NW, Washington, DC 20460, (202) 272-0167, http://water.epa.gov.

Peter Brimblecombe
William A. Atkins, B.B., B.S., M.B.A.

Alcoholism

Definition

Alcoholism is a chronic physical, psychological, and behavioral disorder characterized by the excessive, compulsive, and uncontrolled consumption of alcohol, which is an organic compound in which the hydroxyl functional group (–OH) is bound to a carbon atom (with the carbon center saturated, and having single bonds to three other atoms). Alcoholics have emotional and physical dependence on alcoholic beverages; increased tolerance over time of the effects of alcohol; and withdrawal symptoms if drinking stops. These problems usually cause the alcoholic's health to deteriorate, along with adversely affecting personal relationships, professional obligations, and social responsibilities. Alcoholism is medically considered a neurological disorder.

Risk factors for alcoholism

- **Age:** Beginning drinking at a young age increases the risk of alcohol dependence.
- **Family history:** Children of alcohol-dependent parents are at greater risk of developing alcoholism.
- **Gender:** Males are more likely to become alcohol dependent than females, but women are at an increased risk of developing complications associated with alcoholism, such as liver disease.
- **Length of use:** Regular binge drinking over an extended period of time may result in alcohol dependence.
- **Mental health:** Persons afflicted by mental health disorders such as depression may be more likely to misuse alcohol or other substances.
- **Social and cultural factors:** Being surrounded by friends who routinely drink may increase a person's level of alcohol use. Alcohol consumption in the media may also influence personal drinking habits.

SOURCE: Mayo Clinic, "Alcoholism." Available online at: http://www.mayoclinic.com/health/alcoholism/DS00340 (accessed August 17, 2010).

(Table by PreMediaGlobal. © 2013 Cengage Learning)

Description

Alcoholism is a complex behavioral as well as medical disorder. Its emergence in an individual's life is affected by a number of variables ranging from age, weight, gender, and ethnic background to family history, peer group, occupation, religious preference, and many other categories. Moreover, persons diagnosed with alcoholism may demonstrate considerable variety in their drinking patterns, age at onset of the disorder, and the speed of its progression.

The *Diagnostic and Statistical Manual of Mental Disorders*, 4th edition (DSM–IV), distinguishes between Alcohol Dependence and Alcohol Abuse largely on the basis of a compulsive element in Alcohol Dependence that is not present in Alcohol Abuse. Some psychiatrists differentiate between so-called primary alcoholism, in which the patient has no other major psychiatric diagnosis; and secondary alcoholism, in which the problem drinking is the patient's preferred way of medicating symptoms of another psychiatric disorder, such as depression, schizophrenia, post–traumatic **stress** disorder, or one of the dissociative disorders. Experts in other branches of medicine tend to emphasize patterns of, and attitudes toward, drinking in order to distinguish between nonproblematic use of alcohol and alcohol abuse or dependence. Classification is typically based on the following five categories:

- Social drinkers: Individuals who use alcohol in minimal to moderate amounts to enhance meals or other social activities. They do not drink alone.
- Situational drinkers: These people rarely or never drink except during periods of stress. They are far more likely to drink alone than social drinkers.
- Problem drinkers: These individuals drink heavily, even when they are not under overwhelming stress. Their drinking causes some problems in their lives (e.g., DUI [driving under the influence] arrests), but they are capable of responding to warnings or advice from others.
- Binge drinkers: This type of drinker uses alcohol in an out-of-control fashion at regular intervals. The binges may be planned in advance. This pattern is a problem on many college campuses.
- Alcoholic drinkers: These are drinkers who have no control of any kind over their intake, and find that their lives are unmanageable.

Other factors have complicated definitions of alcoholism in the United States, including: 1) the increasing tendency to combine alcohol with other drugs of abuse, sometimes called "cross-addiction;" and 2) the rising rates of alcohol abuse and dependence among children under 12 years of age.

Origins

The drinking of alcohol has been written about and described as far back as history is recorded. The abuses and dependence of alcohol have also been documented back to this era. German physician Christoph W.F. Hufeland (1762–1836) first used the term *dipsomania* in 1819, for the uncontrolled consumption of alcohol. In 1849, Swedish physician Magnus Huss (1807–1890) first coined the term *alcoholism* to systematically classify the damage that was attributable to the excessive consumption of alcohol. *Alcoholism* replaced *dipsomania* at about that time within the medical literature.

Demographics

The **World Health Organization (WHO)** estimates that some two billion people worldwide consume alcoholic beverages, which can have immediate and long-term consequences on health and social life. According to the **WHO**, 2.5 million people die each year from the harmful consumption of alcohol. In fact, 60 different diseases can result where alcohol has played a significant role. The WHO also states that the worldwide consumption of alcohol annually is equal to 6.13 liters (6.48 quarts) of pure alcohol per person 15 years and older.

According to the U.S. **Centers for Disease Control and Prevention** (**CDC**), 50.9% of American adults 18 years of age and older are regular drinkers of alcohol (that is, they have drunk at least 12 alcoholic beverages over the past year); and 13.6% of adults 18 years of age and over are infrequent drinkers (one to 11 drinks over the past year). The CDC also states that the number of deaths in 2009 from alcoholic liver disease was 15,183, while the number of alcohol-induced deaths (excluding accidents and homicides) was 24,518.

As of 2011, the CDC states that more than 79,000 deaths are attributable to excessive consumption of alcohol each year in the United States. This statistic makes excessive alcohol use the third leading lifestyle-related cause of death in the country. Further, it is responsible for about 2.3 million years of potential life lost annually. In addition, in any given year, more than 1.6 million hospitalizations and emergency room visits occur because of alcohol-related conditions.

According to the 2009 report of the National Survey on Drug Use and Health, 7.8% of Americans aged 12 or older (an estimated 19.3 million people) needed treatment for an alcohol problem in the past year. Of those who needed alcohol treatment, 8.1% received treatment at a specialty substance use treatment facility, 4.5% did not receive treatment but felt they needed it, and 87.4% did not receive treatment and did not perceive a need for it.

Alcohol use by persons under the age of 21 years is an important public health concern. In the United States, alcohol is the most commonly used and abused drug among youth. Although drinking under the age of 21 is against the law, people aged 12 to 20 years drink nearly 20% of all alcohol consumed in the United States. More than 90% of this alcohol is consumed in the form of binge drinking.

According to the National Institute on Alcohol Abuse and Alcoholism (NIAAA), a part of the National Institutes of Health (NIH), the percentage of American adults who had at least one drink over the past year was 59.6% for women and 71.8% for men, while the percentage of women and men who have never drunk alcohol is 22.5% and 11.6%, respectively. Further, the percentages of binge drinkers—whose who consume four or more drinks (for women) and five or more (for men) within a two-hour period at least once over the past year are 28.8% and 43.1%, respectively. On a normal day of the year, 48.2% of the women state they had one drink, 29.9% had two drinks, and 21.9% had three or more drinks. For men, the percentages are 28.7%, 29%, and 42.3%, respectively.

Studies of women alcoholics indicate that women are at higher risk than men for serious health problems related to alcoholism. Because women tend to metabolize alcohol more slowly and have a lower percentage of body water and a higher percentage of body fat than men, they develop higher blood alcohol levels than do men at a given amount of alcohol per pound of body weight. Thus, even though women typically begin to drink heavily at a later age than do men, they often become dependent on alcohol much more rapidly. This relatively speedy progression of alcoholism in women is called "telescoping."

At the other end of the age distribution, alcoholism among the elderly appears to be under-recognized. One-third of older alcoholic persons develop a problem with alcohol in later life, while the other two-thirds grow older with the medical and psychosocial consequences of early-onset alcoholism. Confusion and other signs of intoxication in an elderly person are also often misinterpreted as side effects of other medications. In addition, the effects of alcohol may be increased in elderly patients because of physiological changes associated with **aging**. The elderly are at higher risk for becoming dependent on alcohol than younger people because their bodies do not absorb alcohol as efficiently; a 90-year-old who drinks the same amount of alcohol as a 20-year-old (of the same sex) will have a blood alcohol level 50% higher.

Causes and symptoms

The cause of alcoholism is not well established. However, there is evidence that it may be based on predisposed genetics. Further research is necessary to validate such preliminary data. The symptoms of alcoholism are often seen in the behaviors of the people battling the disease.

Causes

The physical dependence and **addiction** to alcohol occurs gradually. Over time, drinking regularly and excessively alters the balance of chemicals in the part of the brain that controls pleasure and other such emotions. Excessive, long-term drinking affects the balance of these chemicals, which causes the brain to desire more and more alcohol to restore good feelings or to eliminate bad ones.

Symptoms

The symptoms of alcohol intoxication often include talkativeness and a positive mood while the drinker's blood alcohol level is rising, with depression and mental impairment when it is falling. Blood alcohol concentration (BAC) produces the following symptoms of central nervous system (CNS) depression at specific levels:

- 50 milligrams per deciliter (mg/dL): feelings of calm or mild drowsiness
- 50–150 mg/dL: loss of physical coordination. The legal BAC for drivers in most states is 100 mg/dL or lower.
- 150–200 mg/dL: loss of mental faculties
- 300–400 mg/dL: unconsciousness
- Over 400 mg/dL: may be fatal.

The symptoms of long-term heavy consumption of alcohol may take a variety of different forms. In spite of a long history of use for "medicinal" purposes, alcohol is increasingly recognized to be toxic to the human body. It is basically a central nervous system (CNS) depressant that is absorbed into the bloodstream, primarily through the small intestine. Regular consumption of large amounts of alcohol can cause irreversible damage to a number of the body's organ systems, including the cardiovascular system, the digestive tract, the central nervous system, and the peripheral nervous system. Heavy drinkers are at high risk of developing stomach or duodenal ulcers, cirrhosis of the liver, and cancers of the digestive tract. Many alcoholics do not eat properly, and often develop nutritional deficiency diseases as well as organ damage.

In addition to physical symptoms, most alcoholics have a history of psychiatric, occupational, financial, legal, or interpersonal problems as well. Alcohol misuse is the single most important predictor of **violence** between domestic partners as well as intergenerational violence within families. According to the National Highway Traffic Safety Administration, the percentages of drivers involved in fatal crashes with a BAC level of 0.08 or higher, in 2010, were 28% for motorcycle riders, 23% for passenger cars, 22% for light trucks; and 2% for large trucks. According to the Substance Abuse and Mental Health Services Administration, driving while under the influence (DUI) is associated with age. In 2010, the rate was 23.4% for people 21 to 25 years of age; 15.1% for people 18 to 20; and 5.8% for people 16 to 17;. For people over the age of 25 years, the DUI rates shows a general decline with increasing age.

According to the National Highway Traffic Safety Administration, in 2010, fatal crashes involving drunk drivers was 34% for people 21 to 24 years; 30% for those 25 to 34; and 25% for those 35 to 44. Since the early 1990s, most states have passed stricter laws against alcohol–impaired driving. These laws include such provisions as immediate license suspension for the first DWI arrest and lowering the legal blood alcohol limit to 0.08 grams per deciliter (g/dL) for adults and 0.02 g/dL for drivers under the age of 21 years. Penalties for repeated DWI citations include prison sentences; house arrest with electronic monitoring; license plates that identify offending drivers; automobile confiscation; and putting a special ignition interlock on the offender's car.

Diagnosis

The diagnosis of alcoholism is usually based on the patient's drinking history, a thorough physical examination, laboratory findings, and the results of psychodiagnostic assessment.

Examination

A physician who suspects that a patient is abusing, or is dependent on, alcohol should give him or her a complete physical examination with appropriate laboratory tests, paying particular attention to liver function and the nervous system. Physical findings that suggest alcoholism include head injuries after age 18 years; broken bones after age 18; other evidence of blackouts, frequent accidents, or falls; puffy eyelids; flushed face; alcohol odor on the breath; shaky hands; slurred speech or tongue tremor; rapid involuntary eye movements (nystagmus); enlargement of the liver (hepatomegaly); hypertension; insomnia; and problems with impotence (in males). Severe memory loss may point to advanced alcoholic damage to the CNS.

Tests

Several laboratory tests can be used to diagnose alcohol abuse and evaluate the presence of medical problems related to drinking. These tests include:

- Full blood cell count. This test indicates the presence of anemia, which is common in alcoholics. In addition, the mean corpuscular volume (MCV) is usually high in heavy drinkers. An MCV higher than 100 femtoliters (fL) suggests alcohol abuse.
- Liver function tests. Tests for serum glutamine oxaloacetic transaminase (SGOT) and alkaline phosphatase can indicate alcohol-related injury to the liver. A high level (30 units) of gamma–glutamyltransferase (GGT) is a useful marker because it is found in 70% of heavy drinkers
- Blood alcohol levels

- Carbohydrate deficient transferrin (CDT) tests. This test should not be used as a screener but is useful in monitoring alcohol consumption in heavy drinkers (those who consume 60 grams of alcohol per day) When CDT is present, it indicates regular daily consumption of alcohol.

The results of these tests might not be accurate if the patient is abusing or dependent on other substances.

Procedures

Since some of the physical signs and symptoms of alcoholism can be produced by other drugs or disorders, screening tests can also help to determine the existence of a drinking problem. There are several assessment instruments for alcoholism that can be either self-administered or administered by a clinician. The so-called CAGE test (which is abbreviated based on four key terms) is a brief screener consisting of four questions:

- Have you ever felt the need to *cut down* on drinking?
- Have you ever felt *annoyed* by criticism of your drinking?
- Have you ever felt *guilty* about your drinking?
- Have you ever taken a morning *eye opener*?

One "yes" answer should raise a suspicion of alcohol abuse; two "yes" answers are considered a positive screen.

Other brief screeners include the Alcohol Use Disorder Identification Test, or AUDIT, which also highlights some of the physical symptoms of alcohol abuse that doctors look for during a physical examination of the patient. The Michigan Alcoholism Screening Test, or MAST, is considered the diagnostic standard. It consists of 25 questions; a score of five or higher is considered to indicate alcohol dependency. A newer screener, the Substance Abuse Subtle Screening Inventory, or SASSI, was introduced in 1988. It can be given in either group or individual settings in a paper-and-pencil or computerized format. The SASSI is available in an adolescent as well as an adult version from the SASSI Institute.

According to one 1998 study, some brief screeners may be inappropriate for widespread use in some subpopulations because of ethnic and sex bias. The CAGE questionnaire often yielded inaccurate results when administered to African American men and Mexican American women. The AUDIT does not appear to be affected by ethnic or gender biases. Another study of the use of alcohol-screening questionnaires in women found that the AUDIT was preferable to the CAGE questionnaire for both African American and Caucasian women.

Prevention

It is widely recognized that the best **prevention** measure for children is strong parenting. This requires good communication between parents and their kids, so that they may be advised about the dangers of alcoholism and addiction. Prevention initiatives in schools, churches, and the community have also been widely implemented. However, alcoholism prevention remains a difficult issue because the potential for a problem condition is often not recognized at its onset.

Treatment

Because alcoholism is a complex disorder with social and occupational as well as medical implications, treatment plans usually include a mix of several different approaches. The following key issues are usually considered in determining which treatment option is appropriate:

- severity of the problem and evidence to suggest other mental health problems (e.g., depression, suicide attempts)
- staff credentials of those treating the child or teen, and what forms of therapy (e.g., family, group, medications) are to be used
- nature of family involvement
- how education is to be continued during treatment
- if an in-patient program is necessary, what length it should be
- what aftercare is to be provided following discharge
- what portion of treatment is to be covered by health insurance, and what needs to be paid out of pocket

Traditional

Most alcoholics are treated with a variety of psychosocial approaches, including regular attendance at Alcoholics Anonymous (AA) meetings, group therapy, marital or family therapy, community-based approaches, social skills training, relapse prevention, and stress-management techniques. Insight-oriented individual psychotherapy by itself is ineffective with the majority of alcoholics.

The most effective psychosocial treatments of alcohol dependence incorporate a cognitive–behavioral approach. Relapse prevention utilizes cognitive-behavioral approaches to identifying high–risk situations for each patient and restructuring his or her perceptions of the effects of alcohol as well as of the relapse process. Network therapy, which combines individual cognitive–behavioral psychotherapy with the involvement of the patient's family and peers as a group support network, is a newer approach to alcohol dependence. One recent study found that while cognitive–behavioral therapy is effective in treating alcohol dependence, the reasons that are usually offered to explain its effectiveness should be re-examined.

Drugs

Most drugs that are now being used to treat alcoholism fall into one of two groups: those that restrain the desire to drink by producing painful physical symptoms if the patient does drink; and those that appear to reduce the craving for alcohol directly. Several medications in the second category were originally developed to treat addiction to opioid substances (e.g., heroin and morphine).

ALCOHOL–SENSITIZING MEDICATIONS. The most commonly used alcohol-sensitizing agent is disulfiram (Antabuse), which has been used since the 1950s to deter alcoholics from drinking by the threat of a very unpleasant physical reaction if they do consume alcohol. The severity of the disulfiram/ethanol reaction, or DER, depends on the amount of alcohol and disulfiram in the blood. The symptoms of the reaction include facial flushing, rapid heartbeat, palpitations, difficult breathing, lowered blood pressure, headaches, nausea, and vomiting.

A DER results when the drinker consumes alcohol, because disulfiram inhibits the functioning of an enzyme called "aldehyde dehydrogenase." This enzyme is needed to convert acetaldehyde, which is produced when the body begins to oxidize the alcohol. Without the aldehyde dehydrogenase, the patient's blood level of acetaldehyde rises, causing the symptoms associated with DER.

Another alcohol-sensitizing agent is calcium carbimide, which is marketed under the brand name Temposil. Calcium carbimide produces physiological reactions with alcohol similar to those produced by disulfiram, but the onset of action is far more rapid, and the duration of action is much shorter.

ANTI-CRAVING MEDICATIONS. Another medication approved for the treatment of alcoholism is naltrexone, which appears to reduce the craving for alcohol. In addition, an injectable, long-acting form of naltrexone (Vivitrol) is available.

An anti-craving drug that is currently approved for use in the European Community, acamprosate (calcium acetyl–homotaurinate), has no psychotropic side effects nor any potential for abuse or dependence. Acamprosate is also approved in the United States to treat alcohol dependence. It appears to reduce the frequency of drinking, but its effects on enhancing abstinence from alcohol are no greater than those of naltrexone. In addition, acamprosate does not appear to enhance the effectiveness of naltrexone if the drugs are given in combination.

Other medications are available to treat the symptoms of alcohol withdrawal, such as shakiness, nausea, and sweating that occur after someone with alcohol dependence stops drinking.

Alternative

Many clinical trials for the treatment or prevention of alcoholism are currently sponsored by the National Institutes of Health (NIH) and other agencies. In 2012, NIH reported 624 ongoing or recently completed studies, including some in the recruitment stage.

Examples include:

- Alcohol Dependency Study: Combining Medication Treatment for Alcoholism: "The purpose of this study is to learn whether ondansetron and topiramate, either alone or in combination, are safe and effective in the treatment of alcohol dependence. This 13-week outpatient clinical trial is randomized, double-blind, and placebo-controlled. There are post-study follow up visits one, two, and three months after the end of the study. Participants will receive ondansetron and topiramate either alone or in combination or a placebo, coupled with psychotherapy."
- Treatment of Patients With Alcoholism and Attention Deficit Disorder: "This study of persons with both alcoholism and ADHD will determine whether adding the drug methylphenidate to a standard treatment program will decrease alcohol use. In approximately half of patients with ADHD, symptoms persist into adulthood, and the untreated condition is associated with a significantly increased incidence of substance-use disorder. More than one-third of adults with substance use disorder have symptoms of ADHD. This study will evaluate the effectiveness of adding methylphenidate to a standard alcohol treatment program in improving patients' treatment compliance and decreasing adverse consequences of drinking, as well as monitoring their attention deficit/hyperactivity symptoms."
- Effects of Omegas 3 and 6 on Alcohol Dependence: "The treatment of alcoholism is a challenge for psychiatrists and patients. Some studies have shown that alcohol alters the environment of the membranes, mainly by modifying their permeability through the lipid fraction. These lipids are known as essential fatty acids (EFA) because they are obtained only through the diet, as the human body is unable to synthesize them. Linolenic acid (LA), or omega 6, and alpha-linolenic acid (ALA), or omega 3, are polyunsaturated fatty acids (PUFAs). Finally, ethanol changes the absorption and metabolism of PUFAs, and

it's supplementation may be helpful for alcohol dependence recovery."

- Facilitation of NMDA Receptor Function in Patients With Schizophrenia and Co-morbid Alcoholism: "This placebo-controlled study is designed to evaluate the efficacy of glycine, an agonist of the glycine-B co-agonist site of the NMDA receptor, on alcohol consumption and craving as well as negative symptoms in schizophrenia."

Clinical trial information is constantly updated by NIH, and the most recent information on alcoholism trials can be found at: http://clinicaltrials.gov/ct2/results?term=alcoholism.

Prognosis

The prognosis for recovery from alcoholism varies widely. The usual course of the disorder is one of episodes of intoxication beginning in adolescence, with full-blown dependence by the mid-20s to mid-30s. The most common pattern is one of periodic attempts at abstinence alternating with relapses into uncontrolled drinking. On the other hand, it is thought that as many as 20% of persons diagnosed as alcohol-dependent achieve long-term sobriety even without medical treatment. It is difficult to compare the outcomes of the various treatment approaches to alcoholism, in part because their definitions of "success" vary. Some researchers count only total abstinence from alcohol as a successful outcome, while others regard curtailed drinking and better social adjustment as indicators of success. The role of genetic factors in the prognosis is still disputed. Available evidence suggests that such factors as the presence of a spouse, partner, or close friend in the alcoholic's life, or religious commitment, can outweigh genetic vulnerability to the disorder.

Risks

According to the NIAAA, the risk for developing alcoholism seems to run in families. Genetics and lifestyle are both factors. Socializing patterns, the amount of stress in a person's life, and the availability of alcohol are all factors that may increase the risk for alcoholism. In general, more men than women are alcohol dependent. Alcohol problems are highest in the 18–29 age group and lowest among adults aged 65 and older. People who start drinking in their teens are also at much higher risk of developing alcohol problems, compared to people who start drinking at age 21 or older.

Results

The long-term effects of chronic alcohol use are severe damage, possibly both physically and mentally. There is a strong correlation between extreme alcohol consumption and an increased risk of developing alcoholism, along with alcoholic liver disease, **cancer**, cardiovascular disease, chronic pancreatitis, and malabsorption. Chronic alcohol abuse can also damage the central and peripheral nervous systems. Generally, excessive consumption of alcohol over long periods can result in damage to nearly every organ and system in the body.

KEY TERMS

Acamprosate—An anti-craving medication used to reduce the craving for alcohol.

Alcohol Use Disorders Inventory Test (AUDIT)—A test for alcohol use developed by the World Health Organization (WHO). Its ten questions address three specific areas of drinking over a 12-month period: the amount and frequency of drinking, dependence upon alcohol, and problems that have been encountered due to drinking alcohol.

Behavioral therapy—Form of psychotherapy used to treat depression, anxiety disorders, phobias, and other forms of psychopathology.

Binge drinking—Consumption of five or more alcoholic drinks in a row on a single occasion.

CAGE—A four-question assessment for the presence of alcoholism in both adults and children.

Disulfiram—A medication that has been used since the late 1940s as part of a treatment plan for alcohol abuse. Sold under the trade name Antabuse, it produces changes in the body's metabolism of alcohol that cause headaches, vomiting, and other unpleasant symptoms if the patient drinks even small amounts of alcohol.

Ethanol—The chemical name for beverage alcohol. It is also sometimes called "ethyl alcohol" or "grain alcohol" to distinguish it from isopropyl or rubbing alcohol.

Naltrexone—A medication originally developed to treat addiction to heroin or morphine that is also used to treat alcoholism. It works by reducing the craving for alcohol rather than by producing vomiting or other unpleasant reactions.

Withdrawal—The characteristic withdrawal syndrome for alcohol includes feelings of irritability or anxiety, elevated blood pressure and pulse, tremors, and clammy skin.

QUESTIONS TO ASK YOUR DOCTOR

- Can you help me manage my drinking?
- What medications could help me to stop drinking?
- Are any of my current health issues related to drinking?
- What resources are available to me locally? On the Internet?
- What are my treatment options?
- What are the risks associated with treatment?
- How much alcohol consumption is safe for me?
- How long will I be on medication? What are the potential side effects of my medication?

Aftercare

Aftercare from alcoholism is a lifelong process and does not end when a drug/alcohol rehabilitation program is completed. Continuing support is critical to a healthy recovery.

Resources

BOOKS

Benton, Sarah Allen. *Understanding the High-Functioning Alcoholic: Professional Views and Personal Insights.* Westport, CT: Praeger Publishers, 2009.

The Healing Project. *Voices of Alcoholism: The Healing Companion: Stories for Courage, Comfort and Strength.* Brooklyn, NY: LaChance Publishing, 2008.

Hedblom, Jack H. *Last Call: Alcoholism and Recovery.* Baltimore: The Johns Hopkins University Press, 2007.

Jay, Jeff, and Debra Jay. *Love First: A Family's Guide to Intervention.* Center City, MN: Hazelden, 2008.

Kinney, Jean. *Loosening the Grip: A Handbook of Alcohol Information.* New York: McGraw-Hill, 2012.

Maltzman, Irving. *Alcoholism: Its Treatments and Mistreatments.* Hackensack, NJ: World Scientific Publishing, 2008.

Piggott, John, editor. *Alcoholic Beverages: Sensory Evaluation and Consumer Research.* Oxford: Woodhead, 2012.

Tracy, Sarah W. *Alcoholism in America: From Reconstruction to Prohibition.* Baltimore, MD: The Johns Hopkins University Press, 2007.

Watkins, Christine. *Alcohol Abuse.* Detroit: Greenhaven Press, 2012.

WEBSITES

Alcoholism: List Results. ClinicalTrials.gov. http://www.clinicaltrials.gov/ct2/results?term=alcoholism (accessed August 16, 2012).

Alcoholism. Mayo Clinic. (May 6, 2010). http://www.mayoclinic.com/health/alcoholism/DS00340 (accessed August 7, 2012).

Alcoholism. Medline Plus. (August 6, 2012). http://www.nlm.nih.gov/medlineplus/alcoholism.html (accessed August 7, 2012).

Alcohol Use. Centers for Disease Control and Prevention. (January 27, 2012). http://www.cdc.gov/nchs/fastats/alcohol.htm (accessed August 7, 2012).

Faces of Change: Do I Have a Problem with Alcohol or Drugs? Substance Abuse and Mental Health Services Administration. http://www.kap.samhsa.gov/products/brochures/pdfs/TIP35.pdf (accessed August 7, 2012).

Overview of Alcohol Consumption. National Institutes of Health. http://www.niaaa.nih.gov/alcohol-health/overview-alcohol-consumption (accessed August 7, 2012).

Ringold, Sarah. *Alcohol Abuse and Alcoholism.* Journal of the American Medical Association. (May 3, 2006). http://jama.ama-assn.org/cgi/reprint/295/17/2100.pdf (accessed August 7, 2012).

Statistics. Mothers Against Drunk Driving. http://www.madd.org/statistics/ (accessed August 7, 2012).

ORGANIZATIONS

Al-Anon/Alateen, 1600 Corporate Landing Pkwy., Virginia Beach, VA U.S.A. 23454, 1 (757) 563-1600, Fax: 1 (757) 563-1655, (800) 877-1600, wso@al-anon.org, http://www.al-anon.alateen.org/

Alcoholics Anonymous, 475 Riverside Dr. at West 120th St., New York City, NY U.S.A. 10115, 1 (212) 870-3400, http://www.aa.org/

National Council on Alcoholism and Drug Dependence, 217 Broadway, Ste. 712, New York City, NY U.S.A. 10007, 1 (212) 269-7797, Fax: 1 (212) 269-7510, (800) 622-2255, national@ncadd.org, http://www.ncadd.org/

National Institute on Alcohol Abuse and Alcoholism, 1 (301) 443-2857, (888) 696-4222, http://www.niaaa.nih.gov/.

Rebecca J. Frey, PHD
Joan Schonbeck, RN
William A. Atkins, BB, BS, MBA

Allergies

Definition

Allergies are hypersensitive responses by the immune system to otherwise harmless foreign substances.

Demographics

Allergies are among the most common medical disorders. It is estimated that 60 million Americans, or more

Foods that may contain common allergens

Allergen	Food product
Milk	Butter (including butter flavor, butter fat, and butter oil) Buttermilk Casein Casemates Cheese Cream Cottage cheese Custard Ghee Goat milk Milk proteins (lactalbumin, lactalbumin phosphate, lactoglobulin, lactulose) Milk solids Pudding Sour cream Yogurt
Eggs	Albumin or albumen Eggnog Lecithin Lysozyme Marshmallows Marzipan Mayonnaise Meringue Nougat Pasta Surimi (fish product)
Peanuts	Any nut product (including nut butters and oils) Ethnic foods (especially African, Chinese, Indonesian, Mexican, Thai, and Vietnamese dishes) Many candies and baked goods Nougat Sunflower seeds

(Table by PreMediaGlobal. © 2013 Cengage Learning)

than one in every five, suffer from some form of allergy that is pronounced enough to cause symptoms. More than half of all Americans test positive for one or more allergens. Allergies are the third leading cause of chronic disease among American children and the single largest reason for school absences. Allergies are the fifth leading cause of chronic disease among all Americans, accounting for one in nine physician visits and a major source of lost workplace productivity. There are similar proportions of allergy sufferers throughout much of the world.

Among Americans:

- Approximately 36 million suffer from seasonal allergies, with seasonal allergic rhinitis—or hay fever—affecting 20% of all adults and up to 40% of children. Pollen allergies generally develop between the ages of 6 and 13. Other respiratory allergies, such as those to dust, animal dander, and molds, may occur in children as young as two or three.
- Approximately 12 million have food allergies, including 4% of adults and 6-8% of children four years-of-age and under. Approximately 6.9 million Americans are allergic to seafood and 0.4-0.6% are allergic to peanuts and other nuts—the most severe of food allergies.
- Allergic drug reactions account for 5-10% of all adverse drug reactions, with skin reactions being the most common. About one-fifth of all children are allergic to some type of medication, often penicillin, sulfa drugs, or aspirin.
- Although about 15% of adults have mild, localized allergic reactions to insect bites and stings, approximately 3% have serious allergies to the venom of stinging insects, such as honeybees, wasps, hornets, yellow jackets, and fire ants (which are found only in the South). Children rarely experience the severe reactions to venom that sometimes occur in adults.
- Hives affect up to 20% of the population at some point in their lives.
- Skin allergies or allergic contact dermatitis is the most common skin condition in children under age 11.
- Estimates of the prevalence of latex allergy vary from less than 1% to 6%. Healthcare workers are particularly at risk for contact dermatitis from latex gloves.

Almost nine million American children suffer from **asthma**, a chronic disease that causes inflammation of the airways, making it difficult to breathe. Many different allergens can trigger asthma attacks and it is estimated that 50% of adults and more than 80% of children with asthma have associated allergies, especially allergic rhinitis. It is believed that asthma is both under-diagnosed and under-treated in the elderly.

Anaphylaxis or anaphylactic shock is a rare, severe, and potentially fatal allergic reaction that causes blood pressure to drop severely and the airways to swell shut. Among Americans:

- More than 700 die each year from anaphylaxis brought on by an allergic reaction
- Approximately 150–200 die from food-induced anaphylaxis
- Penicillin in its various forms results in about 400 deaths per year in the United States. Worldwide, 32 out of every 100,000 patients exposed to penicillin have an anaphylactic reaction
- Each year 40–100 Americans die from an anaphylactic reaction to insect bites or stings
- There are about 220 cases of anaphylaxis and three deaths annually from latex allergy

The incidence of allergies and asthma is increasing in industrialized countries by about 5% per year and as many as half of all those affected are children. Some of this increase can be attributed to better diagnosis and

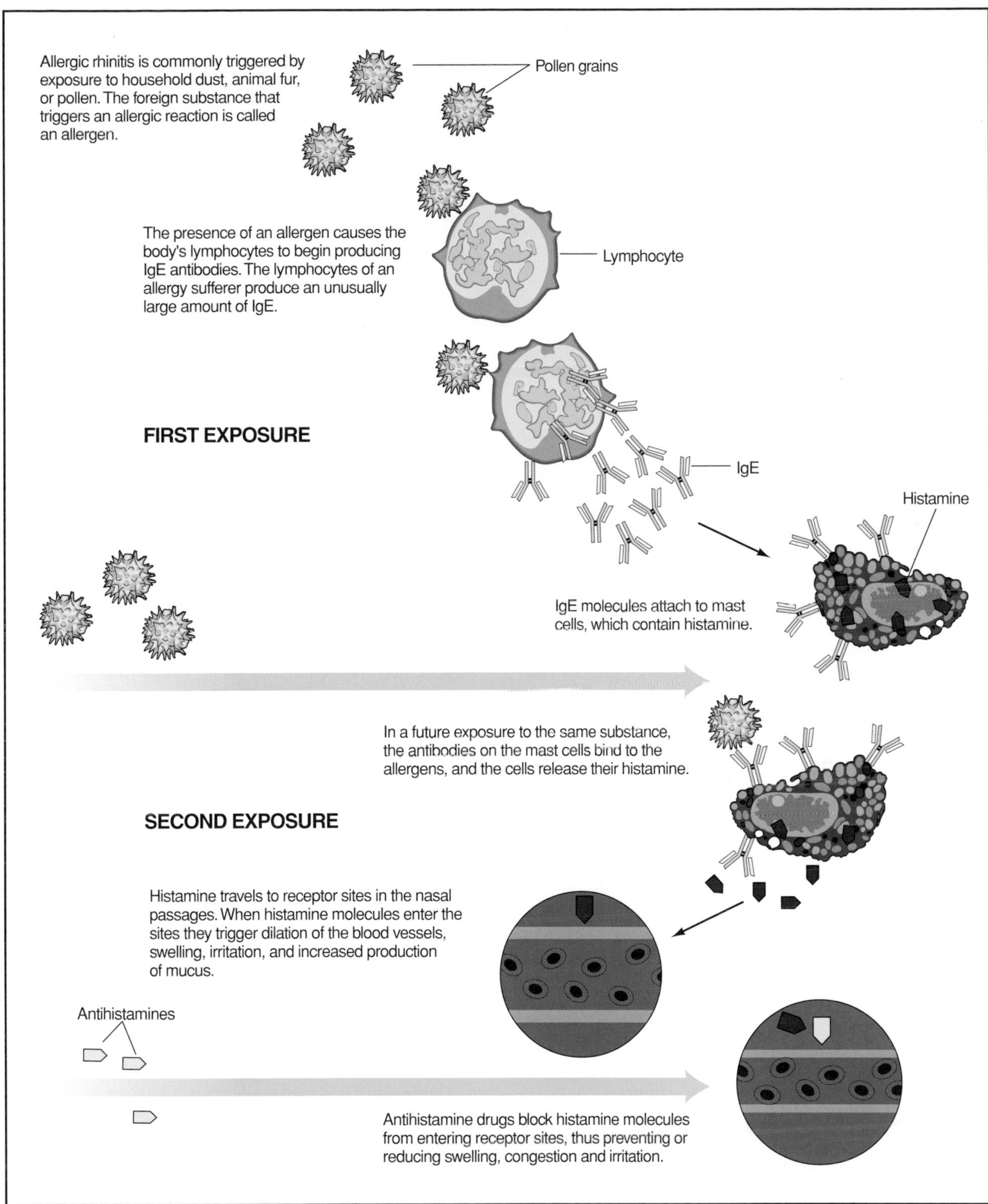

Allergic rhinitis is commonly triggered by exposure to household dust, animal fur, or pollen. The foreign substance that triggers an allergic reaction is called an allergen.
Pollen grains
The presence of an allergen causes the body's lymphocytes to begin producing IgE antibodies. The lymphocytes of an allergy sufferer produce an unusually large amount of IgE.
Lymphocyte
FIRST EXPOSURE
IgE
Histamine
IgE molecules attach to mast cells, which contain histamine.
In a future exposure to the same substance, the antibodies on the mast cells bind to the allergens, and the cells release their histamine.
SECOND EXPOSURE
Histamine travels to receptor sites in the nasal passages. When histamine molecules enter the sites they trigger dilation of the blood vessels, swelling, irritation, and increased production of mucus.
Antihistamines
Antihistamine drugs block histamine molecules from entering receptor sites, thus preventing or reducing swelling, congestion and irritation.

(Illustration by Electronic Illustrators Group. © 2013 Cengage Learning)

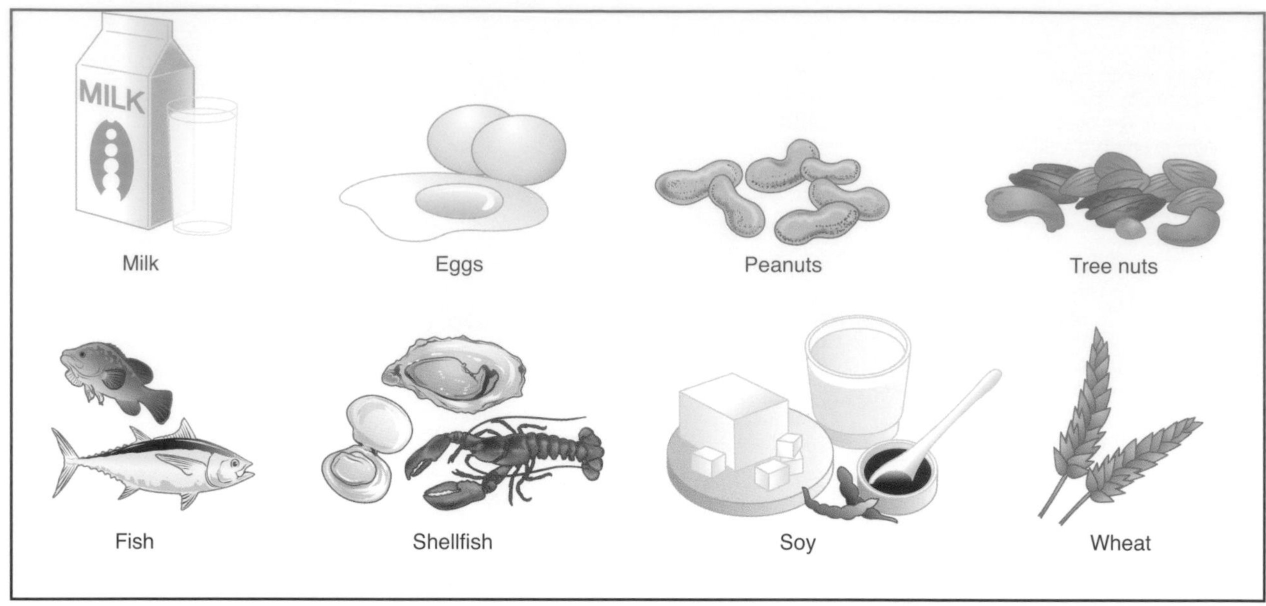

Foods that are known for causing allergic reactions. *(Illustration by Electronic Illustrators Group. © 2013 Cengage Learning)*

reporting. However much of it may be due to lifestyle and environmental factors.

Description

An allergy is a type of immune response. The immune system normally responds to microorganisms, such as bacteria or viruses, or foreign particles by producing specific proteins called antibodies. These antibodies identify and bind to a specific foreign molecule—known as the antigen. The reaction between the antibody and its antigen sets off a series of chemical reactions designed to protect the body from infection. However with allergies, this immune response is triggered by harmless common substances called allergens. Allergens may be inhaled into the lungs (pollen, dust, animal dander, **mold**, pollutants), swallowed (food, drugs), injected (drugs, insect venom), or touched (poisonous plants, latex).

There are two main types of allergic reactions. Immediate hypersensitivity reactions are mediated predominately by a type of immune-system cell called a mast cell and occur within minutes of contact with the allergen. Delayed hypersensitivity reactions are mediated by T cells, a type of white blood cell, and occur hours to days after exposure to the allergen.

In immediate sensitivity reactions allergens bind to a type of antibody called immunoglobulin E or IgE on the surface of mast cells. Mast cells are filled with granules that contain a variety of potent chemicals including histamine. When the IgE on a mast cell binds its specific allergen, the contents of the granules spill out onto neighboring cells. Histamine binds to proteins called histamine receptors on the surfaces of these other cells, causing a chain of reactions that lead to allergy symptoms. Histamine binding to receptors on blood vessels increases leakage, leading to the fluid accumulation, swelling, and redness. In the nasal passages histamine causes swelling, congestion, and increased mucus production. Histamine also stimulates **pain** receptors on nerve cells, causing sensitivity and irritation. These symptoms last from one to several hours following contact with the allergen.

In delayed hypersensitivity reactions roving T cells contact the allergen, setting in motion a more prolonged immune response. This type of allergic response may develop over several days following contact with the allergen and symptoms may persist for a week or more.

Allergens enter the body through four main routes: the airways, the gastrointestinal tract, the circulatory system, and the skin. Inhaled or ingested allergens usually cause immediate hypersensitivity reactions. Allergens on the skin usually cause delayed hypersensitivity reactions.

People are sensitive to different allergens. For example, some people have severe allergic rhinitis but no food allergies, whereas others are extremely sensitive to nuts but not to any other food. Allergies may worsen over time. For example, allergic rhinitis can be either seasonal or chronic and a childhood ragweed allergy may progress to year-round dust and pollen allergies. Conversely, people can lose allergies. Infant or childhood atopic dermatitis, for example, almost always disappears with advancing age. However most often, an apparent loss of sensitivity is due to reduced exposure to the allergen or increased tolerance for the allergy symptoms.

Risk factors

Although allergies to specific allergens are not inherited, the propensity for developing allergies is frequently inherited.

- If neither parent has allergies, the chances of a child developing allergies are approximately 10–20%.
- A child with one allergic parent has a 30–50% chance of developing allergies.
- The likelihood of developing allergies rises to 40–75% if both parents have allergies. However children are not necessarily sensitive to the same allergens as their parents. Since people with allergies tend to produce more IgE than those without allergies, it may be that the tendency to produce more IgE is inherited. High levels of IgE also increase the likelihood of having allergies to multiple allergens.

Other risk factors for the development of childhood allergies include:

- low birth weight
- being born during a high-pollen season
- not being breastfed
- growing up in a home with tobacco smoke
- having a family pet
- having a lower socioeconomic status
- repeated exposure to an allergen or prolonged exposure to a strong allergen

Causes and symptoms

The most common airborne allergens are:

- plant pollens
- animal fur and dander
- body parts from house mites (microscopic creatures found in all houses)
- house dust
- mold spores
- feathers
- cigarette smoke
- chemicals
- solvents
- cleansers

Pollen can cause both seasonal and chronic rhinitis. Seasonal rhinitis occurs at the same time every year and is caused by the pollen of specific plants, especially grasses and trees in the spring and ragweed in the late summer and fall. Allergies tend to worsen as the season progresses because the immune system becomes sensitized to particular antigens and produces a faster, stronger response. Chronic rhinitis can be caused by food as well as airborne allergens.

Airborne allergens cause immediate hypersensitivity reactions in the upper airways and eyes. These include sneezing, runny nose, itchy, watery, and bloodshot eyes, nasal congestion, and scratchy or irritated throat due to postnasal drip. Airborne allergens can also cause inflammation of the thin membrane (conjunctiva) covering the eye, resulting in the redness, irritation, and increased tearing of allergic conjunctivitis or pink eye. Asthma causes wheezing, coughing, and shortness of breath and is associated with exposure to numerous allergens including cockroach allergens.

Common food allergens include:

- cow's milk
- eggs
- grains such as wheat or corn
- nuts, especially peanuts, walnuts, and Brazil nuts
- fish, mollusks, and shellfish
- soy products
- some fruits, especially raw seeded fruit
- some vegetables, especially tomatoes or legumes such as peas or beans
- chocolate
- certain spices
- food additives and preservatives

True food allergies are often confused with intolerance to certain foods. Food allergies, like other types of allergies, are caused by an antibody response, whereas intolerance is due a deficiency in the enzymes needed to digest a certain food. For example, a milk allergy is caused by sensitivity to an allergen (often the protein lactalbumin) in the milk itself. In contrast, people who lack the enzyme lactase have lactose intolerance—the inability to digest one of the sugars in milk—and suffer from gastrointestinal problems when they consume milk or certain milk products.

Symptoms of food allergies depend on the tissues that are most sensitive to the allergen and whether the allergen has spread systemically through the circulatory system. Allergens in food can cause immediate hypersensitivity reactions that include itching, swelling, and/or rashes of the eyes, lips, mouth, and throat. Food allergies can also cause respiratory symptoms. Swelling and irritation of the intestinal lining can cause nausea, vomiting, cramping, diarrhea, and gas. When food allergens enter the bloodstream from the gastrointestinal tract, they can cause hives, atopic dermatitis, or more severe reactions such as angioedema. Some food allergens may cause anaphylaxis, a potentially life-threatening condition marked by tissue swelling, airway constriction, and drop in blood pressure. Reactions to peanuts and other nuts can be so dangerous that physicians recommend caution in giving these foods to infants and children with a family history of allergy. Some school systems are restricting the use of peanuts and peanut butter in lunchrooms or banning them altogether, since even smelling or touching them can cause an allergic reaction in some children.

Drugs that often cause allergic reactions include:

- penicillin and other antibiotics
- flu vaccines
- tetanus toxoid vaccine
- gamma globulin

Insects and other arthropods whose bites or stings may cause an allergic reaction include:

- bees, wasps, and hornets
- mosquitoes
- fleas
- scabies

Injected allergens from drugs or insect bites and stings are introduced directly into the circulation where they can cause both local reactions, such as swelling and irritation at the injection site, and system-wide (systemic) reactions, including anaphylaxis. Symptoms of an allergy to insect venom include:

- hives
- itchy eyes
- a dry cough
- constriction of the throat and chest
- nausea
- dizziness
- abdominal pain

There are three main types of allergic skin reactions:

- atopic dermatitis or eczema
- hives (urticaria)
- contact dermatitis

Atopic dermatitis and eczema are skin reactions to allergens introduced through the airways or gastrointestinal tract. Eczema commonly occurs in infants and children with a family history of allergies and is usually outgrown by the age of six. It generally occurs in cycles, beginning with dry, itchy skin that becomes inflamed when scratched, followed by weeping sores that subsequently crust over. In the chronic stage the affected skin becomes thickened, leathery, and scaly. Eczema appears most often on the cheeks, ears, and neck and the inner folds of elbows and knees, but it may affect other parts of the body as well.

Whole-body or systemic reactions can occur with any type of allergen, but are more common following ingestion or injection of an allergen. Hives are a systemic skin reaction characterized by raised, red, itchy blotches of varying sizes anywhere on the body, but especially on the stomach, chest, arms, hands, and face. Angioedema is a deeper, more extensive, and painful reaction in which fluid accumulation causes recurrent, non-inflammatory swelling of the skin, eyelids, lips, mucous membranes, genitals, other organs, and brain. However it most often occurs on the extremities, fingers, toes, and parts of the head, neck, and face. Hives and angioedema are usually acute conditions, although they can sometimes persist for weeks.

Skin contact with allergens can cause reddening, itching, and blistering, known as contact dermatitis. The dermatitis sometimes has an identifying pattern, such as the outline of an earring or latex glove. Common causes include:

- poison ivy, oak, and sumac
- nickel or nickel alloys
- chemicals
- cosmetics
- latex

Dermatitis can also be caused by non-allergic damage to skin cells arising from irritants such as cold, soap, or chemical agents.

Asthma is a chronic, reversible respiratory disorder caused by obstruction and swelling of the airways to the lungs. An asthma attack begins when the muscles surrounding the bronchial tubes spasm and the tubes narrow. This stimulates increased mucus production, further blocking the airways, and inflammation and swelling, which cause even more congestion and discomfort. Symptoms of asthma include coughing, wheezing, shortness of breath, fatigue, anxiety, and tightness in the chest. Asthma can be triggered by allergens—including pollen, animal dander, dust, and certain foods—and by non-allergenic irritants.

Anaphylaxis is an IgE-mediated hypersensitivity reaction brought about by mediators released by mast cells in the tissues and by immune system cells called basophils in the blood. These can cause airway constriction, blood pressure drop, widespread tissue swelling, heart rhythm abnormalities, and sometimes loss of consciousness. Other symptoms may include dizziness, weakness, seizures, coughing, flushing, or cramping. Symptoms can begin within five minutes after exposure

KEY TERMS

Allergen—Any substance that provokes an allergic response.

Allergenic—Acting as an allergen or inducing an allergic response.

Allergic rhinitis—Inflammation of the mucous membranes of the nose and eyes in response to an allergen. Hay fever is seasonal allergic rhinitis.

Anaphylaxis—Severe, potentially fatal hypersensitivity caused by previous exposure to an allergen that can result in blood vessel dilation and a sharp drop in blood pressure, smooth muscle contraction, and difficulty breathing.

Angioedema—Severe non-inflammatory swelling of the skin, organs, and brain, possibly accompanied by fever and muscle pain.

Antibody—A specific immunoglobulin protein produced by the immune system in response to a specific antigen.

Antigen—A foreign protein or particle that causes the body to produce specific antibodies that bind to it.

Asthma—A lung condition, usually of allergic origin, in which the airways become narrow due to smooth muscle contraction, causing wheezing, coughing, and shortness of breath.

Atopic dermatitis—A skin condition resulting from exposure to airborne or food allergens.

Atopy—Genetic predisposition toward the development of allergies.

Conjunctivitis—Inflammation of the conjunctiva, the membrane covering the white part of the eye.

Contact dermatitis—Skin inflammation resulting from contact with an allergen or other substance.

Delayed hypersensitivity reactions—Allergic reactions mediated by T cells that occur hours to days after exposure to the antigen.

Eczema—An inflammatory skin condition characterized by redness, itching, and oozing lesions, which become crusty, scaly, or hardened.

Epinephrine—Adrenalin; a hormone released into the bloodstream in response to stress. Its many effects include stimulating the heart and increasing blood pressure, metabolic rate, and blood glucose concentration.

Granules—Small packets of reactive chemicals stored within cells.

Histamine—A chemical released by mast cells during an allergic reaction and which has a variety of effects on other cells.

Hives—A raised, itchy area of skin that is usually a sign of an allergic reaction.

Immediate hypersensitivity reactions—Allergic reactions that are mediated by mast cells and occur within minutes of allergen contact.

Immunoglobulin E (IgE)—Antibodies produced in the lungs, skin, and mucous membranes that are responsible for allergic reactions.

Mast cells—A type of immune system cell that displays immunoglobulin E (IgE) on its cell surface and participates in allergic reactions by releasing histamine and other chemicals from intracellular granules. The lining of the nasal passages and eyelids are particularly rich in mast cells.

T cells—Immune system white blood cells that have highly specific antigen receptors on their surfaces. Some T cells stimulate other immune system cells to produce and release antibodies.

to the allergen or up to an hour or more later. Anaphylaxis is most often associated with allergies to foods, medications, and insect venoms.

Genetic profile

The genetic predisposition toward the development of hypersensitivity reactions upon exposure to specific antigens is called atopy. After birth the immune system switches to become either non-allergy prone (TH1) or allergy prone (TH2), depending on an interplay of heredity and environment. TH stands for T-helper white blood cells. TH1 cells fight bacteria and viruses and protect against allergies. TH2 cells fight parasitic infections and promote the production of excessive IgE, increasing the likelihood of developing allergies. TH2 immunity is much more likely to be switched on in children with a family history of allergies.

Over the past four decades atopy has increased significantly, for reasons that are not well understood. In addition to genetic factors, it has been suggested that our environment contains more allergy-inducing substances and that protective factors may have been removed from the environment. There is also some evidence suggesting that the worldwide fight against

infectious disease and increased personal cleanliness may be interfering with immune system function. Global warming—and the accompanying changes in natural vegetation patterns and increased pollen production—may also be affecting atopy.

Diagnosis

Examination

Allergies can often be diagnosed by a careful medical history that matches the onset of symptoms with exposure to possible allergens. Allergy is suspected if the symptoms are characteristic of an allergic reaction and occur repeatedly upon exposure to the suspected allergen, at a certain time of year, or in a particular environment. Although allergy tests can be used to identify potential allergens, their results must be supported by evidence of an allergic response.

Tests

With allergy skin tests a tiny dose of an aqueous extract of the suspected allergen is pricked, scratched, punctured, or patched on the skin. The initial test is usually a prick or patch test on the back, forearm, or top of the thigh. Reactions are usually evaluated about 15 minutes after exposure. An allergen may produce a classic immune wheal-and-flare response—a skin lesion with a raised, white, compressible area surrounded by a red flare. A positive skin reaction will occur even if the allergen is normally encountered in the airways or in food. Skin testing can produce false positives and, occasionally, serious allergic reactions. Intradermal skin tests involve injection of the allergen into the dermis of the skin. These are more sensitive and use smaller amounts of allergen, so they can be used with potentially fatal allergens such as **antibiotics**.

Provocation tests administer the allergen directly through its normal route under medically controlled conditions. Food allergen provocation tests involve the ingestion of a measured amount of the suspected allergen in an opaque capsule after abstinence from the suspected allergen for two weeks or more. The results are compared to the response to ingestion of a placebo. Diagnosis of delayed allergic contact dermatitis involves the application of a skin patch containing the allergen. Provocation tests are never used when a patient's medical history suggests the possibility of anaphylaxis.

Since people with allergies may have a higher level of total IgE in their serum (the portion of the blood that contains antibodies) than those without allergies, total IgE can be measured with a two-site immunometric assay. However there is considerable overlap in serum IgE levels among people with and without allergies. Furthermore other non-allergic conditions—including **smoking**, HIV/AIDS, parasitic infections, and IgE myeloma—can raise IgE levels. However a total serum IgE test is useful for diagnosing some conditions.

With allergen-specific IgE measurements, the suspected allergen is bound to a solid support, such as a cellulose sponge, microtiter plate, or paper disk. A patient's serum is incubated with the allergen. Allergen-specific IgE antibodies will bind to the solid phase and remain there when the serum is washed off. A second labeled antibody that binds to any IgE is added to determine the level of the allergen-specific IgE. The radioallergosorbent test (RAST) uses radioactive anti-IgE antibodies. A newer test called an enzyme-linked immunosorbent assay (ELISA) uses anti-IgE antibodies that are linked to an enyzme. A test called the CAP-RAST measures the amount of IgE in the blood that is specific for a given food.

Attempts are being made to directly measure immune system mediators such as histamine, eosinophil cationic protein (ECP), and mast cell tryptase.

Electrodermal testing or electro-acupuncture allergy testing has been used in Europe, but is somewhat controversial and has not been approved by the U.S. Food and Drug Administration (FDA). An electric potential is applied to the skin and changes in the electrical resistance are measured upon exposure to the suspected allergen.

Procedures

Elimination diets are often used to diagnose food allergies. Suspect foods may be sequentially eliminated from the diet. Alternatively, after several weeks on a diet lacking any of the suspected allergenic foods, each suspected food is reintroduced one at a time and the patient is observed for signs of allergic reaction.

Treatment

Traditional

The most effective allergy treatment is avoiding all allergen exposure. This is usually possible with food allergens but can be very difficult with other types of allergens. Therefore immediate hypersensitivity reactions are usually treated with drugs.

Immunotherapy, usually called allergy shots or desensitization, alters the balance of antibody types in the body. Immunotherapy is generally used when medications cannot relieve symptoms. Extracts of the allergen are injected into the skin in gradually increasing amounts over a period of weeks, months, or years, with occasional booster shots. The amounts of allergen are too small to trigger an allergic response; however patients are monitored closely after each injection because of the small risk of anaphylaxis. Immunotherapy is most effective for hay fever and insect sting allergies, particularly in patients who cannot avoid allergens in the environment and who do not respond to medications. It may also reduce or eliminate the need for medications. While many rhinitis sufferers have been helped by allergy shots, they are costly and time-consuming and are not always effective. It may take up to several years of treatment to fully benefit from immunotherapy and about one in five patients do not respond at all. However some experts recommend preventative immunotherapy for children who have severe reactions to insect stings.

Drugs

There are a large number of prescription and over-the-counter medications for treating immediate hypersensitivity reactions. Most of these work by decreasing the ability of histamine to provoke symptoms. Other drugs counteract the effects of histamine by stimulating other systems or by reducing the general immune response. Medications are available as pills, liquids, nasal sprays, eye drops, and skin creams. The appropriate medication depends on the symptoms and the patient's overall health. A physician may recommend trying a few different medications to determine which ones are most effective with the fewest side effects.

Antihistamines are the most common treatment for rhinitis. They block the histamine receptors in nasal tissue, thereby decreasing the effects of histamine released by mast cells. Antihistamines can be used after symptoms appear, although they may be even more effective when used preventively, before symptoms appear. They help reduce sneezing, itching, and runny nose (rhinorrhea). Antihistamines can also be used to treat other types of allergies.

There are a wide variety of antihistamines available. Older first-generation antihistamines often cause drowsiness as a major side effect. They can also cause dizziness, dry mouth, tachycardia, blurred vision, constipation, and a lowered threshold for seizures. Their effects can be similar to those of alcohol and care should be taken when operating motor vehicles, since individuals may not be aware that they are impaired. These antihistamines include:

- diphenhydramine (Benadryl and generics)
- chlorpheniramine (Chlor-trimeton and generics)
- brompheniramine (Dimetane and generics)
- clemastine (Tavist and generics)

Newer antihistamines that do not cause drowsiness or cross the blood-brain barrier include:

- loratidine (Claritin)
- cetirizine (Zyrtec)
- fexofenadine (Allegra)
- desloratadine (Clarinex)
- azelastin HCl (Astelin)
- astemizole (Hismanal)

Seldane (terfenadine), the original non-drowsy antihistamine, was voluntarily withdrawn from the market by its manufacturer in early 1998 because of its potential for causing serious heart arrhythmias and the availability of the equally effective but safer drug fexofenadine. Hismanal also has the potential for causing heart arrhythmias when taking more than the recommended dose or taking it along with the antibiotic erythromycin, the antifungal drugs ketoconazole or itraconazole, or the antimalarial drug quinine.

Decongestants constrict the blood vessels in the nasopharyngeal and sinus mucosa, reducing swelling and relieving nasal and sinus congestion. Both oral systemic preparations and nasal sprays—which are applied directly to the nasal lining—are available. Decongestants are stimulants and may cause increased heart rate and blood pressure, headaches, insomnia, agitation, and difficulty emptying the bladder. Use of nasal decongestants for longer than several days can result in loss of effectiveness and rebound congestion in which nasal passages become even more swollen.

Cromolyn **sodium** is a nonsteroidal mast cell stabilizer that prevents the release of mast cell granules and thus the release of histamine and other chemicals. It can be started several weeks before the onset of the allergy season as a preventive treatment. It can also be used for year-round allergy **prevention**. Cromolyn sodium is available as a nasal spray that coats the nasal membranes to treat allergic rhinitis and in aerosol form (a suspension of particles in gas) for asthma.

Newer types of allergy medications include:

- the IgE modifier omalizumab (Xolair), which interferes with the action of mast cells
- leukotriene modifiers or antileukotrienes, which block the action of leukotrienes—inflammatory substances released by the immune system during an allergic reaction—and include zafirlukast (Accolate), montelukast (Singulair), and zileuton (Zyflo)
- immunomodulatory topical ointments—which interfere with cell mechanisms that produce inflammatory responses—and include pimecrolimus (Elidel cream) and tacrolimus (Protopic ointment)

Corticosteroids help to prevent and treat the inflammation associated with allergic conditions by reducing the recruitment of inflammatory cells and the synthesis of immune-system chemicals called cytokines. Studies have shown that steroidal nasal sprays are more effective on an as-needed basis for seasonal allergies than antihistamines. Although hives and angioedema are usually treated with antihistamines, cromolyn, or epinephrine, intractable cases may be treated with oral cortisone; however it should be used sparingly and only as a last recourse because of its side effects. Corticosteroids are also used to prevent and control asthma attacks.

Topical corticosteroids reduce mucous membrane and skin inflammations by decreasing the amount of fluid that moves from the vascular spaces into the tissues. Topical corticosteroid creams are effective for contact dermatitis, although overuse can lead to dry and scaly skin. Moderately strong corticosteroids can be applied as a wrap for 24 hours. Short-term oral corticosteroid therapy also may be appropriate for acute contact dermatitis. Side effects are usually mild, but may include headaches, nosebleeds, and unpleasant taste sensations.

Because allergic reactions involving the lungs cause the airways or bronchial tubes to narrow, bronchodilators—which open or dilate the smooth muscle lining the airways—can be very effective for treating asthma attacks. Bronchodilators include:

- adrenaline (epinephrine)
- albuterol (Proventil)
- pirbuterol (Maxair)
- theophylline
- other adrenergic stimulants

Most bronchodilators are administered as aerosols. Theophylline, naturally present in coffee and tea, is usually taken orally, but in a severe asthma attack it may be administered intravenously.

Bronchodilators are often administered via metered-dose inhalers (MDIs):

- The inhaler is shaken and the patient exhales air from the lungs
- The inhaler is placed at least two fingerbreadths in front of the mouth and aimed at the back of the throat
- The inhaler is activated while breathing in slowly for three to four seconds
- The breath is held for at least ten seconds and then expelled
- There should be at least 30–60 seconds before the inhaler is used again
- The mouth should be washed out and the teeth brushed to remove residual medication

Other drugs, including steroids, are used in the long-term management of asthma and to prevent asthma attacks. The anticholinergics ipratropium bromide (Atrovent) and atropine sulfate are also used to treat asthma. Ipratropium is used in emergency situations with a nebulizer.

An anaphylaxis emergency is treated by injection of adrenaline, which relaxes muscles and helps open the airways. People who are susceptible to anaphylaxis because of food or insect allergies often carry an EpiPen—adrenaline in a hypodermic needle. Prompt injection into the thigh can prevent a more serious reaction. The patient should be placed in a recumbent position and vital signs—especially the airway status—determined. If the reaction is the result of an insect sting or injection, a tourniquet may need to be placed proximal to the penetrated area and released for one to two minutes at 10-minute intervals. If the individual does not respond to these interventions, emergency treatment is essential.

Alternative

Any alternative treatment for allergies starts with identifying the allergen and avoiding or eliminating it, although this is not always possible. A physician should be consulted before initiating any alternative therapy. Although alternative remedies may be derived from natural sources, they are still drugs and can have potentially harmful effects.

The following treatments may help relieve symptoms of allergic rhinitis from airborne allergens:

- Traditional Chinese medicine treats allergic rhinitis with various herbs. The patent combination medicines Bu Zhong Yi Qi Wan (Tonify the Middle and Augment the Qi) and Yu Ping Feng San (Jade Windscreen) are used for preventing allergies. Bi Yan Pian (Rhinitis Infusion) is often prescribed for symptoms affecting the nose.
- Acupuncture may be as effective as antihistamine drugs in treating allergic rhinitis. It is also may strengthen the immune system.
- Vitamins A and E are antioxidants and help to promote normal functioning of the immune system.
- Coenzyme Q10 may help promote normal functioning of the immune system.
- Zinc may boost the immune system.
- *Echinacea* spp. may have anti-inflammatory activity and may boost the immune system.
- *Astragalus membranaceus* (milk-vetch root) may help strengthen the immune system.
- Vitamin C has antihistamine and decongestive activities.
- Stinging nettle (*Urtica dioica*) has antihistamine and anti-inflammatory properties. The usual dose is 300 milligrams (mg) four times daily.

- Grape (*Vitis vinifera*) seed extract has antihistamine and anti-inflammatory properties. The usual dose is 50 mg three times daily.
- The bioflavonoid hesperidin may act as a natural antihistamine.
- The dietary supplement N-acetylcysteine may have decongestive activity.
- The homeopathic remedies *Rhus toxicodendron*, *Apis mellifica*, *Nux vomica*, and *Ferrum phosphoricum* alternating with *Kali muriaticum* have decongestant activities when taken internally.
- Licorice (*Glycyrrhiza glabra*) has cortisone-like anti-inflammatory activity, stimulating the adrenals and relieving allergy symptoms. It can be taken as a tea or in 100–300 mg capsules. Long-term use can result in sodium retention or potassium loss.
- Chinese skullcap (*Scutellaria baicalensis*) has bronchodilating activity, is an anti-inflammatory, and can help prevent allergic reactions. It is taken in combination with other herbs.
- The herbal remedies khellin (*Ammi visnaga*) and cramp (*Viburnum opulus*) bark have bronchodilating activity.
- *Ginkgo biloba* seeds are used in Chinese medicine for relief from wheezing and coughing.
- The bioflavonoids quercetin and hesperidin may help stabilize mast cells.
- Although *Ephedra sinicia* (ma huang in traditional Chinese medicine) has anti-inflammatory activity and has proven effective in treating allergies, ephedra should not be used because it can raise blood pressure, cause rapid heartbeat, and interfere with adrenal gland function. The supplement ephedra was banned from sale in the United States in April of 2004 because of severe health risks.

The following homeopathic remedies are taken internally:

- Marsh tea (*Ledum*) for itching insect bites
- *Apis mellifica* for bee stings and hives that are relieved by cold
- Poison ivy (*Rhus toxicodendron*) for hives that are relieved with heat and for poison ivy, oak, or sumac rashes
- Stinging nettle (*Urtica urens*) for hives
- *Croton tiglium* oil for poison ivy, oak, or sumac rashes
- *Anacardium* A qualified homeopathic practitioner should be consulted to match symptoms with the correct remedy.

Various Chinese herbal remedies may be effective in treating atopic dermatitis. A poultice (crushed herbs applied directly to the affected area) made of jewelweed (*Impatiens* spp.) or chickweed (*Stellaria media*) may soothe the skin. A topical cream or wash containing *Calendula officinalis*, a natural antiseptic and anti-inflammatory agent, may help heal rash.

Home remedies

The basic home remedy for allergies is to avoid or eliminate the allergen. This may involve keeping dust under control by cleaning or using air filters, making adjustments in pet ownership, removing items such as feather pillows, and eliminating allergenic foods from the diet. Children with allergies to milk, eggs, fish, or apples who follow an oral desensitization procedure—in which they are exposed to allergenic foods in controlled, but increasing, doses—may develop resistance to the allergen.

Eczema is treated by keeping the skin lubricated with hypoallergenic lotions and gentle soaps. For extremely dry, sensitive skin, Cetaphil lotion may be used as a cleanser instead of soap.

Cold-water compresses and calamine lotion may help reduce the irritation of contact dermatitis. Hydrocortisone ointment or cream or similar preparations can help alleviate itching. Side effects of topical agents may include excessive drying of the skin.

Prognosis

There is no cure for allergies. Although most allergy symptoms can be successfully treated with medications, these cannot prevent future allergic reactions. Some allergies improve over time, but often they worsen. Although severe asthma and anaphylaxis can be life-threatening, learning to recognize and avoid allergy-provoking situations enables most people with allergies to lead normal lives.

Some children outgrow their allergies, meaning that the allergen no longer causes obvious symptoms. Children younger than three who are in danger of anaphylaxis from foods such as milk, eggs, wheat, or soybeans often outgrow their food allergies after several years. Children who develop food sensitivities after three years-of-age are less likely to outgrow them. Allergies to foods such as tree nuts, fish, and seafood are generally lifelong.

More than half of all asthmatic children outgrow the condition completely and another 10% improve to the point where they have only occasional asthma attacks as adults.

Prevention

Avoiding allergens is the first line of defense. By identifying allergens, most people can learn to avoid allergic reactions from food, drugs, and contact allergens such as poison ivy or latex. Many allergenic foods, such as peanuts, eggs, and milk, are used as ingredients in other foodstuffs. Since 2006 food manufacturers in the United States have been required to clearly state if a product contains any of the eight major food allergens that are responsible for more than 90% of allergic food reactions: milk, eggs, peanuts, tree nuts, fish, shellfish, wheat, and soy.

Airborne allergens are more difficult to avoid. Recommendations include:

- avoiding environmental irritants such as tobacco smoke, perfumes, household cleaning agents, paints, glues, air fresheners, and potpourri
- controlling dust mites with allergen-impermeable covers on mattresses and pillows, frequent washing of bedding in hot water, and removal of items that collect dust such as stuffed toys
- vacuuming often keeping windows and doors closed to prevent pollen from entering the home
- reducing growth of mold by lowering indoor humidity, repairing foundations to reduce indoor leakage and seepage, and installing exhaust systems to ventilate areas where steam is generated, such as the bathroom and kitchen
- reducing pet dander, avoiding pet allergens including those in saliva, body excretions, pelts, urine, and feces, and restricting pets to only specific areas of the home
- repairing poorly vented gas and wood-burning stoves and artificial fireplaces because nitrogen dioxide from these has been linked to poor asthma control

Infants appear to be most sensitive to allergens during the first six months of life. Some physicians believe babies are especially vulnerable to allergies because their immune systems are still developing. Breastfeeding is recommended to reduce the likelihood of allergic reactions, since infants are never allergic to their mother's milk. However traces of whatever the mother consumes pass into breast milk, so it is important to be alert to possible connections between a baby's allergic symptoms and foods, medication, or even **vitamins** ingested by the mother.

Rashes in infants under one year of age are likely caused by a food or drug allergy. Physicians often recommend that solid foods be introduced gradually if there is a family history of allergies. New foods can be introduced one at a time with 7–10 days in between. The later a food item is introduced into the diet, the less likely it is to cause an allergic reaction.

Babies and young children can have allergic reactions to ingredients in lotions, soaps, detergents, and baby wipes. Dye- and fragrance-free baby products can help prevent unnecessary exposure to potential allergens.

Toddlers are old enough to become anxious about allergy symptoms, which can trigger further allergic attacks and create a frustrating cycle. Parents should try to avoid conveying their own anxieties about allergy symptoms to the child.

During the preschool years, controlling a child's diet and environment becomes more difficult. Children may feel stigmatized or left out when provided with special foods and denied others. Children also may begin encountering potential allergens, including pet dander, at school and playmates' homes.

Parents of school-age children with allergies need to educate them about their condition and inform teachers and the school nurse of any restrictions and/or emergency procedures. Children are generally not allowed to carry medication, asthma inhalers, or EpiPens in school, so arrangements must be made for the school nurse or other supervising adult to administer emergency medication.

Health care team roles

Diagnosis and effective management of allergy symptoms involves cooperation and collaboration between the patient and an interdisciplinary team of healthcare professionals. The primary-care physician or pediatrician, allergy and immunology specialists, nurses, laboratory technologists, respiratory therapists, and health educators are involved in helping patients and families learn to prevent and effectively manage symptoms. They teach patients how to distinguish mild allergy symptoms from those requiring immediate medical attention. Pharmacists and pharmacy assistants may offer additional instruction about medication use and the importance of adhering to prescribed treatment.

Resources

BOOKS

Gensler, Tracy Olgeaty. *Probiotic and Prebiotic Recipes for Health: 100 Recipes that Battle Colitis, Candidiasis, Food Allergies, and Other Digestive Disorders.* Beverly, MA: Fair Winds Press, 2008.

Kay, A. Barry, et al., eds. *Allergy and Allergic Diseases*, 2 vols. New York: Wiley-Blackwell, 2008.

Lockey, Richard F., and Dennis K. Ledford, eds. *Allergens and Allergen Immunotherapy*, 4th ed. London: Informa Healthcare, 2008.

Mitman, Gregg. *Breathing Space: How Allergies Shape Our Lives and Landscapes*. New Haven, CT: Yale University Press, 2007.
Sutton, Amy L. *Allergies Sourcebook*. Detroit, MI: Omnigraphics, 2007.
Wright, Tanya. *Food Allergies*. London: Class Publishing, 2006.

PERIODICALS

Bakos, N., et al. "Risk Assessment in Elderly for Sensitization to Food and Respiratory Allergens." *Immunology Letters* 107, no. 1 (September 2006): 15–21.
Björkstén, Bengt, et al. "Worldwide Time Trends for Symptoms of Rhinitis and Conjunctivitis: Phase III of the International Study of Asthma and Allergies in Childhood." *Pediatric Allergy and Immunology* (March 2008): 110–124.
Finegold, Ira. "Immunotherapy: When to Initiate Treatment in Children." *Allergy and Asthma Proceedings* (November/December 2007): 698–705.
Green, C. M., C. R. Holden, and D. J. Gawkrodger. "Contact Allergy to Topical Medicaments Becomes More Common with Advancing Age: An Age-Stratified Study." *Contact Dermatitis* 56, no. 4 (April 2007): 229–231.
Hamelmann, E., et al. "Primary Prevention of Allergy: Avoiding Risk or Providing Protection?" *Clinical & Experimental Allergy* (February 2008): 233–245.
Noimark, Lee, and Helen E. Cox. "Nutritional Problems Related to Food Allergy in Childhood." *Pediatric Allergy and Immunology* (March 2008): 188–195.
Pourpak, Zahra, Mohammad R. Fazlollahi, and Fatemeh Fattahi. "Understanding Adverse Drug Reactions and Drug Allergies: Principles, Diagnosis, and Treatment Aspects." *Recent Patents on Inflammation & Allergy Drug Discovery* (January 2008): 24–46.

OTHER

"Allergy Overview." *Asthma and Allergy Foundation of America*. http://www.aafa.org
Pauls, John D. "Seniors and Asthma: Getting the Medication and Dosage Right." *AAAAI*. http://www.aaaai. org/patients/seniorsandasthma/medications_and_dosage.stm
"Tips to Remember: What is an Allergic Reaction?" *AAAAI*. http://www.aaaai.org/patients/publicedmat/tips/whatisallergicreaction.stm

ORGANIZATIONS

American Academy of Allergy, Asthma & Immunology (AAAAI), 555 East Wells Street, Milwaukee, WI 53202-3823, (414) 272-6071, http://www.aaaai.org/
Asthma and Allergy Foundation of America, 8201 Corporate Drive, Suite 1000, Landover, MD 20785, (800) 7-ASTHMA, Info@aafa.org, http://www.aafp.org
Centers for Disease Control and Prevention, 1600 Clifton Road, Atlanta, GA 30333, (888) 232-6348, Fax: (301) 563-6595, cdcinfor@cdc.gov, http://www.cdc.gov
National Institute of Allergy and Infectious Diseases (NIAID), Office of Communications and Public Liaison, 6610 Rockledge Drive, Bethesda, MD 20892-66123, (8660 284-4107, http://www3.niaid.nih.gov
U.S. Food and Drug Administration, 10903 New Hampshire Ave., Silver Spring, MD 20993-0002, (888) INFO-FDA, http://www.fda.gov.

Richard Robinson
Jill Granger, MS
Teresa G. Odle
Tish Davidson, AM
Belinda Rowland
Monique Laberge, PhD
Margaret Alic, PhD

Alternative medicine

Definition

Alternative medicine is the term for treatments that do not follow the conventional method of addressing illnesses through the use of drugs and surgery. This umbrella term encompasses a variety of methods, including herbal medicine, energy medicine, homeopathy, and naturopathy. This article will primarily discuss the last two practices.

Naturopathic medicine is a branch of medicine in which a variety of natural medicines and treatments are used to heal illness. It uses a system of medical diagnosis and therapeutics based on the patterns of chaos and organization in nature. It is founded on the premise that people are naturally healthy and that healing can occur through removing obstacles to a cure and by stimulating the body's natural healing abilities. The foundations of health in natural medicine are diet, **nutrition**, homeopathy, physical manipulation, **stress** management, and exercise.

Homeopathy is often used by naturopaths, those who practice naturopathic medicine. Developed in the late eighteenth century, it is based on the idea that substances that produce symptoms of sickness in healthy people will have a curative effect when given in very diluted quantities to sick people who exhibit those same symptoms. Homeopathic remedies are believed to stimulate the body's own healing processes

Purpose

Naturopathic medicine and homeopathy can be useful for treating chronic as well as acute diseases. Practitioners seek to cure their patients on the physical, mental and emotional levels, and each treatment is tailored to a patient's individual needs, which are determined through extensive interviews and examinations of the patient.

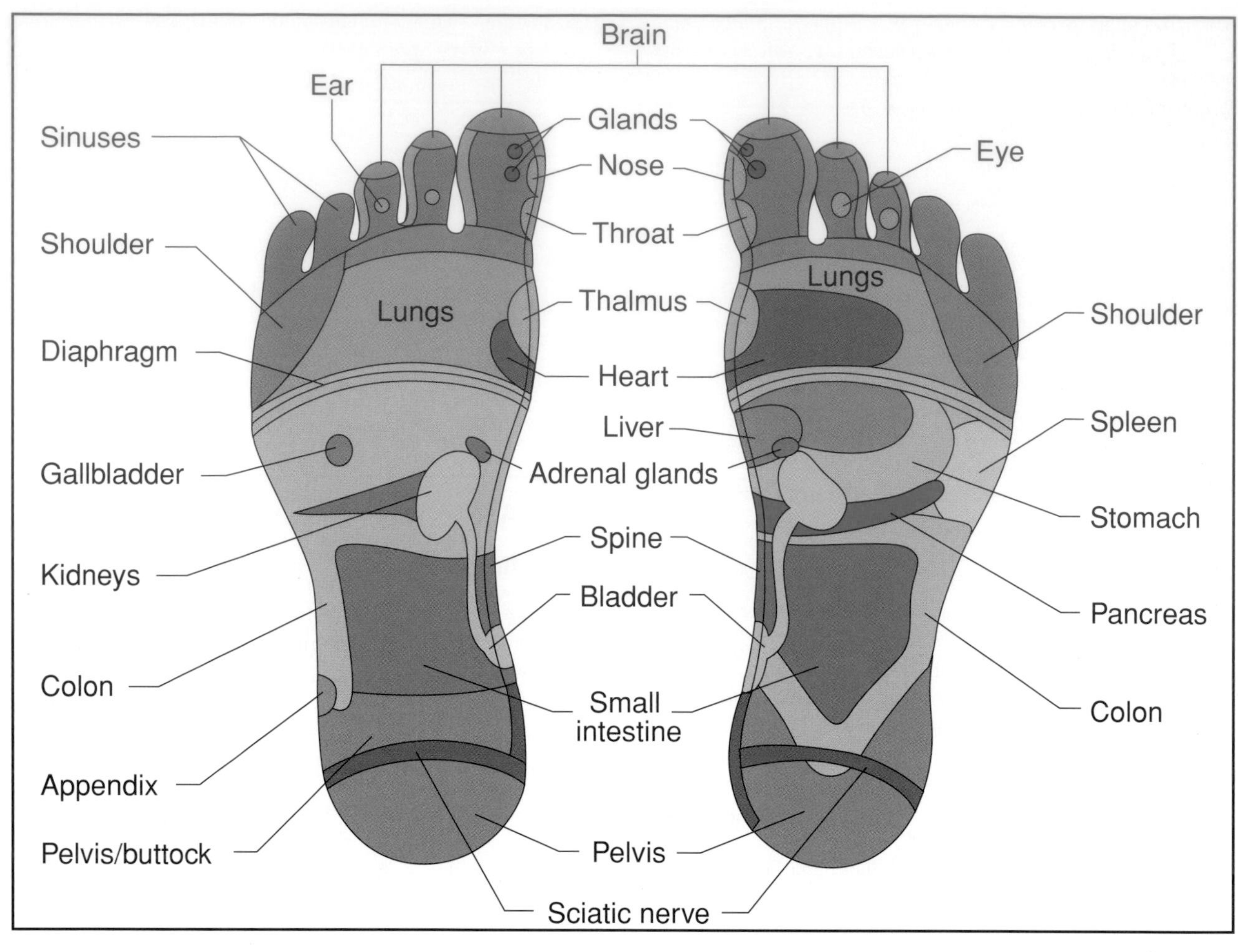

Reflexology employs the principle that the reflex points on the feet, when and pressure is applied, will reflexively stimulate energy to a related muscle or organ in the body and promote healing. *(Illustration by Electronic Illustrators Group. © 2013 Cengage Learning)*

Homeopathic physicians seek to cure their patients on the physical, mental and emotional levels, and each treatment is tailored to a patient's individual needs. Homeopathy is generally a safe treatment, as it uses medicines in extremely diluted quantities, and there are usually minimal side effects. Its non-toxicity makes it a good choice for the treatment of children. Another benefit of homeopathy is the cost of treatments; homeopathic remedies are inexpensive, often a fraction of the cost of conventional drugs.

Homeopathic treatment has been shown effective in treating many conditions. Colds and flu may be effectively treated with aconite and bryonia. **Influenza** sufferers in a double-blind study found that they were twice as likely to recover in 48 hours when they took homeopathic remedies. Studies have been published in British medical journals confirming the efficacy of homeopathic treatment for rheumatoid arthritis. Homeopathic remedies are effective in treating infections, circulatory problems, respiratory problems, **heart disease**, depression and nervous disorders, migraine headaches, **allergies**, arthritis, and diabetes. Homeopathy is a good treatment to explore for acute and chronic illnesses, particularly if these are found in the early stages and where there is no severe damage. Homeopathy can be used to assist the healing process after surgery or chemotherapy. The naturopath often spends more time educating patients in preventive health, lifestyle, and nutrition than most MDs.

Description

Origins

People have always seen a connection between diet and disease, and many therapies are built around special diets. Naturopathy began in the 18th and 19th centuries as the Industrial Revolution brought about unhealthy lifestyles, and the European custom of "taking the cure" at natural spas became popular. Benedict Lust, who

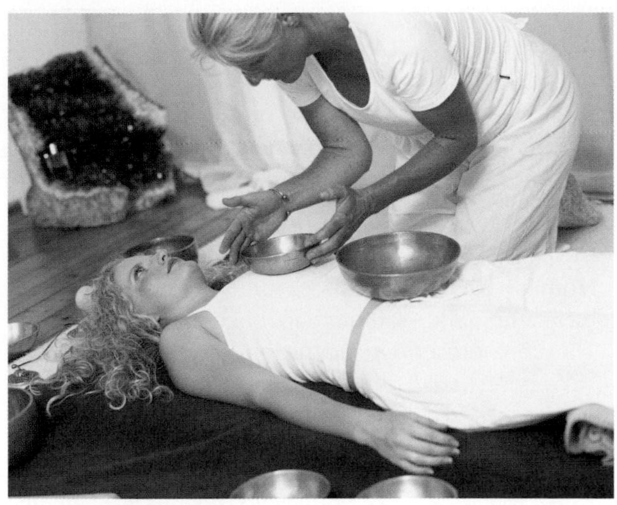

Sound therapy: practitioner using singing bowls to relax and heal her patient. *(© Mauritius, GMBH / Phototake – All rights reserved.)*

believed deeply in natural medicine, organized naturopathy as a formal system of healthcare in the 1890s. By the early 1900s, it was flourishing.

The first naturopaths in the United States emphasized the healing properties of a nutritious diet, as did a number of their contemporaries. In the early 20th century, for instance, John Kellogg, a physician and vegetarian, opened a sanitarium that used healing methods such as hydrotherapy, often prescribed by today's naturopaths. His brother Will produced health foods, such as corn flakes and shredded wheat. The Kellogg brothers helped make naturopathic ideas popular and emphasized the value of whole grains over highly refined ones. They and one of their employees, C.W. Post, eventually went on to start the cereal companies that bear their names.

In the early 1900s, most states licensed naturopaths as physicians. There were 20 medical schools of naturopathic medicine. From early on, naturopathic physicians were considered "eclectic," since they drew on a variety of natural therapies and traditions for treating their patients.

In the 1930s, naturopathy dramatically declined for several reasons. Allopathic medicine finally stopped using therapies such as bloodletting and heavy metal **poisoning** as curatives. New therapies were more effective and less toxic. Allopathic medical schools became increasingly well funded by foundations with links to the emerging drug industry. Allopathic physicians also became much more organized and wielded political clout. Naturopathy has experienced a resurgence over the last 20 years, however. The lay public is aware of the connection between a healthy diet and lifestyle and avoiding chronic disease. In addition, conventional medicine is often unable to treat these chronic diseases. Patients are now health care consumers and will seek their own resolution to health problems that cannot be resolved by conventional physicians. As a result, even medical groups that once considered naturopathy ineffective are now beginning to accept it.

In the early 1900s, homeopathy was popular in the United States, with over 15% of all doctors being homeopathic. There were 22 major homeopathic medical schools, including Boston University and the University of Michigan. However, with the formation of the American Medical Association, which restricted and closed down alternative practices, homeopathy declined for half a century. When the 1960s invigorated back-to-nature trends and distrust of artificial drugs and treatments, homeopathy began to grow again dramatically through the next decades. In 1993, *The New England Journal of Medicine* reported that 2.5 million Americans used homeopathic remedies and that 800,000 patients visited homeopaths in 1990, and these figures have continued to grow. Homeopathy is much more popular in Europe than in the United States. French pharmacies are required to make homeopathic remedies available along with conventional medications. Homeopathic hospitals and clinics are part of the national health system in Britain. Homepathy is also practiced in India and Israel, among other countries.

As with most doctors, treatment by a naturopath or homeopath can range from one office visit to many. Some ailments can be alleviated with one or two visits. Other chronic diseases need regular weekly or monthly attention. Clinical care provided by alternative physicians are covered by insurance in a number of states in the United States.

Preparations

There are about 1,500 naturopathic physicians in the United States practicing; nearly 80% of these practitioners entered the profession following the revival of interest in naturopathy in the late 1970s. Naturopaths are required to graduate from a four-year naturopathic medical school that has been accredited by the Council on Naturopathic Medical Education; as of 2012, five American programs and two Canadian programs had such accreditation. Graduates then take a licensing exam. Seventeen states license naturopathic physicians: Alaska, Arizona, California, Connecticut, Hawaii, Idaho, Kansas, Maine, Minnesota, Montana, New Hampshire, North Dakota, Oregon, Utah, Vermont, Utah, and Washington, as well as Washington, D.C., Puerto Rico and the Virgin Islands, as of 2012.

Precautions

A good naturopath is always willing to work with the patient's other physicians or health care providers. To avoid drug interactions and to coordinate care, it is important for a patient to inform his or her conventional doctor about supplements prescribed by a naturopath. In addition, naturopaths are not licensed to perform major surgery or to prescribe narcotics or antidepressant drugs. They must involve an oncologist when treating a **cancer** patient.

Although homeopathic remedies sometimes use substances that are toxic, they are diluted and prescribed in non-toxic doses. Remedies are regulated by the U.S. Food and Drug Administration and should be prescribed by a homeopathic practitioner. Homeopathic medicine should also be handled with care and should not be touched with the hands or fingers, which can contaminate it.

Side effects

Some alternative medicine remedies have side effects and can interact with prescription medicines. It is important for a patient to inform his or her conventional-medicine practitioner about any natural remedies or herbs a naturopath has prescribed.

The U.S. Food and Drug Administration considers medicinal herbs as dietary supplements, not drugs, and so they are not subject to the same regulations that drugs are. As a result, the active ingredients may not always be in the same concentration from bottle to bottle, because plants naturally vary. To guard against using too little or too much of a natural remedy, use herbs and supplements recommended by a naturopath or those produced by well-respected companies.

Homeopathy is generally a safe treatment, as it uses medicines in extremely diluted quantities, and there are usually minimal side effects. Its non-toxicity makes it a good choice for the treatment of children. Another benefit of homeopathy is the cost of treatments; homeopathic remedies are inexpensive, often a fraction of the cost of conventional drugs. Like naturopathic remedies, it is wise to select homeopathic remedies from those recommended by a trained practitioner or produced by an established firm.

Research and general acceptance

Medical research in naturopathy has increased dramatically in the United States within the last 10 years. Naturopathic research often employs case histories, summaries of practitioners' clinical observations, and medical records. Some U.S. studies have also met today's scientific gold standard; they were double-blind and placebo-controlled. Much naturopathic research has also been done in Germany, France, England, India, and China. Homeopathy is widely used in Europe, particularly in Great Britain.

KEY TERMS

Clinical nutrition—The use of diet and nutritional supplements as a way to enhance health prevent disease.

Herb—In alternative medicine, a plant or plant derivative or extract prescribed for health or healing.

Homeopathy—The use of diluted remedies that have energetic, rather than chemical, properties. They are prescribed according to the axiom that "like cures like."

A recent survey of parents by faculty in the Department of Pediatrics at Harvard Medical School found that 28% of children and adolescents with **autism** spectrum disorder (autism, pervasive developmental disorder (PDD), or Asperger's) had used complementary and alternative medicine. Use was higher among children who experienced seizures, gastrointestinal symptoms, and behavior problems.

Another survey, this one of administrators at United States Veterans Administration Hospitals, found that, among programs to treat **post-traumatic stress disorder**, 96% offered at least one form of complementary and alternative medicine, and 88% of those offered treatments that were not usually a part of conventional PTSD treatment.

Some conventional medical practitioners, especially in the United States, however, remain distrustful of alternative medicine. Part of the difficulty for homeopathy, for example, lies in the fact that the basis tenets of homeopathy run counter to what is currently understood about physics and chemistry.

Resources

BOOKS

Arora, Saurav. *Homeopathic Philosophy, Theory, Doctrines: A Compilation of Key Peer Reviewed Abstracts and References*. Seattle: Amazon Digital Services, 2012.

Hechtman, Leah. *Clinical Naturopathic Medicine*. London: Churchill Livingstone, 2012.

PERIODICALS

Libby, Daniel, Ph.D., et al. "Complementary and Alternative Medicine in VA Specialized PTSD Treatment Programs." *Psychiatric Services*2012 Nov 1;63(11):1134–6.

Perrin, J.M., et al. "Complementary and alternative medicine use in a large pediatric autism sample." *Pediatrics* November 2012: 130.

WEBSITES

"Complementary and Alternative Medcine." Medline Plus. http://www.nlm.nih.gov/medlineplus/complementaryand alternativemedicine.html (accessed November 13, 2012).

ORGANIZATIONS

American Association of Naturopathic Physicians, 4435 Wisconsin Ave., NW, Suite 403, Washington, DC 20016, (202) 237-8150, Fax: (202) 237-8152, (866) 538-2267, member. services@naturopathic.org, http://naturopathic .org/

American Institute of Homeopathy, 801 N. Fairfax St., Suite 306, Alexandria, VA 22314, (888) 445-9988, http://www .homeopathyusa.org

Canadian Association of Naturopathic Doctors, 20 Holly St., Ste. 200, Toronto, Ontario, Canada M4S 3B1, (416) 496-8633, Fax: (416) 496-8634, (800) 551-4381, http://www .cand.ca.

Barbara Boughton
Rebecca J. Frey, PhD
Ken R. Wells
Fran Hodgkins

Amebiasis

Definition

Amebiasis is an **infectious disease** caused by a parasitic one-celled microorganism (protozoan) called *Entamoeba histolytica*. Persons with amebiasis may experience a wide range of symptoms, including diarrhea, fever, and cramps. The disease may also affect the intestines, liver, or other parts of the body.

Description

Amebiasis, also known as amebic **dysentery**, is one of the most common parasitic diseases occurring in humans, with an estimated 500 million new cases each year. It occurs most frequently in tropical and subtropical areas where living conditions are crowded, with inadequate **sanitation**. Although most cases of amebiasis occur in persons who carry the disease but do not exhibit any symptoms (asymptomatic), as many as 100,000 people die of amebiasis each year. In the United States, between one and 5% of the general population will develop amebiasis in any given year, while male homosexuals, migrant workers, institutionalized people, and recent immigrants develop amebiasis at a higher rate.

Human beings are the only known host of the amebiasis organism, and all groups of people, regardless of age or sex, can become affected. Amebiasis is primarily spread in food and **water** that has been contaminated by human feces but is also spread by person-to-person contact. The number of cases is typically limited, but regional outbreaks can occur in areas where human feces are used as fertilizer for crops, or in cities with water supplies contaminated with human feces.

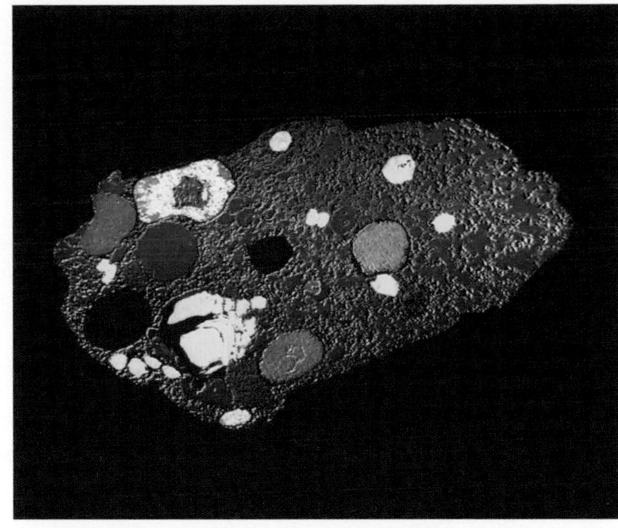

Magnified 1125X, this photomicrograph revealed the presence of a parasitic Entamoeba histolytica trophozoite, which contained vacuolated cytoplasm. *(CDC)*

Causes and symptoms

Recently, it has been discovered that persons with symptom-causing amebiasis are infected with *Entamoeba histolytica*, and those individuals who exhibit no symptoms are actually infected with an almost identical-looking ameba called *Entamoeba dispar*. During their life cycles, the amebas exist in two very different forms: the infective cyst or capsuled form, which cannot move but can survive outside the human body because of its protective covering, and the disease-producing form, the trophozoite, which although capable of moving, cannot survive once excreted in the feces and, therefore, cannot infect others. The disease is most commonly transmitted when a person eats food or drinks water containing *E. histolytica* cysts from human feces. In the digestive tract the cysts are transported to the intestine where the walls of the cysts are broken open by digestive secretions, releasing the mobile trophozoites. Once released within the intestine, the trophozoites multiply by feeding on intestinal bacteria or by invading the lining of the large intestine.

Within the lining of the large intestine, the trophozoites secrete a substance that destroys intestinal tissue and creates a distinctive bottle-shaped sore (ulcer). The trophozoites may remain inside the intestine, in the intestinal wall, or may break through the intestinal wall and be carried by the blood to the liver, lungs, brain, or other organs. Trophozoites that remain in the intestines eventually form new cysts that are carried through the digestive tract and excreted in the feces. Under favorable

KEY TERMS

Ameboma—A mass of tissue that can develop on the wall of the colon in response to amebic infection.

Antibody—A specific protein produced by the immune system in response to a specific foreign protein or particle called an antigen.

Appendicitis—Condition characterized by the rapid inflammation of the appendix, a part of the intestine.

Asymptomatic—Persons who carry a disease and are usually capable of transmitting the disease but who do not exhibit symptoms of the disease are said to be asymptomatic.

Dysentery—Intestinal infection marked by diarrhea containing blood and mucus.

Fulminating colitis—A potentially fatal complication of amebic dysentery marked by sudden and severe inflammation of the intestinal lining, severe bleeding or hemorrhaging, and massive shedding of dead tissue.

Inflammatory bowel disease (IBD)—Disease in which the lining of the intestine becomes inflamed.

Lumen—The inner cavity or canal of a tube-shaped organ, such as the bowel.

Protozoan—A single-celled, usually microscopic organism that is eukaryotic and, therefore, different from bacteria (prokaryotic).

temperature and humidity conditions, the cysts can survive in soil or water for weeks to months, ready to begin the cycle again.

Although 90% of cases of amebiasis in the United States are mild, pregnant women, children under two years of age, the elderly, malnourished individuals, and people whose immune systems may be compressed, such as **cancer** or **AIDS** patients and those individuals taking prescription medications that suppress the immune system, are at a greater risk for developing a severe infection.

The signs and symptoms of amebiasis vary according to the location and severity of the infection and are classified as follows:

Intestinal amebiasis

Intestinal amebiasis can be subdivided into several categories:

ASYMPTOMATIC INFECTION. Most persons with amebiasis have no noticeable symptoms. Even though these individuals may not feel ill, they are still capable of infecting others by person-to-person contact or by contaminating food or water with cysts that others may ingest, for example, by preparing food with unwashed hands.

CHRONIC NON-DYSENTERIC INFECTION. Individuals may experience symptoms over a long period of time during a chronic amebiasis infection and experience recurrent episodes of diarrhea that last from one to four weeks and recur over a period of years. These patients may also suffer from abdominal cramps, fatigue, and weight loss.

AMEBIC DYSENTERY. In severe cases of intestinal amebiasis, the organism invades the lining of the intestine, producing sores (ulcers), bloody diarrhea, severe abdominal cramps, vomiting, chills, and fevers as high as 104–105°F (40–40.6°C). In addition, a case of acute amebic dysentery may cause complications, including inflammation of the appendix (appendicitis), a tear in the intestinal wall (perforation), or a sudden, severe inflammation of the colon (fulminating colitis).

AMEBOMA. An ameboma is a mass of tissue in the bowel that is formed by the amebiasis organism. It can result from either chronic intestinal infection or acute amebic dysentery. Amebomas may produce symptoms that mimic cancer or other intestinal diseases.

PERIANAL ULCERS. Intestinal amebiasis may produce skin infections in the area around the patient's anus (perianal). These ulcerated areas have a "punched-out" appearance and are painful to the touch.

Extraintestinal amebiasis

Extraintestinal amebiasis accounts for approximately 10% of all reported amebiasis cases and includes all forms of the disease that affect other organs.

The most common form of extraintestinal amebiasis is amebic abscess of the liver. In the United States, amebic liver abscesses occur most frequently in young Hispanic adults. An amebic liver abscess can result from direct infection of the liver by *E. histolytica* or as a complication of intestinal amebiasis. Patients with an amebic abscess of the liver complain of **pain** in the chest or abdomen, fever, nausea, and tenderness on the right side directly above the liver.

Other forms of extraintestinal amebiasis, though rare, include infections of the lungs, chest cavity, brain, or genitals. These are extremely serious and have a relatively high mortality rate.

Diagnosis

Diagnosis of amebiasis is complicated, partly because the disease can affect several areas of the body and can range from exhibiting few, if any, symptoms to being severe, or even life-threatening. In most cases, a physician will consider a diagnosis of amebiasis when a patient has a combination of symptoms, in particular, diarrhea and a possible history of recent exposure to amebiasis through travel, contact with infected persons, or anal intercourse.

It is vital to distinguish between amebiasis and another disease, inflammatory bowel disease (IBD) that produces similar symptoms because, if diagnosed incorrectly, drugs that are given to treat IBD can encourage the growth and spread of the amebiasis organism. Because of the serious consequences of misdiagnosis, potential cases of IBD must be confirmed with multiple stool samples and blood tests, and a procedure involving a visual inspection of the intestinal wall using a thin lighted, tubular instrument (sigmoidoscopy) to rule out amebiasis.

A diagnosis of amebiasis may be confirmed by one or more tests, depending on the location of the disease.

Stool examination

This test involves microscopically examining a stool sample for the presence of cysts and/or trophozoites of *E. histolytica* and not one of the many other intestinal amebas that are often found but that do not cause disease. A series of three stool tests is approximately 90% accurate in confirming a diagnosis of amebic dysentery. Unfortunately, however, the stool test is not useful in diagnosing amebomas or extraintestinal infections.

Sigmoidoscopy

Sigmoidoscopy is a useful diagnostic procedure in which a thin, flexible, lighted instrument, called a sigmoidoscope, is used to visually examine the lower part of the large intestine for amebic ulcers and take tissue or fluid samples from the intestinal lining.

Blood tests

Although tests designed to detect a specific protein produced in response to amebiasis infection (antibody) are capable of detecting only about 10% of cases of mild amebiasis, these tests are extremely useful in confirming 95% of dysentery diagnoses and 98% of liver abscess diagnoses. Blood serum will usually test positive for antibody within a week of symptom onset. Blood testing, however, cannot always distinguish between a current or past infection since the antibodies may be detectable in the blood for as long as 10 years following initial infection.

Imaging studies

A number of sophisticated imaging techniques, such as computed tomography scans (CT), magnetic resonance imaging (MRI), and ultrasound, can be used to determine whether a liver abscess is present. Once located, a physician may then use a fine needle to withdraw a sample of tissue to determine whether the abscess is indeed caused by an amebic infection.

Treatment

Asymptomatic or mild cases of amebiasis may require no treatment. However, because of the potential for disease spread, amebiasis is generally treated with a medication to kill the disease-causing amebas. More severe cases of amebic dysentery are additionally treated by replacing lost fluid and blood. Patients with an amebic liver abscess will also require hospitalization and bed rest. For those cases of extraintestinal amebiasis, treatment can be complicated because different drugs may be required to eliminate the parasite, based on the location of the infection within the body. Drugs used to treat amebiasis, called amebicides, are divided into two categories:

Luminal amebicides

These drugs get their name because they act on organisms within the inner cavity (lumen) of the bowel. They include diloxanide furoate, iodoquinol, metronidazole, and paromomycin.

Tissue amebicides

Tissue amebicides are used to treat infections in the liver and other body tissues and include emetine, dehydroemetine, metronidazole, and chloroquine. Because these drugs have potentially serious side effects, patients given emetine or dehydroemetine require bed rest and heart monitoring. Chloroquine has been found to be the most useful drug for treating amebic liver abscess. Patients taking metronidazole must avoid alcohol because the drug-alcohol combination causes nausea, vomiting, and headache.

Most patients are given a combination of luminal and tissue amebicides over a treatment period of seven to ten days. Follow-up care includes periodic stool examinations beginning two to four weeks after the end of medication treatment to check the effectiveness of drug therapy.

Prognosis

The prognosis depends on the location of the infection and the patient's general health prior to infection. The prognosis is generally good, although the mortality rate is higher for patients with ameboma, perforation of the bowel, and liver infection. Patients who develop fulminant colitis have the most serious prognosis, with over 50% mortality.

Prevention

There are no **immunization** procedures or medications that can be taken prior to potential exposure to prevent amebiasis. Moreover, people who have had the disease can become reinfected. **Prevention** requires effective personal and community **hygiene**.

Specific safeguards include the following:

- Purification of drinking water. Water can be purified by filtering, boiling, or treatment with iodine.
- Proper food handling. Measures include protecting food from contamination by flies, cooking food properly, washing one's hands after using the bathroom and before cooking or eating, and avoiding foods that cannot be cooked or peeled when traveling in countries with high rates of amebiasis.
- Careful disposal of human feces.
- Monitoring the contacts of amebiasis patients. The stools of family members and sexual partners of infected persons should be tested for the presence of cysts or trophozoites.

Resources

BOOKS

Friedman, Lawrence S. "Liver, Biliary Tract, & Pancreas." In McPhee, Stephen, and Maxine Papadakis.*Current Medical Diagnosis and Treatment, 2010*, 49th ed. New York: McGraw-Hill Medical, 2009.

Rebecca J. Frey, PhD

American Public Health Association

Definition

The American Public Health Association (APHA) is an association of public health professionals headquartered in Washingon, D.C., with the goal of ensuring that information about the best available public health practices is available to all Americans.

Purpose

The purpose of the APHA is to ensure that all individual Americans and all American communities are protected from preventable health threats and that information about and resources for disease **prevention** are accessible throughout the country. The association strives to achieve this goal both through education programs for the general public and for the profession, as well as through lobbying of decision makers at all levels of government.

Description

The APHA was founded in 1872 by American physician Stephen Smith, a pioneer in the U.S. public health movement. The organization currently claims more than 50,000 members throughout the world. It consists of 29 primary sections that focus on topics such as **Aging** and Public Health; Alcohol, Tobacco, and Other Drugs; Disability; Food and **Nutrition**; Health Administration; Maternal and Child Care; and Social Work. The organization is run by an Executive Board of 24 and a staff of nearly 90 full–time employees. In addition to its primary sections, the APHA works through its 53 state affiliates to provide a number of specialized forums on topics such as Breastfeeding, **Cancer**, Family **Violence** Prevention, and **Genomics**. It has also created special group caucuses, such as the Asian Pacific Islander caucus and women's caucus, as well as a Student Assembly for student members.

The work of the APHA is carried out through a number of programs, initiatives, action programs, and other activities. For example, its Take Action! advocacy program provides a mechanism by which members can lobby the U.S. Congress and state legislatures on matters of interest to public health professionals. The Healthiest Nation in One Generation Program is a comparable activity aimed at encouraging the Congress to expand and improve existing health options for all American citizens. The association also prepares, adopts, and publicizes a number of policy statements each year on topics of concern to public health professionals, such as access to over–the–counter contraception, access of minors to **abortion** services, improved access of all citizens to vision services, and improved housing for farm workers.

An essential part of the APHA program is a collection of ongoing programs on public health topics. For example, the Center for Professional Development, Public Health Systems & Partnerships provides continuing education programs in public health skills, as well as managerial, technical, and administrative aspects of the profession. The Enviromental Public Health Initiative is an educational program designed to provide information for the general public and decision makers on topics such as climate change, food systems, workforce development, and chemical exposure and prevention. The Get Ready Campaign works to help individuals and communities prepare for a whole range of emergencies that might include **pandemic** flu attacks, **natural disasters**, **infectious disease** outbreaks, and other natural and manmade events. The APHA also serves as lead organizer for the annual National Public Health Week which features a variety of events that include contests, speeches, training sessions, webinars, and other events on a number of public health topics.

Professional Publications

One of the APHA's primary publications is "Nation's Health," a newsletter published ten times a year containing information on public health and legislative developments of interest to members (by subscription only). Its other major publication is the monthly *American Journal of Public Health*, a peer-reviewed journal that contains the results of research, reviews, and commentary on public health topics. The APHA, in conjunction with Jones and Bartlett Learning, also publishes a series of textbooks on the Essentials of Public Health, with titles such as *Essentials of Management and Leadership in Public Health* and *Essentials of Global Community Health*. Two other regular online publications available to members are "Inside Public Health," available only to members, and "Public Health Newswire,"available to the general public.

Resources

PERIODICALS

Bryce, Peter H. "History of the American Public Health Association." *American Journal of Public Health* 8, 5. (1918): 327–335.

Glasser, Jay H., Elizabeth Fee, and Theodore M. Brown. "Stephen Smith (1823–1922): Founder of the American Public Health Association." *American Journal of Public Health* 101, 11. (2011): 2058.

Treviño, Fernando M., and Jeff P. Jacobs. "Public Health and Health Care Reform: The American Public Health Association's Perspective.". *Journal of Public Health Policy* 15, 4. (1994): 397–406.

ORGANIZATIONS

American Public Health Association (APHA), 800 I St., N. W., Washington, D.C. USA 20001–3710, (202) 777-APHA, Fax: (202) 777-2534, comments@apha.org, http://www.apha.org/.

David E. Newton, EdD

Anthrax

Definition

Anthrax is an infection caused by the bacterium *Bacillus anthracis* that primarily affects livestock but that can occasionally spread to humans, affecting either the skin, intestines, or lungs. In humans, the infection can often be treated, but it is almost always fatal in animals.

Description

Anthrax is most often found in the agricultural areas of South and Central America, southern and eastern Europe, Asia, Africa, the Caribbean, and the Middle East. In the United States, anthrax is rarely reported; however, cases of animal infection with anthrax are most often reported in Texas, Louisiana, Mississippi, Oklahoma, and South Dakota. The bacterium and its associated disease get their name from the Greek word meaning "coal" because of the characteristic coal-black sore that is the hallmark of the most common form of the disease.

During the 1800s, in England and Germany, anthrax was known either as "wool-sorter's" or "ragpicker's" disease because workers contracted the disease from bacterial spores present on hides and in wool or fabric fibers. Spores are the small, thick-walled dormant stage of some bacteria that enable them to survive for long periods of time under adverse conditions. The first anthrax vaccine was perfected in 1881 by Louis Pasteur.

The largest outbreak ever recorded in the United States occurred in 1957 when nine employees of a goat hair processing plant became ill after handling a contaminated shipment from Pakistan. Four of the five patients with the pulmonary form of the disease died. Other cases appeared in the 1970s when contaminated

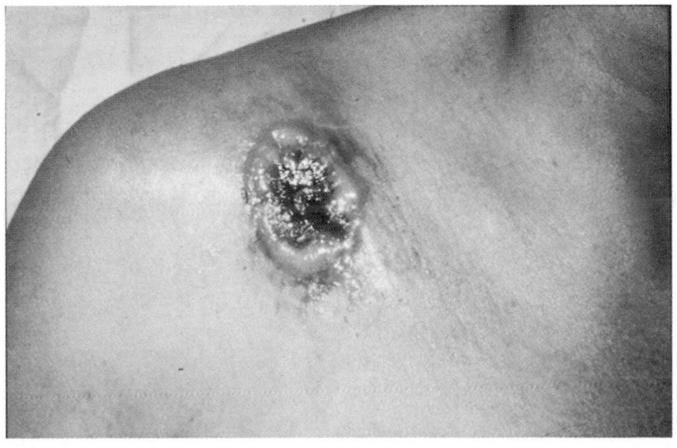

Bacillus Anthracis. *(© Wellcome Image Library / Custom Medical Stock Photo)*

KEY TERMS

Antibody—A specific protein produced by the immune system in response to a specific foreign protein or particle called an antigen.

Antitoxin—An antibody that neutralizes a toxin.

Bronchitis—Inflammation of the mucous membrane of the bronchial tubes of the lung that can make it difficult to breathe.

Cutaneous—Pertaining to the skin

Meningitis—Inflammation of the membranes covering the brain and spinal cord called the meninges.

Pulmonary—Having to do with the lungs or respiratory system.

Spore—A dormant form assumed by some bacteria, such as anthrax, that enable the bacterium to survive high temperatures, dryness, and lack of nourishment for long periods of time. Under proper conditions, the spore may revert to the actively multiplying form of the bacteria.

goatskin drumheads from Haiti were brought into the U.S. as souvenirs.

Today, anthrax is rare, even among cattle, largely because of widespread animal **vaccination**. However, some serious epidemics continue to occur among animal herds and in human settlements in developing countries due to ineffective control programs. In humans, the disease is almost always an occupational hazard, contracted by those who handle animal hides (farmers, butchers, and veterinarians) or sort wool. There are no reports of the disease spreading from one person to another.

Anthrax as a weapon

There has been a great deal of recent concern that the bacteria that cause anthrax may be used as a type of biological warfare, since it is possible to become infected simply by inhaling the spores, and inhaled anthrax is the most serious form of the disease. The bacteria can be grown in laboratories, and with a great deal of expertise and special equipment, the bacteria can be altered to be usable as a weapon.

The largest-ever documented outbreak of human anthrax contracted through spore inhalation occurred in Russia in 1979, when anthrax spores were accidentally released from a military laboratory, causing a regional epidemic that killed 69 of its 77 victims. In the United States in 2001, terrorists converted anthrax spores into a powder that could be inhaled and mailed it to intended targets, including news agencies and prominent individuals in the federal government. Because the United States government considers anthrax to be of potential risk to soldiers, the Department of Defense has begun systematic vaccination of all military personnel against anthrax. For civilians in the United States, the government has instituted a program called the National Pharmaceutical Stockpile program in which **antibiotics** and other medical materials to treat two million people are located so that they could be received anywhere in the country within twelve hours following a disaster or terrorist attack.

Causes and symptoms

The naturally occurring bacterium *Bacillus anthracis* produces spores that can remain dormant for years in soil and on animal products, such as hides, wool, hair, or bones. The disease is often fatal to cattle, sheep, and goats, and their hides, wool, and bones are often heavily contaminated.

The bacteria are found in many types of soil, all over the world, and usually do not pose a problem for humans because the spores stay in the ground. In order to infect a human, the spores have to be released from the soil and must enter the body. They can enter the body through a cut in the skin, through consuming contaminated meat, or through inhaling the spores. Once the spores are in the body, and if antibiotics are not administered, the spores become bacteria that multiply and release a toxin that affects the immune system. In the inhaled form of the infection, the immune system can become overwhelmed and the body can go into shock.

Symptoms vary depending on how the disease was contracted, but the symptoms usually appear within one week of exposure.

Cutaneous anthrax

In humans, anthrax usually occurs when the spores enter a cut or abrasion, causing a skin (cutaneous) infection at the site. Cutaneous anthrax, as this infection is called, is the mildest and most common form of the disease. At first, the bacteria cause an itchy, raised area like an insect bite. Within one to two days, inflammation occurs around the raised area, and a blister forms around an area of dying tissue that becomes black in the center. Other symptoms may include shivering and chills. In most cases, the bacteria remain within the sore. If, however, they spread to the nearest lymph node (or, in rare cases, escape into the bloodstream), the bacteria can cause a form of blood **poisoning** that rapidly proves fatal.

Inhalation anthrax

Inhaling the bacterial spores can lead to a rare, often-fatal form of anthrax known as pulmonary or inhalation anthrax that attacks the lungs and sometimes spreads to the brain. Inhalation anthrax begins with flu-like symptoms, namely fever, fatigue, headache, muscle aches, and shortness of breath. As early as one day after these initial symptoms appear, and as long as two weeks later, the symptoms suddenly worsen and progress to bronchitis. The patient experiences difficulty breathing, and finally, the patient enters a state of shock. This rare form of anthrax is often fatal, even if treated within one or two days after the symptoms appear.

Intestinal anthrax

Intestinal anthrax is a rare, often-fatal form of the disease, caused by eating meat from an animal that died of anthrax. Intestinal anthrax causes stomach and intestinal inflammation and sores or lesions (ulcers), much like the sores that appear on the skin in the cutaneous form of anthrax. The first signs of the disease are nausea and vomiting, loss of appetite, and fever, followed by abdominal **pain**, vomiting of blood, and severe bloody diarrhea.

Diagnosis

Anthrax is diagnosed by detecting *B. anthracis* in samples taken from blood, spinal fluid, skin lesions, or respiratory secretions. The bacteria may be positively identified using biochemical methods or using a technique whereby, if present in the sample, the anthrax bacterium is made to fluoresce. Blood samples will also indicate elevated antibody levels or increased amounts of a protein produced directly in response to infection with the anthrax bacterium. Polymerase chain reaction (PCR) tests amplify trace amounts of DNA to show that the anthrax bacteria are present. Additional DNA-based tests are also currently being perfected.

Treatment

In the early stages, anthrax is curable by administering high doses of antibiotics, but in the advanced stages, it can be fatal. If anthrax is suspected, health care professionals may begin to treat the patient with antibiotics even before the diagnosis is confirmed because early intervention is essential. The antibiotics used include penicillin, doxycycline, and ciprofloxacin. Because inhaled spores can remain in the body for a long time, antibiotic treatment for inhalation anthrax should continue for 60 days. In the case of cutaneous anthrax, the infection may be cured following a single dose of antibiotic, but it is important to continue treatment so as to avoid potential serious complications, such as inflammation of the membranes covering the brain and spinal cord (**meningitis**). In the setting of potential bioterrorism, cutaneous anthrax should be treated with a 60-day dose of antibiotics.

Research is ongoing to develop new antibiotics and antitoxins that would work against the anthrax bacteria and the toxins they produce. One Harvard professor, Dr. R. John Collier, and his team have been testing two possible antitoxins on rats. A Stanford microbiologist and a Penn State chemist have also been testing their new antibiotic against the bacteria that cause **brucellosis** and **tularemia**, as well as the bacteria that cause anthrax. All of these drugs are still in early investigational stages, however, and it is still unknown how these drugs would affect humans.

Prognosis

Untreated anthrax is often fatal, but death is far less likely with appropriate care. Ten to twenty percent of patients will die from anthrax of the skin (cutaneous anthrax) if it is not properly treated. All patients with inhalation (pulmonary) anthrax will die if untreated. Intestinal anthrax is fatal 25-75% of the time.

Prevention

Anthrax is relatively rare in the United States because of widespread animal vaccination and practices used to disinfect hides or other animal products. Anyone visiting a country where anthrax is common or where herd animals are not often vaccinated should avoid contact with livestock or animal products and avoid eating meat that has not been properly prepared and cooked.

Other means of preventing the spread of infection include carefully handling dead animals suspected of having the disease, burning (instead of burying) contaminated carcasses, and providing good ventilation when processing hides, fur, wool, or hair.

In the event that exposure to anthrax spores is known, such as in the aftermath of a terrorist attack, a course of antibiotics can prevent the disease from occurring.

In the case of contaminated mail, as was the case in the 2001 attacks, the U.S. postal service recommends certain precautions. These precautions include inspecting mail from an unknown sender for excessive tape, powder, uneven weight or lumpy spots, restrictive endorsements such as "Personal," or "Confidential," a postmark different from the sender's address, or a sender's address that seems false or that cannot be verified. **Handwashing** is also recommended after handling mail. In order to decontaminate batches of mail before being opened, machines that use bacteria-killing **radiation** could be used to sterilize the mail. These machines are similar to systems already in place on assembly lines for sterile products, such as bandages and medical devices, but this technique would not be practical for large quantities of mail. In addition, the radiation could damage some of the mail's contents, such as undeveloped photographic film. Microwave radiation or the heat from a clothes iron is not powerful enough to kill the anthrax bacteria.

For those in high-risk professions, an anthrax vaccine is available that is 93% effective in protecting against infection. To provide this immunity, an individual should be given an initial course of three injections, given two weeks apart, followed by booster injections at six, 12, and 18 months and an annual **immunization** thereafter.

Approximately 30% of those who have been vaccinated against anthrax may notice mild local reactions, such as tenderness at the injection site. Infrequently, there may be a severe local reaction with extensive swelling of the forearm, and a few vaccine recipients may have a more general flu-like reaction to the shot, including muscle and joint aches, headache, and fatigue. Reactions requiring hospitalization are very rare. However, this vaccine is only available to people who are at high risk, including veterinary and laboratory workers, livestock handlers, and military personnel. The vaccine is not recommended for people who have previously recovered from an anthrax infection or for pregnant women. Whether this vaccine would protect against anthrax used as a biological weapon is, as yet, unclear.

Resources

OTHER

"Anthrax." New York State Department of Health Communicable Disease Fact Sheet. http://www.health.state.ny.us/nysdoh/consumer/anthrax.htm.

"Bacillus anthracis (Anthrax)." http://web.bu.edu/COHIS/infxns/bacteria/anthrax.htm.

Begley, Sharon and Karen Springen. "Anthrax: What You Need to Know: Exposure doesn't guarantee disease, and the illness is treatable." Newsweek October 29, 2001: 40.

Centers for Disease Control. http://www.cdc.gov.

Kolata, Gina. "Antibiotics and Antitoxins." New York Times October 23, 2001: Section D, page 4, second column.

Park, Alice. "Anthrax: A Medical Guide." Time 158, no. 19 (October 29, 2001): 44.

Shapiro, Bruce. "Anthrax Anxiety." The Nation 273, no. 4 (November 5, 2001): 4.

Wade, Nicholas. "How a Patient Assassin Does Its Deadly Work." New York Times October 23, 2001: Section D, page 1.

ORGANIZATIONS

Centers for Disease Control and Prevention (CDC), 1600 Clifton Road, Atlanta, GA 30333, (800) 232-4636, cdcinfo@cdc.gov, http://www.cdc.gov

National Institute of Allergies and Infectious Diseases, 6610 Rockledge Drive, MSC 6612, Bethesda, MD 20892-6612, (301) 496-5717, Fax: (301) 402-3573, (866) 284-4107, ocpostoffice@niaid.nih.gov, http://www.niaid.nih.gov

World Health Organization (WHO), Avenue Appia 201211, Geneva, Switzerland 27, 41 22 791-2111, info@who.int, http://www.who.int.

Carol A. Turkington

Antibiotics

Definition

Antibiotics are drugs that treat infections caused by bacteria. Some antibiotics may have secondary uses, such as the use of demeclocycline (Declomycin, a tetracycline derivative) to treat the syndrome of inappropriate antidiuretic hormone (SIADH) secretion. Other antibiotics may be useful in treating protozoal (another type of single-celled organism) infections.

Purpose

Antibiotics are used for treatment or **prevention** of bacterial infection. Different antibiotics are effective in killing different species of bacteria.

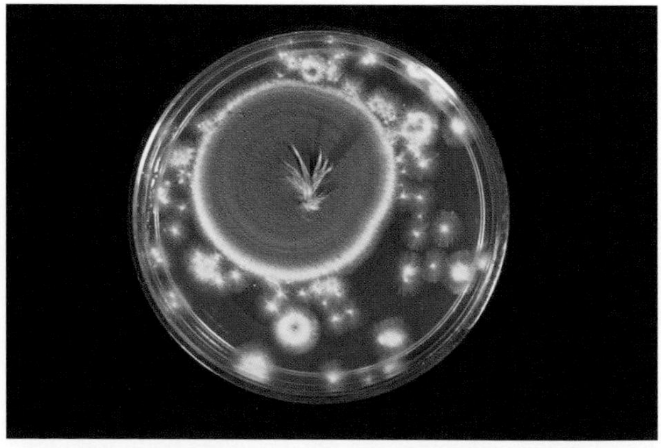

Antibiotic compounds obtained from the mold penicillum notatum and related species. *(Patricia Barber, RBP/Custom Medical Stock)*

Description

There are a very large number of antibiotics approved for use in the United States and Canada, sold under a variety of brand names.

There are several classification schemes for antibiotics. The most useful is based on chemical structure. Antibiotics within a structural class will generally show similar patterns of effectiveness, toxicity, and allergic potential. Additional classification schemes are based on:

- bacterial spectrum—broad spectrum can kill many types of bacteria, whereas narrow spectrum antibiotics specifically target a single class of bacteria
- route of administration—injectable, oral, or topical
- type of activity—bactericidal drugs kill bacteria outright whereas bacteriostatic drugs inhibit bacterial growth

Penicillins

The penicillins are the oldest class of antibiotics. They have a common chemical structure that they share with the cephalopsorins. The two groups are classed as beta-lactam antibiotics, and are generally bacteriocidal—that is, they kill bacteria rather than inhibiting growth. Penicillins are sold under a variety of generic and brand names.

The penicillins can be further subdivided. Natural penicillins are based on the original penicillin G structure; penicillinase-resistant penicillins, notably methicillin and oxacillin, are active even in the presence of the bacterial enzyme that inactivates most natural penicillins. Aminopenicillins such as ampicillin and amoxicillin have an extended spectrum of action compared with natural penicillins. Extended spectrum penicillins are effective against a wider range of bacteria. These generally include coverage for *Pseudomonas aeruginaosa*. The penicillin may be used in combination with a penicillinase inhibitor.

Cephalosporins

Cephalosporins and the closely related cephamycins and carbapenems are the most widely prescribed class of antibiotics in the United States. They were discovered in Italy in 1948 and were first manufactured commercially in the United States in 1964. Like the penicillins, cephalosporins contain a beta-lactam chemical structure. Consequently, bacteria resistant to penicillins are also likely to be resistant to cephalosporins, and people allergic to penicillins are likely to be allergic to cephalosporins.

KEY TERMS

Anaerobic bacteria—Bacteria that grow and reproduce in an oxygen-free environment, such as the bacterium that causes tetanus.

Bacteria—Tiny, one-celled forms of life that cause many diseases and infections.

Blood-brain barrier—A specialized, semi-permeable layer of cells around the blood vessels in the brain that controls which substances can leave the circulatory system and enter the brain.

Inflammation—Pain, redness, swelling, and heat that usually develop in response to injury or illness.

Meningitis—Inflammation of tissues that surround the brain and spinal cord.

Microorganism—An organism that is too small to be seen with the naked eye.

Myasthenia gravis—A muscle weakness that occurs because the body makes antibodies to the natural chemical that facilitates transmission of impulses between the nerve and the muscle.

Pregnancy category—A system of classifying drugs according to their established risks for use during pregnancy. Category A: Controlled human studies have demonstrated no fetal risk. Category B: Animal studies indicate no fetal risk, but no human studies; or adverse effects in animals, but not in well-controlled human studies. Category C: No adequate human or animal studies; or adverse fetal effects in animal studies, but no available human data. Category D: Evidence of fetal risk, but benefits outweigh risks. Category X: Evidence of fetal risk. Risks outweigh any benefits.

The "cepha" drugs are among the most diverse class of antibiotics and are themselves subgrouped into first-, second-, third-, and fourth-generation drugs. Each generation has a broader spectrum of activity than the one before. In addition, cefoxitin, a cephamycin, is highly active against anaerobic bacteria, which makes them a good choice in the treatment of abdominal infections. The fourth-generation cephalosporins (cefepime, cefluprenam, cefozopran, cefpirome, cefquinome) cross the blood-brain barrier and may be used to treat **meningitis** and **encephalitis**.

Fluoroquinolones

The fluoroquinolones are synthetic antibacterial agents, and not derived from bacteria. A related class of antibacterial agents developed earlier, the quinolones, were not well absorbed and could be used only to treat urinary tract infections. The fluoroquinolones, which are based on the older group, are broad-spectrum bactericidal drugs that are chemically unrelated to the penicillins or the cephalosporins. They are well distributed into bone tissue, and so well absorbed that in general they are as effective when given by mouth as by intravenous infusion. Cipro is the brand name of the best-known fluoroquinolone sold in the United States.

Tetracyclines

Tetracyclines got their name because they share a chemical structure that has four rings. They are derived from a species of *Streptomyces* bacteria. As broad-spectrum bacteriostatic agents, the tetracyclines may be effective against a wide variety of microorganisms, including rickettsia and amoebic **parasites**.

Macrolides

The macrolide antibiotics are derived from *Streptomyces* bacteria and got their name because they all have a macrocyclic lactone chemical structure. Erythromycin, the prototype of this class, has a spectrum and use similar to penicillin. Newer members of the group, azithromycin (Zithromax) and clarithyromycin (Biaxin), are particularly useful for their high level of lung penetration. Clarithromycin has been widely used to treat *Helicobacter pylori* infections that cause stomach ulcers.

Others

Other classes of antibiotics include the aminoglycosides, which are particularly useful for their effectiveness in treating *Pseudomonas aeruginosa* infections. Gentamycin (garamycin), polymyxin B sulfate/trimethoprim (Polytrim), and tobramycin (Tobrex) fall into this category. The lincosamindes include clindamycin (Cleocin) and lincomycin (Lincocin), which are highly active against anaerobic pathogens. The sulfonamides include co-trimoxazole (Bactrim) and trimethoprim (Proloprim). There are other individual drugs that have also been useful in treating specific infections.

Recommended dosage

Dosage varies with drug, route of administration, pathogen, site of infection, and severity. Additional considerations include renal function, age of patient, and other factors. Consult manufacturers' recommendations for dose and route.

Precautions

To minimize risk of adverse reactions and development of resistant strains of bacteria, antibiotics should be restricted to use in cases where there is either known or a reasonable presumption of bacterial infection. The use of antibiotics in viral infections such as the **common cold** is to be avoided. Avoid use of fluoroquinolones for trivial infections. Use antibiotics as often as directed and for as long as directed. Although the symptoms may have disappeared, the infection may not clear up completely if the drug is stopped too soon.

In severe infections, therapy with a broad-spectrum antibiotic such as a third or fourth generation cephalosporin may be appropriate. Treatment should be changed to a narrow spectrum agent as soon as the disease-causing bacterium has been identified. After 48 hours of treatment, if there is clinical improvement, an oral antibiotic should be considered.

Side effects

Due to the various types of antibiotics available, there are a variety of side effects possible. The most common problems associated with each type are:

- Penicillins: Allergic reactions may be common, and cross allergenicity with cephalosporins has been reported. Penicillins are classed as category B during pregnancy.
- Cephalopsorins: Several cephalopsorins and related compounds have been associated with seizures. Cefoperazone (Cefobid), cefotetan (Cefotan), and ceftriaxone (Rocephin) may be associated with a decrease in the ability of the blood to clot and other coagulation abnormalities. Some forms of colitis (a serious infection of the large intestine) have been reported with cephalosporins and other broad-spectrum antibiotic use. Some drugs in this class may cause kidney damage. Pregnancy category B.
- Fluoroquinolones: Lomefloxacin (Maxaquin) has been associated with increased photosensitivity. All drugs in this class have been associated with convulsions. Pregnancy category C.
- Tetracyclines: Demeclocycline (Declomycin) may cause increased photosensitivity. Minocycline (Dynacin) may cause dizziness. Oral tetracyclines bind to anions such as calcium and iron. Although doxycycline and minocycline may be taken with meals, patients should take other tetracycline antibiotics on an empty stomach and should not take the drugs with milk or other calcium-rich foods. Expired tetracycline should never be administered. Pregnancy category D.

- Macrolides: Erythromycin may aggravate the weakness of patients with myasthenia gravis. Azithromycin has rarely been associated with allergic reactions, including angioedema, anaphylaxis (life-threatening shock), and skin reactions, including Stevens-Johnson syndrome and toxic epidermal necrolysis. Oral erythromycin may be highly irritating to the stomach and when given by injection may cause severe phlebitis. These drugs should be used with caution in patients with liver dysfunction. Pregnancy category B: Azithromycin, erythromycin. Pregnancy category C: Clarithromycin, dirithromycin, troleandomycin.
- Aminoglycosides: This class of drugs causes kidney damage and damage to the organs of the inner ear. These problems can occur even with normal doses. Dosing should be based on kidney (renal) function, with periodic testing of both kidney function and hearing. Pregnancy category D.

Pediatric

Tetracyclines should not be prescribed for children under the age of eight. They should be specifically avoided during periods of tooth development. In children, these drugs can cause permanent tooth discoloration.

Geriatic

Older patients are more sensitive to the side effects of antibiotics. Since these patients often take multiple medications, their use and possible drug interactions should be carefully monitored by a physician and pharmacist.

Pregnant or breastfeeding

Several antibiotics may impair fetal development. Their use during pregnancy should be discussed with a physician and closely monitored. Generally, breastfeeding is not recommended while taking antibiotics, due to the risk of upsetting the balance of the infant's intestinal bacteria and risk of masking infection in the infant.

The use of tetracyclines should be avoided during pregnancy as it may cause alterations in bone development.

Other conditions and allergies

All antibiotics cause risk of overgrowth by nonsusceptible bacteria. Manufacturers list other major hazards by class; however, the health care provider should review each drug individually to assess the degree of risk.

Excessive or inappropriate use of any antibiotic may lead to the development of antibiotic-resistant strains of bacteria. This has become an increasing concern as antibiotics are routinely added to animal feed and some household cleaning products. A strain that is considered resistant is one that can no longer be treated effectively using the antibiotics commonly prescribed for that type of infection.

Methicillin-resistant *Staphylococcus aureus* (MRSA) is a strain of staphylococcal bacteria that is resistant to the antibiotic methicillin and other common antibiotics that normally control staph infections. Although this strain of staph has existed in hospitals for years, in the 1990s, MRSA began appearing in places other than hospitals. By 2007, two forms of MRSA were recognized, hospital-acquired MRSA (HA-MRSA) and community-acquired MRSA (CA-MRSA). Symptoms of a MRSA infection are similar to other staph infection symptoms, only MRSA is much more dangerous and has a much higher mortality rate because treatment with common antibiotics does not kill the bacterium.

Interactions

The potential for interactions with other drugs and with foods is pronounced with the antibiotic drug group as a whole. Patients should request verbal and written information about the potential of these interactions for every antibiotic they are prescribed.

Resources

BOOKS

Cunha, Burke A. *Antibiotic Essentials 2012*, 11th ed. Sudbury, MA: Jones & Bartlett Learning, 2012.

Gallagher, Jason C., and Conan MacDougall. *Antibiotics Simplified*, 2nd ed. Sudbury, MA: Jones & Bartlett Learning, 2011.

Schlossberg, David, and Rafik Samuel. *Antibiotic Manual: A Guide to Commonly Used Antimicrobials*. Shelton, CT: PMPH-USA, 2012.

PERIODICALS

Jernberg, C., et al. "Long-term Impacts of Antibiotic Exposure on the Human Intestinal Microbiota." *Microbiology* 156, Pt. 11. (2010): 3216–23.

Landers, T.F., et al. "A Review of Antibiotic Use in Food Animals: Perspective, Policy, and Potential." *Public Health Reports* 127, 1. (2012): 4–22.

Liou, A.P., and P.J. Turnbaugh. "Antibiotic Exposure Promotes Fat Gain." *Cell Metabolism* 16, 4. (2012): 408–10.

Zenner, D., and N. Shetty. "European Antibiotic Awareness Day 2011: Antibiotics–A Powerful Tool and a Dwindling Resource." *Family Practice* 28, 5. (2011): 471–3.

OTHER

"Antibiotics." emedicinehealth. http://www.emedicinehealth.com/antibiotics/article_em.htm. Accessed on October 20, 2012.

"Antibiotics". MedlinePlus. http://www.nlm.nih.gov/medlineplus/antibiotics.html. Accessed on October 20, 2012.

"Get Smart: Know When Antibiotics Work." Centers for Disease Control and Prevention. http://www.cdc.gov/getsmart/. Accessed on October 20, 2012.

"Using Antibiotics Wisely. WebMD."http://www.webmd.com/a-to-z-guides/using-antibiotics-wisely-topic-overview. Accessed on October 20, 2012.

ORGANIZATIONS

Alliance for the Prudent Use of Antibiotics (APUA), 300 Harrison Ave., Posner 3 (Business), Boston, MA 02111-1901, (617) 636-0966, Fax: (617) 636-3999, apua@tufts.edu Attn. Kathleen Young, http://www.tufts.edu/med/apua/

Centers for Disease Control and Prevention (CDC), 1600 Clifton Rd., Atlanta, GA 30333, (800) 232–4636, http://www.cdc.gov/cdc-info/requestform.html, http://www.cdc.gov

United States Food and Drug Administration (FDA), 10903 New Hampshire Ave., Silver Spring, MD 20993, (888) INFO-FDA (463-6332), http://www.fda.gov/AboutFDA/ContactFDA/default.htm, http://www.fda.gov.

Samuel D. Uretsky, PharmD
Tish Davidson, AM
Melinda Granger Oberleitner, RN, DNS, APRN, CNS

Antimicrobial resistance

Definition

Antimicrobial resistance (AMR) is the reduced effectiveness of an antibiotic, antimalarial, antifungal, or antiviral prescription medication in treating microorganisms that were previously sensitive to the drug in question. AMR results from the overuse or misuse of antimicrobial agents and emerges as a public health problem when pathogens mutate or develop genetic resistance to these agents.

Description

Antimicrobial resistance is the end result of a combination of natural processes and human behaviors, including the misuse of antimicrobial drugs.

Causes

Biological causes of antimicrobial resistance include:

- Natural resistance. Since the experiments of Joshua and Esther Lederberg in 1952, which demonstrated that penicillin-resistant bacteria existed prior to the discovery and use of penicillin, other naturally resistant microbes have been discovered, including several strains of *Clostridium difficile*. One theory that has been advanced to explain natural antimicrobial resistance is that heavy metals and some pollutants in the soil may select for resistant bacteria, thus providing an ongoing or recurrent population of them in nature.
- Selective pressure. Selective pressure refers to the evolutionary advantages of pathogens that are resistant to antimicrobials. When a patient is treated with an antimicrobial drug, the organisms that are susceptible to the drug are killed, leaving a small number of resistant organisms. These resistant microbes can then multiply, and their offspring are likely to become the dominant type of that particular disease organism.
- Mutation. Disease organisms reproduce rapidly, often within a few hours. Although mutations—spontaneous changes in an organism's genetic material—are thought to occur in only one in a million or one in 10 million pathogens, the sheer speed of replication of these organisms means that mutations appear fairly frequently, and some of these mutations confer resistance to antimicrobial drugs.
- Gene transfer. Bacteria can reproduce by a process called conjugation, which is a form of cell-to-cell contact that allows for the transfer of genetic material between the two organisms. Gene transfer allows a drug-resistant bacterium to transfer genes that encode drug resistance to its partner. Many drug resistance genes are fund on plasmids, which are molecules of DNA that are separate from chromosomes and can replicate independently of chromosomal DNA.

Human behaviors responsible for antimicrobial resistance include the overuse and misuse of antimicrobials:

- Prescribing and taking antibiotics for diseases caused by viruses. Antibiotics are a specific class of antimicrobials intended to treat bacterial diseases. Many people, however, request their doctors to prescribe antibiotics for such viral diseases as flu, most sore throats, and the common cold. Antibiotics are ineffective against viruses and may in fact contribute to the development of drug-resistant bacteria in the patient's body. The reasons for doctors prescribing antibiotics inappropriately are complex: in some cases, the doctor may have misdiagnosed the cause of the patient's illness. In others, the doctor may have been worn down by the patient's insistence on an antibiotic or may fear a malpractice lawsuit. According to the Centers for Disease Control and Prevention (CDC), $1.1 billion is spent each year in the United States on unnecessary antibiotic prescriptions for upper respiratory infections in adults.

- Failure to complete a prescribed course of antibiotics. Many people stop taking their medication as soon as they feel better, but an incomplete course of antibiotics increases the likelihood that drug-resistant organisms will survive and reproduce. In the long run the illness may recur and be harder to treat because the pathogen has become drug-resistant. In addition, a person who harbors drug-resistant bacteria because they did not complete their course of antibiotics may pass on their drug-resistant organisms to family members and friends.
- Poor hand hygiene in hospital staff. One of the most common types of drug-resistant infections is nosocomial or hospital-acquired infections. These are often difficult to treat not only because the disease organisms are drug-resistant but also because the infected patients are weakened by the illness or injury that led to their being hospitalized in the first place.
- Indiscriminate off-label use of antibiotics in animals. Antibiotics have been used not only to treat infections in household pets and farm animals as well as in humans, but have also been added to farm animals' feed to promote growth. This use of medications for reasons other than those approved by the Food and Drug Administration (FDA), or in species other than those approved by the agency, is termed off-label use. Antibiotics added to animal feed can contribute to the development of drug-resistant bacteria in several ways. First, they can enter the soil in animal waste, as about 70% of antibiotics given to animals are not broken down in the body but are discharged through waste products. Second, humans can acquire disease-resistant bacteria from farm animals through consuming their meat. Third, humans can acquire these bacteria through close contact with the animals.

Mechanisms of antimicrobial resistance

Microbes have several different mechanisms for resisting antimicrobial drugs:

- Inactivation. Some species of penicillin-resistant bacteria secrete enzymes that deactivate the drug.
- Alteration of the target site. Most antibiotics work by binding to certain proteins on the surface of the bacterium. Some mutations eliminate or change the target protein so that the drug can no longer bind to the bacterium.
- Alteration of the metabolic pathway. Some antimicrobials work by interfering with the disease organism's metabolism. Certain mutations may enable the organism to change its metabolism.
- Development of efflux mechanisms. Some bacteria develop pumping mechanisms that push the antibiotic back out of the cell so that it never reaches its target inside the cell.

Specific drug-resistant pathogens

Staphylococcus aureus. Staphylococcus aureus, or staph, has become a deadly multidrug-resistant bacterium. As early as 1947, it developed resistance to penicillin. In the early 1960s, strains of methicillin-resistant staph, or MRSA, began to appear in Europe. By the early 2000s, *S. aureus* had developed resistance to tetracycline and erythromycin as well as penicillin and methicillin. That left vancomycin as the sole antibiotic effective against MRSA; however, a vancomycin-resistant strain, or VRSA, appeared in the United States in 2002. Community-acquired MRSA, or CA-MRSA, has become endemic in some urban areas around the world, particularly among homosexual men. Other outbreaks of CA-MRSA have occurred in athletic facilities, military installations, prisons, and newborn nurseries. CA-MRSA is an increasingly common cause of such rapidly progressing and potentially fatal illnesses as necrotizing fasciitis, sepsis, and necrotizing **pneumonia**.

Mycobacterium tuberculosis. M. tuberculosis is a bacterium that causes **tuberculosis**, a severe infection that may affect other organs as well as the lungs. It usually requires treatment with a 6-month course of **antibiotics**. Multidrug-resistant tuberculosis (MDR-TB) is a form of the disease caused by strains of *M. tuberculosis* that are resistant to rifampin and isoniazid, the most common antibiotics used to treat TB. MDR-TB requires up to 2 years of therapy with other antibiotics. Extensively drug-resistant TB (XDR-TB) is resistant to treatment with kanamycin, amikacin, or capreomycin as well as rifampin and isoniazid, and is extremely challenging to treat as of 2012.

Neisseria gonorrhoeae. N. gonorrhoeae, or the gonococcus, is the bacterium responsible for gonorrhea, a sexually transmitted disease (STD). Gonorrhea is the second most common STD in the United States as of 2012. The gonococcus has proved to be unusually competent in developing **drug resistance** through gene transfer and the use of an efflux pump to prevent antibiotics from entering its cell wall. At present, gonorrhea is usually treated with a combination of two antibiotics, a cephalosporin and either doxycycline or azithromycin. There is evidence, however, that *N. gonorrhoeae* is becoming increasingly resistant to all known antibiotics. The first case of a so-called "superbug" form of gonorrhea was diagnosed in a prostitute in Japan in 2009. In June 2012, the **World Health Organization (WHO)** issued a warning that strains of the gonococcus resistant to cephalosporins are now present worldwide.

Enterococcus faecalis. E. faecalis is a gram-positive bacterium that lives in the digestive tracts of humans and other animals. It is also commonly found in root canal-treated teeth. As of 2012, multidrug-resistant *E. faecalis* is often found in hospitals, where it can produce life-threatening **meningitis** and bacteremia as well as urinary tract infections. Penicillin resistance was first noted in *E. faecalis* in 1983, vancomycin resistance in 1987, and linezolid resistance in the 1990s.

Pseudomonas aeruginosa. P. aeruginosa is a pathogen with a high level of resistance to antibiotics due to its frequent mutations, frequent gene transfers, and the low permeability of its cell wall. Pseudomonas infections are common in hospitals because the bacterium can live in or on hospital equipment, including urinary catheters. It is also a frequent cause of lung infections in patients with cystic fibrosis. Pseudomonas infections are also often spread by hospital workers with poor hand **hygiene**.

Clostridium difficile. C. difficile is a gram-positive bacterium that causes diarrheal disease, most often in patients whose normal intestinal flora have been altered by the administration of antibiotics for other illnesses. Diarrhea caused by *C. difficile* is common in hospitals around the world as of 2012. The first outbreaks of clindamycin-resistant *C. difficile* diarrhea first occurred in hospitals in the United States in 1989. As of 2012, the most effective treatments for this bacterium are to discontinue the antibiotics that were first given to the patient, or to administer vancomycin.

Escherichia coli. E. coli is the most common single cause of urinary tract infections. A rod-shaped bacterium that lives in the digestive tract, it can cause disease through **food contamination**; many food product recalls have involved *E. coli*. Some virulent strains of *E. coli* are responsible for bacterial pneumonia, hemolytic-uremic syndrome, peritonitis, and meningitis in newborns. Fluoroquinolone-resistant strains of the bacterium have been present in the United States since 1993.

Demographics

Antimicrobial resistance is a worldwide problem that affects both sexes, all age groups, and all races. In the United States, between 5% and 10% of all hospital inpatients develop nosocomial infections each year. The number of patients who have died from such infections rose from 13,300 in 1002 to 90,000 in 2010.

Worldwide, multidrug resistant tuberculosis (MDR-TB) causes at least 150,000 deaths each year, according to the **World Health Organization** (**WHO**). Other diseases that are becoming increasingly resistant to standard treatments as of 2012 include HIV infection, **malaria**, and gonorrhea. Those at greatest risk include persons with weakened immune systems, those who have had organ transplants, and men who have sex with men.

Effects on public health

The effects of antimicrobial resistance on public health include stepped-up concern for preventive measures in underdeveloped countries that include relieving overcrowding, ensuring supplies of clean **water**, and improving **sanitation** measures. Stronger governmental oversight of access to antibiotics and better surveillance of outbreaks of **infectious disease** would also be beneficial.

Another public health measure that has been suggested is the establishment of an international action network that would track antibiotic resistance around the world, thus allowing public health workers to identify trends and determine whether education programs and other preventive measures are effective.

Costs to society

WHO has noted a number of costs to society resulting from antimicrobial resistance. One is the increase in mortality as noted above. Another is the ever-rising cost of health care, as patients infected by drug-resistant organisms require longer and more expensive courses of treatment. They are also likely to remain infectious longer, thus spreading their diseases to a wider circle of friends, workplace colleagues, and family members. A third cost to society is the increased riskiness of organ transplantation, other complex surgical procedures, and **cancer** treatment due to the rising number of nosocomial infections. Last is the association of drug-resistant infections with international trade and travel. Tourism and international business travel can spread drug-resistant organisms rapidly from country to country and across continents, thus making it impossible to effectively quarantine infectious diseases.

Efforts and solutions

Vaccines. Some infectious diseases, such as **influenza**, can be prevented by administration of vaccines. Flu vaccines, however, must be modified each year because the flu virus mutates so rapidly. Vaccines against *S. aureus* are theoretically possible, but are still in the research and development stage as of 2012.

Phage therapy. Phage therapy refers to the use of bacteriophages—viruses that infect bacteria—to treat bacterial infections. The bacteriophage destroys the bacterium by binding to it and injecting its own genetic material into the bacterium. This process disrupts the bacterium's normal cell processes and forces it to make new virus particles. First used in the former Soviet Union in the 1920s, phage therapy has not been used in the West since the 1930s. The reasons for its disuse have to do with the unavailability of Russian research in the West during

KEY TERMS

Antimicrobial—A general term for any drug that is effective against disease organisms, including bacteria, viruses, fungi, and parasites. Antibiotics, which are used to treat bacterial infections, are one type of antimicrobial.

Bacteremia—The presence of bacteria in the bloodstream.

Bacteriophage—A type of virus that can be used to treat bacterial infections. Bacteriophages (or simply phages) work by injecting their own genetic material into bacteria and forcing the bacteria to produce new virus particles rather than a new generation of bacteria.

Cephalosporins—A class of beta-lactam antibiotics originally derived from the fungus *Acrimonium*, which was previously called *Cephalosporium*.

Conjugation—The transfer of genetic material between two bacteria through cell-to-cell contact.

Fluoroquinolones—A class of synthetic broad-spectrum antibiotics that contain a fluorine atom in addition to the basic quinolone structure. They work by preventing the DNA in bacteria from unwinding and replicating.

Gene transfer—The exchange of genetic material between bacteria during conjugation. It is a common mechanism for developing antimicrobial resistance.

Natural selection—The process by which certain biological traits become either more or less common in the population of a given species as a result of the different rates of reproduction of individuals bearing those traits.

Nosocomial infection—An infection acquired in a hospital during treatment for another condition.

Off-label use—The practice of prescribing a medication for an indication, age group, dosage level, or method of administration unapproved (or not yet approved) by the Food and Drug Administration.

Pathogen—Any microorganism, virus, or other substance that causes disease in another organism.

Plasmid—A small loop of genetic material that is not part of a chromosome and can be easily transferred between bacteria.

Selective pressure—Influence exerted by an antibiotic or other factor on natural selection to promote the survival of one group of organisms over another.

Superbug—An informal term for a bacterium that has become resistant to many different antibiotics. Bacteria that are resistant to several different drugs are also called multidrug-resistant or MDR bacteria.

the Cold War, and the discovery and increasing use of antibiotics to treat bacterial infections after World War II.

New medications. There are relatively few new antimicrobial drugs under research and development. One reason is the rapidly escalating costs of research and development, and the high number of compounds that fail during preclinical studies and clinical trials. It can take as long as 10 years and cost $300 million to bring a new antibiotic to market, while microbial resistance to the new drug can develop in as little as two years. Another reason is that drug companies make most of their profits from drugs to treat chronic diseases and lifestyle issues, and have little motivation to invest money in developing new antimicrobials. One exception is the archaeocins, a promising new class of antibiotics derived from the Archaea, single-celled organisms that used to be classified together with the bacteria but are now considered a distinctive domain of microorganisms. About eight different archaeocins have been identified as of 2012, but it is thought that there may be literally hundreds of these compounds.

Orders of prohibition. An order of prohibition is an official government action prohibiting the use of a certain drug or class of drugs in animals in order to slow down the development of antimicrobial resistance and preserve the effectiveness of the drug(s) in treating humans. In September 2005, the FDA banned the use of fluoroquinolones in poultry because of the emergence of fluoroquinolone-resistant strains of *Campylobacter* in humans. These strains were associated with consumption of poultry meat. On April 6, 2012, the Food and Drug Administration's ban on the use of cephalosporins in cattle, swine, chickens, and turkeys went into effect. The order of prohibition applies to the use of cephalosporins used for the treatment of disease in humans or household pets to prevent or treat disease in farm animals.

Human behavioral changes. These would include limiting the use of existing antibiotics to treat minor illnesses; educating people about the ineffectiveness of antibiotics in treating viral infections; being more careful about hand hygiene at home as well as in hospitals; reducing the use of antibiotics in agriculture; and

QUESTIONS TO ASK YOUR DOCTOR

- When is it appropriate to take an antibiotic for an infection?
- How can I find out more information about antimicrobial resistance in our local area?
- Have you ever treated a patient with a multi-drug-resistant infection? Was the treatment effective?

practicing **safe sex** to reduce the spread of drug-resistant gonorrhea as well as other STDs.

Resources

BOOKS

Keen, Patricia L., and Mark H.M.M. Montforts, eds. *Antimicrobial Resistance in the Environment.* Hoboken, NJ: Wiley, 2012.

Kolendi, Charles L., ed. *Methicillin-resistant Staphylococcus aureus (MRSA): Etiology, At-risk Populations and Treatment.* Hauppauge, NY: Nova Science Publishers, 2010.

Pommerville, Jeffrey. *Fundamentals of Microbiology*, 10th ed. Burlington, MA: Jones and Bartlett Learning, 2013.

Weber, J. Todd, ed. *Antimicrobial Resistance: Beyond the Breakpoint.* New York: Karger, 2010.

PERIODICALS

Breathnach, A.S., et al. "Multidrug-resistant *Pseudomonas aeruginosa* Outbreaks in Two Hospitals: Association with Contaminated Hospital Waste-water Systems." *Journal of Hospital Infection* 82 (September 2012): 19–24.

Capita, R., and C. Alonso-Calleja. "Antibiotic-resistant Bacteria: A Challenge for the Food Industry." *Critical Reviews in Food Science and Nutrition* 53 (January 2013): 11–48.

Castillo Neyra, R., et al. "Antimicrobial-resistant Bacteria: An Unrecognized Work-related Risk in Food Animal Production." *Safety and Health at Work* 3 (June 2012): 85–91.

Goldstein, E., et al. "Factors Related to Increasing Prevalence of Resistance to Ciprofloxacin and Other Antimicrobial Drugs in *Neisseria gonorrhoeae*, United States." *Emerging Infectious Diseases* 18 (August 2012): 1290–1297.

Keshavjee, S., and P. Farmer. "Tuberculosis, Drug Resistance, and the History of Modern Medicine." *New England Journal of Medicine* 367 (September 6, 2012): 931–936.

Nelson, J.M., et al. "Fluoroquinolone-Resistant *Campylobacter* Species and the Withdrawal of Fluoroquinolones from Use in Poultry: A Public Health Success Story." *Clinical Infectious Diseases* 44 (July 2007): 877–980.

Stamino, S., et al. "Retrospective Analysis of Antimicrobial Susceptibility Trends (2000–2009) in Neisseria gonorrhoeae Isolates from Countries in Latin America and the Caribbean Shows Evolving Resistance to Ciprofloxacin, Azithromycin and Decreased Susceptibility to Ceftriaxone." *Sexually Transmitted Diseases* 39 (October 2012): 813–821.

Tamma, P.D., et al. "Combination Therapy for Treatment of Infections with Gram-negative Bacteria." *Clinical Microbiology Reviews* 25 (July 2012): 450–470.

WEBSITES

"Animation of Antimicrobial Resistance." Food and Drug Administration (FDA). This is a 9-minute animation of the development and mechanisms of drug resistance in bacteria. http://www.fda.gov/AnimalVeterinary/SafetyHealth/AntimicrobialResistance/ucm134359.htm (accessed October 14, 2012).

"Antibiotic/Antimicrobial Resistance." Centers for Disease Control and Prevention (CDC). http://www.cdc.gov/drugresistance/index.html (accessed October 14, 2012).

"Antimicrobial Resistance." Food and Drug Administration (FDA). http://www.fda.gov/AnimalVeterinary/SafetyHealth/AntimicrobialResistance/default.htm (accessed October 14, 2012).

"Antimicrobial Resistance." World Health Organization (WHO). http://www.who.int/mediacentre/factsheets/fs194/en/ (accessed October 13, 2012).

"Antimicrobial (Drug) Resistance." National Institute of Allergy and Infectious Diseases (NIAID). http://www.niaid.nih.gov/topics/antimicrobialresistance/Pages/default.aspx (accessed October 14, 2012).

"What Is Antibiotic Resistance and Why Is It a Problem?" Alliance for the Prudent Use of Antibiotics (APUA). http://www.tufts.edu/med/apua/about_issue/antibiotic_res.shtml (accessed October 14, 2012).

ORGANIZATIONS

Alliance for the Prudent Use of Antibiotics (APUA), 200 Harrison Avenue, Posner 3 (Business), Boston, MA United States 02111, (617) 636-0966, Fax: (617) 636-0458, apua@tufts.edu, http://www.tufts.edu/med/apua/

American Public Health Association (APHA), 800 I Street, NW, Washington, DC United States 20001-3710, (202) 777-APHA, Fax: (202) 777-2534, http://apha.org/

Centers for Disease Control and Prevention (CDC), 1600 Clifton Road, Atlanta, GA United States 30333, (800) CDC-INFO (232-4636), http://www.cdc.gov/cdc-info/requestform.html, http://www.cdc.gov/

Food and Drug Administration (FDA), 10903 New Hampshire Ave., Silver Spring, MD United States 20993-0002, (866) INFO-FDA (463-6332), http://www.fda.gov/default.htm

National Institute of Allergy and Infectious Diseases (NIAID), 6610 Rockledge Drive, MSC 6612, Bethesda, MD United States 20892-6612, (301) 496-5717, (866) 284-4107, Fax: (301) 402-3573, ocpostoffice@niaid.nih.gov, http://www.niaid.nih.gov/Pages/default.aspx

World Health Organization (WHO), Avenue Appia 20, Geneva, Switzerland 1211 Geneva 27, +41 22 791 21 11, Fax: +41 22 791 31 11, http://www.who.int/en/.

Rebecca J. Frey, PhD

Asbestosis

Definition

Asbestosis is a chronic, progressive inflammation of the lung caused by prolonged exposure to large quantities of asbestos, a naturally occurring material once widely used in construction, insulation, and manufacturing. Asbestosis can result in shortness of breath, coughing, and permanent lung damage.

Description

Asbestos fibers can enter the air through weathering of natural deposits or from the breakdown of manufactured products containing asbestos. When asbestos is inhaled, fibers penetrate the breathing passages and irritate, inflame, and scar lung tissue. The scar tissue does not expand and contract normally, which interferes with breathing and oxygen transfer. In advanced asbestosis, the lungs shrink, stiffen, and become honeycombed (riddled with tiny holes). The disease tends to progress, even after exposure to asbestos ceases.

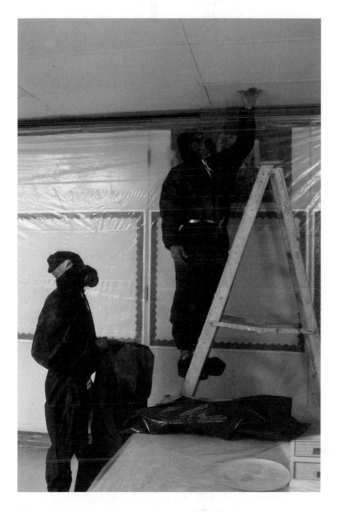

Workers remove asbestos from ceiling tile in a school. *(© Stock Connection Blue / Alamy)*

Regulations, which were first introduced in the 1970s, have reduced use of asbestos in the United States. However, workers who handle automobile brake shoe linings, boiler insulation, ceiling acoustic tiles, electrical equipment, and fire-resistant materials may still be exposed to the substance. Asbestos is also used in the production of paints and plastics. Significant amounts can be released into the atmosphere when old buildings or boats are razed or remodeled.

Risk Factors

Workers who were involved in mining, milling, manufacturing, installation or removal of asbestos products before the late 1970s are at the greatest risk of developing asbestosis. Examples of such occupations include:

- asbestos miners
- aircraft and auto mechanics
- building construction workers
- workers removing asbestos insulation around steam pipes in older buildings
- electricians
- shipyard workers
- boiler operators
- railroad workers

Demographics

In 2010, the **World Health Organization (WHO)** estimated that about 125 million people in the world are exposed to asbestos in the workplace and that more than 107,000 people die each year from asbestos-related lung **cancer**, malignant mesothelioma and asbestosis resulting from occupational exposure. About 2 to 6 million people in the United States are estimated to have had significant levels of exposure. Although high exposures to asbestos ceased in the United States in the late 1970s, given that the latency period between initial exposure and development of asbestos-related diseases is 15 to 20 years or more, asbestosis remained an important public health problem. Between 1999 and 2004, there were 3,211 deaths due to asbestosis in the United States. According to a study by the Environmental Working Group, almost 10,000 deaths per year in the United States, or close to 30 deaths per day, are due to asbestos-related diseases, including malignant mesothelioma, asbestosis, lung cancer and gastrointestinal cancer.

Causes and symptoms

If asbestos fibers are contained to prevent escape into the air, health risks are minimal. Occupational exposure is the most common cause of asbestosis, but the condition can also affect people who inhale asbestos fibers in their homes or who are exposed to waste products from plants near their homes. Family members can develop the disease as a result of inhaling particles of asbestos dust that cling to workers' clothes or by washing clothes contaminated with asbestos fibers.

It is rare for asbestosis to develop in anyone who has not been exposed to large amounts of asbestos on a regular basis for at least ten years. Symptoms of the disease do not usually appear until 15–20 years after initial exposure to asbestos.

The first symptom of asbestosis is usually shortness of breath following exercise or other physical activity. The early stages of the disease are also characterized by a dry cough and a generalized feeling of illness.

As the disease progresses and lung damage increases, shortness of breath occurs even when the patient is at rest. Recurrent respiratory infections and coughing up blood are common. So is swelling of the feet, ankles, or hands. Other symptoms of advanced asbestosis include chest **pain**, hoarseness, and restless sleep. Patients who have asbestosis often have clubbed (widened and thickened) fingers. Other potential complications include heart failure, collapsed (deflated) lung, and pleurisy (inflammation of the membrane that protects the lung).

Diagnosis

Screening of at-risk workers can reveal lung inflammation and lesions characteristic of asbestosis. Patients' medical histories can identify occupations, hobbies, or other situations likely to involve exposure to asbestos fibers. Asbestosis can be difficult to diagnose because the symptoms can be similar to other respiratory diseases.

A battery of tests is used to diagnosis asbestosis. X rays can show shadows or spots on the lungs or an indistinct or shaggy outline of the heart that suggests the presence of asbestosis. Blood tests are used to measure concentrations of oxygen and carbon dioxide. Pulmonary function tests can be used to assess a patient's ability to inhale and exhale, and a computed tomography scan (CT) of the lungs can show flat, raised patches associated with advanced asbestosis.

Treatment

The goal of treatment is to help patients breathe more easily, prevent colds and other respiratory infections, and control complications associated with advanced disease. Ultrasonic, cool-mist humidifiers, controlled coughing, and chest percussion and vibration can loosen bronchial secretions. The patient may require the use of supplemental oxygen by mask or by a plastic piece that fits into the nostrils. Sometimes prescription inhalers, which are used by persons with **asthma**, can aid in treatment. Severe cases of asbestosis may require that the patient have a lung transplant.

Regular exercise helps maintain and improve lung capacity. Although temporary bed rest may be recommended, patients are encouraged to resume their regular activities as soon as they can.

Anyone who develops symptoms of asbestosis should see a family physician or lung disease specialist. A doctor should be notified if someone who has been diagnosed with asbestosis develops the following symptoms:

- coughing up blood
- continued loss of weight
- shortness of breath
- chest pain
- sudden fever of 101°F (38.3°C) or higher
- unfamiliar, unexplained symptoms

Public health role and response

The U.S. government has taken many steps to protect individuals from asbestos exposure:

- In 1989, the U.S. Environmental Protection Agency (EPA) established a ban on new uses of asbestos, although uses established before this date are still allowable.
- EPA regulations require that schools be inspected for asbestos, and if damaged asbestos is found, the schools must eliminate or reduce exposure risk by removing the asbestos or covering it up so that it cannot get into the air. If asbestos is deemed a hazard, a school must develop a management plan. A public health agency reviews the plan and inspects the abatement project as it proceeds.
- The EPA also provides guidance and support for reducing asbestos exposure in other public buildings.
- The EPA regulates the release of asbestos from factories and from building demolition and renovation sites.

KEY TERMS

Asbestos—Asbestos is the commercial name, not a mineralogical term, given to a variety of six naturally occurring fibrous minerals that have been mined for wide use because of their heat resistance and chemical resistance properties. These minerals possess high tensile strength, flexibility, resistance to chemical and thermal degradation, and electrical resistance. These minerals have been used for decades in more than 3,000 types of commercial products, such as insulation and fireproofing materials, automotive brakes, textile products, and cement and wallboard materials. Asbestos has been classified as a known human carcinogen by the U.S. Department of Health and Human Services, the EPA, and the International Agency for Research on Cancer.

Chronic obstructive pulmonary disease (COPD)—Chronic obstructive pulmonary disease (COPD) is a progressive disease that makes it hard to breathe. COPD can cause coughing that produces large amounts of mucus (a slimy substance), wheezing, shortness of breath, chest tightness, and other symptoms. Cigarette smoking is the leading cause of COPD. Most people who have COPD smoke or used to smoke. Long-term exposure to other lung irritants, such as air pollution, chemical fumes, or dust, also may contribute to COPD.

Malignant mesothelioma—Malignant mesothelioma is a rare form of cancer that develops from transformed cells originating in the mesothelium, the protective lining that covers many of the internal organs of the body. It is usually caused by exposure to asbestos. The most common anatomical site for the development of mesothelioma is the pleura (the outer lining of the lungs and internal chest wall), but it can also arise in the peritoneum (the lining of the abdominal cavity), and the pericardium (the sac that surrounds the heart), or the tunica vaginalis (a sac that surrounds the testis).

Pleural effusion—Pleural effusion is excess fluid that accumulates between the two pleural layers, the fluid-filled space that surrounds the lungs. Excessive amounts of such fluid can impair breathing by limiting the expansion of the lungs during ventilation.

Pleural plaques—Pleural plaques are localized scars (fibrosis) consisting of collagen fiber deposits that form as a result of exposure to asbestos. They are the most common manifestation of exposure to asbestos. Normally, pleural plaque is found on the inside of the diaphragm, but in very rare cases it also can be found near the ribcage. Pleural plaques themselves are not associated with any symptoms. However, many people who develop pleural plaques also develop pleural effusion, asbestosis, malignant mesothelioma and other conditions associated with asbestos inhalation.

- The EPA regulates the disposal of waste asbestos materials by requiring the materials to be placed in approved locations.
- The EPA has established a limit of 7 million asbestos fibers per liter on the concentration of long fibers (length greater than or equal to 5 mic) that may be present in drinking water. The major sources of asbestos in drinking water are decay of asbestos cement water mains and erosion of natural deposits.
- The Food and Drug Administration (FDA) regulates the use of asbestos in the preparation of drugs and restricts the use of asbestos in food-packaging materials.
- The National Institute for Occupational Safety and Health (NIOSH) has set recommended inhalation exposure limits.
- The Occupational Safety and Health Administration (OSHA) has established enforceable limits on the average 8-hour daily concentration of asbestos that is allowed in the air in a workplace.

Prognosis

Asbestosis cannot be cured, but its symptoms may be controlled. Doctors do not know why the health of some patients deteriorates and the condition of others remains the same, but many suspect the difference may be due to varying exposures of asbestos. People with asbestosis who smoke are at increased risk for developing lung cancer and are strongly advised to quit **smoking**. Other complications associated with asbestosis include chronic obstructive pulmonary disease (COPD), malignant mesothelioma, pleural effusion, and pleural plaques.

Prevention

Persons can lower their exposure by being aware of sources of asbestos and avoiding those sources. In a home these sources may include damaged or deteriorating asbestos containing insulation or ceiling or floor tiles. The state or local health department should be contacted to learn how to test for asbestos and to aid in locating a company that can remove or contain the asbestos fibers.

If a person lives near asbestos mining or processing sites, exposure can be reduced by frequent hand and face washing, regular cleaning of the home of dust, use of door mats, and removal of shoes when entering the home. Federal laws regulate work practices to limit the amount of asbestos being brought home. These practices may include workers' showering and changing clothes before leaving work, storing street clothes in a separate area of the workplace, and laundering work clothes at work.

Workers in asbestosis-related industries should have regular x rays to determine whether their lungs are healthy. A person whose lung x ray shows a shadow should eliminate asbestos exposure even if no symptoms of the condition have appeared.

People who works with asbestos should wear a protective mask or a hood with a clean-air supply and obey recommended procedures to control asbestos dust. Persons at risk of developing asbestosis should also do the following:

• not smoke
• be vaccinated against influenza and pneumonia
• exercise regularly to maintain cardiopulmonary fitness
• avoid crowds and people who have respiratory infections

Resources

BOOKS

Craighead, John E., and A. R. Gibbs. *Asbestos and Its Diseases*. New York: Oxford, 2008.

Dodson, Ronald F., and Samuel P. Hammar, eds. *Asbestos: Risk Assessment, Epidemiology, and Health Effects, Second Edition.* Boca Raton, FL: CRC Press, 2011.

WEBSITES

Agency for Toxic Substances and Disease Registry. "Asbestos." http://http://www.atsdr.cdc.gov/asbestos/

U.S. National Library of Medicine. "Asbestosis." http://http://http://www.ncbi.nlm.nih.gov/pubmedhealth/PMH0001177/

ORGANIZATIONS

American Lung Association, 1301 Pennsylvania Ave. NW, Ste. 800, Washington, DC 20001, (202) 758-3355, Fax: (202) 452-1805, (800) 548-8252, info@lungusa.org, http://www.lungusa.org.

Judith Sims

Asperger syndrome *see* **Autisim**

Assessment Protocol for Excellence in Public Health (APEX-PH)

Definition

The Assessment Protocol for Excellence in Public Health (APEX-PH) is a joint project of the **American Public Health Association** (APHA), the Association of Schools of Public Health (ASPH), the Association of State and Territorial Health Officials (**ASTHO**), the **Centers for Disease Control and Prevention (CDC)**, the National Association of County and City Health Officials (**NACCHO**), and the United States Conference of Local Health Officers (USCLHO), funded through a Cooperative Agreement between the **Centers for Disease Control and Prevention** and the National Association of County Health Officials in March 1991 to aid in improving the functioning of local public **health departments**.

Purpose

The APEX-PH program had two major objectives: (1) aiding local public health departments in the assessment and improvement of their organizational structure and (2) working with the local community to improve the general health status of all citizens.

Description

APEX-PH is a voluntary program designed to be used by local public health departments in evaluating their own organizational structures and procedures, with a view to making improvements in each department's operation and following up with ongoing evaluation of those changes. The program consists of three parts, the first of which is a review and assessment of the department's organizational capacity. The review examines the legal authority under which the department operates, the ways in which it interacts with the local community, the ways in which policies are developed, and the administrative structure through which actions are taken. The second part of the program is called Community Process. It involves a joint review by members of the local public health staff and members of the general public of the general health of the community and specific health problems that may be present. The review makes use of not only data about public health issues, but also about public perceptions of the general health of the community. Part three of the program is called Completing the Cycle, a stage of the process that depends on findings produced in the first two steps of the program. This final stage of the process involves a discussion of policy development, monitoring of programs and accomplishments, and evaluation of plans developed in phases one and two of the project. The original guidelines developed for the implementation of APEX-PH contained detailed instructions for each of the primary steps. For example, stage one, Organizational Capacity Assessment, consisted of eight discrete steps: prepare for organizational capacity assessment, score indicators for importance and current status, identify strengths and weaknesses, analyze and report strengths, analyze weaknesses, rank problems in order of priority, development and implement action plans, and institutionalize the assessment process.

Public health officials have expressed the view that APEX-PH has been a powerful tool in improving the function of local departments. However, they have also pointed out two major deficiencies in the program. The first is a lack of attention to the importance and role of **environmental health** problems in public health programs. The second was the inattention to strategic planning in APEX-PH. In order to respond to these deficiences, NACCHO and **CDC** have collaborated to produce two additional programs for use with (or in place of) APEX-PH. These are the Protocol for Assessing Community Excellence in Environmental Health (PACE EH) and **Mobilizing for Action through Planning and Partnerships (MAPP)**. This suite of programs now provides a comprehensive mode for approaching the assessment and improvement of public health programs at the local level.

Professional Publications

Most of the original print and electronic material relating to the APEX-PH is no longer generally available. Some basic information about the program is archived at a number of locations, including

- CDC Wonder. Centers for Disease Control and Prevention. http://wonder.cdc.gov/wonder/prevguid/p0000089/p0000089.asp#head002000000000000
- APEXPH. National Association of County & City Health Officials. http://www.naccho.org/topics/infrastructure/APEXPH/index.cfm
- APEXPH, PACE EH, and MAPP: Local Public Health Planning and Assessment at a Glance. National Association of City & County Health Officials. http://www.naccho.org/topics/infrastructure/mapp/upload/MappPaceApex.pdf

Resources

BOOKS

American Public Health Association, et al. *APEXPH: Assessment Protocol for Excellence in Public Health.* Washington, D.C.: National Association of County Health Officials, 1991.

PERIODICALS

McDonald, Tim L., Charles D. Treser, and Jack B. Hatlen. "Development of an Environmental Health Addendum to the Assessment Protocol for Excellence in Public Health." *Journal of Public Health Policy*. 15. 2 (1994): 203–17.

Linnan, Laura, et al. "Planning and the Professional Preparation of Health Educators: Implications for Teaching, Research, and Practice." *Health Promotion Practice*. 6. 3 (2005): 308–19

WEBSITES

Assessment Protocol for Excellence in Public Health (APEXPH). Centers for Disease Control and Prevention. http://wonder.cdc.gov/wonder/prevguid/p0000089/p0000089.asp#head002000000000000. (accessed October 10, 2012).

ORGANIZATIONS

Centers for Disease Control and Prevention, 1600 Clifton Rd., Atlanta, GA USA 30333, (800) 232-4636, cdcinfo@cdc.gov, http://www.cdc.gov/.

David E. Newton, EdD

Association of State and Territorial Health Officials (ASTHO)

Definition

The Association of State and Territorial Health Officials (ASTHO) is a national nonprofit organization that represents public health agencies in the fifty states, six U.S. Territories, and the District of Columbia, as well as the more than 100,000 men and women employed by these agencies.

Purpose

The purpose of the ASTHO is to follow the development of public policy relating to public health issues, to assess those developments, and to transmit to its members information about the way in which these policy changes are likely to impact the work they do. The organization also provides its members with information that will contribute to the general improvement of the citizens with whom their agencies work.

Description

ASTHO traces its history to an 1879 meeting of the Sanitary Council of the Mississippi Valley called to discuss an outbreak of **cholera** in the area. Attendees at the meeting considered the possibility of forming a national organization that could deal with common problems faced by public health officials. The following year, representatives from 19 states met in Detroit to establish such an organization, the National Conferences of State Boards of Health. For the first third of the twentieth century, the organization was concerned primarily with the threat posed to public health by infectious diseases such as **yellow fever** and **diphtheria**. It held annual conferences to discuss ways of better dealing with such threats. After adoption of the Social Security Act of 1935, the organization recognized a need to expand its interests to the growing role of both federal and state government in the operation of local public health agencies. Finally, on March 23, 1942, the organization incorporated itself under its present name to better carry out these objectives. Today, the ASTHO is part of a large network of public health organizations that includes twenty affiliated organizations such as the Association of Health Facility Survey Agencies, Association of **Immunization** Managers, Association of Public Health Laboratories, Council of State and Territorial Epidemiologists, and National Association of Vector-Borne Disease Control Officials.

Today, ASTHO's work is organized around about a dozen major themes that include accreditation and performance, e-health, **environmental health**, health reform, immunization, **infectious disease**, preparedness, and preparation. As an example, the e-health program is designed to help public health agencies use electronic resources to the maximum extent possible for such applications as collecting and interpreting health statistics and safeguarding the privacy of individual health data. The preparedness program aids local public health agencies to develop strategies for dealing with bioterrorist attacks and other threats to public health.

One of the most important functions of ASTHO is to act as an advocate for the public health profession before the U.S. Congress, administrative agencies, and other decision-making organizations. It also acts as an essential source of information for its members about federal and state programs that are available for local public health agencies. An example is the organization's distribution of information about federal aid available to local public health programs for **natural disasters** such as the 2011 tornado that destroyed much of the city of Joplin, Missouri. Under grants from the Robert Wood Johnson Foundation and the **Centers for Disease Control and Prevention**, ASTHO is also developing a comprehensive and sophisticated database of public health activities in the United States and its territories. The organization annually sponsors one major conference and a number of other meetings and webinars that deal with specific topics of interest to public health agencies.

Professional Publications

The ASTHO's major publication is its annual report, which contains an overview of its goals and objectives, its major accomplishments for the year, and a description of its ongoing programs. In addition, the organization publishes a number of reports on specific topics of interest in public health, such as *Health Reform and Public Health*, *State Perspectives on the Use of Fiscal Intermediaries*, *Prescription Drug Overdose: State Health Agencies Respond*, and *2007 Public Health Workforce Report*.

Resources

PERIODICALS

Corso, L. C., et al. "The National Public Health Performance Standards: Driving Quality Improvement in Public Health Systems." *Journal of Public Health Management and Practice*. 16. 1. (2010): 19–23

Gebbie, Kristine. "Public Health Certification." *Annual Review of Public Health*. 30. 1. (2009): 203–10

Kirkwood, J., and P. E. Jarris. "Aligning Health Informatics across the Public Health Enterprise." *Journal of Public Health Management and Practice*. 18. 3. (2012): 288–90

WEBSITES

Association of State and Territorial Health Officials. Centers for Disease Control and Prevention. http://www.cdc.gov/stltpublichealth/partnerships/astho.html (accessed October 10, 2012).

ORGANIZATIONS

Association of State and Territorial Health Officeers, 2231 Crystal Dr., Suite 450, Arlington, VA 22202, (202) 371-9090, Fax: (571) 527-3189, http://www.astho.org/.

David E. Newton, EdD

Asthma

Definition

Asthma is a chronic (long-lasting) inflammatory disease of the airways. In those susceptible to asthma, this inflammation causes the airways to spasm and swell periodically so that the airways narrow. The individual then must wheeze or gasp for air. Obstruction to air flow

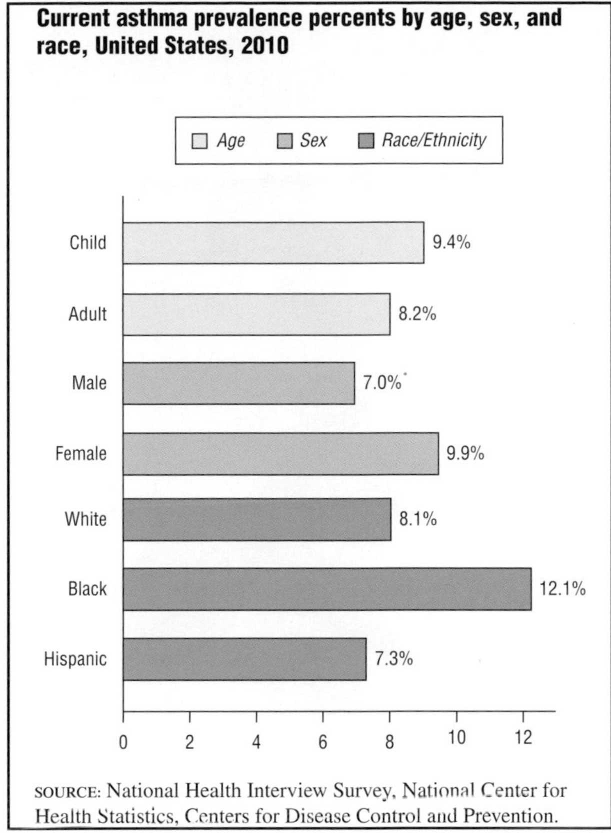

(Table by PreMediaGlobal. © 2013 Cengage Learning)

either resolves spontaneously or responds to a wide range of treatments, but continuing inflammation makes the airways hyper-responsive to stimuli such as cold air, exercise, dust mites, pollutants in the air, and even **stress** and anxiety.

Demographics

Asthma is common in industrialized countries. In the United States, it is estimated to affect between 10% and 15% of the population. This number appears to be both increasing, especially among children under age 6, while at the same time the disease is becoming more severe. Asthma is estimated to cause between 3,500 and 5,000 deaths annually in the United States. In 2007, it was responsible for 217,000 emergency room visits and 10.4 million office visits. Its estimated cost to the United States economy is about $20 billion. Worldwide, asthma is estimated to affect 300 million people.

About two-thirds of all cases of asthma are diagnosed in people under age 18, but asthma also may first appear during adult years. More women than men are diagnosed with adult-onset asthma. While the symptoms may be similar, certain important aspects of asthma differ in children and adults.

Description

The changes that take place in the lungs of people with asthma makes the airways (the "breathing tubes," or bronchi and the smaller bronchioles) hyper-reactive to many different types of stimuli that do not affect healthy lungs. In an asthma attack, the muscle tissue in the walls of bronchi go into spasm, and the cells lining the airways swell and secrete mucus into the airways. Both these actions cause the bronchi to become narrowed (bronchoconstriction). As a result, an asthmatic person has to make a much greater effort to breathe in air and to expel it.

Cells in the bronchial walls, called mast cells, release certain substances that cause the bronchial muscle to contract and stimulate mucus formation. These substances, which include histamine and a group of chemicals called leukotrienes, also bring white blood cells into the area, which is a key part of the inflammatory response. Many individuals with asthma are sensitized to react to such "foreign" substances as pollen, house dust mites, or animal dander; these substances are called allergens. On the other hand, asthma affects many individuals who are not allergic in this way.

Risk factors

Asthma is closely linked to **allergies**; about 75% of people with asthma also have allergies.

Child-onset asthma

About nine million American children have been diagnosed with asthma. Approximately 20% of cases begin in the first year of life. When asthma begins in childhood, it often does so in a child who is likely, for genetic reasons, to become sensitized to common allergens in the environment (an atopic person). When these children are exposed to dust mites, animal proteins (i.e., animal hair, dander), **mold**, or other potential allergens, they produce a type of antibody that is intended to engulf and destroy the foreign materials. This has the effect of making the airway cells sensitive to particular materials. Further exposure can lead rapidly to an asthmatic response. This condition, called atopy, is present in at least one-third and as many as one-half of the general population.

Adult-onset asthma

Allergies also may play a role when adults become asthmatic. Adults who develop asthma may be exposed to allergens in the workplace, such as certain forms of plastic, solvents, and wood dust. Other adults may be sensitive to aspirin, nonsteroidal anti-inflammatory drugs (NSAIDs, such as ibuprofen), or other drugs. Compared to childhood-onset asthma, adult-onset asthma tends to be more continuous, while childhood asthma often is

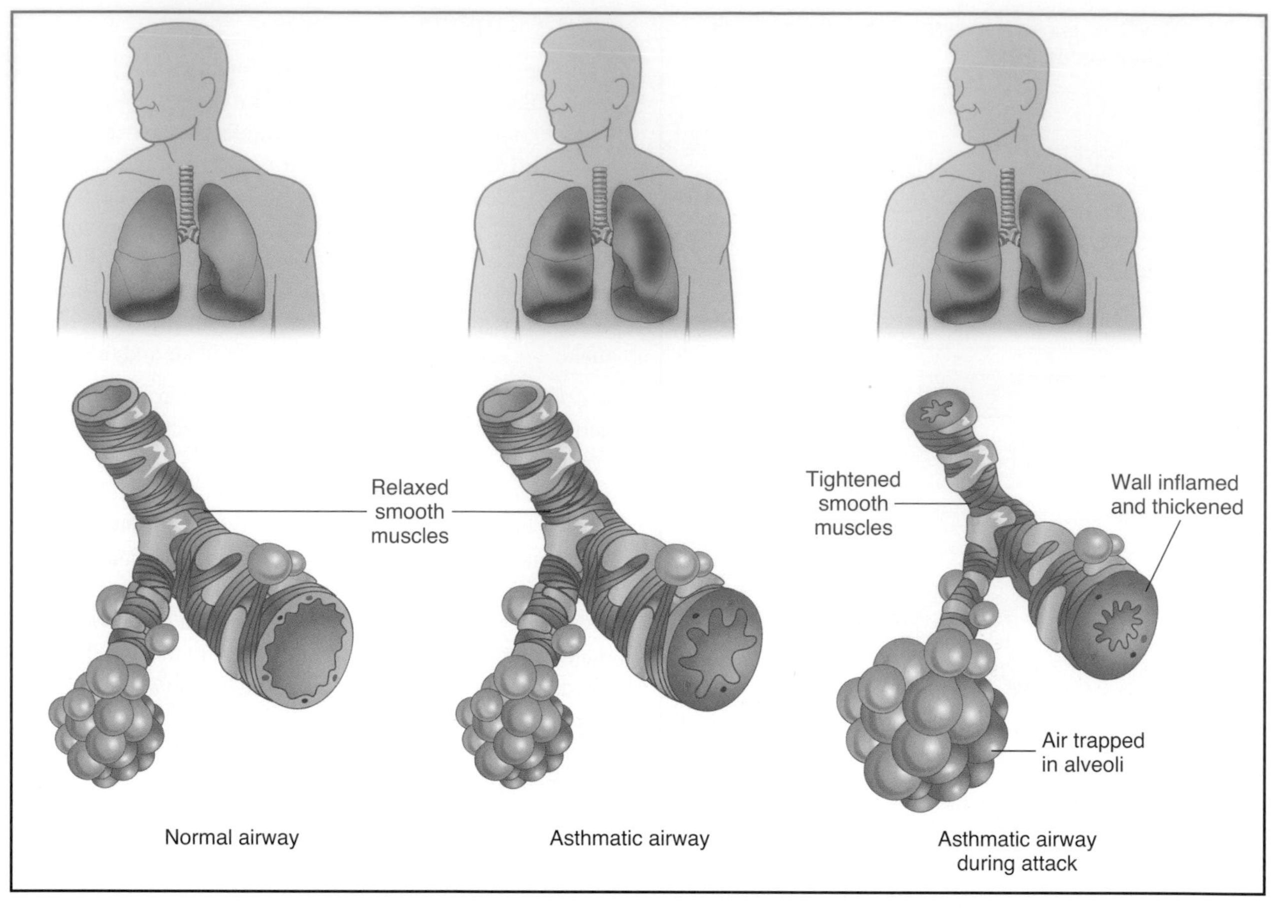

Examples of normal and asthmatic lung airways. *(Illustration by Electronic Illustrators Group. © 2013 Cengage Learning)*

marked by asthmatic episodes followed by asthma-free periods.

Exercise-induced asthma

People who do not have allergies can still develop a form of asthma that is brought on by aerobic exercise. These episodes can last for several minutes and leave the individual gasping for breath. Some estimates suggest that 12–15% of Americans who do not have allergies are susceptible to exercise-induced asthma; rates of 40–90% have been reported in individuals who do have allergies. Inhaling cold air, aerobic exercise lasting more than 10 minutes, or shorter periods of very heavy aerobic exercise, tend to trigger an exercise-induced asthma attack in susceptible individuals. Polluted air and certain chemicals (e.g., chlorine in pools, herbicides on a playing field) appear to increase the likelihood of an asthma episodes in sensitive individuals.

Causes and symptoms

In most cases, asthma is caused by inhaling an allergen to which the individual is hypersensitized. This sets off the chain of biochemical and tissue changes leading to airway inflammation, bronchoconstriction, and wheezing. Avoiding or at least minimizing exposure to asthma triggers is the most effective way of treating asthma, so it is helpful to identify which specific allergen or irritant is causing symptoms in a particular individual. Once asthma is present, symptoms may be triggered or aggravated if the individual also has rhinitis (inflammation of the lining of the nose as from allergies) or sinusitis (sinus inflammation). When stomach acid passes back up the esophagus (acid reflux), this also may worsen asthma symptoms. A viral infection of the respiratory tract (e.g., a cold) also may trigger or worsen an asthmatic reaction. Aspirin, NSAIDs, and beta-blocker drugs also may worsen the symptoms of asthma.

The most common inhaled allergens that trigger asthma attacks are:

- animal dander
- mites in house dust
- fungi (molds) that grow indoors
- cockroach allergens

- pollen
- chemicals, fumes, or airborne industrial pollutants
- smoke

Inhaling tobacco smoke, either by **smoking** or being around people who are smoking, can irritate the airways and trigger an asthmatic attack. Air pollutants such as wood smoke can have a similar effect. In addition, three factors that regularly produce attacks in certain asthmatic individuals, and may sometimes be the sole cause of symptoms are:

- inhaling cold air (cold-induced asthma)
- exercise-induced asthma
- stress or a high level of anxiety

Wheezing is often obvious, but mild asthma attacks may be confirmed only when the physician listens to the individual's chest with a stethoscope. Besides wheezing and being short of breath, the individual may cough and/or may report a feeling of "tightness" in the chest. Wheezing is often loudest when the individual breathes out (exhales) in an attempt to expel air through the narrowed airways. Some people with asthma are free of symptoms most of the time but occasionally may have episodes of shortness of breath. Others spend much of their time wheezing or have frequent bouts of shortness of breath until properly treated. Crying or laughing may bring on an attack. Severe episodes often develop when the individual has a viral respiratory tract infection or is exposed to a heavy load of an allergen or irritant (e.g., breathing in smoke from a campfire). Asthma attacks may last only a few minutes or can continue for hours or even days (a condition called status asthmaticus).

Being short of breath may cause an individual to become visibly anxious, sit upright, lean forward, and use the muscles of the neck and chest wall to help move air in and out of the lungs. The individual may be able to say only a few words at a time before stopping to take a breath. Confusion and a bluish tint to the skin are clues that the oxygen supply is seriously low and that emergency treatment is needed. In a severe attack that lasts for an extended period, some of the air sacs in the lung may rupture so that air collects within the chest. This makes it even harder for the lungs to exchange enough air.

Diagnosis

The physician will ask about a family history of asthma or allergies. A diagnosis of asthma may be strongly suggested when typical signs and symptoms are present. Apart from listening to the individual's chest, the examiner should look for maximum chest expansion while taking in air. Hunched shoulders and contracted neck muscles are other signs of narrowed airways. Nasal polyps or increased amounts of nasal secretions often are noted in asthmatic individuals. Skin changes, such as atopic dermatitis or eczema, are indications that the individual is likely to allergies.

KEY TERMS

Allergen—A foreign substance, such as mites in house dust or animal dander which, when inhaled, causes the airways to narrow and produces symptoms of asthma.

Atopy—A state that makes persons more likely to develop allergic reactions of any type, including the inflammation and airway narrowing typical of asthma.

Beta blockers—Drugs used to treat high blood pressure (hypertension) that limit the activity of epinephrine, a hormone that increases blood pressure.

Hypersensitivity—The state where even a tiny amount of allergen can cause the airways to constrict and bring on an asthmatic attack.

Spirometry—A test using an instrument called a spirometer that shows how difficult it is for an asthmatic individual to breathe. It is used to determine the severity of asthma and to see how well it is responding to treatment.

Tests

A test called spirometry measures how rapidly air is exhaled and how much air is retained in the lungs. Repeating the test after the individual inhales a bronchodilator drug that widens the airways will show whether the airway narrowing is reversible, which is a very typical finding in asthma. Often individuals use a related instrument, called a peak flow meter, to keep track of asthma severity when at home.

It often is difficult to determine what is triggering asthma attacks. Allergy skin testing may be used, although an allergic skin response does not always mean that the allergen being tested is causing the asthma. The body's immune system produces specific antibody to fight off each allergen. Measuring the amount of a specific antibody in the blood may indicate how sensitive the individual is to a particular allergen. If the diagnosis is still in doubt, the individual can inhale a suspect allergen while using a spirometer to detect airway narrowing. Spirometry also can be repeated after a bout of exercise when exercise-induced asthma is suspected. A chest x ray may be done to help rule out other lung disorders.

Treatment

The goals of asthma treatment are to prevent troublesome symptoms, maintain lung function as close to normal as possible, and allow individuals to pursue their normal activities including those requiring exertion. Individuals should periodically be examined and have their lung function measured by spirometry to make sure that treatment goals are being met. The best drug therapy is that which controls asthmatic symptoms while causing few or no side effects. Many people with asthma are treated with a combination of long-acting drugs taken on a regular basis to help prevent asthma attacks and short-acting (quick relief) drugs given by inhaler to reduce the immediate symptoms of an attack.

Drugs

The choice of initial drug treatment often depends on whether the asthma is classified as intermittent, mildly persistent, moderately persistent, or severely persistent, the age of the individual, other medical conditions that may be present, and other drugs the patient may be taking. It make take several attempts to find the best combination of drugs to control the asthma.

BETA-RECEPTOR AGONISTS (BRONCHODILATORS). These drugs, which relax the airways, often are the best choice for relieving sudden attacks of asthma and for preventing attacks of exercise-induced asthma. Some bronchodilators, such as albuterol (Ventolin, Proventil) and levalbuterol (Xopenex), act mainly in lung cells and have little effect on other organs. Bronchodilators occasionally may be taken orally (i.e., pills or liquid), but normally they are administered through inhalers. The inhaled drugs go directly into the lungs and cause fewer side effects. These drugs generally start acting within minutes, but their effects last only four to six hours.

Long-acting beta agonists (LABAs) have been developed that can last up to 12 hours. These include salmeterol (Severent Diskus), fluticasone/salmeterol (Advair Diskus), arformoterol (Brovana), formoterol (Perforomist, Foradil), and budesonide/formoterol (Symbacort). In December 2008, the United States Food and Drug Administration (FDA) issued a warning that LABAs may increase the chance of severe asthma episodes and asthma-caused death, but was divided on whether these drugs should be banned for use in children. As of early 2009, LABAs were not recommended as a first-line treatment for asthma or for use alone (i.e., without inhaled steroids) as an asthma treatment. The FDA strongly recommends that people taking LABAs discuss the risks and benefits with their physician in light of emerging information about their safety.

LEUKOTRIENE RECEPTOR ANTAGONISTS. The leukotriene receptor antagonists such as montelukast (Singulair), zafirlukast (Accolate), and Zyflo (zileuton) control inflammation of the airways by blocking the action of leukotrienes, which are chemicals involved in producing inflammation. These drugs are tablets taken by mouth on a regular basis to treat or prevent symptoms of asthma and exercise-induced asthma. In March 2008, the FDA released a preliminary warning that Singulair might cause behavior and mood changes, suicidal thinking and behavior, and **suicide**. The warning was preliminary, meaning a cause and effect relationship between these adverse reactions and the drug had not been definitely established, and that more information was needed. The FDA recommended that individuals taking Singulair or any other leukotriene receptor antagonist drug should be alert to these behavioral side effects but not stop taking these drugs until they had discussed their condition with a physician.

CORTICOSTEROIDS. These drugs, which resemble natural body hormones, block inflammation and are often effective in relieving symptoms of chronic asthma and preventing asthma episodes, but they generally are not used to treat asthma attacks once they have begun. Examples include fluticasone (Flovent), triamcinolone (Azmacort), and beclomethasone (Vanceril, Beclovent, QVAR) all of which are taken by inhalation. When corticosteroids are taken by inhalation over a long time, asthma attacks become less frequent as the airways become less sensitive to allergens. Prendisone (Deltasone, Orasone, Meticorten) is given by mouth (i.e., pills) to speed recovery after treatment of initial symptoms of an asthma attack and sometimes to treat chronic asthma.

Corticosteroids are strong drugs and usually can control even severe cases of asthma over the long term and maintain good lung function. Corticosteroids may cause numerous side effects, however, including bleeding from the stomach, loss of calcium from bones, cataracts in the eye, and a diabetes-like state. Individuals using corticosteroids for lengthy periods also may have problems with wound healing, may gain weight, and may experience psychological problems. In children, growth may be slowed.

OTHER DRUGS. Cromolyn (Intal) and nedocromil (Tilade) are anti-inflammatory drugs that affect mast cells. They may be used as initial treatment to prevent asthmatic attacks. They may also prevent attacks when given before exercise or when exposure to an allergen cannot be avoided. To be effective, these drugs must be taken regularly even if there are no asthma symptoms. Anticholinergic drugs, such as atropine, may be useful in controlling severe attacks when added to an inhaled beta-receptor agonist. They help widen the airways and suppress mucus production.

Managing asthmatic attacks

A severe asthma attack should be treated as quickly as possible; professional emergency medical assistance may be needed, as an individual experiencing an acute attack may need to be given extra oxygen. Rarely is it necessary to use a mechanical ventilator to help the individual breathe. An inhaler, usually containing a beta-receptor agonist, is inhaled repeatedly or continuously. If the individual does not respond promptly and completely, a corticosteroid may be given. A course of corticosteroid therapy, given after the attack is over, may make a recurrence less likely.

Many asthma experts recommend a device called a "spacer" to be used along with metered-dose inhalers. The spacer is a tube or bellows-like device held in or around the mouth into which the metered-dose inhaler is puffed. This device enables more medication from a metered-dose inhaler to reach the lungs.

Maintaining control

Long-term asthma treatment is based on inhaling appropriate drugs using a special inhaler that meters the dose. Individuals must be instructed in proper use of an inhaler to be sure that it will deliver the right amount of drug. Once asthma has been controlled for several weeks or months, a physician may recommend that the patient gradually cut down on drug treatment. The last drug added usually is the first to be reduced. Individuals should be seen by their physician every one to six months, or as needed, depending on the frequency of asthma episodes.

School-age and older children may also be prescribed peak flow meters, simple devices which measure how easy or difficult it is for a person to exhale. With home peak-flow monitoring, it is possible for many children with asthma to discern at an early stage that a flare-up is just beginning and adjust their medications appropriately.

Individuals with asthma do best when they have a written action plan to follow if symptoms suddenly become worse. This plan should address how to adjust their medication and when to seek medical help. A 2004 report found that individuals with self-management written action plans had fewer hospitalizations, fewer emergency department visits, and improved lung function. They also had a 70% lower mortality rate.

Referral to an asthma specialist should be considered if:

- a life-threatening asthma attack has occurred or if asthma is severe and persistent
- treatment for three to six months has not met its goals
- some other condition, such as nasal polyps or chronic lung disease, is complicating asthma treatment
- special tests, such as allergy skin testing or an allergen challenge, are needed
- intensive long-term corticosteroid therapy has been needed to control asthma.

Special populations

INFANTS AND YOUNG CHILDREN. It is especially important to closely watch the course of asthma in young individuals. Treatment is cut down when possible, and if there is no clear improvement, treatment should be modified. Asthmatic children often need medication at school to control acute symptoms or to prevent exercise-induced attacks. Parents or guardians of these children should consult the school district on their drug policy in order to assure that a procedure is in place to permit their child to carry an inhaler. The health care provider should write an asthma treatment plan for the child's school. Proper management will usually allow a child to take part in play activities. Only as a last resort should activities be limited.

THE ELDERLY. Older persons often have other types of lung disease, such as chronic bronchitis or emphysema. These must be taken into account when treating asthma symptoms. Side effects from beta-receptor agonist drugs (including a speeding heart and tremor) may be more common in older individuals.

Alternative Treatments

Alternative medicine tends to view asthma as the body's protective reaction to environmental agents and pollutants. As such, the treatment goal is often to restore balance to and strengthen the entire body and provide specific support to the lungs and to the immune and hormonal systems. Individuals with asthma can help by keeping a diary of asthma attacks in order to determine environmental and emotional factors that may be contributing to their condition.

Alternative treatments have minimal side effects, are generally inexpensive, and are convenient forms of self-treatment. They also can be used alongside allopathic (traditional drug treatments) treatments to improve their effectiveness and lessen their negative side effects.

DIETARY AND NUTRITIONAL THERAPIES. Some alternative practitioners recommend cutting down on or eliminating dairy products from the diet, as these increase mucus secretion in the lungs and are sources of food allergies. Other recommendations include avoiding processed foods, refined starches and sugars, and foods with artificial additives and sulfites. Beneficial diets should be high in fresh fruits, vegetables, and whole grains, and low in salt. Individuals with asthma should experiment with their diets to determine if food allergies are playing a role in their asthma. Some studies have shown that a sustained vegan diet can be effective in controlling asthma.

Individuals with asthma also should stay well hydrated by drinking plenty of water, as water helps to keep the passages of the lungs moist. Onions and garlic contain quercetin, a flavonoid (a chemical compound/biological response modifier) that inhibits the release of histamine, and should be a part of an asthmatic's diet. Quercetin is also available as a supplement and should be taken with a digestive enzyme to increase its absorption.

As nutritional therapy, **vitamins** A, C, and E have been touted as important treatments for asthma. Also, the B complex vitamins, particularly B_6 and B_{12}, may be helpful for individuals with asthma, as well as magnesium, selenium, and an omega-3 fatty acid supplement such as flaxseed oil. A good multivitamin supplement also is recommended.

Herbal remedies

Chinese medicine has traditionally used *ma huang* for asthma attacks. Ma huang contains ephedrine, a bronchodilator that was once used in many drugs. However, the FDA issued a ban on the sale of ephedra that took effect in April 2004 because it was shown to raise blood pressure and stress the circulatory system, resulting in heart attacks and strokes for some users. Manufacturers of ephedra raised legal challenges to this decision. When the U. S. Supreme Court refused to hear these challenges in 2007, however, the ban on ephedra became permanent.

Another herbal product, ginkgo, has been shown to reduce the frequency of asthma attacks, and licorice is used in traditional Chinese medicine as a natural decongestant and expectorant. There are many formulas used in traditional Chinese medicine to prevent or ease asthma attacks, depending on the specific Chinese diagnosis given by the practitioner.

Other herbs used for asthma include lobelia, also called Indian tobacco; nettle, which contains a natural antihistamine; thyme, mullein, feverfew, passionflower, saw palmetto and Asian ginseng. Coffee and tea have been shown to reduce the severity of asthma attacks because caffeine works as a bronchodilator. Tea also contains minute amounts of theophylline, a drug used to treat asthma. Ayurvedic (traditional East Indian) medicine recommends the herb *Tylophora asthmatica.*

Mind/body approaches

Mind/body medicine has demonstrated that psychological factors play a complex role in asthma. Emotional stress can trigger asthma attacks. Mind/body techniques strive to reduce stress and help asthma sufferers manage the psychological component of their condition. Biofeedback is a treatment method that uses monitors to reveal physiological information to patients, to teach relaxation and deep breathing methods that may help people with asthma. Some other mind/body techniques used for asthma include relaxation methods, meditation, hypnotherapy, mental imaging, psychotherapy, and visualization.

Yoga and breathing methods

Some studies have shown that yoga significantly helps people with asthma by teaching exercises specifically designed to expand the lungs, promote deep breathing, and reduce stress. Pranayama is the yogic science of breathing, which includes hundreds of deep breathing techniques. These breathing exercises may be done daily as part of any treatment program for asthma, as they are an effective and inexpensive measure.

Controlled exercise

Many people believe that people with asthma should not exercise. This belief is especially common among parents of children with asthma. In a 2004 study, researchers reported that 20% of children with asthma do not get enough exercise. Many parents believe it is dangerous for their children with asthma to exercise, but **physical activity** benefits all children, including those with asthma. Parents should work with their children's healthcare providers and any coach or organized sport leader to carefully monitor the children's activities.

Acupuncture

Acupuncture can be an effective treatment for asthma. It is used in traditional Chinese medicine along with dietary changes. Acupressure also can be used as a self-treatment for asthma attacks and **prevention**. The Lung 1 points, used to stimulate breathing, can be easily found on the chest. These are sensitive, often knotted spots on the muscles that run horizontally about an inch below the collarbone, and about two inches from the center of the chest. The points can be pressed in a circular manner with the thumbs, while the head is allowed to hang forward and the individual takes slow, deep breaths.

Reflexology also uses particular acupressure points on the hands and feet that are believed to stimulate the lungs.

Other treatments

Aromatherapists recommend eucalyptus, lavender, rosemary, and chamomile as fragrances that promote free breathing. In Japan, a common treatment for asthma is administering cold baths. This form of hydrotherapy has been demonstrated to open constricted air passages. Massage therapies such as Rolfing can help individuals with asthma as well, as they strive to open and increase circulation in the chest area. Homeopathy uses the remedies *Arsenicum album, Kali carbonicum, Natrum sulphuricum,* and *Aconite*.

Prognosis

More than half of all asthma cases in children resolve by young adulthood, but chronic infection, pollution, cigarette smoke, and chronic allergen exposure are factors which make resolution less likely. Infants and toddlers who have persistent wheezing even without viral infections and those who have a family history of allergies are most likely to continue to have asthma into the school-age years.

Most individuals with asthma respond well once the proper drug or combination of drugs is found, and most asthmatics are able to lead relatively normal, active lives. A few individuals will have progressively more trouble breathing and run a risk of going into respiratory failure, for which they must receive intensive treatment. Asthma causes between 3,500 and 5,000 deaths in the United States each year.

Prevention

Exposure to the common allergens and irritants that provoke asthmatic attacks often can be reduced or avoided by implementing the following:

- If the individual is sensitive to a family pet, remove the animal from the home. If this is not acceptable, keep the pet out of the bedroom (with the bedroom door closed), remove carpeting, and keep the animal away from upholstered furniture.
- To reduce exposure to dust mites, remove wall-to-wall carpeting, keep humidity low, and use special covers for pillows and mattresses. Reduce the number of stuffed toys and wash them weekly in hot water.
- If cockroach allergen is causing asthma attacks, killing the roaches using poison, traps, or boric acid is preferable to using sprayed pesticides. Avoid leaving food or garbage exposed to discourage re-infestation.
- Keep indoor air clean by vacuuming carpets once or twice a week (with the asthmatic individual absent). Avoid using humidifiers and use air conditioning during warm weather so that windows can be kept closed. Change heating and air conditioning filters regularly. High-efficiency particulate air (HEPA) filters are available that are very effective in removing allergens from household air.
- Avoid exposure to tobacco or wood smoke.
- Do not exercise outdoors when air pollution levels are high or when air is extremely cold.
- When asthma is related to exposure at work, take all precautions, including wearing a mask and, if necessary, arranging to work in a safer area. Occupational safety and health (OSHA) regulations limit exposure to certain pollutants and potential allergens in the workplace.

Resources

BOOKS

Allen, Julian Lewis et al. eds. The Children's Hospital of Philadelphia Guide to Asthma: How to Help You Child Live a Healthier Life. Hoboken, NJ: J. Wiley, 2004.

OTHER

"Asthma." *United States Centers for Disease Control and Prevention.* [August 19, 2009]. http://www.cdc.gov/asthma.

"Asthma." *MedlinePlus.* [August 19, 2009]. http://www.nlm.nih.gov/medlineplus/asthma.html.

Morris, Michael. "Asthma." *eMedicine.com.* [August 18, 2009]. http://emedicine.medscape.com/article/296301-overview.

ORGANIZATIONS

Allergy and Asthma Network: Mothers of Asthmatics (AANMA), 2751 Prosperity Ave., Suite 150, Fairfax, VA 22031, (800) 878-4403, Fax: (703) 573-7794, http://www.aanma.org

American Academy of Allergy, Asthma, and Immunology (AAAAI), 555 East Wells Street, Suite 1100, Milwaukee, WI 53202-3823, (414) 272-6071, http://www.aaaai.org

American College of Allergy, Asthma, and Immunology, 85 West Algonquin Road, Suite 550, Arlington Heights, IL 60005, (847) 427-1200, mail@acaai.org, http://www.acaai.org

Asthma and Allergy Foundation of America, 1233 20th Street, NW, Suite 402, Washington, DC 20036, (800) 7-ASTHMA or (800) 727-8462, info@aafa.org, http://www.aafa.org

National Institute of Allergy and Infectious Diseases Office of Communications and Government Relations, 6610 Rockledge Drive, MSC 6612, Bethesda, MD 20892-6612, (301) 496-5717, (866) 284-4107 or TDD: (800)877-8339 (for hearing impaired), Fax: (301) 402-3573, http://www3.niaid.nih.gov.

David A. Cramer, M.D.
Tish Davidson, A.M.

Autism

Definition

Autism is a complex developmental disorder distinguished by difficulties with social interaction, verbal and nonverbal communication, and behavioral problems, including repetitive behaviors and narrow focus of interest.

Description

Autism was first described by Leo Kanner in 1943. He observed and described a group of children with "autistic disturbances of affective contact," impaired communication, and behavioral inflexibility. These children had some unique abilities and did not seem to be emotionally disturbed or mentally retarded. He coined the term "infantile autism" and discussed the causes in terms of biological processes, although at that time, most scientific attention was focused on analytical theories of the disorder. Hans Asperger made the same discoveries in the same year. He also described children with a unique behavioral profile and used the term "Autism" to describe them. His original study was in German and was not translated into English until the late 1980s. Because the children that he identified all had speech, the term Asperger syndrome is often used to label autistic children who have speech.

Classic autism is one of several disorders categorized as autism spectrum disorders (ASD). Other ASDs include Asperger syndrome, Rett syndrome, childhood disintegrative disorder, and pervasive developmental disorder. The diagnostic criteria of autism and autism spectrum disorders are being re–evaluated by the American Psychiatric Association in the fifth edition of the *Diagnostic and Statistical Manual of Mental Disorders* (*DSM*), expected to be finalized and put into practice in 2013. It has been proposed that Asperger syndrome be eliminated as a diagnosis and pervasive developmental disorder not otherwise specified (PPD–NOS) be classified as autism spectrum disorder. This proposal is controversial and remains unresolved as of 2012.

Autism usually manifests before a child is three years old and it continues throughout his/her lifetime. The severity of the condition varies between individuals, ranging from the most severe (extremely unusual, repetitive, self–injurious, and aggressive behavior) to very mild. No one autistic child is alike in the manifestation of their symptoms so treatment options must be devised to treat each autistic child individually. Autism cannot be cured but is treatable. With early diagnosis and intensive therapy, autistic children may be able to lead healthy, full lives.

Risk factors

There appears to be a strong genetic basis for autism. Family studies have shown that identical twins are more likely to both be diagnosed with autism than twins who are fraternal (not genetically identical). In a family with one autistic child, the chance of having another child with autism is about one in 20 or approximately 5%, much higher than in the general population.

Other risk factors associated with autism include:

- Gender. Boys are almost four times more likely to be diagnosed with autism than girls.
- Paternal age. Children born of fathers over age 40 have a greater chance of developing autism than children born to younger fathers. The age of the mother appears to have no effect on autism.
- Certain disorders and diseases. Children who have fragile X syndrome, tuberous sclerosis, Tourette syndrome, and epilepsy are more likely to have autism.

Demographics

As of 2012, the Centers for Disease Control (**CDC**) estimate that about one of every 88 children in the United States are affected by ASD. ASD is almost five times more likely to be diagnosed in males. Autism is a disorder that is found worldwide. In the United Kingdom, one out of every 100 children have autism, with more than half a million total diagnosed as of 2010. Studies conducted in Asia, Europe, and North America report a prevalence rate of approximately one percent. Autism is not specific to any one socio–economic, ethnic, or racial group.

Prevalence of Autism Spectrum Disorders

- On average, an estimated 1 in 110 children in the United States have an Autism Spectrum Disorder (ASD).
- Of the roughly 4 million babies born in the United States each year, approximately 36,500 of those children will eventually be diagnosed with an ASD. If the prevalence rate has stayed constant during the past 20 years, then 730,000 individuals between the ages of 0 to 21 born in the United States currently have an ASD.
- ASDs occur in all racial, ethnic, and socioeconomic groups, but are on average 4 to 5 times more likely to occur in boys than in girls.
- Studies in Asia, Europe, and North America have identified a prevalence of ASDs in 0.6% to more than 1% of individuals.
- Approximately 13% of children have a developmental disability, ranging from mild speech and language impairments to more severe disorders such as cerebral palsy and autism.

SOURCE: Centers for Disease Control and Prevention, "Autism Spectrum Disorders (ASDs): Data & Statistics." Available online at: http://www.cdc.gov/ncbddd/autism/data.html (accessed August 18, 2010).

(Table by PreMediaGlobal. © 2013 Cengage Learning)

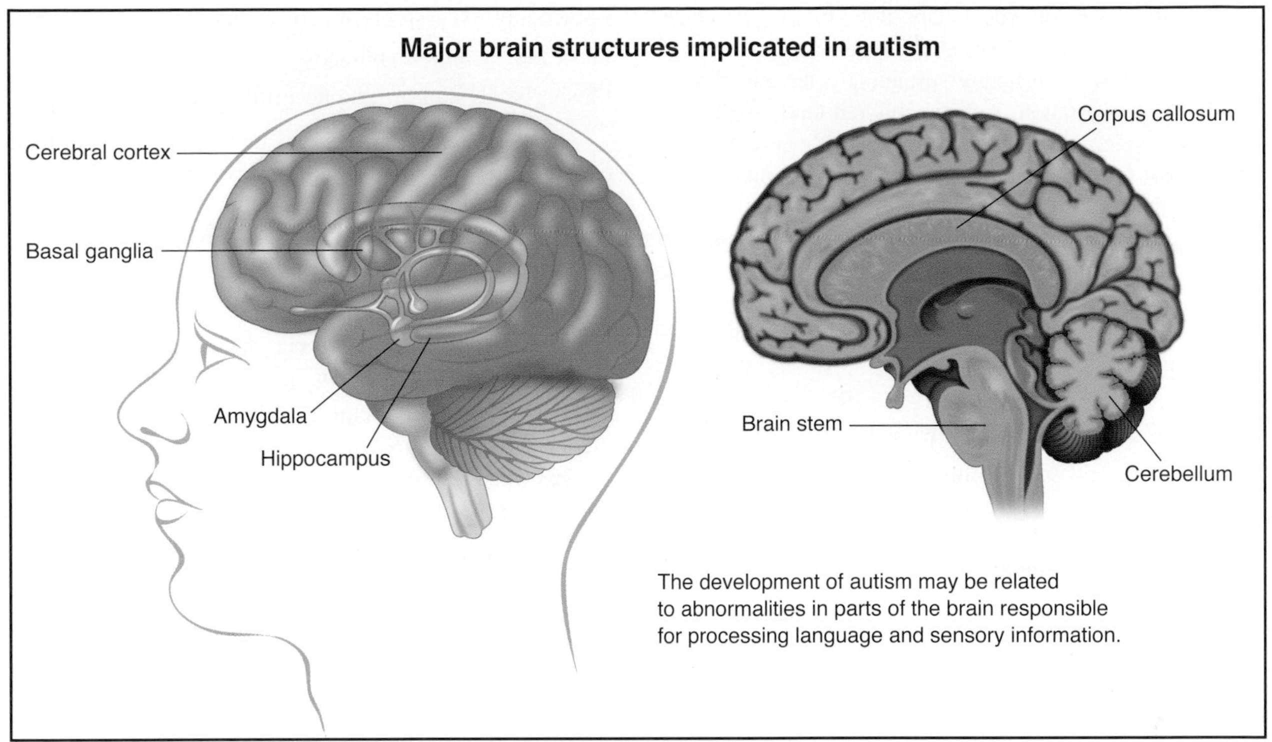

(Illustration by Electronic Illustrators Group. © 2013 Cengage Learning)

Causes and symptoms

Researchers know that autism is a complex brain disorder that affects the way the brain uses or transmits information. Studies have implicated several causes for the disorder including genetic errors and possible environmental triggers, but more investigation is needed. Studies have found abnormalities in several parts of the brain that are believed to have occurred during fetal development. The problem may be centered in the parts of the brain responsible for processing language and information from the senses.

Profound problems with social interaction are the most common symptoms of autism and the most visible. Autistic children have different ways of learning and experiencing the world around them. Often autistic children have more acute reactions to sensory stimulation such as sound and touch. This results in avoidance of eye contact, physical contact, and oftentimes an aversion to music and other sounds. It is perhaps the way autistic children experience their world that causes difficulties with social interaction, language, and nonverbal communication.

Human beings are social and social interaction is present from birth onward. Children with autism have difficulty making social connections. A developmental milestone is when an infant can follow an object or person with his/her gaze. Autistic children tend to avoid eye contact altogether. They do not actively cuddle or hug but rather they passively accept physical contact or they shy away from it. They may become rigid or flaccid when they are held, cry when picked up, and show little interest in human contact. Such a child does not lift his/her arms in anticipation of being picked up. The child may appear to have formed no attachment to his/her parents, and does not learn typical childhood games, such as "peek–a–boo."

Autistic children do not readily learn social cues. They do not know when or how to react to specific social situations or exchanges. Because of this, autistic children tend to look at and respond to different situations similarly. They do not understand that others have different perspectives and, therefore, autistic children seem to lack empathy.

Because of their problems socially and the inability to translate social interactions appropriately, autistic children seem to have uncontrolled emotional outbursts, expressing themselves in a manner that does not suit the specific social situation of the moment.

Language problems

Verbal communication problems vary greatly for autistic children. Some children do not speak at all. Some will only use one or two words at a time. Some autistic children may develop vocabulary only to lose it. Other autistic children may develop an extensive vocabulary; however, they have difficulty sustaining a natural, "back–and–forth" conversation. Autistic children tend to talk in a sing–song voice or more robotically without emotional inflections. Often autistic children do not take body language into consideration and they take what is being said quite literally. Because of their impinged language skills and the inability to express their needs, autistic children seem to act inappropriately to get what they need. They may grab something without asking or blurt out statements.

Restricted interests and activity

Language and social problems inhibit social play for autistic children. Autistic children do not engage in imaginative play and role playing. They focus on repetition, some focusing on a subject of interest very intensely.

Autistic children often stick to a rigid daily routine. Any variance to the routine may be upsetting to them and result in an extreme emotional response. Repetitive physical behaviors such as rocking, spinning, and arm flapping are also characteristic of autism. The repetitive behaviors are often self–soothing responses to sensory stimulation from the outside world.

Sensory problems

The sensory world poses a real problem to many autistic children, who seem overwhelmed by their own senses. A child with autism may ignore objects or become obsessed with them, continually watching the object or the movement of his or her fingers over it. Some children with autism may react to sounds by banging their head or flapping their fingers. Some high–functioning autistic adults who have written books about their childhood experiences report that sounds were often excruciatingly painful to them, forcing them to withdraw from their environment or try to cope by withdrawing into their own world of sensation and movement.

Diagnosis

There is no medical test for diagnosing autism. Diagnosis is made after careful observation and screening by parents, caregivers, and physicians. Early diagnosis is beneficial in treating the symptoms of autism. Some early warning signs are:

- avoiding eye contact
- avoiding physical contact such as hugs
- inability to play make–believe
- not pointing out interesting objects
- not responding to conversation directed at him/her
- practicing excessively repetitive behaviors
- repeating words or phrases
- losing skills and/or language after learning them

Once parents feel there is a problem or their pediatrician has identified developmental problems during well–baby check–ups, they can seek out a developmental pediatrician for further diagnosis. There are several screening tests used. They are:

- Childhood Autism Rating Scale (CARS)—a test based on a 15 point scale where specific behaviors are observed by the physician.
- Checklist for Autism in Toddlers (CHAT)—a test to detect autism in 18–month olds that utilizes questionnaires filled out by both the parents and the pediatrician.
- Autism Screening Questionnaire—a 40–item questionnaire for diagnosing children four and older.
- Screening Test for Autism in Two–Year–Olds—a direct observation of three skill areas including play, motor imitation, and joint attention.

Some children have a few of the symptoms of autism, but not enough to be diagnosed with the "classical" form of the condition. Children who have autistic behavior but no problems with language may be diagnosed with Asperger syndrome by using the Autism Spectrum Screening Questionnaire, the Australian Scale for Asperger syndrome, or the Childhood Asperger Syndrome Test. The American Psychiatric Association may eliminate the diagnosis of Asperger syndrome in 2012. Children who have no initial symptoms but who begin to show autistic behavior as they get older might be diagnosed with childhood disintegrative disorder (CDD), another autistic spectrum disorder. It is also important to rule out other problems that seem similar to autism.

Treatment

Because the symptoms of autism can vary greatly from one person to the next, there is not a single treatment that works for every person. A spectrum of interventions including behavioral and educational training, diet and **nutrition**, **alternative medicine** and therapies, and medication should be utilized and finetuned to treat the individual. The most strongly recommended treatment option is behavioral and educational training. Early intervention and treatment is key to helping autistic children grow into productive adults.

Educational and behavioral treatment

Several educational and behavioral treatments are:

- Applied Behavior Analysis (ABA)
- speech therapy

- occupational therapy, including sensory integration therapy
- social skills therapy, including play therapy

Typically, behavioral techniques are used to help the child respond and decrease symptoms. This might include positive reinforcement to boost language and social skills. This training includes structured, skill–oriented instruction designed to improve social and language abilities. Training needs to begin as early as possible, since early intervention appears to positively influence brain development.

Most autistic children respond to intervention at home as well as at school. Schools focus on areas where the child may be delayed, such as in speech or socialization. As autistic children grow and move to different phases of childhood and adolescence, parents in collaboration with educators and physicians need to adapt the treatment to best suit the needs of their autistic child.

Medication

No single medication treats symptoms of autism; however, some medications have been used to combat specific needs in autistic children. Drugs can control epilepsy, which affects up to 20% of people with autism. Medication can also treat anxiety, depression, and hyperactivity. Medication must be individualized and adjusted as the child develops.

Five types of drugs are sometimes prescribed to help the behavior problems of people with autism are:

- stimulants, such as methylphenidate (Ritalin)
- antidepressants, such as fluvoxamine (Luvox)
- opiate blockers, such as naltrexone (ReVia)
- antipsychotics
- tranquilizers

Alternative treatment

Some parents report success with megavitamin therapy. Some studies have shown that vitamin B_6 with magnesium improves eye contact and speech and lessens tantrum behavior. Vitamin B_6 causes fewer side effects than other medications and is considered safe when used in appropriate doses. However, not many health practitioners advocate its use in the treatment of autism, citing that the studies showing its benefit were flawed.

DMG (dimethylglycine)

This compound, available in many health food stores, is legally classified as a food, not a vitamin or drug. Some researchers claim that it improves speech in children with autism. Those who respond to this treatment will usually do so within a week. Again, many doctors do not feel that the studies are adequate to promote this treatment.

Diet

Many parents have seen beneficial effects from a gluten–free and casein–free diet. Gluten is a substance found in the seeds of cereal plants such as wheat, barley, oats, and rye. Casein is a protein found in milk. Often people have sensitivities to these substances without

KEY TERMS

Antidepressants—A type of medication that is used to treat depression; it is also sometimes used to treat autism.

Asperger syndrome—Children who have autistic behavior but no problems with language and no clinically significant cognitive delay.

Fragile X syndrome—A genetic condition related to the X chromosome that affects mental, physical and sensory development.

Major tranquilizers—The family of drugs that includes the psychotropic or neuroleptic drugs, sometimes used to help autistic people. They carry significant risk of side effects, including Parkinsonism and movement disorders, and should be prescribed with caution.

Opiate blockers—A type of drug that blocks the effects of natural opiates in the system. This makes some people, including some people with autism, appear more responsive to their environment.

Phenylketonuria (PKU)—An enzyme deficiency present at birth that disrupts metabolism and causes brain damage. This rare inherited defect may be linked to the development of autism.

Rubella—Also known as German measles. When a woman contracts rubella during pregnancy, her developing infant may be damaged. One of the problems that may result is autism.

Stimulants—A class of drugs, including Ritalin, used to treat people with autism. They may make children calmer and better able to concentrate, but they also may limit growth or have other side effects.

Tuberous sclerosis—A genetic disease that causes skin problems, seizures, and mental retardation. Autism occurs more often in individuals with tuberous sclerosis.

realizing it. Many foods contain these substances as an ingredient; however, there are growing numbers of gluten–free and casein–free foods available for people that would like to eliminate them from their diets. Parents interested in using diet as a treatment should discuss with their child's doctor how to initiate an elimination diet.

Exercise

One researcher found that vigorous exercise (20 minutes or longer, three or four days a week) seems to decrease hyperactivity, aggression, self–injury and other autistic symptoms.

Public health role and response

A study conducted by Micahel Ganz at the Harvard School of Public Health estimated the cost of taking care of all people with autism over their lifetimes at $35 billion per year. As such, autism has a significant impact on public health and solutions are being actively sought.

One example is the Global Autism Public Health (GAPH) Initiative, sponsored by *Autism Speaks*, an integrated approach that focuses on three goals to improve the health and well–being of children and families affected by autism. These goals are:

- Increasing public and professional awareness of autism spectrum disorders (ASD).
- Increasing research expertise and international collaboration through training of autism researchers, with a focus on epidemiology, screening and early diagnosis, and treatment.
- Enhancing service delivery by providing training and expertise to service providers in early diagnosis and intervention.

Prognosis

Autism is treatable but not curable. With appropriate treatments adjusted to suit the autistic child as he/she grows up, the symptoms of autism improve. Today, parents and caregivers are focused on providing the best therapies possible in order for autistic children to develop to their highest potential. Because the incidence of autism seems to be increasing at a rapid rate worldwide, enough so that the CDC has voiced concern about its prevalence, there is more awareness of autism and more ongoing research efforts. People with autism have a normal **life expectancy** and with proper intervention they can lead full lives.

Prevention

Until the cause of autism is discovered, **prevention** is not possible.

QUESTIONS TO ASK YOUR DOCTOR

- What causes autism?
- By what age can autism be diagnosed?
- What is the purpose of medicating a child with autism?
- How is autism treated?
- Do symptoms of autism change over time?

Resources

BOOKS

Glasberg, Beth. *Stop That Seemingly Senseless Behavior: FBA–Based Interventions for People With Autism.* Bethesda, MD: Woodbine House, 2008.

Grandin, Temple. *Thinking in Pictures, Expanded Edition: My Life with Autism.* London, UK: Vintage (Random House), 2010.

Hughes–Lynch, Claire. Children with High–Functioning Autism: A Parent's Guide. Waco, TX: Prufrock Press, 2010.

Offit, Paul A. *Autism's False Prophets: Bad Science, Risky Medicine, and the Search for a Cure.* New York: Columbia University Press, 2008.

Moor, Julia. Playing, Laughing and Learning with Children on the Autism Spectrum: A Practical Resource of Play Ideas for Parents and Carers. London, UK: Jessica Kingsley Publishers, 2008.

McClannahan, Lynn and Patricia Krantz. Activity Schedules for Children With Autism, Second Edition: Teaching Independent Behavior. Bethesda, MD: Woodbine House, 2010.

PERIODICALS

Andersson, G. W., et al. "Pre–school children with suspected autism spectrum disorders: Do girls and boys have the same profiles?" Research in Developmental Disabilities 34, no. 1 (2012): 413–422.

Bekhet, A. K., et al. "Resilience in family members of persons with autism spectrum disorder: a review of the literature." Issues in Mental Health Nursing 33, no. 10 (2012): 650–656.

Daniels, J. L., et al. "Parental psychiatric disorders associated with autism spectrum disorders in the offspring." Pediatrics 121, no. 5 (May 2008): e1357–e1362.

Gadow, K. D. "Schizophrenia spectrum and attention–deficit/hyperactivity disorder symptoms in autism spectrum disorder and controls." Journal of the American Academy of Child and Adolescent Psychiatry 51, no. 10 (2012): 1076–1084.

Honey, K. "Attention focuses on autism." Journal of Clinical Investigation 118, no. 5 (May 2008): 1586–1587.

Hock, R., and B. K. Ahmedani. "Parent perceptions of autism severity: Exploring the social ecological context." Disability and Health Journal r, no. 4 (2012): 298–304.

Kishida, K. T., et al. "New approaches to investigating social gestures in autism spectrum disorder." Journal of Neurodevelopmental Disorders 4, no. 1 (May 2012): 14.

Nightingale, S. "Autism spectrum disorders."Nature Reviews. Drug Discovery 11, no. 10 (October 2012): 745–746.

Reiersen, A. M., and R. D. Todd. "Co–occurrence of ADHD and autism spectrum disorders: phenomenology and treatment."Expert Review of Neurotherapeutics 8, no. 4 (April 2008): 657–669.

State, M. W., and N. Sestan. "Neuroscience. The emerging biology of autism spectrum disorders."Science 337, no. 6100 (September 2012): 580–587.

Tsai, L. Y. "Sensitivity and Specificity: DSM-IV Versus DSM-5 Criteria for Autism Spectrum Disorder."American Journal of Psychiatry 169, no. 10 (2012): 1009–1011.

WEBSITES

Autism. Mayo Foundation for Medical Education and Research. October 6, 2012. http://www.mayoclinic.com/print/autism/DS00348

Autism. MedlinePlus. October 3, 2012. http://www.nlm.nih.gov/medlineplus/autism.html

Autism Resource Center. American Academy of Child and Adolescent Psychiatry, July 2009. http://www.aacap.org/cs/Autism.ResourceCenter

ORGANIZATIONS

Autism Research Institute/Autism Resource Center, 4182 Adams Avenue, San Diego, CA 92116, English: (866) 366-3361; Spanish: (877) 644-1184 ext. 5, Fax: (619) 563-6840, http://www.autism.com

Autism Society of America, 4340 East–West Hwy, Suite 350, Bethesda, MD (301) 657-0881, (800) 3-AUTISM [(800) 328-8476], http://www.autismsource.org

Autism Speaks, 1 East 33rd Street, 4th Floor, New York, NY 10016, (212) 252-8584, Fax: (212) 252-8676, contactus@autismspeaks.org, http://www.autismspeaks.org.

Carol A. Turkington
Tish Davidson, AM

Avian flu

Definition

Avian **influenza**, known more casually as bird flu, is an **infectious disease** caused by a family of viruses that normally infect birds. Beginning in 1997, a subtype of avian influenza known as Avian influenza A (H5N1), has infected and caused a small number of deaths in humans worldwide.

Demographics

The avian H5N1 influenza virus was first isolated in terns (migratory shore birds) in South Africa in 1961. The virus is highly contagious and sometimes fatal in birds; it did not appear to cause disease in humans until 1997. In that year in Hong Kong, H5N1 bird flu caused 18 confirmed cases of severe respiratory disease in humans, of which six were fatal. All but one of the individuals diagnosed with bird flu in Hong Kong had close contact with infected poultry. The exception was a case in which the disease was transmitted from child to parent but spread no further.

According to the **World Health Organization (WHO)**, between 2003 and 2011, there were 566 laboratory-confirmed cases of avian influenza in humans worldwide resulting in 332 deaths. The disease can affect people of all ages, genders, and ethnicities. Almost all individuals who have developed avian flu were in close contact with infected birds; only a few contracted the disease from extended contact with a sick family member. As of mid-2012, all confirmed cases of avian flu in humans had occurred in Asia or Africa.

Description

There are three types of influenza viruses: types A, B, and C. Only influenza A viruses causes serious, widespread illness in humans. Several different strains or subtypes of influenza A virus cause infection in humans. Other subtypes of influenza A cause disease in birds, pigs, horses, ferrets, whales, and seals. In most cases, the subtypes that cause disease in one species do not spread the disease to other species.

Bird flu was first identified in Italy more than 100 years ago. Avian influenza viruses can infect both domestic and wild birds, including chickens, ducks, geese, turkeys, swans, pheasants, and quail. Although the disease is often fatal in domestic birds (e.g., chickens, turkeys), it often causes less severe illness in wild birds; wild ducks are natural reservoirs of infection. Infected wild birds shed large quantities of virus in their feces but often appear to be relatively unaffected by flu symptoms. During migration, infected wild birds encounter other wild and domestic birds, such as chickens, and spread the disease to them. The virus then kills a large percentage of domestic birds, along with some species of wild birds. There are several subtypes of avian influenza virus, but the one of most concern to human health is called H5N1. Under most circumstances, avian influenza viruses do not infect humans.

Understanding the avian influenza virus

Influenza viruses are protein sacks with a core of eight loosely connected genes. Two proteins spike from the surface of the virus. The most plentiful protein is called haemagglutinin (H). The other surface protein is neuraminidase (N). The job of these proteins is to hook the influenza virus on to the surface of a cell in the animal it has infected and then help get the virus's genes inside that cell. Once inside, the virus gene takes over the host cell and reprograms it to make thousands of copies of the virus.

There are many subtypes of influenza A viruses. These are identified by a series of letters and numbers that refer to two surface proteins, H and N. There are 16 known types of H proteins and nine known types of N proteins of influenza The structure of the genes in the influenza virus allows these viruses to mutate (change) very rapidly. Many combinations of the two proteins can result from these mutations, each representing a new subtype of influenza A.

According to the United States **Centers for Disease Control and Prevention (CDC)** 15 different Influenza A subtypes can infect birds. Normally the subtypes of influenza that infect birds do not harm human, although some can infect pigs. However, the avian influenza virus called H5N1 has mutated in such a way that it is able to infect humans.

Humans and bird flu

When H5N1 avian flu was first discovered to infect humans in Hong Kong in 1997, it was feared that the disease, now called bird flu, would sweep through the community and kill thousands the way another subtype of influenza had swept across the world in 1918 and 1919. That influenza **pandemic** killed between 20 and 100 million people on six continents. To prevent this outcome, Hong Kong health authorities ordered all poultry be killed. Within three days, about 1.5 million birds in Hong Kong were destroyed to prevent further spread of the disease. Hong Kong, a relatively small island, was able to contain the infection.

The next outbreak of avian flu in humans was reported in Asia. From November 2003 through March 2004, a handful of human cases of bird flu were found in China, Vietnam, and Thailand. Meanwhile avian flu was epidemic among the bird populations in Japan, Thailand, Lao People's Democratic Republic (formerly Laos), China, and Indonesia. Millions of birds died from avian flu as the disease spread throughout Southeast Asia, and many of these countries reported a small number of human infections. By 2009, the disease had spread to some parts of the Middle East and northern Africa, where Egypt and Djibouti reported some human cases. As of mid-2012, more than three-fourths of all laboratory-confirmed cases of avian flu in humans had occurred in Southeast Asia; none had been reported in North or South America or Australia.

KEY TERMS

Pandemic—The occurrence of a disease that in a short time infects a large percentage of the population over a wide geographical area.

Secondary or opportunistic infection—An infection by a microbe that occurs because the body is weakened by a primary infection caused by a different kind of microbe.

Risk factors

People at greatest risk of contracting avian flu are those who live or work closely with poultry. Potentially vulnerable people include those working on poultry on farms, in poultry processing plants, and live bird markets. Individuals living with a family member who has avian flu are also at risk of developing the disease. Avian flu does not spread easily to humans, and many people who are exposed to infected birds do not get sick. Travelers to Asia and Africa who expect to handle birds or visit poultry farms should check the **CDC** Travelers' Health website for information on the country to which they are traveling.

Causes and symptoms

An influenza virus that birds carry in their intestines causes avian flu. The virus spreads as infected birds excrete saliva, nasal secretions, and feces. Birds vulnerable to the flu become infected when they come into contact with the excretions or surfaces contaminated by the viruses.

Birds that survive the H5N1 infection can excrete the virus for at least ten days. This allows the H5N1 strain to spread through bird-to-bird contact from wild birds to domestic birds on farms and in live bird markets. The virus can also spread on surfaces, including manure, bird feed, equipment, vehicles, egg flats, and crates, and the clothing and shoes of people who are exposed to the virus. Influenza is a respiratory disease. People must inhale the virus or carry it on their hands to their nose, eyes, or mouth to become sick. People cannot get the disease by eating properly cooked poultry.

In general, people who contract bird flu have symptoms similar to seasonal human influenza, including fever, cough, sore throat, and aching muscles. Other symptoms included eye infections (conjunctivitis), **pneumonia**, acute respiratory distress, and viral pneumonia. Influenza weakens the respiratory system and leaves the lungs more vulnerable to infection. Many people with flu die from pneumonia caused by a secondary bacterial infection. Bacteria are able to grow in the lungs because the body's defenses have been weakened by the flu virus.

Diagnosis

The symptoms of avian flu and seasonal influenza are similar. A physician may suspect avian influenza if an individual showing flu-like symptoms has been in close contact with poultry in an infected area. Nevertheless, laboratory testing is needed to confirm a diagnosis of avian influenza. Symptoms normally develop within seven days of infection.

Tests

Diagnostic tests for human flu are rapid and reliable, according to the **World Health Organization (WHO)**. International laboratories within the WHO global network have high-security facilities and experienced staff to test samples of suspected avian flu sent from around the world. Test methods include a viral culture that analyzes a blood sample and swabbing from the nose or throat. Other testing can be done on respiratory secretions.

In April 2009, the U.S. Food and Drug Administration (FDA) approved a rapid detection test for the H5N1 strain of bird flu. The test is manufactured by Arbor Vita Corporation of California. All it requires is a swab from the nose or throat of an ill individual. This test produces results in about 40 minutes. Previous bird flu tests took at minimum four hours to complete.

Treatment

Drugs

Some antiviral drugs appear to be partially effective against avian flu viruses if they are administered promptly, usually within 48 hours after the start of symptoms. These drugs do not cure flu, but lessen its symptoms and duration. In the United States, four drugs have been approved by the U.S. Food and Drug Administration (FDA) for the treatment of influenza A viruses in otherwise healthy adults. These are amantadine (Symmetrel), rimantadine (Flumadine), oseltamivir (Tamiflu), and zanamivir (Relenza). Research indicates that the avian H5N1 virus is resistant to amantadine and rimantadine; therefore, the drugs of choice for treating bird flu are oseltamivir and zanamivir.

Antibiotics may be needed to treat secondary bacterial infections. Acetaminophen may be used to control fever and reduce aches.

Alternative treatment

In March 2005, people in South Korea began eating more kimchi to ward off avian flu infection, according to the reports from the British Broadcasting Company and other news organizations. The public turned to the spicy vegetable dish after scientists at Seoul National University announced that kimchi aided in the recovery of 11 out of 13 infected chickens. The scientists fed the birds an extract of kimchi, a dish made by fermenting cabbage with red peppers, radishes, and large amounts of garlic and ginger. A week later, all but two birds showed signs of recovery. The researchers acknowledged that their study was unscientific. At that time, they were not sure how or why kimchi was related to the recovery. However, the announcement led people again to regard kimchi as a health remedy.

Home remedies

Much of the treatment for influenza is supportive and consists bed rest, drinking plenty of fluids to stay hydrated, and using a humidifier to relieve nasal congestion and ease breathing.

Prognosis

Approximately 60% of individuals who develop avian influenza die. The rest typically recover completely.

Prevention

Although avian influenza has been confirmed in fewer than 500 individuals worldwide, scientists at WHO, the CDC, and public health agencies of many other countries are concerned about the deadly consequences that could occur if H5N1 mutated into a virus subtype that could spread easily from one human to another. A strain of bird flu spread by human-to-human contact could cause an influenza pandemic and sicken millions. WHO and CDC experts believe that the question is not if another influenza epidemic will occur, but when it will happen and how severe it will be. For this reason, **prevention** strategies and pandemic planning are extremely important.

In the United States, the CDC is among the organizations preparing for a possible outbreak of bird flu in humans. In addition to laboratories equipped to test for bird flu, the CDC recommends precautions to prevent the spread of flu and other respiratory infections. Precautionary measures include restricting birds from coming into the United States from infected countries, testing poultry for avian flu viruses, and euthanizing infected birds. People with symptoms of respiratory infection are advised to cover their mouths or use facial tissues when coughing or sneezing. After coughing or

QUESTIONS TO ASK YOUR DOCTOR

- How is avian flu different from regular seasonal flu?
- If I work with birds, am I likely to get avian flu?
- Are there specific symptoms associated with avian flu that I should watch for?
- If I contract avian flu, can I pass it on to other family members?

sneezing, individuals should wash their hands well with soap and water, alcohol-based hand rub, or antiseptic handwash.

As of 2012, bird flu was primarily a risk for people in infected areas who work with poultry. People working with birds in locations such as commercial poultry facilities, veterinary offices, and live bird markets should wear protective clothing. That equipment includes boots, coveralls, face masks, gloves, and headgear, according to the United States Department of Agriculture (USDA).

Furthermore, poultry producers should implement security measures to prevent the outbreak of a highly pathogenic virus. Those actions include keeping flocks away from wild or migratory birds and providing clothing and disinfectant facilities for employees. Plastic crates are recommended for use at live bird markets because they are easier to clean than wood crates. Cleaning and disinfecting areas are also important for preventing an outbreak. Infected birds must be quarantined or destroyed.

In July 2007, FDA approved a vaccine for use against H5N1 bird flu. As of mid-2012, the vaccine is not available to the public because no serious outbreaks of avian flu have occurred. Because the avian influenza virus mutates rapidly (a new variant, called a clade was recognized in February 2011), the vaccine may not be highly effective in preventing the disease. As of mid-2012, the threat to public health from avian influenza was considered very low.

Resources

BOOKS

Scoones, Ian, ed. *Avian Influenza: Science, Policy and Politics*. Washington, DC: Earthscan, 2010.

Sipress, Alan. *The Fatal Strain: On the Trail of Avian Flu and the Coming Pandemic*. New York: Viking, 2009.

WEBSITES

Centers for Disease Control and Prevention (CDC). "Information on Avian Influenza." http://www.cdc.gov/flu/avianflu (accessed September 21, 2012).

MedlinePlus. "Bird Flu." http://www.nlm.nih.gov/medlineplus/birdflu.html (accessed September 21, 2012).

World Health Organization (WHO). "Avian Influenza in Humans." http://www.who.int/influenza/human_animal_interface/avian_influenza/en (accessed September 21, 2012).

ORGANIZATIONS

Centers for Disease Control and Prevention (CDC), 1600 Clifton Rd., Atlanta, GA 30333, (404) 639-3534, (800) CDC-INFO (800-232-4636), (888) 232-6348, inquiry@cdc.gov, http://www.cdc.gov

World Health Organization (WHO), Avenue Appia 20, 1211 Geneva 27, Switzerland, +22 41 791 21 11, Fax: +22 41 791 31 11, info@who.int, http://www.who.int.

Tish Davidson, AM

B

Bedbug infestation

Definition

Bedbug infestation is the contamination of bedding, clothing, and household furnishings with the small nocturnal parasitic insects of the family *Cimicidae*, commonly known as bed bugs. Bedbugs feed on the blood of humans and other warm-blooded animals. Bedbug bites can result in skin rashes and sores, psychological effects, and allergic reactions.

Description

Bedbugs have been recognized as human **parasites** for thousands of years. The development of the pesticide DDT eliminated bedbugs from most developed countries by the early 1940s. However, after DDT use was banned because of its harmful effects on the environment, bedbugs returned. Bedbug infestation is relatively common in developed countries and very common in developing countries. Bedbugs spread easily, often carried by international travelers or by the exchange of secondhand furnishings and other items among households. Bed bugs are difficult to exterminate because of insecticide resistance and use of pest control methods that do not affect bed bugs because these chemicals have less toxic, less persistent, chemical-active ingredients and formulations.

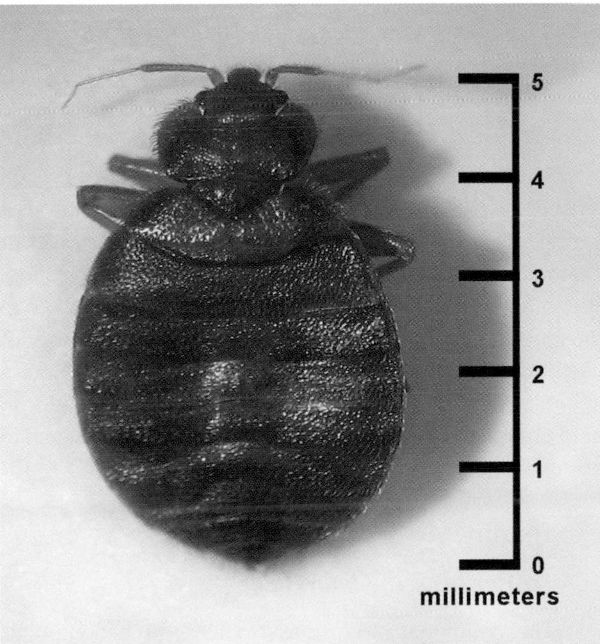

A dorsal view of an adult Cimex lectularius bed bug. *(CDC/CDC-DPDx; Blaine Mathison)*

Generally, adult bed bugs are .25–.5 in (4–5 mm) long, brown in color, with a flat, oval-shaped body. Young bed bugs (also called nymphs) are smaller and lighter in color. They are primarily nocturnal, feeding on the blood of birds and mammals at night. When they bite, they inject an anesthetic and an anticoagulant that prevents a person from feeling the bite. Because bites usually occur while people are sleeping, most people do not realize they have been bitten until marks appear. Bed bugs are attracted to their hosts by carbon dioxide, blood, and warmth. During the day, they hide in mattress seams, cracks in bed frames or other furniture, behind loose wallpaper, and in bedding and clothing. Females lay from one to five eggs a day, or up to 500 in a lifetime. The eggs hatch in seven to ten days. Adults can live for months without feeding.

Bedbug bites are painless, but the bites can cause an allergic reaction after a few days, resulting in an itchy, red rash. Although bedbug bites are rarely medically dangerous, they can become infected through scratching. A bedbug infestation can also cause emotional distress, resulting in anxiety, **stress**, and disruption of sleep.

Risk factors

People often associate bed bugs with poor or dirty living conditions, but bed bugs can be found in pristine environments. In the early 2000s, complaints about bed bugs in both budget and first-class hotels increased.

The risk of exposure to bed bugs increases with certain activities including the following:

- international travel
- frequent overnight stays in hotels and motels
- living in refugee camps or homeless shelters
- living in apartment buildings (bed bugs are efficient crawlers and can move through cracks from apartment to apartment)
- living in military barracks or academic dormitories

In 2010, a survey conducted by the U.S. National Pest Management Association and the University of Kentucky found that calls to exterminators in the United States increased 57% nationwide in the previous five years. More than 95% of 519 U.S. exterminators participating in the survey reported finding at least one bed bug infestation in the previous year. The number of exterminators reporting doing more than 100 bedbug jobs a year increased more than three-fold, from 6% in 2008 to 20% just two years later, the survey found. Seven percent reported doing more than 500 bedbug jobs in the previous year. According to the Vector Biology and Zoonotic Disease at SRI International, more than 95% of U.S. pest control agencies reported bed bugs as a priority in 2010, thus superseding termites as the number one urban pest. The number of reported bedbug **infestations** in the United States in single family homes, hotel rooms, and multiunit housing has increased 10- to 100-fold since those recorded in 1990. This survey also included international exterminators. Of the international exterminators participating in the study, high frequencies of exterminators encountering a bedbug infestation in the previous year were reported for Canada (98%), Europe (92%) and Africa/Middle East (90%). The majority of respondents also encountered bedbugs during the past year in Mexico/Central America (80%), Asia (73%), and South America (59%).

Terminix, a pest control provider, releases annually a Most Bedbug-Infested U.S. Cities ranking, based on an evaluation of service calls and confirmed cases by service professionals. In 2012, the top 15 most bedbug-infested cities were:

- Philadelphia
- Cincinnati
- New York City
- Chicago
- Detroit
- Washington, DC
- Columbus, Ohio
- San Francisco
- Denver
- New Haven, Connecticut
- Dallas
- Houston
- Indianapolis
- Miami
- Cleveland

Causes and symptoms

The bite of a bed bug causes an allergic reaction in most people that can be difficult to differentiate from skin reactions caused by other bites or **allergies**. The rash caused by bed bugs is red and itchy and typically darker in the center of the bite. Often, but not always, bites form lines or groups of three, sometimes called "breakfast," "lunch," and "dinner." Although bed bugs will bite any exposed skin, bites are most often found on the face, neck, arms, and hands.

The time it takes a bedbug rash to appear is variable, ranging from as long as ten days to less than one minute. Generally, the more frequently a person is exposed to bed bugs, the shorter the time it takes for the rash to appear. In rare cases, some individuals can have an extreme, life-threatening allergic reaction to bedbug bites called anaphylaxis or anaphylactic shock.

A bedbug infestation can also cause anxiety for weeks or months, depending on the person and the severity of the infestation. Shame and embarrassment are also common among bedbug sufferers, mostly because of social stigma against bed bugs and other insects. It is a misconception that a bedbug infestation is the result of poor housekeeping.

Diagnosis

Medical diagnosis is not always necessary; an individual can make the diagnosis based on their past experience with bed bugs and recent history of travel or examination of their bedding for signs of infestation. When a medical diagnosis is sought, it is made based on the appearance of the rash along with a detailed history of recent travel and hotel stays. The doctor may also inquire about any drugs, herbs, or supplements being taken to help eliminate other possible causes of the rash. There are no tests to diagnose bedbug bites.

Treatment

Treatment of the individual

The symptoms and rash associated with bedbug bites go away on their own, usually within a week to ten days. An over-the-counter skin cream containing hydrocortisone may be applied to reduce itching. An over-the-counter antihistamine containing diphenhydramine (e.g., Benadryl) may also help reduce itching. Parents of affected infants and children or pregnant and breastfeeding women should consult an appropriate healthcare professional before using these medications. In addition, if a person is experiencing distress, anxiety, or insomnia, a healthcare professional may be helpful. There is also an online support forum available through http://bedbugger.com.

Treatment of the infested environment

Ridding an infested environment of bed bugs is considerably more difficult than treatment of the individual. A professional exterminator experienced with bedbug elimination may be required. Because bed bugs can hide in small cracks in furniture, mattresses, and box springs, vacuuming will not remove all of them. Special mattress covers can be purchased to lock out bed bugs, but it may be more effective to purchase a new mattress and box springs. Bed bugs can live for 9–12 months without feeding.

Bed bugs can be killed by heat. Bedding and clothing should be washed in hot water and dried at very hot temperatures. The temperature must reach at least 120°F (49°C). Items that cannot be washed can be put in sealed plastic bags and placed in a car with the windows rolled up in the summer when the temperature will reach 120 degrees or more inside the car. Freezing is less effective. Items must be left at temperatures below 32°F (0°C) for several days to kill bed bugs.

Insecticides effective against bed bugs include pemethrin and diethyltoulamide. Pemethrin spray can be used on clothing. Diethyltoluamide in high concentrations can be toxic to infants and children, so a doctor should be consulted before use. The use of a professional exterminator is the safest way to rid the environment of bed bugs.

Fumigation, the process of sealing infested areas and applying a gas that is registered for use by the federal and state governments can control live insects and bedbug eggs. Fumigation has a long history of success against insects, including bed bugs. Sulfuryl fluoride is the most common fumigant used to control bed bugs. This material is a gas and is released into an infested area or materials using very controlled procedures. Homeowners cannot purchase sulfuryl fluoride. It can only be used by a properly licensed company that has specially trained technicians. Fumigation usually requires vacating the property several days while the structure is being fumigated. When fumigating, the gas penetrates all cracks and crevice in the fumigated area. After the fumigation is complete, the area is aired out and monitored for residual gas. Another method of fumigation is to remove belongings that are infested to a chamber. These infested items are then fumigated and returned to the rooms. Precautions must be taken so that infested items do not spread bed bugs when they are removed and relocated. Fumigation does not provide any residual protection, although it does penetrate all accessible areas, including cracks and crevices. It will not prevent bedbug infestation and reinfestation can occur after treatment.

Room foggers and sprays against mosquitoes and ticks are ineffective against bed bugs. Many treatments for the elimination or of bed bugs are sold over the Internet. These vary considerably in cost and effectiveness, so it is important to research products before buying them.

Bed bugs pose both a social and economic threat to owners and residents of apartment buildings, hotels, and public buildings. Economic losses from health care, lost wages, lost revenue and reduced productivity can be significant. The cost of effectively eliminating bed bugs may be significantly more than the cost of eliminating other pests because bedbug control usually requires multiple visits from a licensed pest control operator and diligence on the part of those who are experiencing the infestation. Control in multifamily homes is much more difficult than in single family homes because bed bugs frequently travel between units, either via direct transport by humans or through voids in the walls. There are additional costs and complexities associated with coordinating and encouraging participation from multiple residents. According to staff associated with the New York State Integrated Pest Management program at Cornell University, a family can spend $5,000 or more on inspections, exterminator fees, cleaning and storage. Landlords of large apartment buildings have been known to spend as much as $80,000 to get rid of bed bugs.

Public health response

State, tribal, and local government agencies and **health departments** play a critical role in protecting the public from bed bugs. Public health departments serve on the front lines, providing information on prevention and control of bed bugs through various programs to the public and private sector. The community, together with local health agencies, must be involved in the control and management of bedbug populations and must be provided with the knowledge of best practices to prevent and control bedbug infestations. In some cases, a coordinated community control program may be necessary to reduce or eliminate bedbug populations.

The U.S. **Centers for Disease Control and Prevention (CDC)** and the U.S. **Environmental Protection Agency (EPA)** have identified challenges

KEY TERM

Anaphylaxis—Also called anaphylactic shock; a severe allergic reaction characterized by airway constriction, tissue swelling, and lowered blood pressure.

that the public health community faces when trying to control bedbug infestations. These challenges include the following:

- Local public health departments have very limited resources to combat the problem and bed bugs frequently are not seen as a priority.
- Municipal codes struggle to identify those responsible for control of bedbug infestations. Tenants and landlords often dispute who is ultimately responsible for the cost of control and treatment. Treatment costs are high, and transient populations make it difficult or impossible to assign responsibility.
- Pesticide resistance and limited control choices make treatment even more difficult. Some bedbug populations are resistant to almost all pesticides registered to treat them. Residents may use over-the-counter or homemade preparations that are ineffective (or even dangerous) and may promote further resistance.
- Pesticide misuse is also a potential public health concern. Because bedbug infestations are so difficult to control and are such a challenge to mental and economic health, residents may resort to using pesticides that are not intended for indoor residential use and may face serious health risks as a result. Additionally, residents may be tempted to apply pesticides registered for indoor use, but at greater application rates than the label allows. Doing so results in a much greater risk of pesticide exposure for those living in the home. Pesticides must always be used in strict accordance with their labeling to ensure that the residents and applicators are not exposed to unsafe levels of pesticide residues.

Prognosis

Almost everyone recovers from bedbug bites within two weeks. Complications may arise from scratching the bites so that they become infected. If infection occurs, then an antibiotic may be prescribed. Bed bugs have been shown to be able to be infected by at least 28 human pathogens, but no study has clearly found that the insect is able to transmit the pathogen to humans.

QUESTIONS TO ASK YOUR DOCTOR

- Can you prescribe a medicine to treat my irritating or infected bedbug bits?
- What can I do to protect my children from bedbug bites?

Prevention

Prevention is difficult. Avoiding secondhand furniture, couches, bed frames, mattresses, and beds is helpful. Birds and bats can carry bed bugs, so they should be eliminated from attics and eaves. Reducing clutter in the home reduces hiding places for bed bugs. The use of a protective cover that encases mattresses and box springs will eliminate many hiding spots. The light color of the encasement makes bed bugs easier to see. A high quality encasement that will resist tearing should be used. The encasements should be checked regularly for holes.

When traveling, checking the seams of mattresses for dark specks of bedbug excrement in hotels is helpful but not foolproof. Use luggage racks to hold luggage when packing or unpacking rather than setting the luggage on the bed or floor. Upon returning home, unpack directly into a washing machine and inspect the luggage carefully.

The Bed Bug Registry (http://bedbugregistry.com) is a free, public database of user-submitted bedbug reports from across the United States and Canada. Founded in 2006, the site has collected more than 20,000 reports covering 12,000 locations. This resource can be checked before booking a hotel room or renting an apartment.

Resources

BOOKS

Pinto, Larry, Richard Cooper, and Sandy Kraft. *Bed Bug Handbook: The Complete Guide to Bed Bugs and Their Control.* Mechanicsville, MD: Pinto & Associates, 2007.

WEBSITES

"Bed Bug Guide (A Resource Site)." 2010. http://www.bedbugsguide.com

"Bedbugs." Foundation for Medical Research and Education MayoClinic.com. http://www.mayoclinic.com/health/bedbugs/ds00663.

"Insect Bites and Stings." MedlinePlus. http://www.nlm.nih.gov/medlineplus/insectbitesandstings.html

Schwartz, Robert A. "Bedbug Bites." eMedicine.com. March 24, 2010. http://emedicine.medscape.com/article/1088931-overview

ORGANIZATIONS

Centers for Disease Control and Prevention (CDC), 1600 Clifton Rd., Atlanta, GA 30333, (404) 639-3534, (800) CDC-INFO (232-4636). TTY: (888) 232-6348, inquiry@cdc.gov, http://www.cdc.gov

National Institute of Allergy and Infectious Diseases, Office of Communications and Government Relations, 6610 Rockledge Dr., MSC 6612, Bethesda, MD 20892-6612, (301) 496-5717, (866) 284-4107 or TDD: (800)877-8339 (for hearing impaired), Fax: (301) 402-3573, http://www3.niaid.nih.gov.

Judith Sims, AM

Behavioral health

Definition

Behavioral health is a discipline that includes mental health services such as psychiatric care, marriage and family counseling, and treatment for addictions. Services are provided by mental health professionals including psychiatrists, psychologists, social workers, neurologists, counselors, and physicians. The disorders treated include anxiety disorder, mood disorders, impulse-control disorders, and substance abuse disorders. These conditions may be present acutely on a short-term basis or may be chronic, long-term issues.

Description

Behavioral health services are provided by mental health professionals to help individuals who have mental health or substance abuse disorders. It is not uncommon for the diagnosis to begin with the primary care provider. In persons who have mental illness, 42% of individuals with clinical depression and 47% with generalized anxiety disorder (GAD) were first diagnosed by their primary care physician. Given these statistics, it is clear that primary care physicians are a critical aspect of behavioral health care.

The National Survey on Drug Use and Health reported that, in 2009, more than 60% of adults and 70% of children who had a diagnosable behavioral health disorder requiring treatment did not receive care. Studies consistently show that the main obstacle for receiving treatment is cost.

Providers

Specialists that treat behavioral health issues include the following:

- Psychiatrist—physician (MD or DO) who diagnoses and treats behavioral health disorders. A psychiatrist may treat individuals in a clinical setting and is licensed to prescribe medications. He or she may also function in a research setting. A sub-specialty of psychiatry is addiction psychiatry.
- Neurologist—A physician (MD or DO) who specializes in the treatment of neurological disorders. A clinical neuropsychologist is a physician who specializes in treating conditions related to the brain as well as behaviors. The American Board of Clinical Neuropsychology provides board certification for medical specialists in this field.
- Psychologist—Possesses an advanced degree (doctorate required for clinical psychologist) and works in a private practice setting or along with others on a healthcare team, or may work in a research setting. Clinical psychologists determine the cause and effect of a behavioral health condition. They focus on the prevention and treatment of emotional conflicts, personality disturbances, psychopathology, and seek to work with clients to correct these issues. Tools used may include psychotherapy, group therapy, behavior therapy, marital and family counseling, biofeedback, and cognitive retraining. A licensed is required in all states.
- Primary care physician—A physician (MD or DO) who treats individuals through a practice in internal medicine, family medicine, pediatrics, gerontology, or other discipline that focuses on medical conditions affecting the entire body. In the United States, the primary care physician often diagnoses and provides treatment for behavioral health conditions.
- Social workers—The largest segment of behavior health practitioners belongs to clinical social workers. They work in mental health centers, hospitals, substance abuse programs, schools, and a variety of other public assistance settings. In order to be a Qualified Clinical Social Worker (QCSW), an individual must have a master's degree, post-degree professional education, experience, a state social work license, and must adhere to National Association of Social Work (NASW) standards.
- Counselor—A counselor may provide marriage and family counseling or related services. Behavioral health professionals with varying backgrounds may specialize in counseling for couples or other demographic groups. Groups such as the American Association for Marriage and Family Therapy offer accreditation.

According to the National Survey on Drug Use and Health, the behavioral health treatments used in 2009 fit into the following categories:

- prescription medications only—40%
- outpatient therapy and prescription medications—32%
- outpatient therapy only—13%

- inpatient and outpatient treatment and prescription medications—3%
- inpatient treatment only—2%
- inpatient and outpatient treatments—1%

Diagnoses

Behavioral health diagnoses can be categorized as follows, according to the National Institute of Mental Health:

- Anxiety disorders—people with these disorders experience anxiety that impedes their ability to complete routine tasks. The types of disorders in this category are generalized anxiety disorder (GAD), obsessive-compulsive disorder (OCD), panic disorder, post-traumatic stress disorder, and social anxiety disorder.
- Attention deficit hyperactivity disorder (ADHD or ADD)—common disorder in childhood, which may continue into adolescence and beyond. Classic sign is an inability to keep attention focused.
- Autism spectrum disorders—developmental brain disorders with varying levels of impairment. The five disorders in this category are Autism disorder, Asperger's disorder, Pervasive developmental disorder not otherwise specified, Rett's disorder, and Childhood disintegrative disorder.
- Bipolar disorder—also known as manic depressive disorder, this condition creates mood shifts that impair an individual's ability to complete routine tasks. This condition most often develops in late teens or young adulthood.
- Borderline personality disorder—this form of mental illness is characterized by instability in moods, behaviors, and relationships with others. Individuals with this condition tend to also have other disorders such as depression, substance abuse issues, anxiety, and eating disorders. They may exhibit suicidal behaviors.
- Depression—feelings of sadness that impair activities of daily life and negatively impact a person and others around that person.
- Eating disorders—types of illnesses that disrupt normal eating patterns. In many cases, other behavioral health illnesses, such as depression, substance abuse or anxiety, are also present.
- Schizophrenia—chronic, serious brain disorder that is disabling. Approximately 1% of Americans suffer from schizophrenia.
- Substance abuse disorders—addiction disorder that manifests in excessive use of alcohol or drugs.

Demographics

In the United States and Canada, mental illness and substance abuse constitute the top five causes of disability in persons ages 15 to 44 years (excluding disability caused by communicable diseases).

According to the National Comorbidity Study-Replication, nearly one-third of adults meet the diagnostic criteria for a behavioral health condition, and more than 50% will meet these criteria at some point during their lives.

Children experience behavioral health issues as well. In that population, the most common issues are mood disorders such as depression, as well as anxiety, oppositional defiant disorder, **eating disorders**, attention deficit/hyperactivity disorder, and substance abuse issues. These conditions may persist into adulthood or may resolve as the child ages.

Individuals in lower economic groups are more commonly found to have behavioral health disorders when compared with persons in higher income categories. Men and women tend to be equally affected overall. However, some conditions tend to be more common in one gender over the other. For example, depression is more common in women while substance abuse more often affects men.

KEY TERMS

Comorbidity—Diagnosis of two or more illnesses at the same time. It is common in behavioral health for adults to have more than one disorder simultaneously.

Effects on Public Health

Behavioral health experts predict that by 2020 behavioral health issues will exceed all physical disease as the major causes of illness around the world.

Costs to society

Public sources of funding pay a larger portion of behavioral health costs than they do for other types of health services. Medicare covers 26% of behavioral health costs while Medicaid covers only 7% of these costs. When compared to overall health care costs, local and state funding pay a larger portion of behavioral health costs.

Resources

BOOKS

Suls, Jerry M., PhD, Karina W. Davidson, PhD, Robert M. Kaplan, PhD, Eds. *Handbook of Health Psychology and Behavioral Medicine*. New York: The Guilford Press, 2010.

PERIODICALS

Gantner, Leigh A., and Christine M. Olson. "Evaluation of Public Health Professionals' Capacity to Implement Environmental Changes Supportive of Healthy Weight." *Evaluation and Program Planning* 35, no. 3 (2012): 407.

Rosenberg, Linda. "Behavioral Disorders: The New Public Health Crisis" *Journal of Behavioral Health Services & Research* 39, no. 1: (January 2012).

WEBSITES

American Board of Professional Psychology. http://www.abpp.org/i4a/pages/index.cfm?pageid=3304 (accessed September 28, 2012).

An Employer's Guide to Behavioral Health Services. Center for Prevention and Health Services. https://www.businessgrouphealth.org/pdfs/fullreport_behavioralhealthservices.pdf (accessed September 28, 2012).

Mental Health Financing in the United States. http://www.kff.org/medicaid/upload/8182.pdf (accessed September 28, 2012).

National Association of Social Workers. http://www.socialworkers.org/practice/standards/naswclinicalswstandards.pdf (accessed September 28, 2012).

National Institute of Mental Health. http://www.nimh.nih.gov/statistics/Dashboard-Resources.shtml (accessed September 28, 2012).

Society of Clinical Psychology. http://www.apa.org/divisions/div12/aboutcp.html (accessed September 28, 2012).

Rhonda Cloos, RN

Biodiversity *see* **Global Public Health**

Bird flu *see* **Avian flu**

Domestic violence *see* **Domestic abuse**

Birth defects

Definition

Birth defects are structural, functional, or metabolic abnormalities that are present at birth; they are also called congenital abnormalities. More than 4,000 different congenital abnormalities have been identified as of 2012. Birth defects range from minor problems to life-threatening conditions; they are the leading cause of death during the first year of life.

Description

Birth defects are found in 3% of all newborn infants in North America, according to the American Congress of Obstetricians and Gynecologists (ACOG); the **Centers for Disease Control and Prevention (CDC)** gives a figure of one in every 33 babies. This rate doubles in the first year and reaches 10% by age five, as more defects become evident and can be diagnosed. Almost 20% of deaths in newborns are caused by birth defects.

Birth defects can affect any major organ, body system, or part of the body. Major defects are structural abnormalities that affect the way a person looks and require medical and/or surgical treatment. The most common category of structural birth defects is heart defects, which affect 1 in every 150 newborns. Most metabolic birth defects, which affect the infant's body chemistry, are major birth defects. Although metabolic defects occur in only 1 in 3,500 infants, they are often incurable or fatal conditions. Minor defects are abnormalities that do not cause serious health or social problems for the growing child. When multiple birth defects occur together and have a similar cause, they are called syndromes. If two or more defects tend to appear together but do not share the same cause, they are called associations.

Demographics

According to the March of Dimes, the rate of birth defects worldwide is 6%, double the 3% rate reported for the United States and Canada. This difference may be due to higher rates of exposure to **environmental toxins** during pregnancy in less developed countries; poor or no prenatal care; and malnutrition. It is estimated that 3.3 million children in underdeveloped countries die each year as the result of birth defects.

There are differences among racial and ethnic groups in the United States and Canada with regard to the relative frequency of specific birth defects. For example, African American infants have a higher risk of trisomy 18 (Edwards syndrome), tetralogy of Fallot, and leg defects, but a lower risk of cleft palate, esophageal atresia, gastroschisis, and Down syndrome. Conversely, Hispanic babies have a higher risk of gastroschisis, Down syndrome, anencephaly, and spina bifida, but a lower risk of tetralogy of Fallot, esophageal atresia, and cleft palate. Asian and Native American babies have a relatively high risk of cleft palate.

Causes and symptoms

The specific cause of most congenital abnormalities (about 60% of cases) is unknown; most of the remaining 40% however, are thought to result from the interaction of environmental and genetic factors. Some risky personal behaviors or treatments associated with pregnancy and delivery can increase the risk of birth defects.

Teratogens

Any substance that can cause abnormal development of the fetus in the mother's womb is called a teratogen. In the first two months after conception, the developing

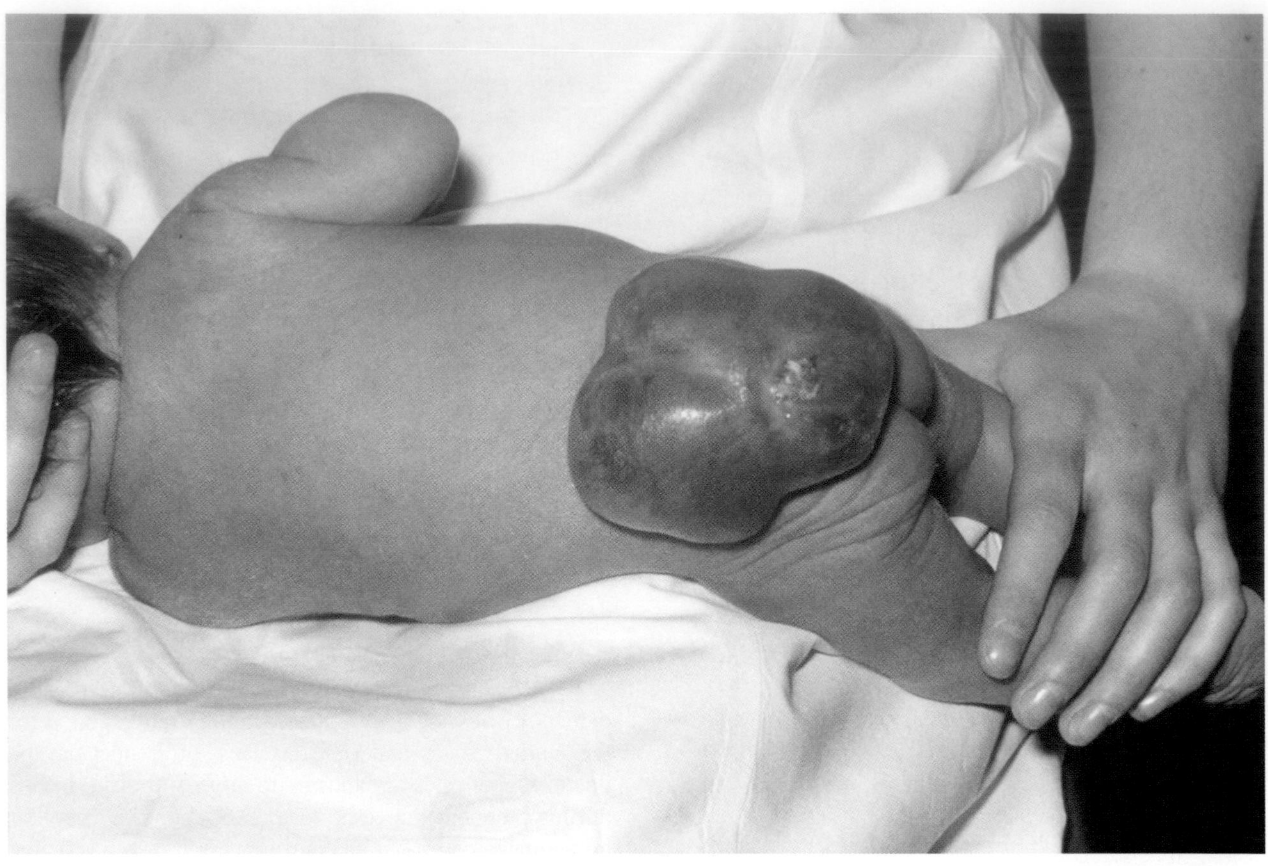

Infant with spina bifida. *(Biophoto Associates/Photo Researchers, Inc.)*

organism is called an embryo; from two months to birth, the conceptus is called a fetus. Growth is rapid, and each body organ has a critical period in which it is especially sensitive to outside influences. About 7% of all congenital defects are caused by exposure to teratogens.

DRUGS. Most commonly prescribed drugs do not cause birth defects, but some have the potential to cause harm. For example, a 2003 study found that use of topical (local) corticosteroids in the first trimester of pregnancy may be associated with cleft lip. Isotretinoin, a drug used to treat severe acne, is known to cause visual or hearing problems or mental retardation if taken during pregnancy or even shortly before conception. Thalidomide is known to cause defects of the arms and legs; several other drugs also cause problems, such as:

- Alcohol. Drinking large amounts of alcohol while pregnant causes a cluster of defects called fetal alcohol syndrome (FAS), which includes mental retardation, heart problems, and growth deficiency. Binge drinking early in pregnancy is dangerous even if the woman quits drinking after the first trimester.
- Antibiotics. Certain antibiotics are known teratogens. Tetracycline affects bone growth and discolors the teeth. Drugs used to treat tuberculosis can lead to hearing problems and damage to a nerve in the head (cranial damage).
- Anticonvulsants. Drugs given to prevent seizures can cause serious problems in the developing fetus, including mental retardation and slow growth. Studies in the United Kingdom and Australia have tracked the percentage of birth defects caused by certain antiepileptic drugs.
- Antipsychotic and antianxiety agents. Several drugs given for anxiety and mental illness are known to cause specific birth defects.
- Antineoplastic agents. Drugs given to treat cancer can cause major congenital malformations, especially central nervous system defects. They also may be harmful to a health care worker who is giving them while she is pregnant.
- Hormones. Male hormones may cause masculinization of a female fetus. Diethylstilbestrol (DES), a synthetic estrogen given in the 1940s and 1950s to prevent miscarriage or premature birth, caused an increased risk of cancer in the adult female children of the mothers who received the drug.

- Narcotic pain relievers. Prescription opioids are associated with an increased risk of heart defects and spina bifida in newborns, particularly in those born to mothers who take these pain medications during the first trimester of pregnancy.
- Recreational drugs, including tobacco. Such drugs as LSD have been associated with arm and leg abnormalities and central nervous system problems in infants. Crack cocaine also has been associated with birth defects, as have ecstasy and marijuana. Heavy smoking has been linked to an increased risk of structural heart defects in newborns. Since drug abusers tend to use many drugs and have poor nutrition and prenatal care, it is not always easy to determine the effects of individual drugs.

CHEMICALS. Such environmental chemicals as fungicides, **food additives**, heavy metals like lead or mercury, and pollutants are suspected of causing birth defects, though the connections are sometimes difficult to prove. Exposure to chlorinated organic solvents during pregnancy, however, has been shown to be associated with an increased risk of heart defects in newborns.

RADIATION. Exposure of the mother to high levels of **radiation**, as for example with **cancer** therapy, can cause small skull size (microcephaly), blindness, spina bifida, and cleft palate. The severity of the defect depends on the duration and timing of the exposure.

INFECTIONS. Three viruses are known to harm a developing baby: **rubella** (German **measles**), **cytomegalovirus** (CMV), and **herpes** simplex. *Toxoplasma gondii,* a parasite that can be contracted from undercooked meat, from dirt, or from handling the feces of infected cats, causes serious problems. Untreated **syphilis** in the mother also is harmful.

Genetic factors

A gene is a small molecular unit of heredity containing information (DNA) that guides the formation and functioning of the body. Each individual inherits tens of thousands of genes from each parent, arranged on 46 chromosomes. Genes control all aspects of the body, how it works, and all its unique characteristics, including eye color and body size. Genes are influenced by chemicals and radiation, but sometimes changes (mutations) in the genes are spontaneous and unexplained accidents. Each child gets half of its genes from each parent. In each pair of genes, one will take precedence (dominance) over the other (recessive) in determining each trait, or characteristic. Birth defects caused by dominant inheritance include a form of dwarfism called achondroplasia; high cholesterol; Huntington's disease, a progressive nervous system disorder; Marfan syndrome, which affects connective tissue; some forms of glaucoma, and polydactyly (extra fingers or toes).

If both parents carry the same recessive gene, they have a one-in-four chance that the child will inherit the disease. Recessive diseases are severe and may lead to an early death. They include sickle cell anemia, a blood disorder that commonly affects persons of African descent; and Tay-Sachs disease, which causes mental retardation in people of Eastern European Jewish or Cajun (French-Acadian) heritage. Two recessive disorders more common in Caucasians are cystic fibrosis, a lung and digestive disorder, and phenylketonuria (PKU), a metabolic disorder. If only one parent passes along the genes for the disorder, the normal gene received from the other parent will prevent the disease, but the child will be a carrier. Having the gene is not harmful to the carrier, but there is a 25% chance of the genetic disease showing up in the children of two carriers.

Some disorders are linked to the sex-determining chromosomes passed along by parents. The genes for hemophilia, a condition that prevents blood from clotting, and Duchenne muscular dystrophy, which causes muscle weakness, are carried on the X chromosome. Genetic defects also can take place when the egg or sperm are forming if the mother or father passes along some faulty genetic material. This type of occurrence is more common in older mothers. The most common defect of this kind is Down syndrome, a pattern of mental retardation and physical abnormalities, often including heart defects, caused by inheriting three copies of a chromosome rather than the normal pair.

A less well understood cause of birth defects is the interaction of genes from one or both parents with environmental influences. Defects in this category are thought to include:

- Cleft lip and palate, which are malformations of the mouth.
- Clubfoot, an abnormality in which the baby's foot is twisted or misshapen.
- Spina bifida, an open spine caused when the neural tube, a structure in the embryo that gives rise to the brain and spinal cord, does not close properly.
- Water on the brain (hydrocephalus), which causes brain damage.
- Diabetes mellitus, an abnormality in sugar metabolism that appears later in life.
- Heart defects.
- Some forms of cancer.

A serious illness in the mother, such as an underactive thyroid, or **diabetes mellitus**, in which her body cannot process sugar, also can cause birth defects in the child. It has been shown that babies of diabetic mothers are five times as likely to have structural heart defects as other babies. An abnormal amount of amniotic fluid may indicate or cause birth defects. Amniotic fluid is the liquid that surrounds and protects the unborn child in the uterus. Too little of this fluid can interfere with lung or limb development. Too much amniotic fluid can accumulate if the fetus has a disorder that interferes with swallowing. Obese women are about three times more likely to have an infant with spina bifida or omphalocele (protrusion of part of the intestine through the navel) than women of average weight. Women who are overweight or classified as obese also are twice as likely to have an infant with a heart defect or multiple birth defects than women classified as average weight.

Assisted reproduction

One technological factor associated with an increased risk of birth defects is assisted reproductive technologies, particularly intracytoplasmic sperm injection (ICSI). In-vitro fertilization (IVF) has also been linked to a higher incidence of birth defects in children conceived by this method. The reason for this association is not known as of 2012.

Diagnosis

Screening and diagnostic tests can be performed during pregnancy to gain information about the health of the baby. These tests are recommended for all women over 35; women who have a personal or family history of birth defects; women who have given birth to a previous child with a birth defect; women who have type 1 or type 2 diabetes; women who drink alcohol or use street drugs; and women who have a body mass index (BMI) of 30 or higher. Specific screening and more detailed diagnostic tests include:

- Blood tests in the first trimester of pregnancy. There are two blood tests performed during this period. The first test is for the presence of pregnancy-associated plasma protein A (PAPP-A); a low level of this protein may indicate that the fetus has Down syndrome. The second blood test measures the presence of human chorionic gonadotropin (hCG), a hormone that is produced during pregnancy.
- A blood test that is usually done in the second trimester of pregnancy is the alpha-fetoprotein or AFP test. This is a simple blood test that measures the level of a substance called alpha-fetoprotein that is associated with some major birth defects. An abnormally high or low level may indicate the need for further testing.
- Ultrasound. The use of sound waves to examine the shape, function, and age of the fetus is a common procedure. It can be performed during the first trimester to measure the thickness at the back of the neck of the fetus to screen for Down syndrome. This type of ultrasound is called nuchal translucency screening. Ultrasound also can detect such malformations as anencephaly, spina bifida, limb defects, and heart and kidney problems.
- Amniocentesis. This is a diagnostic test that is usually performed between the 13th and 15th weeks of pregnancy. A small sample of amniotic fluid is withdrawn through a thin needle inserted into the mother's abdomen. Chromosomal analysis can rule out Down syndrome and other genetic conditions.
- Chorionic villus sampling (CVS). This diagnostic test can be done as early as the ninth week of pregnancy to identify chromosome disorders and some genetic conditions. A thin needle is inserted through the abdomen, or a slim tube is inserted through the vagina that takes a tiny tissue sample for testing.

If a birth defect is suspected after a baby is born, then confirmation of the diagnosis is very important. The patient's medical records and medical history may hold essential information. A careful physical examination and laboratory tests should be done. Special diagnostic tests also can provide genetic information in some cases. The March of Dimes, a nonprofit organization, recommends that every baby born in the United States receive at minimum screening for the same core group of birth defects, including phenylketonuria, congenital adrenal hyperplasia (an inherited disorder of the adrenal gland), congenital hypothryroidism, biotinidase deficiency, and others. As of 2012, most states in the United States routinely screen African American newborns for sickle cell anemia. The goal of the recommendations is to unify screening procedures across the United States.

Prevention

Pregnant women should eat a nutritious diet. Taking folic acid supplements before and during pregnancy reduces the risk of having a baby with neural tube defects. It is also important to avoid any teratogen that can harm the developing baby, including alcohol and drugs. Women who have not had rubella as children should be vaccinated against it; however, rubella vaccine should not be administered during pregnancy.

When there is a family history of congenital defects in either parent, genetic counseling and testing can help parents plan for future children. Often, counselors can determine the risk of a genetic condition occurring and the availability of tests for it. Talking to a genetic counselor after a child is born with a defect can provide parents with information about medical management and available community resources.

KEY TERMS

Anencephaly—A birth defect in which the baby is born without a forebrain and with part of the skull and scalp missing. Babies with this defect either are stillborn or die shortly after birth.

Atresia—A condition in which a body orifice or passage is abnormally closed or absent. In esophageal atresia, the esophagus is closed before it reaches the stomach.

Biotinidase deficiency—An inherited metabolic disorder in which biotin (vitamin B_7 is not released from proteins in the diet during digestion, leading to a deficiency of this vitamin.

Congenital—Present at birth.

Edwards syndrome—A genetic disorder caused by an extra copy (trisomy) of chromosome 18. It is characterized by heart abnormalities, kidney malformations, and disorders of other internal organs; few newborns survive past the first week of life. The syndrome is named for John H. Edwards (1928–2007), a British geneticist who first described it in 1960.

Gastroschisis—A birth defect in which there is an opening in the abdominal wall (usually to the right of the umbilicus) that allows the intestines to protrude through it.

Neural tube—A structure in the human embryo that is the forerunner of the brain and spinal cord. Neural tube defects are responsible for such congenital abnormalities as anencephaly and spina bifida.

Teratogen—Any agent that can cause the malformation of a fetus.

Tetralogy of Fallot—A congenital heart condition characterized by four separate anatomical abnormalities in the baby's heart. It is named for Arthur Fallot (1850–1911), a French physician who described it in detail in 1888.

Trisomy—A chromosomal disorder in which there are three copies of a chromosome in each body cell instead of the normal two copies. The most common trisomies are trisomy 21 (Down syndrome) and trisomy 18 (Edwards syndrome).

Umbilicus—The medical term for the navel or belly button.

Treatment

Treatment depends on the type of birth defect and how serious it is. When an abnormality has been identified before birth, delivery can be planned at a health care facility that is prepared to offer any special care needed. Some abnormalities can be corrected with surgery. Experimental procedures have been used successfully in correcting some defects, like excessive fluid in the brain (hydrocephalus), even before the baby is born. Early reports have shown success with fetal surgery on spina bifida patients. By operating on these fetuses while still in the womb, surgeons have improved outcomes at birth for many newborns and prevented the need for shunts in later childhood. However, long-term studies still are needed. Patients with complex conditions usually need the help of experienced medical and educational specialists with an understanding of the specific disorder.

Prognosis

The prognosis for a congenital disorder varies with the specific condition.

Costs to society

Birth defects are costly to society, not only in terms of the financial costs of treating or caring for children with severe metabolic or structural defects, but also in terms of the emotional **pain** for the parents and other family members. In many cases, families with children with severe birth defects find support groups more helpful than their healthcare providers in caring for the child. According to the **CDC**, children with birth defects have an increased risk of long-term chronic illness or disability as adults. They are also at greater risk of mental health problems—particularly anxiety disorders and depression—during adolescence and adult life.

Although the economic costs of all children born with major birth defects in any one year in the United States would be difficult to calculate because of the need to decide on the specific conditions to be included in the estimate, the CDC did make one attempt in 1992 to calculate the costs of children born with cerebral palsy and 17 other severe birth defects. Adding together the costs of hospital services, outpatient treatment, medications, special education, long-term care, and caregiver expenditures, the CDC arrived at a total of $8 billion per year (in 1992 dollars). The birth defects with the highest cost per case at the time the estimate was made were cerebral palsy ($503,000 per case), Down syndrome ($451,000), and spina bifida ($294,000).

Efforts and solutions

Efforts and solutions to lower the incidence of birth defects include the following:

- Fortification of certain foods with folic acid. Since 1998, the Food and Drug Administration (FDA) has required the addition of folic acid to enriched breads, cereals, flours, corn meals, pastas, rice, and other grain products. This supplementation has reduced the number of neural tube defects in American newborns.
- Education programs and outreach to teenagers and other underserved women to help them prepare for a healthy pregnancy; in particular, to warn them about the dangers of smoking, drinking, and drug use during pregnancy.
- Improving states' monitoring and recording of birth defects. A report issued by the Trust for America's Health in 2002 found that many states do not keep accurate records of the number and type of birth defects in newborns. Accurate tracking of birth defects is a necessary first step toward a better understanding of their true frequency and possible causes.
- Further research into the role of environmental pollutants and toxins in causing birth defects.
- Ongoing genetic research. The National Human Genome Research Institute (NHGRI) of the National Institutes of Health (NIH) is the central facility for advanced genetic research in the United States. The institute has a special section that investigates genetic factors that affect birth defects and other health problems in minority populations.
- Studies of the ethical, legal, and social issues involved in genetic testing and research involving birth defects. The NHGRI has a research program devoted to questions concerning the possible abuses of genetic testing and genetic counseling as well as their benefits. In addition to potential violations of patient confidentiality, other issues of concern include pregnancy termination (specifically whether women carrying a child diagnosed with a birth defect should be advised, or even forced, to terminate the pregnancy); rationing of health care for infants born with birth defects; and similar topics.

Resources

BOOKS

Judd, Sandra J., ed. *Genetic Disorders Sourcebook*, 4th ed. Detroit, MI: Omnigraphics, 2010.

Levino, Kenneth J., senior editor. *Williams Manual of Pregnancy Complications*, 23rd ed. New York: McGraw-Hill Professional, 2013.

Louis, Germaine Buck, and Robert Platt, eds. *Reproductive and Perinatal Epidemiology*. New York: Oxford University Press, 2011.

Moore, Keith L., T.V.N. Persaud, and Mark G. Torchia. *Before We Are Born: Essentials of Embryology and Birth Defects*, 8th ed. Philadelphia: Saunders/Elsevier, 2013.

PERIODICALS

Brennan, M.C., and W.F. Rayburn. "Counseling about Risks of Congenital Anomalies from Prescription Opioids." *Birth Defects Research, Part A. Clinical and Molecular Teratology* 94 (August 2012): 620–625.

Davies, M.J., et al. "Reproductive Technologies and the Risk of Birth Defects." *New England Journal of Medicine* 366 (May 10, 2012): 1803–1813.

Forand, S.P., et al. "Adverse Birth Outcomes and Maternal Exposure to Trichloroethylene and Tetrachloroethylene through Soil Vapor Intrusion in New York State." *Environmental Health Perspectives* 120 (April 2012): 616–621.

Gilboa, S.M., et al. "Association between Maternal Occupational Exposure to Organic Solvents and Congenital Heart Defects, National Birth Defects Prevention Study, 1997–2002." *Occupational and Environmental Medicine* 69 (September 2012): 628–635.

Janvier, A., et al. "The Experience of Families with Children with Trisomy 13 and 18 in Social Networks." *Pediatrics* 130 (August 2012): 293–298.

Milstein, J.M., et al. "A Piece of My Mind. A Path to Wholeness." [article is about the loving care provided for a baby born with trisomy 18 who lived only 19 days, and the wider importance of compassion in medicine.] *Journal of the American Medical Association* 308 (September 12, 2012): 985–986.

Parker, S.E., et al. "Updated National Birth Prevalence Estimates for Selected Birth Defects in the United States, 2004–2006." *Birth Defects Research, Part A. Clinical and Molecular Teratology* 88 (December 2010): 1008–1016.

Patel, S.S., et al. "Analysis of Selected Maternal Exposures and Non-syndromic Atrioventricular Septal Defects in the National Birth Defects Prevention Study, 1997–2005." *American Journal of Medical Genetics. Part A* 158A (October 2012): 2447–2455.

WEBSITES

"Birth Defects." Centers for Disease Control and Prevention (CDC).http://www.cdc.gov/ncbddd/birthdefects/index.html (accessed October 16, 2012).

"Birth Defects." Lucile Packard Children's Hospital at Stanford. http://www.lpch.org/DiseaseHealthInfo/HealthLibrary/genetics/bdefects.html (accessed October 18, 2012).

"Birth Defects." Nemours Foundation. http://kidshealth.org/parent/system/ill/birth_defects.html (accessed October 18, 2012).

"Frequently Asked Questions: Reducing Your Risk of Birth Defects." American Congress of Obstetricians and Gynecologists (ACOG). www.acog.org/~/media/For Patients/faq146.pdf (accessed October 18, 2012).

"Frequently Asked Questions: Screening for Birth Defects." American Congress of Obstetricians and Gynecologists (ACOG). www.acog.org/~/media/For Patients/faq165.pdf (accessed October 18, 2012).

"Genetic Testing." National Human Genome Research Institute (NHGRI). http://www.genome.gov/10002335 (accessed October 17, 2012).

ORGANIZATIONS

American Congress of Obstetricians and Gynecologists (ACOG), P.O. Box 70620, Washington, DC United States 20024-9998, (202) 638-5577, (800) 673-8444, http://www.acog.org/

Centers for Disease Control and Prevention (CDC), National Center on Birth Defects and Developmental Disabilities (NCBDDD), 1600 Clifton Road, MS E-87, Atlanta, GA United States 30333, (800) CDC-INFO (232-4636), cdcinfo@cdc.gov, http://www.cdc.gov/

March of Dimes, 1275 Mamaroneck Avenue, White Plains, NY United States 10605, (914) 997-4488, http://www.marchofdimes.com/contactus/contactus.html, http://www.marchofdimes.com/default.html

National Human Genome Research Institute (NHGRI), Building 31, Room 4B09, 31 Center Drive, MSC 2152, 9000 Rockville Pike, Bethesda, MD United States 20892-2152, (301) 402-0911, Fax: (301) 402-2218, http://www.genome.gov/.

Karen Ericson, RN
Teresa G. Odle
Rebecca J. Frey, PhD

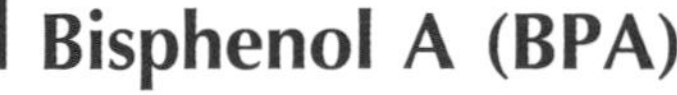

Bisphenol A (BPA)

Definition

Bisphenol A (BPA) is an organic substance used in the manufacture of polycarbonate plastics and epoxy resins. Commonly found in household products and food containers, BPA has been a topic of concern since the 1990s for potential public health hazards.

Description

Bisphenol A (BPA) is usually a cream or white crystal or flake. BPA is used in creating the polycarbonate plastics that are found in many household items, including: plastic baby bottles, plastic **water** bottles, food containers, the lining of food and beverage cans, reusable plastic cups and utensils, CD and DVD cases, the shells of household electronic and medical devices, refrigerator shelves, flooring, artificial teeth, nail polish, some dental sealants, car parts, flame retardants, eyeglass lenses, thermal copying paper (receipts), fax paper, self-adhesive labels, and some toys.

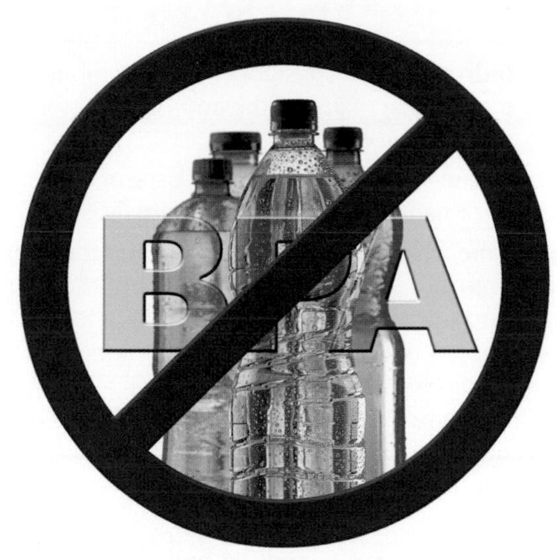

Anti-bisphenol A sign. *(© monticello/Shutterstock.com)*

Exposure to BPA comes from consuming food or liquid that was in a container made with Bisphenol A, touching or inhaling BPA during manufacturing, or coming in contact with water, air, or soil where BPA has leaked as a result of manufacturing processes. Containers are more susceptible to leaking BPA when they are scratched, washed in dishwashers at high temperatures, otherwise heated to high temperatures, or filled with hot or acidic liquids.

BPA is found in some, but not all, of recyclable plastics in the United States that are labeled with the number 3 or the number 7 in a triangle.

Origins

Bisphenol A was first synthesized by Russian chemist, Alexksandr Dianin, in 1891, though some sources list Germany's Thomas Zincke as discovering the substance in 1905.

BPA—an organic monomer that is used to construct larger polymers—consists of two phenol groups linked by a propane (3-carbon). BPA is known by the International Union of Pure and Applied Chemistry (IUPAC) as 4,4-dihyrdoxy-2, 2-diphenylpropane.

In the 1950s, production methods were developed to mass-produce plastics using BPA, at which point BPA began to be produced on an industrial scale. As of 2002, the estimated production of Bisphenol A was almost

KEY TERMS

Anti-androgen—A substance that inhibits the body's reception of any of the androgen hormones, such as testosterone.

Carcinogen—A substance that causes or increases the risk of cancer in humans or animals.

Endocrine disruptor—A foreign chemical that, when introduced into the body, acts on it similarly to a naturally-occurring hormone. In addition to Bisphenol A, other endocrine disruptors include dichlorodiphenyltrichloroethane (DDT)—which is an insecticide now banned in the US, and polychlorinated biphenyl (PCBs)—which are toxic and commonly found in coolants and pesticides.

Endocrine system—Glandular body system which dispatches hormones to regulate body functions. The endocrine system includes the thyroid, adrenal glands, and hypothalamus. This system affects other organs including the liver, pancreas, and kidneys and manages hormones like estrogen, testosterone, cortisol, and insulin.

Monomer—A molecule that can be bound to other similar molecules in order to make a polymer.

Polycarbonate plastics—With a variety of household and industrial uses, these plastics are clear, hard, and incredibly durable. These plastics are subject to breakdown and chemical degradation under high temperatures.

Polymer—A natural or synthetic substance composed of multiple monomers.

three million tons worldwide. The **Environmental Protection Agency (EPA)** classifies BPA as a high production volume (**HPV**) chemical. Bisphenol A is a suspected carcinogen, potentially acting as a contributing factor in breast and prostate cancers.

BPA is a known endocrine disruptor, and when in the body, it mimics the effects of estrogen. This interaction with the human endocrine system could potentially change the metabolism and functionality of certain cells. Despite binding to the same cell receptors as estrogen, BPA binds to these receptors more weakly than estrogen. BPA has also been shown to inhibit estrogen from binding to cell receptors and is an anti-androgen. Since the 1930s, BPA has been known to possess properties similar to estrogen but it was only in the 1990s that BPA began to cause widespread public health concerns.

Research

Research surrounding the effects of BPA is varied and does not easily lead to conclusions because most research is done using rodents and results cannot be directly correlated to human physiology. In addition, research has tended to suggest a bias—tests funded by industry groups tend to suggest no harm in BPA exposure while tests funded by independent non-profit or government organizations suggest potential harm.

The Environmental Working Group (EWG), a non-profit research and lobbying organization dealing with public and **environmental health** has conducted numerous studies relating to the effects of BPA. Of the foods tested for an EWG study in 2007, 10% of canned foods tested and 33% of infant formula tested contained sufficient BPA to expose an adult or child to levels of BPA 200 times greater than the exposure levels determined to be safe by the government. An EWG study in July of 2010 found high levels of BPA on 40% of receipts from major U.S. businesses including McDonalds, CVS, Whole Foods, Wal-Mart, and the United States Postal Service.

Research on aquatic organisms suggests that bisphenol A biodegrades easily and does not accumulate in tissues.

A 2011 Korean study published in *Toxicology* showed that when female mice were exposed to consistent levels of BPA during pregnancy, after birth, their offspring were unable to regenerate hippocampus cells normally and demonstrated issues with memory retention. Multiple studies of pregnant rats exposed to BPA have shown that in rats, BPA can be continually reintroduced to the fetus through the placenta and amniotic fluid, explaining the adverse affects on the offspring when the mothers were exposed to BPA during pregnancy.

Despite some previous suspicion, a 2011 Swedish study showed no correlation between BPA or phthalates and coronary problems in the elderly.

Risks

In addition to being an endocrine disruptor, Bisphenol A is suspected to have the potential to cause a number of other health concerns. From 2003-2004, the **Centers for Disease Control and Prevention (CDC)** conducted the National Health and **Nutrition** Examination Survey (NHANES III), in which they found detectable levels of BPA in 93% of over 2500 urine samples collected from individuals six years of age and older. This study, which is likely to represent the exposure levels of the general population in the United States, demonstrates that exposure is widespread—whether exposure poses any substantial health risks is still being debated.

As of 2012, there is insufficient data to positively link BPA with any adverse health conditions in humans. Most research studying BPA in rodents, however, shows negative health effects. There has been research to suggest that exposure to Bisphenol A may contribute to the following conditions:

- breast and prostate cancers
- early onset puberty in girls
- type 2 diabetes
- obesity
- attention deficit disorders
- brain functionality
- behavior
- thyroid function

There is evidence in rodent studies that a mother's exposure to Bisphenol A during pregnancy leads to adverse health conditions in the mother's offspring. As a result of these studies and the rapid development and cell growth that children undergo as fetuses, as infants, and during their early childhood—there is special concern about potential risks of BPA exposure during those times. In adults, BPA seems to degrade relatively quickly and is processed by the liver and expelled in urine.

Effects on Public Health

Though research is still largely inconclusive, if Bisphenol A is found to be dangerous to humans, its widespread presence in common products—particularly food packaging and storage containers—would be a great public health concern.

In 2007, the National Institutes of Health (NIH) conducted a census through the National Toxicology Program Center for the Evaluation of Risks to Human Reproduction (NTP-CERHR). This survey determined that, on average, most Americans were exposed to levels of Bisphenol A that were higher than the levels leading to harmful effects in animal experiments. The results of the survey were divided into five levels of concern:

- serious concern
- concern
- some concern
- minimal concern
- negligible concern

Effects of BPA on the brain, behavior, and prostate glands of fetuses, infants, and children were placed in the category of *some concern*. Effects of BPA on the mammary glands and earlier onset puberty in girls were placed in the category of *minimal concern*. Effects of BPA exposure on pregnant women causing fetal or newborn death, **birth defects**, low birth weight, or stunted growth were placed in the *negligible concern* category. The study authors made no conclusions about the effects of BPA exposure on **obesity**, type 2 diabetes, thyroid function, or **cancer**. The study also did not consider effects of exposure past early childhood.

The tolerable daily intake (TDI)—level of BPA deemed safe internationally—is 0.5 mg per kg of body weight.

Efforts and Solutions

United States

As a result of public concern regarding the potential health effects of Bisphenol A, in 2009, the top six manufacturers of baby bottles in America voluntarily stopped using BPA. These manufacturers, which represent more than 90% of the U.S. market include such brand names as: Avent, Doctor Brown's Natural Flow, Evenflow, First Essentials, Gerber, Munchkin, Nuk, and Playtex. Other baby and child items such as pacifiers, infant cups, and teething rings are also now available in BPA-free forms. Multiple container companies, including Rubbermaid, Tupperware, Eco, Thermos, and Nalgene have created BPA-free plastic products including food storage containers, water bottles, and food wrappers.

Some states and localities have banned the use of BPA in infant products or containers for children's food. Some major retail chains including Wal-Mart and Toys"R"Us have stopped carrying bottles, children's cups, and other food containers containing Bisphenol A.

The National Institute of Environmental Health Sciences (NIEHS) has invested approximately $30 million on research regarding the potential health effects of BPA. This funding from a variety of sources is part of a five-year initiative in conjunction with the U.S. Food and Drug Administration (FDA)'s National Center for Toxicological Research.

The FDA is taking multiple steps to minimize BPA exposure including: supporting a stop to the production of baby bottles and infant cups containing BPA in the U.S., assisting in the development of BPA-free linings for baby formula containers, and encouraging efforts to replace and minimize BPA levels in the lining of other food containers. The FDA is also working on developing a better regulatory system for monitoring BPA as well as soliciting public comment and scientific research regarding BPA. As of 2000, through the Food Contact Notification Program, the FDA regulates the use of BPA in food containers, its potential health concerns, and maintains a contingency plan for public safety in the event of amassing sufficient scientific evidence to suggest BPA-related health risks.

As of 2012, the **EPA** does not plan on taking regulatory action regarding Bisphenol A under the Toxic Substances Control Act.

International

In 2003, Japan stopped using epoxy linings containing BPA in its food cans. In October 2008, Canada banned the use of BPA in baby bottles and formula products in addition to putting Bisphenol A on its toxic substances list. Australia, New Zealand, and the European Union have declared that products containing BPA are safe as long as consumers adhere to manufacturers' instructions regarding proper use.

Precautions

Despite the inconclusive evidence of adverse health effects in humans as a result of Bisphenol A exposure, many consumers are still concerned about the potential health risks of BPA. If there is a concern about BPA, precautions can be taken to minimize exposure.

For Infants and Children

- Look for bottles and containers labeled "BPA-Free" or use glass bottles.
- Breastfeed until at least the age of 12 months when possible to provide the best possible nutrition for a child as well as greatly reducing the likelihood of BPA exposure.
- Use powdered formula instead of canned formula, if possible. Powdered formula usually has no detectable levels of BPA.
- If using canned formula, serve at room temperature or warm slightly by running bottle under warm water.
- Do not heat canned formula on a stove or in boiling water.
- Do not heat baby bottles in a microwave oven.
- Before adding water to formula, boil the water in a non-BPA container and allow it to cool.
- Sterilize and clean bottles according to instructions. Bottles should always be cooled to room temperature before using.
- Discard scratched baby bottles and infant cups—the scratches allow germs to collect and make BPA more likely to leach into the contents.

For Older Children and Adults

- Follow instructions on all food containers. Only put items labeled "microwave safe" in a microwave and those labeled "dishwasher safe" in a dishwasher.
- Use steel or BPA-free water bottles.
- Avoid heating food in plastic containers.
- Use plastic products containing U.S. recycle numbers 1, 2, 4, 5, or 6, which do not contain BPA.
- Do not put hot or acidic liquids in plastic containers—these liquids accelerate the breakdown of the plastic and increase the likelihood of BPA leaking into the contents.
- Look for BPA-free food storage containers and wrappers.

Resources

BOOKS

"Bisphenol A." *The Gale Encyclopedia of Children's Health: Infancy through Adolescence.* Ed. Jacqueline L. Longe. Vol. 1 2nd ed. Detroit: Gale, 2011. 326-29. *Gale Virtual Reference Library.* Web. June 29, 2012.

"Bisphenol-A" *The Encyclopedia of Poisons and Antidotes.* Carol Turkington and Deborah Mitchell. 3rd ed. New York: Facts on File, 2010. 37. Facts on File Library of Health and Living. *Gale Virtual Reference Library.* Web. June 29, 2012.

Blankenship, Alan L, and Katie Coady. "Bisphenol A." *Encyclopedia of Toxicology.* Ed. Philip Wexler, et al. 2nd ed. Vol. 1. Oxford, United Kingdom: Elsevier, 2005. 314-7. *Gale Virtual Reference Library.* Web. June 29, 2012.

Krishnan, Lalitha. "Bisphenol A (BPA)." *Salem Health: Cancer.* Ed. Jeffrey A. Knight. Vol. 1. Pasadena, CA: Salem Press, 2009. 149-50. *Gale Virtual Reference Library.* Web. June 29, 2012.

McIntosh, Philip. "Bisphenol A." *Food: In Context.* Ed. Brenda Wilmoth Lerner and K. Lee Lerner. Vol 1:Advertising Food to International Fund for Agricultural Development. Detroit: Gale, 2011. 81-83. *Gale Virtual Reference Library.* Web June 29, 2012.

Toxicological and Health Aspects of Bisphenol A: Report of Joint FAO/WHO Expert Meeting 2-5 November 2010 and Report of Stakeholder meeting on Bisphenol A 1 November 2010. World Health Organization. Geneva, Switzerland: WHO Press, 2011. http://whqlibdoc.who.int/publications/2011/97892141564274_eng.pdf Accessed June 29, 2012.

PERIODICALS

"High dose bisphenol A impairs hippocampal nerogenesis in female mice across generations." *Toxicology* 296.1-3 (2012): 73+. *Health Reference Center Academic.* Web. June 29, 2012.

Lind, Lars, P. Monica Lind, and Lena Olsen. "Associations between circulating levels of bisphenol A and phthalate metabolites and coronary risk in the elderly." *Ecotoxicology and Environmental Safety* 80 (2012): 179+. *Health Reference Center Academic.* Web. June 29, 2012.

"Placental Transfer of Conjugated Bisphenol A and Subsequent Reactivation in the Rat Fetus" *Children's Environmental Health News.* September (2010). *Children's Environ mental Health International Initiatives.* Web. June 29, 2012.

WEBSITES

Centers for Disease Control and Prevention. "Bisphenol A (BPA) Factsheet" http://www.cdc.gov/biomonitoring/BisphenolA_FactSheet.html Accessed June 29, 2012.

Environmental Working Group. “Bisphenol-A.” http://www.ewg.org/chemindex/chemicals/bisphenolA Accessed June 29, 2012.

National Institute of Environmental Health Sciences. “Since You Asked - Bisphenol A (BPA).” http://www.niehs.nih.gov/news/sya/sya-bpa/Accessed June 29, 2012.

U.S. Department of Health & Human Services. “Bisphenol A (BPA) Information for Parents.” http://www.hhs.gov/safety/bpa/ Accessed June 29, 2012.

U.S. Food and Drug Administration. “Bisphenol A (BPA): Use in Food Contact Application.” http://www.fda.gov/newsevents/publichealthfocus/ucm064437.htm Accessed June 29, 2012.

United States Environmental Protection Agency. “Bisphenol A (BPA) Action Plan Summary.” http://www.epa.gov/oppt/existingchemicals/pubs/actionplans/bpa.html Accessed June 29, 2012.

ORGANIZATIONS

The Environmental Working Group, 1436 U Street NW, Suite 100, Washington, DC USA 20009, 1 (202) 667-6982, www.ewg.org

U.S. Food and Drug Administration, 10903 New Hampshire Avenue, Silver Spring, MD USA 20993, (1-888) INFO-FDA (463-6332), www.fda.gov

World Health Organization, Avenue Appia 20, 1211 Geneva 27, Switzerland, 41 22 791 21 11, Fax: 41 22 791 31 11, www.who.int.

Andrea Nienstedt, MA

Black lung disease

Definition

Black lung disease is a respiratory illness caused by the inhalation of dust from coal, graphite, or man-made carbon. The amount of dust inhaled will determine the length of time required to cause noticeable symptoms of the disease. It is also known by the names coalworkers' pneumoconiosis (CWP), miners' **asthma**, and anthracosis. The main cause is workplace exposure incurred by coalmine workers who breathe the dust in underground mines. Coalworkers' pneumoconiosis is known as black lung disease, because the color of the lungs turns from the normal, healthy pink to black. The debilitating disease damages the lungs through inflammation of the lungs; air sacs, and scarring and thickening of lung tissue. It is potentially fatal.

Description

Black lung disease is one of a group of lung diseases called pneumoconioses. Black lung disease results from the inhalation of coal dust, which is generated during underground coalmining operations. Other types of pneumoconioses include **asbestosis** and byssinosis, which result from the inhalation of asbestos fibers and cotton dust, respectively. Black lung disease is considered preventable, provided that coalmine workers are afforded and take all of the necessary precautions to prevent the breathing of the dust in underground mines.

Black lung disease comes in two forms: simple CWP and complicated CWP. Those with simple CWP may experience no symptoms at all, but others may have a persistent cough. Simple CWP may progress to complicated CWP, which is also known as progressive massive fibrosis (PMF). Individuals with PMF experience more severe coughing, shortness of breath, or difficulty breathing, and in some cases, failure of the right side of the heart, which is the side that pumps blood to the lungs.

Origins

As far back as 1813, autopsies were revealing the presence of black lungs in coal miners in Great Britain. A subsequent medical report there in 1822 described coal miners' asthma, followed by numerous other reports about lung diseases among miners in Great Britain. The disease was quickly attributed to the inhalation of coal dust.

As coal mining increased in the United States, the prevalence of black lung disease also rose. The vast majority of these cases were among older miners who had been breathing coal dust for many years. Following the Federal Coal Mine Health and Safety Act of 1969 and the implementation of improved working conditions, black lung disease showed a steady decline over the next three decades. In 2000, however, the disease began a resurgence. This rise was accompanied by an increase in the number of severe cases of CWP in young miners.

Demographics

The national prevalence of black lung disease is 3.2%. According to the United Mine Workers of America, about 1,500 workers per year die as a result of black lung disease. CWP mainly affects underground coal-mine workers, typically those 50 years of age or older. It is, therefore, most common in those regions with active coal-mining operations. Besides coal miners, persons in certain other occupations that expose them to coal dust are at risk. These include individuals involved in storage; the mining or milling of graphite; or the manufacture of carbon electrodes or carbon black. Uses for carbon electrodes include arc welding, and as components in some large furnaces. Carbon black uses include pigment in inks and other similar products, and reinforcing material in rubber goods.

Causes and Symptoms

Causes

CWP results from the long-term inhalation of coal dust. As the dust accumulates in the lungs, symptoms begin to appear.

Symptoms

Symptoms typically do not appear until after many years of exposure. When enough dust has accumulated in the lungs, an individual will begin to experience coughing and shortness of breath, the symptoms of CWP. Symptoms vary depending on the individual's exposure to coal dust. Patients with the severe form of CWP get progressively worse and develop complications, such as chronic bronchitis, chronic obstructive pulmonary disease (COPD), respiratory failure, failure of the right side of the heart (cor pulmonale), lung **cancer**, and pulmonary **tuberculosis**.

Diagnosis

After obtaining a patient's history, and performing a physical exam that includes the use of a stethoscope to listen to the lungs, the doctor may suspect CWP. To help confirm the diagnosis, the doctor will typically order radiological imaging that may be in the form of an x-ray or computed tomography scan of the chest. The doctor may also order additional lung-function tests.

Treatment

No specific treatments are available for CWP, but patients do receive treatment for the symptoms of the disease, and for the symptoms of the various complications that may occur with PMF.

Prognosis

The prognosis for individuals with the simple form of CWP is good, and the disease rarely causes disability or death. For individuals with complicated CWP, the disease may progress and cause disability, complications, and possibly death.

Prevention

The best way to prevent the disease is to avoid long-term exposure to coal dust. Occupational exposure is the primary cause of CWP, so workers should take precautions to avoid inhalation of the dust. Precautions include wearing an approved mask, washing skin contaminated with coal dust, removing dust from and properly washing clothing, and refraining from eating or drinking in areas where coal dust may be present. By law, employers must supply protective equipment to their employees who may be exposed to coal dust.

Effects on Public Health

Long on the decline, black lung disease has made a resurgence in the 2000s. According to an investigation conducted by the Center for Public Integrity and National Public Radio (NPR), "the disease is now being diagnosed in younger miners and evolving more quickly to complicated stages." The report noted that the number of black lung cases doubled from 2002–2012, and men in their 40s were now developing PMF, whereas previously PMF affected men in their 50s and older. The report also noted that autopsies of victims of the mine explosion at the Massey Energy's Upper Big Branch mine revealed that 71 % showed signs of CWP, and some of them were in their 20s. Some blame the increases on improved production methods that can produce more coal dust, longer work weeks, and loopholes in and/or noncompliance with federal restrictions on coal-dust exposure levels.

Costs to Society

The U.S. Black Lung Benefits Act helps to ensure that payments are made to and medical treatments are provided for coal miners who are completely disabled from CWP. This condition is the result of working in and around underground coal mines. Payments must be made to survivors (spouses and children) of miners that died from CWP. The mine owners or operators are responsible for making such payments. In the event a miner's company is no longer in business, that individual may receive compensation from the Black Lung Disability Trust Fund, which is funded through taxes paid by coal operators.

From 1970–2011, according to the Mine Safety and Health Administration, government and industry have paid out more than $45 million in compensation.

Efforts and Solutions

The National Institute for Occupational Safety and Health (NIOSH), which is part of the **Centers for Disease Control and Prevention (CDC)**, operates the Coal Workers' Health Surveillance Program. Mandated by the 1969 Federal Coal Mine Health and Safety Act, the program is designed to monitor the health of coal workers in the United States. Through the statistics gathered, it was noted that the number of CWP cases was rising overall, and the number of severe CWP cases was also increasing among young coal miners.

NIOSH's Office of Mine Safety and Health Research conducts research to improve dust control and monitoring methods and instrumentation that the mining industry can

QUESTIONS TO ASK YOUR DOCTOR

- If I quit my job now, will I completely recover from my CWP?
- I work in a coal mine. Am I putting my family in danger for CWP? What precautions should they be taking, if any?
- I am a coal miner. What precautionary tests can you offer so that I will know if I may be getting CWP?

use to reduce exposure to coal dust. A NIOSH publication titled "Best Practices for Dust Control in Coal Mining" summarizes state of the art dust suppression technologies available to mine operators. In addition, the Office of Mine Safety and Health Research presents information through dust-control workshops and videos.

As of 2012, workers typically do not have immediate access to data about coal dust in the air they are breathing. To address this delay in providing dust-sampling findings to workers, the Office of Mine Safety and Health Research has developed the personal dust monitor (PDM), a device that provides real time dust exposure data to miners. Information like this can be important for modifying protective technologies and operating practices in the mines to lessen the risk of coal dust exposure.

Resources

WEBSITES

Berkes, Howard. "As Mine Protections Fail, Black Lung Cases Surge." National Public Radio. http://www.npr.org/2012/07/09/155978300/as-mine-protections-fail-black-lung-cases-surge (accessed September 11, 2012).

"End Black Lung: Act Now!" Mine Safety and Health Administration, U.S. Department of Labor. http://www.msha.gov/S&HINFO/BlackLung/homepage2009.asp (accessed September 11, 2012).

"Black Lung." United Mine Workers of America. http://www.umwa.org/?q=content/black-lung (accessed September 11, 2012).

"Black Lung Benefits Act." U.S. Department of Labor. http://www.dol.gov/compliance/laws/comp-blba.htm (accessed September 11, 2012).

"Coal worker's pneumoconiosis." PubMedHealth, U.S. National Library of Medicine. http://www.ncbi.nlm.nih.gov/pubmedhealth/PMH0001187/ (accessed September 11, 2012).

"Pneumoconiosis (Black Lung Disease)." PubMedHealth, American Lung Association. http://www.lung.org/lung-disease/pneumoconiosis/ (accessed September 11, 2012).

"Trend in Black Lung Cases Concerns NIOSH Researchers." U.S. Centers for Disease Control and Prevention. http://www.cdc.gov/niosh/mining/news/blacklung.htm (accessed September 11, 2012).

OTHER

Colinet, Jay F. et al. "Best Practices for Dust Control in Coal Mining." Pittsburgh, PA: U.S. Department of Health and Human Services, Public Health Service, Centers for Disease Control and Prevention, National Institute for Occupational Safety and Health, DHHS (NIOSH). Publication No. 2010-110, Information Circular 9517, 2010 Jan;:1-76.

ORGANIZATIONS

American Lung Association, 1301 Pennsylvania Ave. NW, Suite 800, Washington, DC 20004, (202) 785-3355, http://www.lung.org/.

Mine Safety and Health Administration, 1100 Wilson Boulevard, 21st Floor, Arlington, VA 22209-3939, (202) 693-9400, http://www.msha.gov/.

United Mine Workers of America (UMWA), 18354 Quantico Gateway Dr., Suite 200, Triangle, VA 22172-1179, (703) 291-2400, http://www.umwa.org/.

Leslie Mertz, Ph.D.

Bovine spongiform encephalopathy

Definition

Bovine spongiform encephalopathy (BSE) is a disease of cattle. Often called mad cow disease, it is a progressive disorder that affects the nervous system and ultimately leads to death. Scientists believe the disease is transmitted to humans through the ingestion of BSE-contaminated cow products. Called variant Creutzfeldt-Jakob disease, the human disease has no cure and is fatal. BSE also has no cure and is fatal.

Description

BSE is associated with an accumulation of agents known as BSE prions, which are misfolded and pathogenic forms of normal proteins. The prions cause lesions in the brain and spinal cord. The deterioration gives the brain a spongy appearance, and is reflected in the disease's name of bovine spongiform encephalopathy, which means cow sponge-like brain disease. The disease develops slowly, and from three–six years following infection, symptoms appear. Symptoms progressively worsen, and death follows about four–six months later, sometimes earlier.

Variant Creutzfeldt-Jakob disease (vCJD) is the human form of the disease. People can contract the illness by eating contaminated beef products, primarily those containing brain or nervous tissue from an infected

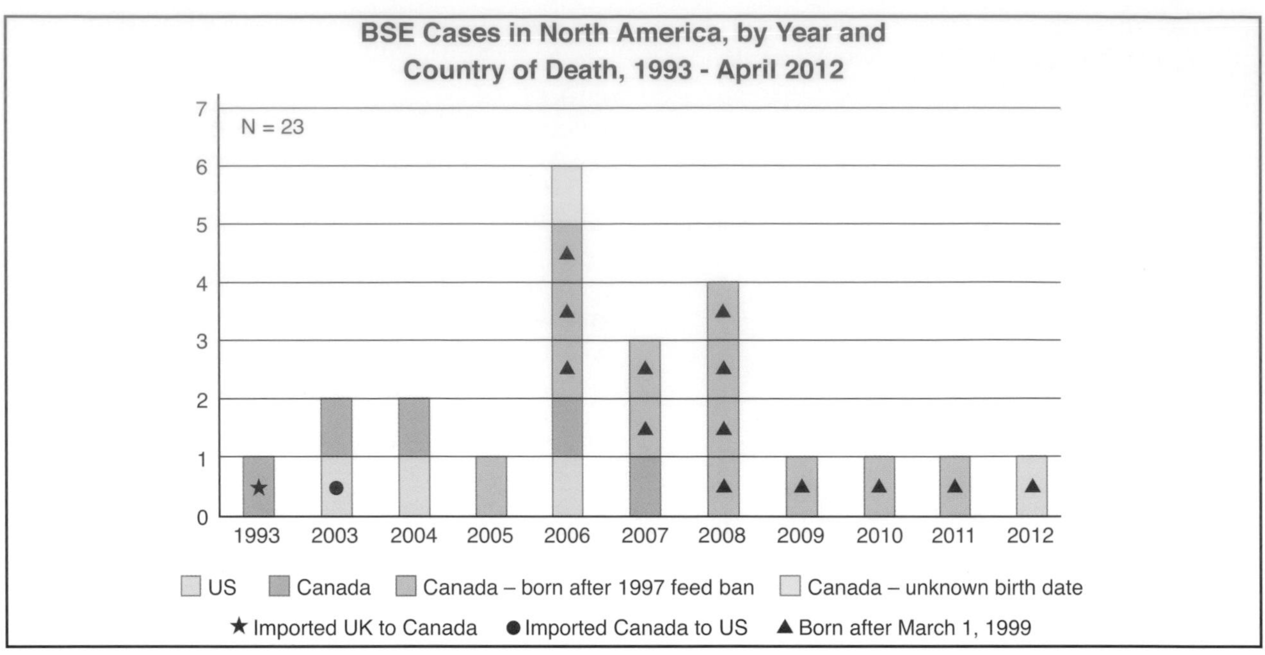

(Illustration by Electronic Illustrators Group. © 2013 Cengage Learning)

cow. Since most U.S. slaughterhouses remove those tissues and do not incorporate them in products slated for human consumption, combined with the significant decline in number of BSE cases overall, the risk of a person contracting vCJD is extremely low. Symptoms in humans include a range of neurologic problems, such as loss of coordination and steadiness (ataxia); loss of memory and confusion (dementia); and involuntary muscle contractions or twitching (myoclonus). vCJD is fatal.

Origins

Bovine spongiform encephalopathy is one of a number of prion diseases that infect animals. One of these diseases, called scrapie, has been known in sheep for about three centuries. In the mid-1980s, some cows in the United Kingdom began showing signs of a neurologic disease. Medical study of these cows ultimately revealed that they had spongy brain features like those seen in sheep that had scrapie, and the disease was named bovine spongiform encephalopathy.

BSE took on epidemic proportions by the early 1990s, peaking in January 1993 with almost 1,000 new cases reported every week in the United Kingdom, according to the U.S. **Centers for Disease Control and Prevention (CDC)**. Cattle feed was identified as the cause of the outbreak, and through feed changes, the number of BSE cases have dropped dramatically since then. According to the World Organisation for Animal Health, the United Kingdom experienced just 12 cases of BSE in 2009, 11 cases in 2010, and seven cases in 2011. This compares to 1991, 1992, and 1993 BSE totals in the UK of 25,359, 37,280, and 35,090, respectively.

In 1995, the first case of vCJD occurred, also in the United Kingdom. This illness was distinguished from previously known instances of CJD, a rare illness that typically affected individuals who were older than 60. vCJD not only had a different disease course (14 months compared to five months for CJD), but it also affected much younger people. The median age at death for CJD patients is 68 years old, while the median age at death for a vCJD patient is 28. According to the United Kingdom Food Standards Agency, a total of 176 cases of vCJD had been diagnosed in the UK as of January 2012, and more than 80% of those occurred before 2005.

Demographics

The vast majority of BSE cases occurred in the United Kingdom. BSE cases have also been reported in the European and Asian countries of Austria, Belgium, Denmark, Finland, France, Germany, Greece, Ireland, Israel, Italy, Liechtenstein, Luxembourg, Portugal, Spain, Switzerland, the Czech Republic, the Netherlands, Slovakia, Slovenia, and Japan.

Canada and the United States have also had BSE cases. In North America, the number of BSE cases from 2003–2011 totaled 21, and just three of the affected cattle were in the United States. As of April 24, 2012, one additional case of BSE had been reported for the 2012 year in North America, and that was an infected dairy cow in California.

Only one case of vCJD has been reported in the United States as of 2012. This was a woman who likely contracted the disease while previously living in the United Kingdom.

Causes and Symptoms

Causes

BSE is part of a family of diseases known as the transmissible spongiform encephalopathies, several of which occur in the United States. These include scrapie in sheep and goats; chronic wasting disease in deer and elk; feline spongiform encephalopathy in cats; and transmissible spongiform encephalopathy in minks.

As of 2012, evidence suggests that BSE has two forms: typical BSE strain, and atypical BSE strain.

The typical BSE strain was behind the outbreak of mad cow disease in the United Kingdom. It is sometimes called transmissible BSE. Researchers suspect that the typical BSE strain originated as a result of cattle feed that included meat-and-bone meal contaminated with scrapie-infected sheep products or with cow products that were infected with the atypical strain of BSE. (The practice of including mammalian meat, bone, and blood products in feed was common in Europe at that time.)

This typical strain is also responsible for most of the BSE cases in Canada, but as of April 2012, it has not been associated with any BSE cases in United States-born cattle, according to the **CDC**. The typical strain, which can be prevented by ceasing the use of BSE-contaminated feed, is linked to vCJD in humans.

The UK Spongiform Encephalopathy Advisory Committee proposed in 2007 that atypical BSE may be a distinct strain of prion disease that arises spontaneously, albeit rarely, in cattle. The United States beef industry, which overwhelmingly uses grain feed for cattle, did not experience the typical BSE strain. As of April 2012, four U.S.-born cattle have contracted infection with the atypical strain.

The atypical BSE strain has been divided into two forms: the H-type and the L-type. Both the H-type and L-type atypical BSE strains have caused disease in North American cattle.

BSE is not contagious, and cannot spread from contact with an infected animal. The only known means of transmission of typical BSE is through the ingestion of contaminated feed.

Symptoms

The first symptoms of BSE usually occur 2.5–8 years following the initial infection, and the typical age is between 3 and 6 years. Once symptoms appear, the disease progresses rapidly, usually resulting in death within six months.

Symptoms include:

- difficulty standing
- weight loss
- nervous or aggressive behavior
- twitching and tremors
- decreased milk production

Diagnosis

The rapid onset and progression of symptoms helps to diagnose BSE. Autopsy examinations of brain tissue confirms the diagnosis.

Treatment

No treatment exists for BSE, or for vCJD. Both are fatal.

Prevention

The most effective preventive measure against BSE infection is the elimination of mammalian products from cattle feed.

Effects on Public Health

The human disease vCJD has been linked to the ingestion of BSE-contaminated beef. No treatment and no cure are available for vCJD. It is fatal.

Costs to Society

Identification of BSE in cattle can lead to costly import bans on that country's beef. For example, the outbreak of BSE in the United Kingdom led to the European Union banning exports of UK beef from 1996–2006. In addition, reports of BSE (or vCJD) can cause

KEY TERMS

Encephalitis—An inflammation and swelling of the brain, usually due to infections with bacteria, viruses, or other agents. It may be contracted through contaminated foods or drinks, from insect or tick bites, or by other means.

Prion—An infectious agent composed of a protein that has been folded in an abnormal manner. Prions are believed to be responsible for various neurodegenerative diseases, including bovine spongiform encephalitis (mad cow disease).

extreme responses from consumers, and these can result in reduced beef purchases, regardless of assurances of beef safety from health and agricultural officials.

Efforts and Solutions

The U.S. Food and Drug Administration (FDA) issued a 1997 ban on the use of mammalian proteins in the feed for ruminants, including cattle, and in October 2009, enhanced that feed ban. With this enhanced ban, the feed-control measures in the United States and Canada work together to help eliminate BSE in cattle.

On a global scale, the World Organisation for Animal Health has developed criteria that it uses to classify each country's risk for BSE, and provides guidelines that countries may use to determine the policies regarding their beef imports.

In addition, countries have developed targeted surveillance programs to identify and act on incidences of BSE in their cattle herds, and to monitor cattle feed.

Resources

WEBSITES

"Bovine Spongiform Encephalopathy (BSE) Fact Sheet." Alberta Agriculture and Rural Development. http://www1.agric.gov.ab.ca/$department/deptdocs.nsf/all/cpv8104 (accessed November 8, 2012).

"Bovine Spongiform Encephalopathy—'Mad Cow Disease'" U.S. Department of Agriculture Food Safety and Inspection Service. http://www.fsis.usda.gov/FACTSheets/Bovine_Spongiform_Encephalopathy_Mad_Cow_Disease/index.asp (accessed November 8, 2012).

"Bovine Spongiform Encephalopathy." World Health Organization. http://www.who.int/mediacentre/factsheets/fs113/en/ (accessed November 8, 2012).

"Bovine Spongiform Encephalopathy." World Organisation for Animal Health. http://www.oie.int/index.php?id=169&L=0&htmfile=chapitre_1.11.5.htm (accessed November 8, 2012).

"BSE and other Transmissible Spongiform Encephalopathies." U.K. Food Standards Agency. http://www.food.gov.uk/policy-advice/bse/#.UJ_wkOOe9AM (accessed November 8, 2012).

"BSE (Bovine Spongiform Encephalopathy, or Mad Cow Disease)." U.S. Centers for Disease Control and Prevention. http://www.cdc.gov/ncidod/dvrd/bse/ (accessed November 8, 2012).

"Making Sense of Mad Cow Disease." University of Maryland Medical Center. http://www.umm.edu/features/madcow.htm (accessed November 8, 2012).

"Number of cases of bovine spongiform encephalopathy (BSE) reported in the United Kingdom." World Organisation for Animal Health (OIE). http://www.oie.int/en/animal-health-in-the-world/bse-specific-data/number-of-cases-in-the-united-kingdom/ (accessed November 6, 2012).

ORGANIZATIONS

Centers for Disease Control and Prevention (CDC), 1600 Clifton Road, Atlanta, GA 30333, (800) 232-4636, cdcinfo@cdc.gov, http://www.cdc.gov/std/

U.S. Food and Drug Administration (FDA), 10903 New Hampshire Avenue, Silver Spring, MD 20993, (888) 463-6332, http://www.fda.gov/

World Organization for Animal Health (OIE), 12, rue de Prony, Paris, France 75017, 33 (0) 1 44 15 18 88, oie@oie.int, http://www.oie.int.

Leslie Mertz, Ph.D.

Breast feeding *see* **Maternal health**

Brucellosis

Definition

Brucellosis is a bacterial disease caused by members of the *Brucella* genus that can infect humans but primarily infects livestock. Symptoms of the disease in humans include intermittent fever, sweating, chills, aches, and mental depression. The disease can become chronic and recur, particularly if untreated.

Description

Also known as undulant fever, Malta fever, Gibraltar fever, Bang's disease, or Mediterranean fever, brucellosis is most likely to occur among those individuals who regularly work with livestock. The disease originated in domestic livestock but was passed on to wild animal species, including the elk and buffalo of the western United States. In humans, brucellosis continues to be spread via unpasteurized milk obtained from infected cows or through contact with the discharges of cattle and goats during miscarriage. In areas of the world where milk is not pasteurized, such as in Latin America and the Mediterranean, the disease is still contracted by ingesting unpasteurized dairy products. However, in the United States, the widespread **pasteurization** of milk and nearly complete eradication of the infection from cattle has reduced the number of human cases from 6,500 in 1940 to fewer than 100 today. The **World Health Organization (WHO)**, however, estimates that about half a million cases of brucellosis occur worldwide every year, making it the most important of all zoonotic diseases.

Causes and symptoms

The disease is caused by several different species of parasitic bacteria of the genus Brucella. *B. abortus* is

KEY TERMS

Antibody—A specific protein produced by the immune system in response to a specific foreign protein or particle called an antigen.

Chronic—Disease or condition characterized by slow onset over a long period of time.

Parasite—An organism living in or on, and obtaining nourishment from, another organism.

Pasteurization—The process of applying heat, usually to milk or cheese, for the purpose of killing, or retarding the development of, pathogenic bacteria.

Zoonotic—Referring to a disease that occurs primarily in animals.

found in cattle and can cause cows to abort their fetuses. *B. suis* is most often found in hogs and is more deadly when contracted by humans than the organism found in cattle. *B. melitensis* is found in goats and sheep and causes the most severe illness in humans. *B. rangiferi* infects reindeer and caribou, and *B. canis* is found in dogs.

A human contracts the disease by coming into contact with an infected animal and either allowing the bacteria to enter a cut, breathing in the bacteria, or consuming unpasteurized milk or fresh goat cheese obtained from a contaminated animal. In the United States, the disease is primarily confined to slaughterhouse workers.

Scientists do not agree as to whether brucellosis can be transmitted from one person to another, although some people have been infected from a tainted blood transfusion or bone marrow transplant. Newborn babies have also contracted the illness from their mothers during birth. Currently, it is believed that brucellosis can also be transmitted sexually.

The disease is not usually fatal, but the intermittent fevers (a source of its nickname, "undulant fever") can be exhausting. Symptoms usually appear between five days and a month after exposure and begin with a single bout of high fever accompanied by shivering, aching, and drenching sweats that last for a few days. Other symptoms may include headache, poor appetite, backache, weakness, and depression. Mental depression can be so severe that the patient may become suicidal.

In rare, untreated cases, the disease can become so severe that it leads to fatal complications, such as **pneumonia** or bacterial **meningitis**. *B. melitensis* can cause miscarriages, especially during the first three months of pregnancy. The condition can also occur in a chronic form, in which symptoms recur over a period of months or years.

Diagnosis

Brucellosis is usually diagnosed by detecting one or more *Brucella* species in blood or urine samples. The bacteria may be positively identified using biochemical methods or using a technique whereby, if present in the sample, the brucellosis bacteria are made to fluoresce. Brucellosis may also be diagnosed by culturing and isolating the bacteria from one of the above samples. Blood samples will also indicate elevated antibody levels or increased amounts of a protein produced directly in response to infection with brucellosis bacteria.

Treatment

Prolonged treatment with **antibiotics**, including tetracyclines (with streptomycin), co-trimoxazole, and sulfonamides, is effective. Bed rest is also imperative. In the chronic form of brucellosis, the symptoms may recur, requiring a second course of treatment.

Prognosis

Early diagnosis and prompt, treatment is essential to prevent chronic infection. Untreated, the disease may linger for years, but it is rarely fatal. Relapses may also occur.

Prevention

There is no human vaccine for brucellosis, but humans can be protected by controlling the disease in livestock. After checking to make sure an animal is not already infected, and destroying those that are, all livestock should be immunized. Butchers and those who work in slaughterhouses should wear protective glasses and clothing, and protect broken skin from infection.

Some experts suggest that a person with the disease refrain from engaging in unprotected sex until free of the disease. The sexual partners of an infected person should also be closely monitored for signs of infection.

Resources

BOOKS

Choffnes, Eileen R., et al., eds. *The Causes and Impacts of Neglected Tropical and Zoonotic Diseases: Opportunities for Integrated Intervention Strategies: Workshop Summary*. Washington, DC: National Academies Press, 2011.

Petersen, Eskild, Lin Hwei Chen, and Patricia Schlagenhauf, eds. *Infectious Diseases: A Geographic Guide*. New York: Wiley-Blackwell, 2011.

PERIODICALS

"Human Exposures to Marine Brucella Isolated from a Harbor Porpoise—Maine, 2012." *MMWR Morbidity and Mortality Weekly Report.* 61, 25. (2012): 461–3.

"Laboratory-acquired Brucellosis–Indiana and Minnesota, 2006." *MMWR Morbidity and Mortality Weekly Report* 57, 2. (2008): 39–42.

OTHER

"Brucellosis." Centers for Disease Control and Prevention. http://www.cdc.gov/ncidod/dbmd/diseaseinfo/brucellosis_g.htm. Accessed on October 21, 2012.

"Brucellosis." PubMedHealth. http://www.ncbi.nlm.nih.gov/pubmedhealth/PMH0001623/. Accessed on October 21, 2012.

"Brucellosis." World Health Organization. http://www.who.int/zoonoses/diseases/brucellosis/en/. Accessed on October 21, 2012.

ORGANIZATIONS

Centers for Disease Control and Prevention (CDC), 1600 Clifton Rd., Atlanta, GA 30333, (800) 232-4636, cdcinfo@cdc.govhttp://www.cdc.gov/email.do?url=http%3A//www.cdc.gov/contact/, http://www.cdc.gov.

Carol A. Turkington

Bullying

Definition

Bullying is a persistent pattern of threatening, harassing, or aggressive behavior directed toward another person or persons who are perceived as smaller, weaker, or less powerful. Although often thought of as a childhood phenomenon, bullying can occur wherever people interact, most often observable in the workplace and in the home in adults. Bullying is also called "harassment."

Demographics

Bullying in children

Bullying among children is a persistent and substantial problem that requires serious attention. According to a study published in 2001 by the Kaiser Family Foundation and Nickelodeon Television, 55% of 8-11-year-olds and 68% of 12-15-year-olds said that bullying is a "big problem" for people their age. Seventy-four percent of the 8-11-year-olds and 86% of the 12-15-year-olds also reported that children were bullied or teased at their school. These statistics were essentially unchanged in 2011. Children at greatest risk of being bullied are those who are perceived as social isolates or outcasts by their peers, have a history of changing schools, have poor social skills or a desire to fit in "at any cost," are defenseless, or are viewed by their peers as being different.

A study of more than 16,000 children in the sixth through tenth grades conducted for the National Institute of Child Health and Human Development found that nearly 60% of the children responding had been victims of rumors. More than 50% of the children reported that they had been the victims of sexual harassment. A Canadian study reported in 2010 that cyberbullying is also a common problem, with 49% of children in a sample of 2,200 students reporting having been bullied on the Internet and 34% admitting to having bullied others online.

The National Center for Education Statistics (NCES) of the U.S. Department of Education found that white, non-Hispanic children were more likely to report being the victims of bullying than black or other non-Hispanic children. Younger children were more likely to report being bullied than older children, and children attending schools with gangs were more likely to report being bullied than children in schools without a major gang presence. No differences were found in these patterns between public and private schools. Fewer children reported bullying in schools that were supervised by police officers, security officers, or staff hallway monitors. Victims of bullying were more likely to be criminally victimized at school than were other children. Victims of bullying were more afraid of being attacked both at school and elsewhere and more likely to avoid certain areas of school (for example, the cafeteria, hallways or stairs, or restrooms) or activities where bullying was more likely to take place. Significantly, victims of bullies were more likely to report that they carried weapons to school for protection.

Children who are identified as bullies by the time they are eight years of age are six times more likely than other children to have a criminal conviction by the time they are 24 years old. Bullying behavior may also be accompanied by other inappropriate behavior, including criminal, delinquent, or gang behavior.

Bullying in the workplace

Although research has been conducted on workplace bullying in Europe for some time, the topic has only recently become of interest in the United States. The nonprofit Workplace Bullying Institute conducted two surveys in 2010 with more than 6,000 respondents. It defined workplace bullying as "repeated mistreatment: sabotage by others that prevented work from getting done, verbal abuse, threatening conduct, intimidation and

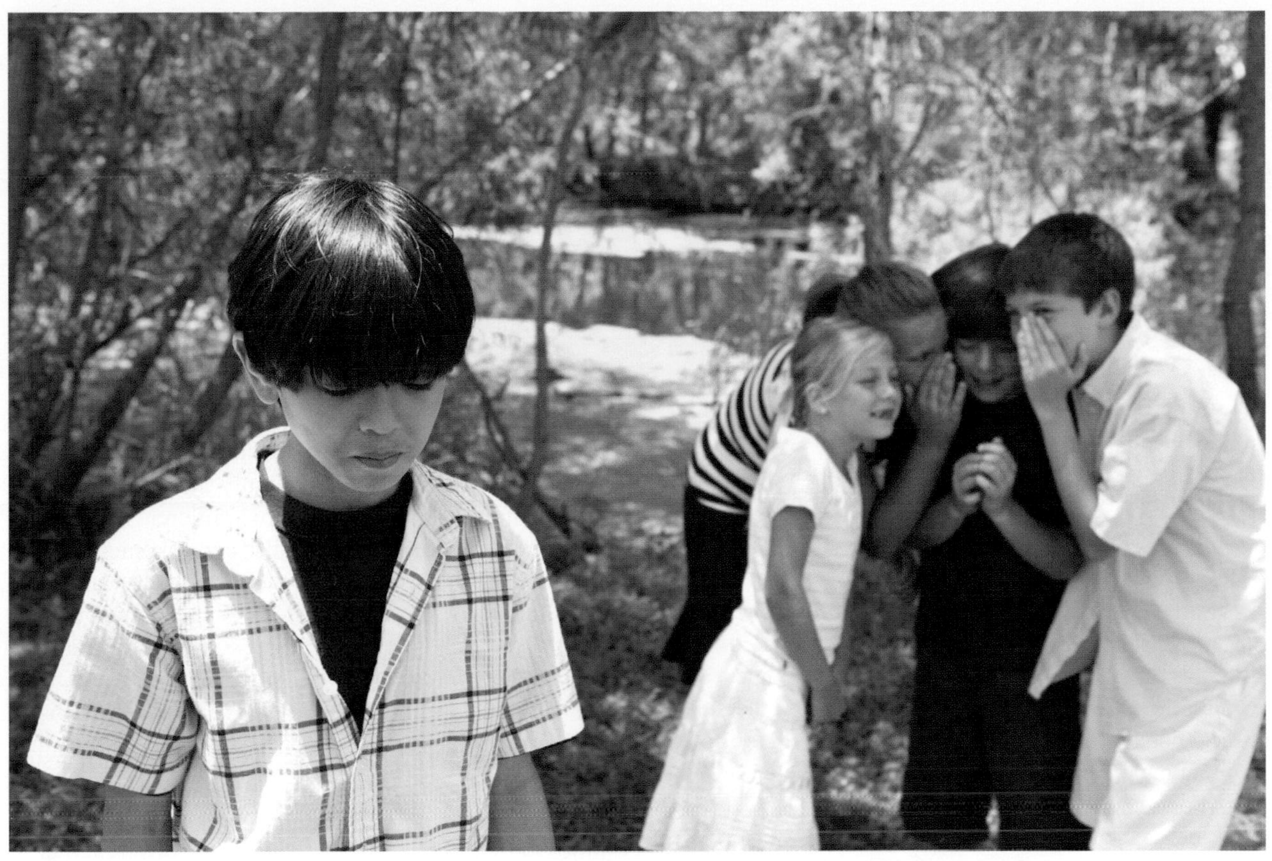

Children ganging up against a classmate: classic bullying behavior. *(© iStockphoto.com/Ana Abejon)*

humiliation" and compared statistics to its 2007 survey. The 2010 survey found that 35% of workers have experienced bullying first hand (37% in 2007); 62% of bullies are men and 58% of targets are women; women bullies target women in 80% of cases; and the majority (68%) of bullying is same-gender harassment.

Description

There are many forms of bullying in both children and adults. Bullies may intimidate or harass their victims physically through hitting, pushing, or other physical **violence**; verbally through such actions as threats or name calling; or psychologically through spreading rumors (either live or online), making sexual comments or gestures, or excluding the victim from desired activities.

There are many reasons to stop bullying. Bullying interferes with school performance, and children who are afraid of being bullied are more likely to miss school or drop out. Bullied children frequently experience developmental harm and fail to reach their full physiological, social, and academic potentials. Children who are bullied grow increasingly insecure and anxious and have persistently decreased self-esteem and greater depression than their peers, often even as adults. Children and adolescents have even been known to commit **suicide** as a result of being bullied; this tragic outcome has been referred to by some writers as "bullycide."

People who are bullies as children often become bullies as adults. Bullying behavior in the home is called "child abuse" or "spousal abuse." Bullying also occurs in prisons, churches, summer camps, college or boarding school dormitories, and other social groups or group living situations.

Recently, attention has been turned to the topic of bullying in the workplace, defined as occurring when bosses and organizational peers bully those whom they perceive as weaker or inferior. Those bullied at work often become perceived as ineffective, thus abrogating their career success and influencing their earning potential. Victims of workplace bullying often change jobs in search of a less hostile environment because organizations are frequently not sensitive to the issue of workplace bullying or are not equipped to deal with it adequately or justly.

Cyberbullying

Bullying does not need to occur in person: cyberbullying is a persistent pattern of threatening, harassing, or aggressive behavior carried out online. The widespread popularity of cell phones and other mobile devices means that cyberbullying can be carried out anonymously without the need for a computer. Cyberbullying can take a number of different forms:

- sending hurtful or threatening messages directly to the victim via e-mail or phone texting
- spreading rumors about the victim to others via e-mail or other forms of messaging
- setting up websites, posting videos, or creating pages on social media to hurt or humiliate the victim

Cyberbullying is increasingly considered a particularly damaging form of bullying because it can be carried on at all times, can be shared with a wide number of people (for example, a video that "goes viral" on YouTube), and is hard to undo due to a number of online services that archive Internet sites.

Some researchers maintain that cyberbullies fall into several different categories and do not necessarily resemble the classic schoolyard bully. While some cyberbullies are power-hungry or vengeful, others may just be bored and looking for something to do for online entertainment. Another common type of cyberbully is the inadvertent bully, typically an adolescent who doesn't think before sending a message or who is so invested in online role-playing that he or she fails to understand that the recipient of such a message may take it seriously.

Another reason for concern about cyberbullying is that electronic communication itself has the potential to intensify situations that are already touchy, because the absence of face-to-face contact makes it harder for the cyberbully to "see" the humanity of the victim. E-mail messages and texting lack vocal tone, making it easier to increase the hostility and aggressiveness of text messages. There have been several notable cases of electronic messaging escalating into real-world violence, such as the "Facebook murder" that occurred in Florida in April 2011, in which a 15-year-old boy was lured into an ambush by his former girlfriend via text messages.

Risk factors

Warning signs and factors that may indicate risk for being or becoming a bully include:

- lack of impulse control (frequent loss of temper, extreme impulsiveness, easily becoming frustrated, extreme mood swings)
- family factors (physical abuse or violence within the family, substance or alcohol abuse within the family, overly permissive parenting, lack of clear limits, inadequate parental supervision, harsh or even corporal punishment, child abuse, inconsistent parenting)
- behavioral symptoms (gang affiliation, name calling or abusive language, carrying a weapon, hurting animals, abusing alcohol or drugs, making serious threats, vandalizing or damaging property, frequent physical fighting)

Causes and symptoms

There is no evidence to support the theory that there is a genetic component to bullying behavior. Particularly in children, bullying appears to result from the bully's copying the actions of role models who bully others. According to the **Centers for Disease Control and Prevention (CDC)**, this pattern frequently occurs when bullies come from a home in which one parent bullies another, or one or both parents bully the children. When such behavior is modeled for children with such personality traits as lack of impulse control or aggression, they are particularly prone to bullying behavior, which often continues into adulthood.

Bullying in children

According to the U.S. **Department of Health and Human Services**, children who have dominant personalities and who are more impulsive and active are more prone to becoming bullies than children without these traits. Bullies also often have a history of emotional or behavioral problems. Victims of bullying, on the other hand, tend to be more anxious, insecure, and socially isolated than their peers and often lack age-appropriate social skills. The probability of victimization can be compounded when the victim has low self-esteem due to physical characteristics (for example, the victim believes her/himself to be unattractive, is disfigured in some way, or is outside the normal range for height or weight) or personal problems (for example, health problems or physical or mental disability).

Symptoms or indications that a child may be being bullied include:

- social withdrawal or isolation (few or no friends; feeling isolated, sad, and alone; feeling picked on or persecuted; feeling rejected or not liked; having poor social skills)
- somatic complaints (frequent complaints about illness; displaying victim body language, including hanging head, hunching shoulders, and avoiding eye contact)
- avoidant behavior (not wanting to go to school, skipping classes or school)
- affective reactions (crying easily; having mood swings; talking about hopelessness, running away, or suicide)
- physical clues (bringing home damaged possessions or reporting that belongings were "lost")

KEY TERMS

Bullycide—Suicide attributed to the victim's having been bullied.

Cyberbullying—The use of electronic devices, including computers, cell phones, and other mobile devices, to bully by means of hurtful messages, spreading rumors, or misusing social media.

- behavior changes (changes in eating or sleeping patterns)
- aggressive behavior (threatening violence to self or others, taking or attempting to take a weapon to school)

Each child will react to bullying in a different manner, and some children will react with only a few of these symptoms. These differences, however, do not mean that bullying is not severe or that intervention is not needed.

Bullying in the workplace

Bullying in the workplace is usually motivated by political rather than personal reasons. Workers may compete for promotions, raises, and other honors. In an attempt to climb the ladder of success, some individuals do what they can to not only present themselves in a good light to their superiors, but also to make one or more coworkers seem unworthy or inept. Bullying bosses demonstrate poor leadership styles and poor motivational skills, frequently attempting to further either their own or the company's agenda through harassment, belittling, or other negative behaviors.

Common tactics used by workplace bullies include:

- discounting or belittling the victim in public (making statements such as "that's silly" in response to the victim's ideas, disregarding evidence of satisfactory or superlative work done by victim, taking credit for victim's work)
- making false accusations (rumors about victim, lies about victim's performance)
- harassing the victim (verbal putdowns based on gender, race, disability)
- isolating the victim (encouraging others to turn against the victim, socially or physically isolating the victim from others)
- nonverbal aggression (staring, glaring, silent treatment)
- sabotaging the victim's work
- unequal treatment (retaliating against victim who files a complaint, making up arbitrary rules for victim to follow, assigning undesirable work as a punishment, making unreasonable or unreachable goals or deadlines for victim, performing a constructive discharge of duties)

Diagnosis

Bullying, in itself, is not a mental disorder, although aggressive or harassing behavior may be symptomatic of a number of disorders, particularly antisocial personality disorder. There are, however, a number of criteria to help determine whether someone is a bully. First, to qualify as bullying, the bully's behavior must be intended to cause physical or psychological harm to the other person. Second, bullying behavior is not an isolated incident but results in a consistent pattern of such behavior over time. Third, bullying occurs where there is an imbalance of power whereby the bully has more physical or psychological power than the victim. Harassing behavior is not considered to be bullying if it occurs between individuals of equal strength and status or if it is a one-time event.

Bullying behavior in children can include any of the following behaviors:

- dominance (enjoying feeling powerful and in control, seeking to dominate or manipulate others, being a poor winner or loser)
- lack of empathy (deriving satisfaction from the fears, pain, or discomfort of others; enjoying conflict between others; displaying intolerance of, or prejudice toward, others)
- negative emotions or violence (displaying uncontrolled anger or a pattern of impulsive and chronic hitting, intimidating, or aggressive behavior)
- lack of responsibility (blaming others for his/her problems)
- other behaviors (using drugs or alcohol, hiding bullying behavior from adults, having a history of discipline problems)

Victims of bullying, whether children or adults, may need to be assessed and treated if they need help responding to, or recovering from, bullying.

Treatment

If bullying behavior is symptomatic of an underlying mental disorder such as conduct disorder or antisocial personality disorder, treatment should first address the underlying disorder. For situations in which bullying behavior is not part of a pattern associated with an underlying mental disorder, treatment and establishing organizational or familial processes for addressing it are required.

Bullying in children

If parent(s) suspect that their child is a bully, help can be sought from mental health professionals and school counselors. Taking the child to a child psychologist and participating in family therapy as appropriate can

QUESTIONS TO ASK YOUR DOCTOR

- I didn't grow up with cell phones and social media. What should I tell my children to help them protect themselves against cyberbullying?
- Have you ever treated a child or teenager who developed a physical or mental disorder because of bullying? What was the outcome?
- Have you ever treated or referred an adult who was suffering from workplace bullying?

help teach a bully better interpersonal skills. Contacting the school counselor or a child psychologist is also an appropriate step in helping the victims of bullies.

If parents suspect that their child may be being bullied, they should make sure that he or she understands that the problem is not his or her fault and that he or she does not have to face the situation alone. Parents can discuss ways to deal with bullies, including walking away, being assertive, and getting help. Parents should also encourage the child to report bullying behavior to a teacher, counselor, or other trusted adult. Parents should not try to resolve the situation themselves, but should contact the school to report the behavior and to seek recommendations for further assistance.

Dealing with cyberbullying

Cyberbullying requires some different approaches than face-to-face bullying, because of the nature of electronic messages and also because it can involve legal penalties for the bully. Some practical tips for dealing with cyberbullying include:

- saving evidence of harassing e-mails and other forms of cyberbullying. These can be forwarded to a parent or trusted friend, or saved on a flash drive.
- Reporting cyberbullying to the service provider. Many social networking sites as well as phone companies and e-mail providers take reports of cyberbullying seriously and will block the bully's account.
- Using the block setting on cell phones or other mobile devices to stop the cyberbully from sending messages.
- Using passwords to protect online e-mail accounts and cell phones, and changing the passwords frequently.

Bullying in the workplace

Bullying in the workplace can be minimized if the organization develops and enforces antiharassment policies and procedures. These should include a stated definition on what constitutes harassment, creating and implementing a disciplinary system to punish the bully rather than the victim, and instituting a formal grievance system to report workplace bullying. Other measures that can be taken include inclusiveness and harassment training, awareness training to educate employees on how to spot bullying behavior, and offering courses in conflict resolution, anger management, or assertiveness training.

Bullies are not the only ones needing help. The intention of a bully is to harm the other person; victims, therefore, may experience a number of negative consequences from being the victim of a bully. If the behavior associated with being a victim persists after the bullying situation has been resolved, or if the situation continues without just resolution, victims should be assessed for depression and/or an anxiety disorder (if their symptoms warrant) and should receive the appropriate treatment. Though the relationship between bullying and post–traumatic stress disorder (PTSD), has not been widely studied, a 2012 Norwegian study suggests that this connection, may be strong, especially for students. The results of the study of students in grades 8 and 9 showed PTSD symptoms within the clinical range in 27.6% of bullied boys and 40.5% of bullied girls. Though this study represents a small demographic, its results suggest the importance of bullying victims being accurately assessed by a mental health professional.

Costs to society

As bullying becomes more widely–studied, its long-term effects become better understood. The societal effects of bullying can be seen in bullies and their victims. The cycles of abuse that lead the bullied to become bullies themselves, as well as predisposing childhood bullies to criminal activity later in life, allow the effects of bullying on society to be seen outside of the original act. From domestic violence and **child abuse** to juvenile and adult criminal records, bullies become very much an issue for society at large. Additionally, the psychological effects of bullying on its victims which can lead to lifelong battles with depression, anxiety, PTSD, and even suicide, show the far-reaching effects of bullying for the bullies, their victims, and the rest of society.

Prevention

To help keep a child from becoming a bully, it is important to be a role model for nonviolent behavior. Parents should also clearly communicate to the child that bullying behavior is not acceptable—clear limits should be established for acceptable behavior, and consequences for ignoring the limits should be defined. Teaching good social skills, including efficacious conflict-resolution skills and anger management skills, can also help potential bullies learn alternative socially acceptable behaviors.

Recent attention in the media to student suicides related to bullying as well as school shootings and similar acts of violence has prompted a search for new approaches to the problem. One approach involves making it easier for students to break the "code of silence" that makes them reluctant to inform on their peers. Safe2Tell is an anonymous 24/7 hotline that some communities have set up that allows students to report bullying, plans to attack the school, and other forms of violent behavior.

A more comprehensive approach is the Olweus (pronounced ohl-VAY-us) Bullying Prevention Program (OBBP), a systems-change approach designed by a Norwegian educator named Dan Olweus in 1983 and tested in both Norway and the United States for over 25 years. The program is designed to improve peer relations and make schools safer, more positive places for students to learn and develop. Goals of the program include reducing existing bullying problems among students, preventing new bullying problems, and achieving better peer relations at school. As of 2011, the OBBP approach had been used with over 40,000 students in both countries and was reported to have reduced bullying rates by up to 50%. Designed for long-term use in elementary, middle, and junior high schools, the program includes a questionnaire about bullying for students to answer as well as training for teachers, school administrators, parents, and community leaders. The program does not utilize conflict-resolution or peer-mediation techniques, because it believes that these approaches assume that the parties involved are equal in power or status, whereas bullying is based on power imbalances. According to proponents of the Olweus program, it reduces vandalism as well as bullying and other forms of antisocial behavior in the schools where it has been tried. It has also been successfully used in summer camps, sports teams, and other organizations for children and adolescents.

Efforts and solutions

The U.S. Department of Health & Human Services maintains a website—stopbullying.gov—dedicated to providing resources to help stop bullying and support those who have been bullied, as well as documenting ongoing efforts on the state and national levels to address bullying. In December 2010, the U.S. Department of Education examined existing laws and found eleven "key components" within those laws that apply to bullying. Forty–two states and Puerto Rico have both anti–bullying laws and policies in effect, eight states have anti–bullying measures in effect in law only, and Montana has anti–bullying measures in effect in policy only. In June 2012, the District of Columbia signed into law The Youth Bullying Prevention Act of 2012. Updates on relevant news, and changes to state and federal laws can be obtained from stopybullying.gov. In addition to these resources, through the Stop Bullying website, the U.S. Department of Health & Human Services offers webinars (instructional online videos) on various forms of bullying and bullying prevention, and participates in the annual Federal Partners in Bullying Prevention Summit, which began in 2010.

Resources

BOOKS

Hamilton, Jill, ed. *Bullying and Hazing*. Detroit, MI: Greenhaven Press, 2008.

Monks, Claire P., and Iain Coyne, eds. *Bullying in Different Contexts*. New York: Cambridge University Press, 2011.

Olweus, Dan, et al. *Olweus Bullying Prevention Program: Schoolwide Guide*. Center City, MN: Hazelden, 2007.

Pennsylvania Bar Institute. *Surviving the Schoolyard Battlefield*. Mechanicsburg, PA: PBI, 2008.

Spivet, Bonnie. *Stopping Cyberbullying*. New York: PowerKids Press, 2012.

PERIODICALS

Blosnich, J., and R. Bossarte. "Low-level Violence in Schools: Is There an Association between School Safety Measures and Peer Victimization?" *Journal of School Health* 81 (February 2011): 107–113.

Centers for Disease Control and Prevention (CDC). "Bullying among Middle School and High School Students—Massachusetts, 2009." *Morbidity and Mortality Weekly Report* 60 (April 22, 2011): 465–471.

Dyregrov, Atle, Ella Cosmovici Idsoe, and Thormod Idsoe. "Bullying and PTSD Symptoms." *Journal of Abnormal Child Psychology* 40.6 (2012): 901–911.

Johnson, S.L. "An Ecological Model of Workplace Bullying: A Guide for Intervention and Research." *Nursing Forum* 46 (April 2011): 55–63.

Meloni, M., and M. Austin. "Implementation and Outcomes of a Zero Tolerance of Bullying and Harassment Program." *Australian Health Review* 35 (February 2011): 92–94.

Mishna, F., et al. "Cyber Bullying Behaviors among Middle and High School Students." *American Journal of Orthopsychiatry* 80 (July 2010): 362–374.

Olweus, D., and S.P. Limber. "Bullying in School: Evaluation and Dissemination of the Olweus Bullying Prevention Program." *American Journal of Orthopsychiatry* 80 (January 2010): 124–134.

Payne, S.R., and D.S. Elliott. "Safe2Tell(®): An Anonymous, 24/7 Reporting System for Preventing School Violence." *New Directions for Youth Development* 129 (March 2011): 103–111.

Stagg, S.J., and D. Sheridan. "Effectiveness of Bullying and Violence Prevention Programs." *Journal of the American Association of Occupational Health Nurses* 58 (October 2010): 419–424.

Waasdorp, T.E., et al. "A Multilevel Perspective on the Climate of Bullying: Discrepancies Among Students, School Staff, and Parents." *Journal of School Violence* 10 (January 1, 2011): 115–132.

Wang, J., et al. "Cyber and Traditional Bullying: Differential Association with Depression." *Journal of Adolescent Health* 48 (April 2011): 415–417.

WEBSITES

ABC News. "Teen Triangle and Facebook Feud Lead to Murder of 15-Year-Old Florida Boy." http://abcnews.go.com/US/teen-triangle-leads-vicious-murder-15-year-florida/story?id=13422887 (accessed May 24, 2011).

American Academy of Child and Adolescent Psychiatry (AACAP) Facts for Families. "Bullying." http://www.aacap.org/cs/root/facts_for_families/bullying (accessed May 23, 2011).

Hazelden Foundation. "An Overview of the Olweus Bullying Prevention Program" (10-minute video). http://www.youtube.com/watch?v=P9C5wJ6uAk0 (accessed May 23, 2011).

Olweus Bullying Prevention Program. "What Is Bullying?" http://www.olweus.org/public/bullying.page (accessed May 22, 2011).

StopBullying.gov Home Page. http://www.stopbullying.gov (accessed August 2, 2012).

STOP Cyberbullying. "What Methods Work with the Different Kinds of Cyberbullies?" http://www.stopcyberbullying.org/parents/howdoyouhandleacyberbully.html (accessed May 22, 2011).

TeensHealth. "Cyberbullying." http://kidshealth.org/teen/school_jobs/bullying/cyberbullying.html (accessed May 22, 2011).

TeensHealth. "Dealing with Bullying." http://kidshealth.org/teen/your_mind/problems/bullies.html (accessed May 22, 2011).

Workplace Bullying Institute Home Page. http://www.workplacebullying.org (accessed May 22, 2011).

ORGANIZATIONS

Act Against Bullying, PO Box 57962, London, United Kingdom W4 2TG, 44 020 8995 9500, info@actagainstbullying.org, http://www.actagainstbullying.org/index.htm

American Academy of Child and Adolescent Psychiatry (AACAP), 3615 Wisconsin Avenue, NW, Washington, DC United States, 20016-3007, (202) 966-7300, Fax: (202) 966-2891, http://www.aacap.org

Hazelden Foundation, PO Box 11, Center City, MN United States, 55012-0011, (651) 213-4200, (800) 257-7810, info@hazelden.org, http://www.hazelden.org

Olweus Bullying Prevention Program, (800) 328-9000, olweusinfo@hazelden.org, http://www.olweus.org/public/index.page

STOP Cyberbullying, (201) 463-8663, parry@aftab.com, http://www.stopcyberbullying.org/index2.html

Workplace Bullying Institute (WBI), PO Box 29915, Bellingham, WA United States, 98228, http://www.workplacebullying.org.

Ruth A. Wienclaw, Ph.D.
Rebecca J. Frey, Ph.D.
Andrea Nienstedt, MA

Burns

Definition

Burns are injuries to tissues caused by heat, friction, electricity, **radiation**, or chemicals.

Description

Burns are characterized by degree, based on the severity of the tissue damage. A first-degree burn causes redness and swelling in the outer layer of skin (epidermis). A second-degree burn involves redness, swelling, and blistering, and the damage may involve the outer layer of skin and the layer underneath. A third-degree burn, also called a full-thickness burn, destroys the entire depth of skin and may affect the underlying fat, muscle, or bone tissues.

The severity of the burn is also judged by the amount of body surface area (BSA) involved. Health care workers use the "rule of nines" to determine the percentage of BSA affected in patients more than nine years old: each arm with its hand is 9% of BSA; each leg with its foot is 18%; the front of the torso is 18%; the back of the torso, including the buttocks, is 18%; the head and neck are 9%; and the genital area (perineum) is 1%. This rule cannot be applied to a young child's body proportions, so BSA is estimated using the palm of the patient's hand as a measure of 1% area.

The severity of the burn will determine not only the type of treatment, but also where the burn patient should receive treatment. Minor burns may be treated at home or in a doctor's office. These are defined as first- or second-degree burns covering less than 15% of an adult's body or less than 10% of a child's body, or a third-degree burn on less than 2% BSA. Moderate burns should be treated at a hospital. These are defined as first- or second-degree burns covering 15%-25% of an adult's body or 10%-20% of a child's body, or a third-degree burn on 2%-10% BSA. Critical, or major, burns are the most serious and should be treated in a specialized burn unit of a hospital. These are defined as burns to the the face, feet, hands, ears, eyes, or genitals, or as first- or second-degree burns covering more than 25% of an adult's body or more than 20% of a child's body, or a third-degree burn on more than 10% BSA. Other factors influence the level of treatment needed, including associated injuries such as bone fractures and smoke inhalation, presence of a chronic disease, or a history of physical abuse. Children and the elderly are more vulnerable to complications from burn injuries and require more intensive care.

Causes and symptoms

Burns may be caused by even a brief encounter with heat greater than 120°F (49°C). The source of this heat

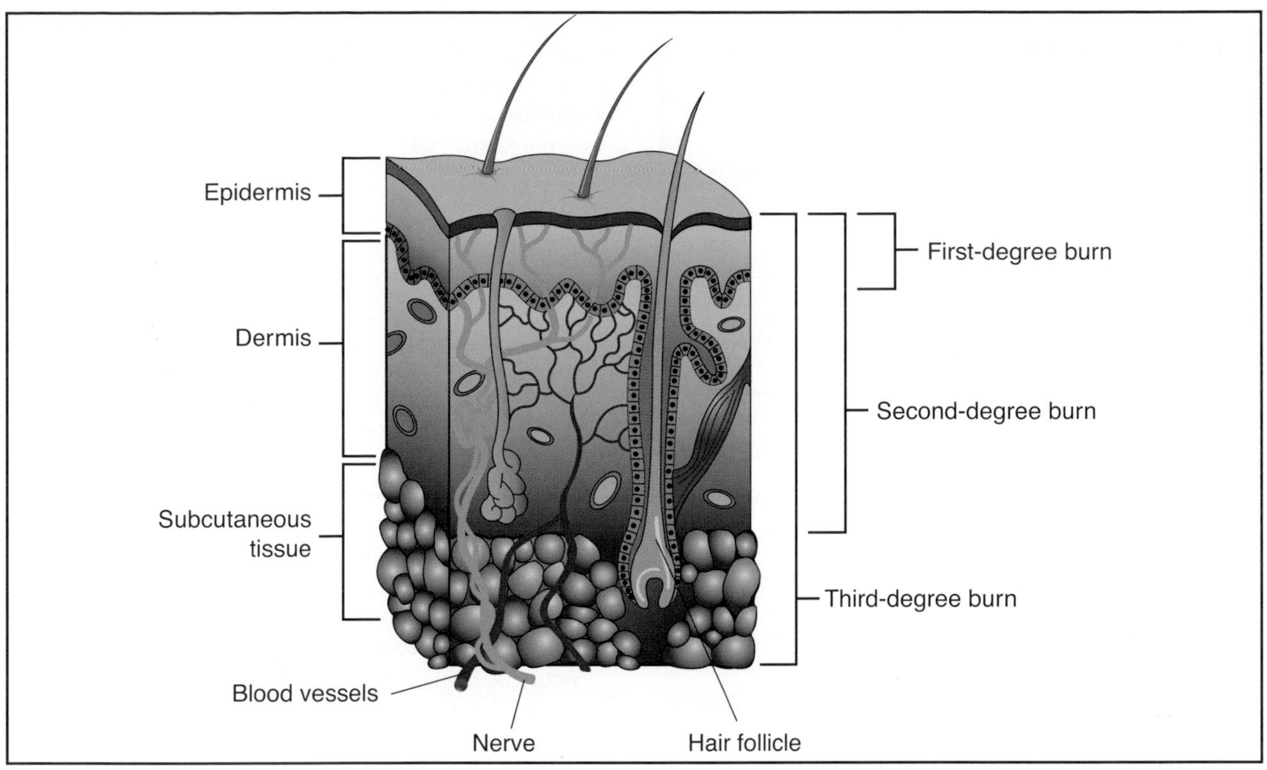

Degrees of burns. *(Illustration by Electronic Illustrators Group. © 2013 Cengage Learning)*

may be the sun (causing a sunburn), hot liquids, steam, fire, electricity, friction (causing rug burns and rope burns), and chemicals (causing a caustic burn upon contact).

Signs of a burn are localized redness, swelling, and **pain**. A severe burn will also blister. The skin may also peel, appear white or charred, and feel numb. A burn may trigger a headache and fever. Extensive burns may induce shock, the symptoms of which are faintness, weakness, rapid pulse and breathing, pale and clammy skin, and bluish lips and fingernails.

Diagnosis

A physician will diagnose a burn based upon visual examination, and will also ask the patient or family members questions to determine the best treatment. He or she may also check for smoke inhalation, **carbon monoxide poisoning**, cyanide **poisoning**, other event-related trauma, or, if suspected, further evidence of physical abuse.

Treatment

Burn treatment consists of relieving pain, preventing infection, and maintaining body fluids, electrolytes, and calorie intake while the body heals. Treatment of chemical or electrical burns is slightly different from the treatment of thermal burns, but the objectives are the same.

Thermal burn treatment

The first act of thermal burn treatment is to stop the burning process. This may be accomplished by letting cool water run over the burned area or by soaking it in cool (not cold) water. Ice should never be applied to the burn. Cool (not cold) wet compresses may provide some pain relief when applied to small areas of first- and second-degree burns. Butter, shortening, or egg whites should never be applied to the burn because they can lead to infection.

If the burn is minor, it may be cleaned gently with soap and water. Blisters should not be broken. If the skin of the burned area is unbroken, and it is not likely to be further irritated by pressure or friction, the burn should be left exposed to the air to promote healing. If the skin is broken or apt to be disturbed, the burned area should be coated lightly with an antibacterial ointment and covered loosely with a sterile gauze bandage. Aspirin, naproxen (Aleve), acetaminophen (Tylenol), or ibuprofen (Advil) may be taken to ease pain and relieve inflammation. A doctor should be consulted if there is increased warmth, redness, pain, or swelling; pus or similar drainage from the wound; swollen lymph nodes; or red streaks

Classification of burns

First-degree burn	The burned area is painful. The outer skin is reddened. Slight swelling is present.
Second-degree burn	The burned area is painful. Deeper layers of skin (the dermis) are affected. Blisters may form. The area may have a wet, shiny appearance because of exposed tissue.
Third-degree burn	The burned area is insensitive due to the destruction of nerve endings. Skin is destroyed. Muscle tissue and bone underneath may be damaged. The area may be charred, white, or grayish in color.

(Table by PreMediaGlobal. © 2013 Cengage Learning)

spreading away from the burn, as these are signs of infection.

In situations where a person has received moderate or critical burns, lifesaving measures take precedence over burn treatment, and emergency medical assistance must be called. A person with serious burns may stop breathing, and artificial respiration (also called mouth-to-mouth resuscitation or rescue breathing) should be administered immediately. Also, a person with burns covering more than 12% BSA is likely to go into shock; shock may be prevented by laying the person flat and elevating the feet about 12 in (30 cm). Burned arms and hands should also be raised higher than the person's heart.

In rescues, a blanket may be used to smother any flames as the person is removed from danger. The person whose clothing is on fire should "stop, drop, and roll" or be assisted in lying flat on the ground and rolling to put out the fire. Afterwards, only burnt clothing that comes off easily should be removed; any clothing embedded in the burn should not be disturbed. Removing any smoldering apparel and covering the person with a light, cool, wet cloth, such as a sheet but not a blanket or towel, will stop the burning process.

At the hospital, the staff will provide further medical treatment. A tube to aid breathing may be inserted if the patient's airways or lungs have been damaged, as can happen during an explosion or a fire in an enclosed space. Also, because burns dramatically deplete the body of fluids, replacement fluids will be administered intravenously. The patient will also be given **antibiotics** intravenously to prevent infection, and he or she may also receive a **tetanus** shot, depending on his or her **immunization** history. Once the burned area is cleaned and treated with antibiotic cream or ointment, it is covered in sterile bandages, which are changed two to three times a day. Surgical removal of dead tissue (debridement) also takes place. As the burns heal, thick, taut scabs (eschar) form, and the doctor may have to cut them to improve blood flow to the more elastic healthy tissue beneath. The patient will also undergo physical and occupational therapy to keep the burned areas from becoming inflexible and to minimize scarring.

In cases where the skin has been so damaged that it cannot properly heal, a skin graft is usually performed. A skin graft involves taking a piece of skin from an unburned portion of the patient's body (autograft) and transplanting it to the burned area. When doctors cannot immediately use the patient's own skin, a temporary graft is performed using the skin of a human donor (allograft), either living or deceased, or the skin of an animal (xenograft), usually that of a pig.

The burn victim also may be placed in a hyperbaric chamber, if one is available. In a hyperbaric chamber (which can be a specialized room or enclosed space), the patient is exposed to pure oxygen under high pressure, which can aid in healing. However, for this therapy to be effective, the patient must be placed in a chamber within 24 hours of being burned.

Chemical burn treatment

Burns from liquid chemicals must be rinsed with cool water for at least 15 minutes to stop the burning process. Any burn to the eye must be similarly flushed with water. In cases of burns from dry chemicals such as lime, the powder should be completely brushed away before the area is washed. Any clothing that may have absorbed the chemical should be removed. The burn should then be loosely covered with a sterile gauze pad, and the person taken to the hospital for further treatment. A physician may be able to neutralize the chemical with another before treating the burn like a thermal burn of similar severity.

Electrical burn treatment

Before electrical burns are treated at the site of the accident, the power source must be disconnected if possible, and the victim moved away from it to protect aid givers from being electrocuted. Lifesaving measures again take priority over burn treatment, so breathing must be checked and assisted if necessary. Electrical burns should be loosely covered with sterile gauze pads, and the person taken to the hospital for further treatment.

Alternative treatment

In addition to the excellent treatment of burns provided by traditional medicine, some alternative approaches may be helpful, though major burns should always be treated by a medical practitioner.

KEY TERMS

Debridement—The surgical removal of dead tissue.

Dermis—The basal layer of skin; it contains blood and lymphatic vessels, nerves, glands, and hair follicles.

Epidermis—The outer portion of skin, made up of four or five superficial layers.

Shock—An abnormal condition resulting from low blood volume due to hemorrhage or dehydration. Signs of shock include rapid pulse and breathing, and cool, moist, pale skin.

The homeopathic remedies *Cantharis* and *Causticum* can assist in burn healing. A number of botanical remedies, applied topically, can also help burns heal, especially aloe (*Aloe barbadensis*). Oil of St. St. John's wort (*Hypericum perforatum*), calendula (*Calendula officinalis*), comfrey (*Symphytum officinale*), and tea tree oil (*Melaleuca* spp.) can also be helpful.

Researchers in New Zealand and Europe are investigating medicinal-grade honey, which has been effective in China as a treatment; however, use of this treatment requires considerable experience. The dietary supplements vitamin C, vitamin E, and zinc can also benefit wound healing.

Prognosis

The prognosis is dependent upon the degree of the burn, the amount of body surface covered, whether critical body parts were affected, any additional injuries or complications (such as infection), and the promptness of medical treatment. Minor burns may heal in 5 to 10 days with no scarring. Moderate burns may heal in 10–14 days and may leave scarring. Critical or major burns take more than 14 days to heal and will leave significant scarring. Scar tissue may limit mobility and functionality, but physical therapy may overcome these limitations. In some cases, additional surgery may be advisable to remove scar tissue and restore appearance. Pigment changes may occur in the healed area, leaving it a different color from the surrounding skin. Burned tissue should be protected after healing by wearing sunscreen for at least a year.

Prevention

Burns are commonly received in residential fires. Properly placed and working smoke detectors in combination with rapid evacuation plans will minimize a person's exposure to smoke and flames in the event of a fire. Children must be taught never to play with matches, lighters, fireworks, gasoline, or cleaning fluids.

Burns caused by scalding with hot water or other liquids may be prevented by setting the water heater thermostat no higher than 120°F (49°C), checking the temperature of bath water before getting into the tub, and turning pot handles on the stove so they are out of the reach of children. Care should be used when removing covers from pans of steaming foods and when uncovering or opening foods heated in a microwave oven.

Thermal burns are often received from electrical appliances. Care should be exercised around stoves, space heaters, clothes irons, and curling irons.

Sunburns may be avoided by the liberal use of a sunscreen containing either an opaque active ingredient, such as zinc oxide or titanium dioxide, or a nonopaque active ingredient, such as PABA (para-aminobenzoic acid) or benzophenone. Hats, loose clothing, and umbrellas also provide protection, especially between 10 a.m. and 3 p.m., when the most damaging ultraviolet rays are present in direct sunlight.

Electrical burns may be prevented by covering unused electrical outlets with safety plugs and keeping electrical cords away from infants and toddlers who might chew on them. Persons should also seek shelter indoors during a thunderstorm to avoid being struck by lightning.

Chemical burns may be prevented by wearing protective clothing, including gloves and eyeshields. Chemical agents should always be used according to the manufacturer's instructions and properly stored when not in use.

Resources

WEBSITES

"Burns." MedlinePlus. http://www.nlm.nih.gov/medlineplus/burns.html (accessed November 4, 2012).

"Burns: First aid." MayoClinic.com. http://www.mayoclinic.com/health/first-aid-burns/FA00022 (accessed November 4, 2012).

"Aloe vera."National Center for Complementary and Alternative Medicine. http://nccam.nih.gov/health/aloevera (accessed November 4, 2012).

"Condition Care Guide: Burns." http://www.drweil.com/drw/u/ART02917/Burns.html (accessed November 4, 2012).

ORGANIZATIONS

Shriners Hospitals for Children, 2900 Rocky Point Drive, Tampa, FL 33607, (813) 281-0300, http://www.shrinershq.org/Hospitals/Main.

Bethany Thivierge
Fran Hodgkins

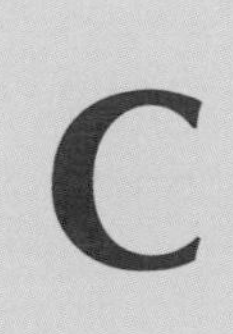

Campylobacteriosis

Definition

Campylobacteriosis refers to infection by the group of bacteria known as *Campylobacter*. The term comes from the Greek word meaning "curved rod" referring to the bacteria's curved shape. The most common disease caused by these organisms is diarrhea, which most often affects children and younger adults. *Campylobacter* infections account for a substantial percent of food-borne illness encountered each year.

Description

There are more than 15 different subtypes, all of which are curved Gram-negative rods. *C. jeuni* is the subtype that most often causes gastrointestinal disease. However, some species such as *C. fetus* produce disease outside the intestine, particularly in those with altered immune systems, such as people with **AIDS**, **cancer**, and liver disease.

Campylobacter are often found in the intestine of animals raised for food products and pets. Infected animals often have no symptoms. Chickens are the most common source of human infection. It is estimated that 1% of the general population is infected each year.

Causes and symptoms

Improper or incomplete food preparation is the most common way the disease is spread, with poultry accounting for over half the cases. Untreated **water** and raw milk are also potential sources.

The incubation period after exposure is from one to 10 days. A day or two of mild fever, muscle aches, and headache occur before intestinal symptoms begin. Diarrhea with or without blood and severe abdominal cramps are the major intestinal symptoms. The severity of symptoms is variable, ranging from only mild fever to dehydration and rarely death (mainly in the very young or old). The disease usually lasts about one week, but persists longer in about 20% of cases. At least 10% will have a relapse, and some patients will continue to pass the bacteria for several weeks.

Complications

Dehydration is the most common complication. Especially at the extremes of age, this should be watched for and treated with either Oral Rehydration Solution or intravenous fluid replacement.

Infection may also involve areas outside the intestine. This is unusual, except for infections with *C. fetus*. *C. fetus* infections tend to occur in those who have diseases of decreased immunity such as AIDS, cancer, etc. This subtype is particularly adapted to protect itself from the body's defenses.

Areas outside the intestine that may be involved are:

- Nervous system involvement either by direct infection of the meninges (outer covering of the spinal cord and brain) or more commonly by producing the Guillain-Barré syndrome (progressive and reversible paralysis or weakness of many muscles). In fact, *Campylobacter* may be responsible for 40% of the reported cases of this syndrome.
- Joint inflammation can occur weeks later (leading to an unusual form of arthritis).
- Infection of vessels and heart valves is a special characteristic of *C. fetus*. Immunocompromised patients may develop repeated episodes of passage of bacteria into the bloodstream from these sites of infection.
- The gallbladder, pancreas, and bone may be affected.

Diagnosis

Campylobacter is only one of many causes of acute diarrhea. Culture (growing the bacteria in the laboratory)

KEY TERMS

Antibiotic—A medication that is designed to kill or weaken bacteria.

Anti-motility medications—Medications such as loperamide (Imodium), dephenoxylate (Lomotil), or medications containing codeine or narcotics which decrease the ability of the intestine to contract. This can worsen the condition of a patient with dysentery or colitis.

Fluoroquinolones—A relatively new group of antibiotics that have had good success in treating infections with many Gram-negative bacteria. One drawback is that they should not be used in children under 17 years of age, because of possible effect on bone growth.

Food-borne illness—A disease that is transmitted by eating or handling contaminated food.

Gram-negative—Refers to the property of many bacteria that causes them to not take up color with Gram's stain, a method which is used to identify bacteria. Gram-positive bacteria which take up the stain turn purple, while Gram-negative bacteria which do not take up the stain turn red.

Guillain-Barré syndrome—Progressive and usually reversible paralysis or weakness of multiple muscles usually starting in the lower extremities and often ascending to the muscles involved in respiration. The syndrome is due to inflammation and loss of the myelin covering of the nerve fibers, often associated with an acute infection.

Meninges—Outer covering of the spinal cord and brain. Infection is called meningitis, which can lead to damage to the brain or spinal cord and even death.

Oral Rehydration Solution (ORS)—A liquid preparation developed by the World Health Organization that can decrease fluid loss in persons with diarrhea. Originally developed to be prepared with materials available in the home, commercial preparations have recently come into use.

Stool—Passage of fecal material; a bowel movement.

of freshly obtained diarrhea fluid is the only way to be certain of the diagnosis.

Treatment

The first aim of treatment is to keep up **nutrition** and avoid dehydration. Medications used to treat diarrhea by decreasing intestinal motility, such as Loperamide or Diphenoxylate are also useful, but should only be used with the advice of a physician. **Antibiotics** are of value, if started within three days of onset of symptoms. They are indicated for those with severe or persistent symptoms. Either an erythromycin type drug or one of the fluoroquinolones (such as ciprofloxacin) for five to seven days are the accepted therapies.

Prognosis

Most patients with *Campylobacter* infection rapidly recover without treatment. For certain groups of patients, infection becomes chronic and requires repeated courses of antibiotics.

Prevention

Good hand washing technique as well as proper preparation and cooking of food is the best way to prevent infection.

Resources

ORGANIZATIONS

Centers for Disease Control and Prevention (CDC), 1600 Clifton Road, Atlanta, GA 30333, (800) 232-4636, cdcinfo@cdc.gov, http://www.cdc.gov.

David Kaminstein, MD

Cancer

Definition

Cancer is not just one disease, but a large group of more than 100 diseases. Its two main characteristics are uncontrolled growth of the cells in the human body, and the ability of these cells to migrate from the original site and spread to distant sites. If the spread is not controlled, cancer can result in death.

Demographics

The American Cancer Society estimated that more than 1.6 million Americans received a cancer diagnosis in 2012. (This total includes melanomas, but does not include basal and squamous cell skin cancers.) The ACS

Cancer incidence and mortality, 2010[1]

Type of cancer	Number of new diagnoses	Number of deaths
Breast cancer	207,090	39,840
Cervical cancer[2]	12,200	4,210
Colorectal cancer	142,570	51,370
Lung cancer	222,520	157,300
Non-Hodgkin lymphoma	65,540	20,210
Ovarian cancer	21,880	1,385
Prostate cancer	217,730	32,050
Skin cancer, melanoma	68,130	8,700
Skin cancer, non-melanoma	2,000,000	2,000
Testicular cancer	8,480	350

[1]Numbers are estimates
[2]Invasive

SOURCE: American Cancer Society.

(Table by PreMediaGlobal. © 2013 Cengage Learning)

Common pathogens and associated cancers

Causative agent	Type(s) of cancer
Viruses	
Epstein-Barr virus	Burkitt's lymphoma
Hepatitis B	Liver cancer
Hepatitis C	Liver cancer
Human immunodeficiency virus (HIV)	Kaposi's sarcoma, lymphoma
Papillomaviruses	Cervical cancer
Bacteria	
Helicobacter pylori	Stomach cancer, lymphomas

(Table by PreMediaGlobal. © 2013 Cengage Learning)

also estimated that more than 557,000 people in the United States would die of cancer in 2012. This equates to more than 1,500 deaths from cancer per day. One out of every four deaths in the United States is from cancer, making cancer second only to **heart disease** as a cause of death overall in the United States.

On the positive side, the five-year relative survival rate for all cancers diagnosed has increased substantially over the past three decades. From 1975–1977, the survival rate was 49%. This compares to 67% in 2001–2007, according to the ACS. It credits the increase to an increasing ability to diagnose certain cancers at an earlier stage (the stage is a description of the spread of the disease at the time of diagnosis: stage I is the earliest stage, stage IV is the most advanced), and to improvements in treatment.

Since the occurrence of cancer increases as individuals age, most of the cases are seen in adults, middle-aged or older. Among males, the most common cancers are prostate (241,740 estimated new cases in 2012); lung and bronchus (116,470); and colon and rectum (73,420). Among women, the most common cancers are breast (226,870 estimated new cases in 2012); lung and bronchurs (109,690); and colon and rectum (70,040). Among both men and women, lung and bronchus cancer caused the most deaths in 2012: 87,750 for men, and 72,590 for women. Childhood cancer is much more rare.

Although most cancer occurs in adults, cancer does occur in children. In 2012, the American Cancer Society estimated 12,060 new cases would be diagnosed. About 1,340 children aged 0–14 years died of cancer in the U.S. in 2012. In general, children respond better to cancer treatment than adults do. Advances in treatment have resulted in better outcomes and increased long-term survival rates for children. Approximately 83% of children newly diagnosed with cancer now live at least five years compared to less than 60% in the mid-1970s. However, the American Cancer Society notes that childhood cancer incidence had increased slightly—at a rate of about 0.5% each year—since 1975.

Description

Cancer, by definition, is a disease of the genes. A gene is a small part of DNA, which is the master molecule of the cell. Genes make proteins, which are the ultimate workhorses of the cells. These proteins allow the body to carry out all the many processes that permit an individual to function—to breathe, to think, and to move.

Throughout people's lives, the cells in their bodies are growing, dividing, and replacing themselves. Many genes produce proteins that are involved in controlling the processes of cell growth and division. Certain alterations (mutations) to the DNA molecule can disrupt the genes and produce faulty proteins that can remove a cell's restraints on growth. This abnormal cell begins to divide uncontrollably and eventually forms a new growth known as a tumor or neoplasm (medical term for cancer meaning "new growth").

In a healthy individual, the immune system typically recognizes the neoplastic cells and destroys them before they get a chance to divide. However, some mutant cells may escape immune detection and survive to become tumors or cancers.

Tumors are of two types, benign or malignant. A benign tumor is not considered cancer. It is typically slow-growing, does not spread or invade surrounding tissue, and once it is removed, does not usually recur.

Breast cancer

- An estimated 207,090 **female** breast cancer cases were diagnosed in 2010.
- An estimated 1,970 **male** breast cancer cases were diagnosed in 2010.
- The lifetime risk of developing invasive breast cancer is 1 in 8 in females and 1 in 1,000 in males.
- In 2010, there were more than **2.5 million** breast cancer survivors living in the United States.

SOURCE: American Cancer Society, "What are the key statistics about breast cancer?" and "What are the key statistics about breast cancer in men?" Available online at http://www.cancer.org/index (accessed August 23, 2010).

(Table by PreMediaGlobal. © 2013 Cengage Learning)

Recommendations for cancer screening

Procedure	Frequency
Chest x ray	Not recommended on a routine basis
Sputum cytology	Not recommended on a routine basis
Fecal occult blood testing (FOBT) or slgmoidoscopy	Yearly after age 50
Papanicolaou (Pap) smear	Every 3 years from onset of sexual activity to age 65
Mammography alone or mammography and breast physical examination	Yearly mammograms starting at age 40. Clinical breast exam every three years for women in their 20s and 30s; every year for women 40 and older.

SOURCE: American Cancer Society.

(Table by PreMediaGlobal. © 2013 Cengage Learning)

A malignant tumor, by contrast, is cancer. It invades surrounding tissue and spreads to other parts of the body. If the cancer cells have spread to the surrounding tissues, it can recur even after the malignant tumor is removed.

Several different types of cancer exist:

- Carcinomas are cancers that arise in the epithelium (the layer of cells covering the body's surface and lining the internal organs and various glands). Carcinomas can be subdivided into adenocarcinomas, which are those that develop in an organ or a gland, and squamous cell carcinomas, which are those that originate in the skin.
- Melanomas also originate in the skin, usually in the pigment cells (melanocytes).
- Sarcomas are cancers of the supporting tissues of the body, such as bone, muscle, and blood vessels.
- Cancers of the blood and lymph glands are called leukemias and lymphomas, respectively.
- Gliomas are cancers of the nerve tissue.

Causes and symptoms

CAUSES. A majority of cancers are caused by changes in the cell's DNA that are related to environmental factors. These factors, called carcinogens, are responsible for causing the initial mutation in the DNA, and they come in many types.

Some cancers have a genetic or inherited basis. In other words, individuals can inherit faulty DNA from a parent. This faulty DNA can predispose the person to getting cancer. Numerous cancers are linked to both environmental and hereditary factors, but fewer than 10% of all cancers are strictly linked to hereditary factors. Cancers that are known to have a hereditary link are breast cancer, colon cancer, ovarian cancer, and uterine cancer. Certain inherited physiological traits may also contribute to cancers. For example, inheriting fair skin makes a person more likely to develop skin cancer, but only if that person also has prolonged exposure to intensive sunlight. This is one of many examples of inherited and environmental factors both affecting a person's risk of developing cancer.

The major risk factors for cancer are related to: tobacco and alcohol use, dietary factors, sexual and reproductive behavior, exposure to infectious agents, family history, occupation, and environmental factors including pollution.

- Smoking. Eighty to 90% of lung cancer cases occur in smokers. Smoking has also been shown to be a contributory factor in cancers of the upper respiratory tract, esophagus, larynx, bladder, pancreas, and probably liver, stomach, breast, and kidney as well. Secondhand smoke (or passive smoking) can increase one's risk of developing cancer.
- Alcohol. Excessive consumption of alcohol is a risk factor in certain cancers, such as liver cancer. Alcohol, in combination with tobacco, significantly increases the chances that an individual will develop mouth, pharynx, larynx, and esophageal cancers.
- Diet and exercise. About a third of all cancer deaths in the United States are due to poor nutrition, excess weight, and lack of exercise, according to the American Cancer Society. Excessive intake of fat leading to obesity has been associated with cancers of the breast, colon, rectum, pancreas, prostate, gall bladder, ovaries, and uterus.
- Sexual and reproductive behavior. The human papillomavirus (HPV), which is sexually transmitted, has been shown to cause cancer of the cervix. Having multiple sexual partners and becoming sexually active at an early age have been shown to increase one's chances of

JANET D. ROWLEY (1925–)

Janet Davison Rowley was born in New York City on April 5, 1925, to Ethel Mary (Ballantyne) and Hurford Henry Davison. Rowley attended the University of Chicago, earning her B.S. degree in 1946 and her M.D. degree in 1948. She also married Donald A. Rowley in 1948, and the couple ultimately had four sons. Rowley completed both her internship and residency at Chicago hospitals before returning to the University of Chicago Medical School where she conducted research from 1962–1969. She became an associate professor, and finally, in 1977, earned her position as a full professor.

Rowley's research has focused on understanding cancer, with special emphasis on its cytogenetic causes. Her development and use of Giemsa and quinacrine stains enabled Rowley to discover oncogenes and to ultimately show a consistent shifting or translocation of genetic material in chronic myeloid leukemia cells. Rowley's discoveries and continued research have shown that malignant cells in humans undergo this translocation and deletion of genes that cause tumors to grow. Her research has given oncologists new pathways to explore concerning gene therapies for the treatment of cancer.

Co-editor and co-founder of the journal, *Genes, Chromosomes and Cancer*, Rowley has published an abundance of materials including *Chromosome Changes in Leukemia* (1978), *Genes and Cancer* (1984), and *Advances in Understanding Genetic Changes in Cancer* (1992). Rowley has also received many awards and honors for her work and research.

In 1984, Dr. Rowley was made the Blum-Riese Distinguished Service Professor at the University of Chicago, a position she still holds, as well as serving as the interim deputy dean for science since 2001. In 1998, she was one of three scientists awarded the prestigious Lasker Award for their work on translocation. She has published more than 400 articles and continues her research at the University of Chicago.

contracting HPV. HPV is also linked to other cancers, such as cancers of the oral cavity and pharynx (oropharyngeal cancers). (From 1999–2008, HPV-related oropharyngeal cancers increased by 4.4% per year for white men and 1.9% per year for white women, but other ethnic groups did not see increases.) In addition, it has also been shown that women who do not have children or have children later in life have an increased risk for both ovarian and breast cancer.

- Infectious agents. The World Health Organization (WHO) estaimates that about 18% of the world's cancer cases (about two million cases each year) result from chronic infections with such infectious agents as HPV, hepatitis B and C viruses, Epstein-Barr virus, and human immunodeficiency virus.
- Family history. Certain cancers such as breast, colon, ovarian, and uterine cancer recur generation after generation in some families, and the inheritance of particular genes may make a person susceptible to certain cancers.
- Occupational hazards. Persons in certain professions have shown an increased incidence for some cancers. The National Institute for Occupational Safety and Health (NIOSH) maintains a list of more than 100 substances it considers to be potential occupational carcinogens.
- Environmental factors. One environmetal factor that causes cancer is radiation. A 2012 study published in the journal of Energy & Aneironmental Science, estimated that as many as 2,500 cases of cancer, and up to 1,300 deaths, may result from radiation fallout from the 2011 disaster at the Fukushima Dai-Ichi nuclear plant in Japan. Ultraviolet radiation from the sun accounts for a majority of melanoma deaths. Other sources of radiation are x rays, radon gas, and ionizing radiation from nuclear material.

Symptoms

Cancer is a progressive disease and goes through several stages. Each stage may produce a number of symptoms. Some symptoms are produced early and may occur due to a tumor that is growing within an organ or a gland. As the tumor grows, it may press on the nearby nerves, organs, and blood vessels. This causes **pain** and some pressure, which may be the earliest warning signs of cancer.

Despite the fact that more than 100 different types of cancers exist, and they produce very different symptoms, the American Cancer Society lists the following as possible warning signals of cancer:

- unexplained weight loss
- unexplained fever
- chronic fatigue
- chronic headache or other pain
- changes in the size, color, or shape of a wart or a mole, or other changes in the skin (reddening, yellowing, darkeing, itching, excessive hair growth)
- a sore that does not heal

KEY TERMS

Benign—Mild, nonmalignant. Recovery is favorable with treatment.

Biopsy—The surgical removal and microscopic examination of living tissue for diagnostic purposes.

Bone marrow—Spongy material that fills the inner cavities of the bones. The progenitors of all the blood cells are produced in this bone marrow.

Carcinogen—Any substance capable of causing cancer by mutating the cell's DNA.

Chemotherapy—Treatment with certain anticancer drugs.

Epithelium—The layer of cells covering the body's surface and lining the internal organs and various glands.

Hormone therapy—Treatment of cancer by inhibiting the production of hormones such as testosterone and estrogen.

Immunotherapy—Treatment of cancer by stimulating the body's immune defense system.

Malignant—A general term for cells and the tumors they form that can invade and destroy other tissues and organs.

Metastasis—The spread of cancer from one part of the body to another.

Radiation therapy—Treatment using high-energy radiation from x-ray machines, cobalt, radium, or other sources.

Sore—An open wound, bruise, or lesion on the skin.

Tumor—An abnormal growth resulting from a cell that lost its normal growth control restraints and started multiplying uncontrollably.

X rays—High-energy radiation used in high doses, either to diagnose or treat disease.

- persistent cough, hoarseness, or sore throat
- a lump or thickening in the breast or elsewhere
- unusual bleeding or discharge
- chronic indigestion or difficulty in swallowing
- any change in bowel or bladder habits
- white patches or spots in the mouth or on the tongue

Many other diseases besides cancer can produce the same symptoms. However, individuals who have any of these symptoms should have them checked as soon as possible, especially if they linger. The earlier a cancer is diagnosed and treated, the better the chance of cure. Many cancers such as breast cancer may not have any early symptoms. Routine screening tests such as breast self-exams and mammograms are, therefore, critical in identifying these silent diseases.

Diagnosis

EXAMINATION. Diagnosis of many cancers begins with a thorough physical examination and a complete medical history. The doctor will observe, feel, and palpate (apply pressure by touch) different parts of the body in order to identify any variations from the normal size, feel, and texture of the organ or tissue. For instance, the doctor may palpate the lymph nodes in the neck, under the arms, and in the groin, because many illnesses and cancers cause a swelling of the lymph nodes.

Tests

The doctor may order diagnostic tests if an abnormality has been detected on physical examination, or if the patient has some symptom that could be indicative of cancer. For example, the doctor may order laboratory studies of sputum (sputum cytology), blood, urine, and stool to detect abnormalities that may indicate cancer. Imaging tests such as computed tomography scans (CT scans), magnetic resonance imaging (MRI), ultrasound, and fiberoptic scope examinations help the doctors determine the location of the tumor even if it is deep within the body. Conventional x rays are often used for initial evaluation because they are relatively cheap, painless, and easily accessible. In order to increase the information obtained from a conventional x ray, air or a dye (such as barium or iodine) may be used as a contrast medium to outline or highlight parts of the body.

The most definitive diagnostic test is the biopsy, wherein a piece of tissue is surgically removed for microscope examination. Besides confirming a cancer, the biopsy also provides information about the type of cancer, the stage it has reached, the aggressiveness of the cancer, and the extent of its spread. Since a biopsy provides the most accurate analysis, it is considered the gold standard of diagnostic tests.

Treatment

Treatment and **prevention** of cancers continues to be the focus of a great deal of research as of 2012.

Research into new cancer therapies includes cancer-targeting gene therapy, cancer vaccines, and other targeted therapies such as monoclonal antibodies. Most new therapies take years of clinical testing and research.

The aim of cancer treatment is to remove all or as much of the tumor as possible and to prevent the recurrence or spread of the primary tumor. While devising a treatment plan for cancer, the likelihood of curing the cancer has to be weighed against the side effects of the treatment. If the cancer is very aggressive and a cure is not possible, then the treatment should be aimed at relieving the symptoms and controlling the cancer for as long as possible.

Cancer treatment can take many different forms, and is typically tailored to the individual patient. The decision as to which type of treatment is the most appropriate depends on the type and location of cancer, the extent to which it has already spread, the patient's age, sex, general health status, and personal treatment preferences. The major types of treatment are: surgery, **radiation**, chemotherapy, biological therapy, targeted therapy, hormone therapy, and bone-marrow and stem cell transplantation.

Surgery

Surgery is the removal of a visible tumor and is the most frequently used cancer treatment. It is most effective when a cancer is small and/or confined to one area of the body. Along with the cancer, some part of the normal surrounding tissue is also removed to ensure that no cancer cells remain in the area. Since cancer usually spreads via the lymphatic system, adjoining lymph nodes may be examined and sometimes are removed as well. In some cases, the doctor may recommend surgery to treat symptoms associated with a tumor. For instance, surgery may not cure a case of advanced cancer, but it may alleviate symptoms caused by a large tumor.

Preventive surgery is another option in some cases. Preventive or prophylactic surgery involves removal of tissue that is likely to become malignant over time. For example, women have cancer in one breast and who are at high risk of developing breast cancer in the other due to a genetic predisposition for the disease, may opt to have a double mastectomy rather than wait and worry about getting the disease in the second breast.

Radiation therapy

Radiation kills tumor cells. Radiation is used alone in cases in which a tumor is unsuitable for surgery. More often, it is used in conjunction with surgery and chemotherapy. Radiation can be either external or internal. In the external form, the radiation is aimed at the tumor from outside the body. In internal radiation (also known as brachytherapy), a radioactive substance in the form of pellets or liquid is placed at the cancerous site by means of a pill, injection, or insertion in a sealed container.

Chemotherapy

Chemotherapy is the use of drugs to kill cancer cells. It destroys the hard-to-detect cancer cells that have spread and are circulating in the body. Chemotherapeutic drugs can be given in many forms. The most common administration methods include oral (by mouth) or intravenous administration. Chemotherapy may be given alone or in conjunction with surgery, radiation, or both.

When chemotherapy is used before surgery or radiation, it is known as primary chemotherapy or neoadjuvant chemotherapy. An advantage of neoadjuvant chemotherapy is that since the cancer cells have not been exposed to anti-cancer drugs, they are especially vulnerable. It can, therefore, be used effectively to reduce the size of the tumor for surgery or target it for radiation. The more common use of chemotherapy is adjuvant therapy, which is given to enhance the effectiveness of other treatments. For example, after surgery, adjuvant chemotherapy is given to destroy any cancerous cells that still remain in the body.

Biological and targeted therapies

Biological and targeted therapies use the body's own immune system to destroy cancer cells. These include:

- nonspecific immunomodulating agents, which are drugs that stimulate the immune sustem to fight cancer, as well as infections
- biological response modifiers, including interferons, interleukins, monoclonal antibodies, and vaccines, that work by enhancing the ability of the immune system to target disease cells.

Hormone therapy

Hormone therapy is standard treatment for some types of cancers that are hormone-dependent and grow faster in the presence of particular hormones. These include cancer of the prostate, breast, and uterus. Hormone therapy may involve blocking the production or action of these hormones, or surgically removing the hormone-producing gland altogether. These actions can slow the growth of the tumor, and in some cases, can halt the progression of the disease for many years.

Bone marrow, stem cell, and cord-blood transplantation

The bone marrow is the tissue within the bone cavities that contains blood-forming cells. Healthy bone marrow tissue constantly replenishes the blood supply and is essential to life.

A bone marrow transplant is the removal of marrow from one person and the transplant of the blood-forming cells either to the same person or to someone else. Bone-marrow transplantation, while not a therapy in itself, is often used to "rescue" patients, by allowing those with cancer to undergo aggressive therapy. Stem cell transplants have been performed to replace bone marrow that has been destroyed by cancer, chemotherapy, or radiation therapy. Stem cells are specialized cells in the bone marrow from which the body receives a constant source of blood cells. Stem cells may also be harvested from umbilical cords, a process that is referred to as a cord blood transplant. Some cancers in which stem cell transplants may be used include leukemia, lymphoma, and multiple myeloma.

Cancer treatment team

Many different specialists generally work together as a team to treat cancer patients. An oncologist is a physician who specializes in cancer care. The oncologist provides chemotherapy, hormone therapy, and any other non-surgical treatment that does not involve radiation. The oncologist often serves as the primary physician and coordinates the patient's treatment plan.

The radiation oncologist specializes in using radiation to treat cancer, whereas the surgical oncologist performs the operations needed to diagnose or treat cancer. Gynecologist-oncologists and pediatric-oncologists, as their titles suggest, are physicians involved with treating women's and children's cancers, respectively. Many other specialists also may be involved in the care of a cancer patient. For example, radiologists specialize in the use of x rays, ultrasounds, CT scans, MRI imaging and other techniques that are used to diagnose cancer. Hematologists specialize in disorders of the blood and are consulted in case of blood cancers and bone marrow cancers. The samples that are removed for biopsy are sent to a laboratory, where a pathologist examines them to determine the type of cancer and extent of the disease. There are many other specialties, and virtually any type of medical or surgical specialist may become involved with care of the cancer patient should it become necessary.

Prognosis

Many cancers are curable if detected and treated in their early stages. A cancer patient's prognosis is affected by many factors, particularly the type of cancer the patient has, the stage of the cancer, the extent to which it has metastasized, and the aggressiveness of the cancer. In addition, the patient's age, general health status, and the effectiveness of the treatment being pursued are important factors.

Prevention

Screening examinations conducted regularly by healthcare professionals can result in the detection of a wide variety of cancers at early stages, when treatment is more likely to be successful. These include breast, colon, rectum, cervix, prostate, testis, tongue, mouth, and skin cancer. Some of the routine screening tests recommended by the ACS are:

- Breast cancer: yearly mammograms for women beginning at age 40; and clinical breast exam every three years for women in their 20s and 30s, and every year for women aged 40 and older.
- Colon cancer: flexible sigmoidoscopy, double-contrast barium, or CT (virtual) colonography every five years; or colonoscopy every five years; or colonoscopy every 10 years.
- Cervical cancer: Pap test every three years for women aged 21–29; and Pap test and HPV test every five years for women aged 30–65.

As of 2012, the American Cancer Society recommends that men talk to their doctor about whether to be tested for prostate cancer because, "Research has not yet proven that the potential benefits of testing outweigh the harms of testing and treatment."

In addition, self-examinations for cancers of the breast, testis, mouth, and skin can also help in detecting the tumors before the symptoms become serious.

A revolution in molecular biology and cancer genetics has contributed a great deal to the development of several tests designed to help predict whether a person will develop cancer. These new techniques include genetic testing, in which molecular probes are used to identify mutations in certain genes that have been linked to particular cancers. The American Society of Clinical Oncology recommends that physicians offer genetic testing under these conditions: if the patient has a personal or family history that suggests a genetic cause of cancer; if the test can be adequately interpreted; and if the results of the genetic test will be helpful for the diagnosis, treatment or management of the patient, as well as family members who are also at risk for cancer.

Individuals can also take steps on their own to reduce their risks of developing cancer. These include:

- eating plenty of vegetables and fruits
- exercising vigorously for at least 30 minutes, and preferably 45–60 minutes, on five or more days every week.
- avoiding excessive weight gain
- avoiding tobacco (even secondhand smoke)
- decreasing or avoiding consumption of animal fats and red meats
- avoiding excessive amounts of alcohol
- avoiding the midday sun (between 11 a.m. and 3 p.m.) when the sun's rays are the strongest
- avoiding risky sexual practices
- avoiding known carcinogens in the environment or workplace

Effects on public health

It is a very rare individual who has not been touched by the disease either through a personal illness, or the illness of a family member or friend. According to the American Cancer Society, an estimated 12.7 million cases of cancer were diagnosed in 2008, and about 60 percent of the cancer-related deaths occurred in low- and middle-income countries that often had limited medical resources available to its citizens. In addition, it predicted approximately 21.4 million new cancer cases and 13.2 million cancer deaths in the year 2030. The increase is due to the global **population** boom, as well as the **aging** of the overall population. Because cancer is such a widespread disease, the medical profession, as well as government and other public and private agencies have placed a major emphasis on the importance of cancer prevention, early diagnosis, new treatment options, and cancer research.

Costs to society

In 2007 (the latest data available as of 2012), the National Institutes of Health (NIH) estimated that the overall costs of cancer were $226.8 billion. That total included $103.8 billion for direct medical costs, and $123.0 billion for indirect costs (costs related to lost productivity due to premature death).

Efforts and solutions

Governments, as well as public and pirvate organizations have mounted numerous campaigns to help prevent cancer. These include campaigns warning of the increased risk of lung cancer associated with tobacco use, encouraging the use of sunscreen to prevent skin cancer, and promoting the importance of a diet and exercise to stave off many types of cancer and other diseases. At the same time, treatments and preventative measures are improving and evolving as researchers discover most about the different types of cancer, why they begin, how they develop, and how they spread.

Resources

BOOKS

Mukherjee, Siddhartha. The Emporer of All Maladies: A Biography of Cancer. New York: Scribner, 2010.

PERIODICALS

Hoeve, John E. Ten, and Mark Z. Jacobson. "Worldwide Health Effects of the Fukushima Daiichi Nuclear Accident." *Energy & Environmental Science* 5, no. 9(2012): 8743–8757.

WEBSITES

"American Cancer Society Guidelines for the Early Detection of Cancer." American Cancer Society. http://www.cancer.org/Healthy/FindCancerEarly/CancerScreeningGuidelines/american-cancer-society-guidelines-for-the-early-detection-of-cancer (accessed October 5, 2012).

"Cancer Facts & Figures." American Cancer Society. http://www.cancer.org/acs/groups/content/@epidemiology surveilance/documents/document/acspc-031941.pdf (accessed October 5, 2012).

"Charting the Path From Infection to Cancer." National Cancer Institute, U.S. National Institutes of Health. http://www.cancer.gov/aboutnci/ncicancerbulletin/archive/2009/092209/page5 (accessed October 5, 2012).

"Genetic Testing." American Society of Clinical Oncology. http://www.cancer.net/all-about-cancer/genetics/genetic-testing (accessed October 5, 2012).

"HPV and Cancer." National Cancer Institute, U.S. National Institutes of Health. http://www.cancer.gov/cancertopics/factsheet/Risk/HPV (accessed October 5, 2012).

"Infectious Agents and Cancer." National Cancer Institute, U.S. National Institutes of Health. http://epi.grants.cancer.gov/infectious-agents/ (accessed October 5, 2012).

"Occupational Cancer: Carcinogen List." U.S. Centers for Disease Control and Prevention. http://www.cdc.gov/niosh/topics/cancer/npotocca.html (accessed October 5, 2012).

"Stem Cell Transplant, Peripheral Blood, Bone Marrow, and Cord Blood Transplants." American Cancer Society. http://www.cancer.org/acs/groups/cid/documents/webcontent/003215-pdf.pdf (accessed October 5, 2012).

ORGANIZATIONS

American Cancer Society, 250 Williams Street NW, Atlanta, GA 30303, (800) 227-2345, https://www.cancer.org/

National Cancer Institute, 6116 Executive Blvd., Suite 300, Bethesda, MD 20892-8322, (800) 422-6237, http://www.cancer.gov

National Coalition for Cancer Survivorship, 1010 Wayne Avenue, Suite 770, Silver Spring, MD 20910, (877) 622-7937, http://www.canceradvocacy.org/.

Rosalyn Carson-DeWitt, M.D.
Teresa G. Odle
Melinda Oberleitner, R.N., D.N.S.
Leslie Mertz, Ph.D.

Car seats

Definition

"Car Seats" is the term commonly used to denote child safety seats. Car seats are seats specifically designed to help protect and restrain children riding in automobiles. Car seats come in multiple forms in order to best protect children at different stages of growth. In addition to various relevant safety features, car seats come in a variety of colors, fabrics, and shapes to appeal to consumers.

Origins

The first car seat was designed by the Bunny Bear Corporation in 1933. Early car seats were designed to keep a child stationary in the vehicle as well as to raise them high enough to be seen by adults in the front seat of the vehicle. The first car seat designed to function as a safety device appeared in 1962—this seat was the invention of Jean Ames of England and featured a Y-shaped harness.

Purpose

Car accidents are the leading cause of death for children aged 1-12 years old. Since Ames' invention in the 1960s, car seats have continually evolved in order to protect children riding in cars, especially in the event of an accident. When a car is in an accident, the car stops abruptly, but unrestrained objects continue on the car's original trajectory until stopped by a hard surface. The end of this trajectory could be hitting the dashboard, window, a seat or other interior car surface, or the ground if ejected from the vehicle. The faster the car is going at the time of impact, the greater the risk for injury or death. Children are at high risk for injury or death due to their small size, proportionally larger heads, and underdeveloped bones.

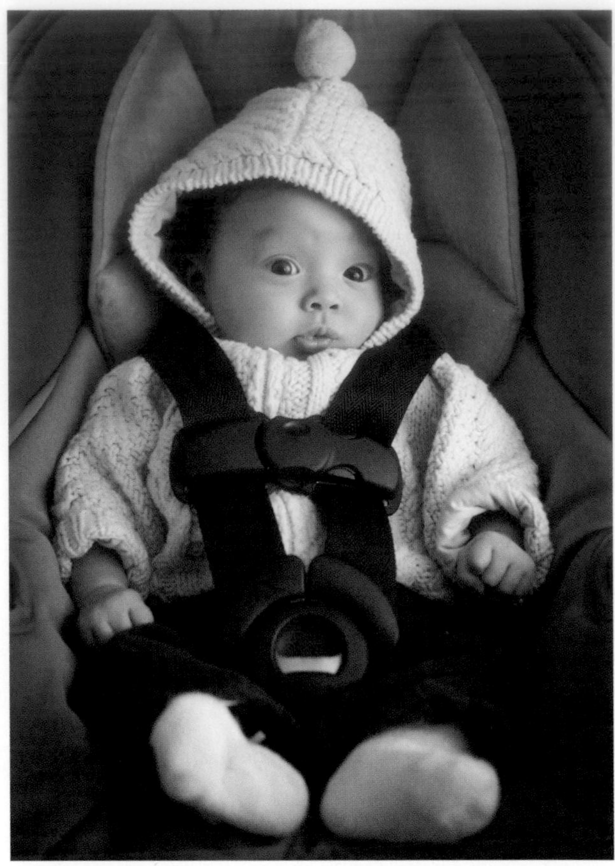

Infant strapped properly into a car seat. *(Michael Pettigrew/Shuterstock.com)*

Car seats help to properly restrain children to minimize unnecessary injury. Car seats for older children, called "booster seats", help maximize efficacy of a vehicle's seatbelts, which are designed for adults. Since seatbelts are designed for adults, children wearing seatbelts without the aid of a car seat or booster seat are not properly protected and are susceptible to additional injuries.

Description

Car seats are usually made of polypropylene—a durable plastic that is flexible under pressure but does not crack easily. The fabrics and foams of car seats are usually treated with flame retardants and should only be hand washed with water and mild soap. Government regulations (Federal Motor Vehicle Safety Standards 213) help determine how car seats are constructed, but the particulars of many car seats vary aesthetically.

There are three primary types of car seats: rear-facing seats, forward-facing seats, and booster seats. Whether a child is in one of these types of seats or using

KEY TERMS

Car Bed—A type of car seat, most commonly used for infants born prematurely. A car bed allows the child to be securely fastened while lying down as opposed to being in a seated position. As a result of frequently having underdeveloped respiratory systems, many premature babies have serious difficulty breathing in a traditional seated car seat.

Polysomnography—Monitoring of respiratory, cardiac, brain, muscular, and ocular function simultaneously during sleep. This form of monitoring is often used to diagnose sleep apnea.

Trajectory—The path of an object in motion.

a seatbelt, there should never be more than one child or person per car seat or seatbelt. The safest place for all car seats and all children under 13 years of age is in the back seat. It is critical that car seats be correctly installed in a vehicle—improperly installed car seats could result in serious injury or even the child and seat being ejected from the car in the event of an accident. For the same reasons, it is also essential that children be correctly buckled into their car seats. Recommendations for which seat is safest for a child's age change over time, therefore government agencies, child safety organizations, and American Academy of Pediatrics (AAP) suggest following manufacturers' instructions based on weight and height. This method has proven to be much safer than "graduating" a child to another seat based on their age. Age requirements are a general guideline, but may not be appropriate given an individual child's weight and height. As of April 2011, the AAP also recommends keeping children in rear-facing seats until the age of two to minimize injury. Injury for children between the ages of one and two years old is 500% greater in forward-facing seats as opposed to rear-facing seats.

Rear-Facing Seats

These seats are usually used for infants from birth to approximately 20 lb. Straps should always be fit snugly to the child. Since bulky garments like coats can inhibit the proper fastening of straps, these types of items should be removed prior to buckling. The strap clips for a rear-facing seat should be roughly lined up with the infant's underarms and the harness slots should be flat and fall approximately at the infant's shoulder level.

Rear-facing car seats need to be properly adjusted to cradle the infant's head without it flopping forward. Car seats often come with instructions to help determine the proper angle based on a child's age, and sometimes a rolled blanket may help prevent the infant from sliding down or to the side of the seat. Padding (whether it is part of the car seat or added for comfort and security) should never be placed behind or under the baby.

Studies done on healthy, full-term infants suggest that riding in rear-facing seats in a seated position does not significantly reduce oxygen levels. Studies on pre-term infants, however, suggest that car seats utilizing a seated position can cause severe breathing difficulty. A polysomnographic exam in the seated position can help parents and doctors determine which car seat is appropriate for pre-term babies. Car beds, which restrain the child in a recumbent position, are often used for pre-term infants.

Most rear-facing seats are designed to carry a child to and from the car and have some sort of handle to that end. Despite the ease of keeping a child in the car seat, the seat should not be used as a crib or chair, and the child should be taken out of the seat when not driving. Studies have shown that the car seat could interfere with a child's breathing when used in this manner. Children should also not be left in car seats unattended.

Forward-Facing Seats

These seats face the front of the car and are usually used for children until they weigh approximately 40 lb. These seats usually have a five-point harness system. The straps on a forward-facing seat should always lie flat and be snug against the child. The harness slots should fall approximately at the child's shoulders. As with rear-facing seats, bulky clothing can inhibit a child from being properly secured in a forward-facing seat, and such items should be removed before buckling the child.

Booster Seats

There are two types of booster seats: those with and without high backs. As its name implies, a booster seat "boots" the child in the seat so that the seat belt fits and protects the child properly. Booster seats should be used until the child is four feet and nine inches tall or between eight and twelve years old. The use of a booster seat as opposed to just a seat belt reduces the risk of injury by 59% for children from four to eight years of age. It is critical when using a booster seat that the child's seatbelt is fastened properly, with the lap belt across the child's thighs and the shoulder band diagonally across the child's torso. When a child is fastened improperly or only using a lap belt, they are susceptible to an additional set of injuries.

A child should not stop using a booster seat until the child has reached the weight and height limits of the booster seat; the child's legs should also be able to bend over the edge of the seat while keeping his or her back flat against the back of the seat. When children meet the requirements to stop using booster seats, their lap and shoulder bands should always be securely fastened and they should continue to ride in the back seat until they are 13 years old. Children should be secured into high-backed boosters when travelling in cars with low seatbelts or cars without headrests.

LATCH

As of September 2002, all American-made vehicles and car seats come equipped with lower anchors and tethers for children (LATCH). The LATCH system consists of metal anchors in the seats of vehicles and specialized straps on car seats to attach to these anchors. The LATCH system was designed in response to frequent consumer difficulty in properly securing car seats with seatbelts. LATCH components can be purchased for cars that were manufactured without LATCH anchors.

Buying and installing car seats

When buying a car seat, it is important to get the appropriate seat for the child's age, size, and the type of vehicle to be used. The latest recommendations and regulations, available from the National Highway Traffic Safety Administration (NHTSA), should be consulted before purchasing a case seat. The NHTSA also provides car seat ratings, and car seat recalls can be obtained from the Consumer Product Safety Commission.

When selecting a car seat, fit is most important and buyers should be sure that the seat fits the child correctly. Buyer' should also make sure that the car seats can be properly installed in their cars. The NHTSA has a list of specialists and locations certified to check the proper installation of car seats—using this type of service ensures that the seat is properly fitted and that the owner knows how to install it in the future.

It is not advisable to purchase a secondhand car seat. Used car seats may have been in an accident, have missing or outdated parts, have hidden damage, or may be worn out. Additionally, the car seat may have been recalled.

According to the *Encyclopedia of Children's Health,* after a car seat has been in a moderate or severe accident, seats should only be reused if all of the following conditions are met:

- The vehicle was driven away from the accident.
- No one in the vehicle was injured.
- The air bags did not inflate.
- The door closest to the safety seat was undamaged.
- The car safety seat has no visible signs of damage.

Car seats should always be placed in the back seat, in the middle away from airbags, when possible. The car seat should be attached using a LATCH system if possible, and with seatbelts when a LATCH system is not in place. The car seat should be secure and should not move to either side or the front more than 1 inch. A vehicle's operating manual should be consulted to be certain of the best car seat placement for that vehicle.

Demographics

- Only 21% of children between the ages of four and eight use a booster seat even occasionally.
- Only 55% of children between the ages of four and eight always use a booster seat when other children are in the car.
- More than 10% of all children under 80 lb. are not placed in any restraints in the car, including seatbelts.
- The NHTSA estimates that proper use of car seats reduces the risk of dying in a crash by 71% for infants and 54% for toddlers. For children big enough to use seatbelts, proper seatbelt use reduces the risk of injury by approximately 50% and the risk of death by 45%.
- According to the NHTSA in 2008, only 86% of children under one year old, less than 75% of toddlers, and about 55% of children aged four to seven were correctly restrained.

Legislation

Tennessee passed the first child passenger safety law in 1978 and by 1984 all states and Washington, D.C. had some sort of child passenger safety law. As of 2012, all 50 states, the District of Columbia, Guam, and the Virgin and Mariana Islands all require child safety seats for infants and children but the specific requirements vary widely from state to state. Additionally, some states require that another traffic violation be made before a police officer can pull over and ticket a driver for seatbelt (including car seat) violations. Not all state laws follow the scientific evidence and recommendations of government agencies, medical associations, and child safety organizations. For example, Florida only requires a car seat for children three years old or younger, and children aged four or older may wear an adult seat belt with no booster seat. Many state laws are based on age, and not the weight and height of the child. State laws do not always represent the optimal safety standards; therefore, it is safest for children if parents and caregivers err on the side of caution and follow the weight and height restrictions on car seats and booster seats, keep children in booster seats until they are four feet and nine inches tall, and keep all children under 13 properly buckled in a back seat.

Effects on public health

Since car accidents are the leading cause of death among children and car accidents result annually in hundreds of thousands of injuries to children, car seats and their proper use are important public health issues.

There are multiple obstacles to improved car seat use. Varied state legislation—including some states which do not ticket out-of-state drivers for car seat violations—makes it harder to establish national standards and guidelines. Many consumers assume that following state law is sufficient, when in many cases, it may not be sufficient protection for children.

There is an economic disparity in the use of car seats, especially the use of booster seats, with lower income children being less likely to be adequately restrained. Some state Medicaid programs offer discounts or free car seats and booster seats to eligible participants. Programs which combine education with free booster seats or discounts on booster seats have been particularly effective for four to eight year olds.

One of the biggest challenges with car seats is their proper use. Even well-informed parents may have inappropriately sized car seats, they may have the car seats improperly installed, or they may be improperly buckling in their children. Even though 96% of parents and caregivers think that they have properly installed and fastened car seats, 70% of children are in seats that are either improperly installed or improperly fastened.

Efforts and solutions

In order to address the difficulty of installing and using car seats, the NHTSA released a study in December 2009 that monitored and surveyed parents and caregivers as they installed and fastened car seats. The study recommended updating and clarifying the language and location of instructions and labels in car seats, vehicles, and their corresponding manuals.

SaferCar.Gov has a variety of public service announcements and graphics in English and Spanish to help communicate not only the importance of car seats but how frequently they are incorrectly installed and used. This website also offers recommended guidelines for selecting and installing car seats and booster seats.

The American Academy of Pediatrics continues to update their suggestions based on new research and they make this research and the subsequent recommendations available to the public and relevant government agencies.

Resources

BOOKS

Greenspan, Alrene I. "Car Safety for Infants and Children." *Encyclopedia of Lifestyle Medicine & Health.* Ed. James M. Rippe. Vol. 1. Thousand Oaks, CA: Safe Reference, 2012. 184-7. *Gale Virtual Reference Library.* Web. June 30, 2012.

Holmes, Gillian S. "Child Safety Seat." *How Products Are Made: An Illustrated Guide to Product Manufacturing.* Ed. Jacqueline L. Longe. Vol. 5. Detroit: Gale Group, 2000. 80-5. *Gale Virtual Reference Library.* Web. June 30, 2012.

Roehler, Douglas R., David A. Sleet, and Ann M. Dellinger. "Preventing Traffic Inujuries" *Encyclopedia of Lifestyle Medicine & Health.* Ed. James M. Rippe. Vol. 2. Thousand Oaks, CA: Sage Reference, 2012. 951-6. *Gale Virtual Reference Library.* Web. June 30, 2012.

"Your Baby's Car Seat." *Babycare: Everything you need to know.* Ann Peters. New York: DK Publishing, 2011. 170-1. *Gale Virtual Reference Library.* Web. June 30, 2012.

PERIODICALS

Anderson, Jane. "Booster seat use inconsistent." *Pediatric News*Feb. 2012: 30. *Health Reference Center Academic.* Web. June 30, 2012.

Anderson, Jane. "Guidelines: rear-facing seats for first 2 years." *Family Practice News* 1 Apr. 2011: 5. *Health Reference Center Academic.* Web. June 30, 2012.

Bass, Joel., et al. "Comparison of respiratory physiologic features when infants are placed in car safety seats or car beds." *Pediatrics* Aug. 2006: 522+. *Health Reference Center Academic.* Web. June 30, 2012.

Hirasawa, Kyoko, et al. "Effect of sitting position on respiratory status in preterm infants." *Journal of Prenatal Medicine* 37.4 (2009): 407+. *Health Reference Center Academic.* Web. June 30, 2012.

Tucker, Miriam E. "Medicaid benefit: car seats for kids a wise move; vehicle restraint system distribution was found to be more cost effective than most administered vaccines." *Family Practice News* Dec. 2005: 68. *Health Reference Center Academic.* Web. June 30, 2012.

"Warning about car seats." *Family Practice News* 1 Jan. 2007: 44. *Health Reference Center Academic.* Web. June 30, 2012.

WEBSITES

GHSA.gov. "State Child Passenger Safety Laws." http://www.ghsa.org/html/stateinfo/laws/childsafety_laws.html. Accessed July 5, 2012.

NHTSA.gov. "Drivers' Mistakes When Installing Child Seats." www.nhtsa.gov/DOT/NHTSA/NVS/Crash%20Avoidance/Technical%20Publications/2009/811234.pdf. Accessed June 30, 2012.

NHTSA.gov. "Child Seats" http://www.nhtsa.gov/Safety/CPS. Accessed July 5, 2012.

Safercar.gov. "Car Seats." http://www.safercar.gov/parents/CarSeats.htm. Accessed July 5, 2012.

ORGANIZATIONS

National Highway Traffic Safety Association, 1200 New Jersey Avenue, SE, West Building, Washington, DC USA 20590, (888) 327-4236, www.nhtsa.gov

American Academy of Pediatrics, 141 Northwest Point Boulevard, Elk Grove Village, IL USA 60007-1098, (847) 434-4000, (800) 433-9016, Fax: (847) 434-8000, www.aap.org.

Andrea Nienstedt, MA

Carbon monoxide poisoning

Definition

Carbon monoxide (CO) **poisoning** occurs through the inhalation of carbon monoxide gas. CO poisoning causes headache, nausea, convulsions, and finally death by asphyxiation.

Origins

Carbon monoxide, sometimes called coal gas, has been known as a toxic substance since the third century B.C. It was used for executions and suicides in early Rome. Today it is the leading cause of accidental poisoning in the United States.

Description

Produced by incomplete combustion, CO is a colorless, odorless, highly poisonous gas. It is found in automobile exhaust fumes, faulty stoves and heating systems, fires, and cigarette smoke. Other sources include wood-burning stoves, kerosene heaters, improperly ventilated **water** heaters and gas stoves, and blocked or poorly maintained chimney flues. CO interferes with the ability of the blood to carry oxygen.

Anyone who is exposed to CO will become sick, and the entire body is involved in CO poisoning. A developing fetus can also be poisoned if a pregnant woman breathes CO gas. Infants, people with heart or lung disease, or those with anemia may be more seriously affected. People such as underground parking garage attendants who are exposed to car exhausts in a confined area are more likely to be poisoned by CO. Firemen also run a higher risk of inhaling CO.

DEMOGRAPHICS. All people, as well as pets and other animals, are at risk for CO poisoning. Especially susceptible populations include unborn babies, infants, and people who have chronic **heart disease**, anemia, or respiratory problems. Annually, more than 20,000 Americans visit the emergency room each year due to CO poisoning, more than 4,000 are hospitalized, and about 400 die from unintentional CO poisoning. Deaths are most common among Americans 65 and older.

Causes and symptoms

Causes

Normally, when a person breathes fresh air into the lungs, the oxygen in the air binds with a molecule called hemoglobin (Hb) that is found in red blood cells. This allows oxygen to be moved from the lungs to every part of the body. When the oxygen/hemoglobin complex reaches a muscle where it is needed, the oxygen is released. Because the oxygen-binding process is reversible, hemoglobin can be used over and over again to pick up oxygen and move it throughout the body.

Inhaling carbon monoxide gas interferes with this oxygen-transport system. In the lungs, CO competes with oxygen to bind with the hemoglobin molecule. Hemoglobin prefers CO to oxygen and accepts it more than 200 times more readily than it accepts oxygen. Not only does the hemoglobin prefer CO, it holds onto the CO much more tightly, forming a complex called carboxyhemoglobin (COHb). As a person breathes CO-contaminated air, more and more oxygen transportation sites on the hemoglobin molecules become blocked by CO. Gradually, the sites available for oxygen become fewer and fewer in number. All cells need oxygen to live. When they do not get enough oxygen, cellular metabolism is disrupted, and eventually cells begin to die.

Symptoms

The symptoms of CO poisoning and the speed with which they appear depend on the concentration of CO in the air and the rate and efficiency with which a person breathes. Heavy smokers can start off with up to 9% of their hemoglobin already bound to CO, which they regularly inhale in cigarette smoke. This makes them much more susceptible to environmental CO.

With exposure to 200 ppm for two to three hours, a person begins to experience headache, fatigue, nausea, and dizziness. These symptoms correspond to 15–25% COHb in the blood. When the concentration of COHb reaches 50% or more, death results in a very short time.

The symptoms of CO poisoning in order of increasing severity include:

- headache
- shortness of breath
- dizziness
- fatigue
- mental confusion and difficulty thinking
- loss of fine hand-eye coordination
- nausea and vomiting
- rapid heart rate
- hallucinations

- inability to execute voluntary movements accurately
- collapse
- lowered body temperature (hypothermia)
- coma
- convulsions
- seriously low blood pressure
- cardiac and respiratory failure
- death

In some cases, the skin, mucous membranes, and nails of a person with CO poisoning are cherry red or bright pink. Because the color change does not always occur, it is an unreliable symptom to rely on for diagnosis.

Although most CO poisoning is acute, or sudden, it is possible to suffer from chronic CO poisoning. This condition exists when a person is exposed to low levels of the gas over a period of days to months. Symptoms are often vague and include (in order of frequency) fatigue, headache, dizziness, sleep disturbances, cardiac symptoms, apathy, nausea, and memory disturbances. Little is known about chronic CO poisoning, and it is often misdiagnosed.

Diagnosis

The main reason to suspect CO poisoning is evidence that fuel is being burned in a confined area. Examples include: a car running inside a closed garage, a charcoal grill burning indoors, and an unvented kerosene heater in a workshop. Under these circumstances, one or more persons suffering from the symptoms listed previously strongly suggests CO poisoning. In the absence of some concrete reason to suspect CO poisoning, the disorder is often misdiagnosed as migraine headache, **stroke**, psychiatric illness, food poisoning, alcohol poisoning, or heart disease.

Concrete confirmation of CO poisoning comes from a carboxyhemoglobin test. This blood test, for which blood is drawn as soon after suspected exposure to Co as possible, measures the amount of CO that is bound to hemoglobin in the body.

Other tests that are useful in determining the extent of CO poisoning include measurement of other arterial blood gases and pH; a complete blood count; measurement of other blood components such as **sodium**, potassium, bicarbonate, urea nitrogen, and lactic acid; an electrocardiogram (ECG); and a chest x ray.

Treatment

Immediate treatment for CO poisoning is to remove the victim from the source of carbon monoxide gas and get him or her into fresh air. If the victim is not breathing and has no pulse, cardiopulmonary resuscitation (CPR) should be started. Depending on the severity of the poisoning, 100% oxygen may be given with a tight-fitting mask as soon as it is available.

When combined with other symptoms of CO poisoning, COHb levels of more than 25% in healthy individuals, more than 15% in patients with a history of heart or lung disease, and more than 10% in pregnant women usually indicate the need for hospitalization. In the hospital, fluids and electrolytes are given to correct any imbalances that have arisen from the breakdown of cellular metabolism.

In severe cases of CO poisoning, patients receive hyperbaric oxygen therapy. This treatment involves placing the patient in a chamber breathing 100% oxygen at a pressure greater than one atmosphere (the normal pressure the atmosphere exerts at sea level). The increased pressure forces more oxygen into the blood. Hyperbaric facilities are specialized and are usually available only at larger hospitals.

Prognosis

The speed and degree of recovery from CO poisoning depend on the length and duration of exposure to the gas. The half-life of CO in normal room air is four to five hours. This means that, in four to five hours, half of the CO bound to hemoglobin will be replaced with oxygen. At normal atmospheric pressures, but breathing 100% oxygen, the half-life for the elimination of CO from the body is 50–70 minutes. In hyperbaric therapy at three atmospheres of pressure, the half-life is reduced to 20–25 minutes.

Although the symptoms of CO poisoning may subside in a few hours, some patients show memory problems, fatigue, confusion, and mood changes for two to four weeks after their exposure to the gas.

Prevention

Carbon monoxide poisoning is preventable. Particular care should be paid to situations where fuel is burned in a confined area. Inexpensive, portable, and permanently installed carbon-monoxide detectors that sound a warning similar to smoke detectors are available. Specific actions that will prevent CO poisoning include:

- stopping smoking, because smokers have less tolerance to environmental CO
- having heating systems and appliances installed by a qualified contractor to ensure that they are properly vented and meet local building codes
- inspecting and properly maintaining heating systems, chimneys, and appliances

KEY TERMS

Carboxyhemoglobin (COHb)—Hemoglobin that is bound to carbon monoxide instead of oxygen.

Hemoglobin (Hb)—A molecule that normally binds to oxygen in order to carry it to our cells, where it is required for life.

Hypothermia—Development of a subnormal body temperature.

pH—A measurement of the acidity or alkalinity of a fluid. A neutral fluid, neither acid nor alkali, has a pH of 7.

- not using a gas oven or stove to heat the home. According to the U.S. Environmental Protection Agency, the average level of CO in a home without a gas stove is 0.5–5 parts per million (ppm), and levels near properly operating gas stoves are often 5-15 ppm. Poorly adjusted stoves, however, may be 30 ppm or higher.)
- not burning charcoal indoors
- making sure that good ventilation accompanies the use of a kerosene heater indoors
- not leaving cars or trucks running inside the garage
- keeping car windows rolled up when stuck in heavy traffic, especially if inside a tunnel
- installing a carbon monoxide detector

Effects on public health

Carbon monoxide is insidious because it is odorless and colorless, so individuals do not realize that they are breathing CO-laden air. In addition, the initial symptoms, such as headache and nausea, can be attributed to other causes. For that reason, people do not realize they are being poisoned. Once the symptoms do become severe, individuals may already be too incapacitated to act and may therefore ultimately die.

Costs to society

Unintentional carbon monoxide poisoning results in hundreds of deaths every year in the United States. These often occur in the homes of persons who are economically disadvantaged and use improper or improperly adjusted fuel-burning devices in the home for heat.

Efforts and solutions

Some municipalities and other government agencies now require the installation of carbon monoxide detectors in homes or in certain residential buildings. In addition, the Occupational Safety and Health Administration (OSHA) has established a maximum permissible exposure level of 50 parts per million (ppm) over eight hours.

Resources

WEBSITES

"An Introduction to Indoor Air Quality (IAQ): Carbon Monoxide (CO)." U.S. Environmental Protection Agency. http://www.epa.gov/iaq/co.html (accessed November 10, 2012).

"Carbon Monoxide Indoors"American Lung Association. http://www.lung.org/healthy-air/home/resources/carbon-monoxide-indoors.html (accessed November 10, 2012).

"Carbon Monoxide Poisoning." U.S. Occupational Safety and Health Administration (OSHA), U.S. Department of Labor. http://www.osha.gov/OshDoc/data_General_Facts/carbon monoxide-factsheet.pdf (accessed November 10, 2012).

"Carbon Monoxide Poisoning." U.S. Centers for Disease Control and Prevention. http://www.cdc.gov/co/faqs.htm (accessed November 10, 2012).

"Carbon Monoxide Questions and Answers." U.S. Consumer Product Safety Commission. http://www.cpsc.gov/cpscpub/pubs/466.html (accessed November 10, 2012).

"Carbon Monoxide Detectors—Safe, Affordable, and Now the Law." Los Angeles Fire Department. http://lafd.blogspot.com/2011/07/carbon-monoxide-detectors-safe.html (accessed November 10, 2012).

ORGANIZATIONS

Centers for Disease Control and Prevention (CDC), 1600 Clifton Road, Atlanta, GA 30333, (800) 232-4636, cdcinfo@cdc.gov, http://www.cdc.gov/std/

American Lung Association, 1301 Pennsylvania Avenue NW, Suite 800, Washington, DC 20001, (202) 758-3355, (800) 548-8252, info@lungusa.org, http://www.lungusa.org/

U.S. Department of Labor Occupational Safety and Health Administration (OSHA), 200 Constitution Avenue, Washington, DC 20210, (800) 321-6742, http://www.osha.gov/.

Tish Davidson, A.M.
Teresa G. Odle
Leslie Mertz, Ph.D.

Centers for Disease Control and Prevention (CDC)

Definition

The Centers for Disease Control and Prevention (CDC) is one of the lead agencies of the United States government for the promotion of good health practices, the prevention of disease and injuries, and preparedness for threats to the health and safety of citizens of the nation.

Purpose

The CDC has a number of major goals and objectives, including monitoring the health of the American public, detecting and investigating health problems, conducting research that will lead to more effective programs of prevention and cure, developing and implementing sound programs for good health, implementing strategies for the prevention of disease and injury, promoting healthy behaviors in the everyday lives of citizens, fostering safe and healthful living and working environments, and providing training and leadership in public health practices.

Description

The CDC traces its beginnings to World War II when it was established as the Office of National Defense **Malaria** Control Activities, with the task of eradicating the mosquitoes responsible for malaria in the United States. At the time, the agency was a division of the U.S. Public Health Service with a staff of only seven medical officers out of a total of about 400 employees, the vast majority of whom were engineers and entomologists. The agency occupied a single floor on the sixth floor of a small building in Atlanta, Georgia. Over the years, the mission of the CDC expanded to include other infectious diseases, then the greater scope of disease and injury in general. Its name changed a number of times, to the Office of Malaria Control in War Areas in 1942, the Communicable Disease Center in 1946, the National Communicable Disease Center in 1967, the Center for Disease Control in 1970, the Centers for Disease Control in 1980, and, finally, the Centers for Disease Control and Prevention in 1992. Each name change reflected a widening in the scope of the agency's responsibilities.

The CDC's mission includes a wide variety of health–related topics that fall under seven major rubrics: public health preparedness and response; state, tribal, local, and territorial support; surveillance, **epidemiology**, and laboratory services; noncommunicable diseases, injuries, and **environmental health**; infectious diseases; global health; and occupational safety and health. Each of these major divisions is divided, in turn, into more specific categories. The Office of Surveillance, Epidemiology, and Laboratory Services, for example, includes the National Center for Health Statistics, the Laboratory Science Policy and Practice Program Office, the Public Health Informatics and Technology Program Office, the Public Health Surveillance Program Office, the Epidemiology and Analysis Office, and the Scientific Education and Professional Development Office.

CDC programs and activities cover the full range of public health challenges ranging from the design and implementation of programs to protect the nation against terrorist attacks to recommendations for protecting visitors to a state fair from animal–borne diseases. The agency is the central clearinghouse for information and data about outbreaks of disease in the United States, identification and analysis of the disease agents, and distribution of materials and personnel for dealing with those outbreaks. During the first decade of the twenty–first century, it was the lead agency for dealing with a number of natural and manmade disasters, including the attack on the World Trade Center in 2001, the **West Nile virus** epidemic in 2002, the response to hurricanes Charley and Frances in 2004, **Salmonella** and *E. coli* outbreaks in 2008, the Haitian earthquake in 2010, and the Japan earthquake and tsunami in 2011. In 2012, the agency was involved in a number of **infectious disease** outbreaks such as Salmonella infections from small turtles in March and from live poultry in June, a pertussis epidemic in Washington state in March, a new spread of the West Nile virus in Texas in August, and an outbreak of Salmonella in cantaloupes in August.

In addition to its data collection and distribution activities, the CDC operates an extensive training and education program that consists of conferences, webcasts and webinars, instructor–led sessions, and a host of print and electronic materials on health–related issues. In 2012, a diverse array of topics included in the CDC educational program included conferences on **autism**; health data and statistics; health communication and marketing; **cancer**; **occupational health** and safety; the leptospira vaccine; **immunization** practices; and food, **nutrition**, and **physical activity** as they relate to cancer. As of late 2012, the CDC had also developed three programs for specific groups: travelers' health; life stages and populations; and state, tribal, local, and territorial issues. The Life Stages and Populations topic area, for example, provides extensive information on a number of topics within this area, such as infants and toddlers, children, adolescents, adults, and older adults and seniors, as well as special groups such as at risk populations; families; immigrants and refugees; gay, lesbian, bisexual, and transgender individuals; people who use drugs; and women.

Professional publications

The CDC publishes two major journals, *Emerging Infectious Diseases* and *Preventing Chronic Disease*, as well as the essential weekly newsletter, *Morbidity and Mortality Weekly Report*, widely known simply as *MMWR*. In addition, the agency publishes a host of reports and other publications such as *Health Information for International Travel* (the so–called Yellow Book), and brochures, fact sheets, pamphlets, and other publications on topics including cancer, lead **poisoning**, diabetes, HIV/AIDS, oral health, and sexually transmitted infections.

Resources

BOOKS

Centers for Disease Control and Prevention: Agency Leadership Taking Steps to Improve Management and Planning, But Challenges Remain: Report to the Director of the Centers for Disease Control and Prevention. United States General Accounting Office. Washington, D.C.: U.S. General Accounting Office, 2004.

PERIODICALS

Messonnier, M. L. "Economics and Public Health at CDC." *MMWR. Morbidity and Mortality Weekly Report* 55. Suppl 2. (2006): 17–19

Sadler, J. H. "Centers for Disease Control and Prevention: A Clinician's View of the Past, Present, and Future." *Seminars in Dialysis.* 13, 2, (2000): 68–70

WEBSITES

Centers for Disease Control and Prevention. The Body. http://www.thebody.com/content/art17026.html (accessed October 10, 2012).

Centers for Disease Control and Prevention. USA Today. http://content.usatoday.com/topics/topic/Organizations/Government+Bodies/Centers+for+Disease+Control+and+Prevention (accessed October 10, 2012).

ORGANIZATIONS

Centers for Disease Control and Prevention, 1600 Clifton Rd., N.E., Atlanta, GA 30333, (800) 232-4636, cdcinfo@cdc.gov., www.cdc.gov.

David E. Newton, EdD

Chagas disease

Definition

Chagas disease is named after Brazilian physician Carlos Ribeiro Justiniano Chagas who first found the organism responsible for the disease in the early 1900s. The disease may affect the nerves that control the heart, digestive, and other organs, and eventually lead to damage to these organs. Worldwide, as many as 11 million people may have Chagas disease, and more than 10,000 die from it each year.

Description

Chagas disease is caused by infection with a parasite, a protozoan of the species *Trypanosoma cruzi*, that is transmitted to humans by certain insects that live in the Americas. For this reason, Chagas disease is also known as American trypanosomiasis. Once infected, individuals experience a mild, short-lived period of acute illness that may include fever; followed by a long period without symptoms. After the symptom-free period, which typically lasts many years, the more serious effects of the infection start to appear. These frequently involve the heart, esophagus, and colon, which become unable to contract properly, and begin to stretch or dilate.

Causes and symptoms

CAUSES. Certain insects from the Reduviidae family carry the parasite that causes Chagas disease. Most of the reduviid insects are predatory, but some use their beaks to penetrate human skin—especially the soft skin around the eyes and lips—and suck blood. Called "kissing bugs" and sometimes "barber bugs," "cone-nosed bugs," or "blood suckers," they include several species in the subfamily Triatominae, and are prevalent in Central and South America, where they inhabit poorly constructed houses and huts.

Although the insects bite humans, the primary way that humans acquire the parasite is from exposure to the waste products of the insects, which contain the **parasites**. The parasites may enter the individual through a cut or via the eyes or mouth. An individual may also become infected via a contaminated blood transfusion or transplantation of an organ from an infected donor, by eating uncooked or contaminated food or drinking contaminated liquids, or through breastfeeding. Kissing bugs, in turn, become infected with the parasite by biting infected animals and humans.

Symptoms

The disease has three phases:

- Acute phase. This lasts about two months, and patients experience non-specific symptoms of low-grade fever, headache, fatigue, and enlarged liver or spleen.
- Indeterminate phase. This phase lasts 10–20 years, during which time the patient experiences no symptoms. The parasites are reproducing in various organs during this time.
- Chronic phase. In this stage, symptoms related to damage of major organs (heart, esophagus, colon) begin.

Chronic-phase symptoms associated with the cardiovascular system include may include irregularities of heart rhythm, heart failure, and blood clots that can cause weakness, fainting, and even sudden death.

Esophageal symptoms are related to difficulty with swallowing and chest **pain**. Because the esophagus does not empty properly, food regurgitates into the lungs causing cough, bronchitis, and repeated bouts of **pneumonia**. Inability to eat, weight loss, and malnutrition become significant factors in affecting survival.

Involvement of the large intestine (colon) causes constipation, distention, and abdominal pain.

Origins

Chagas disease has plagued humans for thousands of years, as has been shown in several studies. A 2009 study in the journal Memórias do Instituto Oswaldo Cruz, for instance, verified the presence of the disease in prehistoric remains excavated from archeological sites on the border between Texas and Mexico, and in the state of Minas Gerais, in the Brazilian cerrado, or savannah.

Despite the long history of the disease, it was the early 1900s before Brazilian physician Carlos Chagas discovered the cause. Chagas already had participated in treating and controlling **malaria**, which is also caused by a parasite, when he began studying another disease that was making railroad workers ill at the South American Port of Santos. That illness would eventually become known as Chagas disease. In 1909, he correctly made the connection between kissing bugs and Chagas disease, and upon dissecting the bugs, identified the protozoan *T. cruzi* as the responsible agent.

Demographics

The kissing bugs live throughout much of Mexico, Central America, and South America, where approximately 8–11 million people are infected, according to the **Centers for Disease Control and Prevention (CDC)**. The insects thrive in areas with poor housing conditions, such as homes built with mudded walls and thatched roofs that are common to rural areas.

Although 11 different species of kissing bugs occur in the United States, only rare vector-borne cases of Chagas disease have been documented. Nonetheless, the **CDC** estimates that more than 300,000 U.S.-living immigrant persons are infected, and most of them acquired the disease in their home countries. More than 10,000 people die due to Chagas disease a year.

Diagnosis

The best way to diagnose acute infection is to identify the parasites in tissue or blood. Occasionally, it is possible to culture the organism from infected tissue, but this process usually requires too much time to be of value. In the chronic phase, antibody levels can be measured. Efforts to develop new, more accurate tests are ongoing.

If the disease is progressed beyond the acute phase, the doctor may order other tests to determine whether the disease has affected the heart, colon, or other organs.

KEY TERMS

Achalasia—An esophageal disease of unknown cause, in which the lower sphincter or muscle is unable to relax normally, and leads to the accumulation of material within the esophagus.

Endoscopy—Exam using an endoscope (a thin, flexible tube equipped with a lens or miniature camera to view various areas of the gastrointestinal tract). When the procedure is performed to examine certain organs such as the bile ducts or pancreas, the organs are not viewed directly, but rather indirectly through the injection of x ray.

Parasite—An organism that lives on or in another and takes nourishment (food and fluids) from that organism.

Treatment

If the diagnosis of Chagas disease is made soon after infection and at the onset of the acute phase of the illness, the antiparasitic drugs benznidazole and nifurtimox are nearly 100% effective in curing the disease, according to the **World Health Organization**. Although neither drug is FDA-approved for use in the United States, the CDC does make them available under investigational protocols.

The further into the disease course, the less effective the drugs, so the earliest possible treatment is best. Patients should consult with their medical professionals to weigh the benefits of the drugs against their possible side effects, which increase with age.

Beyond these medications, a healthcare professional may recommend specific therapies to treat symptoms. For instance, cardiac effects are managed with pacemakers and medications. Esophageal complications require either endoscopic or surgical methods to improve esophageal emptying. These methods are similar to those used to treat the disorder known as achalasia. Constipation is treated by increasing fiber and bulk laxatives, or removal of diseased portions of the colon.

CONTRAINDICATIONS. Women who are pregnant and those who are breastfeeding, and any individuals who have liver or kidney failure should not take the drugs. Persons with a history of neurological or psychiatric disorders should also consult their physician about Nifurtimox, which may not be a good choice.

RECOMMENDED DOSAGE. According to the CDC, the recommended oral dosages per day are:

- For benznidazole, 10 mg/kg in two divided doses for 60 days for those who are younger than 12 years of age;

QUESTIONS TO ASK YOUR DOCTOR

- Given my general state of health, and the stage of Chagas disease, can you weigh the possible advantages vs. the disadvantages of taking the antiparasitic drugs?
- How long will I have to take this medication?
- What side effects can I expect, and which side effects are cause for alarm?
- What should I do if I miss a dose?
- Do I have to worry about passing this parasite to the other members of my family, and if so, can I take any preventative measures?

and 5–7 mg/kg in two divided doses for 60 days for those 12 years old and older.

- For nifurtimox, 15–20 mg/kg in three or four divided doses for 90 days for those 10 years old and younger; 12.5–15 mg/kg in three or four divided doses for 90 days in those 11–16 years old; and 8–10 mg/kg in three or four divided doses for 90 days for those older than 16.

SIDE EFFECTS. Both benznidazole and nifurtimox have numerous common side effects, including anorexia, weight loss, and various neuropathies. Nifurtimox may also cause nausea and/or vomiting; headache; and dizziness or vertigo.

Prognosis

Early treatment with antiparasitic drugs can cure a patient of the disease. Those patients with gastrointestinal complications often respond to some form of treatment. Cardiac problems are more difficult to treat, particularly since transplant would rekindle infection.

Prevention

Visitors traveling to areas of known infection should avoid staying in mud, adobe, or similar huts. Mosquito nets and insect repellents are useful in reducing contact with the bugs.

In 2010, the U.S. Food and Drug Administration approved a second test to screen blood, tissue and organ donors for *T. cruzi*. This test is called Abbott Prism Chagas [*T. cruzi* (*E. coli*, Recombinant) Antigen]. The previously approved test is called the *T. cruzi* Whole Cell Lysate Antigen.

As of 2012, research at the University of Georgia was under way to develop a vaccine for pets with the hope of reducing the spread of the disease to humans.

Effects on public health

Between 8 and 11 million people worldwide have Chagas disease. Up to 30% of these will experience associated cardiac disorders, and as many as one in 10 will experience digestive, neurological, or other health issues. As the disease progresses, especially in older individuals, the disease can lead to heart failure and sudden death. More than 10,000 people die each year from Chagas disease.

Although Chagas disease has been primarily limited to Latin America, it is now appearing elsewhere in the world due to the movement of people from these areas and around the world.

Costs to society

Individuals often become infected at a young age. In fact, Chagas disease is a primary cause of cardiac lesions in young adults in Latin America. This has numerous negative consequences for economic productivity. Not only can this disease dampen these individuals' potential contributions to the community, but it can also affect the financial state of their immediate and extended families. This becomes a particular problem because the infections are more common among poorer, rural families who have little, if any, financial buffer.

Efforts and solutions

Since the 1990s, a number of multinational initiatives have been organized to reduce the incidence of Chagas disease and to promote early diagnosis and treatment. One method that has proven particularly successful is the screening of donor blood and organs for the parasites, thereby reducing transmission by that vector.

Resources

BOOKS

Delaporte, François. *Chagas Disease: History of a Continent's Scourge.* Bronx, NY: Fordham University Press, 2012.

Telleria, Jenny, and Michel Tibayrenc (eds.). *Trypanosomiasis: Chagas Disease One Hundred Years of Research.* Burlington, MA: Elsevier, 2010.

PERIODICALS

Araújo, A., A.M. Jansen, K. Reinhard, and L.F. Ferreira. "Paleoparasitology of Chagas Disease—A Review." *Memórias do Instituto Oswaldo Cruz* 104, suppl. 1 (2009): 9–16.

WEBSITES

"Chagas disease (American Trypanosomiasis)." World Health Organization. http://www.who.int/mediacentre/factsheets/fs340/en/index.html (accessed November 2, 2012).

Hataway, James. University of Georgia "UGA animal vaccine may slow deadly spread of Chagas disease." http://news.uga.edu/releases/article/uga-animal-vaccine-may-slow-deadly-spread-of-chagas-disease/ (accessed November 2, 2012).

MedlinePlus. "Chagas disease (American Trypanosomiasis)." U.S. National Library of Medicine, National Institutes of Health. http://www.nlm.nih.gov/medlineplus/chagasdisease.html (accessed November 2, 2012).

"Parasites—American Trypanosomiasis (Also Known as Chagas Disease). Antiparasitic Treatment." Centers for Disease Control and Prevention. http://www.cdc.gov/parasites/chagas/health_professionals/tx.html (accessed November 2, 2012).

Pottinger, Paul, M.D. Infectious Disease and Antimicrobial Agents, Antimicrobe. "History of Chagas Disease" http://www.antimicrobe.org/history/chagas_disease.asp (accessed November 2, 2012).

ORGANIZATIONS

Centers for Disease Control and Prevention (CDC), 1600 Clifton Road, Atlanta, GA 30333, (800) 232-4636, cdcinfo@cdc.gov, http://www.cdc.gov/std/

The Chagas Disease Foundation, 1191 DaAndra Drive, Watkinsville, GA 30677, (641) 715-3900 ext.46250#, chagasfoundation@gmail.com, http://www.chagasfound.org/.

David Kaminstein, M.D.
Leslie Mertz, Ph.D.

Chemical poisoning

Definition

Chemical **poisoning** is a major public health concern. Approximately 95% of all accidental or intentional poisonings are due to chemicals. Nearly 90% of these cases occur at home. Infants, toddlers, and small children are at the greatest risk for accidental (acute) poisoning. In 2012, poison control centers received about 2.5 million calls about poison exposures, more than a million of which involved children younger than age six. Chronic exposure is chemical poisoning that occurs slowly and insidiously over a prolonged period of time. Many chronic, degenerative diseases have been linked to environmental pollution or poisoning. The list may include **cancer**, memory loss, **allergies**, multiple chemical sensitivity, chronic fatigue syndrome, **infertility** in adults, learning and behavioral disorders, developmental abnormalities, and **birth defects**.

Description

Of the millions of natural and synthetic chemicals in existence, approximately 3,000 are known to cause significant health problems. In many cases, the type and severity of danger posed by a chemical is a matter of dispute among experts. Accidental acute chemical poisoning involving common household or garden products is easy to diagnose and treat, as long as it is recognized early enough. By contrast, chronic poisoning due to daily exposure to chemicals is more difficult to diagnose and the extent of damage is more difficult to assess. Toxic chemicals can be found anywhere—in homes, around homes on private property, at work, on the playground—even in foods and **drinking water**. Some result from illegal dumping. However, many chemical poisonings occur insidiously by the supposedly harmless chemicals that people bring into their homes or office to make their lives more comfortable.

Household poisons

Because of the huge amounts of toxic chemicals that can be found inside homes, scientists have come to believe the home—not the office or the freeway—is the most contaminated place of all. Any chemicals found inside the house can be accidentally ingested by small children. Daily exposure to chemicals indoors may also cause significant health risks. Major chemical poisons inside homes include volatile organic compounds, lead, radon, carbon monoxide, and the various substances in household cleaners and carpet.

VOLATILE CHEMICALS. Indoor **air pollution** is caused by volatile chemicals, those which evaporate at room temperature. When people use products that contain these volatile substances, the chemicals are trapped inside their homes, and they can reach levels thousands of times higher than exist outdoors in the air. Chronic exposure to polluted air may cause lung infections, headaches, nausea, mental confusion, fatigue, depression, and memory loss. In addition, it may cause damage to an unborn fetus and increase the risk of developing cancer. The following are some of the most common volatile substances found inside the home:

- trichloroethane (spray cans, insulation, spot removers)
- tetrachloroethylene (dry-cleaning solutions)
- formaldehyde (glue, foam, preservatives, plywood, fabrics, insulation)
- para-dichlorobenzene (pDCB) (mothballs, air fresheners)
- toluene (solvents, cleaning fluids, wood finishing products)
- benzene (gasoline)
- xylene (paints, finishing products)
- acetone (nail polish remover)
- styrene (foam, carpets, adhesives)
- carbon tetrachloride (dry cleaning solutions, paint removers)
- perchloroethylene (cleaning solvents)

LEAD AND OTHER HEAVY METALS. Lead is a very toxic chemical, especially to small children. Lead poisoning can cause learning disabilities and behavioral problems in children. Lead poisoning in pregnant women can cause fetal abnormalities, brain damage, and impaired motor skills in their babies. Lead is found in leaded paint (in old houses) and is sometimes present in pesticides, pottery and china, artists' paint, and products used for hobbies and crafts. Also harmful are other heavy metals, such as mercury and cadmium.

RADON. Radon is an odorless gas produced from the radioactive decay of uranium. It is believed to be the most common cause of lung cancer second only to **smoking**. Outdoors, radon gas is usually too well-dispersed to reach dangerous levels. It is far more dangerous indoors, where ventilation tends to be inadequate, as in places such as basements where radon can seep from the soil and accumulate to dangerous concentrations. Radon testing is the only way to discover if a home is contaminated.

CARBON MONOXIDE. In closed areas, carbon monoxide (CO) is the most lethal gas produced by a burning heat source. Sources of CO are gas heat, fireplaces, or idling cars. A CO detector is needed in all homes because this gas is odorless, colorless, and deadly.

CHEMICALS TRAPPED INSIDE CARPETS. Carpets contain many chemicals capable of causing nerve damage. These neurotoxic chemicals include acetone, benzene, toluene, phenol, xylene, decane, and hexane.

HOUSEHOLD CLEANERS. The following are neurotoxic chemicals commonly found in household cleaners:

- chlorine (dishwasher detergents)
- ammonia (antibacterial cleaning agents)
- petroleum (dish soaps, laundry detergents, floor waxes)

MEDICINES. Medicines are one of the most common causes of accidental and intentional (**suicide**) poisonings. Drugs most commonly involved are aspirin, acetaminophen, sedatives; any psychoactive drug if the patient is prone to impulsive, suicidal action (e.g., antidepressants); antiseizure drugs; iron pills; vitamins/mineral supplements containing iron; and cardiac drugs, such as digoxin and quinidine.

Yard chemicals

Yard materials that can be toxic to humans and pets include:

- Insecticides: Toxic chemicals that can be found in insecticide preparations include lindane, arsenic, lead, malathion, diazinon, and nicotine.
- Rodenticides (chemicals that kill mice or rats): Rodenticides often contain highly toxic chemicals, such as sodium fluoroacetate, phosphorus, thallium, barium, strychnine, methyl bromide, and cyanides.
- Herbicides (chemicals that kill weeds): Herbicides contain carbaryl and diazinon, which increase the risk of childhood brain cancer.

The regulatory status of some of these chemicals varies from country to country and state to state. Critics often call for a ban on chemicals that are especially toxic or otherwise dangerous. For example, by 2009, lindane was approved for use in the United States and many other countries. However, a worldwide campaign was working to have the chemical banned because of its toxicity.

Occupational hazards

Workers are often exposed to toxic effects of various chemicals in their working environment:

- polluted air: affecting workers in poorly ventilated plants that manufacture paints, insecticides, fungicides, pesticides
- radiation: affecting workers in poorly constructed nuclear chemical plants
- contaminated environment: affecting miners who labor underground
- obnoxious fumes: affecting fire fighters who are exposed to toxic fumes
- skin contact with toxic chemicals: affecting crop pickers who have exposure to sprayed insecticides

Toxic chemicals in foods

Highly processed or prepackaged foods use various chemical additives to make these foods look more attractive, taste better, or store for longer periods of time. Harmful substances that can be found in foods include:

- Monosodium glutamate (MSG), a common flavoring agent: Excessive consumption of MSG may cause hyperactivity, memory loss, or other types of brain damage. It is often associated with the so-called Chinese restaurant syndrome characterized by headaches, nausea, vomiting, palpitations, and flushing of skin, due to the MSG content in the food.
- Artificial sweeteners, such as aspartame or saccharin: These sweeteners can cause a variety of health problems, including headaches (migraines included), dizziness, seizures, depression, nausea, and vomiting, and abdominal cramps. Their use may be associated with hyperactivity in children. Whether they increase risk of cancer was unknown as of 2012. Pregnant women should avoid using these sweeteners.
- Artificial colors: Color additives can be found in a variety of foods, including cereals, juices, candy, frozen foods, ice cream, cookies, pizza, salad dressings, and soft drinks. Children and adults alike may be exposed to cancer-causing artificial colors such as red numbers 8, 9, 19, and 37, or orange number 17.
- Preservatives: Many of the preservatives found in foods are hazardous. Nitrates, common preservatives in cured and

luncheon meats and canned products, are known to cause cancer. In addition, pregnant women who consume large amounts of nitrates (for example, through eating hot dogs or salami) unknowingly increase risk of brain damage in their unborn child. Synthetic antioxidants are used in prepackaged foods to prevent food spoilage. Common synthetic antioxidants, such as butylated hydroxyanisole (BHA) and butylated hydroxytoluene (BHT), can be found in cereals, baking mixes, or instant potatoes. These products are known to cause brain, liver, and kidney damage, as well as respiratory problems.

- Food contaminants: Health-promoting foods such as fruits and vegetables may contain dangerous herbicide and pesticide residues on their surfaces. Fish in contaminated lakes or rivers may contain mercury, dioxin, PCBs, or other harmful chemicals. Babies of mothers who consume contaminated fish during pregnancy have lower birth weight, smaller heads, developmental delays, and lower scores on tests of baby intelligence.

Air pollution and environmental contamination

Air pollution can cause or worsen lung or heart diseases and increase risk of cancer. Chemicals that most often cause pollution in the air and **water** supply are fine particles, ozone, asbestos, carbon monoxide, lead, nitrogen oxides, halogenated hydrocarbons, and pesticides.

Demographics

According to the National Capital Poison Center, chemical poisoning is common and the second leading cause of injury and death in the United States. In 2008, more than 41,000 people died as a result of poisoning, and poisoning became the leading cause of injury death for the first time since at least 1980. The poisoning death rate nearly tripled over the past 30 years and the percentage of poisoning deaths that were caused by drugs increased from about 60% to about 90%. Nearly 9 out of 10 poisoning deaths are caused by drugs, and opioid **pain** medications were involved in more than 40% of all 2008 drug and chemical poisoning deaths, up from about 25% in 1999. According to the **CDC**, about 76% of poisoning deaths were unintentional, 16% were suicides, and 8% were of undetermined intent.

Causes and symptoms

Acute poisoning

The following events are possible causes for acute poisoning:

- Accidental ingestion of household products. This problem primarily affects children under the age of five.
- Medication errors. Such errors occur most often among elderly people. Sometimes hospital staff make the error; at other times, the patient gets confused about or cannot read directions regarding the identity or dosage of drugs.
- Suicide.
- Excessive alcohol or drug abuse.

The following signs and symptoms indicate the possibility of acute chemical poisoning:

- difficulty breathing
- changes in skin color
- headaches or blurred vision
- irritated eyes, skin, or throat
- sweating
- dizziness
- breath odor, including bitter almond (cyanide poisoning) or garlic odor (arsenic poisoning)
- nausea, vomiting, diarrhea
- unusual behavior
- difficulty walking or standing straight

Chronic poisoning

COMMON ROUTES OF EXPOSURE. Individuals may accumulate toxic amounts of a chemical in their body through daily exposure to the chemical. Common routes of exposure include:

- inhalation of the poisonous gas
- consumption of contaminated food, water, or medications
- contact with toxic or caustic chemicals in the eyes, skin, or through contaminated clothing
- pregnant mother's exposure to toxic chemicals during pregnancy, especially during the first trimester

EFFECTS OF TOXIC CHEMICALS ON THE YOUNG. Toxic chemicals can have devastating effects on developing fetuses and children. The following diseases and conditions are linked to chronic exposure to home and environmental pollution:

- miscarriages and spontaneous abortions
- low birth weight
- premature births
- stillbirths
- birth defects
- sudden infant death syndrome (SIDS)
- developmental delays
- poor motor coordination
- attention-deficit hyperactivity disorder (ADHD)
- aggressive behavior
- learning disabilities

- speech and language problems
- autism
- sensory deficits
- allergies and chemical sensitivity in childhood and in later years
- asthma, hay fever, and sinusitis
- cancer in childhood, adulthood, and in subsequent generations
- poorly functioning organs and systems
- weakened immune system and increased risk of infections

The following chronic diseases and conditions may occur in adults as a result of cumulative chemical poisoning:

- fatigue
- headaches
- skin rashes
- aches and pains
- generalized weakness
- asthma
- increased risk of infection
- depression and irritability
- liver diseases, such as jaundice (yellowing of the skins and eyes), inflammation of the liver (hepatitis), and cirrhosis (a chronic degenerative disease of the liver)
- lung diseases
- heart diseases
- cancer
- decreased life expectancy
- sick building syndrome
- Gulf War syndrome (due to nerve agent and pesticide exposure)

Diagnosis

Acute poisoning

In many cases, the identity of the poison is known to the patient or the parents of the affected child. The role of the physician is to determine what treatment (if any) is necessary based on the type and amount of toxic substance exposure, the identity of the chemical, and patient's signs and symptoms.

Chronic poisoning

Chronic environmental poisoning is more difficult to diagnose. To find out if environmental pollution is causing an illness, a physician conducts a thorough physical exam of the patient. The doctor also obtains a thorough medical history with detailed information concerning the food and water sources, as well as the nature of the patient's work or place of residence. Laboratory tests may include blood and urine tests and hair sample analysis. In addition, liver and kidney function tests are conducted to see if these organs are affected. The doctor also inquires about other diseases the patient may have developed in the recent past.

Treatment

Alternative treatments are not appropriate for acute chemical poisoning. When an emergency poisoning occurs, especially in children, parents are encouraged to call a toll-free hotline that is staffed 24 hours a day at 1-800-222-1222. However, alternative treatments may be useful in treating chronic exposure to toxic chemicals. The specific treatment plan depends on the type of poison by which a person is affected. Generally speaking, most treatments involve identifying the offending chemical and avoiding future exposures to it. A healthy diet, nutritional supplements and/or detoxification therapy are also helpful. Detoxification therapy is especially effective for the liver, which is the organ that metabolizes most toxins.

Detoxification diet

Naturopaths sometimes recommend patients suspected of chronic chemical poisoning to follow a detoxification (detox) diet for at least several months. Pregnant women, small children, or very frail people should avoid taking this diet. Medical experts see little harm in these diets but find little evidence that they are effective. A detox diet has the following characteristics:

- Low fat intake to increase fat mobilization (moving fat from storage to be used for energy). Limited consumption of olive oil and vegetable oils is allowed.
- Limited intake of sugar and highly processed foods and avoidance of alcohol, caffeine, and tobacco.
- High fiber consumption to absorb the toxic chemicals and eliminate them from the body.
- Limited consumption of red meat. The bulk of protein intake should come from vegetable sources, such as legumes and tofu, as well as fish from unpolluted waters.
- Strong emphasis on organic fruits and vegetables (and their juices) with detoxification effects. These include papayas, apples, pears, strawberries, dark green leafy vegetables, carrots, beets, and garlic. Antioxidant foods, such as broccoli, cauliflower, kale, yams, tomatoes, peaches, watermelon, hot peppers, green tea, red grapes, citrus fruits, soybeans, and whole grains are also recommended.
- Increased water intake to at least eight glasses of water per day to help eliminate waste from the body.
- Dietary supplementation with high potency multivitamin/mineral products.

Exercise

Exercise to the point of perspiration helps eliminate toxins from the body. Daily walking for 30 minutes is helpful and appropriate for most people.

Herbal therapy

Milk thistle (*Silybum mariannum*) is a powerful antioxidant that protects the liver and assists in the detoxification process by increasing glutathione supply in the liver. Glutathione is the enzyme primarily involved in the detoxification of many toxic chemicals in the environment, such as solvents, pesticides, and heavy metals.

Traditional Chinese medicine

Depending on a patient's specific condition, an expert Chinese herbalist may prescribe herbal remedies that can help remove toxins from the body and improve liver function.

Homeopathy

For homeopathic therapy, patients should consult a homeopathic physician who can prescribe specific remedies based on knowledge of the underlying cause.

Fasting

Fasting is an ancient way of detoxification and is also very efficient. During three-day fasting, patients take supplements and drink four glasses of juice a day to assist the cleansing process and to prevent exhaustion. Supplements recommended are those that include antioxidants, such as **vitamins** C and E, selenium, zinc, and magnesium. For patients suspected of significant poisoning, a naturopath may also prescribe milk thistle to aid the detoxification process and provide support for the body. The patient may also consider a food fast, where only food that is simple to digest is consumed. For example, ultra-clear hydrolyzed rice is simple to digest and is also hypo-allergenic.

Allopathic treatment

Acute poisoning

For acute poisoning, individuals should call 911, a local poison control center, or 1-800-222-1222 immediately. The toll-free number is a national hotline begun in 2002 by the American Association of Poison Control Centers to provide 24-hour poison treatment and **prevention** services. If a child is suspected of eating or drinking hazardous chemicals, parents should look for the container and call for instructions. Patients or parents of the poisoned child should wait for instructions before administering syrup of ipecac, activated charcoal, or anything else by mouth. Treatment of a particular poison depends on the identity of the poison and how the poison is absorbed by the body.

INHALED POISONS. Treatment of inhaled poison includes bringing the patient out and away from the area contaminated with poisonous gas. The patient should be given oxygen and other respiratory support as necessary.

SKIN AND EYE CONTAMINATION. If a person's skin comes into contact with toxic chemicals, the contaminated clothing should be removed, the chemical carefully brushed off the skin, and the body flushed with running water to dilute the poison. The wounds, if any, should be covered with sterile gauze or cloth and the patient transferred to the hospital for treatment of chemical burn. If toxic or caustic chemicals get in the eyes, the affected person should remove glasses or any contact lenses immediately, rinse the eyes well with clean water or normal saline solution, and go to the emergency room for further treatment or observation.

INGESTED POISONS. Depending on the specific type of ingested poisons, syrup of ipecac, activated charcoal, and/or gastric lavage (stomach pumping) can be used.

In many cases of accidental poisoning, syrup of ipecac can be used effectively. When swallowed, it irritates the stomach and induces vomiting. As of 2012, syrup of ipecac was considered the safest drug for treating poisoning and was often the most effective. Syrup of ipecac can be used for most ingested poisons. However, syrup of ipecac should not be used if the suspected poison is strychnine, a corrosive substance (strong acids or lye), petroleum products (gasoline, kerosene, paint thinner, or cleaning fluids), or certain prescription drugs, such as antidepressants or sustained-release theophylline. In addition, it should not be used in patients who are unconscious or seizing.

Activated charcoal is also an effective treatment for many chemical poisons. It absorbs poisons quickly and in large amounts. In addition, it is nontoxic, may be stored for a long time, and can be conveniently administered at home. Charcoal works by absorbing irritating or toxic substances in the stomach and intestines. This action prevents the toxic drug or chemical from spreading throughout the body. The toxic drug or chemical and the activated charcoal are excreted in the stools without harming the body.

If both syrup of ipecac and charcoal are recommended for treatment of the poison, ipecac should be given first. Charcoal should not be given for at least 30 minutes after ipecac or when vomiting from ipecac stops. Activated charcoal is often mixed with a liquid before being swallowed or put into the tube leading to the stomach. Activated charcoal is available in liquid form in 30 g bottles. It is also available in 15 g container sizes, and as slurry of charcoal premixed in water or as a container to which water or soda pop is added.

Charcoal should not be used to treat poisoning caused by corrosive products, such as lye or other strong acids or petroleum products such as gasoline, kerosene, or cleaning fluids. Charcoal may make the condition worse and delay the diagnosis and treatment. In addition, charcoal is not effective if the poison is lithium, cyanide, iron, ethanol, or methanol.

Gastric lavage may also be used to treat chemical poisoning. This procedure is performed by medical professionals in emergency rooms only. Lavage fluids (saline water or water) are given through a large tube down the patient's throat and the stomach contents are pumped out. This procedure is repeated until most of the toxic substance is removed. Then a specific antidote for the chemical or activated charcoal is given to absorb the rest.

Sometimes, antidotes are available to neutralize poison and render it harmless. The following are common antidotes:

- naloxone: for morphine, methadone, or heroin overdose
- atropine: for organophosphate (insecticide) poisoning
- acetylcysteine: for acetaminophen (Tylenol) toxicity
- digoxin immune fab (Digibind): for digoxin toxicity

Chronic chemical poisoning

Treatment of chronic chemical poisoning involves identifying and eliminating the source of poison from the patient's environment, followed by symptomatic treatment of the condition. Chelation therapy can be used to remove heavy metals, such as lead, iron, mercury, copper, nickel, zinc, cadmium, beryllium, and arsenic. This treatment uses chelating agents, such as ethylenediamine tetraacetic acid (EDTA) and dimethylsuccinate (DMSA) to bind and precipitate metals and remove them from the body.

Expected results

Depending on the severity of the poisoning, the affected person may have total or partial recovery. If the rescue effort comes too late, a patient may die of acute chemical or drug poisoning. For those affected by chronic exposure to environmental poisoning, recovery depends on the severity of the poisoning, the ability to stay away from the offending agent, and appropriate diagnosis and treatment. Total recovery can occur in many patients.

Prevention

Some strategies for avoiding poisoning are:

- Avoiding eating contaminated fish, especially that which comes from known contaminated areas or a lot of big fish, such as shark, swordfish, or tuna, which tend to contain higher amounts of mercury than smaller fish. Pregnant women should not consume more than 7 oz of tuna per week. Mercury can cause brain damage in the developing fetus.
- Not painting or remodeling a home while pregnant or when children are still small. Paint may contain chemicals that can harm a fetus and cause learning disabilities in small children.
- Limiting use of chemicals inside the house as much as possible and instead using natural benign alternatives, such as baking soda (as cleaner, deodorizer), distilled white vinegar (as cleaner), essential oils (as fragrances), lemon juice (as cleaner), and liquid soaps (as detergents).
- Increasing ventilation of the house.
- Considering installing tile or wood floors in new homes instead of new carpet.
- Having the house tested for radon.
- Eating organic foods. Otherwise, to better remove toxins, washing fruits and vegetables carefully before eating with a mild acid solution, such as diluted vinegar.
- Avoiding toxic chemical exposure as much as possible if pregnant.
- Keeping all medications, petroleum products, cleaning products locked and away from small children. Installing child-proof locks or gates to prevent children from finding poisons.
- Avoiding mixing household cleaning products. Non-toxic chemicals when mixed together can release toxic gases or cause an explosion.
- Keeping all chemicals in original containers, properly identified and stored away from foods.
- Only using chemicals in well-ventilated areas to avoid breathing in fumes. Using adequate skin, eye, and respiratory protection.

KEY TERMS

Antidote—A remedy to counteract a poison.

Cumulative—Increasing in effects or quantity by successive additions.

Detoxification—A structured program for removing stored toxins from the body.

Diazinon—A member of the organophosphate family of pesticides. This chemical causes nerve and reproductive damage.

Insecticides—Any substance used to kill insects.

Pesticides—Chemicals used to kill insects.

QUESTIONS TO ASK YOUR DOCTOR

- How do you treat most chemical poisonings?
- What are the survival rates for someone exposed to hazardous chemicals?
- Does chemical poisoning pose any other health risks?
- Are some chemical more harmful than others?

- Never putting household chemicals in food or beverage containers.
- Avoiding smoking or lighting a candle near household chemicals, such as cleaning solutions, hair spray, paints or paint thinner, or pesticides.
- Disposing all hazardous chemicals properly according to the manufacturer's instructions.

Public health role and response

The **World Health Organization** has established poison centers to deal with chemical poisoning. They are a specialized unit that advises on, and assists with, the prevention, diagnosis and management of poisoning. The structure and function of poisons centers varies around the world, however, at a minimum a poisons center is an information service. Some poisons centers may also include a toxicology laboratory and/or a clinical treatment unit.

A poisons center answers enquiries about exposure to chemical agents, including products, pharmaceuticals, natural toxins, pesticides and industrial chemicals. It provides an assessment of whether a particular exposure is hazardous, and information on the need for treatment and the kind of treatment that should be given. Poisons centers aim to promote the evidence-based, cost-effective management of poisoning and to ensure that unnecessary or ineffective treatment is avoided.

Poisons centers offer a service to health professionals and also, in many countries, to the general public. Other users include the emergency services, government bodies, regulatory agencies and education services. They are uniquely centralized repositories of data about human exposures to chemicals, including information about the agents involved, the circumstances giving rise to exposure, and the health effects of exposure. These data can be used to help reduce the incidence of poisoning by identifying emerging toxicological hazards (a process known as toxicovigilance), stimulating preventive measures by manufacturers and regulators and assessing the efficacy of such measures. Poisons center data also contribute to improving knowledge about the human health effects of chemicals.

Resources

BOOKS

Aulakh, S. K. "Carbon Monoxide Poisoning." In *Ferri's Clinical Advisor 2012: 5 Books in 1*, 187–88. Philadelphia: Mosby Elsevier, 2012.

Howd, Robert A., and Anna M. Fan. *Risk Assessment for Chemicals in Drinking Water.* New York: Wiley Interscience, 2007.

McGuigan M. A. "Chronic Poisoning: Trace Metals and Others." In *Cecil Medicine,* edited by Lee Goldman and Andrew I. Schafer. 23rd ed. Philadelphia: Saunders Elsevier, 2008.

Stranks, Jeremy. *The A–Z of Food Safety.* Abingdon, UK: Thorogood, 2007.

Van Leeuwen, C. J., and T. G. Vermeire, eds. *Risk Assessment of Chemicals: An Introduction.* New York: Springer, 2007.

PERIODICALS

Bronstein, A. C., D. A. Spyker, L. R. Cantilena, J. L. Green, et al. "2008 Annual Report of the American Association of Poison Control Centers' National Poison Data System (NPDS): 26th Annual Report." *Clinical Toxicology* 47 (2009): 911–1084

Isman, Murray B. "Botanical Insecticides: for Richer, for Poorer." *Pest Management Science* (January 2008): 8–11.

Peter, John Victor, John L. Moran, and Petra L. Graham. "Advances in the Management of Organophosphate Poisoning." *Expert Opinion on Pharmacotherapy* (July 2007): 1451–64.

Schier, Joshua G., et al. "Strategies for Recognizing Acute Chemical-Associated Foodborne Illness." *Military Medicine* (December 2006): 1174–80.

WEBSITES

"Case Definitions for Chemical Poisoning." Centers for Disease Control and Prevention. http://www.bt.cdc.gov/chemical/casedef.asp. (accessed August 31, 2012).

"Chemical Poisoning and Syrup of Ipecac." University of Maryland Medical Center. January 25, 2008. http://www.umm.edu/non_trauma/chempois.htm. (accessed September 1, 2012).

ORGANIZATIONS

Agency for Toxic Substances and Disease, 1825 Century Blvd., Atlanta, GA 30345, (800) 232-4636, http://www.atsdr.cdc.gov

American Academy of Environmental Medicine., 6505 E Central Ave., No. 296, Wichita, KS 67206, (316) 684-5500, http://www.aaemonline.org

American Association of Poison Control Centers., 3201 New Mexico Ave., Ste. 330, Washington, DC 20016, (800) 222-1222, http://www.aapcc.org

Environmental Protection Agency, Ariel Rios Bldg. 1200 Pennsylvania Ave. NW, Washington, DC 20460, (202) 260-7751, http://www.epa.gov.

Mai Tran
Teresa G. Odle
David Edward Newton, Ed.D.
Karl Finley

Child abuse

Definition

Child abuse, sometimes called child maltreatment, describes four types of actions toward children: physical abuse, sexual abuse, psychological abuse, and neglect. In many cases, the same child experiences more than one type of abuse. The abusers can be parents or other family members, caregivers such as teachers or babysitters, acquaintances (including other children), and (in very rare instances) strangers.

Demographics

Child abuse was once viewed as a minor social problem affecting only a handful of American children. However, in the late twentieth century, issues of child welfare came under scrutiny by the media, law enforcement, and the helping professions. This increase in public and professional awareness led to a sharp rise in the number of reported cases of child abuse. Today, child abuse is recognized as a problem that occurs among households of all racial, ethnic, and income levels, although the incidence of reported cases is higher in low-income households where adult caregivers experience greater financial **stress** and social difficulties, have less education and less understanding of child development, and may have less access to social services. In addition, children of parents who are substance abusers are more likely to experience abuse than children living in households where there is no substance abuse. Many child abusers were themselves abused as children.

Statistically, it is difficult to find reliable national figures for cases of child abuse because each state keeps its own records and has its own definitions of what constitutes abuse. Child abuse almost always occurs in private, and because it often is hidden from view, and its victims may be too young or too frightened to speak out, experts suggest that its true prevalence is probably greater than the official data indicate. However, based on information states reported to the United States **Department of Health and Human Services** Administration for Children and Families, during 2010 (the most recent data available) Child Protective Services (CPS) investigated 3.3 million reports of alleged maltreatment, in reference to approximately 5.9 million children. Of these, approximately 794,000 children were documented victims. More than 78% were victims of neglect, 17.6% of physical abuse, 9.2% of sexual abuse, 4.2% of psychological maltreatment, less than 1% of medical neglect, and approximately 754,000 were victims of multiple maltreatments. Victims were split almost evenly between girls and boys, but boys had a higher child fatality rate.

Of 891,218 duplicate perpetrators, 81.2% were parents of the victim, and another 6.1% were other relatives of the victim. One-fifth, or 18.5% of victims were abused by both parents. In addition, the National Child Abuse and Neglect Data System (NCANDS) reported that an estimated 1,760 children (2.35 children per 100,000) died from an injury where abuse or neglect was the cause or a contributing factor. Of these, more than 75% were under age 4, with the largest number of deaths occurring in infants under one year old.

Description

Physical abuse

Physical abuse is nonaccidental infliction of physical injury to a child. Legal definitions of physical child abuse vary from state to state, but injuries requiring medical attention typically are regarded as abusive. Physical abuse takes many forms, including cuts, bruises, **burns**, broken bones, **poisoning**, and internal injuries. Nonetheless, difficulties associated with defining the line between discipline and abuse are well known. Many states explicitly note that spanking "when administered in a reasonable manner" does not constitute abuse. Thus, how severely parents can inflict physical punishment upon their children without it being considered abusive remains subject to interpretation.

In confirmed cases of abuse in the most recent data from CPS, 45.2% of unique perpetrators were male and 53.6% were female. The injuries can be inflicted by punching, kicking, biting, burning, beating, or use of a weapon such as a baseball bat or knife. One rare form of physical abuse is Munchausen syndrome by proxy, in which a caregiver (most often the mother) seeks attention by intentionally making the child sick or appear to be sick.

Sexual abuse

Children are sexually abused when they experience contact that is for the sexual gratification of an adult or a

Child abuse signs and symptoms

Although these signs do not necessarily indicate that a child has been abused, they may help adults recognize that something is wrong. The possibility of abuse should be investigated if a child shows a number of these symptoms, or any of them to a marked degree:

Sexual abuse

Being overly affectionate or knowledgeable in a sexual way inappropriate to the child's age
Medical problems such as chronic itching, pain in the genitals, or venereal diseases
Other extreme reactions, such as depression, self-mutilation, suicide attempts, running away, overdoses, or anorexia
Personality changes, such as becoming insecure or clingy
Regressing to younger behavior patterns such as thumb sucking or bringing out discarded cuddly toys
Sudden loss of appetite or engaging in compulsive eating
Being isolated or becoming withdrawn
Inability to concentrate
Lack of trust or fear toward someone they know well, such as not wanting to be alone with a babysitter or specific family member
Starting to wet the bed again or having nightmares
Anxiety about clothing being removed
Suddenly starting to draw sexually explicit pictures
Trying to be "ultra-good" or perfect; overreacting to criticism

Physical abuse

Unexplained recurrent injuries or burns
Improbable excuses or refusal to explain injuries
Wearing clothes to cover injuries, even in hot weather
Refusal to undress for gym
Bald patches
Chronic running away
Fear of medical help or examination
Self-destructive tendencies
Aggression toward others
Fear of physical contact; shrinking back if touched
Admitting that they are punished, but the punishment is excessive (such as a child being beaten every night to make him/her study)
Fear of suspected abuser being contacted

Psychological abuse

Physical, mental, and psychological developmental lags
Sudden speech disorders
Continual self-depreciation (e.g., "I'm stupid, ugly, worthless," etc.)
Overreaction to mistakes
Extreme fear of any new situation
Inappropriate response to pain (e.g., "I deserve this")
Neurotic behavior (e.g., rocking, hair twisting, self-mutilation)
Extremes of passivity or aggression

Neglect

Constant hunger
Poor personal hygiene
No social relationships
Constant tiredness
Poor state of clothing
Compulsive scavenging
Emaciation
Untreated medical problems
Destructive tendencies

A child may be subjected to a combination of different kinds of abuse. It is also possible that a child may show no outward signs and hide what is happening from everyone.

(Table by PreMediaGlobal. © 2013 Cengage Learning)

significantly older or dominant child when they are younger than the legal age of consent or at a stage of development at which they do not possess sufficient maturity to understand the nature of the acts and therefore to provide informed consent. Abusers may use coercion or deceptive manipulation, but often physical force is not necessary, since the perpetrator is likely to be someone with whom the child has a trusting relationship and who is in a position of authority over the child. In many states, sexual activity is automatically assumed to be abuse when a defined age difference exists between the older abuser and the younger (minor) victim, independent of any consent the victim may have given.

Sexual behaviors can include touching breasts, genitals, and buttocks while the victim is either dressed or undressed. Sexual-abuse behavior also includes cunnilingus, fellatio, or penetration of the vagina or anus with sexual organs or objects. Sexual abuse does not have to involve any actual touching. Children can be coerced into disrobing and exposing themselves or watching adults disrobe or engage in sexual activity. Pornographic photography or videography containing children also are forms of sexual abuse of children.

The U.S. Department of Justice estimates that one in six victims of a **sexual assault** is under age 12. Sexual abuse victims can be either boys or girls. Most, but not all, perpetrators are male. Despite publicity surrounding cases where a child is sexually assaulted by a stranger, almost all sexual abuse against children is perpetrated by a family member (e.g., father, stepfather, uncle, aunt, sibling, cousin) or family intimate (e.g., live-in lover or friend of the parent). Perpetrators go to great lengths to conceal sexual abuse. Children who have been sexually abused might not report the behavior due to threats, shame, or a lack of understanding of what has happened.

Rape is the most violent form of sexual abuse. It is the perpetration of an act of sexual intercourse when:

- will is overcome by force or fear (from threats, use of weapons, or use of drugs).
- mental impairment renders the victim incapable of rational judgment.
- the victim is below the legal age established for consent.

According the U.S. Department of Justice, 54% of all rapes are of women under age 18.

Psychological abuse

Abuse of children is not limited to the physical body. Psychological abuse encompasses rejecting, ignoring, criticizing, belittling, humiliating, threatening the child with **violence**, or otherwise terrorizing the child, all of which have the effect of eroding the child's self-esteem and sense of security. It also can include isolating the child from friends or other family members or destroying the child's property.

Psychological abuse may be the result of actions not directed specifically at the child. The prevalence of domestic violence exposes children to intimidating and frightening scenes every day. Many children live in homes where domestic violence is an ongoing problem that they witness regularly, often as a result of being "caught in the middle" of a parental altercation. Children who observe violence react with many of the same psychological symptoms as children who have experienced it directly. Psychological abuse often accompanies other types of abuse. It is difficult to prove and is rarely reported.

Neglect

Neglect is the failure to satisfy a child's basic needs. About 60% of cases of maltreatment documented by CPS involve neglect. Neglect can assume many forms. Physical neglect is the failure (beyond the constraints imposed by **poverty**) to provide adequate food, clothing, shelter, or supervision. Children may live in filthy conditions or situations where food is not provided, or where they develop infections or other medical conditions that go untreated. Failure to send children to school or otherwise provide for their education may also be considered neglect. Psychological neglect is the failure to satisfy a child's normal psychological needs and/or behavior that damages a child's normal psychological development (e.g., permitting drug abuse in the home, having the child witness domestic violence).

Risk factors

The greatest risk factor for abuse is being young. According to the most recent data from the Department of Health and Human Services, 34% of victims of maltreatment were under age four, while another 23.4% were between ages four and seven. The death rate from abuse is skewed even more heavily toward the young, with 79.4% of fatalities resulting from abuse or neglect occuring in children younger than four years old.

Children who are handicapped and those who are nonrhythmic (that is, with unpredictable eating and sleeping patterns) are more likely to be abused. Similarly, children who are distractible or impulsive, or who have high activity levels are more likely to experience physical abuse.

Causes and symptoms

Sociocultural factors contributing to abuse

Poverty is the sociocultural factor most strongly linked to abuse. Although physical abuse occurs at all income levels, it happens more often in very poor families. It is true that in middle-class families, child injuries are treated by a sympathetic personal physician who may be less likely to diagnose and report abuse-related injuries than the physician in the emergency room who is more likely to treat poor families. Even with such reporting bias, however, poverty seems strongly linked to abuse. It seems that the frustrating effects of poverty on parents are instrumental in creating situations for parents' abuse.

Physical crowding, more likely to occur in poverty, is also associated with abuse. If too many people share a small living space, severe punishment of children as a means of maintaining control is more likely.

Job loss and dissatisfaction are often associated with child abuse. Higher rates of abuse exist in military, as compared to non-military, families. It is generally felt that the link between these environmental stressors and abuse is strengthened by the absence of social support networks that might otherwise buffer the family against adversity. Having no one to assist with child care and no one to question the use of severe discipline increases the chance that a parent may injure a child.

Pedophiles exist in all economic and cultural groups. Psychologically, however, they share certain traits. Pedophiles often have a history of being abused themselves, and abusing other children seems to be triggered by increased life stressors, such as marital problems, job layoffs, or abuse of drugs.

Caregiver factors

Parents who were themselves abused as children are more likely to abuse their own children. However, not every parent who was abused becomes an abuser; some parents go to great lengths to insure that they never harm their children.

Parents who abuse their children are likely to be younger than the average parent. They also are more likely to be single parents. Having mental illness, such as depression, or abusing drugs or alcohol also makes a parent more likely to abuse a child.

Abusive parents socialize differently from nonabusive parents. Nonabusive parents tend to use ignoring or time-out procedures, whereas abusive parents tend to shout, threaten, and spank. Some forms of child abuse escalate over time, with the parent spanking harder and more frequently to get the same effect, or resorting to abuse to get results. Female caregivers inflict more soft-tissue injuries, broken bones, and internal injuries than male caregivers. Severe injuries from a single, explosive incident in which the child is shaken, thrown, or struck are more likely to involve male caregivers.

Abusive parents often expect the child to perform behaviors he or she is not yet capable of performing. Parents who abuse their young children expect them to be able to control their impulses, recall and obey complex parental rules, and perform mature chains of behavior such as getting up, washing, and getting dressed by themselves. Nonabusive parents recognize that toddlers and preschool children are incapable of such behaviors. Understanding the limitations of a young child's memory, ability to be controlled by words, impulse control, and attention span is essential to developing reasonable expectations for the child. Parents who expect behavior the child cannot deliver are apt to increase their control techniques progressively in order to get the child to comply.

Abusive discipline is often the result of the belief that the young child is capable of better behavior and that he or she is deliberately misbehaving to cause the parent difficulty. Such parents often claim that their 18-month-old could stay clean if she wanted to but that she dirties her pants just to make more work for the mother. Abusive parents who believe that a child has chosen to misbehave inflict more punishment on their children than parents who accurately recognize when a child's behavior is not intentional.

Such abusive parents also often believe that effective parenting involves maintaining tight control over the child. A mother who can toilet train her child early and keep the child in line at the grocery store is viewed by abusive parents as a "good" mother. Closely tied to beliefs about the importance of control are aphorisms such as "spare the rod, spoil the child" and "respect comes through fear," which indicate that children learn best through the application of force.

Another belief that abusive parents often hold is that their children should engage in reciprocal parenting. They believe that if they sometimes comfort, wait on, and take care of the child, the child should do the same for them. Such beliefs fit with abusive parents' lack of awareness of children's developmental capabilities and may also stem from the parents' own immaturity and lack of support from other adults. Regardless of the source, when the child does not meet such expectations, the parent often responds with anger and hostility.

Emotion

Anger is the most frequent trigger for parental abuse. Abusive parents appear to have a lower threshold for childish behaviors than do average parents. Abusive parents are more upset by the same child cues than are nonabusive parents. Thus, child behaviors that are merely irritating to average parents are infuriating to abusive parents. Finally, abusive parents may have less control over their anger than may nonabusive parents, either because they are unaware of their level of anger, because they are chronically angry, or because they lack anger-management skills.

When considering how emotion influences child abuse, it seems important to consider positive emotions as well. Abusive parents experience their children as less rewarding than do nonabusive parents. In observation, abusive parents touch their children less, cuddle them less, less frequently call them affectionate names ("honey," "sweetheart"), and smile less at them. Nonabusive parents respond flexibly to their children, letting the child lead the play interaction. Even in play, abusive parents have expectations that their children seem unable or unwilling to fulfill, making play a disagreeable chore rather than a rewarding endeavor. Abusive parents seem trapped by their own lack of skills, limited developmental understanding, inappropriate expectations, high negative emotion, and low enjoyment of their children.

Symptoms

Although these signs do not necessarily indicate that a child has been abused, they may help adults recognize that something is wrong. The possibility of abuse should be investigated if a child shows a number of these symptoms, or any of them to a marked degree:

Sexual Abuse

- Being overly affectionate or knowledgeable in a sexual way inappropriate to the child's age
- Medical problems such as chronic itching, pain in the genitals, venereal diseases
- Other extreme reactions, such as depression, self-mutilation, suicide attempts, running away, overdoses, anorexia
- Personality changes such as becoming insecure or clingy
- Regressing to younger behavioral patterns such as thumb sucking or bringing out discarded cuddly toys
- Sudden loss of appetite or compulsive eating
- Being isolated or becoming withdrawn
- Inability to concentrate
- Lack of trust or fear of someone they know well, such as not wanting to be alone with a babysitter or specific family member
- Starting to wet the bed again, day or night/nightmares
- Becoming worried about clothing being removed
- Suddenly starting to draw sexually explicit pictures
- Trying to be "ultra-good" or perfect; over-reacting to criticism

Physical Abuse

- Unexplained recurrent injuries or burns
- Improbable excuses or refusal to explain injuries
- Wearing clothes to cover injuries, even in hot weather
- Refusal to undress for gym
- Bald patches
- Chronic running away
- Fear of medical help or examination
- Self-destructive tendencies
- Aggression toward others
- Fear of physical contact; shrinking back if touched
- Admitting that they are punished, but the punishment is excessive (such as a child being beaten every night to make him or her study)
- Fear of suspected abuser being contacted

Psychological Abuse

- Physical, mental, and psychological developmental lags
- Sudden speech disorders
- Continual self-depreciation (e.g., "I'm stupid, ugly, worthless")
- Overreaction to mistakes
- Extreme fear of any new situation
- Inappropriate response to pain (e.g., "I deserve this")
- Neurotic behavior (e.g., rocking, hair twisting, self-mutilation)
- Extremes of passivity or aggression

Neglect

- Constant hunger
- Poor personal hygiene
- No social relationships
- Constant tiredness
- Poor state of clothing
- Compulsive scavenging
- Emaciation
- Untreated medical problems
- Destructive tendencies

A child may be subjected to a combination of different kinds of abuse. It is also possible that a child will show no outward signs and hide what is happening from everyone.

Diagnosis

Doctors and many other professionals who work with children are required by law to report suspected abuse to their state's CPS agency. Abuse investigations often are a group effort involving medical personnel, social workers, police officers, and others. Some hospitals and communities maintain child protection teams that respond to cases of possible abuse. Careful questioning of the parents is crucial, as is interviewing the child (if he or she is capable of being interviewed). Trained investigators must ensure, however, that their questioning does not further traumatize the child and also that their style of questioning does not prompt the child to give the answers the child thinks the questioner wants rather than accurate answers. A physical examination for signs of physical or sexual abuse or of neglect is necessary and may include x rays, blood tests, and other procedures.

KEY TERM

Pedophile—A person who sexually abuses children.

Treatment

Notification of the appropriate authorities, treatment of the child's injuries, and protecting the child from further harm are the immediate priorities in abuse cases. If the child does not require hospital treatment, protection often involves placing him or her with relatives, in a group home, or in foster care. Once the immediate concerns are addressed, it becomes essential to determine how the child's long-term medical, psychological, educational, and other needs can best be met. This process involves evaluating not only the child's needs but also those of the family (e.g., drug abuse counseling, parental skills training, anger-management training). The authorities also must determine whether other children living in the same household also have been abused. On investigation, signs of physical abuse are discovered in about 20% of other children living in the abused child's household.

Prognosis

Child abuse often has lifelong consequences. Research shows that abused children and adolescents are more likely to do poorly in school and experience depression, extreme anger, antisocial personality traits, and other psychiatric problems. They also are more likely to become promiscuous, abuse drugs and alcohol, run away, and attempt **suicide**. As adults, they often have trouble establishing intimate relationships.

Most children who have been abused experience some symptoms of **post-traumatic stress disorder** (PTSD). PTSD in children and adolescents may be acute or delayed, that is, the child may experience symptoms immediately or after a period of time has passed, perhaps when the child feels safe. Symptoms may include re-experiencing the abusive episodes at some level, feeling emotionally numb, or becoming physiologically aroused (e.g., elevated heart rate and respiration). Children may experience disassociation and appear to "space out" when reminded of the abuse or perpetrator. They may have physical symptoms. They may become enraged or feel guilt at having provoked the episodes or survived them. They may have invasive memories, repeated behaviors, or fears related to the abusive situations. They may act out some of their issues in play—punishing the bad guy or victimizing another character while playing with dolls or action figures. In severe cases of chronic trauma, the child may develop serious or prolonged disassociation or depression. Severe and chronic abuse has also been implicated in cases of multiple personality disorder.

Once the abuse has stopped, some of these symptoms can be treated with some form of counseling or therapy. Some have argued that full recovery is a lifelong task. Adults who have been abused as children may have to face issues long after the abuse has stopped, when they enter into their own sexual relationships or when they raise their own children. Long-term therapy by a professional trained in working with abused children and adults offers the best chance of overcoming childhood abuse.

Prevention

There are many barriers to changing abusive parental behavior. Most parents' own history suggests that strong physical discipline is the preferred model of parenting. Further, most abusive parents live in families and neighborhoods in which violence is not only condoned but also viewed as a necessary vehicle for interpersonal influence. The stresses that are omnipresent in abusive parents' lives assist in maintaining high levels of anger and depression, which block the positive enjoyment of the child. When the parent responds with strong physical discipline, the child's misbehavior typically stops, for that moment at any rate. Thus, the parent is intermittently rewarded for responding abusively. Thus, changing abusive parenting is a challenging task.

It may be preferable to prevent the development of abusive parenting by early interventions to give skills, alter developmental knowledge, change unreasonable parenting expectations, and block the steady build-up of anger and extinguishing of affection for the child. **Prevention** programs now target teenagers before pregnancy as well as young mothers to try to break the cycle of abuse.

Government efforts to prevent abuse include home-visitor programs aimed at high-risk families, and school based efforts to teach children how to respond to attempted sexual abuse. Psychological abuse prevention has been promoted through the media.

When children reach age three, parents should begin teaching them about "bad touches" and about confiding in a suitable adult if they are touched or treated in a way that makes them uneasy. Parents also need to exercise caution in hiring babysitters and other caregivers. Anyone who suspects abuse should report those suspicions to the police or his or her local CPS agency. Prevent Child Abuse America (listed in references) is an excellent source of information about the many support groups and other organizations that help abused and at-risk children and their families. One of these organizations, Parents Anonymous, sponsors local self-help groups throughout the United States, Canada, and Europe.

Resources

AMERICAN HELP HOTLINES

Childhelp National Child Abuse Hotline 1-800-4-A-CHILD. TDD for the Deaf 1-800-2-A-Child. Help for children who are being abused or adults who are concerned that a child they know is being abused or neglected.

Rape, Abuse and Incest National Network (RAINN) Online hotline http://www.rainn.org/get-help/national-sexual-assault-online-hotline or telephone: 1-800-656-HOPE. Online counseling and referral to local rape crisis centers using anonymous instant messaging or telephone counseling and referrals to local crisis center.

BOOKS

U.S. Department of Health and Human Services, Administration for Children and Families, Administration on Children, Youth and Families, Children's Bureau. (2011). *Child Maltreatment 2010.*

OTHER

"Child Abuse." *MedlinePlus, National Institutes of Health.* http://www.nlm.nih.gov/medlineplus/childabuse.html Accessed November 11, 2012.

"Child Welfare Information Gateway." *United States Department of Health and Human Services.* http://www.childwelfare.gov Accessed November 11, 2012.

ORGANIZATIONS

Parents Anonymous, 675 W. Foothill Blvd., Suite 220, Claremont, CA 91711-3475, (909) 621-6184, Fax: (909) 625-6304, http://www.parentsanonymous.org

Prevent Child Abuse America, 500 North Michigan Avenue, Suite 200, Chicago, IL 60611-3703, (312) 663-3520, 1-800-CHILDREN, Fax: (312) 939-8962, mailbox@preventchildabuse.org, http://www.preventchildabuse.org/index.shtml.

Tish Davidson, A.M.
Andrea Nienstedt, MA

Child care *see* **Children's health**

Child labor laws

Definition

Child labor refers to the use of minors (persons under 18 years of age) for any type of commercial work. Child labor laws regulate the use of child labor and the parameters under which it can be utilized. Some states also regulate child labor in relation to nonprofit organizations.

Description

In the United States, in 1832, more than 40% of mill workers were boys under the age of 12. Over the course of American history, child labor has been used in many industries including: textiles, domestic service, tobacco farming, glass making, and coal mining. Child laborers were often overworked and underpaid, if they were paid at all. Child laborers were also frequently susceptible to physical abuse and corporal punishment. During the early years of the United States, the government did not keep records of child workers, but conditions for child laborers in the United States were believed to be much more favorable than those of child laborers in Great Britain.

Like many civil rights movements in American history, there was a movement toward rights for child workers before there was corresponding legislation, and even when there was legislation, there was not necessarily enforcement. As the abuse of child labor became a more transparent issue in the mid–to late nineteenth century, states began making some legislative efforts to protect children. There were laws passed regarding child labor as early as 1813. These efforts included dictating minimum levels of education and minimum employment ages. These laws were often not enforced and as late as the early twentieth century, there were many child laborers working full-time jobs in factories. Some important figures in the early American movement for the rights of child workers include John Peter Altgeld, who was the governor of Illinois. Altgeld appointed Florence Kelley to help regulate and monitor issues and legislation related to child labor. Kelley went on to become the director of the National Consumers League in New York where she continued her efforts on behalf of working children. Kelley worked with other advocates for child laborers including Jane Addams and Lewis Hine who were connected with the National Child Labor Committee. Hine was known for documenting the plight of working children through candid photographs. Hine's photographs showed the dire situation of child workers.

In 1919, Congress passed the Child Labor Tax Law (40 Stat. 1057) which put an excise tax on employers that employed children younger than 14 years of age, or those between 14 and 16 years of age who worked more than eight hours per day or more than six days per week. In 1922, however, the U.S. Supreme Court declared the law unconstitutional with the *Baily v. Xrexel Furniture Co.* ruling.

In addition to the federal law regulating child labor, individual states often have their own regulations. In some states, each child under a certain age that is to be employed must have a corresponding employment certificate filled out by the employer. These certificates often outline the parameters of the children's working conditions, and their specific duties. Improper completion of this certificate or lack of a certificate can render the employment illegal.

Though child labor laws have greatly helped regulate child labor in the United States, abuse of child labor remains a large problem globally and is at the forefront of many **human rights** battles.

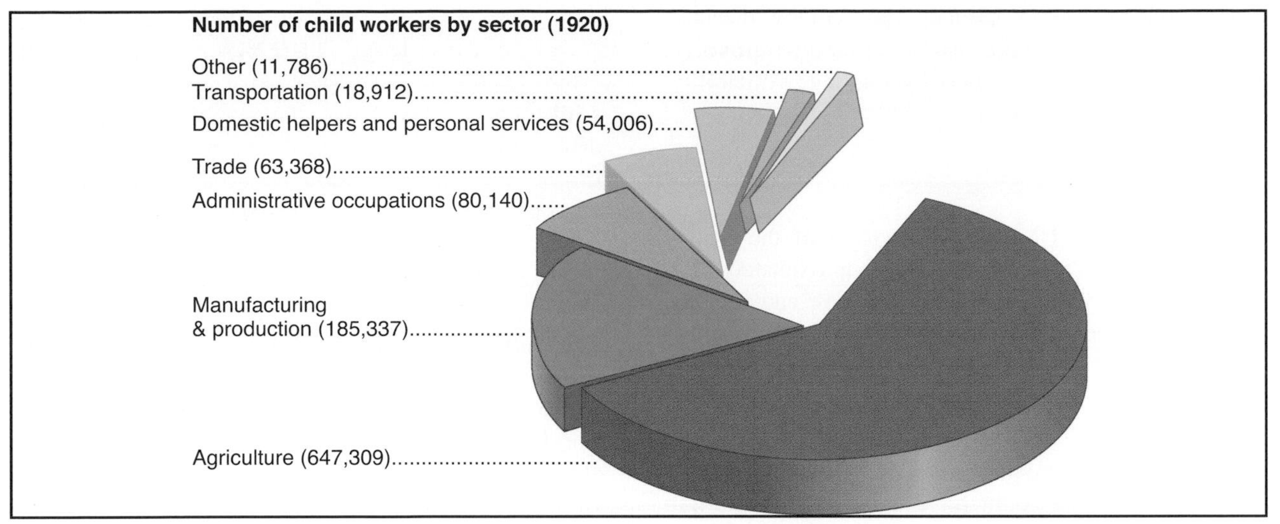

Number of child workers in the United States in 1920, before laws were inacted to regulate. *(Illustration by Electronic Illustrators Group. © 2013 Cengage Learning)*

Exploitative child labor makes children much more susceptible to chronic health problems, often prevents their ability to complete their education, and often limits their future economic opportunities. Child labor problems affect many facets of a child's development and also severely limit the opportunities for girls and women.

Even in developed countries where child labor practices are fairly well-regulated, the employment of minors still poses risks. Minors are often not able to solve problems, assess situations, or assert themselves in the same way as adults. As a result, young workers can be taken advantage of, sexually harassed, or otherwise manipulated more easily than many adult workers. A reasonable job in a healthy environment can, however, help a young person gain valuable life skills and a sense of independence, both of which can contribute to the individual's success as an adult. It is important for parents to carefully assess the safety of their children's potential job environment and help them to understand their rights in the workplace.

Origins

Children and young people have been a part of the workforce for at least hundreds of years, if not longer. Traditionally, children helped their families by working in farming or around the house. With the advent of the Industrial Revolution in Great Britain, and eventually Europe and the United States, the nature of child labor changed drastically. Children went from working with their families in agrarian situations to working outside the home under the often lax care of strangers.

As children began to work in industrial settings, they were often outside the care of family members working in factories, mills, and mines. During the Industrial Revolution in Great Britain, children represented approximately one half of the workforce in textile mills alone. The conditions of these facilities were usually unhealthy and dangerous; however, children were able to help support their families by being viable wage earners. Children's small size and agility made them especially useful for certain tasks that were more difficult for adults to perform, but children were easier to manipulate in terms of wages, hours, and working conditions.

The first movement to limit child labor came in Great Britain, but not without much controversy. Members of Parliament who were interested in protecting child workers compiled reports called Blue Books or the Sadler Reports which documented the treatment of child workers and their environments through interviews with child workers, their parents, overseers, factory owners, and physicians. The results of these reports painted a grim picture including serious verbal and physical abuse, sometimes ending in permanent injury or maiming. In 1802, Great Britain passed the first child labor law, the First Factory Act, which limited children to 12 hour work days. The act also improved conditions at cotton mills, though not in textile mills due to difficulties with enforcement. A series of child labor laws followed over the next decades, including the Regulation of Child Labor Law in 1833, which lowered the work day to nine hours for children, forbade night work, and allowed inspections. The law also included fines for employers found to be in violation of the law.

Scholars continue to debate the reasons for the historically widespread use of child labor in Great Britain and the United States. Some of the potential causes posited are: demand, particularly because children could be paid less than adults; **poverty**; **population** expansion; poor schooling availability; and technological changes.

Demographics

According to UNICEF (a division of the United Nations), in developing nations, approximately 150 million children between the ages of five and fourteen are presently involved in child labor. This number represents about 16% of all children in this age group.

Statistics regarding gender and child labor can be deceiving because many of the types of work that young girls are put into are invisible, or not easily tracked. Women and girls account for roughly 80% of **human trafficking**, much of which is for sexual exploitation.

UNICEF estimates that 90% of children involved in domestic labor are girls.

Costs to Society

Modern child labor—especially in the international arena—is a complex issue and its effects are widespread. Child labor affects the children and their families most immediately, but it also has significant effects on the child's community, society, and local and international economies. The complexity of global child labor has made solutions difficult to implement, though a variety of international organizations fight continuously for the rights of child laborers.

Patterns of child labor contribute to transgenerational cycles of poverty. Child labor in many areas also helps to enforce discrimination—children of lower social classes or indigenous groups are more likely to be forced or compelled into labor, thereby being more likely to drop out of school, and limiting their chances for economic stability or social mobility. Migrant children are especially vulnerable to the effects of child labor.

Efforts and Solutions

As of 2012, the federal law that regulates child labor in the United States is the Fair Labor Standards Act of 1938 (FLSA). This law—part of the New Deal legislation program introduced by President Roosevelt—is enforced by the United States Labor Department Wage and Hour Division. FLSA regulates parameters for all workers in the United States, and includes specific requirements for child workers. FLSA includes provisions for restrictions on age of child workers, working hours, minimum wage, occupational restrictions, and industry restrictions. Additionally, each state has its own child labor laws which may further restrict the parameters under which children are able to work.

In 1999, President Clinton signed Executive Order 13,126, or the "Prohibition of Acquisition of Products Produced by Forced or Indentured Child Labor." This action was aimed against sweatshops—particularly those in foreign countries, whose goods were imported for sale and use in the United States.

Half the Sky Movement is an organization that started in the 2010s with a book published by Pulitzer Prize-winning journalists, Nicholas Kristof and Sheryl WuDunn. The movement looks to end oppression of women and girls around the globe through education, advocacy, and local charitable organizations. Half the Sky works against multiple forms of oppression, including the exploitation of children through sex trafficking. Half the Sky also works to create entrepreneurial opportunities for women in developing countries. These types of opportunities can diversify local economies and workforces, minimizing or eliminating the need for exploitative child labor.

The regulation of children's work on family farms has been an issue of debate between voters and lawmakers since at least the 1920s. In May of 2012, this debate flared up again when the U.S. Department of Labor attempted to restrict children under the age of 12 from certain types of work (including working with

KEY TERMS

Child Labor Tax Law—Passed by Congress in 1919, this law put an excise tax on companies that employed children younger than 14 years of age, or those between 14 and 16 years of age who worked more than eight hours per day or more than six days per week. The Supreme Court declared this law unconstitutional in 1922.

Fair Labor Standards Act (FLSA)—Passed in 1938 as part of President Roosevelt's New Deal, FLSA provided regulations for employers to improve conditions of workers. The FLSA included certain statutes that applied specifically to the employment of minors. FLSA continues to be the primary federal law governing child labor in the United States.

Sweatshop—According to the United States Department of Labor, a workplace is considered a sweatshop if it violates two or more basic labor laws, including (but not limited to): child labor, fire safety, minimum wage, or overtime pay.

types of heavy machinery) and exposure to chemicals often involved in farming (such as pesticides). Like many global child labor issues, this proposition is complicated. On one hand, the Labor Department sought to protect children, who often miss school, to engage in yearly harvesting. These activities can often be grueling manual labor, and every year, children are injured or killed in these types of work during the harvest season. On the other hand, as opponents argued, the government is interfering in the way parents raise their children and operate their own private family farms. Due to the public opposition to the proposed restrictions, President Obama's administration and the Labor Department retracted the potential changes, leaving the regulations for child labor in agriculture much more lax than other industries.

Resources

BOOKS

"Child Labor." *Historical Encyclopedia of American Business.* Ed. Richard L. Wilson. Vol. 1. Pasadena, CA: Salem Press, 2009.

"Child Labor and Child Labor Laws in Early Industrial Great Britain." *World History Encyclopedia.* Ed. Alfred J. Andrea and Carolyn Neel. Vol. 15: Era 7: The Age of Revolutions, 1750–1914. Santa Barbara, CA: ABC–CLIO, 2011.

"Child Labor Laws." *Gale Encyclopedia of American Law.* Ed. Donna Batten. 3rd ed. Vol. 2. Detroit: Gale, 2010.

Pantea, Maria-Carmen. "Child Labor." *Encyclopedia of Women in Today's World.*Ed. Mary Zeiss Stange, Carol K. Oyster, and Jane E. Sloan. Vol. 1. Thousand Oaks, CA: Sage Reference, 2011.

PERIODICALS

Coursen-Neff, Zama. "Labor Department abandons child farmworkers." *Human Rights Watch.* www.hrw.org. Accessed September 23, 2012.

Wood, Marjorie Elizabeth. "Pitting Child Safety Against the Family Farm." *The New York Times.* www.nytimes.com. Accessed September 23, 2012.

WEBSITES

Half the Sky Movementhttp://www.halftheskymovement.org/ Accessed September 23, 2012.

UNICEF. "Child protection from violence, exploitation and abuse."http://www.unicef.org/protection/57929_57977.html Accessed September 23, 2012.

ORGANIZATIONS

United States Department of Labor, Frances Perkins Building, 200 Constitution Avenue, N.W., Washington, DC USA 20210, (866) 487-9243, www.dol.gov.

Andrea Nienstedt, MA

Child safety seats *see* **Car seats**

Risks associated with childhood obesity

- ✓ Cardiovascular disease
- ✓ Degenerative joint disease
- ✓ Depression
- ✓ Early puberty and early start of menstruation in girls
- ✓ Eating disorders
- ✓ Exposure to social prejudice and discrimination
- ✓ Fat accumulation in the liver (fatty liver/liver disease)
- ✓ Gallbladder disease
- ✓ High cholesterol
- ✓ Hypertension
- ✓ Increased anxiety and stress
- ✓ Joint pain
- ✓ Low self-esteem
- ✓ Sleep apnea
- ✓ Type 2 diabetes mellitus

(Table by PreMediaGlobal. © 2013 Cengage Learning)

Childhood obesity

Definition

Childhood **obesity** is the condition of being severely overweight between the ages of two and 19 years. The U.S. **Centers for Disease Control and Prevention** defines overweight as "having an excess body weight for a particular height." The excess weight can come from bone, fat, muscle, **water**, or a combination of all four. Obesity is defined as "having excess body fat."

Demographics

There is no doubt that American children are getting heavier. In 2008, the **CDC** estimated that one-third of American children and adolescents were overweight or obese. Other surveys have found the total obesity rate among American children and adolescents to be between 21% and 24%. Although the problem of excessive weight is growing fastest in the United States, the trend toward heavier children is occurring in most developed countries.

In the United States, the National Center for Health Statistics has tracked children's weight for several decades and recorded the following changes in the percent of children who are obese:

- Children ages 2–5: 1976 5.0%, 2008 10.4%
- Children ages 6–11: 1976 6.5%, 2008 19.6%
- Children ages 12–19: 1976 5.0%, 2008 18.1%

The number of children who are overweight or obese differs significantly among different races and ethnic groups. Significantly more Hispanic-American boys are obese than non-Hispanic black or white boys. Significantly more Hispanic American girls and non-Hispanic black girls are obese than white girls. Native American and Native Hawaiian children also have higher rates of obesity than whites.

Description

Childhood obesity is of increasing concern as a public health problem in the United States. Most healthcare professionals calculate obesity using the body mass index (BMI). BMI is a calculation that compares a person's weight and height to arrive at a specific number.

BMI for children is calculated the same way it is for adults, but, unlike for adults, age and gender are taken into consideration. The BMIs of children between the ages of 2 and 19 are compared against growth charts based on age and gender, referred to as BMI-for-age percentiles. A child's percentile indicates how his or her weight compares to other children who are the same age and gender. For example, if a boy is in the 65th percentile for his age group, 65 of every 100 children who are his age weigh less than he does and 35 of every 100 weigh more than he does.

The BMI weight categories for children are:

- below the 5th percentile: underweight
- 5th to less than the 85th percentile: healthy weight
- 85th to less than the 95th percentile: overweight
- 95th percentile and above: obese

In the early 2000s, many health organizations avoided applying the term "obese" to children. Children between the 85th and 95th percentile were classified as "at risk for overweight" and children above the 95th percentile were called "overweight." No child was labeled obese, in part because of the social stigma the word carries.

Children who are classified in the top 15th percentile are at risk of developing weight-related health problems. However, one criticism of BMI is that it does not take into consideration factors like muscle mass. Certain adolescent athletes, such as wrestlers or weightlifters, may be categorized as overweight or obese when using BMI calculations, even if they are fit and in good health.

Causes and symptoms

At its simplest, obesity is caused by taking in more calories than the body uses. This difference is called the "energy gap." A 2006 study done by the Harvard School of Public Health and published in the journal *Pediatrics* found that, on average, American children consumed between 110 and 165 more calories every day than they used. Over a 10-year period, these extra calories add 10 lb. to their weight. However, already overweight teens took in an average of 700–1,000 extra calories every day, resulting in an average of 58 extra pounds.

Causes

There are many reasons why the energy gap exists. These reasons are related to both increased food intake and decreased energy use. Food intake reasons include:

- increased consumption of sugary beverages, and along with this, a decreased consumption of milk
- tendency to supersize portions. In some fast food restaurants portions have almost tripled since the 1970s
- more meals eaten away from home
- more use of prepared foods in the home
- increased snacking between meals along with fewer meals eaten together as a family
- heavy advertising of high-sugar, high-fat foods to children
- decrease in children carrying their lunch to school from home
- poor eating habits such as skipping breakfast and later snacking on high-fat, sugary foods

Inadequate energy use reasons include:

- more time spent watching television, playing video games, or using the computer than playing outside
- fewer physical education requirements at school—many schools do not require or provide a regularly scheduled recess
- fewer children walking to school—in 1969, half of all schoolchildren walked or biked to school, but by 2003 (the date of the most recent CDC study), the rate had dropped to 15%
- fear of crime, which limits outdoor activities of children and walking to school
- more affluence—teen access to cars has increased over the past 30 years

According to a 2012 study published in the *Journal of Teaching in Physical Education*, only six states required at least 150 minutes of **physical activity** in elementary schools and only two states required 225 minutes in middle schools, the amounts recommended by the National Association of Sport and Physical Education. No states met the guidelines for high schools, which were also 225 minutes of activity per week. The U.S. Centers for Disease Control and **Prevention** recommends that children 6–17 participate in at least one hour of physical activity each day.

Other factors that affect childhood obesity include an inherited tendency toward weight gain; mental illness; binge eating disorder; eating in response to **stress**, boredom or loneliness; poor sleeping habits; and having at least one obese parent.

In rare cases, medical or genetic disorders can cause obesity. For example, Prader-Willi syndrome is a genetic disorder that causes an uncontrollable urge to eat. The only way to prevent a person with Prader-Willi disorder from constant eating is to keep them in an environment where they have no free access to food. Other genetic and hormonal disorders (e.g., hypothyroidism) can cause obesity. Certain medications also can cause weight gain (e.g., cortisone, tri-cyclic antidepressants), but these situations are the exception. Researchers estimate that fewer than 10% of cases of childhood obesity are associated with hormonal or genetic causes. Most children are too heavy because they eat too much and/or exercise too little.

Symptoms

The most obvious symptom of obesity is an accumulation of body fat. Other symptoms involve changes in body chemistry. Some of these changes cause disease in children, while others put the child at risk for developing health problems later in life. Children who are obese are at increased risk of:

- type 2 diabetes; this disease is appearing in adolescents and young adults at an alarmingly high rate, whereas in the past, it was usually seen in older adults.
- high blood pressure (hypertension)
- fat accumulation in the liver (fatty liver/liver disease)
- sleep apnea
- early puberty; early start of menstruation in girls
- eating disorders
- joint pain
- depression
- increased anxiety and stress
- low self-worth
- exposure to social prejudice and discrimination

Diagnosis

Diagnosis of obesity is usually made based on the child's BMI. To better assess the problem, the physician will take a family history and a medical history and do a complete physical examination, including standard blood and urine tests. A thyroid hormone test may be done to rule out hypothyroidism as the cause of obesity. Based on the physician's findings, other tests may be performed to rule out medical causes of obesity.

Treatment

Obese children and their parents may be referred to a registered dietitian or nutritionist who can help them develop a plan to replace high-fat/energy foods with nutrient-rich, low-calorie foods. **Nutrition** education usually involves the entire family. Children may be asked to keep a food diary to record everything that they eat in order to determine what changes in behavior and diet need to be made. Typically, children are encouraged to increase their level of physical activity rather than to drastically reduce calorie intake.

Drug therapy and weight-loss surgery are very rarely used in children, except in the most extreme cases of health-threatening obesity when other methods of weight control have failed. Some teenagers may benefit from joining a structured weight-loss program such as Weight Watchers or Jenny Craig. They should check with their physician before joining.

Nutrition and dietary concerns

Teaching children how to eat a healthy diet sets a framework for their lifetime eating habits. A nutritionist or dietitian can help families to understand how much and what kinds of food are appropriate for their child's age, weight, and activity level.

The American Heart Association has adapted the following dietary suggestions for children over the age of two. Separate guidelines exist for infant nutrition.

- For children over the age of three, limit fat intake to 25%–30% of total calories. Fat sources should be low in saturated and *trans* fats.
- Consume a variety of colorful fruits and vegetables daily, but limit fruit juice due to its sugar content.
- Select high-fiber, whole-grain cereals and breads.
- Limit sugary drinks and foods, such as carbonated soft drinks, candy, and baked goods.
- Drink fat-free or low-fat milk after age two. Children younger than two have higher energy requirements and need the benefits of dietary fat, including improved absorption of fat-soluble vitamins, for proper growth and development of the nervous system. Other good sources of calcium include low-fat or fat-free yogurt and cottage cheese.
- Eat a variety of foods, including fish and shellfish; oily fish such as salmon provide healthy fats.
- Do not add extra salt to foods and reduce overall sodium intake.
- Balance calories consumed with regular physical activity to help maintain a healthy weight.

It is often difficult for parents to understand how much food their child should eat at a particular age. Parents tend to overestimate the amount of food small children need. The daily amounts of some common foods that meet the American Heart Association guidelines for different ages

KEY TERMS

Body Mass Index (BMI)—Also known as BMI, the index determines whether a person is at a healthy weight, underweight, overweight, or obese. The BMI can be calculated by converting the person's height into inches. That amount is multiplied by itself and then divided by the person's weight. That number is then multiplied by 703. The metric formula for the BMI is the weight in kilograms divided by the square of height in meters.

Cognitive behavioral therapy—A type of psychotherapy in which people learn to recognize and change negative and self-defeating patterns of thinking and behavior.

are listed below. These amounts are based on children who are sedentary or physically inactive. Active children will need more calories and slightly larger amounts of food. Calorie and serving recommendations are as follows:

- children ages 2–3—total daily calories, 1,000; milk, 2 cups; lean meat or beans, 2 ounces; fruits, 1 cup; vegetables, 1 cup; grains, 3 ounces
- girls ages 4–8—total daily calories, 1,200; milk, 2 cups; lean meat or beans, 3 ounces; fruits, 1.5 cups; vegetables, 1 cup; grains, 4 ounces
- boys ages 4–8—total daily calories, 1,400; milk, 2 cups; lean meat or beans, 4 ounces; fruits, 1.5 cup; vegetables, 1.5 cups; grains, 5 ounces
- girls ages 9–13—total daily calories, 1,600; milk, 3 cups; lean meat or beans, 5 ounces; fruits, 1.5 cups; vegetables, 2 cups; grains, 5 ounces
- boys ages 9–13—total daily calories, 1,800; milk, 3 cups; lean meat or beans, 5 ounces; fruits, 1.5 cups; vegetables, 2.5 cups; grains, 6 ounces
- girls ages 14–18—total daily calories, 1,800; milk, 3 cups; lean meat or beans, 5 ounces; fruits, 1.5 cups; vegetables, 2.5 cups; grains, 6 ounces
- boys ages 14–18 years—total daily calories, 2,200; milk, 3 cups; lean meat or beans, 6 ounces; fruits, 2 cups; vegetables, 3 cups; grains, 7 ounces

Therapy

Children who are overweight or obese may have accompanying psychological and social problems that may be helped with psychotherapy in addition to nutritional counseling. Cognitive-behavioral therapy (CBT) is designed to confront and change thoughts and feelings about one's body and behaviors toward food. CBT is relatively short-term and does not address the origins of those thoughts or feelings. CBT may include strategies to maintain self-control with regard to food. Family therapy may help children who overeat for emotional reasons related to conflicts within the family. Family therapy teaches strategies for reducing conflict, disorder, and stress that may be factors in triggering emotional eating.

Prognosis

The younger the child is when weight control strategies begin, the better the chance that the child will be able to maintain a normal weight. When it comes to weight control, one advantage children have over adults is that they grow. If a child can maintain his weight without gaining, he may grow into a normal weight as he becomes taller.

Parents need to be careful about how they approach weight loss in children. Critical comments about weight from parents or excess zeal in putting their child on a rigorous diet can trigger **eating disorders** such as anorexia nervosa or bulimia nervosa in some children, especially adolescent girls. Instead of placing their child on a diet, parents should promote healthy eating and prepare meals that include lots of fruits and vegetables, whole grains, and low-fat dairy and protein. It is helpful for parents to lead by example, so that the child does not feel isolated. Criticism and focus on losing weight as opposed to getting healthy may lead to a negative body image.

Children who remain overweight or obese have a much greater likelihood of being overweight or obese adults with all the health problems that obesity brings. Studies have found that 26–41% of preschoolers who are obese become obese adults. In school-aged children, 42–63% of children with obesity become obese adults. The relationship between obesity in early life and adulthood is strongest for adolescents, so it is important to deal with childhood obesity as soon as possible.

Prevention

Parents must take the lead in preventing obesity in children. Starting good eating habits in children when they are young may help them carry such practices into adult life. Some of the ways parents can promote healthy habits are:

- serve a healthy variety of foods; keep healthy snacks on hand
- choose low-fat cooking methods such as broiling or baking

QUESTIONS TO ASK YOUR DOCTOR

- To what degree is my child overweight or obese?
- Should my child be on a formal diet?
- Can you recommend a nutritionist or dietitian to help our family eat better?
- Would behavioral therapy help my child handle his/her food issues better?
- In what ways is my child's weight affecting his/her health?

- eliminate high-fat and high-calorie snack food and sugary beverages from the house; this removes temptation and eliminates the need to nag
- eat meals together as a family rather than grabbing something quick on the run
- limit visits to fast-food restaurants
- limit television, computer and video game time
- plan family activities that involve physical activity, such as hiking, biking, or swimming
- encourage children to become more active in small ways such as walking to school, biking to friends' houses, or doing chores such as walking the dog or mowing the lawn
- avoid using food as a reward
- pack healthy homemade lunches on school days
- encourage school officials to eliminate soda machines on campus, bake sales, and fundraising with candy and cookies
- set realistic goals for weight control and reward children's efforts (but not with food)
- model the eating behaviors and active lifestyle you would like your child to adopt

Resources

BOOKS

Fletcher, Anne M. *Weight Loss Confidential: How Teens Lose Weight and Keep It Off—And What They Wish Parents Knew.* Boston: Houghton Mifflin Harcourt, 2008.

Hassink, Sandra. ed. *A Parent's Guide to Childhood Obesity: A Road Map to Health.* Elk Grove Village, IL: American Academy of Pediatrics, 2006.

Okie, Susan. *Fed Up!: Winning the War Against Childhood Obesity.* Washington, DC: Joseph Henry Press, 2005.

Schumacher, Donald, and J. Allen Queen. *Overcoming Obesity in Childhood and Adolescence: A Guide for School Leaders.* Thousand Oaks, CA: Corwin Press, Sage, 2007.

Waters, Elizabeth. *Preventing Childhood Obesity: Evidence Policy and Practice (Evidence-Based Medicine).* Hoboken, NJ: Blackwell, 2010.

PERIODICALS

Kakinami, Lisa, et al. "Association Between Different Growth Curve Definitions of Overweight and Obesity and Cardiometabolic Risk in Children." *Canadian Medical Association* 184, no. 10 (2012): E539–E550. http://dx.doi.org/10.1503/cmaj.110797 (accessed July 11, 2012).

McCullick, Bryan A., et al. "An Analysis of State Physical Education Policies." *Journal of Teaching in Physical Education* 31, no. 2 (2012): 200–210.

Park, M.H., et al. "The Impact of Childhood Obesity on Morbidity and Mortality in Adulthood: A Systematic Review." *Obesity Reviews* (June 26, 2012): e-pub ahead of print. http://dx.doi.org/10.1111/j.1467-789X.2012.01015.x (accessed July 11, 2012).

Sanchez-Villegas, Almudena, et al. "Perceived and Actual Obesity in Childhood and Adolescence and Risk of Adult Depression." *Journal of Epidemiology & Community Health* (July 5, 2012): e-pub ahead of print. http://dx.doi.org/doi:10.1136/jech-2012-201435 (accessed July 11, 2012).

Verstraeten, Roosmarijn, et al. "Effectiveness of Preventive School-Based Obesity Interventions in Low- and Middle-Income Countries: A Systematic Review." *American Journal of Clinical Nutrition* (July 3, 2012): e-pub ahead of print. http://dx.doi.org/10.3945/ajcn.112.035378 (accessed July 11, 2012).

OTHER

American Heart Association. *Understanding Childhood Obesity: 2011 Statistical Sourcebook.* Dallas: AHA and American Stroke Association, 2011. http://www.heart.org/idc/groups/heart-public/@wcm/@fc/documents/downloadable/ucm_428180.pdf (accessed July 11, 2012).

U.S. Department of Agriculture and U.S. Department of Health and Human Services. *Dietary Guidelines for Americans, 2010.* 7th ed. Washington, DC: U.S. Government Printing Office, December 2010. http://health.gov/dietaryguidelines (accessed February 22, 2012).

WEBSITES

American Heart Association. "Dietary Recommendations for Healthy Children." http://www.heart.org/HEARTORG/GettingHealthy/NutritionCenter/Dietary-Recommendations-for-Healthy-Children_UCM_303886_Article.jsp (accessed July 11, 2012).

Mayo Clinic staff. "Childhood Obesity." MayoClinic.com. http://www.mayoclinic.com/health/childhood-obesity/DS00698 (accessed July 9, 2012).

MedlinePlus. "Obesity in Children." U.S. National Library of Medicine, National Institutes of Health. http://www.nlm.nih.gov/medlineplus/obesityinchildren.html (accessed July 9, 2012).

National Heart, Lung, and Blood Institute. "How Are Overweight and Obesity Diagnosed?" U.S. National Institutes of Health. http://www.nhlbi.nih.gov/health/health-topics/topics/obe/diagnosis.html (accessed July 10, 2012).

Schwartz, Steven M. "Obesity in Children." Medscape Reference. January 26, 2012. http://emedicine.medscape.com/article/985333-overview (accessed July 9, 2012).

U.S. Centers for Disease Control and Prevention. "BMI Percentile Calculator for Child and Teen." http://apps.nccd.cdc.gov/dnpabmi/Calculator.aspx (accessed July 9, 2012).

U.S. Centers for Disease Control and Prevention. "Childhood Overweight and Obesity." http://www.cdc.gov/obesity/childhood (accessed July 9, 2012).

U.S. Centers for Disease Control and Prevention. "How Much Physical Activity Do Children Need?" http://www.cdc.gov/physicalactivity/everyone/guidelines/children.html (accessed July 9, 2012).

ORGANIZATIONS

American Academy of Pediatrics (AAP), 141 Northwest Point Blvd., Elk Grove Village, IL 60007, (847) 434-4000, (800) 433-9016, Fax: (847) 434-8000, http://www.aap.org

Academy of Nutrition and Dietetics, 120 South Riverside Plz., Ste. 2000, Chicago, IL 60606-6995, (312) 899-0040, (800) 877-1600, amacmunn@eatright.org, http://www.eatright.org

Center for Nutrition Policy and Promotion, U.S. Department of Agriculture, 3101 Park Center Drive, 10th Fl., Alexandria, VA USA, (703) 305-7600, Fax: (703) 305-3300, support@cnpp.usda.gov, http://www.cnpp.usda.gov

Centers for Disease Control and Prevention, 1600 Clifton Rd. NE, Atlanta, GA 30333, (800) CDC-INFO (232-4636), (888) 232-6348, cdcinfo@cdc.gov, http://www.cdc.gov

The Obesity Society, 8757 Georgia Ave., Ste. 1320, Silver Spring, MD 20910, (301) 563-6526, Fax: (301) 563-6595, http://www.obesity.orghttp://www.obesity.org/resources-for/consumer.htm

Weight-Control Information Network (WIN), 1 WIN Way, Bethesda, MD 20892-3665, (202) 828-1025, (877) 946-4627, Fax: (202) 828-1028, win@http://win.niddk.nih.gov, http://win.niddk.nih.gov.

Tish Davidson, AM

Children's health

Definition

Children's health encompasses the physical, mental, emotional, and social well-being of children from infancy through adolescence.

Description

All children should have regular well-child check-ups according to the schedule recommended by their physician or pediatrician. The American Academy of Pediatrics (AAP) advises that children be seen for well-baby checks at two weeks, two months, four months, six months, nine months, twelve months, fifteen months, and eighteen months. Well-child visits are recommended at ages two, three, four, five, six, eight, 10, and annually thereafter through age 21. Well-baby and well-child check-ups assess the child physically, behaviorally, developmentally, and emotionally and are important in spotting developmental delays or behavioral abnormalities early. Well-child check-ups usually include reviewing medical history, measuring height, weight, blood pressure, and temperature, vision, hearing, reflex screening, a developmental/behavioral assessment, physical examination, immunizations, guidance about developmental milestones, **nutrition**, injury **prevention**, and referrals as needed to a pediatric dentist or other pediatric specialists. The **Centers for Disease Control and Prevention** has estimated that about 30% of children under the age of two in the United States in 2011 without any form of health insurance failed to get regular well-child checkups, compared to about 12% with public insurance and 10% with private insurance. The comparable figures for children age three to four were 42%, 16%, and 14%; for children age five to 11 were 55%, 22%, and 22%; and for children age 12 to 17, 60%, 27%, and 28%.

Immunization to protect against specific diseases is an important part of a child's healthcare program. Vaccines must be administered within certain time limits. When multiple doses are needed, a certain amount of time must elapse between doses. As of 2012, the American Association of Pediatrics (AAP) and the **Centers for Disease Control and Prevention (CDC)** recommended these childhood immunizations:

- Hepatitis B vaccine. Three doses, beginning at birth and completed no later than 18 months with at least four weeks between doses.
- Rotavirus vaccine. Two or three doses depending on vaccine with the first dose given beginning no earlier than 6 weeks and no later than 14 weeks and the final dose completed no later than eight months.
- Diphtheria, Tetanus, and Pertussis (DTaP) vaccine. Doses at two and six months with a final dose between four and six years of age. A booster is given at 11–12 years of age.
- *Haemophilus influenzae* type b (Hib) vaccine. Three doses beginning no earlier than two months with a booster at 12–15 months.
- Pneumococcal conjugate vaccine. Doses at 2, 4, 6, and 12–15 months. High-risk children may require additional doses of related vaccine.
- Inactivated Polio vaccine. Doses at 2, 4, 6–18 months and 4–6 years.

- Influenza vaccine. Two doses every year for children under age nine. Single dose every year through adulthood.
- Measles, Mumps, Rubella (MMR) vaccine. Two doses, the first no earlier than one year, the second between ages four and six years.
- Varicella (chickenpox) vaccine. Two doses, the first no earlier than one year, the second usually between ages four and six years.
- Hepatitis A vaccine. Two doses, the first no earlier than one year, the second six months later. High risk children may require additional doses during adolescence.
- Meningococcal vaccine. One dose between the ages of 11 and 18 years. High risk children only may require dose between the ages of two and 10 years.
- Human papillomavirus (HPV) vaccine. Girls only, three doses beginning at age 11. Older unvaccinated females may be vaccinated up to age 26.

Mental health

Children who have difficulty in areas of language acquisition, cognitive (mental) development, and behavior control may have a mental health disorder. Mental health problems that arise in children include:

- Attention deficit hyperactivity disorder (ADHD). ADHD is estimated to affect 3–7% of school-age children in the United States and is 3–5 times more common in boys than in girls. It is a disorder characterized by excessive motor activity, distractibility, and poor impulse control.
- Learning disorders. Learning disabilities affect one in 10 school children in the United States.
- Depression, anxiety, and bipolar disorder. Affective, or mood, disorders are now more commonly recognized in children than in the past.
- Eating disorders. Anorexia nervosa, bulimia nervosa, and binge eating disorder frequently occur in adolescent girls. It is estimated that one out of every 100–200 adolescent girls meets all the diagnostic criteria for anorexia.
- Schizophrenia. A disorder characterized by bizarre thoughts and behaviors, paranoia, impaired sense of reality, and psychosis may be diagnosed in childhood or adolescence.
- Obsessive-compulsive disorder (OCD). Symptoms often begin in childhood or adolescence.
- Autism and pervasive developmental disorder. Severe developmental disabilities that cause a child to become withdrawn and unresponsive.
- Mental retardation. Children under age 18 with an IQ of 70 or below and impairments in adaptive functioning are considered mentally retarded.

Emotional and social health

Children take their first significant steps toward socialization and peer interaction when they begin to engage in cooperative play at around age four. Their social development progresses throughout childhood and adolescence as they expand their social contacts, develop friendships, start to be influenced by their peers, and begin to show interest in the opposite sex. In adolescence, there is a strong, but normal, trend away from involvement with family and toward establishing their own identity and values.

Several factors may have a negative impact on the emotional and social well-being of children:

- Violence. Bullying can cause serious damage to a child's sense of self-esteem and personal safety, as can experiences with community violence.
- Family turmoil. Divorce, domestic abuse, death of a family member, and other life-changing events that alter the family dynamic can have a serious impact on a child. Even a positive event such as the birth of a sibling or a move to a new city and school can put emotional strain on a child.
- Stress. The pressure to perform well academically and in extracurricular activities such as sports can be overwhelming to some children. Emphasis on physical appearance also creates stress that can lead to eating disorders.
- Peer pressure. Although it can have a positive impact, peer pressure is often a source of significant stress for children. This is particularly true in adolescence when "fitting in" is important to most teens.
- Drugs and alcohol. Curiosity is intrinsic to childhood, and more than 30% of children have experimented with alcohol by age 13. Open communication with children that sets forth parental expectations about drug and alcohol use is essential.
- Negative sexual experiences. Sexual abuse and assault can emotionally scar a child and instill negative feelings about sexuality and relationships. Early and/or indiscriminate sexual relationships can cause emotional harm and increase the likelihood of pregnancy and sexually transmitted diseases.

Causes and symptoms

Childhood health problems may be congenital (i.e., present at birth) or acquired through infection, immune system deficiency, or another disease process. They may also be caused by physical trauma (e.g., a car accident or a playground fall), exposure to a toxic substance (e.g., drug allergy, or exposure to poisonous chemical), or triggered by a genetic factor (e.g., celiac disease, sickle

DR. BENJAMIN SPOCK (1903–1998)

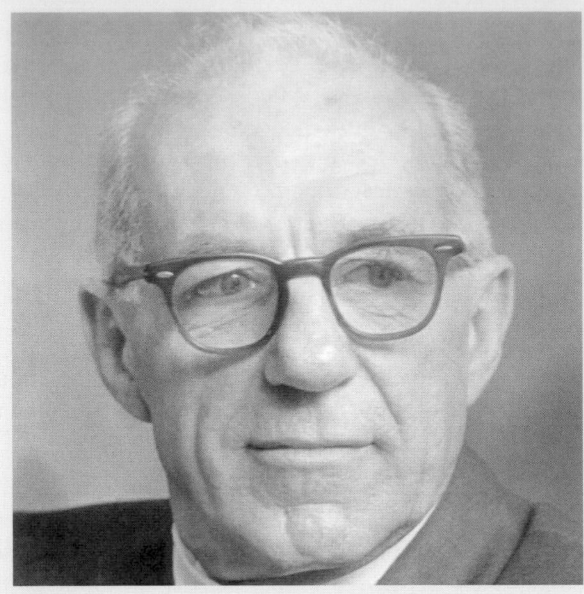

(© Bettmann/CORBIS)

Benjamin Spock, pediatrician and political activist, was most noted for his authorship of *Baby and Child Care*, which significantly changed predominant attitudes toward the raising of infants and children. He began medical school at Yale University in 1925, and transferred to Columbia University's College of Physicians and Surgeons in 1927. Spock had decided well before starting his medical studies that he would "work with children, who have their whole lives ahead of them" and so, upon taking his M.D. degree in 1929 and serving his general internship at the prestigious Presbyterian Hospital, he specialized in pediatrics at a small hospital crowded with children in New York's Hell's Kitchen area.

On a summer vacation in 1943 he began to write his most famous book and he continued to work on it from 1944 to 1946 while serving as a medical officer in the Navy. The book sharply broke with the authoritarian tone and rigorous instructions found in earlier generations of baby-care books, most of which said to feed infants on a strict schedule and not to pick them up when they cried. Spock, who spent ten years trying to reconcile his psychoanalytic training with what mothers were telling him about their children, told his readers, "You know more than you think you do.... Don't be afraid to trust your own common sense.... Take it easy, trust your own instincts, and follow the directions that your doctor gives you." The response was overwhelming. *Baby and Child Care* rapidly became America's all-time best-seller except for Shakespeare and the Bible; by 1976 it had also eclipsed Shakespeare.

Spock prided himself in keeping up with the times, a fact that's reflected in the many revisions of *Baby and Child Care* in which he incorporated the latest medical developments and dealt with emerging social issues such as working mothers, daycare centers, and single parenthood.

cell anemia) or environmental factors (e.g., dust mite **allergies**, pollen allergies).

Physical and mental health problems in childhood can cause a wide spectrum of symptoms. The following behaviors suggest a larger emotional, social, or mental disturbance that may need to be evaluated by a health care professional.

- signs of alcohol and drug use
- suddenly falling grades or school avoidance
- lack of interest in activities that were previously enjoyable
- excessive anxiety
- persistent, prolonged depression
- withdrawal from friends and family
- involvement with violence or vandalism
- extreme or irrational perfectionism
- repeated, aggressive confrontations with authority figures
- age-inappropriate temper tantrums or inappropriate displays of anger
- self-inflicted injury
- bizarre behavior and/or speech
- trouble with the police
- sexual promiscuity
- prolonged, unexplained fatigue
- suicide threats or attempts

The causes of developmental disorders and delays and learning disabilities are not always fully understood. Pervasive developmental disorder (PDD) and autistic spectrum disorder (more commonly known as **autism**) are characterized by unresponsiveness and severe impairments in one or more of these areas:

- Social interaction. Autistic children often have difficulty interpreting social cues and are unaware of acceptable social behavior. They tend to be withdrawn and socially isolated. They frequently reject physical contact.

KEY TERMS

Bipolar disorder—Formerly called manic-depressive disorder. A mood disorder characterized by alternating periods of overconfidence and activity (manic highs) and depressive lows.

Child development—The process of physical, intellectual, emotional, and social growth that occurs from infancy through adolescence. Erik Erikson, Margaret Mahler, Sigmund Freud, and Jean Piaget are among the best known child development theorists.

Immunization—Administering a vaccine that stimulates the body to create antibodies to a specific disease (immunity) without causing symptoms of the disease.

Learning disabilities—An impairment of the cognitive processes of understanding and using spoken and written language that results in difficulties with one or more academic skill sets (e.g., reading, writing, mathematics).

Motor skills—Controlled movement of muscle groups. Fine motor skills involve tasks that require dexterity of small muscles, such as buttoning a shirt. Tasks such as walking or throwing a ball involve the use of gross motor skills.

Obsessive-compulsive disorder (OCD)—An anxiety disorder in which a person cannot prevent himself from dwelling on unwanted thoughts, acting on urges, or performing repetitious rituals, such as washing one's hands or checking to make sure lights have been turned off.

Psychological tests—Written, verbal, or visual tasks that assess psychological functioning, intelligence, and/or personality traits.

Type 1 diabetes—A chronic immune system disorder in which the pancreas does not produce sufficient amounts of insulin, a hormone that enables cells to use glucose for energy. Also called juvenile diabetes, it must be treated with insulin injections.

- Communication and language. A child with autism or PDD may not speak or may display limited or immature language skills.
- Behavior. Autistic or PDD children may have difficulty dealing with anger, can be self-injurious, and may display obsessive behavior.

Autism is associated with brain abnormalities, but the exact mechanisms that trigger the disorder are yet to be determined. Research suggests that it may be linked to certain congenital conditions such as neurofibromatosis, fragile X syndrome, and phenylketonuria (PKU). Despite much speculation, no well-designed, controlled studies have shown any link between autism and childhood vaccinations.

Diagnosis

Physical, intellectual, emotional, and social maturation are all-important markers of a child's overall health and well being. When evaluating children, pediatricians and child-care specialists assess related skill sets, such as a child's acquisition and use of language, fine and gross motor skills, cognitive growth, socialization, and achievement of certain milestones in these areas. A developmental milestone is a task or skill set that a child is expected to reach at a certain age or stage of life. For example, by age one, most children have achieved the physical milestone of walking with the assistance of an adult. Developmental disorders may be identified and/or diagnosed by physicians, teachers, child psychologists, therapists, counselors, and other professionals who interact with children on a regular basis.

It is important to remember that all children are unique and develop at different paces within this broad framework. Reaching a milestone early or late does not necessarily indicate a developmental problem. However, if a child is consistently lagging in achieving milestones or has a significant deficit in one developmental area, he or she may be experiencing developmental delays that warrant professional evaluation.

Pediatricians and other medical professionals typically diagnose physical illness and disease in children as well as provide preventative health care. In cases of illness and injury, children will undergo a thorough physical examination and patient history. Diagnostic tests may be performed as appropriate. In cases of mental or emotional disorders, a psychologist or psychiatrist will meet with the patient to conduct an interview and take a detailed social and medical history. Interviews with a parent or guardian and teacher may also be part of the diagnostic process. The physician may also administer one or more psychological tests (also called clinical inventories, scales, or assessments).

Treatment

Medications may be prescribed to treat certain childhood illnesses. Proper dosage is particularly important with infants and children, as medications such as acetaminophen can be toxic in excessive amounts. Parents and caregivers should always follow the instructions for use that accompany medications, and inform the child's pediatrician if the child is taking any other drugs or **vitamins** to prevent potentially negative drug interactions. Any side effects or adverse reactions to medication should be reported to the child's physician. If **antibiotics** are prescribed, the full course should always be taken. Parents should be especially careful when using herbal medicine or dietary supplements, as the pediatric doses for these treatments often have not been established.

Other treatments for childhood illness and/or injuries include, but are not limited to, nutritional therapy, physical therapy, respiratory therapy, medical devices (e.g., hearing aids, glasses, braces), and in some cases, surgery.

Counseling is typically a first treatment for psychological disorders. Therapy approaches include psychotherapy, cognitive therapy, behavioral therapy, family counseling, and group therapy. Therapy or counseling may be administered by social workers, nurses, licensed counselors and therapists, psychologists, or psychiatrists. Psychoactive medication may be prescribed by a psychiatrist for symptom relief in children and adolescents with mental disorders.

Support groups may provide emotional support for children with chronic illnesses or mental disorders. This approach, which allows individuals to seek advice and counsel from others in similar circumstances, can be extremely effective, especially in older children who look toward their peers for guidance and support. Support groups for family members often help adults and siblings cope with a chronically ill child.

Speech therapy may help children with developmental delays in language acquisition. Children with learning disorders can benefit from special education classes and accommodations arrived at through professional evaluation and the creation of an individualized educational plan (IEP).

Alternative

Therapeutic approaches that encourage self-discovery and empowerment may be useful in treating some childhood emotional traumas and mental disorders. Art therapy, the use of the creative process to express and understand emotion, encompasses a broad range of humanistic disciplines, including visual arts, dance, drama, music, film, writing, literature, and other artistic genres. It can be particularly effective in children who may have difficulty gaining insight about emotions and thoughts they are otherwise incapable of expressing.

Certain mild herbal remedies may also be safely used with children, such as ginger (*Zingiber officinale*) tea for nausea and aloe vera salve for **burns**. Parents and caregivers should always consult their healthcare provider before administering herbs to children, as certain herbs may affect children differently than they do adults.

Prognosis

The prognosis for childhood health problems varies widely. In general, early detection and proper treatment can greatly improve the odds of recovery from many childhood illnesses and disabilities. Early intervention is key in helping a child with disabilities reach his or her full potential.

Some learning disabilities and mild developmental disorders can be overcome or greatly improved through appropriate therapies. As of 2012, there were no known medical treatments or pharmacological therapies that eliminate all of the symptoms associated with pervasive developmental disorder (PDD), autism spectrum disorder, and mental retardation. Mental illnesses such as schizophrenia and bipolar disorder are chronic, lifelong disorders, although their symptoms can often be controlled with medication.

Prevention

Parents can take precautions to ensure the safety of their children. Childproofing the home, following a recommended immunization schedule, educating children on safety, learning first aid, and taking children for regular well-child check-ups can help to protect against physical harm. In addition, encouraging open communication with children can help them grow both emotionally and socially. Providing a loving and supportive home environment can help to nurture an emotionally healthy child who is independent, self-confident, socially skilled, insightful, and empathetic toward others.

Because they are still developing motor skills, children may be particularly accident prone. Observing the following safety guidelines may help protect children from injury:

- Helmets and padding. Children should always wear a properly fitted helmet and appropriate protective gear when riding a bike, scooter, or similar equipment or participating in sports. They should ride on designated bike paths whenever possible, and learn bicycle safety rules (e.g., ride with traffic, use hand signals).
- Playground safety. Swing sets and other outdoor play equipment should be well-maintained, have at least 12 in (30 cm) of loose fill materials (e.g., sand, wood chips) underneath to cushion falls, and children should be properly supervised at play.
- Staying apprised of recalls. Children's toys, play equipment, and care products are frequently involved in product recalls. The U.S. Consumer Safety Products Commission (CSPC) is the agency responsible for tracking these recalls.
- Staying safe in the car. Up to 85% of children's car seats are improperly installed and/or used. Infants

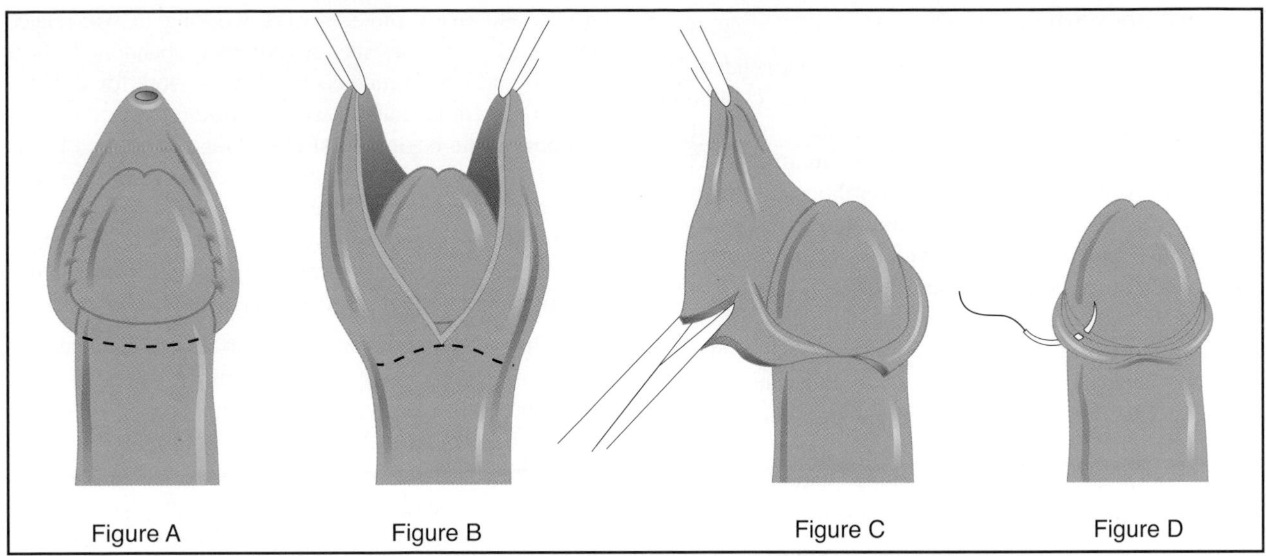

The process of circumcision. *(Illustration by Electronic Illustrators Group. © 2013 Cengage Learning)*

should always be in a rear-facing car seat until they are over 12 months of age and weigh more than 20 lbs (9 kg). An infant or car seat should never be put in a front passenger seat that has an air bag. Once they outgrow their forward-facing car seats, children between the ages of four and eight who weigh between 40 and 80 lbs (18 to 36 kg) should ride in a booster seat. Every child over this age and weight who rides in a car should use a properly fitted lap and shoulder belt.

- Teaching children pedestrian safety. Young children should never be allowed to cross the street by themselves. Older children should know to follow traffic signs and signals, cross the street at the corner, and look both ways before stepping off the curb.
- Teaching children about personal safety. Children should know what to do in case they get lost or are approached by a stranger. It is also imperative that parents talk openly with their children about their body and sexuality, and what behavior is inappropriate, to protect them against sexual predators.

Childproofing the household is an important step toward keeping children healthy. To make a house a safe home, parents and caregivers should:

- Keep guns away from children. Accidental shootings in the home injure an estimated 1,500 children under age 14 each year. If a gun must be in the home, it should be securely locked in a tamperproof gun safe with the ammunition kept locked in a separate place.
- Keep matches, lighters, and flammable materials properly stored and out of the reach of children.
- Make sure hot water heaters are set to 120°F (49°C) or below to prevent scalding injuries.
- Equip the home with working fire extinguishers and smoke alarms; teach children what to do in case of fire.
- Secure all medications (including vitamins, herbs, and supplements), hazardous chemicals, and poisonous substances (including alcohol and tobacco) in ways that they cannot be accessed by children.
- Do not smoke. Aside from causing cancer and other health problems in smokers, second-hand smoke is hazardous to a child's health (e.g., increases their risk of developing allergies).
- Keep small children away from poisonous plants outdoors; remove any indoor plants that are toxic.
- Post the phone numbers of poison control and the pediatrician near the phone; teach children how to dial 9-1-1 and report an emergency.
- Children under age five should never be left alone in the bathtub or wading pool, or near any standing water source (including an open toilet). Fence all swimming pools, and install a self-latching gate. Drowning is the leading cause of death by injury for children between the ages of one and four in the United States.
- Remove lead paint. Lead is a serious health hazard for children and can cause cognitive retardation. Houses built before 1978 should be tested for lead paint. If lead is found, the paint should be removed using the appropriate safety precautions.
- Be alert to coins, small play pieces, and similar items that are choking hazards for small children.

Circumcision

One procedure that is sometimes recommended for the prevention of medical conditions during childhood and adult years is circumcision, the surgical removal of the prepuce (foreskin) of the penis. Circumcision has been performed in human societies for thousands of years for social, medical, cultural, and religious reasons. Today, the practice varies widely from country to country. Once a routine operation in the United States, encouraged by pediatricians and obstetricians for newborns, circumcision has become an elective option that parents make for their sons on an individual basis. (Female circumcision is also conducted in many societies, although it is generally strongly opposed in the United States and most other developed nations.) Among the potential benefits of male circumcision are:

- Reduced likelihood of phimosis (inability to retract foreskin normally), paraphimosis (painful inability to restore foreskin to its normal position), and balanoposthitis (inflammation of the glans and foreskin);
- Reduced risk of urinary tract infections;
- Reduced risk of HIV and sexually transmitted infections transmission;
- Reduced risk of cervical cancer in sexual partners;
- Reduced risk of penile cancer.

In spite of these potential benefits, medical organizations have tended to take a neutral view of the procedure. In 2012, for example, the American Academy of Pediatrics (AAP) issued a position statement noting that the benefits of circumcision tended to outweigh the risks of the procedure but that the decision as to whether to circumcise babies should be left to individual families. The AAP statement was later endorsed by the American College of Obstetricians and Gynecologists. Much stronger opposition to male circumcision has been expressed throughout history and also in recent years by individuals who see the practice as an unnecessary violation of the human body. Such opponents have sometimes sought to have laws adopted prohibiting the practice, although such laws have not yet been adopted in any part of the United States.

Day Care Centers

Day care centers are facilities that provide supervision of preschool children, generally while their parent(s) are at work. Day care centers are hardly a modern concept, as most societies throughout history have found ways of caring for very young children when their parents were too busy, for a variety of reasons, to provide that care. During World War II, for example, the federal government provided care centers for more than 400,000 children, primarily because fathers were usually in the military service, and many mothers were working in war-related jobs. After the war, the government abandoned these efforts because most mothers had left the work force; fewer than 10 percent of married women were employed outside the home at the beginning of the 1950s. As women began to return to the work force over the next few decades, day care once more became a necessity in most communities. In 2011, 60.6 percent of women with children under the age of three were employed outside the home, making day care an important part of American society once more.

While day care centers are an essential aspect of American society today, these facilities do pose some health problems for young children. These risks arise partially because of the close contact among children and staff that occur in day care centers, as well as the fact that young children tend to be less observant of good **hygiene** practices than are older children and adults. They may, for example, be less inclined to wash their hands after using the toilet. As a consequence, children who attend day care centers tend to be at greater risk for a number of infectious diseases than are children in the general population, diseases such as gastroenteritis, diarrhea, ear infections, respiratory infections, **hepatitis** A, head lice and scabies, and giardia.

Governmental licensing agencies generally establish fairly rigorous standards to ensure that day care centers are maintained under conditions that protect the health of their young clients. Those standards generally require that a day care facility meet all relevant state and local health requirements, that they have a nurse on site for at least part of the day, that they have immediate access to a licensed physician, and that they provide a full-time food service employee where appropriate. They may also include a number of more detailed requirements, such as

- A tuberculin test for all employees
- A record of rubella vaccination for all female employees of child-bearing age
- An up-to-date vaccination record for all children
- A pre-admission physical examination for all children
- An annual lead screening for all attendees
- First aid equipment available on site
- An instructional poster on choke prevention
- Injury reports and records
- Regular fire drills
- Posted evacuation plans
- An on-site no-smoking policy
- A strictly enforced handwashing policy for staff, along with handwashing instruction for children
- An appropriate nutritional and menu program appropriate for children of all ages in attendance at the center.

Resources

BOOKS

American Public Health Association and American Academy of Pediatrics. *Caring for Our Children: National Health and Safety Performance Standards: Guidelines for Early Care and Early Education Programs*, 3rd ed. Elk Grove Village, IL: American Academy of Pediatrics, 2011.

Marotz, Lynn R. *Health, Safety, and Nutrition for the Young Child*, 8th ed. Belmont, CA: Wadsworth Publishing, 2011.

Sears, William, et al. *The Portable Pediatrician: Everything You Need to Know About Your Child's Health*. Boston: Little, Brown, 2011.

PERIODICALS

Bernstein, A.S., and S.S. Myers. "Climate Change and Children's Health." *Current Opinion in Pediatrics* 23, 2. (2011): 221–6.

Liu, L., et al. "Global, Regional, and National Causes of Child Mortality: An Updated Systematic Analysis for 2010 with Time Trends since 2000." *Lancet* 379, 9832. (2012): 2151–61.

McCurdy, L.E., et al. "Using Nature and Outdoor Activity to Improve Children's Health." *Current Problems in Pediatric and Adolescent Health Care* 40, 5. (2010): 102–17.

OTHER

"Children's Health" Mayo Clinic. http://www.mayoclinic.com/health/childrens-health/MY00383. Accessed on October 20, 2012.

"Children's Health." WebMD. http://children.webmd.com/. Accessed on October 20, 2012.

"Kids Health." http://kidshealth.org/. Accessed on October 20, 2012.

ORGANIZATIONS

Academy of Nutrition and Dietetics, 120 South Riverside Plaza, Suite 2000, Chicago, IL 60605, (800) 877-1600, http://www.eatright.org/media/content.aspx?id=6442467512#.UIMqo8UqY1I, http://www.eatright.org

American Academy of Child and Adolescent Psychiatry, 3615 Wisconsin Ave., NW, Washington, DC 20016-3007, (202) 966-7300, Fax: (202) 966-2891, http://www.aacap.org/cs/root/contact_us/contact_us, http://www.aacap.org

American Academy of Family Physicians, P.O. Box 11210, Shawnee Mission, KS 66207, (913) 906-6000, (800) 274-2237, Fax: (913) 906-6075, http://www.aafp.org/online/en/home/aboutus/theaafp/contact.html#Parsys71461, http://www.aafp.org

American Academy of Pediatrics, 141 Northwest Point Blvd., Elk Grove Village, IL 60007-1098, (847) 434-4000, http://www2.aap.org/visit/contact.htm, http://www.aap.org

National Eating Disorders Association, 603 Stewart St., No. 803, Seattle, WA 98101, (206) 382-3587, info@NationalEatingDisorders.org, http://www.nationaleatingdisorders.org

National Institute of Child Health and Human Development (NICHD), P.O. Box 3006, Rockville, MD 30847, (800) 370-2943, TTY: (800) 320-6942, Fax: (866) 760-5947, NICHDInformationResourceCenter@mail.nih.gov, http://www.nichd.nih.gov

Project EAT, Eating Among Teens, University of Minnesota, 1300 S. Second St., Suite 300, Minneapolis, MN 55454, (612) 624-1818, http://www.epi.umn.edu/research/eat/index.shtm.

Tish Davidson, AM
Paula Anne Ford-Martin
Teresa G. Odle
Laura Jean Cataldo, RN, EdD

Chlorination

Definition

Chlorination is the process of adding a chlorine mixture to a substance (usually **water**) for the purposes of disinfecting that substance. Chlorination is also used to remove color from fabrics, sanitize surfaces, disinfect the water of swimming pools, and to reduce odors.

Description

Chlorine (CL_2) is a greenish-yellow gaseous element, originally discovered by Swedish chemist, Carl Wilhelm Scheele, in 1774 during a chemical reaction. In 1810, Sir Humphrey Davey named chlorine after insisting it was an element. Chlorine has been used in the United States as a disinfectant since the early twentieth century. Chlorine is found in a combined state, usually with some type of **sodium**, such as common salt (NaCl), carnallite ($KMgCL_36H_2O$), and sylvite (KCl). Chlorine is highly toxic, especially as a gas. It is also quite corrosive.

Chlorine is the most commonly used disinfectant in water treatment. Chlorination is a process used in wastewater and **drinking water** treatment plants. Chlorine helps kill pathogens, control troublesome microorganisms, and it works as an oxidant on wastewater. Bacteria are easier to kill with chlorine—eradicating viruses usually requires higher levels of chlorine than for bacteria. Chlorine is able to remove iron, manganese, nitrogen (in the form of ammonia), and eliminate tastes and odors from the wastewater.

Drinking water often contains naturally-occurring microorganisms that can cause disease or illness. Drinking water can also become contaminated by chemicals that seep into the water table or water source. The process of disinfection makes water safer for human consumption. Chemicals used to disinfect water, however, can also undergo chemical reactions with the

Pros and Cons of Chlorination
The benefits of chlorination are:
• Proven reduction of most bacteria and viruses in water
• Residual disinfectant protection against recontamination
• Ease-of-use and acceptability
• Proven reduction in occurrence of diarrheal disease
• Scalability and low cost
The drawbacks of chlorination are:
• Relatively low protection against protozoa
• Lower disinfection effectiveness in turbid waters
• Potential taste and odor objections
• Must ensure quality control of solution
• Potential long-term effects of chlorination by-products
SOURCE: Centers for Disease Control and Prevention

(Table by PreMediaGlobal. © 2013 Cengage Learning)

components already in the drinking water, resulting in additional, dangerous (and even cancerous) byproducts. Chlorine can react with organics or inorganics in the water, creating byproducts like trihalomethanes (THMs) and haloacetic acids. In tests on laboratory animals, these byproducts have caused **cancer** as well as developmental and reproductive problems.

In 1974, scientific papers first suggested that halogenated methanes were formed during the chlorination process. After these papers were published, the **Environmental Protection Agency (EPA)** conducted surveys of drinking water in the United States. The two studies conducted by the **EPA** were called the National Organics Reconnaissance Survey and the National Organics Monitoring Survey. The purpose of these studies was to test for the presence of trihalomethanes (THMs) and other halogenated organic compounds. The result of these studies was that drinking water is the primary method of exposure to THMs for Americans, and that these compounds were the most commonly found synthetic organic chemicals in U.S. drinking water.

Proper disinfection of drinking water has helped nearly eliminate many illnesses, especially in the developing world, that used to be common and claim many lives. Diseases that have been nearly eliminated through water disinfection include: **cholera**, Pontiac fever, **dysentery**, **polio**, and **typhoid fever**.

Some water treatment plants will add chlorine to the water to be treated and then dechlorinate the water before discharge into mains for delivery to customers. As a result of the potentially harmful side effects from the chlorination process, many major U.S. cities are moving away from chlorination and using alternative methods of disinfection or are adding ammonia to help prevent the formation of harmful byproducts.

A 2011 study out of Hong Kong suggests that the ability of chlorine to remove some of the most common **antibiotics** from the drinking water effectively is dependent upon the pH level of the water.

Demographics

According to Water.Org, an international non-profit dedicated to providing safe drinking water around the world, 780 million people globally do not have access to safe drinking water (equivalent to roughly two and a half times the U.S. **population**). Additionally, Water.Org estimates that 3.4 million people die annually from a water-related disease. According to Water.Org, in 2009, a child died every 15 seconds from a water-related disease. As of 2012, that has improved to one child every 21 seconds. Many of these deaths could be preventable with access to chlorinated drinking water and chlorinated wastewater. Water.Org states that the primary cause of infection worldwide is lack of **sanitation**.

Costs to society

In 1993, there was a waterborne Cryptosporidium outbreak in Milwaukee, Wisconsin that was believed to have been caused by problems with the chlorination process of drinking water. The illnesses of over 400,000 people, more than 100 deaths, and roughly $96.2 million in costs related to illnesses were attributed to this outbreak.

Efforts and solutions

The **CDC** and **Pan American Health Organization (PAHO)** developed the Safe Water System (SWS) in the 1990s. The SWS was created as a response to an epidemic of cholera in South America. The SWS allowed consumers to treat their own water—this was especially important in areas without access to chlorinated municipal water supplies. The SWS uses locally-manufactured sodium hypochlorite (chlorine bleach) solutions. Consumers are given a ratio of chlorine to water (based on whether the water is clear or murky—they then mix the chlorine into the water, agitate, and wait roughly 30 minutes before drinking. This method has proven effective against many diarrhea-causing bacteria, but it is not effective against Cryptosporidium. This method is relatively cost-effective—10 U.S. cents for enough hypochlorite to treat 1,000 liters of water—and requires less infrastructure than setting up municipal treatment facilities, making it quicker and less susceptible to geo-political difficulties.

The United States **Environmental Protection Agency** (EPA) regulates all disinfection byproducts (including those from chlorination). As a result, the EPA has set standards for safe levels of these byproducts. For example, the maximum allowable annual average is

KEY TERMS

Haloacetic acids (HAA5)—a group of five chemicals that are potentially formed when organic matter in drinking water reacts with chlorine during the chlorination disinfection process. The five Haloacetic acids are: monochloroacetic acid, dichloroacetic acid, thrichloroacetic acid, monobromoacetic acid, and dibromoacetic acid. These chemicals are potentially harmful to human health and are thus regulated by the Environmental Protection Agency (EPA).

Microorganism—A microscopic organism made up of one cell or a small cluster of cells. There are many different types of microorganisms and they can be helpful or benign to human health, however, some microorganisms like certain bacteria and fungi can be dangerous to human health.

Trihalomethanes (THMs)—a group of organic chemicals that often occur in drinking water that has been treated through chlorination. THMs are categorized by the Environmental Protection Agency as probable human carcinogens. The THMs are chloroform, bromodichloromethane, dibromochloromethane, and bromoform. The most common THM is chloroform.

Wastewater treatment—the process by which human waste or sewage is filtered, disinfected, and purified, making it safe to reintroduce into the environment.

80 parts per billion for trihalomethanes and 60 parts per billion for haloacetic acids.

Advances in artificial intelligence may help scientists predict—based on factors like water pH, temperature, and length of contact—the formation of chlorination byproducts: trihalomethanes. This development could potentially help eliminate the dangers of the chlorination process.

Chlorine comes in many forms, and not all of them have the same byproducts. Chloramines, compounds of chlorine and ammonia, are more stable than chlorine. As a result, chloramines do not react to organic matter in the water as frequently as chlorine does. Since chloramines produce fewer potentially-dangerous byproducts and are generally more stable, the use of chloramines to disinfect water is gaining popularity in the United States. The ammonia in chloramines is neutralized by the human digestive system, but is toxic to fish.

Resources

BOOKS

Boardman, Gregory D. "Chlorination." *Environmental Encyclopedia.*4th ed. Vol. 1. Detroit: Gale, 2011.

"Disinfection by Chlorination." *Kirk-Othmer Encyclopedia of Chemical Technology.* 5th ed. Vol. 8. Hoboken, NJ: Wiley-Interscience, 2007.

Jarvie, Michelle Edith. "Chlorination By-Products." *Green Health: An A–to–Z Guide.*Ed. Oladele Ogunseitan and Paul Robbins. Thousand Oaks, CA: Sage Reference, 2011.

Thomas, Nicholas C. "Clorination." *Encyclopedia of Environmental Issues, Rev ed.*Ed. Craig W. Allin. Vol. 1. Pasadena, CA: Salem Press, 2011.

PERIODICALS

Gupta, Shikha, and Kunwar P. Singh. "Artificial intelligence based modeling for predicting the disinection by-products in water." *Chemometrics and Intelligent Laboratory Systems*114(2012).

Li, Bing, and Tong Zhang. "pH significantly affects removal of trace antibiotics in chlorination of municipal wastewater." *Water Research*46.11 (2012).

WEBSITES

CDC "The Safe Water System." http://www.cdc.gov/safewater/chlorination.htmlSeptember 20, 2012.

EPA"Disinfection Byproducts: A Reference Resource." http://www.epa.gov/enviro/html/icr/gloss_dbp.htmlSeptember 20, 2012.

USGS "Wastewater Treatment Water Use." http://ga.water.usgs.gov/edu/wuww.htmlSeptember 20, 2012.

Water.gov "Water Facts." http://water.org/water-crisis/water-facts/water/September 20, 2012.

ORGANIZATIONS

U.S. Environmental Protection Agency, Ariel Rios Building 1200 Pennsylvania Avenue, N.W., Washington, DC USA 20460, 1 (202) 272-0165, www.epa.gov.

Andrea Nienstedt, MA

Cholera

Definition

Cholera is a serious, acute, **infectious disease** characterized by watery diarrhea that is caused by the bacterium *Vibrio cholerae.*

Description

The bacterium *Vibrio cholerae* was first identified by Robert Koch in 1883 during a cholera outbreak in Egypt. The name of the disease comes from a Greek

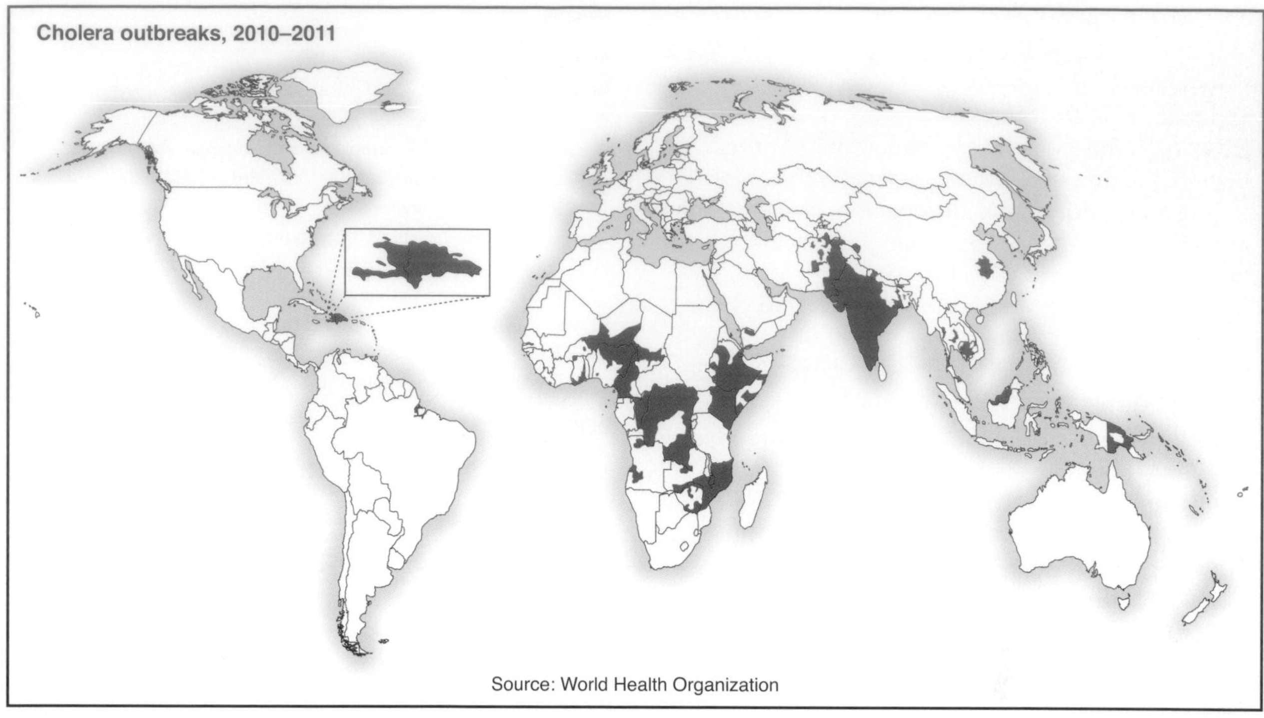

(Illustration by Electronic Illustrators Group. © 2013 Cengage Learning)

word meaning "flow of bile." Cholera typically occurs in major outbreaks or epidemics, often after **natural disasters** such as hurricanes or tsunamis during which **water** supplies are contaminated. Seven pandemics (countrywide or worldwide epidemics) of cholera have been recorded between 1817 and 2010.

Cholera is spread by eating food or drinking water that has been contaminated with *V. cholerae*. Contamination usually occurs when human feces from a person who has the disease seeps into a community water supply. Fruits and vegetables can be contaminated in areas where crops are fertilized with human feces. Cholera bacteria live in warm, brackish water and can infect persons who eat raw or undercooked seafood obtained from such waters. Cholera is rarely transmitted directly from one person to another. The disease is both preventable and treatable. Deaths usually occur in developing countries due to lack of access to hospitals and treatment.

Risk factors

The extensive system of sewage and water treatment in the United States, Canada, Europe, Japan, and Australia, has virtually eliminated concern for visitors and residents of these countries. People visiting or living in other parts of the world, particularly the Indian subcontinent and in parts of Africa and South America, should be aware of the potential for contracting cholera and practice **prevention**.

Some people are at greater risk of having a severe case of cholera if they become infected. These risk factors include:

- Use of proton pump inhibitors, histamine (H2) blockers, or antacids to control acid indigestion. Stomach acid often kills the *V. cholerae* bacterium, so a drug that decreases the acidity of the stomach increases the risk of developing cholera.
- Chronic gastritis caused by infection with *Helicobacter pylori*.
- Partial gastrectomy (surgical removal of a portion of the stomach).

Demographics

Although cholera was a public health problem in the United States and Europe a hundred years ago, modern **sanitation** and the treatment of drinking water have virtually eliminated the disease in developed countries. In 2005 the **World Health Organization (WHO)** reported 12 cases of cholera in the United States. Of these, eight were brought in by travelers and four were attributed to improperly cooked seafood in Louisiana following hurricanes Katrina and Rita. As of 2012, only a few cases are imported into the United States by travelers each year.

Serious cholera outbreaks continue to occur in less developed countries, particularly following natural disasters when water supplies become contaminated

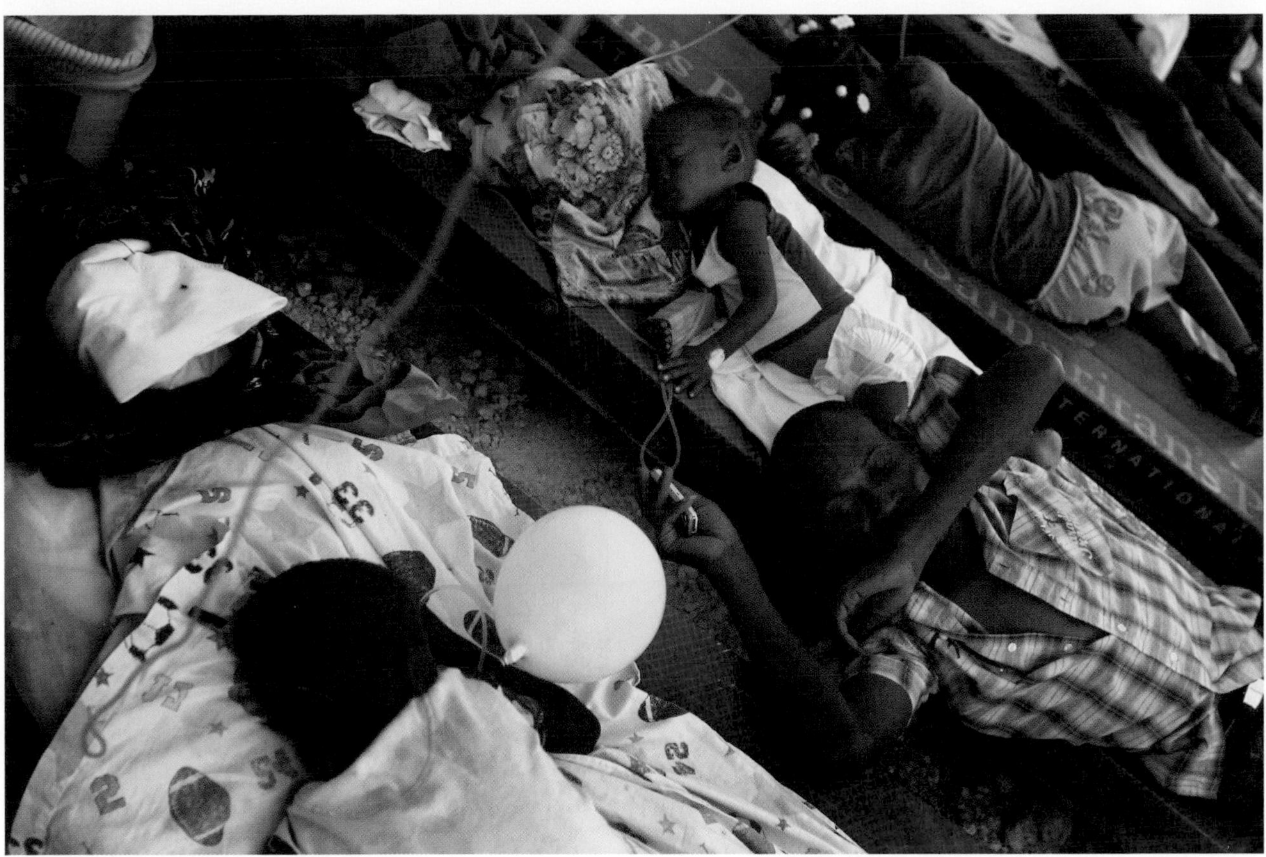

Patients being treated during a Cholera outbreak in Haiti. *(Photo by Joe Raedle/Getty Images)*

and sanitation is compromised. **WHO** estimates that during any cholera epidemic, approximately 0.2–1% of the local **population** will contract the disease and about 2.25% of affected people will die.

In 2010, 317,534 cases of cholera were reported to WHO, up from 221,226 cases in 2009. However, WHO recognizes that only a small percentage of cases are reported. WHO estimates that there are 3–5 million cholera cases resulting in 100,000–130,000 deaths per year. Of reported cases, more than half occurred in the Americas (primarily in Haiti), and about 36% occurred in Africa. In areas where cholera occurs, it is the most feared epidemic diarrheal disease because people can die from dehydration that results from severe diarrhea within hours of infection.

Anyone can contract cholera, but infants, children, pregnant women, and the elderly are more likely to die from the disease because they become dehydrated faster. There is no particular season in which cholera is more likely to occur.

Causes and symptoms

Cholera is caused by the bacterium *V. cholerae*. This bacterium is a gram-negative aerobic bacillus, or rod-shaped bacterium. It has two major biotypes: classic and 01, also called El Tor. El Tor is the biotype responsible for most of the cholera outbreaks reported from 1961 through the 2000s.

V. cholerae is sensitive to acid, so most cholera–causing bacteria die in the acidic environment of the stomach. However, when a person has ingested food or water containing large amounts of cholera bacteria, some survive to infect the intestines. Antacid usage or the use of any medication that blocks or reduces acid production in the stomach allows more bacteria to survive and cause infection.

In the small intestine, the rapidly multiplying bacteria produce a toxin that causes a large volume of water and electrolytes to be secreted into the bowels and then to be abruptly eliminated in the form of watery diarrhea. Vomiting may also occur. Symptoms appear between one and three days after contaminated food or water has been ingested.

Most cases of cholera are mild, but about one in 20 patients experience severe, potentially life-threatening symptoms. In severe cases, fluids can be lost through diarrhea and vomiting at the rate of one quart per hour. This loss of fluid can produce a dangerous state of dehydration unless the lost fluids and electrolytes are rapidly replaced.

JOHN SNOW (1813–1858)

British physician John Snow is called the "father of epidemiology" (the prevention and control of disease) because of his innovative investigative methods. Living in England's Victorian era, he gained prominence as one of the first physicians to use anesthesia. During a cholera epidemic of 1854, he revealed that the disease was caused by waterborne microorganisms.

John Snow was born in York, England on March 15, 1813, the oldest of nine children. His father, William Snow, was an unskilled laborer, and his family lived in one of the poorest sections of York, which was an industrial shipping area located on the River Ouse. Until he was 14, Snow was educated at a common day school for poor families. In 1827, he traveled to Newcastleupon-Tyne, 80 miles from his home, where he began serving a six-year apprenticeship in medicine under surgeon William Hardcastle. From Hardcastle, Snow learned the daily realities of running a medical practice. The apprenticeship included attending lectures at the Newcastle Infirmary. During this apprenticeship, which lasted until 1833, Snow became a vegetarian as well as a total abstainer of alcohol.

While in Newcastle, Snow was employed as one of three surgeon apothecaries at the Lying-In Hospital. He also worked as a secretary. In addition, he held an appointment as mining doctor at the Killingworth Colliery. Through this appointment, he came to know George and Robert Stephenson, the father and son team of locomotive engine designers who hailed from the area. In 1827, they were listed as patients in Snow's practice. During the cholera epidemic that lasted from 1831 to 1832 that hit a coal mining region near Newcastle, Snow worked as a colliery surgeon and unqualified assistant, treating victims. Cholera caused diarrhea and vomiting and, at the time, was fatal in about fifty percent of all cases. Victims usually died within two or three days, from dehydration. From the 1830s through the 1850s, Snow would come in close contact with the devastation the disease caused, and later in his career he would become keenly interested in preventing its outbreak.

As a physician, Snow treated patients from a range of social backgrounds, and he frequently practiced medicine in the poorest sections of London, providing good medical care to those who could least afford it. In 1852, the Medical Society of London (previously the Westminster Medical Society), chose Snow to be its orator for the coming year. In 1853, he moved his home and practice to 18 Sackville Street. On March 10, 1855, he was inducted as the Medical Society's president. Snow also was a member of the Royal Medical Chirurgical Society and the Pathological Society. In 1854, he served as president of the Physiological Society. In 1857, he was president of the Epidemiological Society.

In 1849, he published a pamphlet, "On the Mode of Communication of Cholera," which countered the conventional thinking regarding the disease. In the pamphlet, Snow remarked how the disease had a tendency to occur in the late summer, most often in the poorest sections of England, and in localized and isolated areas. He determined that cholera was a contagious disease caused by a poison that reproduces in the human body and is found in the vomitus and stools of cholera patients. Further, he suspected that cholera was spread through the microorganism contamination of food and water, but the foremost manner of transmission, he stated, was water contaminated with the poison. According to the prevailing theory, diseases such as cholera were transmitted by breathing in "miasmas," or contaminated vapors.

Despite contradicting the commonly held theory, Snow's pamphlet did not generate any great controversy, as many other theories about cholera were being advanced at the time. Still, he received a good deal of positive notoriety for his work, even though he had no way to prove his theory. However, another outbreak provided Snow the opportunity to prove that his ideas were indeed correct. In 1854, another severe cholera epidemic struck London, in a small area in Soho, where more than six hundred people died. Snow immediately began investigating water sources in the area. He was able to demonstrate by thoroughly documenting, correlating, and comparing locations of cholera cases among the customer's of London's two water companies that a higher concentration of incidents occurred among customers of one water company, the Southwark and Vauxhall. The company got its water from the downstream part of the Thames river, an area that was contaminated with London sewage. The other company got its water upstream from the main part of the city, where it was less likely to be contaminated. Snow's evidence was very strong, and it changed many minds.

Signs of dehydration include intense thirst, little or no urine output, dry skin and mouth, an absence of tears, glassy or sunken eyes, muscle cramps, weakness, and rapid heart rate. The fontanelle (soft spot on an infant's head) will appear sunken or drawn in. Dehydration occurs most rapidly in the very young and the very old because they have fewer fluid reserves. A doctor should be consulted immediately any time signs of severe dehydration occur. Immediate replacement of lost fluids and electrolytes is necessary to prevent kidney failure, coma, and death.

Diagnosis

Tests

Rapid diagnosis of cholera can be made by examining a fresh stool sample under the microscope for the presence of *V. cholerae* bacteria. Cholera can also be diagnosed by culturing a stool sample in the laboratory to isolate the cholera-causing bacteria. In addition, a blood test may reveal the presence of antibodies against the cholera bacteria. In areas where cholera occurs often, patients are usually treated for diarrhea and vomiting symptoms as if they had cholera without laboratory confirmation because the onset of life-threatening dehydration is rapid.

Treatment

Traditional

Preventing dehydration by replacing fluids and electrolytes lost through diarrhea and vomiting is key for treating cholera. The discovery that rehydration can be accomplished orally revolutionized the treatment of cholera and similar diseases by making this simple, cost-effective treatment widely available throughout the world. WHO has developed an inexpensive oral rehydration solution (ORS) containing appropriate amounts of water, sugar, and salts that is used worldwide. In cases of severe dehydration, replacement fluids must be given intravenously. Patients are encouraged to drink when they can keep liquids down and eat when their appetite returns. Recovery generally takes three to six days.

KEY TERMS

Antibody—A specific protein produced by the immune system in response to a specific foreign protein or particle called an antigen.

Bacillus—A rod-shaped bacterium. The organism that causes cholera is a gram-negative bacillus.

Biotype—A variant strain of a bacterial species with distinctive physiological characteristics.

Electrolytes—Salts and minerals that ionize in body fluids. Common human electrolytes include sodium, chloride, potassium, and calcium. Electrolytes control the fluid balance of the body and are important in muscle contraction, energy generation, and almost all major biochemical reactions in the body.

Endemic—Occurring naturally and consistently in a particular area.

Epidemic—An outbreak of disease where the number of cases exceeds the usual (endemic) or typical number of cases.

Pandemic—A widespread epidemic that affects whole countries or the entire world.

Toxin—A poison. In the case of cholera, a poison secreted as a byproduct of the growth of the cholera bacteria in the small intestine.

Drugs

Adults may be given the antibiotic tetracycline to shorten the duration of the illness and reduce fluid loss. WHO recommends this antibiotic treatment only in cases of severe dehydration. If **antibiotics** are overused, the cholera bacteria may develop resistance to the drug, making the antibiotic ineffective in treating even severe cases of cholera. Tetracycline and doxycycline are not given to children whose permanent teeth have not come in because it can cause the teeth to become permanently discolored.

Other antibiotics used to speed up the clearance of *V. cholerae* from the body include azithromycin (Zithromax), doxycycline (Bio–Tab, Doryx, Vibramycin), ciprofloxacin (Cipro), and erythromycin.

Alternative and complementary treatment

The **Centers for Disease Control and Prevention (CDC)** reported that the administration of zinc along with rehydration therapy and antibiotic therapy significantly shortens the duration and severity of diarrhea in children with cholera and several other diarrhea-causing diseases. The **CDC** recommends the use of zinc as a complementary treatment generally in children with significant diarrhea.

Public health role and response

The public health role in controlling cholera in the developed world is primarily preventive. Public health agencies are responsible for testing water supplies and assuring that sewage is adequately treated and not discharged into the waterways. Should a sewage spill occur or sewage treatment be disrupted by a natural disaster, public health agencies issue warnings and instructions on avoiding contaminated drinking water and contaminated rivers, streams, and beaches. Bottled water is often provided by a public agency until a clean water supply can be restored.

In developing countries, the public health challenge is much greater. Preventive measures following natural disasters include guaranteeing the purity of community drinking water, either by large-scale **chlorination** and boiling, or by bringing in bottled or purified water from the outside. Other important preventive measures at the community level include provision for the safe disposal of human feces and good food **hygiene**. However, these measures are difficult to implement after natural disasters in less developed and less accessible parts of the world. Organizations such as WHO devote large amounts of money and staff to cholera prevention and treatment, especially providing supplies of ORS, during cholera outbreaks.

A notable recent cholera outbreak occurred in Haiti in January 2010. After a major earthquake, water and sanitation supplies were severely disrupted. The number of cholera cases climbed. As of mid-2012, cholera continues to be a major public health problem in Haiti where the infrastructure elements needed to treat water and sewage have not been restored. It is suspected that two different strains of the cholera bacterium are present in Haiti, and that becoming infected with one strain does not provide immunity against the other strain, increasing the chance of infection and making it harder to control the disease. Haiti continues to be the focus of efforts to control cholera both by global and local public health agencies and non-governmental aid agencies.

Prognosis

Cholera is a very treatable disease so long as resources are available for rehydration. Patients with mild cases of cholera usually recover on their own in three to six days without additional complications. They may eliminate the bacteria in their feces for up to two weeks. Chronic carriers of the disease are rare. With prompt fluid and electrolyte replacement, the death rate in patients with severe cholera is less than one percent. Untreated, the death rate can be greater than 50%. The difficulty in treating severe cholera lies in getting medical care to the sick in developing areas of the world where medical resources are limited.

Prevention

The best form of cholera prevention is to establish good sanitation and waste treatment systems. In the absence of adequate sewage treatment, the following guidelines should be followed to reduce the possibility of infection:

- Boil water. Drink and brush teeth only with water that has been boiled or treated with chlorine or iodine tablets. Safe drinks include coffee and tea made with boiling water or carbonated bottled water and carbonated soft drinks.
- Cook foods. Eat only thoroughly cooked foods, and eat them while they are still hot. Avoid eating food from street vendors.

QUESTIONS TO ASK YOUR DOCTOR

- I am traveling to an area where cholera is present. What are the advantages and disadvantages of receiving the cholera vaccine before I go?
- How can I protect my young children from cholera when our family travels to an area where cholera is known to exist?
- Should I take oral hydration solution (ORS) with me if I am living in a cholera-plagued area?

- Peel foods. Eat only fruit or nuts with a thick intact skin or shell that is removed immediately before eating.
- Avoid raw foods. Do not eat raw foods such as oysters or ceviche. Avoid salads and raw vegetables. Do not use untreated ice cubes in otherwise safe drinks.
- Avoid polluted water. Do not swim or fish in polluted water.

Cholera is one of the few infectious diseases that can be spread by human remains (through fecal matter leaking from corpses into the water supply). During natural disasters, emergency workers who handle human remains are at increased risk of infection. It is considered preferable to bury corpses rather than to cremate them, however, and to allow survivors time to conduct appropriate burial ceremonies or rituals. The remains should be disinfected prior to burial, and buried at least 90 ft (30 m) away from sources of drinking water.

Two cholera vaccines exist, but both have limitations. An older vaccine, Dukoral, is licensed in 60 countries. It is given orally in two doses and provides incomplete (roughly 25–50%) immunity for 4–6 months. The other vaccine, ShanChol is licensed in India and as of 2012 was awaiting prequalification by WHO. It provides the advantages of longer protection and lower cost. As of 2012, the CDC does not recommend routine cholera **vaccination** for travelers. Residents of cholera-plagued areas should discuss the value of the vaccine with their doctor.

Resources

BOOKS

Hamlin, Christopher. *Cholera: The Biography.* New York: Oxford University Press, 2009.

Hempel, Sandra. *The Strange Case of the Broad Street Pump: John Snow and the Mystery of Cholera.* Berkeley, CA: University of California Press, 2007.

WEBSITES

"Cholera: General Information." U.S. Centers for Disease Control and Prevention (CDC).February 24, 2011. http://www.cdc.gov/cholera/index.html (accessed October 13, 2012).

Thaker, Vidhu, V. "Cholera." Medscape.com. July 19, 2011. http://emedicine.medscape.com/article/962643-overview#a0156 (accessed October 13, 2012).

World Health Organization. "Cholera." August 2011. http://www.who.int/mediacentre/factsheets/fs107/en/index.html (accessed October 13, 2012).

ORGANIZATIONS

U.S. Centers for Disease Control and Prevention (CDC), 1600 Clifton Rd., Atlanta, GA 30333, (404) 639–3534, (800) CDC–INFO (232–4636), cdcinfo@cdc.gov, http://www.cdc.gov

World Health Organization (WHO), Avenue Appia 20, 1211 Geneva 27, Switzerland, 22 41 791 21 11, Fax: 22 41 791 31 11, info@who.int, http://www.who.int.

Tish Davidson, AM
Rebecca J. Frey, PhD
Tish Davidson, AM

Circumcision *see* **Children's health**

Clostridium

Definition

Clostridium is a genus of rod-shaped bacteria that can cause a number of illnesses in humans, ranging from food **poisoning** to gas gangrene and **tetanus**. These bacteria are present in the soil. Some are also part of the normal flora, which is the collection of bacteria that live within the average person's body.

Description

The *Clostridium* genus includes dozens of species, but four are of primary interest from a health perspective are:

- *C. botulinum*, which produces the toxin that causes botulism, a dangerous type of food poisoning. It can also cause wound botulism, in which the bacteria grow in a wound, move into the bloodstream, and infect other parts of the body.
- *C. difficile*, which can cause diarrhea and inflammation of the colon. *C. difficile* is often abbreviated to C. diff.
- *C. perfringens*, which can cause mild or severe gastroenteritis (inflammation of the stomach and small intestine), or enteritis necroticans. Enteritis necroticans is also known as pig-bel disease or clostridial necrotizing enteritis.
- *C. tetani*, which can cause the serious illness known as tetanus.

Origins

Scientists identified *C. tetani* in 1884 as the agent responsible for tetanus; *C. perfringens* (once known as *C. welchii* in 1892 as the cause of gas gangrene; *C. botulinum* in 1895 as responsible for botulism food poisoning; and *C. difficile* in 1978 as the major cause of antibiotic-associated diarrhea. Infant botulism was first recognized in 1976. Infant botulism occurs when children a year old or younger eat food contaminated with the spores of *C. botulinum*.

Demographics

C. BOTULINUM. *C. botulinum* is found in soils around the world, and its spores often find their way into foods. In the United States, about 116 cases of botulism food poisoning are reported each year. About four-fifths are cases of infant botulism. Of the remaining 20%, many occur in outbreaks resulting from contaminated foods served at restaurants, banquet halls, or other venues, or from home-canned foods that were improperly prepared. Anyone is susceptible to botulism food poisoning.

C. DIFFICILE. *C. difficile* has been mainly associated with older people who have taken **antibiotics** and are receiving care in hospitals, or in nursing homes and other long-term care facilities, although it is becoming more common in individuals who have had no hospital stays. Because of its connection to healthcare facilities, C. diff is known as a healthcare-associated infection. The U.S. **Centers for Disease Control and Prevention (CDC)** credits C. diff with about 337,000 reported cases and 14,000 deaths annually. A 2012 Mayo Clinic study noted that the number of C. diff infections has been rising in recent years. According to the study, the incidence of infections in children jumped from 2.6 cases per 100,000 in the period 1991–1997 to 32.6 cases per 100,000 from the period 2004–2009.

C. PERFRINGENS. *C. perfringens* is the second-leading bacterial cause of foodborne illness in the United States (behind *Salmonella* food poisoning), and results in approximately 966,000 cases of food poisoning each year. Outbreaks may occur when contaminated food is distributed to the public through grocery stores, restaurants, or other venues.

In some cases, a more dangerous illness, called enteritis necroticans, may arise. Rare in the United States, enteritis necroticans mainly occurs in developing countries. It causes an estimated 26 deaths per year in the United States.

C. TETANI. *C. tetani* produces a toxin that causes tetanus, a dangerous condition that can be fatal. About three to four dozen reports of tetanus occur annually in the United States, and all of them are among individuals who lack up-to-date tetanus vaccinations (including regular booster vaccinations). Tetanus occurs more often among persons 60 years old and older, among individuals who are Hispanic, among those who have diabetes, and among those who use injection drugs.

Neonatal tetanus is a particular problem in developing countries where deliveries may be carried out in non-hygienic conditions. Newborns and their mothers (who have not been properly immunized) are at risk for infection through the cut umbilical cord. Neonatal tetanus is rare in the United States.

Causes and symptoms

CAUSES. Botulism food poisoning occurs when a person eats food that has been contaminated with *C. botulinum* (often by its spores), or that contains neurotoxin that the bacteria has already produced. Botulism often results from improper food handling, preparation, cooking, or storage. Rarely, botulism may also result from two other types of bacteria: *C. baratii* or *C. butyricum*.

C. diff infections are typically associated with antibiotic use and with stays in hospitals or long-term care facilities. Two 2012 Mayo Clinic studies, however, noted an increase in the number of C. diff infections that were "community-acquired," meaning that the patients had not been hospitalized for at least four weeks prior to contracting the infection. One study reported that 40% of C. diff infections were community-acquired. The other reported a higher incidence—75%—of community-acquired C. diff infections among children. Beyond antibiotic use, other individuals who are more susceptible for C. diff infections include persons who have used chemotherapy drugs or other medications that weaken the immune system, who have had surgery recently, or who have previously had pseudomembranous colitis (an infection of the colon).

Infections with *C. perfringens* result from the ingestion of contaminated food. Although proper cooking kills most of the bacteria in foods, the bacterial spores can survive. If food is not stored promptly and properly, these spores can germinate and the resulting new bacteria can multiply to levels that can lead to food poisoning.

Infections with *C. tetani* usually occur when the bacteria, which is present in the soil, enters the body through a cut, deep puncture, or other wound on the skin. Individuals who are up to date on their tetanus vaccinations experience no problems, but those who are not properly immunized can develop an infection and the ensuing illness called tetanus.

Symptoms

Botulism is a potentially life-threatening neuroparalytic illness. Generally, symptoms begin 18–36 hours after eating contaminated food, but in some cases symptoms may begin as early as six hours after exposure, or as late as 10 days after eating the contaminated food. Symptoms may include: double or blurred vision, slurred speech, difficulty swallowing, and muscle weakness. One of the primary symptoms of infant botulism is lethargy. Babies seem weak, have little interest in feeding, cry feebly, have poor muscle tone, and appear tired. Left untreated, all cases of botulism—infant or otherwise—can progress to paralysis of the limbs, trunk, and respiratory muscles.

The bacterium *C. difficile* is the primary cause of infectious diarrhea among hospitalized patients. Symptoms of C. diff infection include: watery diarrhea (often occurring several times per day), urge to have a bowel movement, abdominal cramps, abdominal tenderness, fever, blood in the stool, nausea, appetite and weight loss, and dehydration.

C. perfringens infection is food-borne, and symptoms usually begin about 16 hours after eating. The infection has two forms: a milder one that causes gastroenteritis, and a more serious one that causes enteritis necroticans. The gastroenteritis-related infection has symptoms of watery diarrhea and mild abdominal cramps that typically last no more than 24 hours. (Symptoms may last longer in infants and in individuals who are elderly.) The symptoms of enteritis necroticans include abdominal **pain**, bloated belly, diarrhea that may be bloody, nausea, and the presence of abnormal structures known as pseudomembranes on the surface of the colon or rectum.

In addition to food-borne illness, *C. perfringens* may infect wounds, including surgical incisions, and cause gas gangrene. Symptoms of gas gangrene infections are typically sudden and worsen rapidly. They include pain and the presence of an air pocket beneath the skin at the site of the wound; brownish-red blisters; odorous discharge; fever; and jaundice. Left untreated, gas gangrene can progress to coma and death.

Tetanus, which results from infection with *C. tetani*, is a dangerous condition that causes muscles fibers to contract. Tetanus is also known as lockjaw (trismus), because some of the first skeletal muscles to noticeably spasm are those of the jaw. Muscle contractions can be sudden, powerful, and painful, and may result in muscle tears and even bone fractures. Death results, often from respiratory failure, in about 10–20% of individuals who develop tetanus.

Diagnosis

Medical professionals use patient history, including a review of recently eaten foods, and an evaluation of symptoms to help diagnose botulism food poisoning. They may also order tests to rule out other illnesses that have similar symptoms associated with them, or may order tests to analyze blood, stool, or vomit for evidence of the bacterial toxin to confirm a diagnosis.

To diagnose C. diff, medical professionals may conduct immunoassays that can identify the bacteria in the stool, or other highly sensitive tests to confirm the presence of the bacteria. A colonoscopy or sigmoidoscopy may also detect signs of infection through the presence of pseudomembranes on the rectum or colon.

For *C. perfringens* food poisoning, medical professionals may order laboratory tests that can check the feces to detect the toxin, or can identify an abnormally large number of the bacteria spores.

The diagnosis of tetanus is based on a combination of a physical exam; appearance of muscle spasms, stiffness, and pain indicative of the illness; a review of a patient's **immunization** history; and patient reports of recent wounds.

Prevention

For most types of *Clostridium*-caused food poisoning, the best way to avoid infection is through proper food handling and cooking of foods. People who engage in home canning should be sure to read and follow instructions to ensure that their canned goods are safe. Prompt storage of cooked foods is also important to prevent food poisoning.

To help avoid infant botulism, the U.S. Food and Drug Administration, the **Centers for Disease Control and Prevention**, and the American Academy of Pediatrics all recommend that honey be eliminated from the diets of infants. This reason is that *C. botulinum* often exists as spores that may be present in honey. Once ingested, the spores can germinate, reproduce and lead to the production of toxins inside the baby's intestinal tract, and cause serious illness.

Methods to prevent the C. diff infection include avoiding individuals who have a C. diff infection; frequent and thorough washing of hands with soap and **water**; and cleaning of contaminated surfaces. The latter hygienic precautions are especially important within healthcare facilities, as well as in homes in which an infected person is residing. Individuals should also avoid the overuse of antibiotics, especially those of the broad-spectrum variety. This is because the overuse of antibiotics eliminates the easier-to-kill bacteria, and provides a competition-free environment where antibiotic-resistant bacteria can flourish.

A vaccine is available for tetanus. It is often combined with vaccines for **diphtheria** and/or pertussis. The vaccines are known as DTaP, Tdap, DT, and Td. Specific vaccines are given to individuals at different stages of their lives. For instance, children receive five does of DTap, four of them by the time they reach 18 months old, and one more between the ages of 4–6 years old. Td is a booster shot for adolescents and adults, and is administered at 10-year intervals.

Treatment

Botulism treatment varies depending on the severity of symptoms. Medical professionals may induce vomiting or administer enemas to more speedily remove contaminated food from the digestive system. Patients may also receive injected antitoxin that eliminates further impact from the botulism toxin. For more severe cases, patients may require a ventilator to help them breathe, as well as additional intensive medical and nursing care, often over an extended period of time, to recover.

Treatment for C. diff infections may begin with a review of the patient's current medication regimen, and possible elimination or replacement of some medications. One often-used treatment drug is metronidazole (Flagyl), an antibiotic to help to fight the infection.

Treatment for *C. perfringens* includes rehydration, usually with fluids administered by mouth. In severe cases, patients may receive fluids as well as electrolyte replacement intravenously. Additional care may be necessary.

For tetanus, medical professionals may administer antitoxin to prevent further damage from the toxin, and antibiotics to fight the *C. tetani* bacteria. Additionally, if symptoms have progressed, doctors may prescribe sedatives, morphine, magnesium sulfate, beta blockers, or other medications to help with muscle spasms, and to treat respiration and heart issues. Patients with advanced symptoms typically require many months of intensive care, possibly including the use of a ventilator.

Prognosis

Infections with *Clostridium* bacteria range from mild to severe. With most cases of *Clostridium*-caused food poisoning, individuals recover within a day or so. The more severe infections may require medical attention possibly including hospital care, and some fatalities do occur.

About 10-20% of individuals who have tetanus die from the illness. C. diff infections can be severe, and result in about 14,000 deaths annually in the United States.

Effects on public health

Foodborne botulism can become a public health emergency because outbreaks can and do occur, frequently as a result of improperly home-canned foods. If these foods are served at a restaurant or large gathering, many people can become seriously ill.

C. diff infections are becoming a growing concern. Originally, the infections appeared to be mainly confined to healthcare facilities, but reports in 2012 indicated that the infections may also occur outside these locations. The typically affected individual is one who is taking antibiotics. These bacteria are antibiotic-resistant, and therefore difficult to treat. According to the **CDC**, deaths related to C. diff increased 400% between 2000 and 2007, and that was due in part to a more-resistant strain of the bacteria. In addition, C. diff infections spread quickly, which is a particular issue for healthcare facilities.

Infection with *C. perfringens* is a public-health concern because it is one of the most common causes of foodborne illness in the United States, affecting nearly one million people per year.

In 1988, the **World Health Organization (WHO)** put the number of deaths from neonatal tetanus worldwide at 787,000. The majority of the fatalities occurred in developing countries, where often-unhygienic conditions present during delivery led to infections with *C. tetani*, and medical care was lacking for babies who developed neonatal tetanus.

Costs to society

For all foodborne illnesses, the cost in medical expenses and lost productivity totals about $5–6 billion per year. *C. perfringens* poisoning is the second leading cause of reported foodborne illnesses in the United States, accounting for about 969,000 cases each year. Fortunately, the mortality rate for *C. perfringens* food poisoning is low. In contrast, botulism poisoning is rare in the United States, but the mortality rate is high if it is left untreated.

C. diff infections are costly. According to a study reported in a 2012 issue of *Clinical Microbiology and Infection*, the annual economic burden in the United States of C. diff infections is at least $796 million.

KEY TERMS

Colonoscopy—A medical procedure that allows a doctor to examine the interior lining of the rectum and colon for abnormalities. It is typically used as a screening test for colon cancer.

Gas Gangrene—A potentially fatal form of gangrene (tissue death) caused by a bacterial infection. Gas gangrene usually occurs at the site of a wound, including a surgical incision.

Immunoassay—A laboratory test that uses an antigen-antibody response to determine the presence of a bacterium or other substance in a patient sample.

Sigmoidoscopy—A medical procedure that allows a doctor to examine the interior lining of the lower part of the colon and rectum. It provides a less-complete view of the colon than a colonoscopy does.

Efforts and solutions

FOOD POISONING. As of 2012, the national Food Safe Families public-service campaign—an effort of the Ad Council, the U.S. Department of Agriculture's **Food Safety** and Inspection Service, the U.S. Food and Drug Administration (FDA), and the CDC—was continuing to raise awareness about the risks of food poisoning, and to provide education about reducing or eliminating those risks through proper food-handling methods. In addition, the CDC is always on the lookout for food-poisoning outbreaks. When one occurs, it goes to work to track the origin of the contaminated food and limit its spread, and to provide announcements as necessary to help keep the general public safe.

C. DIFF. In the United States, the Emerging Infections Program (part of the National Center for Emerging and Zoonotic Infectious Diseases) is monitoring the incidence of C. diff infections to determine the scope of illness and trends over time; to identify the proportion of infections that are associated with medical care, including the use of specific antibiotics; and to determine which strains of the bacteria are causing the most illness. State agencies are assisting the effort by tracking C. diff infections in their states and reporting the data to the CDC's National Healthcare Safety Network. In addition, the CDC recommends that healthcare facilities utilize approved spore-killing disinfectants in rooms where patients with C. diff infections have stayed; and notify other healthcare facilities when they are transferring any C. diff patients to them.

QUESTIONS TO ASK YOUR DOCTOR

- When was my last tetanus shot? Do I need a booster?
- When should my child get the initial tetanus vaccine?
- My child has been sick. Should he still get a tetanus vaccine now?
- My child had a bad reaction to the initial tetanus vaccine. Should she still get the next scheduled tetanus shot?
- I am going into the hospital for surgery. Should I take any precautions to help me avoid C. diff infection?
- Is this prescribed antibiotic necessary? Is it making me more susceptible to antibiotic-resistant bacteria?

TETANUS. Following WHO's estimation of 787,000 neonatal-tetanus deaths per year, WHO's decision-making body (the World Health Association) along with the United Nations Children's Fund (UNICEF) and the United Nations **Population** Fund (UNFPA) took action. In 1989, they set a goal of eliminating maternal and neonatal tetanus. The elimination program is called the Maternal and Neonatal Tetanus (MNT) Elimination Initiative. Since then, the number of deaths had dropped to 59,000 in 2008 (the latest data available). The initiative is still active, especially in the 34 countries that had not eliminated MNT as of 2012.

Resources

BOOKS

Center for Food Safety and Applied Nutrition, U.S. Food and Drug Administration, U.S. Department of Health and Human Services. *Bad Bug Book: Foodborne Pathogenic Microorganisms and Natural Toxins Handbook.* 2nd ed., 2012. Published online at http://www.fda.gov/downloads/Food/FoodSafety/FoodborneIllness/FoodborneIllnessFoodbornePathogensNaturalToxins/BadBugBook/UCM297627.pdf (accessed September 4, 2012).

PERIODICALS

Khanna, Sahil. "The Epidemiology of Community-Acquired *Clostridium difficile* Infection: A Population-Based Study." *American Journal of Gastroenterology—Drug Targets.* 107, no. 1 (2012): 89–95.

S. M. McGlone, et al. "The Economic Burden of *Clostridium difficile*." *Clinical Microbiology and Infection.* 18, no. 3 (2012): 282–289.

WEBSITES

Burnham, Ted. "Dangerous Gut Bacteria Move Outside Hospitals, Infect Kids." National Public Radio. http://www.npr.org/blogs/health/2012/05/22/153314338/dangerous-gut-bacteria-move-outside-hospitals-infect-kids (accessed September 4, 2012).

"*Clostridium*." Medical Microbiology Site, Center for Environmental Health and Safety, Southern Illinois University Carbondale.http://www.cehs.siu.edu/fix/medmicro/clost.htm (accessed September 4, 2012).

"*Clostridium botulinum*". Fact Sheets, Foodborne Illness and Disease. Food Safety and Inspection Service, U.S. Department of Agriculture. http://www.fsis.usda.gov/FACTSheets/Clostridium_botulinum/index.asp (accessed September 4, 2012) (accessed September 4, 2012).

"*Clostridium difficile* Infection." U.S. Centers for Disease Control and Prevention. http://www.cdc.gov/hai/organisms/cdiff/cdiff_infect.html (accessed September 4, 2012) (accessed August 29, 2012).

Kendall, P. "Botulism." Colorado State University Extension.http://www.ext.colostate.edu/pubs/foodnut/09305.html (accessed September 4, 2012).

"Maternal and Neonatal Tetanus (MNT) Elimination." World Health Organization. http://www.who.int/immunization_monitoring/diseases/MNTE_initiative/en/index.html (accessed September 4, 2012).

"Tetanus." MedLinePlus, U.S. National Library of Medicine, National Institutes of Health. http://www.nlm.nih.gov/medlineplus/tetanus.html (accessed September 4, 2012).

ORGANIZATIONS

Centers for Disease Control and Prevention (CDC), 1600 Clifton Road, Atlanta, GA 30333, (800) 232-4636, cdcinfo@cdc.gov, http://www.cdc.gov

Food Safety and Inspection Service, U.S. Department of Agriculture, 1400 Independence Avenue, S.W., Washington, DC 20250-3700, (888) 674-6854, MPHotline.fsis@usda.gov, http://www.fsis.usda.gov/Home/index.asp.

Leslie Mertz, Ph.D.

Coal worker's pneumoconiosis *see* **Black lung disease**

Common cold

Definition

The common cold is a viral infection of the upper respiratory system, including the nose, throat, sinuses, eustachian tubes, trachea, larynx, and bronchial tubes. Although more than 200 different viruses can cause a cold, 30–50% are caused by a group known as rhinoviruses. Almost all colds clear up in less than two weeks without complications.

Common cold remedies and side effects

	Symptoms	Side effects
Antihistamines	Congestion Itchy eyes Runny nose Sneezing Stuffy nose	Drowsiness Dry mouth and eyes
Decongestants	Congestion Stuffy nose	Insomnia Rapid heartbeat Stimulation

(Table by PreMediaGlobal. © 2013 Cengage Learning)

Description

Colds, sometimes called rhinovirus or coronavirus infections, are the most common illness to strike any part of the body. It is estimated that the average person has more than 50 colds during a lifetime. Anyone can get a cold, although pre-school and grade-school children catch them more frequently than adolescents and adults. Repeated exposure to viruses causing colds creates partial immunity.

Although most colds resolve on their own without complications, they are a leading cause of visits to the doctor and of time lost from work and school. Treating symptoms of the common cold has given rise to a multimillion dollar industry in over-the-counter medications.

Cold season in the United States begins in early autumn and extends through early spring. Although it is not true that getting wet or being in a draft causes a cold (a person has to come in contact with the virus to catch a cold), certain conditions may lead to increased susceptibility. These include:

- fatigue and overwork
- emotional stress
- poor nutrition
- smoking
- living or working in crowded conditions

Colds make the upper respiratory system less resistant to bacterial infection. Secondary bacterial infection may lead to middle ear infection, bronchitis, **pneumonia**, sinus infection, or strep throat. People with chronic lung disease, **asthma**, diabetes, or a weakened immune system are more likely to develop these complications.

Causes and symptoms

Colds are caused by more than 200 different viruses. The most common groups are rhinoviruses and coronaviruses. Different groups of viruses are more infectious at different seasons of the year, but knowing the exact virus causing the cold is not important in treatment.

People with colds are contagious during the first two to four days of the infection. Colds pass from person to person in several ways. When an infected person coughs, sneezes, or speaks, tiny fluid droplets containing the virus are expelled. If these are breathed in by other people, the virus may establish itself in their noses and airways.

Colds may also be passed through direct contact. If a person with a cold touches his runny nose or watery eyes, then shakes hands with another person, some of the virus is transferred to the uninfected person. If that person then touches his mouth, nose, or eyes, the virus is transferred to an environment where it can reproduce and cause a cold.

Finally, cold viruses can be spread through inanimate objects (e.g., door knobs, telephones, toys) that become contaminated with the virus. This is a common method of transmission in child care centers. If a child with a cold touches her runny nose, then plays with a toy, some of the virus may be transferred to the toy. When another child plays with the toy a short time later, he may pick up some of the virus on his hands. The second child then touches his contaminated hands to his eyes, nose, or mouth and transfers some of the cold virus to himself.

Once acquired, the cold virus attaches itself to the lining of the nasal passages and sinuses. This causes the infected cells to release a chemical called histamine. Histamine increases the blood flow to the infected cells, causing swelling, congestion, and increased mucus production. Within one to three days, the infected person begins to show cold symptoms.

The first cold symptoms are a tickle in the throat, runny nose, and sneezing. The initial discharge from the nose is clear and thin. Later, it changes to a thick yellow or greenish discharge. Most adults do not develop a fever when they catch a cold. Young children may develop a low fever of up to 102°F (38.9°C).

In addition to a runny nose and fever, signs of a cold include coughing, sneezing, nasal congestion, headache, muscle ache, chills, sore throat, hoarseness, watery eyes, fatigue, and lack of appetite. The cough that accompanies a cold is usually intermittent and dry.

Most people begin to feel better four to five days after their cold symptoms become noticeable. All symptoms are generally gone within ten days, except for a dry cough that may linger for up to three weeks.

Colds make people more susceptible to bacterial infections such as strep throat, middle-ear infections, and sinus infections. A person whose cold does not begin to improve within a week; or who experiences chest **pain**,

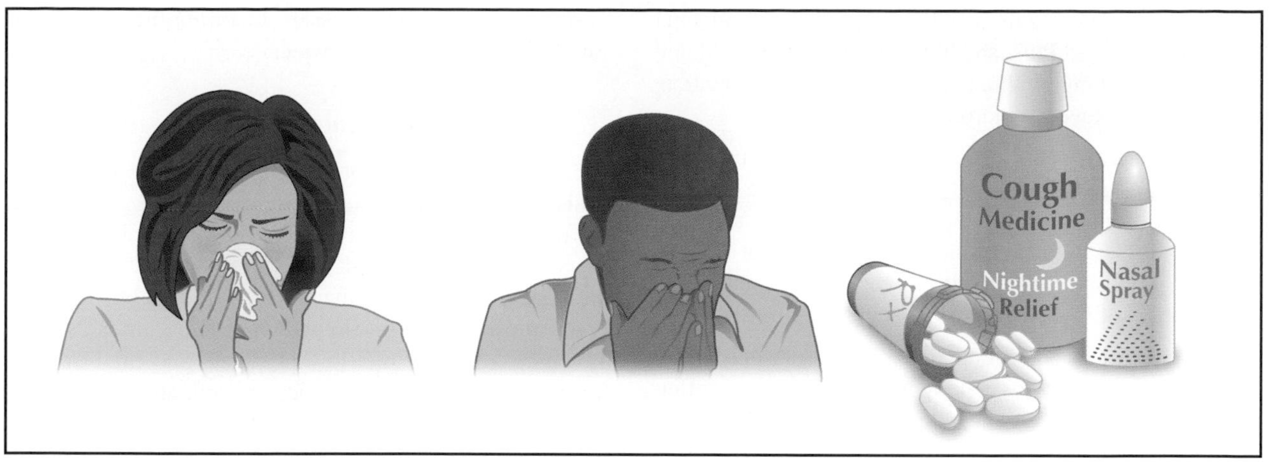

(Illustration by Electronic Illustrators Group. © 2013 Cengage Learning)

fever for more than a few days, difficulty breathing, bluish lips or fingernails, a cough that brings up greenish-yellow or grayish sputum, skin rash, swollen glands, or whitish spots on the tonsils or throat should consult a doctor to see whether he or she has acquired a secondary bacterial infection that needs to be treated with an antibiotic.

People who have emphysema, chronic lung disease, diabetes, or a weakened immune system—either from diseases such as **AIDS** or leukemia, or as the result of medications, (e.g., corticosteroids, chemotherapy drugs)—should consult their doctor if they get a cold. People with these health problems are more likely to get a secondary infection.

Diagnosis

Colds are diagnosed by observing a person's symptoms. There are no laboratory tests readily available to detect the cold virus. However, a doctor may do a throat culture or blood test to rule out a secondary infection.

Influenza is sometimes confused with a cold, but flu causes much more severe symptoms and generally a fever. **Allergies** to molds or pollens also can make the nose run. Allergies are usually more persistent than the common cold. An allergist can run tests to determine whether the cold-like symptoms are being caused by an allergic reaction. Some people get a runny nose when they go outside in winter and breathe cold air. This type of runny nose is not a symptom of a cold.

Treatment

There are no medicines that will cure the common cold. Given time, the body's immune system will make antibodies to fight the infection, and the cold will be resolved without any intervention. **Antibiotics** are useless against a cold. However, a great deal of money is spent by pharmaceutical companies in the United States promoting products designed to relieve cold symptoms. These products usually contain antihistamines, decongestants, and/or pain relievers.

Antihistamines block the action of the chemical histamine that is produced when the cold virus invades the cells lining the nasal passages. Histamine increases blood flow and causes the cells to swell. Antihistamines are taken to relieve the symptoms of sneezing, runny nose, itchy eyes, and congestion. Side effects are dry mouth and drowsiness, especially with the first few doses. Antihistamines should not be taken by people who are driving or operating dangerous equipment. Some people have allergic reactions to antihistamines. Common over-the-counter antihistamines include Chlor-Trimeton, Dimetapp, Tavist, and Actifed. The generic name for two common antihistamines are chlorpheniramine and diphenhydramine.

Decongestants work to constrict the blood flow to the vessels in the nose. This can shrink the tissue, reduce congestion, and open inflamed nasal passages, making breathing easier. Decongestants can make people feel jittery or keep them from sleeping. They should not be used by people with **heart disease**, high blood pressure, or glaucoma. Some common decongestants are Neo-Synepherine, Novafed, and Sudafed. The generic names of common decongestants include phenylephrine, phenylpropanolamine, and pseudoephedrine, and in nasal sprays, naphazoline, oxymetazoline, and xylometazoline.

Many over-the-counter medications are combinations of both antihistamines and decongestants; an ache and pain reliever, such as acetaminophen (Datril, Tylenol, Panadol) or ibuprofen (Advil, Nuprin, Motrin, Medipren); and a cough suppressant (dextromethorphan). Common combination medications include Tylenol Cold and Flu, Triaminic, Sudafed Plus, and Tavist D. Aspirin should not be given to children with a cold because of its association with a risk of Reye's syndrome, a serious disease.

Nasal sprays and nose drops are other products promoted for reducing nasal congestion. These usually contain a decongestant, but the decongestant can act more quickly and strongly than ones found in pills or liquids because it is applied directly in the nose. Congestion returns after a few hours.

People can become dependent on nasal sprays and nose drops. If used for a long time, users may suffer withdrawal symptoms when these products are discontinued. Nasal sprays and nose drops should not be used for more than a few days. The label lists recommendations on length and frequency of use.

In 2004, scientists reported the possibility of a new oral drug for use in relieving common cold symptoms. Called pleconaril, it inhibited viral replication in at least 90% of rhinoviruses if taken within 24 hours of onset.

People react differently to different cold medications and may find some to be more helpful than others. A medication may be effective initially, then lose some of its effectiveness. Children sometimes react differently than adults. Over-the-counter cold remedies should not be given to infants without consulting a doctor first.

Care should be taken not to exceed the recommended dosages, especially when combination medications or nasal sprays are taken. Individuals should determine whether they wish to use any of these drugs. None of them shortens or cures a cold. At best, they help a person feel more comfortable. People who are confused about the drugs in any over-the-counter cold remedies should ask their pharmacist for an explanation.

In addition to the optional use of over the counter cold remedies, there are some self-care steps that people can take to ease their discomfort. These include:

- drinking plenty of fluids, but avoiding acidic juices, which may irritate the throat
- gargling with warm salt water—made by adding one teaspoon of salt to 8 oz of water—for a sore throat
- not smoking
- getting plenty of rest
- using a cool-mist room humidifier to ease congestion and sore throat
- rubbing Vaseline or other lubricant under the nose to prevent irritation from frequent nose blowing
- for babies too young to blow their noses, the mucus should be suctioned gently with an infant nasal aspirator. It may be necessary to soften the mucus first with a few drops of salt water.

Alternative treatment

Alternative practitioners emphasize that people get colds because their immune systems are weak. They point out that everyone is exposed to cold viruses, but that not everyone gets every cold. The difference seems to be in the ability of the immune system to fight infection. **Prevention** focuses on strengthening the immune system by eating a healthy diet low in sugars and high in fresh fruits and vegetables, practicing meditation to reduce **stress**, and getting regular moderate exercise.

Once cold symptoms appear, some naturopathic practitioners believe the symptoms should be allowed to run their course without interference. Others suggest the following:

- Inhaling a steaming mixture of lemon oil, thyme oil, eucalyptus, and tea tree oil (*Melaleuca* spp.). (Aromatherapy)
- Gargling with a mixture of water, salt, and turmeric powder or astringents such as alum, sumac, sage, and bayberry to ease a sore throat. (Ayurvedic medicine)
- Taking coneflower or goldenseal (*Hydrastis canadensis*). Other useful herbs to reduce symptoms include yarrow (*Achillea millefolium*), eyebright (*Euphrasia officinalis*), garlic (*Allium sativum*), and onions (*Allium cepa*). (Herbal)
- Microdoses of *Viscue album*, *Natrum muriaticum*, *Allium cepa*, or *Nux vomica*. (Homeopathy)
- Taking yin chiao (sometimes transliterated as yinquiao) tablets that contain honeysuckle and forsythia when symptoms appear. Natural herb loquat syrup for cough and sinus congestion and Chinese ephedra (*ma-huang*) for runny nose. (Chinese traditional medicine)
- The use of zinc lozenges every two hours along with high doses of vitamin C is suggested. Some practitioners also suggest eliminating dairy products for the duration of the cold. (Nutritional therapy).

The use of zinc lozenges may be moving toward acceptance by practitioners of traditional medicine. In 1996, the Cleveland Clinic tested zinc gluconate lozenges and found that using zinc in the first 24 hours after cold symptoms occurred shortened the duration of symptoms. The mechanism by which zinc worked was not clear, but additional studies are underway.

At one time, the herb (*Echinacea* spp.) was touted as a remedy to relieve cold symptoms. However, a study published in 2004 reported that the herb failed to relieve cold symptoms in 400 children taking it and caused skin rashes in some children.

KEY TERMS

Bronchial tubes—The major airways to the lungs and their main branches.

Coronavirus—A genus of viruses that cause respiratory disease and gastroenteritis.

Corticosteroids—A group of hormones produced naturally by the adrenal gland or manufactured synthetically. They are often used to treat inflammation. Examples include cortisone and prednisone.

Eustachian tube—A thin tube between the middle ear and the pharynx. Its purpose is to equalize pressure on either side of the eardrum.

Rhinovirus—A virus that infects the upper respiratory system and causes the common cold.

Prognosis

Given time, the body will make antibodies to cure itself of a cold. Most colds last a week to 10 days. Most people start feeling better within four or five days. Occasionally, a cold will lead to a secondary bacterial infection that causes strep throat, bronchitis, pneumonia, sinus infection, or a middle-ear infection. These conditions usually clear up rapidly when treated with an antibiotic.

Prevention

It is not possible to prevent colds because the viruses that cause colds are common and highly infectious. However, there are some steps that individuals can take to reduce their spread. These include:

- washing hands well and frequently, especially after touching the nose or before handling food
- covering the mouth and nose when sneezing
- disposing of used tissues properly
- avoiding close contact with someone who has a cold during the first two to four days of their infection
- not sharing food, eating utensils, or cups with anyone
- avoiding crowded places where cold germs can spread
- eating a healthy diet and getting adequate sleep

Costs to Society

The common cold is usually more of a nuisance than a formidable health threat, and as such, it is often dismissed. Though the common cold does not generally pose serious health risks, according to a study by the University of Michigan, this innocuous seasonal virus costs the United States approximately 40 billion dollars annually. This estimate includes costs associated with treatments for the illness and lost productivity. Additionally, the study estimates that the common cold results in 100 million annual doctor visits totalling at least 7.7 billion dollars.

Resources

PERIODICALS

Hagen, Carrie. "Economic impact of cold virus to be more expensive than asthma, heart failure." *The University Record Online.*http://www.ur.umich.edu/0203/Mar10_03/15.shtml. Accessed November 11, 2012.

"Study: Echinacea Is Ineffective." *Chain Drug Review* February 16, 2004: 25.

Zepf, Bill. "Pleconaril for Treatment of the Common Cold?" *American Family Physician* February 1, 2004: 703.

WEBSITES

Centers for Disease Control and Prevention. "Common Cold and Runny Nose." http://www.cdc.gov/getsmart/antibiotic-use/URI/colds.html Accessed November 12, 2012.

Tish Davidson, A.M.
Teresa G. Odle
Andrea Nienstedt, MA

Community development workers

Definition

One definition that has been proposed for the field of community development is that it constitutes a series of actions that make it possible for groups and networks of people to work together to take joint actions on matters that concern them for the public good.

Purpose

The purpose of community development is to provide the members of a local community an opportunity to work together, generally with the help of outside experts in the field, to identify common social, political, economic, and other problems faced by the community and then to develop programs and activities that will help with the solution of those problems.

Description

In one sense, community development activities have existed as long as human societies have existed in that people in almost all cases attempt to establish the structure and procedures that will produce the greatest good for the greatest number of individuals in a society. More formal community development programs can be traced, however, to the nineteenth century, when a number of utopian thinkers, such as Robert Owen, attempted to design new communities that were designed "from the ground up" to achieve these objectives. In the early twentieth century, similar efforts were made in parts of Africa by colonial rulers who wanted to modernize and make more efficient the native communities for which they had become responsible. In the United States, community development first became widely popular in the 1960s with efforts to renew run–down urban areas that had become virtually unlivable for inhabitants. Today, the term *community development* refers to activities directed at the improvement of both urban and rural communities, although the methodologies used in each case are somewhat different from each other.

In the most general sense, community development involves a series of steps that usually begins with a group of interested individuals coming together to attack a perceived problem about a specific community, such as a town in rural Africa or a deteriorated neighborhood in downtown Chicago. The individuals involved in this activity include both residents of the community and individuals from outside the community with some specialized knowledge in dealing with community problems. The outside individuals may be highly trained experts with college training in the field or volunteers who join a program with little or no previous training, and individuals who fall anywhere between these two extremes. The first stage in a community development program consists of identifying the problems that the community development team hopes to solve. The team next reviews the assets and resources available within the community that can be brought to bear in dealing with these problems. Outside experts may then help local participants to develop the knowledge and skills they will need in using their resources to attack community problems. Finally, the community development team will attempt to lay out a plan of attack that will make progress in dealing with the problems it has identified. At the conclusion of these actions, efforts are usually made to evaluate the success of the program and to suggest future efforts to maintain the progress that has been made or to design additional efforts at dealing with other community problems. A successful community development program involves not only the solution of specific community problems, but also the development of personal skills, such as leadership, cooperation, initiative, and participation, that will strengthen the community overall.

Community development workers come from a very wide diversity of backgrounds. Some institutions of higher education now offer courses or degrees in community development that provide an individual with deep and broad experience in the issues faced in community development programs. The University of Alaska at Fairbanks, for example, offers a master's degree in community development that prepares individuals to work in both rural and urban settings. Other community development workers come to the field with backgrounds in other areas, such as sociology, nursing, economics, medicine, or information technology (a field of growing value in many community development programs). Many men and women with no experience at all in community development also volunteer to work in the field and receive the preparation they need in specialized courses on–site or even through on–the–job training on–site. Among the skills that community development workers require, no matter their level of training, are the ability to communicate clearly with others (which involves listening as well as talking), knowing how to build organizations and networks, understanding how to evaluate the results of an activity or program, being able to mediate between individuals, appreciating and taking advantage of cross–cultural and other differences among individuals, patience and flexibility, and understanding how communities can make use of the resources they have to solve their problems.

Resources

BOOKS

DeFilippis, James, and Susan Segert. *The Community Development Reader*. New York: Routledge, 2008.

Robinson, Jerry W., and Gary P. Green. *Introduction to Community Development: Theory, Practice, and Service-learning*. Los Angeles: SAGE, 2011.

PERIODICALS

McArdle, Karen. "What Makes a Successful Rural Regeneration Partnership? The Views of Successful Partners and the Importance of Ethos for the Community Development Professional." *Community Development*. 43. 3. (2012): 333–345.

Matarrita-Cascante, David, and Mark A. Brennan. "Conceptualizing Community Development in the Twenty-first Century." *Community Development*. 43. 3. (2012): 293–305.

WEBSITES

Community Development Alliance (Scotland). http://www.iacdglobal.org/files/WhatCommunityDevelopmentDoes.pdf (accessed October 10, 2012).

Community Development Careers. http://www.kelloggforum.org/community-development-careers/. (accessed October 10, 2012).

Training for Rural Community Development Activities in Rural United Kingdom and Ireland. http://www.iacdglobal.org/files/rpt190406RuralTrainingForCommunityDevelopmentActivists.pdf. (accessed October 10, 2012).

ORGANIZATIONS

National Community Development Association (NCDA), 522 21st St., N.W., #120, Washington, DC 20006, (202) 293-7587, Fax: (202) 887-5546, ncda@ncdaonline.org, http://www.ncdaonline.org/.

David E. Newton, EdD

Community health

Definition

Community health is that field of public health whose purpose it is to identify and solve public health problems, such as the spread of disease, and to provide for the general well–being of members of the community.

Purpose

The purpose of a community health program is to provide mechanisms by which professionals in the field of public health can work with members of the community to initiate and sustain programs and activities that contribute to the maintenance of good health practices for individuals of all ages. This objective includes not only providing essential health procedures for members of the community, but also maintaining a program of information and education about current best practices in the field of public health.

Description

Beyond its more general definition given above, the term *community health* often has a more specific meaning as a program or series of activities that attempts to meet the health needs of low–income families and individuals, those who lack medical insurance, or other vulnerable adults and children. In Great Britain, the first community health centers were established by the Public Health Act of 1848. In addition to establishing the community health centers, the act also established the General Board of Health, the first such institution in the world, with the task of overseeing and administering public health policies and practices throughout the nation. The act also provided for the collection of public health data which recorded information on a number of health variables, most importantly the incidence and prevalence of communicable diseases. In the United States, the federal government first became involved with community health as part of the so–called War on **Poverty** of the 1960s. In 1967, the administration of President Lyndon Johnson established the first two community health clinics (then called neighborhood health clinics) in Boston, Massachusetts, and Mound Bayou, Mississippi, for the purpose of providing health care to otherwise underserved communities. The federal community health program gradually expanded over time until, as of late 2012, there were more than 1,150 community health centers in the United States serving more than 17 million adults and children. These centers are located in areas where individuals are unable to get adequate primary health care because of geographical, financial, cultural, language, or other reasons. In order to qualify for federal funding, a community health center must:

- be located in a medically underserved area (MUA) or serve a medically underserved population (MUP)
- have a nonprofit, public, or tax–exempt status
- provide comprehensive primary health care with the availability of referrals to specialized care
- have a governing board, the majority of which consists of clients of the center
- provide service to anyone who needs and requests it without regard to their income

Some examples of the types of services typically offered by a community health service include:

- diagnosis and treatment of illness
- health screenings, such as mammographies and prostate screenings
- immunizations
- family planning and contraceptive advice
- management of chronic diseases, such as diabetes and asthma
- prenatal care
- dental programs
- behavioral health programs

To a large extent, the United States followed the British example with regard to the creation of boards of health. During the first three decades of the nineteenth century, only five cities had such boards, organized to provide general guidance for the maintenance of good health practices among citizens, especially those with low income, the unemployed, or immigrants. The establishment of the New York Metropolitan Board of Health in 1866, however, provided a stimulus for the creation of similar bodies throughout the United States, with new boards being established in nine states and the District of Columbia over the next decade. To a large extent, the growth of the concept of boards of health was based on the influx of immigrants who often had little or no access to even the most basic of health care services.

Today, boards of health at the state, county or parish, and local levels have general responsibility for all public health issues for their localities. The responsibilities include the setting of health care policy for the region in addition to providing for a host of specific programs that may include administration of animal bite programs, beekeeping inspection programs, inspection of **water** quality, issuing of birth and death certificates, breast **cancer** screeing programs, collection and analysis of health data, provision of contraceptives and contraceptive information, inspection and approval of child care facilities, promotion of farm to fork food programs, administration of **immunization** programs, provision of **food safety** education courses, provision of HIV testing services, administration of mosquito control efforts, surveillance for indoor pollution problems, and inspection of restaurants and other food outlets, to mention only a selection of all possible responsibilities.

A key element of the community health program for any state, county, town, or city is the community health survey. Many governmental units conduct such surveys on a regular basis, every year, two years, three years, or the like. Board of health or other decision–making bodies use the results of these surveys to establish, modify, or revise strategic health care plans for the region, shifting resources to health areas for which there appears to be greater need or demand. The specifics of community health surveys differ from locality to locality, but generally include questions about topics such as:

- demographics (age, education, employment, income, ethnicity, etc.)
- reported physical health status
- mental health status
- chronic health conditions
- weight (overweight and obesity)
- physical activity
- diet and nutrition
- health insurance status
- prescription use
- access to health care
- seat belt use
- tobacco use
- alcohol use
- use of illegal drugs
- vaccination status
- screenings for cancer and other diseases
- HIV/AIDS status
- contraceptive use

Professional publications

In the United States, funding for community health centers is provided by the Health Resources and Services Administration (HRSA) of the **Department of Health and Human Services**. HRSA provides a directory of available community health services at its interactive website at http://findahealthcenter.hrsa.gov/Search_HCC.aspx. The professional organization of community health centers is the National Association of Community Health Centers (NACHC), which also provides links to its state members at its website at http://www.nachc.com/nachc-pca-listing.cfm.

Resources

BOOKS

Hansen, Melissa. *Community Health Centers*. Denver: National Conference of State Legislatures, 2011.

Hing, Esther, and Roderick S. Hooker. *Community Health Centers: Providers, Patients, and Content of Care*. Hyattsville, MD: Centers for Disease Control. National Center for Health Statistics, 2011.

Lefkowitz, Bonnie. *Community Health Centers: A Movement and the People Who Made It Happen*. New Brunswick, NJ: Rutgers University Press, 2007.

PERIODICALS

Dievler, A., and T. Giovannini. "Community Health Centers: Promise and Performance." *Medical Care Research and Review*. 55. 4. (1998): 405–31

Fertig, A. R., P. S. Corson, and D. Balasubramaniam. "Benefits and Costs of a Free Community-based Primary Care Clinic."*Journal of Health and Human Services Administration*. 34. 4. (2012): 456–70.

Gurewich, D., et al. "Achieving Excellence in Community Health Centers: Implications for Health Reform." *Journal of Health Care for the Poor and Underserved*. 23. 1. (2012): 446–59.

WEBSITES

Taylor, Jessamy. "The Fundamentals of Community Health Centers." http://www.nhpf.org/library/background-papers/BP_CHC_08-31-04.pdf (accessed October 10, 2012).

"What Is a Health Center?"Health Resources and Services Administration. http://bphc.hrsa.gov/about/ (accessed October 10, 2012).

ORGANIZATIONS

National Association of Community Health Centers (NACHC), 7501 Wisconsin Ave., Suite 1100W, Bethesda, MD 20814, (301) 347-0400, http://www.nachc.com/contact-us.cfm, http://www.nachc.com/.

David E. Newton, EdD

Community health assessment

Definition

The National Association of County & City Health Officials (**NACCHO**) defines **community health** assessment (CHA) as "a process that uses quantitative and qualitative methods to systematically collect and analyze data to understand health within a specific community."

Purpose

The purpose of a community health assessment procedure is to determine the current status of health conditions within a community, a process that makes it possible then to identify and prioritize specific health issues, to recognize the resources available for dealing with those issues and to develop a program for solving critical health problems.

Description

For nearly a century, the public health community in the United States has been struggling to better articulate its basic mission and the strategies needed for accomplishing this mission. One of the most important documents in that long struggle was a 1988 report prepared by the Committee for the Study of the Future of Public Health of the Institute of Medicine (IOM). That report was issued in the form of a book, *The Future of Public Health*, whose fundamental premise was that public health activities rely on three fundamental elements: assessment, policy development, and assurance. Later reports from IOM and other committees described in more detail the meaning of these terms and how they could be used to drive public health policies and practices. In the ensuing decades, public health experts have been working to refine and develop the concept of community health assessment.

As a consequence of this effort, various public health authorities and agencies use the term *community health assessment* in somewhat different ways. In general, however, there appear to be certain common themes in most interpretations of the phrase. The CHA developed by the State of New York Department of Health contains most of these themes in its ten-step approach to community health assessment projets. Those steps are as follows:

- Creation of the assessment team, which involves identifying the individuals who will be part of the team and obtaining commitments from them for their participation;
- Identifying and securing resources, which includes identifying and securing financial resources needed to conduct the project;
- Identifying and engaging community partners, which extends to every corner of the community, including corporations, parents, students, nonprofit agencies, governmental bodies, and health care professionals;
- Collecting, analyzing, and presenting data, which is generally available from a variety of sources, including local, county, state, and federal public and non-public organizations and agencies;
- Setting health priorities, which also includes developing a protocol by which such priorities can be established;
- Clarifying the issue, which involves developing and testing hypotheses about possible causes and contributing factors for the health issue under consideration;
- Setting goals and objectives, a process that should include consideration and adaptation of existing goals and objectives set by other federal and state agencies, along with specific performance-based methods of measuring achievement of those goals and objectives;
- Choosing strategies, a process that should also draw on previous experiences of other public health agencies, as well as the development of a system of evaluation for

KEY TERMS

Community—All those individuals within a geographical area with common social, cultural, racial, religious, socioeconomic, and other characteristics.

Community partnerships—All of those relationships among individuals, groups, and agencies within a community among whom are shared common goals, responsibilities, resources, and accountability for public health policies and practices.

Demographic characteristics—Population measures, such as age, gender, race, and ethnicity.

Geographic information system (GIS)—Any program or process that makes use of computer technology to capture, store, analyze, interpret, and report geographic data.

Health assessment—The process of collecting, analyzing, assessing, and disseminating data and information about health status, risk factors, resource availability, individual concerns, environmental health factors, and any and all other factors impacting public health issues in a community.

used in measuring progress toward the achievement of goals and objectives;

- Developing the Community Health Assessment document, a specific form required by the State of New York which is comparable to similar summary statements required by other state and local governmental bodies; and
- Managing and sustaining the process, an indication that CHA is an on-going process in which goals and objectives, strategies, and accomplishments are continuously evaluated, reassessed, and revised according to the process described here.

Community health assessment has now become a fundamental part of many public health programs at both the state and local level. Many state public **health departments**, for example, have developed protocols or "toolkits" for use by local public health departments in carrying out the assessment process in their own communities. Other nonprofit and for-profit organizations have also developed similar programs that are available at no cost or for a fee.

Resources

BOOKS

Committee for the Study of the Future of Public Health. Institute of Medicine. *The Future of Public Health.* Washington, D.C.: National Academy Press, 1988.

Issel, L. Michele. *Health Program Planning and Evaluation: A Practical, Systematic Approach for Community Health*, 2nd ed. Sudbury, MA: Jones and Bartlett Learning, 2009.

PERIODICALS

Friedman, Daniel J., and Roy Gibson Parrish. "Is Community Health Assessment Worthwhile?." *Journal of Public Health Management and Practice* 15, 1. (2009): 3–9.

Graham, Sara R., et al. "The Benefits of Using Geographic Information Systems as a Community Assessment Tool." *Public Health Reports* 126, 2. (2011): 298–303

Running, Alice, Kathlee Martin, and Lauren Woodward Tolle. "An Innovative Model for Conducting a Participatory Community Health Assessment." *Journal of Community Health Nursing* 24, 4. (2007): 203–13.

WEBSITES

"ACHI Community Health Assessment Toolkit." hospitalconnect.com. http://www.assesstoolkit.org/. Accessed on September 27, 2012.

Ahari, Saeid S., et al."Community Based Needs Assessment in an Urban Area; A Participatory Action Research Project." BMJ Public Health. http://www.biomedcentral.com/content/pdf/1471-2458-12-161.pdf. Accessed on September 27, 2012.

"Community Health Assessment aNd Group Evaluation (CHANGE): Building a Foundation of Knowledge to Prioritize Community Needs." Centers for Disease Control and Prevention. http://www.cdc.gov/healthycommunitiesprogram/tools/change.htm. Accessed on September 27, 2012.

"2005 - 2010 Community Health Assessment (CHA) Definition and Purpose." New York State Department of Health. http://www.health.ny.gov/statistics/chac/cha05_intro.htm. Accessed on September 27, 2012.

ORGANIZATIONS

National Association of County and City Health Officials (NACCHO), 1100 17th St., N.W., 17th floor, Washington, DC USA 20036, 1 (202) 783–5550, Fax: 1 (202) 783–1583, info@naccho.org, www.naccho.org/.

David E. Newton, Ed.D.

Community health improvement process (CHIP)

Definition

A **community health** improvement process (CHIP) is a system for monitoring overall health matters in a community and addressing specific health issues.

Purpose

The purpose of a CHIP is to provide a community with a method for developing shared community goals for health improvement and the development and implementation of a method for accomplishing those goals.

Description

The principle behind a community health improvement process dates to at least the 1930s, as public health officials began to think about ways in which community health leaders could assemble, identify essential health issues, and develop programs for dealing with those issues. Over the decades, that effort has taken a number of forms, the most recent of which was the system now described as the community health improvement process (CHIP). That system was developed by the Committee on Using Performance Monitoring to Improve Community Health (CUPMICH) of the U.S. Institute of Medicine and published in 1997 by the U.S. National Academies Press as *Improving Health in the Community: A Role for Performance Monitoring*. A critical element in the most recent expression of this movement has been the involvement of performance-based assessments, the development of specific tests that allow one to determine how effectively a program is actually meeting its stated objectives.

Although somewhat complex in its details, a CHIP can be envisioned as a pair of intersecting cycles, both of which involve a process of analysis, action, and measurement. The first cycle involves Problem Identification and Prioritization. The first step within this cycle involves the formation of a community health coalition that includes stakeholders from all elements within the community who have an interest in health issues. This coalition then collects and analyzes data on various health issues within the community and establishes a list of priorities among these issues. Although stated in this form, the Problem Identification and Prioritization cycle can begin at any point within the process with, for example, the rise of some major health issue acting as the impetus for creating a coalition of stakeholders. It should be noted that this process can occur on almost any level. It might involve health leaders in a small town, representatives from a major urban area, or even health organizations across a whole state or region. The strength of this process also rests to some extent on the longevity of the coalition. That is, health improvement programs are likely to be more successful if coalitions survive over extended periods and continue to monitor and revise the process of goal selection and program development and evaluation.

The second cycle of the CHIP process is called the Analysis and Implementation Cycle, which involves seven steps:

- Analysis of health issues. Members of the coalition with expertise in health issues begin this process by identifying important health issues within the community, along with demographic, geographic, economic, social, and other factors that may impact these issues.
- Inventory of resources. All communities have at least some resources from a variety of disciplines that can be brought to bear in the solution of health issues. The coalition needs to identify those resources at this point in the process.
- Develop a health improvement strategy. The next logical step is to decide how available resources within a community can be brought to bear in the solution of a health issue.
- Establish accountability for health improvement activities. The CUPMICH committee identifies this step as a key part of the CHIP strategy since it specifically identifies individuals and organizations that are responsible for various aspects of carrying out activities designed to achieve the designated goals.
- Develop a set of performance indicators. Another key feature of the CHIP strategy is identifying very specific ways in which progress towards the accomplishment of goals can be checked. In some ways, this stage of the process sets the CHIP process off from similar efforts at solving community health problems since it demands that specific performance objectives be met along the way to resolving such issues.
- Implement the improvement strategy. At this point, all of the elements for the actual process are in place, and individuals and agencies can identify the specific actions they will need to take to accomplish the goals set in the first cycle of the CHIP process.
- Monitor process and outcomes of the improvement strategy. The final stage of the CHIP process involves collection of data and observations to determine whether and to what extent the strategy that has been put into place has produced progress towards achiving the goals established for the improvement program.

Recent reviews suggest that some public health agencies have adopted elements of the CHIP program but that, overall, it is not widely used in the United States or other parts of the world.

KEY TERMS

Community coalition—A group of individuals and/ or agencies with common interests in some particular issue, such as a health problem of concern to them all.

Performance-based objective—An objective that is measured by some type of action and defined by the results of that action.

Stakeholder—An individual or organization with an interest in or concern for some specific topic or problem.

Resources

BOOKS

Durch, Jane S., Linda A. Bailey, and Michael A. Stoto, eds. *Improving Health in the Community: A Role for Performance Monitoring*. Washington, DC: National Academies Press, 1997.

PERIODICALS

Layde, P. M., et al. "A Model to Translate Evidence-based Interventions into Community Practice." *American Journal of Public Health*. 102, 4. (2012): 617–24.

Sanders, J., and M. J. Baisch. "Community-based Participatory Action: Impact on a Neighborhood Level Community Health Improvement Process." *Progress in Community Health Partnerships* 2, 1. (2008): 7–15.

WEBSITES

"Community Health Improvement Process and Community Health Assessment Resources." Centers for Disease

Control and Prevention. http://www.cdc.gov/ai/resources/popular/chip.html. Accessed on September 26, 2012.

"Institute of Medicine's Community Health Improvement Process." The Community Tool Box. http://ctb.ku.edu/en/tablecontents/chapter2_section6_tools.aspx. Accessed on September 26, 2012.

ORGANIZATIONS

Centers for Disease Control and Prevention (CDC), 1600 Clifton Rd., N.E., Atlanta, GA USA 30333, 1 (800) 232–4636, cdcinfo@cdc.gov., www.cdc.gov.

David E. Newton, Ed.D.

Food-mood connection

Nutrient	Food sources	Proposed effects
B vitamins (6, 12, and folic acid)	Asparagus, orange juice, spinach	Reduce depression
Choline (B-complex vitamin)	Eggs, wheat germ	Improved memory, mood
Complex carbohydrates	Beans, starchy vegetables, whole grains	Promotes calmness, relaxation
Omega-3 fatty acids	Flax seeds, oily fish (e.g., salmon), walnuts	Supports cognitive functions, positive mood
Protein	Beans, dairy, eggs, lean meats and poultry	Improved concentration, energy

SOURCE: Cleveland Clinic, "Food and Mood," *Be Well Magazine* (Winter 2010), http://cchealth.clevelandclinic.org/cover/food-and-mood, and Goldberg, Katherine Briggs, "The Food and Mood Connection," University of Michigan Depression Center, http://depressiontoolkit.org/news/food_and_mood_connection.asp.

(Table by PreMediaGlobal. © 2013 Cengage Learning)

Community mental health

Definition

Community mental health is an approach to providing access to professional mental health care in local communities. It includes services offered through public mental health programs, public **health departments**, community mental health centers, private programs, medical clinics, hospitals, religious organizations, colleges and other educational institutions, and neighborhood centers. Community mental health assessment has evolved into a field of research called "psychiatric epidemiology," which determines the prevalence of various mental disorders in specific communities, with the goal of developing appropriate community mental health programs and evaluating their effectiveness.

Purpose

The primary purpose of community mental health is to decrease the need for inpatient and hospital-based mental health services as well as to supplement those services, and to help patients become successfully reintegrated into society. Community mental health services are generally dispersed among a variety of local facilities and programs, rather than isolating patients from their communities by segregating them in centralized hospitals. The goal of community mental health programs is to be more responsive to local needs and more accessible to more people. They also help alleviate "psychiatric boarding," in which patients with mental illnesses are confined in overcrowded hospital emergency departments. Community mental health centers (CMHCs) provide valuable services to people who otherwise might not have access to mental health care, especially low-income youth and families in urban and rural areas throughout the United States.

Community mental health can address a wide range of problems. Many programs, including residential, day, and outpatient treatment, are involved in transitioning patients from institutions or from parents' homes to independent or semi-independent living situations. Some programs provide diagnostic and treatment services for a wide variety of mental disorders. Others refer clients to psychologists or psychiatrists. Community mental health may provide emergency care for suicidal patients, for patients with acute panic disorder, or for victims and witnesses of **natural disasters** and other violent or traumatic events. Some community mental health programs provide substance abuse treatment. However, the high demand for community mental health services and the lack of adequate funding have meant that patients might not have timely access to the community-based care that they require.

Demographics

There is a tremendous need for community mental health services throughout the United States. This need skyrockets in times of economic **stress** and recession. In most states, the primary clients of community mental health services are Medicaid recipients. However, it has been estimated that as many as two-thirds of American children and teens—more than six million children—do not receive the mental health services that they need. A survey of juvenile detention facilities found that two-thirds were holding children who were awaiting community mental health services. Some of these children were as young as seven. Over a six-month period, almost 15,000 young people were being held in detention until community mental health services became available, at a very high cost to American taxpayers. These detention facilities are generally not equipped to provide care for mentally ill youth, some of whom may pose a danger to themselves or others.

Community mental health, particularly when it is integrated into other community-based organizations, can be particularly relevant for racial and ethnic minorities in the United States. African Americans are much more likely to turn to family or to their religious or social communities for emotional support than to seek professional help. African Americans also generally have less access to mental health care, even though they are disproportionately more likely to experience circumstances that increase the risk of developing a mental illness. These circumstances include homelessness, exposure to **violence**, and children in foster care or otherwise in the child welfare system.

Asian Americans and Pacific Islanders have higher rates of depressive symptoms than white Americans but have the lowest rates of utilization of mental health services. Southeast Asians, especially refugees, have particularly high rates of depression and **post-traumatic stress disorder** (PTSD). Their need for outpatient mental health services is twice that of the general Asian American population.

Latinos are also at higher risk for depression, anxiety, and substance abuse. American-born Latinos and long-term residents have significantly higher rates of psychiatric disorders, especially substance abuse, compared with recent immigrants. Like African Americans, Latinos are far less likely than others to seek mental health services, especially from specialized mental health facilities. In part, this appears to be related to the severe shortage of Latino and Spanish-speaking mental health care providers.

Description

The services included in community mental health programs depend on the state and local area. The focus of community mental health is on preventing psychiatric hospitalization and in assisting in the transition out of inpatient care. Some states offer only very limited community mental health services. Others offer a wide range of services for children, adults, and families. These may include mental health screening and assessment, psychological testing, psychiatric evaluations, individual psychotherapy, group psychotherapy, psychiatric medications, family and couples therapy, family psychological and educational counseling, peer support programs, respite care, case management, jail diversion, integrated treatment for co-existing disorders, crisis interventions, and grief counseling. Some community mental health programs provide supportive housing, supported employment, and even longer-term and inpatient care. A 24-hour crisis hotline or emergency psychiatric services are important components of community mental health. These may be provided in conjunction with a local hospital.

Community mental health services may be available for severely emotionally disturbed youth or for those who have been traumatized by sexual abuse or violence and require specialized interventions. Juveniles suspected of mental illness may be referred to community mental health programs by the courts. Community mental health also may include multidisciplinary assessments of parents with mental illness who are suspected of, or have been accused of, child maltreatment. Some programs include victims' services for child and adult crime victims and their families.

Some community mental health programs include intensive case management services for ending chronic homelessness and substance abuse. These services may include job and life-skills training, employment referrals, housing options, meals, substance abuse treatment, and other rehabilitation services. Special services may also be available for older adults, including adult day respite, home-meal delivery, housekeeping, and emergency home response, as well as screenings for nursing home placement or veterans' services, and assistance in transitions from nursing homes to independent- or assisted-living arrangements.

Community mental health centers may also provide grief counseling, a form of therapy designed to help individuals having to deal with unusually stressful events in their lives, such as a divorce, the loss of a child, the death of a loved one, loss of a job, stress from economic and financial problems, or even the loss of a loved pet. In such circumstances, individuals may be unable to call on their normal psychological mechanisms for dealing with such events and may feel deep depression, anxiety, anger, helplessness, confusion, isolation, or other psychological responses for which they may require specialized help. An unfortunately increasingly common need for grief counseling arises when whole communities are exposed to extraordinary psychological stress, as when a person kills and/or wounds a number of individuals in a mass attack on a school, post office, office building, store, or other facility. In such cases, community mental health agencies may provide trained counselors from a variety of professional fields to help the survivors of such events to understand what has happened and to develop coping mechanisms that allow them to get on with their lives.

CARL GUSTAV JUNG (1875–1961)

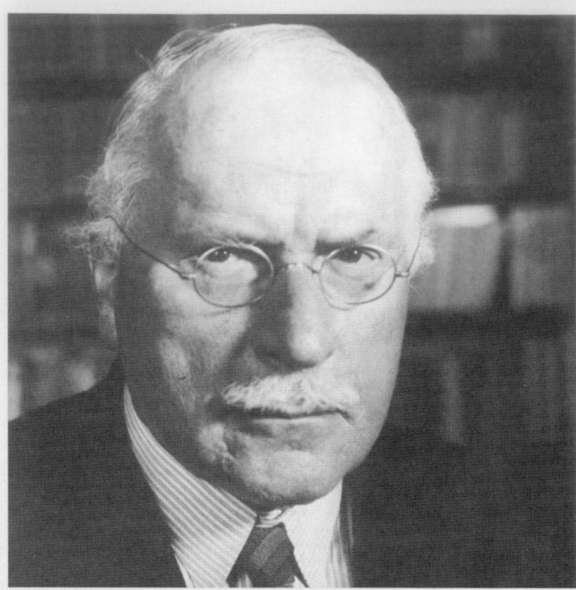

(© Bettmann/CORBIS)

Carl Gustav Jung was born in Kesswil, Switzerland, on July 26, 1875, to a Protestant clergyman who moved his family to Basel when Jung was four. While growing up, Jung exhibited an interest in many diverse areas of study but finally decided to pursue medicine at the University of Basel and the University of Zurich, earning his degree in 1902. He also studied psychology in Paris. In 1903, Jung married Emma Rauschenbach, his companion and collaborator. The couple had five children.

Jung's professional career began in 1900 at the University of Zurich where he worked as an assistant to Eugene Blueler in the psychiatric clinic. During his internship, he and some co-workers used an experiment that revealed groups of ideas in the unconscious psyche which he named *complexes*. Jung sent his publication *Studies in Word Association* (1904) to Sigmund Freud after finding his own beliefs confirmed by Freud's work. Jung and Freud became friends and collaborators until 1913 when Jung's ideas began to conflict with Freud's. During the time following this split, Jung published *Two Essays on Analytical Psychology* (1916, 1917) and *Psychological Types* (1921). Jung's later work developed from the concepts in his *Two Essays* publication and he became known as a founder of modern depth psychology.

In 1944, Jung gave up his psychological practice and his explorations after he suffered a severe heart attack. Jung received honorary doctorates from numerous universities and in 1948 he founded the C. G. Jung Institute in Zurich. Jung died on June 6, 1961.

CMHC programs may include the training of community mental health professionals. In addition to these specialists, community mental health may involve psychiatrists, including child and geriatric psychiatrists, clinical psychologists, clinical social workers, nurse practitioners, psychiatric nurses, counselors, clergy, recreational and occupational therapists, and assertive community treatment (ACT) teams. ACT is a community-based treatment approach for assisting in the recovery and rehabilitation of patients with severe and persistent mental illnesses.

Although some community mental health programs are based in stand-alone CMHCs, programs located within community groups or churches can reach populations that might not otherwise seek mental health services. They also can increase awareness of mental health issues and resources and reduce stigmas associated with mental disorders. Some community mental health programs are school-based, linking mental health providers with teachers and family advocates for treating children with disruptive behavior disorders. Community mental health can also be associated with:

- outpatient psychiatric clinics
- community rehabilitation programs
- community support programs
- adult daycare centers
- day treatment centers
- home health agencies
- club programs
- foster care programs
- sheltered workshops
- group and private homes

Eligibility for community mental health services varies by state and local area. In general, people in crises and children and adults with severe mental illnesses are given first priority. During times of budgetary restraint, the first to be cut from community mental health services are often those who are not enrolled in Medicaid, so as to preserve federal Medicaid matching funds. Approximately 2% of public mental health funding comes from Medicare, which, in addition to senior citizens, serves younger people with disabilities. Unlike Medicaid, Medicare does not cover many community-based services and requires co-payments for outpatient mental health treatment. In addition to **Medicaid and Medicare**, community mental health services may accept private insurance or offer a sliding fee scale based on ability to pay. The State **Children's Health** Insurance Program (SCHIP) may or may not provide the same range of mental health services as Medicaid, depending on the state. Some county and municipal local governments administer and partially fund community mental health services for their residents.

Origins

During the 1960s, in response to the increased availability of psychiatric medications and an outcry over involuntary commitments, public psychiatric hospitals began reducing their populations or closing completely. Mentally ill patients were released into the community to live independently. The Community Mental Health Centers Act of 1963 aimed to create a comprehensive community mental health system to serve this population, providing **prevention**, early treatment, and continuity of care within larger communities and promoting the social integration of people with mental health needs. However, the programs were never adequately funded, and many planned community mental health services never materialized.

Initially, CMHCs provided outpatient care to people with less severe, episodic, or acute mental health problems. Soon they were also caring for the deinstitutionalized chronically mentally ill. With the repeal of the Mental Health Systems Act and with federal funding for CMHCs replaced by block grants to the states in the early 1980s, the system deteriorated further. Subsequent programs to provide for community mental health were relatively short-lived and impacted only a few urban centers. As a result, vast numbers of persons with mental illness have become homeless or incarcerated in prisons.

As of the early twenty-first century, the U.S. Substance Abuse and Mental Health Services Administration was continuing to fund the Comprehensive Community Mental Health Services for Children and Their Families Program. This community mental health program provides youth (from birth through age 21) and their families with cultural- and language-appropriate evidence-based mental health services and support. The National Council for Community Behavioral Healthcare advocates for improved public policies in mental and **behavioral health**, and offers state-of-the-science education and practice improvement resources for the personnel of community mental health programs. It has also pioneered the implantation of Mental Health First Aid USA to educate the public about the signs and symptoms of mental disorders.

KEY TERMS

Assertive community treatment (ACT)—A service-delivery model for providing comprehensive, highly individualized, locally based treatment directly to patients with serious, persistent mental illnesses.

Community Mental Health Clinic (CMHC)—A community-based provider of limited or comprehensive mental health services; usually at least partially publicly funded.

Epidemiology—A field of medical science dealing with the incidence, distribution, and control of disease in a population.

Grief counseling—A form of psychotherapy designed to help people cope with emotional responses to extraordinarily stressful events in their lives, such as the death of a loved one or long-term unemployment.

Medicaid—A joint state and federal program for providing medical care for low-income children and families.

Medicare—The U.S. government healthcare system for those aged 65 and over.

Post-traumatic stress disorder (PTSD)—A psychological response to a highly stressful event; typically characterized by depression, anxiety, flashbacks, nightmares, and avoidance of reminders of the traumatic experience.

Psychiatric boarding—The practice of holding mentally ill patients in emergency department corridors and waiting areas, because of the lack of hospital beds or other facilities.

Respite care—Temporary care of a patient to provide caregivers with a period of physical, mental, and emotional rest.

State Children's Health Insurance Program; SCHIP; CHIP—A state-administered health insurance program for lower- and middle-income children who are without private health insurance and whose family incomes are above the Medicaid eligibility limits.

Common problems

In the early 2010s, states and the federal government are attempting to address economic problems and massive budget deficits in part by further slashing community mental health funding and restricting eligibility for services. At the same time, the demand for

QUESTIONS TO ASK YOUR DOCTOR

- Would community mental health services be helpful for me?
- What type of community mental health services should I pursue?
- What community mental health services are available in my area?
- Am I eligible for community mental health?
- What type of community mental health provider will I be able to see?

mental health services is rising dramatically. Increasingly, law enforcement agencies are forced to provide emergency services for the mentally ill—services that had previously been provided by community mental health programs. In addition, managed behavioral health care and the strict use of medical management techniques is decreasing access to community care, resulting in more patients in crisis and increased utilization of hospital emergency departments. Low reimbursement rates under Medicaid and Medicare further reduce community mental health services. Coverage for antipsychotic drugs are reduced or eliminated. Some experts warn that the entire mental health system in the United States is on the verge of collapse. However, in light of the mass shooting at the elementary school in Newtown, CT in late 2012, the United States and its leaders are aware that something must be done to improve the system so people don't fall through the cracks.

Resources

BOOKS

Brown, Louis D. *Consumer-run Mental Health: Framework for Recovery*. New York: Springer, 2012.

Maller, Doreen. *The Praeger Handbook of Community Mental Health Practice*. Santa Barbara, CA: Praeger, 2013.

Rosenberg, Jessica, et al. *Community Mental Health: Challenges for the 21st Century*. New York: Routledge, 2013.

Thompson, Neil. *Grief and Its Challenges*. Houndmills, Basingstoke, Hampshire; New York: Palgrave Macmillan, 2012.

Yeager, Kenneth, et al. *Modern Community Mental Health: An Interdisciplinary Approach*. Oxford: Oxford University Press, 2013.

PERIODICALS

Cleek, E.N., et al. "The Family Empowerment Program: An Interdisciplinary Approach to Working with Multi-stressed Urban Families." *Family Process* 51, 2. (2012): 207–17.

Koegl, C.J., and B.R. Rush. "Need and Use of Services by Persons with Co-occurring Substance Use and Mental Disorders within a Community Mental Health System." *Mental Health and Substance Use: Dual Diagnosis* 5, 1. (2012): 4–19.

Lewis, S.E., K. Hopper, and E. Healion. "Partners in Recovery: Social Support and Accountability in a Consumer-run Mental Health Center." *Psychiatric Services* 63, 1. (2012): 61–5.

Slyter, M. "Creative Counseling Interventions for Grieving Adolescents." *Journal of Creativity in Mental Health* 7, 1. (2012): 17–34.

WEBSITES

"African American Community Mental Health Fact Sheet." National Alliance on Mental Illness. http://www.nami.org/Template.cfm?Section=Fact_Sheets1&Template=/ContentManagement/ContentDisplay.cfm&ContentID=53812 (accessed November 3, 2012).

"Coping with Grief and Loss." Helpguide.org. http://www.helpguide.org/mental/grief_loss.htm. Accessed on November 3, 2012.

Kortrijk, H.E., et al. "Treatment Outcome in Patients Receiving Assertive Community Treatment." *Community Mental Health Journal* 46, no. 4 (August 2010). http://www.springerlink.com/content/510q277x50364725/full text.html (accessed November 3, 2012).

National Alliance on Mental Illness. "Assertive Community Treatment (ACT)." About Treatments & Supports. http://www.nami.org/Template.cfm?Section=About_Treatments_and_Supports&template=/ContentManagement/ContentDisplay.cfm&ContentID=8075 (accessed November 3, 2012).

ORGANIZATIONS

American Psychiatric Association, 1000 Wilson Blvd., Ste. 1825, Arlington, VA 22209-3901, (703) 907-7300, apa@psych.org, http://www.psych.org

National Alliance on Mental Illness, 3803 N. Fairfax Dr., Ste. 100, Arlington, VA 22203, (703) 524-7600, (800) 950-NAMI (6264), Fax: (703) 524-9094, http://www.nami.org/Content/NavigationMenu/Contact_Us/NAMI_National_Staff/NAMIStaffDirectory2012.pdf, http://www.nami.org

National Council for Community Behavioral Healthcare, 1701 K St. NW, Ste. 400, Washington, DC 20006, (202) 684-7457, Fax: (202) 386-9391, communications@thenationalcouncil.org, http://www.TheNationalCouncil.org

National Institute of Mental Health, 6001 Executive Blvd., Room 8184, MSC 9663, Bethesda, MD 20892-9663, (301) 443-4513, (866) 615-6464, Fax: (301)443-4279, nimhinfo@nih.gov, http://www.nimh.nih.gov

Substance Abuse and Mental Health Services Administration, 1 Choke Cherry Rd., Rockville, MD 20857, (877) SAMHSA-7 (726-4727), Fax: (240) 221-4292, SAMHSAInfo@samhsa.hhs.gov, http://www.samhsa.gov.

Michael Polgar, PhD
Emily Jane Willingham, PhD
Margaret Alic, PhD

Concussion

Definition

A concussion, also called a brain concussion, is a trauma-induced change in mental status—often caused by a blow to the head or a sudden jolt or shaking of the head. When it occurs, a concussion often brings with it confusion, disorientation, and amnesia (memory loss). Severe cases can cause loss of consciousness. Concussions, a type of traumatic brain injury (TBI), frequently occur when participating in sports or recreational events, especially if the activity involves full-contact activities such as football, soccer, and hockey. Whether caused by a sports collision, car accident, or some other kind of impact, concussions cause a substantial number of deaths and permanent disabilities each year, resulting in a serious public health problem in the United States.

Description

A concussion occurs when the head hits or is hit by an object, or when the brain is jarred against the skull, with sufficient force to cause temporary loss of function in the higher centers of the brain. The injured person may remain conscious or lose consciousness briefly, and is disoriented for some minutes after the blow. A TBI may be mild, with only a brief disruption in mental state or consciousness, or severe, with a lengthy period of unconsciousness followed by amnesia and other alterations of mental status.

While concussion usually resolves on its own without lasting effect, it can cause a much more serious condition. Second impact syndrome occurs when a person with a concussion, even a very mild one, suffers a second blow before fully recovering from the first. The brain swelling and increased intracranial pressure that can result are potentially fatal. Numerous such cases have been reported since the syndrome was first described in 1984. Fitness, sports, and exercise experts are becoming more concerned about concussions as a serious problem that may occur during physical activities.

Demographics

The **Centers for Disease Control and Prevention (CDC)** estimate that there are approximately 1.7 million TBIs per year in the United States, with most of these reported injuries receiving medical attention. About three-quarters of TBIs that occur annually in the country are concussions or other types of mild TBIs. While these concussions are mild and do not cause any permanent injury or health concerns, about 10% cause disability or death.

Statistics collected by the **CDC** between 2002 and 2006 (the most recent data available as of August 2012) showed that of the 1.7 million people who suffer a concussion annually, about 1.365 million are treated and released from an emergency department, 275,000 are hospitalized, and 52,000 die. The CDC also reported that TBIs are contributing factors in about one-third of all injury-related deaths in the United States each year. As of July 2007, the CDC reported that U.S. emergency departments annually treat about 135,000 sports-related and recreation-related TBIs among children from the ages of 5 to 18 years. In addition, the CDC estimates that about 300,000 sports-related concussions (those that result in unconsciousness) occur each year in the United States. The CDC admits that the true number is probably higher than these figures suggest due to underreporting.

Causes and symptoms

Causes

Playing contact sports is a risk factor for experiencing one or more concussions. About 300,000 people report sustaining mild to moderate sports-related brain injuries each year; such concussions are widely thought to be underreported. This is largely due to athletes not wanting to be medically disqualified from continuing to play their sport. Most sports-related brain injuries occur in young men between the ages of 16 and 25 years. Sports or fitness activities with high incidences of concussions include football, hockey, soccer, and cycling.

The risk of concussion from football is extremely high, especially at the high school level. Studies show that approximately one in five players suffer a concussion or more serious brain injury during their brief high-school careers. The rate at the collegiate level is approximately one in twenty. Rates for hockey players are less clear, but are believed to be similar. A study conducted at the University of Michigan in 2007 found that 20.2% of retired NFL football players who had sustained three or more concussions had bouts of depression after their playing days were over. That percentage is approximately three times the rate of football players who had not sustained any concussions while playing the game. A similar study in 2009 found that memory problems within former NFL players, such as Alzheimer's disease and other types of dementia, were 19 times more prevalent than in the average male population 30 to 49 years of age.

Concussion and lasting brain damage is an especially significant risk for boxers, since the goal of the sport is, in fact, to deliver a concussion to the opponent. For this reason, the American Academy of Neurology and other such organizations have called for a ban on boxing because the goal of a boxer is to knock out the opponent; that is, make a foe unconscious by giving him/her a TBI. Repeated concussions over months or years can cause cumulative head injury. The cumulative brain injuries experienced by most boxers can lead to permanent brain damage. Multiple blows to the head can cause "punch-drunk" syndrome or dementia pugilistica, as evidenced by Muhammad Ali (born Cassius Clay, Jr. in 1942), whose parkinsonism is a result of his career in the boxing ring.

Falls, such as when playing, account for the greatest number of concussions in children ages 0–4 years. People over the age of 65 years also are at high risk of falling and sustaining a concussion. Individuals over age 75 have the greatest rate of hospitalization and death from concussions.

Though concussions are often associated with motor vehicle accidents and playing sports, those are not the only possible causes. Domestic **violence**, in addition to being a significant public health concern, is another contributing cause to concussions or TBIs. Domestic violence, is an umbrella term that describes multiple types of abuse that might occur between intimate partners or parents and children. As domestic violence is better understood, it has become clear that it can affect all genders, ethnicities, and ages. The abuser can be be male or female, parent or child, and domestic violence can range from verbal and emotional abuse to physical assault. Punches or other strikes to the face, as well as attempts at strangulation, may result in a concussion. Intimate partner violence (IPV), represents domestic violence between intimate partners of any age or sex, regardless of level of sexual intimacy. Teens are increasingly at risk for IPV, so it is important for parents and caretakers to be aware of the signs of concussion and TBI. It is important for all victims of domestic violence or IPV to seek help, even if they are unwilling to go to the police. In the case of physical assaults, if abuse to the head and neck continues, the victim is more likely to sustain long-term brain damage.

Symptoms

Symptoms of concussion include:

- headache
- disorientation as to time, date, or place
- confusion
- dizziness
- vacant stare or confused expression
- inability to be roused or woken
- incoherent or incomprehensible speech
- incoordination or weakness
- amnesia for the events immediately preceding the blow
- nausea or vomiting
- double vision
- ringing in the ears

These symptoms may last from several minutes to several hours. More severe or longer-lasting symptoms may indicate more severe brain injury. The person with a concussion may or may not lose consciousness from the blow. A period of prolonged unconsciousness indicates a more severe brain injury.

The severity of concussion is graded on a three-point scale, and is used as a basis for treatment decisions. The three grades are:

- Grade 1: No loss of consciousness, transient confusion, and other symptoms that resolve within 15 minutes.
- Grade 2: No loss of consciousness, transient confusion, and other symptoms that require more than 15 minutes to resolve.
- Grade 3: Loss of consciousness for any period.

Days or weeks after the accident, the person may show symptoms of a condition called post-concussion syndrome. Signs of post-concussion syndrome include:

- headache
- poor attention and concentration
- memory difficulties
- anxiety
- depression
- sleep disturbances
- light and noise intolerance

Diagnosis

Concussions can occur while playing sports and other recreational pursuits. Consequently, all parents of children participating in such activities, along with coaches, athletes, and spectators, should be aware of the signs and symptoms of a concussion. Due to the risk of IPV among young adults, parents and family members should also be aware of the signs of concussion, even if their loved one is not participating in sports.

Examination

It is very important for those attending a person with concussion to pay close attention to the person's symptoms and progression immediately after the accident. The duration of unconsciousness and degree of confusion are important indicators of the severity of the injury and help guide the diagnostic process and treatment decisions.

A doctor, nurse, or emergency medical technician may make an immediate assessment based on the severity of the symptoms; a neurologic exam of the pupils, coordination, and sensation; and brief tests of orientation, memory, and concentration. Those with very mild concussions may not need to be hospitalized or have expensive diagnostic tests.

Tests

Questionable or more severe cases may require computed tomography (CT) scans or magnetic resonance imaging (MRI) scans to look for brain injury. More extensive neuropsychologic testing may be done, especially on athletes who are at risk for repeat concussions.

Treatment

The symptoms of concussion usually clear up quickly and without lasting effect, if no further injury is sustained during the healing process. Guidelines for returning to sports activities are based on the severity of the concussion.

Traditional

A grade 1 concussion can usually be treated with rest and continued observation. The person may return to sports activities that same day, but only after examination by a trained professional, and after all symptoms have completely resolved. If the person sustains a second concussion of any severity that same day, he or she should not be allowed to continue contact sports until he or she has been symptom-free, during both rest and activity, for one week.

A person with a grade 2 concussion must discontinue sports activity for the day, should be evaluated by a trained professional, and should be observed closely throughout the day to make sure that all symptoms have completely cleared. Worsening of symptoms, or continuation of any symptoms beyond one week, indicates the need for a CT or MRI scan. Return to contact sports should only occur after one week with no symptoms, both at rest and during activity, and following examination by a physician. Following a second grade 2 concussion, the person should remain symptom-free for two weeks before resuming contact sports.

A person with a grade 3 concussion (involving any loss of consciousness, no matter how brief) should be examined by a medical professional either on the scene or in an emergency room. More severe symptoms may warrant a CT or MRI scan, along with a thorough neurological and physical exam. The person should be hospitalized if any abnormalities are found or if confusion persists. Prolonged unconsciousness and worsening symptoms require urgent neurosurgical evaluation or transfer to a trauma center. Following discharge from professional care, the patient is closely monitored for neurological symptoms, which may arise or worsen. If headaches or other symptoms worsen or last longer than one week, a CT or MRI scan should be performed. Contact sports are to be avoided for one week following unconsciousness of only a few seconds, and for two weeks if the unconsciousness lasted a minute or more.

For someone who has sustained a concussion of any severity, it is imperative that he or she avoid the possibility of another blow to the head until well after all symptoms have cleared to prevent second-impact syndrome. The guidelines for returning to sports are designed to minimize the risk of this syndrome. A person receiving a second grade 3 concussion should avoid contact sports for at least a month after all symptoms have cleared, and then only with the approval of a physician. If signs of brain swelling or bleeding are seen on a CT or MRI scan, the athlete should not return to the sport for the rest of the season, or even indefinitely until cleared by a physician.

KEY TERMS

Amnesia—A loss of memory that may be caused by brain injury, such as concussion.

Parkinsonism—A neurological disorder that includes a fine tremor, muscular weakness and rigidity, and an altered way of walking.

Prognosis

About 90% of concussions leave no lasting neurological problems. For the most part, concussions do not result in death. However, lasting problems caused by concussions can be serious. Symptoms of post-concussion syndrome may last for weeks or even months. The older the individual, the more likely the symptoms will last longer, especially if other medical conditions are also present.

Studies of concussion in contact sports have shown that the risk of sustaining a second concussion is even greater than it was for the first concussion if the person continues to engage in the sport. Athletes who have sustained concussions are more likely to have increased risk with physical and mental problems later in life.

Prevention

Many cases of concussion can be prevented by using appropriate protective equipment. This includes seat belts and air bags in automobiles, and helmets in all contact sports. Helmets should also be worn when bicycling, skiing, skateboarding, or horseback riding. Soccer players should avoid heading the ball when it is kicked at high velocity from close range. Playground equipment should be underlaid with soft material—either sand or special matting.

The value of high-contact sports such as boxing, football, or hockey should be weighed against the high risk of brain injury during a young person's participation in the sport. Steering a child's general enthusiasm for sports into activities less apt to produce head impacts may reduce the likelihood of brain injury.

The National Football League (NFL) is especially conscious of the danger of concussions to its players. In the 2010 NFL season, medical personnel began using standardized concussion assessment packages on the sidelines of each game to evaluate any player thought to have sustained a concussion while playing. The package includes a symptom checklist and a neurological examination, which includes a cognitive evaluation (e.g.: "Are you thinking clearly?") and a balance assessment ("Can you touch your nose with your forefingers on your left and right hands?"). The NFL requires football players who show concussion symptoms to sit out the rest of the game or practice and to be analyzed by an independent neurologist before returning to play.

For children participating in high-impact sports, parents should be aware of concussion policies for the organization sponsoring the sport, such as a school district. The policies should:

- emphasize safety as its most important goal
- clearly state that players are not allowed to play after sustaining a concussion
- detail when athletes are allowed to return to play after full recovery from a concussion
- include all steps taken when concussions occur

In addition, a health care professional should evaluate each concussion before any player is allowed to return to the game.

All athletes and parents (in the case of children) should read, understand, and sign a concussion policy statement at the beginning of each season. These should not be signed if there is any problem or concern remaining and children should not be allowed to participate under such conditions. Knowledge and active involvement in sports is a good way to prevent concussions from happening and, when they do occur, to minimize their severity.

Through better societal awareness of domestic violence and its signs, those in abusive situations might be more able and willing to seek help, and other instances of domestic violence can be prevented. A reduction in or **prevention** of domestic violence would have many public health benefits, including a reduction in injuries like concussions and TBIs. The CDC asserts that the key to preventing domestic violence is "first-time preparation"—which stresses taking action the first time someone hurts his or her partner. The CDC is continually working on better understanding domestic violence, its causes, and the efficacy of existing social programs.

QUESTIONS TO ASK YOUR DOCTOR

- What is the best way to avoid a concussion in a contact sport?
- How concerned should I be if I sustain a concussion?
- How old should a child be they are allowed to play tackle football or other contact sports?
- What should I do if my son or daughter wants to continue playing football (or other contact sport) with a serious injury, such as a concussion?
- Should I allow my children to play contact sports in the backyard or elsewhere without adequate protection?
- What should I do if I have symptoms of a concussion?

Effects on public health

The medical costs of concussions and TBIs on the public health are great. The CDC tallies together the direct costs of medical expenses related to concussion as well as indirect costs like loss in productivity because of work time missed. As of August 2012, the most recent data available from the CDC is from 2000, which estimates the costs associated with concussion and TBIs at approximately $76.5 billion. As of August 2012, the CDC's most recent domestic violence and intimate partner violence (IPV) statistics are from 2003. At this time, the overall cost of IPV in the U.S.—including direct medical expenses and mental health services for all types of injuries—totalled $4.1 billion.

Resources

BOOKS

Knoop, Kevin J., et al., editors. *Atlas of Emergency Medicine*, 3rd ed. New York: McGraw-Hill Professional, 2009.

Micheli, Lyle J., editor. *Encyclopedia of Sports Medicine*. Thousand Oaks, CA: SAGE, 2011.

Moorman III, Claude T., and Donald T. Kirkendall, eds. *Praeger Handbook of Sports Medicine and Athlete Health*. Santa Barbara, CA: Praeger, 2011.

Rich, Brent E., and Mitchell K. Pratte. *Tarascon Sports Medicine Pocketbook.* Sudbury, MA: Jones and Bartlett Publishers, 2010.

WEBSITES

Benhardt, David T. *Concussion.* eMedicine.com. (November 16, 2010). http://emedicine.medscape.com/article/92095-overview (accessed October 23, 2012).

Concussion. Mayo Clinic. (February 22, 2011). http://www.mayoclinic.com/health/concussion/DS00320 (accessed October 23, 2012).

Concussion. MedlinePlus. (June 21, 2011). http://www.nlm.nih.gov/medlineplus/concussion.html (accessed October 23, 2012).

National Coalition Against Domestic Violence*Domestic Violence Fact Sheet.*http://www.ncadv.org/files/DomesticViolenceFactSheet%28National%29.pdf (accessed October 23, 2012).

U.S. Centers for Disease Control and Prevention *Intimate Partner Violence.*http://www.cdc.gov/ViolencePrevention/intimatepartnerviolence/index.html (accessed October 23, 2012).

U.S. Centers for Disease Control and Prevention *Traumatic Brain Injury.*http://www.cdc.gov/TraumaticBrainInjury/statistics.html (accessed October 23, 2012).

Healthwise. *Concussion.* WebMD. (July 23, 2010). http://www.webmd.com/brain/tc/traumatic-brain-injury-concussion-overview (accessed October 23, 2012).

ORGANIZATIONS

American Academy of Neurology, 1080 Montreal Ave., St. Paul, MN 55116, (651) 695-2717, Fax: (651) 695-2791, http://www.aan.com

Brain Injury Association of America, 1608 Spring Hill Rd., Suite 110, Vienna, VA 22182, (703) 761-0750, Fax: (703) 761-0755, (800) 444-6443, braininjuryinfo@biausa.org, http://www.biausa.org

National Coalition Against Domestic Violence, One Broadway, Suite B210, Denver, CO 80203, (303) 839-1852, Fax: (303) 831-9251, mainoffice@ncadv.org, http://www.ncadv.org/.

Richard Robinson
Tish Davidson, AM
William Atkins, BB, BS, MBA
Andrea Nienstedt, MA

Condoms *see* **Safe sex**

Consumer safety

Definition

Consumer safety involves keeping the public safe and protected from the risk of injury or death due to the use of a consumer product.

Description

Each year, consumer products are responsible for the injury or death of thousands of individuals in the United States. Consumer safety regulations work with manufacturers and consumers to assure that products are safely made and properly used. According to product safety author Timothy A. Pine, the only true way to achieve product safety is through designing products in such a way that defects do not occur.

The Consumer Product Safety Commission (CPSC) aims to protect consumers of any age. Special programs are in place to protect children, as they are considered more vulnerable to flaws in safety. The agency has identified senior citizens over the age of 75 as being second to children in terms of vulnerability to product safety flaws. Although persons age 75 and up constitute only 13% of the American population, this group suffers 60% of deaths due to consumer products. CPSC data indicate that death or injury from consumer products increases significantly beginning at age 75. The rate of injuries for persons age 75 and up treated in emergency centers is double that of persons ages 65 to 74. Senior citizens are particularly prone to injury or death from falls and fires.

Origin

The CPSC was formed in 1972 after passage of the Consumer Product Safety Act, which protects consumers from "against reasonable risks of injuries associated with consumer products." The agency is independent, and therefore, it does not report to a federal department. Engineers and technical experts are employed by the agency, which helps its efforts to identify potential hazards that are headed to market.

Motivation for forming the CPSC consisted of several factors including a need to develop uniform standards, eliminate requirements that conflicted with one another, and assure that states could not overrule CPSC jurisdiction.

The CPSC has the authority to make decisions regarding the safety of 15,000 products in three categories: school or household use, sports, and recreation. Items under the agency's jurisdiction may be small items such as toys to large structures such as swimming pools.

Consumer advocate Ralph Nader heightened awareness of consumer product safety beginning in 1965, when he wrote *Unsafe at Any Speed.* The book covered automobile safety, bringing that topic into the news. He went on to investigate safety in food products, **vitamins**, appliances, consumer loans, and other products and services.

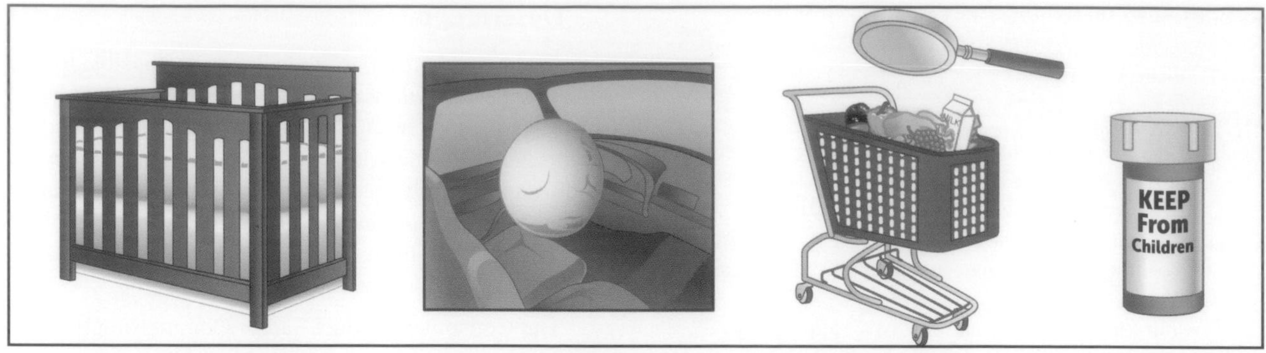

Important consumer safety concerns. *(Illustration by Electronic Illustrators Group. © 2013 Cengage Learning)*

Product safety issues

The CPSC informs consumers of important safety features to consider when making a purchase, evaluates products as they enter the country, and helps manufacturers by publicizing recalls.

In 2007, more than 25 million toys were recalled, along with household items, cribs, and other consumer products. For that reason, 2007 is sometimes called "the year of the recall." When an item is recalled, the product may still be useful with the addition of a simple part, or it may need to be exchanged for an safer version. Some common reasons for recall include:

- Levels of lead
- Fire danger
- Choking hazards

Toys

The most common safety issue regarding toys involves choking. The CPSC reports that a minimum of 41 children aspirated or died from choking between 2005 and 2009. The biggest culprits were balloons, toys, or toy parts.

In addition to choking, other hazards exist for children.

- Magnets—The danger occurs if a child swallows more than one magnet, as the magnets may be attracted to each other in the child's body, causing complications that may be life-threatening.
- Watch batteries that are button-type—Battery acid can result in fatal internal injuries.
- Objects that make noise—Loud toys may damage a child's sensitive ears.
- Strangulation dangers—Items such as mobiles, cords, and drawstrings should not be within a child's reach.
- Lead and other toxic chemicals—Lead and phthalates were being phased out of toy production starting in 2009 but toys made prior to that date may contain these harsh toxins. PVC plastic may contain toxic phthalates.

Toys manufactured after December 31, 2011, and intended for children ages 12 years and younger must be tested by a third party laboratory and must be certified. Toys intended for children ages 14 years and up must comply with safety standards but do not need to be tested by a third party laboratory. Toys and their special features and related materials requiring third party testing fall into the following categories:

- Toy chests
- Surface coating materials
- Liquids, pastes, putties, gels, and powders (not cosmetics)
- Stuffing materials
- Toys that produce sounds
- Objects that are small
- Accessible edges
- Wires or rods
- Nails and fasteners
- Packaging film
- Hinges or mechanisms that fold
- Cords, straps, elastics
- Stability and overload requirements
- Simulated protective devices
- Pacifiers with rubber nipples
- Toy pacifiers
- Teething toys and teethers
- Rattles that have ends that are almost spherical, hemispherical, or with circular flared ends
- Toys that will be attached to a crib or playpen
- Stuffed toys and beanbag toys
- Certain toys with spherical ends
- Pompoms
- Toy gun marking

- Objects with a hemispheric shape
- Yo-Yo tether toys
- Magnets
- Jaw entrapment handles and steering wheels

Cribs

Crib deaths have declined since the CPSC issued standards regarding them. The CPSC offers these suggestions for assuring that a crib is safe:

- Mattress should be firm and fit tight so that the baby cannot become trapped between the mattress and the crib.
- There should be no loose, missing, broken, or improperly installed screws, or other hardware in or on the crib.
- The crib slats should not be more than 2 3/8 inches apart, which is approximately the width of a can of soda. The baby's body should not fit through the slats. Slats should be in perfect condition, with no missing or cracked slats.
- Corner posts should not be more than 1/16 inches high so that the baby's clothing cannot get caught on them.
- There should be no spaces cut out in the headboard or footboard. Such spaces could entrap a baby's head.

Fireworks

Fireworks pose dangers to consumers, particularly to the hands, head, face, and ears. In 2011, four consumers died while using homemade or professionally produced fireworks and approximately 9,600 consumers were injured while using them. Sixty-five percent of these injuries typically occur within 30 days of the July 4th holiday.

The CPSC issues these suggestions to use fireworks safely:

- Consumers should make sure that fireworks are legal in their community prior to using them.
- Young children should never be allowed to play with or set off fireworks. This includes sparklers, which burn at extremely hot temperatures (hot enough to melt metal).
- If older children use fireworks, they should always be closely supervised by a responsible adult.
- Consumers should not purchase fireworks in brown paper packaging as this indicates that they were produced for a professional display and are dangerous for consumers.
- A person should never be positioned directly over a fireworks device while lighting the fuse. He or she should get back to a safe distance immediately after the fireworks are lit.
- A water hose or bucket filled with water should be nearby in case a fire develops.
- Malfunctioning fireworks should never be relit. They should be soaked with water and thrown away.
- Fireworks should never be pointed at another person.
- Fireworks should be lit one at a time, and the person lighting them should step back quickly.
- Fireworks should never be placed in a person's pocket or shot off in metal or glass containers.
- When fireworks have finished burning, they should be doused with a lot of water from a bucket or hose before they are discarded. This will prevent a fire in the trash.

Deaths, injuries and damages to property from fireworks result in costs to the United States of more than $900 billion each year.

Helmets

Wearing a helmet can enhance the safety of a number of activities including bicycle riding, motorcycle riding, skiing, and playing team sports such as football or baseball. Keeping the head covered in a helmet has been shown to lower the risk of a serious head injury or death. If a person falls or experiences a collision while engaging in an activity, the impact energy will be absorbed by the helmet rather than by the person's head and brain.

All helmets are not created equal, and have been designed for specific activities. The design of a particular helmet was created to protect the head from the most common impacts that occur while engaging in a specific activity. It is very important for individuals to wear the helmet designed for their activity. There are a few exceptions to this rule, such as the CPSC-compliant bicycle helmet that may be also be used for recreational roller skating, in-line skating, or while riding a nonpowered scooter.

Bicycle and motorcycle helmets must be in compliance with mandatory federal safety standards. Each bicycle helmet made after 1999 must meet the U.S. CPSC bicycle helmet standard. This standard assures that the helmet provides substantial protection to the head if used correctly. The chin strap must have enough strength so that the helmet stays on the head, in the correct position, if a fall or collision occurs.

According to the CPSC, helmets should be worn during these activities:

- Bicycling—Helmet should be warn flat on the head, not tilted back, should fit snugly, and should not block vision in any way. The chin strap should fit securely with the buckle remaining fastened while riding.
- Roller skating, in-line skating, and skateboarding—Skateboard type helmet.

- BMX cycling—BMX helmet.
- Downhill mountain bike racing—Downhill helmet.
- ATV riding, dirt- and mini-bike riding, motorcrossing—Motorcross or motorcycle helmet
- Karting and go-karting—Karting or motorcycle helmet.
- Moped or powered scooter riding—Moped or motorcycle helmet.
- Horseback riding—Equestrian helmet.
- Rock and wall climbing—Mountaineering helmet.
- Baseball, softball, and T-ball—Baseball batter's or catcher's helmet.
- Football—Football helmet.
- Ice hockey—Hockey helmet.
- Lacrosse—Lacrosse helmet.
- Skiing and snowboarding—Ski helmet.
- Snowmobiling—Snowmobile helmet.
- Ice skating and sledding—Bicycle, skateboard, or ski helmet.

Activities during which a helmet should not be worn include playing on playgrounds or climbing trees. During these activities, the chin strap of the helmet could become caught on the equipment or a tree, creating a chance for strangulation to occur. Also, the helmet may present danger of entrapment if worn during these activities.

Amusement parks

As of 2012, 44 states have regulations in place regarding amusement parks. The states without such regulations are Alabama, Mississippi, Nevada, South Dakota, Wyoming, and Utah, which have few (if any) amusement parks. In 1981, Congress took away the CPSC's authority to regulate rides at fixed sites. However, the CPSC does regulate ride safety at mobile sites.

According to the International Association of Amusement Parks and Attractions (IAAPA), the risk of serious injury on an amusement park ride at a fixed-site park in the United States is one in 1.9 million. In 2010, there were 1,207 injuries related to rides at fixed-site parks. Of those, 59 required overnight treatment in a hospital.

The IAAPA offers these safety tips for guests of amusement parks:

- Restrictions regarding age, height, weight, and health must be observed.
- All ride safety rules must be observed.
- Arms, hands, legs, and feet should always be positioned inside the ride.
- Guests should stay seated until the ride is completely stopped and personnel instruct the guests to exit.
- All verbal instructions or recorded announcements should be observed.
- Safety equipment must always be used and guests should never try to move out of these restrains or loosen them.
- Parents should always make sure that their children comprehend the ride rules and behavior.
- No one, especially a child, should be forced to ride an attraction if he or she does not want to do so.
- Any unsafe behavior should be reported to a supervisor or manager at once.

Efforts and solutions

The Consumer Product Safety Improvement Act (CPSIA) of 2008, sometimes called the "toy bill" established new testing and regulation requirements for children's and non-children's products. The act affected a number of products for infants, including items for the nursery. These items must be in compliance with the new safety rules, must be tested by a laboratory that is approved by the CPSC, and must contain a written Children's Product Certificate, which proves that the item is in compliance. The law also created a searchable database, which is available to consumers and lists the harm as well as the risk of harm that could be caused by a consumer product.

The CPSC operates a hotline (800-638-CPSC), which is available for persons who speak English or Spanish. The purpose of the hotline is for consumers to report a product that is not safe, report an injury related to a product, or determine if a product has been recalled. The website version of the hotline is www.SaferProducts.gov.

According to a statement paper released in 2012 by Robert S. Adler, Commissioner of the CPSC, the rate of deaths and injuries due to consumer products fell 30% between 1982 and 2012. He specifically pointed out the decline in childhood deaths and injuries:

- 92% reduction in children's poisoning
- 92% drop in crib deaths
- 100% decrease in child suffocations from refrigerators that have been abondoned
- 88% drop in injuries from baby walkers
- 92% decrease in deaths from electrocutions
- 46% drop in deaths from residential fires

Adler estimated that the decreases in deaths from electrocutions and residential fires lead to a $16 billion decrease in costs to society.

KEY TERMS

ASTM—ASTM International, previously the American Society for Testing and Materials, develops standards for product quality and safety.

Phthalates—Toxic chemical that may be present in toys and may lead to development dangers.

In the early 2000s, the CPSC found hundreds of problems in samples of consumer products that were imported. Because of this, a division was created to focus on compliance from manufacturers in other countries. CPSC staff are now in place at 15 ports of entry to the United State. In 2012, because of these efforts, 6,600 samples were screened (nearly 10 times the number screened in 2007) and more than 1 million units were not granted entry into the United States.

In October 2012, the United States experienced a multistate **meningitis** outbreak of **fungal infections** among patients who received a steroid injection of a potentially contaminated product into the spinal area. The **CDC** and other agencies conducted investigations of liquid steroids sent pharmaceutical suppliers. According to the CDC, several patients also suffered strokes that are believed to have resulted from their infection. The investigation also included fungal infections associated with injections in a peripheral joint space, such as a knee, shoulder or ankle. Some of the patients recieiving infected shots died from meningitis complications.

Resources

BOOKS

Pine, Timothy. *Product Safety Excellence: The Seven Elements Essential for Product Liability Prevention.* Milwaukee, WI: American Society for Quality, Quality Press: 2012.

PERIODICALS

Adler, Robert S. "Oversight of the Consumer Product Safety Commission" *U.S. Consumer Product Safety Commission* August 2, 2012.

WEBSITES

Amusement ride safety tips. International Association of Amusement Parks and Attractions. http://www.iaapa.org/pressroom/Amusement_Ride_Safety_Tips.asp (accessed September 29, 2012).

The Nader Page. ttp://nader.org/ (accessed September 29, 2012).

Saferproducts.gov http://www.saferproducts.gov/Default.aspx (accessed September 29, 2012).

USRecallNews.com http://www.usrecallnews.com/2008/05/us-consumer-product-safety-commission-cpsc.html (accessed September 29, 2012).

ORGANIZATIONS

Consumer Product Safety Commission, 4330 East West Highway, Bethesda, MD 20814, (800) 595-7054, www.cpsc.gov.

Rhonda Cloos, RN

Contraception and birth control

Definition

Contraception (birth control) prevents pregnancy by interfering with the normal process of ovulation, fertilization, and implantation. Different kinds of birth control act at different points in the process.

Purpose

Every month, a woman's body begins the process that can potentially lead to pregnancy. An egg (ovum) matures, the mucus that is secreted by the cervix (a cylindrical-shaped organ at the lower end of the uterus) changes to be more inviting to sperm, and the lining of the uterus grows in preparation for receiving a fertilized egg. Any sexually active woman who wants to prevent pregnancy must use a reliable form of birth control.

Birth control (contraception) is designed to interfere with the normal process and prevent the pregnancy that

Effectiveness of contraceptives: Percentage of women experiencing an unintended pregnancy within first year of typical[1] and perfect[2] contraceptive use

Form of birth control	Typical use	Perfect use
Birth control pills	8.0%	0.3%
Condom, female	21.0%	5.0%
Condom, male	15.0%	2.0%
Depo-Provera® (injection)	3.0%	0.3%
Diaphragm	16.0%	6.0%
Intrauterine devices (IUDs)	0.8%	0.6%
Spermicides	29.0%	18.0%

[1]Effectiveness based on average or typical usage.
[2]Effectiveness based on perfect or correct usage.

SOURCE: Centers for Disease Control and Prevention, "U.S. Medical Eligibility Criteria for Contraceptive Use, 2010," *Morbidity and Mortality Weekly Report*, vol. 59 (May 28, 2010). Available online at: http://www.cdc.gov/mmwr/pdf/rr/rr59e0528.pdf (accessed August 18, 2010).

(Table by PreMediaGlobal. © 2013 Cengage Learning)

could result. Different types of birth control act at different points in the process, from ovulation, through fertilization, to implantation. Each method has its own side effects and risks. Some methods are more reliable than others.

Description

More varieties of birth control are available today than ever before. They can be divided into groups based on how they work. These groups include:

- Hormonal methods—These use medications (hormones) to prevent ovulation. Hormonal methods include birth control pills (oral contraceptives); minipill, which contains only progestin; injections such as Depo Provera and Lunelle; implants in the arm; and hormone delivery via patch, such as Ortho Evra.
- Barrier methods—These methods work by preventing the sperm from reaching and fertilizing the egg. Barrier methods include the condom, diaphragm, cervical cap, and Lea Shield. The condom is the only form of birth control that also protects against sexually transmitted diseases, including HIV (the virus that causes AIDS).
- Spermicides—These medications kill sperm on contact. Most spermicides contain nonoxynyl-9. Spermicides come in many different forms, such as jelly, foam, tablets, and even a transparent film. All are placed in the vagina. Spermicides work best when they are used at the same time as a barrier method.
- Intrauterine devices—Intrauterine contraceptive devices (IUDs) are inserted into the uterus, where they stay from five to 10 years. An IUD prevents the fertilized egg from implanting in the lining of the uterus and may have other effects as well. The IUD may work through causing an inflammation within the uterus (copper IUD) or by releasing hormones (hormonal IUD).
- Tubal sterilization—Tubal sterilization is a permanent form of contraception for women. Each fallopian tube is either tied or burned closed. The sperm cannot reach the egg, and the egg cannot travel to the uterus.
- Fallopian tube coil—The fallopian tube coil, under the brand name Essure, is a form of permanent birth control in which a tiny coil is inserted into each fallopian tube, causing the formation of scar tissue, which prevents the sperm from making contact with the egg. This form of birth control cannot be reversed.
- Vasectomy—is the male form of sterilization and should also be considered permanent. In this procedure, the vas deferens, the tiny tubes that carry the sperm into the semen, are cut and tied off. Thus, no sperm can get into the semen.
- Emergency contraception—A somewhat controversial form of birth control, there are two forms of emergency contraception: contraceptive pills, which are sometimes referred to as "morning-after pills." and a copper intrauterine device. There are four types of emergency contraceptive pills. One contains progestin and is available over the counter in the United States for men and women ages 17 and up. The second form of contraceptive pill is made from ulipristal acetate and may only be obtained in the United States and Europe by prescription. The third type contains both progestin and estrogen. The fourth type contains mifepristone and is only available in China, Russia, and Vietnam. As a form of emergency contraception, the copper intrauterine device may be inserted up to five days after intercourse to prevent a pregnancy. This device, known as the Copper-T-IUD, lowers the risk of pregnancy by more than 99% and is more effective than any of the four types of emergency contraceptive pills.

Unfortunately, there is no perfect form of birth control. Only abstinence (not having sexual intercourse) can protect against unwanted pregnancy with 100% reliability. The failure rates, which means the rates of pregnancy, for most forms of birth control are quite low. However, some forms of birth control are more difficult or inconvenient to use than others. In actual practice, the birth control methods that are more difficult or inconvenient have much higher failure rates because they are not used regularly or as prescribed.

The methods of birth control differ from each other in the timing of when they are used. Some methods of birth control must be used specifically at the time of sexual intercourse (condoms, diaphragm, cervical cap, spermicides). Emergency contraception must be started as soon as possible after intercourse. All other methods of birth control (hormonal methods, IUDs, tubal sterilization) must be working all the time to provide protection. To provide education regarding emergency contraception, the Association of **Reproductive Health** Professionals and the Office of Population Research at Princeton University provide the Emergency Contraception Website (www.not-2-late.com). Each month, the site attracts more than 150,000 visitors.

Risks

There are risks associated with certain forms of birth control. Some of the risks of each method appear in the following list:

- Birth control pills—The hormone (estrogen) in birth control pills can increase the risk of heart attack in women over 35, particularly those who smoke. Certain women cannot use birth control pills. Use of oral contraceptives may also increase the risk of certain cancers (cervical and liver cancers), but it may also lower the risk of other cancers, such as ovarian and endometrial cancers. Birth control pills may also cause blood pressure to rise. Women age 35 years and up who smoke have a higher risk of heart disease if they take birth control pills. The minipill contains only progestin and is estrogen-free. While the minipill does not have the risks associated with estrogen use, out of 100 women who take the minipill, it is estimated that one to 13 will become pregnant during the first year of use. The minipill also has side effects, such as ovarian cysts, tender breasts, and acne.

- IUD—The copper IUD may cause anemia, back pains, bleeding between periods, uterine cramping, vaginitis, painful intercourse, heavy menstrual periods and severe pain during menstruation, and vaginal discharge. Risks of the hormonal IUD include acne, headache, tender breasts, amenorrhea (no periods), breakthrough bleeding, changes in moods, weight gain, cysts of the ovary, and pain in the abdomen or pelvis.
- Tubal sterilization—"Tying the tubes" is a surgical procedure and has all the risks of any other surgery, including those associated with anesthesia, as well as infection and bleeding.
- Fallopian tube coils—The Essure system has risks such as pain in the pelvis, infection, uterine perforation or fallopian tube perforation, and blockage of the fallopian tubes on one side. Once a woman has had Essure implants, she may not be able to have certain electrosurgical procedures such as endometrial ablation. This is because the metal implants are able to conduct electricity, which may damage the tissue.
- Emergency contraceptive pills or IUD—These methods of birth control should not be used regularly for birth control. They can interrupt the menstrual cycle and are not 100% effective. If the emergency contraception fails, an ectopic pregnancy can occur. They can also cause other side effects, such as nausea and vomiting.
- Vasectomy—A man may experience scrotal symptoms such as swelling, bruising, or bleeding. There may also be blood in the semen or an infection at the site where surgery was performed.

Preparation

No specific preparation is needed before using most forms of contraception. However, a woman must be sure that she is not already pregnant before using a hormonal method or having an IUD placed. Surgical forms of contraception, such as fallopian tube coils, tubal sterilization, and vasectomy, require pre-operative preparation.

Women who select the fallopian tube coil, or Essure system, sometimes take a hormonal form of contraception prior to insertion of the coil. The hormone regime thins the lining of the uterus, giving the health care provider an unobstructed view into the openings of the tubes, which aids in the insertion of the coils.

Prior to a vasectomy procedure, a health care provider may tell the patient to stop taking aspirin or other blood thinners and wash the surgical area or shave it. The provider may also prescribe a sedative to relax the patient before surgery.

Demographics

In developing countries, more than 215 million women need an effective method of contraception. In countries with solid family-planning programs in place, the use of contraceptives has increased significantly since the 1980s; however, in sub-Saharan Africa, the use of contraceptives is very low and hardly changed in the first decade of the twenty-first century. In these areas, selection of contraceptives is limited via acts of politicians, health care providers, cost, and availability of effective methods. A study that included 88 developing countries found that family-planning programs are available to women, and are affordable, in only 14 of these nations.

Cost to society

The lack of effective contraceptive methods in developing countries results in significant financial cost. According to the United Nations Population Fund (UNPFA), every dollar allocated toward contraception will reduce medical spending by $1.40. This is because such an investment would decrease the need to spend money on unintended births and abortions.

Efforts and solutions

In 2012, the London Summit on Family Planning, hosted by the government of the United Kingdom and the Bill & Melinda Gates Foundation, along with other partner organizations, provided resources and policies that will bring contraceptive education, supplies, and family-planning services to young women and girls who live in impoverished parts of the world. The summit resulted in pledges of $4.6 billion toward family-planning services in developing countries between 2012 and 2020. Organizers of the meeting announced that these funds will be sufficient to provide access to contraception for women who otherwise had no access to birth control education or services. The goal of the summit is to enable 120 million more women and girls to utilize contraceptives by the year 2020. The intended outcome is to save the lives of 200,000 women and girls who die while they are pregnant or while giving birth as well as almost 3 million infants who die before they reach one year of age.

KEY TERMS

Fallopian tubes—The thin tubes that connect the ovary to the uterus. Ova (eggs) travel from the ovary to the uterus. If the egg has been fertilized, it can implant in the uterus.

Fertilization—The joining of the sperm and the egg; conception.

Implantation—The process in which the fertilized egg embeds itself in the wall of the uterus.

Ovulation—The release of an egg (ovum) from the ovary.

The specific objectives of the summit were to:

- Raise demand and support for family planning
- Improve supply, service delivery, and systems related to contraceptive care
- Obtain the materials that countries need to provide effective contraceptives
- Develop innovative ways to address the complexities of family planning
- Foster accountability by monitoring and evaluating the programs

The UNFPA is also working toward increasing access to contraception in developing countries. Among the group's goals is promotion of the reproductive rights of women. The UNFPA works with the governments of developing nations to enhance contraceptive education and usage.

In 2008, 17.4 million women in the United States needed public funding to obtain contraceptives. Of these, 12.4 million were impoverished, and 5 million were younger than 20 years of age. Title X of the Public Health Service Act is the only federal program entirely dedicated to family-planning services. This source of funding provides family-planning centers throughout the nation. Still, Medicaid is the largest source of financial support for family planning. In 2010, family planning centers obtained 37% of their support from Medicaid, and 22% from Title X funding.

In developing countries, only 43% of woman of child-bearing age use contraception, compared to 62% in developing nations. Of the women living in **poverty** in developing countries, only 35% use birth control.

There is no perfect form of birth control. Every method has a small failure rate and side effects. Some methods carry additional risks. However, every method of birth control can be effective if used properly.

Resources

BOOKS

World Bank. *Healthy Partnerships: How Governments Can Engage the Private Sector to Improve Health in Africa*, The World Bank, Washington, D.C., 20011.

PERIODICALS

"Contraception; Overview." *NWHRC Health Center–Contraception*. March 9, 2004.

"Ectopic Pregnancy Is a Possibility When Emergency Contraception Fails." *Health & Medicine Week*. March 15, 2004: 222.

Creanga, Andreea A., Duff Gillespie, Sabrina Karklins, and Amy O. Tsui."Low Use of Contraception Among Poor Women in Africa: An Equity Issue." *Bulletin of the World Health Organization*. 89 (2011): 258–266.

WEBSITES

IRIN Globalhttp://www.irinnews.org/Report/95860/HEALTH-Family-planning-summit-focuses-on-mother-and-child-survival (accessed September 18, 2012)

Mayo Clinic. http://www.mayoclinic.com/health/essure/MY00999 (accessed September 19, 2012)

Princeton University Emergency Contraception Website http://ec.princeton.edu/emergency-contraception.html (accessed September 18, 2012)

ORGANIZATIONS

American Pregnancy Association, 1425 Greenway Drive, Suite 440, Irving, TX 75038, (972) 550-0140, Questions@AmericanPregnancy.org, http://www.americanpregnancy.org

Guttmacher Institute, 125 Maiden Lane, 7th Floor, New York, NY 10038, (212) 248-1111, http://www.guttmacher.org

United Nations Population Fund, 605 Third Avenue, New York, NY 10158, (212) 297-5000, hq@unfpa.org, http://www.unfpa.org.

Amy B. Tuteur, MD
Teresa G. Odle
Rhonda Cloos

Correctional health

Definition

Correctional health refers to health services made available to men and women who are incarcerated in prisons or jails.

Purpose

The purpose of correctional health services is to ensure that men and women who are serving time in correctional institutions receive an adequate level of physical and mental health care, at least equivalent to that of non-incarcerated individuals.

Description

Concern about the health status of prisoners is a relatively new phenomenon. Throughout most of human history, men and women who were sentenced to prison terms were generally not thought to be worthy of even the most basic medical attention. This attitude is reflected in the old maxim in which the goal of law enforcement was sometimes seen as having to put a person in jail and "throw away the key." In fact, incarceration was often a guarantee of worsened health and even death for prisoners. They were consigned to living conditions that were far inferior to those of the outside world, involving close confinement with individuals having a range of chronic and acute health conditions. In some cases, a prison sentence also proved to be a death sentence.

Demographics

A number of studies have shown that prisoners often receive medical and health care at least as good as that of many individuals living outside the walls of jails and prisons. A 2004 study by the U.S. Department of Justice (DOJ), for example, found that 44 percent of state inmates and 39 percent of federal inmates reported some type of current medical problem more serious than a cold or viral infection. The most common of those ailments were arthritis (15 percent of state inmates and 12 percent of federal inmates) and hypertension (state: 14 percent; federal: 13 percent). Seventy percent of state inmates and 76 percent of federal inmates reported having seen a health professional about their medical problem. Learning impairments were also common among inmates, with 23 percent of state inmates and 13 percent of federal inmates reporting such a problem. Injuries incurred within the prison setting are also a health issue. Almost a quarter (22 percent) of state inmates reported having been injured in an accident and 16 percent, in a fight. Comparable figures for federal inmates was 23 percent injured in an accident and eight percent in a fight. Research suggests that the rate of chronic health conditions is somewhat higher among prisoners than among the general **population** for conditions such as arthritis, **asthma**, **hepatitis**, hypertension, and cervical **cancer**, but not for other conditions, such as angina, diabetes, myocardial infarction, and **obesity**.

The DOJ study also provided valuable information on health care available in jails and prisons. It found that about 90 percent of all inmates received some type of health intake interview at the time of their arrival, and about three quarters of all inmates reported receiving regular health checkups and services of one kind or another, including **tuberculosis** and HIV testing, counseling for **suicide** concerns, routine health and dental care, and surgical procedures when needed. In all, the study seemed to suggest that inmates in both state and federal prisons receive as much health and medical care as do many comparable populations of non-incarcerated women and men.

History

The modern U.S. program of health care for incarcerated individuals dates to the early 1970s when the American Medical Association (AMA) conducted a study of American penal institutions and found that health and medical care in such institutions was deficient in both quantity and quality. Of special concern to the AMA was the lack of any type of national standards against which the medical and health services in any penal institution could be compared. In the early 1980s, the AMA, in collaboration with other organizations, attempted to resolve that problem by establishing the National Commission on Correctional Health Care (NCCHC), whose mission it was to evaluate the existing status of care in prisons and to recommend improvements in health and medical programs. The NCCHC continues to operate today with similar objectives. It publishes and Standards for Health Care and Mental Health which serve as the guidelines for health and medical care in the vast majority of state and federal penal institutions. It also provides educational programs for such institutions as are attempting to improve the quality of their own services, and it offers accreditation, on a voluntary basis, to institutions who seek that recognition of their efforts.

Legal

Also during the 1970s, the professional concerns exhibited by the AMA study of prison health programs received legal support from a number of court decisions that affirmed the right of prisoners to the same level of health and medical care as was available to non-prisoners. The key decision during that era was the 1976 U.S. Supreme Court decision in *Estelle v. Gamble*. In that case, a Texas prisoner, J. W. Gamble, was injured while on a work detail, and was unable to get the medical assistance needed to deal with that injury. His attorney sued the state of Texas in a case that eventually worked its way to the Supreme Court, which eventually ruled that "an inmate must rely on prison authorities to treat his medical needs; if the authorities fail to do so, those needs will not be met. In the worst cases, such a failure may actually produce physical torture or a lingering death." The Court's decision thereby established a new and rigorous standard for prisoner medical care that has only

> **KEY TERMS**
>
> **Coorectional institution**—A prison or jail.
>
> **Equivalent care**—The concept that a prisoner is legally eligible for a level and health and medical care equivalent to that of a non-incarcerated person.

be reaffirmed on many occasions in the ensuing three decades of jurisprudence.

International Perspectives

Concerns about prison health and medical issues in other parts of the world have been somewhat more recent than in the United States. In 1995, the **World Health Organization (WHO)** established a special bureau to deal with this issue, the Health in Prisons Programme (HIPP), designed to assist member nations in dealing with prison health problems. HIPP now coordinates a 44-nation network (all of whose members are in Europe) working to improve health and medical conditions in national prisons. The primary focus of the network is a group of specific health problems indigenous to prisons: tuberculosis, HIV/AIDS, drugs, mental health, women, and **nutrition**. One of its key publications is a 2007 report (updated in 2011), *Health in Prisons. A WHO Guide to the Essentials in Prison Health.*

Resources

BOOKS

Delgado, Melvin, and Denise Humm-Delgado. *Health and Health Care in the Nation's Prisons: Issues, Challenges, and Policies*. Lanham, MD: Rowman and Littlefied, 2008.

Ruddell, Rick, and Mark Tomita, eds. *Issues in Correctional Health Care*. Regina, SK: Newgate Press, 2008.

Sanchez-Castro, Raquel. *Greed Versus Love: An Inconvenient Truth About the Privatization of Correctional Health Care*. Philadelphia: Xlibris, 2010.

PERIODICALS

Binswanger, I. A., P. M. Krueger, and J. F. Steiner. "Prevalence of Chronic Medical Conditions among Jail and Prison Inmates in the USA Compared with the General Population." *Journal of Epidemiology and Community Health* 63, 11. (2009): 912–19.

Dumont, D. M., et al. "Public Health and the Epidemic of Incarceration." *Annual Review of Public Health* 33 (2012): 325–29.

Wilper, A. P., et al. "The Health and Health Care of US Prisoners: Results of a Nationwide Survey." *American Journal of Public Health* 99, 4. (2009): 666–72.

WEBSITES

Conway, Craig A. "A Right of Access to Medical and Mental Health Care for the Incarcerated." http://www.law.uh.edu/healthlaw/perspectives/2009/(CC)%20Prison%20Health.pdf. Accessed on September 27, 2012.

"National Commission on Correctional Health Care." http://www.ncchc.org/. Accessed on September 27, 2012.

"Prisons and Health." World Health Organization. http://www.euro.who.int/en/what-we-do/health-topics/health-determinants/prisons-and-health/activities. Accessed on September 27, 2012.

"Title." URL HERE. Accessed on September 11, 2012.

ORGANIZATIONS

Acadeny of Correctional Health Professionals, P.O. Box 11583, Chicago, IL USA 60611, (877) 549–2247, Fax: 1 (773) 880–2424, academy@correctionalhealth.org, http://www.correctionalhealth.org/index.asp.

David E. Newton, Ed.D.

Creutzfeldt-Jakob disease

Definition

Creutzfeldt-Jakob disease (CJD) is a transmissible, rapidly progressing, neurodegenerative disorder called a spongiform degeneration related to "mad cow disease."

Description

Before 1995, Creutzfeldt-Jakob disease was not well known outside the medical profession. Even within it, many practitioners did not know much about it. Most doctors had never seen a case. With the recognition of a so-called "new variant" form of CJD and the strong possibility that those with it became infected simply by eating contaminated beef, CJD has become one of the most talked-about diseases in the world. Additionally, the radical theory that the infectious agent is a normal protein that has been changed in its form also has sparked much interest.

First described in the early twentieth century independently by Creutzfeldt and Jakob, CJD is a neurodegenerative disease causing a rapidly progressing dementia ending in death, usually within eight months of symptom onset. It also is a very rare disease, affecting only about one in every million people throughout the world. In the United States, CJD is thought to affect about 250 people each year. CJD affects adults primarily between ages 50 and 75.

Spongiform encephalopathies

The most obvious pathologic feature of CJD is the formation of numerous fluid-filled spaces in the brain (vacuoles) resulting in a sponge-like appearance. CJD is one of several human "spongiform encephalopathies," diseases that produce this characteristic change in brain tissue. Others are kuru; Gerstmann-Straussler-Scheinker disease, a genetic disorder predominantly characterized by cerebellar ataxia (a kind of movement disorder); and fatal familial insomnia, with symptoms of progressive sleeplessness, weakness, and dysfunction of the nervous system that affects voluntary and involuntary movements and functions.

Kuru was prevalent among the Fore people in Papua, New Guinea, and spread from infected individuals after their deaths through the practice of ritual cannibalism, in which the relatives of the dead person honored him by consuming his organs, including the brain. Discovery of the infectious nature of kuru won the Nobel Prize for Carleton Gadjusek in 1976. The incubation period for kuru was between four to 30 years or more. While kuru has virtually disappeared since these cannibalistic practices stopped, several new cases continue to arise each year.

Cases of CJD have been grouped into three types: familial, iatrogenic, and sporadic.

- Familial CJD, representing 5–15% of cases, is inherited in an autosomal dominant manner, meaning that either parent may pass along the disease to a child, who then may develop CJD later in life.
- Iatrogenic CJD occurs when a person is infected during a medical procedure, such as organ donation, blood transfusion, or brain surgery. The rise in organ donation has increased this route of transmission; grafts of infected corneas and dura mater (the tissue covering the brain) have been shown to transmit CJD. Another source is hormones concentrated from the pituitary glands of cadavers, some of whom carried CJD, for use in people with growth hormone deficiencies. Iatrogenic infection from exposure to nerve-containing tissue represents a small fraction of all cases. The incubation period after exposure to the infectious agent is very long and is estimated to be from less than 10 to more than 30 years. It remains unlikely, but not impossible, that blood from patients with CJD is infectious to others by transfusion.
- Sporadic CJD represents at least 85% of all cases. Sporadic cases have no identifiable source of infection. Death usually follows first symptoms within eight months.

Animal forms and "mad cow disease"

Six forms of spongiform encephalopathies are known to occur in other mammals: scrapie in sheep, recognized for more than 200 years; chronic wasting disease in elk and mule deer in Wyoming and Colorado; transmissible mink encephalopathy; exotic ungulate encephalopathy in some types of zoo animals; feline spongiform encephalopathy in domestic cats; and **bovine spongiform encephalopathy** (BSE) in cows.

BSE was first recognized in Britain in 1986. Besides the spongiform changes in the brain, BSE causes dementia-like behavioral changes—hence the name "mad cow disease." BSE was thought to be an altered form of scrapie, transmitted to cows when they were fed sheep offal (slaughterhouse waste) as part of their feed, but researchers believe it is a primary cattle disease spread by contaminated feed.

The use of slaughterhouse offal in animal feed has been common in many countries and has been practiced for at least 50 years. The trigger for the BSE epidemic in Great Britain seems to have come in the early 1980s, when the use of organic solvents for preparation of offal was altered there. It is possible that these solvents had been destroying the agent called a prion, thereby preventing infection, and that the change in preparation procedure opened the way for the agent to "jump species" and cause BSE in cows that consumed scrapie-infected meal. The slaughter of infected (but not yet visibly sick) cows at the end of their useful farm lives, and the use of their carcasses for feed, spread the infection rapidly and widely. For at least a year after BSE was first recognized in British herds, infected bovine remains continued to be incorporated into feed, spreading the disease still further. Although milk from infected cows never has been shown to pass the infectious agent, passage from infected mother to calf may have occurred through unknown means. Researchers also have tried to confirm how to stop infection of the human food chain once the disease spread among cows. In 2003, a study reported that it spread through nervous system tissue in processed meat and that proper temperature and pressure controls could help ensure safety of commercial beef.

Beginning in 1988, the British government took steps to stop the spread of BSE, banning the use of bovine offal in feed and other products and ordering the slaughter of infected cows. By then, the slow-acting agent had become epidemic in British herds. In 1992, it was diagnosed in more than 25,000 animals (1% of the British herd). By mid-1997, the cumulative number of BSE cases in the United Kingdom had risen to more than 170,000. The feeding ban stemmed the tide of the epidemic; however, the number of new cases each week fell from a peak of 1,000 in 1993 to less than 300 two years later.

The export of British feed and beef to member countries was banned by the European Union, but cases of BSE had developed in Europe by then as well;

however, by mid-1997, only about 1,000 cases had been identified. In 1989, the United States banned import of British beef and began monitoring United States herds in 1990. In December 2003, the first case of BSE was discovered in the United States. This prompted recommendations of new safeguards to prevent further spread. Among these were regulations banning animal blood in cattle feed.

Variant CJD: The human equivalent of mad cow disease

From the beginning of the BSE epidemic, scientists and others in Britain feared that BSE might jump species again to infect humans who had consumed infected beef. This, however, had never occurred in scrapie from sheep, a disease known for hundreds of years. In 1996, the first report of this possibility occurred and the fear seemed to be realized with the first cases of a new variant of Creutzfeldt-Jacob disease, termed nvCJD, now just vCJD. Its victims are much younger than the 60–65 year old average for CJD, and the time from symptom onset to death has averaged 12 months or more instead of eight. The disease appears to cause more psychiatric symptoms early on. EEG abnormalities characteristic of CJD are not typically seen in vCJD.

By early 2004, CJD had claimed 143 victims in Great Britain and 10 in other countries. It is of major concern that the number of cases per year seems to be increasing by a factor of 1.35 each year. The only known case in the United States to date had been acquired while the person had been in Great Britain.

Evidence is growing stronger that vCJD is in fact caused by BSE:

- almost all of the cases so far have occurred in Great Britain, the location of the BSE epidemic
- BSE injected into monkeys produces a disease very similar to vCJD
- BSE and vCJD produce the same brain lesions after the same incubation period when injected into laboratory mice
- brain proteins isolated from vCJD victims, but not from the other forms of CJD, share similar molecular characteristics with brain proteins of animals that died from BSE

Researchers now treat the BSE-vCJD connection as solidly established.

Assuming that BSE is the source, the question that has loomed from the beginning has been how many people will eventually be affected. Epidemiological models once placed estimates at tens of thousands, but in 2003, scientists predicted a quicker end to the epidemic and have substantially lowered the numbers expected to contract the disease. The exact incubation period of vCJD in humans is about 10 to 20 years or longer, so it is more difficult to predict the number of cases. Researchers know that some people are more susceptible to vCJD, including young people age 10 to 20 years old.

Causes and symptoms

Causes

It is clear that Creutzfeldt-Jakob disease is caused by an infectious agent, but it is not yet clear what type of agent that is. Originally assumed to be a virus, evidence is accumulating that, instead, CJD is caused by a protein called a prion (PREE-on, for "proteinaceous infectious particle") transmitted from victim to victim. The other spongiform encephalopathies also are hypothesized to be due to prion infection.

If this hypothesis is proven true, it would represent one of the most radical new ideas in biology since the discovery of deoxyribonucleic acid (DNA). All infectious diseases, in fact all life, use nucleic acids—DNA or ribonucleic acid (RNA)—to code the instructions needed for reproduction. Inactivation of the nucleic acids destroys the capacity to reproduce. However, when these same measures are applied to infected tissue from spongiform encephalopathy victims, infectivity is not destroyed. Furthermore, purification of infected tissue to concentrate the infectious fraction yields protein, not nucleic acid. While it remains possible that some highly stable nucleic acid remains hidden within the purified protein, this is seemingly less and less likely as further experiments are done. The "prion hypothesis," as it is called, is now widely accepted, at least provisionally, by most researchers in the field. The most vocal proponent of the hypothesis, Stanley Prusiner, was awarded the Nobel Prize in 1997 for his work in the prion diseases.

A prion is an altered form of a normal brain protein. The normal protein has a helical shape along part of its length. In the prion form, a sheet structure replaces the helix. According to the hypothesis, when the normal form interacts with the prion form, some of its helical part is converted to a sheet, thus creating a new prion capable of transforming other normal forms. In this way, the disease process resembles crystallization more than typical viral infection, in which the virus commands the host's cellular machinery to reproduce more of the virus. Build-up of the sheet form causes accumulation of abnormal protein clumps and degeneration of brain cells, which is thought to cause the disease.

The brain protein affected by the prion, called PrP, is part of the membrane of brain cells, but its exact function is unknown. Exposure to the infectious agent is, of course, still required for disease development. Prion diseases are not contagious in the usual sense, and transmission from an infected person to another person requires direct inoculation of infectious material.

Familial CJD, on the other hand, does not require exposure, but develops through the inheritance of other, more disruptive mutations in the gene for the normal PrP protein. The other two inherited human prion diseases, Gerstmann-Straussler-Scheinker disease and fatal familial insomnia, involve different mutations in the same gene.

The large majority of CJD cases are sporadic, meaning they have no known route of infection or genetic link. Causes of sporadic CJD are likely to be diverse and may include spontaneous genetic mutation, spontaneous protein changes, or unrecognized exposure to infectious agents. It is highly likely that future research will identify more risk factors associated with sporadic CJD.

Symptoms

About one in four people with CJD begin their illness with weakness, changes in sleep patterns, weight loss, or loss of appetite or sexual drive. A person with CJD may first complain of visual disturbances, including double vision, blurry vision, or partial loss of vision. Some visual symptoms are secondary to cortical blindness related to death of nerve cells in the occipital lobe of the brain responsible for vision. This form of visual loss is unusual in that patients may be unaware that they are unable to see. These symptoms may appear weeks to months before the onset of dementia.

The most characteristic symptom of CJD is rapidly progressing dementia, or loss of mental function. Dementia is marked by:

- memory loss
- impaired abstraction and planning
- language and comprehension disturbances
- poor judgment
- disorientation
- decreased attention and increased restlessness
- personality changes and psychosis
- hallucinations

Muscle spasms and jerking movements, called myoclonus, are also a prominent symptom of CJD. Balance and coordination disturbance (ataxia), is common in CJD, and is more pronounced in nvCJD. Stiffness, difficulty moving, and other features representing Parkinson's disease are seen and can progress to akinetic mutism, which is a state of being unable to speak or move.

KEY TERMS

Autosomal dominant inheritance—A pattern of inheritance in which a trait will be expressed if the gene is inherited from either parent.

Encephalopathy—Brain disorder characterized by memory impairment and other symptoms.

Iatrogenic—Caused by a medical procedure.

Nucleic acids—The cellular molecules DNA and RNA that act as coded instructions for the production of proteins and are copied for transmission of inherited traits.

Diagnosis

CJD is diagnosed by a clinical neurological exam and electroencephalography (EEG), which shows characteristic spikes called triphasic sharp waves. Magnetic resonance imaging (MRI) or computed tomography scans (CT) should be done to exclude other forms of dementia, and in CJD typically shows atrophy or loss of brain tissue. Lumbar puncture, or spinal tap, may be done to rule out other causes of dementia (as cell count, chemical analysis, and other routine tests are normal in CJD) and to identify elevated levels of marker proteins known as 14-3-3. Another marker, neuron-specific enolase, may also be increased in CJD. CJD is conclusively diagnosed after death by brain autopsy. Scientists are investigating whether testing lymphatic tissue such as the tonsil may be an early tool in vCJD diagnosis. Additionally, recent studies have suggested that other blood tests may be useful as well.

Treatment

There is no cure for CJD, and no treatment that slows the progression of the disease. Drug therapy and nursing care are aimed at minimizing psychiatric symptoms and increasing patient comfort. However, the rapid progression of CJD frustrates most attempts at treatment, since decreasing cognitive function and more prominent behavioral symptoms develop so quickly. Despite the generally grim prognosis, a few CJD patients progress more slowly and live longer than the average; for these patients, treatment will be more satisfactory. Scientists are investigating whether some medicines that can "break" the abnormal protein form may be useful and whether a vaccine could help.

Prognosis

Creutzfeldt-Jakob disease has proven invariably fatal, with death following symptom onset by an average of eight months. About 5% of patients live longer than two years. Death from vCJD has averaged approximately 12 months after onset. However, in 2003, clinicians reported improvement in a patient with vCJD who received a new experimental drug called Pentosan.

Prevention

There is no known way to prevent sporadic CJD, by far the most common type. Not everyone who inherits the gene mutation for familial CJD will develop the disease, but at present, there is no known way to predict who will and who will not succumb. The incidence of iatrogenic CJD has fallen with recognition of its sources, the development of better screening techniques for infected tissue, and the use of sterilization techniques for surgical instruments that inactivate prion proteins. Fortunately, scientists are making progress. In 2003, researchers announced that they had uncovered the basis for diagnosing, treating and possibly preventing prion diseases such as vCJD. Their research possibly could lead to a vaccine and immunotherapy drugs.

Strategies for **prevention** of vCJD are a controversial matter, as they involve a significant sector of the agricultural industry and a central feature of the diet in many countries. The infectious potential of contaminated meat is unknown, because the ability to detect prions within meat is limited. Surveillance of North American herds strongly suggests there is no BSE here, and strict regulations on imports of European livestock make future outbreaks highly unlikely. Therefore, avoidance of all meat originating in North America, simply on grounds of BSE risk, is a personal choice unsupported by current data.

Resources

PERIODICALS

Brown, Paul, et al. "Ultra-high Pressure Inactivation of Prion Infectivity in Processed Meat: A Practical Method to Prevent Human Infection." *Proceedings of the National Academy of Sciences of the United States* May 13, 2003: 6093–6095.

"GP Sees Patient with vCJD Improve." *Pulse* June 23, 2003: 12.

Kaye, Donald. "FDA Launches New Mad Cow Rules to Protect U.S. Food, Feed." *Clinical Infectious Diseases* March 15, 2004: 3–5.

"Large Human Mad Cow Epidemic Unlikely—Scientists." *Clinical Infectious Diseases* April 15, 2003: i.

"Report Appears to Confirm Blood-borne Transmission of Creutzfeldt-Jakob Disease." *Blood Weekly* January 8, 2004: 28.

"Researchers Discover Possible Diagnosis, Treatment, Vaccine." *Immunotherapy Weekly* June 25, 2003: 2.

"Scientists Predict Swift End to vCJD Epidemic." *British Medical Journal* May 24, 2003: 1104–1111.

"U.S. Lawmakers Want Increase in Mad Cow Testing." *Healthcare Purchasing News* March 2004: 85.

Larry I. Lutwick, MD
Teresa G. Odle

Cytomegalovirus

Definition

Cytomegalovirus, or CMV, is a common virus that infects many people during their lives. Symptoms are generally mild and similar to mononucleosis, and some people never have symptoms at all. CMV infection is more serious in people who have compromised immune symptoms, and in infants, who can become infected during delivery, and may have serious effects, including liver, lung, and spleen problems.

Description

CMV is a herpesvirus, so it is related to other herpes viruses, such as **herpes** simplex virus, which can cause cold sores and fever blisters on the mouth and lips. Other herpesviruses include those responsible for chickenpox, **shingles**, and infectious mononucleosis. Like these other herpesviruses, CMV infection is common.

CMV is not highly contagious, and only rarely spreads from one person to another through casual contact. Rather, the virus spreads when an individual comes into contact with an infected person's bodily fluids, such as saliva, blood, or urine, which have the virus present within them. CMV may also be present in the semen, and can be sexually transmitted. Transplanted organs and blood transfusions from an infected person can also spread the virus. CMV may also spread from mother to child through her infected breast milk, or by transmission from a pregnant woman to her unborn child.

Origins

In 1881, German scientists found unusual masses, called inclusion bodies, in the nuclei of cells of infants and children. Their observations are believed to be the first descriptions of cytomegalovirus within human cell nuclei. In 1925, researchers concluded the culprit was one of a group of viruses that today is known as the herpesvirus family. In the mid-1950s, researchers first isolated and grew CMV from human cells. That allowed the preparation of an antigen to the virus, and that antigen served as a test for the infection. Eventually, scientists developed methods to measure intact virus and specific immunity to the virus. These advancements have allowed the collection of data on the incidence and prevalence of CMV infection.

Demographics

The **CDC** reported the following statistics regarding CMV infection in the United States:

- Between 50–80% of Americans are infected with CMV by the time they reach 40 years of age.
- CMV is the most common congenital viral infection.
- Approximately 30,000 children (about one in 150) per year have a congenital CMV infection. Of those, 80% never have any symptoms or health problems.
- Among women who are infected with CMV before becoming pregnant, about 1% transmit the infection to their fetuses.
- Approximately 30–50% of pregnant women have never been infected with CMV; and about 1–4% of them experience their initial, or primary, CMV infection during their pregnancy. About a third of these newly infected women transmit the infection to their fetuses.

Causes and symptoms

CAUSES. CMV infections result from the transmission of the cytomegalovirus. This may occur from close contact with infected bodily fluids from another individual. Pregnant women may transmit the virus to their fetuses during delivery. Breast milk provides another route for viral transmission.

SYMPTOMS. The initial, or primary, infection of a healthy person may result in no symptoms, or in mild symptoms that include fever, sore throat, swollen glands, and fatigue. Some, however, may experience symptoms similar to mononucleosis with a long-lasting fever and mild **hepatitis**.

Once a person has been infected with CMV, the virus remains in the body for life. There, the virus usually remains dormant, but it can reactivate intermittently. Reactivation rarely causes symptoms, and when it does, they are typically mild.

Infection in immune-compromised patients

The primary infection with CMV can be dangerous for immunocompromised patients, and can cause a variety of health conditions, some of which can be life-threatening. They include: **pneumonia**, diarrhea, ulcers, hepatitis, visual impairment, blindness, **encephalitis**, seizures, and coma. These patients may also undergo behavioral changes due to the infection. In this **population**, reactivation of the virus can also cause illness.

Congenital CMV infection

Four out of five babies with congenital CMV infection never develop any symptoms. Of the remaining infants, most will not have symptoms immediately, but rather begin to show signs at 2 years old or older. Evidence of CMV infection at birth may include: premature birth; small birth size; small head size (microcephaly); seizures; enlarged liver (hepatomegaly) or spleen (splenomegaly); jaundice; rash (petechiae); or lung problems. Health issues that may develop over time include: loss of hearing or vision; mental disability in varying degrees; lack of coordination; and seizures. Death is rare, but does occur.

Diagnosis

Medical professionals will test the blood to determine whether a patient has ever been infected by the virus. To do this, they use a specific antigen that identifies CMV antibodies in the blood. This blood test does not distinguish between dormant and active infections. To determine whether the patient has an active CMV infection, however, they may look for substantial (fourfold) increases in antibodies or for especially strong binding of the antigen to antibodies (high avidity) to indicate an active CMV infection. Other reliable tests sample bodily fluids or tissues for the active virus.

In addition, a healthcare provider may conduct tests, such as bilirubin level and blood tests for liver function, a computed tomography (CT) scan or ultrasound of the head, examination of the retina and other structures in the posterior of the eye, or a chest X-ray.

Prevention

Because CMV infections are common (at least half of the U.S. population is infected by age 40), and

KEY TERMS

Herpesvirus—Any one of a large family of viruses (Herpesviridae) that cause diseases in humans and other animals.

Congenital—A condition that is present at birth.

Petechiae—Tiny red or purple spots on the skin.

typically result in no symptoms in otherwise healthy individuals, the CDC recommends no special efforts to prevent transmission among healthy individuals. As such, it recommends neither screening of children for CMV infection, nor excluding infected children from school or other settings.

Infected infants often have CMV in their urine for several months after becoming infected. Despite the multitude of diaper changes conducted by parents, less than 20 percnt; become infected over the course of a year. The CDC recommends the following measures to reduce a parent's exposure to CMV:

- Frequent and thorough washing of the hands, especially following changing diapers, feeding a young child, wiping a young child's nose or mouth, and handling children's toys, which may be contaminated.
- Refraining for sharing a young child's food, drinks, eating utensils, or toothbrush.
- Cleaning surfaces, as well as toys, that may have come into contact with a child's bodily fluids, including saliva.

The CDC notes that although CMV can be shed in a mother's milk, lactation-related infections in infants usually do not cause symptoms or disease, and no recommendations against breastfeeding exist for this reason. However, it recommends that parents of very premature infants and babies having low birth weights, who are more susceptible to CMV-associated problems, ask the advice of their healthcare providers when weighing the benefits of breastfeeding vs. the risk of disease.

Treatment

Healthy people require no treatment. Symptoms, if present, are minor and these individuals usually recover on their own.

CMV does, however, cause serious symptoms in some patients. As of 2011, four antiviral drugs had been licensed for the treatment of CMV infections. They are cidofovir, foscarnet, ganciclovir and valganciclovir. No antiviral drugs have been approved for the treatment of congenital CMV infections. Healthcare providers can, however, render a valuable service by monitoring these babies for hearing and vision problems as they grow, because early detection can be useful in their care. Physical therapy can also assist children with psychomotor developmental issues.

Prognosis

Most individuals who are infected with CMV show no symptoms, and many never know they carry the infection. According to the CDC, about 20% of children with congenital CMV infection experience developmental disabilities, **hearing loss**, or other permanent health issues.

QUESTIONS TO ASK YOUR DOCTOR

- Do I have a choice in how the CMV antiviral medication administered?
- How long must I take the CMV antiviral medication?
- What are the side effects of this medication?
- How can I help monitor my (or my child's) vision or hearing to identify any problems as early as possible?
- I was infected by CMV earlier in my life and am now pregnant. What can I do to prevent the transmission of this virus to my fetus?

Effects on public health

CMV infection is typically a non-issue for most healthy individuals, who experience no symptoms or mild symptoms from which they can recover without medical care.

Congenital CMV infection is not a threat to most babies, as 80 percent of them have no symptoms. CMV does, however, pose a problem for the remaining 20 percent of infants who have symptoms. This subpopulation of about 5,000 children per year may experience developmental disabilities, hearing loss, or other permanent health issues. That 5,000-plus total is more than the number of children afflicted annually with the following conditions: fetal alcohol (about 5,000 per year), Down syndrome (about 4,000), and spina bifida/anencephaly (about 3,000). CMV infection also has a impact on those individuals who have suppressed immune systems. This includes individuals who have human immunodeficiency virus (HIV), who are undergoing or have undergone various **cancer** therapies, or who have had an organ transplantation.

Costs to society

The annual cost of healthcare for CMV infections was estimated at approximately $4 billion per year as of 2000, according to *Vaccines for the 21st Century: A Tool for Decisionmaking.*

Efforts and solutions

As of 2012, no vaccines were available to prevent CMV infections. Research is under way on new treatment options for those experiencing illness as a result of CMV infection. According to a 2012 article in *Expert Opinion on Pharmacotherapy*, "All current drugs available for systemic treatment, including ganciclovir (GCV), valganciclovir, foscarnet and cidofovir, are hampered by dose-related toxicities and the emergence of resistance," but new antiviral compounds, such as artesunate, leflunomid, letermovir and maribavir, are undergoing clinical studies. The article describes these compounds as being less toxic and providing potential new treatment strategies.

In 2012, the U.S. Food and Drug Administration approved the first DNA test to assist with CMV therapy in organ-transplant patients. This test, called the COBAS AmpilPrep/COBAS TaqMan CMV test, determines how much CMV is present in the body, which helps healthcare providers adjust the patient's antiviral treatment.

Resources

PERIODICALS

Ahmed, Amina. "Antiviral Treatment of Cytomegalovirus Infection." *Infectious Disorders—Drug Targets.* 11, no. 5 (2011): 475–503.

Härter, Georg and Detlef Michel. "Antiviral Treatment of Cytomegalovirus infection: An Update." *Expert Opinion on Pharmacotherapy.* 13, no. 5 (2012): 623–7.

Ho, Monto. "The History of Cytomegalovirus and Its Diseases."*Medical Microbiology and Immunology* 197, no. 2 (2008): 65–73.

WEBSITES

Congenital Cytomegalovirus. PubMed Health, U.S. National Library of Medicine.http://www.ncbi.nlm.nih.gov/pubmedhealth/PMH0002319/ (accessed August 29, 2012).

Cytomegalovirus (CMV) and Congenital CMV Infection. U.S. Centers for Disease Control and Prevention. http://www.cdc.gov/cmv/index.html (accessed August 29, 2012).

"Cytomegalovirus." AIDS.org. http://www.aids.org/topics/cytomegalovirus-cmv/ (accessed August 29, 2012).

ORGANIZATIONS

Brendan B. McGinnis Congenital CMV Foundation, P.O. Box 1718, Wheat Ridge, CO 8003401718.mcginnis@cmvfoundation.org, http://cmvfoundation.org/

Centers for Disease Control and Prevention (CDC), 1600 Clifton Road, Atlanta, GA 30333, (800) 232-4636, cdcinfo@cdc.gov, http://www.cdc.gov

Congenital CMV Foundation, 12801 Crossroads Parkway South, Suite 200, City of Industry, CA 91746, http://www.congenitalcmv.org

STOP COMV—The CMV Action Network, P.O. Box 6221, Sunnyvale, CA 94088-2214.email@stopcmv.org, http://www.stopcmv.org/.

Leslie Mertz, Ph.D.

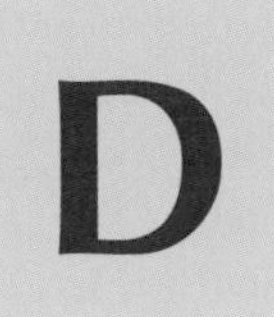

Defibrillation

Definition

Defibrillation is a process in which an electronic device—which may be an external or an implantable device called a "defibrillator"—sends an electric shock to the heart to stop an extremely rapid irregular heartbeat, or to restore the normal heart rhythm. It is often used for such medical problems as cardiac dysrhythmias, ventricular fibrillation, and pulseless ventricular tachycardia. Some external defibrillators, called "automated external defibrillators" (AEDs), automatically diagnosis the heart problem so that non-medical personnel can successfully use them with little or no training.

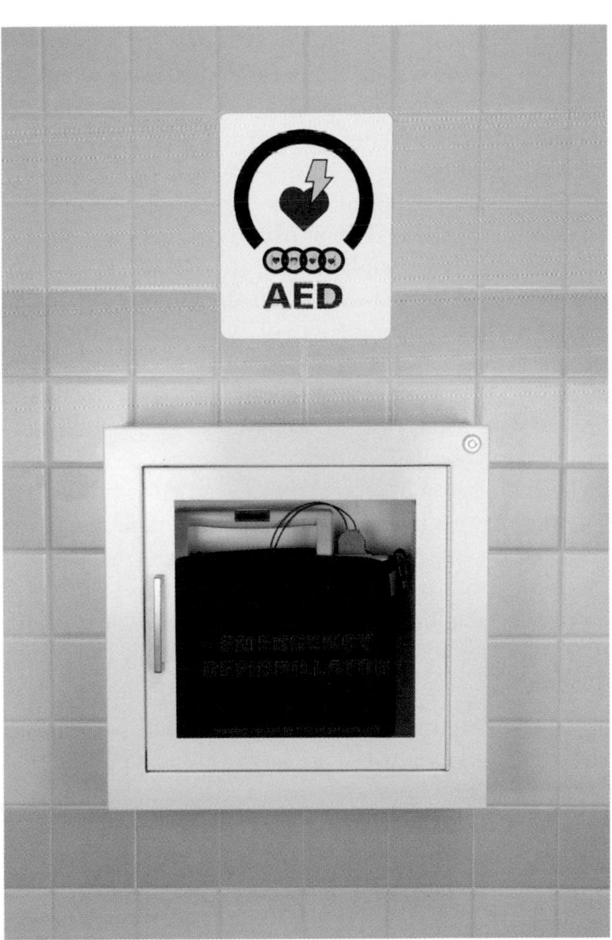

Emergency defibrillator in a wall case. *(© iStockphoto.com/ Captain1854)*

Description

The use of defibrillators was first attempted in 1899, when two Swiss physiologists, Jean-Louis Prévost (1838–1927) and Frederic Batelli, demonstrated them on dogs. In 1947, American cardiac surgeon Claude Schaeffer Beck (1894–1971) was the first to use a defibrillator on a human when he successfully applied it to a 14-year-old male during surgery. Irish physician and cardiologist Frank Pantridge (1916–2004) introduced the portable defibrillator in the early 1960s. The implantable defibrillator device, known as an "implantable cardioverter-defibrillator" (ICD) was developed at Sinai Hospital in Baltimore, Maryland. It was patented in 1980, after over 11 years of development.

Defibrillation may be used for normal and abnormal heart rhythms, and under emergency situations.

Normal and abnormal heart rhythms

Normal heart rhythm is established by the sinoatrial node (SAN), a group of cells located in the wall of the right atrium (upper chamber) of the heart near the entry of the superior vena cava. The superior vena cava is a major vein that carries deoxygenated blood from the upper part of the body to the heart. The SAN, sometimes called the "body's natural pacemaker," discharges electrical impulses at the rate of 60–100 per minute that trigger the contractions of the heart muscle (myocardium). It is the regular contractions of the myocardium that enable blood to be pumped efficiently throughout the rest of the body.

The contractions of the heart muscle result from depolarization, which is the change in a cell's membrane potential, making its electrical charge either more positive or less negative. The electrical impulses discharged by the sinoatrial node produce a wave of depolarization that moves from the right atrium to the left atrium and causes these two upper chambers of the heart to contract. The impulses then travel to another node in the heart known as the "atrioventricular node" or AV node. The AV node functions as a timing device that delays the conduction of the electrical impulses to the ventricles (lower chambers), thus preventing the atria and the ventricles from contracting at the same time. At the end of the cycle, the ventricles of the heart repolarize in preparation for the next heartbeat.

Sudden cardiac arrest (SCA) is an electrical problem caused by a heart rhythm disorder called ventricular fibrillation (VF). Ventricular fibrillation is a medical emergency in which the muscle of the ventricles twitches randomly rather than contracting in a coordinated manner from the apex of the heart to the outflow of the ventricles. It causes the heart to stop pumping blood into the arteries and general body circulation, leading to brain damage and/or cardiac arrest. The mechanisms leading to ventricular fibrillation are not completely understood, as of 2012, and research into this type of cardiac emergency is ongoing. Most episodes of fibrillation occur in diseased or damaged hearts; however, others occur in so-called normal hearts. According to the Heart Rhythm Foundation (HRF), sudden cardiac death accounts for anywhere from 325,000 to 450,000 deaths per year in the United States, of which about 75–80% are due to ventricular fibrillation. Ventricular fibrillation is linked to more deaths each year in North America than lung **cancer**, breast cancer, or **AIDS**. The American Heart Association states that approximately 88% of all sudden cardiac arrest, which happens outside of a hospital, occurs in the home. However, the survival rate for those who experience SCA outside of a hospital is less than 8%.

Emergency defibrillation

About 10% of the ability to restart the heart is lost with every minute that the heart stays in fibrillation. Irreversible brain damage leading to death can occur within three to five minutes unless the normal heart rhythm is restored through defibrillation. Because immediate defibrillation is crucial to the patient's survival, the American Heart Association (AHA) has called for the integration of defibrillation into an effective emergency cardiac care system. The system should include early access, early cardiopulmonary resuscitation, early defibrillation, and early advanced cardiac care.

The AHA has also drawn up guidelines for advanced cardiac life support (ACLS), a set of interventions for cardiac arrest and other heart-related medical emergencies. Only qualified health care providers can supply ACLS when needed, as the guidelines require the ability to manage the patient's airway, initiate intravenous treatment, read and interpret electrocardiograms (EKGs), and understand emergency drug administration. The present ACLS provider course requires about 14 hours of classroom work, including simulations, and the successful completion of a written examination.

How defibrillators work

Defibrillators deliver a brief electric shock to the heart, which enables the heart's natural pacemaker to regain control and establish a normal heart rhythm. The defibrillator is an electronic device with electrocardiogram leads and paddles. During defibrillation, the paddles are placed on the patient's chest, caregivers stand back, and the electric shock is delivered. The patient's pulse and heart rhythm are continually monitored. Medications to treat possible causes of the abnormal heart rhythm may be administered. Defibrillation continues until the patient's condition stabilizes, or the procedure is ordered to be discontinued.

Some patients with a history of ventricular tachycardia or ventricular fibrillation may benefit from an implantable cardioverter-defibrillator or ICD. ICDs, in use since 1980, are small battery-powered devices similar to pacemakers implanted by the surgeon in the patient's heart. It is estimated that over one million of these devices have been implanted as of 2010. ICDs continuously monitor the patient's heart rhythm and deliver an electrical shock when the rate of electrical activity in the patient's heart exceeds a preset number. The newest ICDs are programmed to detect the differences among a normal fast heart rhythm, ventricular tachycardia, and ventricular fibrillation. They can correct ventricular tachycardia before it progresses to ventricular fibrillation. The very newest ICDs are implanted under the skin of the patient's rib cage near the heart. Known as "subcutaneous ICDs," these devices can deliver enough electricity to correct an abnormal heart rhythm without the need for wires or electrodes placed in or on the heart itself, thus lowering the risk of infection.

Early defibrillators, about the size and weight of a car battery, were used primarily in ambulances and hospitals. The newer automated external defibrillators (AEDs) are smaller, lighter, less expensive, and easier to use than the early defibrillators. They are computerized to provide simple verbal instructions to the operator and to make it impossible to deliver a shock to a patient whose heart is not fibrillating. The placement of public-access AEDs, urged by the American Heart Association, has expanded to cover many public locations in Canada and the United States, as of 2012, including corporate and government offices, shopping centers, airports, casinos, hotels, sports arenas, universities, community centers, fitness centers, health clubs, and even some workplaces. Public-access AEDs often are brightly colored to increase their visibility, and they are mounted in protective cases near the entrances of buildings. The use of AEDs is now taught in first aid, first responder, and basic life support (BLS) level CPR classes as well as in military combat and front line hospitals.

Demographics

Sudden cardiac arrest can happen to anyone. For many, there are no warning signs prior to the incident. Medical data on external defibrillators show that the sooner a defibrillator is used on a patient during cardiac arrest, the better that person has to survive. In fact, according to the American Heart Association, survival rates decrease by 7% to 10% for each one minute after the start of cardiac arrest in which a defibrillator (and cardiopulmonary resuscitation [CPR]) is not used.

Purpose

Defibrillation is performed to correct life-threatening fibrillations of the heart or such other arrhythmias as ventricular tachycardia that may result in cardiac arrest. It should be performed immediately after identifying that the patient is experiencing a cardiac emergency, has no pulse, and is unresponsive.

Causes and symptoms

The causes and symptoms relating to defibrillation are described below.

Causes

A defibrillation is needed when sudden cardiac arrest occurs. The cause of sudden cardiac arrest is usually an abnormality in a person's heart rhythm (arrhythmia), which is the result of a malfunction in the electrical system of the heart.

Symptoms

The symptoms of SCA, which usually are sudden, include no breathing, no pulse, sudden collapse, or loss of consciousness. Other symptoms, which may come on gradually, include blackouts, dizziness, chest **pain**, fatigue, fainting, palpitations, shortness of breath, weakness, or vomiting. In many cases, no symptoms happen.

KEY TERMS

Arrhythmia—Any of a number of conditions in which there is abnormal electrical activity in the heart. Some arrhythmias are minor, while others are potentially life-threatening. They are also called "cardiac dysrhythmias."

Automated external defibrillator (AED)—A portable electronic device that automatically diagnoses potentially life-threatening cardiac arrhythmias (ventricular fibrillation and ventricular tachycardia) and is able to treat them through defibrillation.

Cardiac arrest—A condition in which the heart stops functioning. Fibrillation can lead to cardiac arrest if not corrected quickly.

Depolarization—A change in a cell's membrane potential, making its electrical charge more positive or less negative. Defibrillation essentially depolarizes a portion of the heart muscle, allowing the heart's natural pacemaker to reestablish normal heart rhythm.

Myocardium—The medical term for the specialized involuntary muscle tissue found in the walls of the heart.

Pacemaker—A surgically implanted electronic device that sends out electrical impulses to regulate a slow or erratic heartbeat.

Sinoatrial node (SAN)—The heart's natural pacemaker, a group of cells located in the wall of the right atrium (upper chamber) of the heart near the entry of the superior vena cava, a major vein that carries deoxygenated blood from the upper part of the body to the heart.

Ventricular fibrillation—Uncoordinated contraction of the muscle in the ventricles (lower chambers) of the heart.

Ventricular tachycardia—An abnormally rapid heartbeat originating in one of the lower chambers of the heart. It can lead to ventricular fibrillation.

Prognosis

If a defibrillator is used within the first five to seven minutes of cardiac arrest, the survival rate is at least 49%.

Precautions

Defibrillation should not be performed on a patient who has a pulse or is alert, as this could cause a lethal heart rhythm disturbance or cardiac arrest. The paddles used in the procedure should not be placed on a woman's breasts or over a pacemaker.

Preparation

After help is called for, the emergency response team begins cardiopulmonary resuscitation (CPR) and continues until the defibrillator arrives. Electrocardiogram leads are attached to the patient's chest. Gel or paste is applied to the defibrillator paddles, or two gel pads are placed on the patient's chest. The caregivers verify lack of a pulse and select a charge.

Preparation for the implantation of an ICD includes an electrocardiogram (EKG) and a series of other tests of the heart's function to determine what type of arrhythmia the patient is experiencing and whether he or she can benefit from an implanted device. As with most other procedures requiring general anesthesia, the patient will be asked not to eat or drink anything for a minimum of eight hours before the surgery.

Risks

Skin **burns** from the defibrillator paddles are the most common complication of defibrillation. Other risks include injury to the heart muscle, abnormal heart rhythms, and blood clots.

The risks of ICD placement include infection; swelling or bruising at the site of implantation; bleeding around the heart, a potentially life-threatening complication; and damage to the vein where the ICD leads are placed.

Aftercare

After defibrillation, the patient's cardiac status, breathing, and vital signs are monitored until he or she is stable. Typically, this monitoring takes place after the patient has been removed to an intensive care or cardiac care unit in a hospital. An electrocardiogram and chest x ray are taken. The patient's skin is cleansed to remove gel or paste, and, if necessary, ointment is applied to burns. An intravenous line provides additional medication, as needed.

Patients who have received an ICD usually remain in the hospital for one or two days after the procedure so that doctors can test the device for proper functioning. They may need to use over-the-counter pain relievers for several days or weeks to relieve soreness after returning home. While patients with ICDs can lead relatively normal lives, they should avoid sports that involve vigorous movements of the shoulder, arm, or torso close to the implant site. They must also avoid equipment that uses large magnets or produces intense magnetic fields. Such equipment includes magnetic resonance imaging (MRI) devices.

QUESTIONS TO ASK YOUR DOCTOR

- How reliable are defibrillators?
- Will an implantable-cardioverter defibrillator cure my heart rhythm problem?
- Is an ICD appropriate for me?
- Do shocks from a defibrillator hurt?
- Where will an implantable defibrillator be placed?
- What type of surgery is used to implant a defibrillator?
- How is a ICD powered?

Resources

BOOKS

Ellenbogen, Kenneth A., et al., editors. *Clinical Cardiac Pacing, Defibrillation and Resynchronization.* Philadelphia: Elsevier/Saunders, 2011.

Jevon, Phil. *Advanced Cardiac Life Support: A Guide for Nurses*, 2nd ed. Ames, IA: Wiley-Blackwell, 2010.

Le Baudour, Christopher, and J. David Bergeron. *Emergency Medical Responder: First On Scene*. Upper Saddle River, NJ: Pearson, 2012.

Sankaranarayanan, Rajiv, Hanney Gonna, and Michael James. *Treatment of Ventricular Fibrillation*. Hauppauge, NY: Nova Science, 2009.

Valentinuzzi, Max E. *Cardiac Fibrillation-defibrillation: Clinical and Engineering Aspects*. New Jersey: World Scientific, 2011.

PERIODICALS

Adams, B.D., et al. "Cardiopulmonary Resuscitation in the Combat Hospital and Forward Operating Base: Use of Automated External Defibrillators." *Military Medicine* 174 (June 2009): 584–87.

Andresen, D., et al. "Public Access Resuscitation Program Including Defibrillator Training for Laypersons: A Randomized Trial to Evaluate the Impact of Training Course Duration." *Resuscitation* 76 (March 2008): 419–24.

Hoadley, T.A. "Learning Advanced Cardiac Life Support: A Comparison Study of the Effects of Low- and High-fidelity Simulation." *Nursing Education Perspectives* 30 (March-April 2009): 91–95.

Moss, A.J., et al. "Cardiac-Resynchronization Therapy for the Prevention of Heart-Failure Events." *New England Journal of Medicine* 361 (October 1, 2009): 1329–38.

Stewart, G.C., et al. "Patient Expectations from Implantable Defibrillators to Prevent Death in Heart Failure." *Journal of Cardiac Failure* 16 (February 2010): 106–113.

WEBSITES

ACLS Course Materials. American Heart Association. http://www.heart.org/HEARTORG/CPRAndECC/HealthcareTraining/AdvancedCardiovascularLifeSupportACLS/Advanced-Cardiovascular-Life-Support-ACLS_UCM_001280_SubHomePage.jsp (accessed August 7, 2012).

Implantable Cardioverter-Defibrillators (ICDs). Mayo Clinic. (November 19, 2010). http://www.mayoclinic.com/health/implantable-cardioverter-defibrillator/MY00336 (accessed August 7, 2012).

Normal Sinus Rhythm Animation. WebMD. (October 29, 2008). http://www.webmd.com/heart-disease/healthtool-heart-rhythm-disorders-illustrated-guide (accessed August 7, 2012).

Sudden Cardiac Arrest Key Facts. Heart Rhythm Foundation. http://www.heartrhythmfoundation.org/facts/scd.asp (accessed August 16, 2012).

Ventricular Fibrillation. Mayo Clinic. (November 1, 2011). http://www.mayoclinic.com/health/ventricular-fibrillation/DS01158 (accessed August 7, 2012).

Zevitz, Michael E. *Ventricular Fibrillation*. eMedicine (October 12, 2011). http://emedicine.medscape.com/article/158712-overview (accessed August 7, 2012).

ORGANIZATIONS

American Heart Association, 7272 Greenville Ave., Dallas, TX U.S.A. 75231, (800) 242-8721, http://www.heart.org.

American Medical Association, 515 N. State St., Chicago, IL U.S.A. 60654, (800) 621-8335, http://www.ama-assn.org/.

National Heart, Lung and Blood Institute, PO Box 30105, Bethesda, MD U.S.A. 20824-0105, 1 (301) 592-8573, Fax: 1 (240) 629-3246, nhlbiinfo@nhlbi.nih.gov, http://www.nhlbi.nih.gov/.

World Medical Association, 13, ch. Du Levant, Ferney-Voltaire, France 01210, +33 4 (50) 40 75 75, Fax: +33 4 (50) 40 59 37, wma@wma.net, http://www.wma.net/en/.

Lori De Milto
Rebecca J. Frey, Ph.D.
Brenda W. Lerner
William A. Atkins, B.B., B.S., M.B.A.

Dengue fever

Definition

Dengue fever is a disease caused by any of four closely related dengue viruses (DENV 1, DENV 2, DENV 3, or DENV 4) that are carried by mosquitoes. These mosquitoes then transmit the virus to humans.

Description

Dengue used to be called "break–bone" fever as it sometimes results in severe joint and muscle **pain**. Health experts have long known about dengue fever. The first record of a case of dengue fever occurs in a very old Chinese medical encyclopedia (265–420 AD). The first recognized Dengue epidemics occurred at about the same time in Asia, Africa, and North America in the 1780s. The disease was named dengue in 1779 with Benjamin Rush describing the first case report in 1789.

Before 1970, only nine countries had experienced severe dengue epidemics. Dengue is now endemic in more than 100 countries in Africa, the Americas, the Eastern Mediterranean, South-east Asia and the Western Pacific with South-east Asia and the Western Pacific being the most seriously affected.

The viruses that causes dengue fever are arboviruses, which stands for arthropod-borne virus. Mosquitoes are a type of arthropod. In a number of regions, mosquitoes carry this virus and are responsible for passing it along to humans.

In order to understand how dengue fever is transmitted, several terms need to be defined. The word "host" means an animal (including a human) that can be infected with a particular disease. The word "vector" means an organism that can carry a particular disease–causing agent (like a virus or bacteria) without actually developing the disease. The vector can then pass the virus or bacteria on to a new host.

Many of the common illnesses in the United States (including the **common cold**, many viral causes of diarrhea, and **influenza** or "flu") are spread because the viruses that cause these illness can be passed directly from person to person. However, dengue fever cannot be passed directly from one infected person to another. Instead, the virus responsible for dengue fever requires an intermediate vector, a mosquito, that carries the virus from one host to another. In the Western Hemisphere, the *Aedes aegypti* mosquito is the most important transmitter or vector of dengue viruses, although a 2001 outbreak in Hawaii was transmitted by *Aedes albopictus*.

Risk factors

Dengue occurs primarily in areas where *Aedes aegypti* or *Aedes albopictus* mosquitoes are found, including most tropical urban areas of the world. Dengue viruses may be introduced into new areas by travelers who become infected while visiting other areas of the tropics where dengue outbreaks commonly occur.

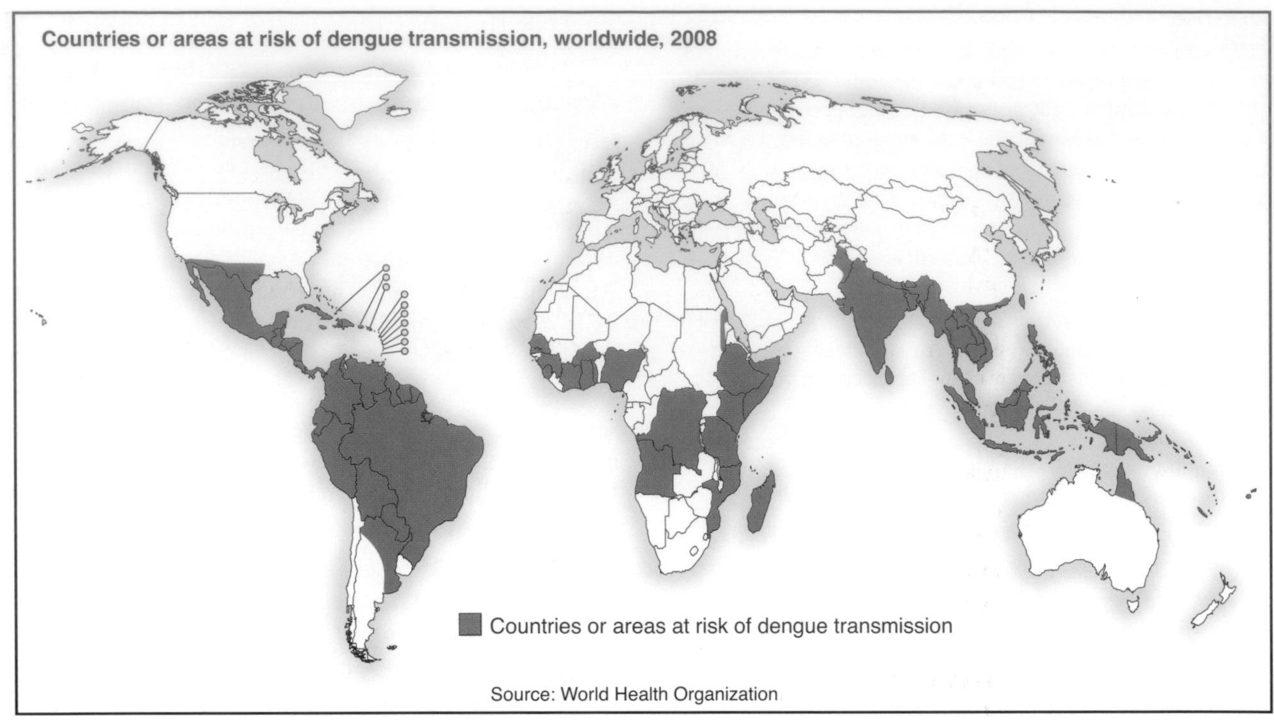

(Illustration by Electronic Illustrators Group. © 2013 Cengage Learning)

Demographics

As of 2013, the Centers for Disease Control (**CDC**) estimates that more than one–third of the world's **population** live in areas at risk for dengue in the tropics and subtropics. In these regions, the dengue fever arbovirus is endemic, meaning that the virus naturally and consistently lives in these areas. Some 100 million people are infected each year. Dengue rarely occurs in the continental United States, where 100 to 200 cases a year occur, mostly in people who have recently traveled abroad. However, it is endemic in Puerto Rico, and in several tourist destinations in Latin America and Southeast Asia. Outbreaks periodically occur in Samoa and Guam. The most common victims are children younger than 10 years of age.

Causes and symptoms

Dengue fever can occur when a mosquito carrying the arbovirus bites a human, passing the virus on to the new host. Once in the body, the virus travels to various glands where it multiplies. The virus can then enter the bloodstream. The presence of the virus within the blood vessels, especially those feeding the skin, causes changes to these blood vessels. The vessels swell and leak. The spleen and lymph nodes become enlarged, and patches of liver tissue die. A process called disseminated intravascular coagulation (DIC) occurs, where chemicals responsible for clotting are used up and lead to a risk of severe bleeding (hemorrhage).

After the virus has been transmitted to the human host, a period of incubation occurs. During this time (lasting about five to eight days) the virus multiplies. Symptoms of the disease appear suddenly and include high fever, chills, headache, eye pain, red eyes, enlarged lymph nodes, a red flush to the face, lower back pain, extreme weakness, and severe aches in the legs and joints.

This initial period of illness lasts about two or three days. After this time, the fever drops rapidly and the patient sweats heavily. After about a day of feeling relatively well, the patient's temperature increases again, although not as much as the first time. A rash of small red bumps begins on the arms and legs, spreading to the chest, abdomen, and back. It rarely affects the face. The palms of the hands and the soles of the feet become swollen and turn bright red. The characteristic combination of fever, rash, and headache are called the "dengue triad." Most people recover fully from dengue fever, although weakness and fatigue may last for several weeks. Once a person has been infected with dengue fever, his or her immune system keeps producing cells that prevent reinfection for about a year.

More severe illness may occur in some people. These people may be experiencing dengue fever for the first time. However, in some cases a person may have already had dengue fever at one time, recovered, and then is reinfected with the virus. In these cases, the first infection teaches the immune system to recognize the presence of the arbovirus. When the immune cells encounter the virus during later infections, the immune system over–reacts. These types of illnesses, called dengue hemorrhagic fever (DHF) or dengue shock syndrome (DSS), involve more severe symptoms. Fever and headache are the first symptoms, but the other initial symptoms of dengue fever are absent. The patient develops a cough, followed by the appearance of small purplish spots (petechiae) on the skin. These petechiae are areas where blood is leaking out of the vessels. Large bruised areas appear as the bleeding worsens and abdominal pain may be severe. The patient may begin to vomit a substance that looks like coffee grounds. This is actually a sign of bleeding into the stomach. As the blood vessels become more damaged, they leak more and continue to increase in diameter (dilate), causing a decrease in blood flow to all tissues of the body. This state of low blood flow is called shock. Shock can result in damage to the body's organs (especially the heart and kidneys) because low blood flow deprives them of oxygen.

Diagnosis

Diagnosis should be suspected in endemic areas whenever a high fever goes on for two to seven days, especially if accompanied by a bleeding tendency. Symptoms of shock should suggest the progression of the disease to DSS.

The arbovirus causing dengue fever is one of the few types of arbovirus that can be isolated from the serum of the blood. The serum is the fluid in which blood cells are suspended. Serum can be tested because the phase in which the virus travels throughout the bloodstream is longer in dengue fever than in other arboviral infections. A number of tests are used to look for reactions between the patient's serum and laboratory–produced antibodies. Antibodies are special cells that recognize the markers (or antigens) present on invading organisms. During these tests, antibodies are added to a sample of the patient's serum. Healthcare workers then look for reactions that would only occur if viral antigens were present in that serum.

Treatment

There is no treatment available to shorten the course of dengue fever, DHF, or DSS. Medications can be given to lower the fever and to decrease the pain of muscle aches and headaches. Fluids are given through a needle in a vein to prevent dehydration. Blood transfusions may be necessary if severe hemorrhaging occurs. Oxygen should be administered to patients in shock.

KEY TERMS

Endemic—Naturally and consistently present in a certain geographical region.

Host—The organism (such as a monkey or human) in which another organism (such as a virus or bacteria) is living.

Vector—A carrier organism (such as a fly or mosquito) that delivers a virus (or other agent of infection) to a host.

Public health role and response

Dengue fever now represents one of the most important public health issues in tropical developing countries and also has a major economic and societal impact. In the Western hemisphere, the estimated economic burden of dengue is about $2.1 billion per year. The incidence of dengue has dramatically increased worldwide in recent decades. Over 2.5 billion people (40% of the world's population) are now at risk from dengue and the **World Health Organization (WHO)** estimates that there may be 50–100 million dengue infections worldwide every year. The number of dengue cases is clearly increasing as the disease spreads to new areas, and explosive outbreaks are now observed. Dengue outbreaks are now possible in Europe with local transmission reported for the first time in France and Croatia in 2010.

WHO has responded as follows:

- Supporting countries in the confirmation of outbreaks through its collaborating network of laboratories;
- Providing technical support and guidance to countries for the effective management of dengue outbreaks;
- Developing new tools, including insecticide products and application technologies;
- Gathering official records of dengue and severe dengue from over 100 Member States.

Prognosis

The prognosis for uncomplicated dengue fever is very good, and almost 100% of patients fully recover. However, as many as 6–30% of all patients die when DHF occurs. The death rate is especially high among the youngest patients (under one year old). In places where excellent medical care is available, very close

QUESTIONS TO ASK YOUR DOCTOR

- What causes dengue fever?
- How does dengue fever spread?
- How is dengue fever treated?
- What medications are used for dengue?

monitoring and immediate treatment of complications lowers the death rate among DHF and DSS patients to about 1%.

Prevention

There is no vaccine for preventing dengue. **Prevention** of dengue fever means decreasing the mosquito population. Any sources of standing **water** (buckets, vases, etc.) where the mosquitoes can breed must be eliminated. Mosquito repellant is recommended for those areas where dengue fever is endemic. To help break the cycle of transmission, sick patients should be placed in bed nets so that mosquitoes cannot bite them and become arboviral vectors.

Resources

BOOKS

Rothman, Alan L., ed. *Dengue Virus.* New York, NY: Springer, 2009.

Russell, Jesse and Ronald Cohn. *Dengue Fever.* Great Malvern, UK: Book on Demand Ltd., 2012.

Toll, Aaron P., ed. *Dengue Fever.* St. Paul, MN: Ceed Publishing, 2012.

PERIODICALS

Pye, J. "Raising awareness of dengue fever."Nursing Standard 26, no. 51 (August 2012): 53–56.

Rajapakse, S., et al. "Treatment of dengue fever."Infection and Drug Resistance 5 (2012): 103–112.

Roberts, C. H., et al. "Dengue fever: a practical guide."British Journal of Hospital Medicine 73, no. 14 (April 2012): C60–C64.

Tantawichien, T. "Dengue fever and dengue haemorrhagic fever in adolescents and adults." Pediatrics and International Child Health 32, suppl. 1 (May 2012): 22–27.

WEBSITES

Dengue. Centers for Disease Control. June 21, 2012. http://www.cdc.gov/dengue/

Dengue Fever. Medline Plus, 27 September 2012. http://www.nlm.nih.gov/medlineplus/ency/article/001374.htm

Dengue Fever. NIAID Health and Research. October 9, 2012. http://www.niaid.nih.gov/topics/DengueFever/Understanding/Pages/overview.aspx

ORGANIZATIONS

Centers for Disease Control and Prevention (CDC), 1600 Clifton Road, Atlanta, GA 30333, (800) 232-4636, cdcinfo@cdc.gov, http://www.cdc.gov.

Rosalyn Carson-DeWitt, MD

Dental health

Definition

Dental health is the proper care and functioning of the teeth and gums, which should remain healthy throughout one's lifetime.

Description

Dental health includes good oral **hygiene**, which is the practice of keeping the mouth clean and healthy by brushing and flossing to prevent bacteria build-up, which can result in tooth decay and gum disease. Sometimes bacteria from the mouth can also make their way into the bloodstream and cause other illnesses. Regular visits to the dentist can keep oral hygiene on track and can identify potential problems in plenty of time to provide proper treatment.

Teeth and gums

A tooth is made up of four main parts: the enamel, which is the outer, white, visible layer; the cementum,

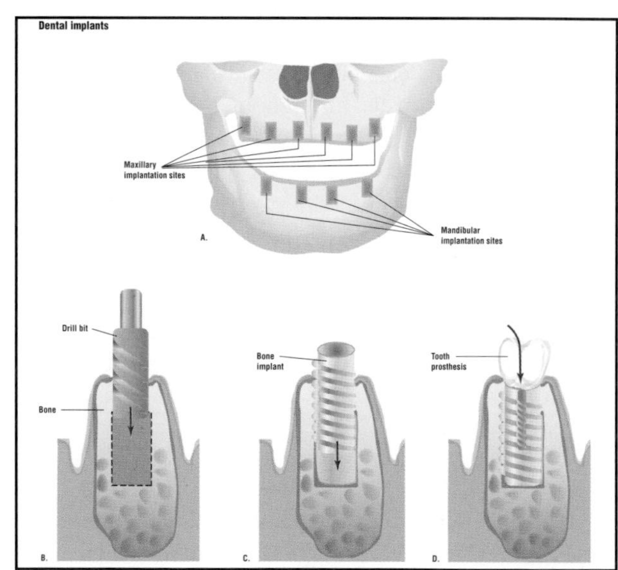

(Illustration by Electronic Illustrators Group. © 2013 Cengage Learning)

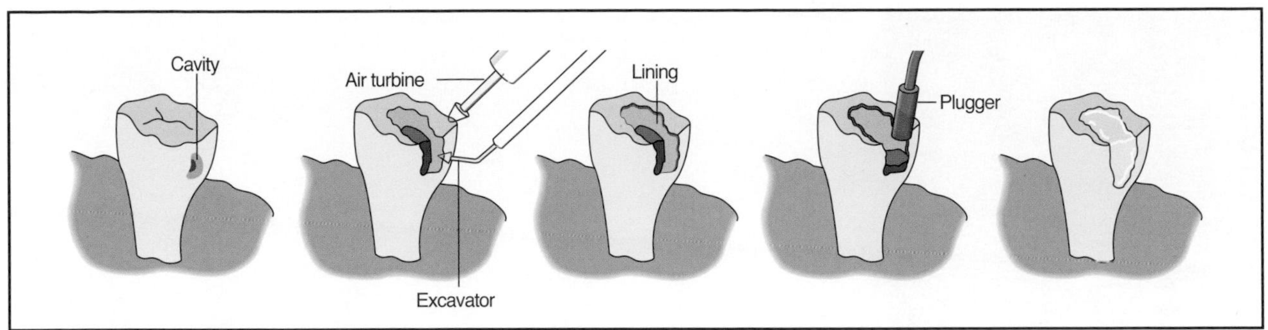

Process of filling a cavity. *(Illustration by Electronic Illustrators Group. © 2013 Cengage Learning)*

which is the tooth's outer layer that is below the gum and covers the root; the dentin, which lies beneath the enamel and cementum in the inner tooth; and the pulp, which is located at the center of the tooth. The soft tissue that surrounds the teeth is the gums, also known as the "gingiva." Good dental health involves both the teeth and the gums.

Common problems

Common dental and gum problems include:

- Cavities, or dental caries, which typically result from a bacterial infection that decays the enamel and dentin. The bacteria and the acids, together with bits of food and saliva, together form plaque, which sticks to teeth and ultimately eats through the enamel and into the dentin to cause a cavity.
- Periodontal disease, which results from plaque and tartar. Plaque becomes tartar, a hard substance, that builds up at the base of the tooth. Plaque and tartar cause both irritation and inflammation of the gums, and they also produce toxins that can further infect gums. Gingivitis is an early form of periodontal disease. It is characterized by inflammation of the gums with painless bleeding during brushing and flossing. This common condition is reversible with proper dental care but if left untreated, it will progress into a more serious periodontal disease, known as "periodontitis." Periodontitis destroys the structures supporting the teeth, including bone. Untreated, the inflammation can lead to loose teeth or lost teeth.
- Chronic bad breath, which usually results from a dental condition, such as bacteria present in the mouth, gum disease, or cavities.
- Tooth sensitivity, in which a patient experiences pain or discomfort from sweets, cold or hot foods, contact with a toothbrush or string of floss, or even cold air that passes by a tooth.
- Oral cancer, which is highly curable if caught and treated early in its progression. Oral cancer includes cancers of the oral cavity (the mouth area, including the lips) and the oropharynx (the throat at the back of the mouth).

Origins

The origin of the modern profession of dentistry is often linked to the start of the first dental school, which opened in 1828 in Ohio. The first dental college, the Baltimore College of Dental Surgery, followed in 1840. Since then, trained dentists have become commonplace around the world. Specialties have also arisen. These include endodontics (associated with root canals), periodontics (gingivitis), and orthodontics (braces).

Demographics

Tooth cavities are very common, affecting more than one-quarter of U.S. children aged 2–5 years; and about half of those aged 12–15 years, according to the **Centers for Disease Control and Prevention**. About three-quarters of American adults have some form of gum disease, and 4–12% of U.S. adults have advanced gum disease. Most gum disease among Americans is related to **smoking**, according to the **CDC**. Smokers are three times more likely to have gum disease than people who have never smoked.

As of 2013, the percentage of U.S. adults aged 65 years or older who had lost all of their teeth was about 25%. The CDC also reported that more than 7,800 Americans die from oral and pharyngeal cancers each year. Approximately 36,500 new cases of those cancers were diagnosed in 2011.

Causes and symptoms

Causes

Most dental problems, such as cavities and gum disease, arise as a result of bacterial growth. Dentists can identify most of these and other dental-related problems through regular check-ups. The causes of oral **cancer**

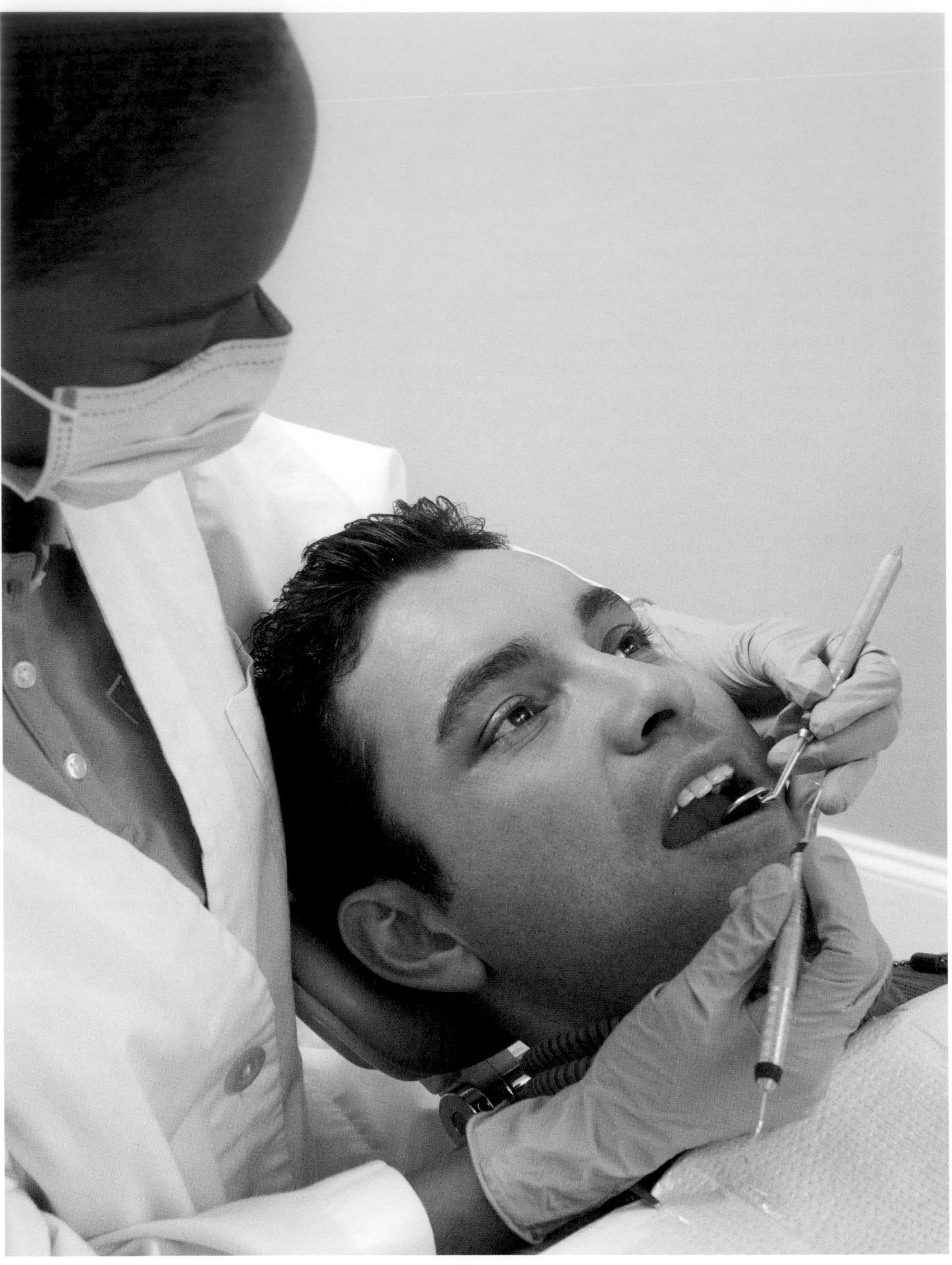

Dentist examining a patient. *(bikeriderlondon/Shutterstock.com)*

may include smoking or chewing tobacco, especially when combined with heavy alcohol use; and sun exposure (lip cancer). In addition, human papillomavirus (**HPV**) infection may be associated with increased oral-cancer risk.

Symptoms

Symptoms vary by type of condition.

- Cavities. Symptoms might not occur. If they do, they can include pain and/or sensitivity at and around the site of the cavity.
- Gum disease. Symptoms can include chronic bad breath; gums that are red, swollen, tender, and/or bleeding; pain when chewing; teeth that are loose; tooth sensitivity; and gum recession.
- Oral cancer. Symptoms can include abnormal thick, swelled, or crusty spots on the lips or inside the mouth; a lip or mouth sore that does not heal; lumps in the oral cavity; white and/or red patches inside the mouth; a lump or lumps in the oral cavity or oropharynx; the impression of something being lodged at the back of the throat; unexplained bleeding, numbness, or tenderness in the mouth, face, or neck; swelling in the jaw or neck; chronic sore throat; hoarseness or other voice change; or difficulty chewing or swallowing food.

Diagnosis

Diagnoses of many oral conditions are made during routine dental examinations. A typical dental visit will include a patient's report of any problems or changes; a tooth cleaning to remove plaque, tartar, and any other stains on the teeth; an evaluation of the mouth for decay, gum disease, and signs of oral cancer; a check of the jaw and bite for potential problems; and administration of dental x rays and other diagnostic tests, as necessary. Additional tests for suspected oral cancer may include a biopsy that removes tissue samples for examination; and a computed tomography (a CT or CAT) scan, ultrasonography, or magnetic resonance imaging to detect possible abnormalities.

Treatment

Treatments vary with the condition. For dental cavities, the dentist will typically remove the decayed portion of the tooth and replace it with a filling, or if the decay is extensive, with a crown that covers all or a portion of the tooth. The dentist will perform a root canal when a tooth has damage to the pulp or has infection of the tooth nerve. If left untreated, this can cause a serious and usually very painful abscess. For a root-canal procedure, the dentist (or a dental specialist such as an endodontist) removes the pulp of the tooth all the way into the tooth's roots.

KEY TERMS

Enamel—The hard, white, outer layer of the tooth.

Fluoride—A compound believed to combat cavities in teeth.

Gingivitis—Inflammation of the gums, seen as painless bleeding during brushing and flossing.

Periodontal—Pertaining to the gums.

Plaque—A thin, sticky, colorless film of bacteria that forms on teeth.

Tartar—A hardened yellow or brown mineral deposit from unremoved plaque; also called "calculus."

For gingivitis, the main goal is to eliminate the gum inflammation. This typically involves the removal of the plaque and tartar buildup on teeth, which may be accomplished through a regular dental cleaning. For more serious periodontal disease, the teeth receive a deep cleaning, known as 'scaling' and "root planing." These procedures involve scraping and/or using a laser to remove plaque and tartar from above and below the gum line. The dentist or specialist may also prescribe medications to help combat bacteria and maintain healthy gums. Additional surgical treatments, including bone grafts, may be helpful.

The treatment for oral cancer depends on the location of the tumor(s) and the progression of the disease. Treatment options include surgery to remove the tumor and possibly additional tissue or bone; **radiation** treatment; and chemotherapy.

Teeth whitening

Teeth whitening is a cosmetic process that uses bleach or other materials to make teeth look whiter by removing stains or other discoloration from the tooth surface. Teeth whitening is not safe or effective for everyone, so a person should have a dental exam before starting treatment. The dentist can advise the patient about the most appropriate procedure and about associated precautions. The oral health professional will also discuss the expected results of treatment, which may fall somewhat short of the gleaming white that patients anticipate.

Prevention

Regular dental checkups and proper dental hygiene are critical for good dental health.

QUESTIONS TO ASK YOUR DENTIST

- Is teeth whitening right for me? What results can I expect?
- We live in an area that does not have fluoridated water. Beyond fluoride toothpaste, what other options are available to give my teeth added protection against cavities?
- How am I doing with tooth brushing and flossing? Am I missing any spots?
- What foods should I avoid to improve my oral health?
- When I am at work, or my child is at school and cannot brush after a meal, what can we do to keep our teeth clean?

Effects on Public Health

Good oral health is important to many everyday functions, including chewing and swallowing, speaking, tasting, and conveying emotions through facial expressions. Most people, however, have had at least one dental-related disease. Few people have not had a cavity, which is actually considered a disease, and a quarter of all Americans aged 65 or older no longer have any of their teeth. In addition, new cases of oral cancer are diagnosed every day.

Costs to Society

Americans make about a half billion visits to dentists every year, according to the CDC. In 2010, it reported that an estimated $108 billion went to dental services.

Efforts and Solutions

Fluoride has been shown to improve dental health, and many water-treatment facilities around the country add fluoride to their **water** for this reason. The CDC provides national leadership in assessing fluoride use and works with state agencies and other organizations to improve the quality of water fluoridation and to implement water fluoridation in those communities that do not yet utilize it.

Beyond this effort, individual states are taking action to improve dental health for their populations. Many states, for instance, are promoting the use of dental sealants in school children. Dental sealants are plastic coatings that are placed on the chewing surfaces of teeth, where school children get up to 90% of decay. Colorado's Be Smart & Seal Them! Program, for instance, has a goal of sealing the teeth of all of the state's children at greatest risk of dental disease. Arkansas is another example. Its Office of Oral Health is working with other organizations to improve oral-health education, **prevention**, and treatment for the state's neediest citizens.

Resources

WEBSITES

"Dental Sealants: Is My Child a Candidate?" Academy of General Dentistry. http://www.knowyourteeth.com/infobites/abc/article/?abc=C&iid=296&aid=1189 (accessed September 20, 2012).

"Oral Cancer." Wexner Medical Center, Ohio State University. http://medicalcenter.osu.edu/patientcare/healthcare_services/mens_health/oral_cancer/pages/index.aspx (accessed September 21, 2012).

"Oral Cancer Facts." Oral Cancer Foundation.http://www.oralcancerfoundation.org/facts/ (accessed September 21, 2012).

"Oral Health: Preventing Cavities, Gum Disease, Tooth Loss, and Oral Cancers at a Glance 2011." Centers for Disease Control and Prevention.http://www.cdc.gov/chronicdisease/resources/publications/aag/doh.htm (accessed September 21, 2012).

"Periodontal (Gum) Disease: Causes, Symptoms, and Treatments." National Institute of Dental and Craniofacial Research. http://www.nidcr.nih.gov/OralHealth/Topics/GumDiseases/PeriodontalGumDisease.htm (accessed September 21, 2012).

PubMed Health"Fact Sheet: Keeping Teeth and Gums Healthy." U.S. National Library of Medicine. http://www.ncbi.nlm.nih.gov/pubmedhealth/PMH0016281/ (accessed September 4, 2012) (accessed September 20, 2012).

PubMed Health"Gingivitis." U.S. National Library of Medicine. http://www.ncbi.nlm.nih.gov/pubmedhealth/PMH0002051/ (accessed September 4, 2012) (accessed September 20, 2012).

"Types of Gum Disease." American Academy of Periodontology. http://www.perio.org/consumer/2a.html (accessed September 21, 2012).

ORGANIZATIONS

Academy of General Dentistry, 211 E. Chicago Ave., Suite 900, Chicago, IL 60611, http://www.knowyourteeth.com/aboutagd/

American Academy of Peridontology, 737 N. Michigan Avenue, Suite 800., Chicago, IL 60611-6660, (312) 787-5518, http://www.perio.org/

American Dental Association, 211 E. Chicago Avenue, Chicago, IL 60611-2678, (312) 440-2500, http://www.ada.org

Centers for Disease Control and Prevention (CDC), 1600 Clifton Road, Atlanta, GA 30333, (800) 232-4636, cdcinfo@cdc.gov, http://www.cdc.gov

National Institute of Dental and Craniofacial Research, 31 Center Drive, MSC 2190, Building 31, Room 5B55, Bethesda, MD 20892-2190, (866) 232-4528, nidcrinfo@mail.nih.gov, http://www.nidcr.nih.gov/

Oral Cancer Foundation, 3419 Via Lido # 205, Newport Beach, CA 92663, (949) 646-8000, info@oralcancerfoundation.org, http://www.oralcancerfoundation.org/.

Leslie Mertz, Ph.D.

Department of Health and Human Services

Definition

The U.S. Department of Health and Human Services (HHS) is the primary federal agency responsible for protecting the health of American citizens and for providing the range of human services for those who are least able to care for themselves.

Purpose

The purpose of HHS is to carry out such activities as it deems necessary to maintain the general health of all U.S. citizens by providing information and services to anyone in need of such services, especially those who are of low–income status, those who are disabled, the unemployed, legal immigrants, and other underserved populations.

Description

The U.S. Department of Health and Human Services (HHS) was established as a cabinet–level department on April 11, 1953 as the Department of Health, Education, and Welfare (HEW). The Department of Education Organizing Act of 1979 removed education from HEW, leading to the formation of the current agency, whose purview was then limited to health and human services. HEW was originally created through the amalgamation of a number of preexisting agencies, such as the Public Health Service (PHS), the National Institutes of Health (NIH), the Food and Drug Administration (FDA), the Indian Health Service (IHS), and the **Centers for Disease Control and Prevention (CDC)**. These agencies are now all divisions within HHS, along with a number of newer divisions, such as the Administration for Children and Families, the Administration for Community Living, the Substance Abuse and Mental Health Services Administration, the Agency for Toxic Substances and Disease Registry, the Agency for Healthcare Research and Quality, and perhaps most notably, the Centers for Medicare and Medicaid Services. (The most notable change in HHS structure in recent history was the separation of social security responsibilities into a new and independent agency, the Social Security Administration, in 1995.) HHS has become a gigantic agency, responsible for about a quarter of all federal non-defense spending. It issues more federal grants than all other federal agencies combined, and its Medicare program alone handles more than a billion claims a year. In addition to its own programs, HHS delegates many of its legislated responsibilities to state, county, tribal, and local agencies through eight divisions within the U.S. Public Health Service and three human services agencies. HHS has ten regional offices across the country in addition to its main headquarters in Washington, D.C., the **CDC** in Atlanta, the Baltimore, Maryland campus for Medicare and Medicaid services, the Bethesda, Maryland campus for the NIH, and the White Oak, Maryland campus for the FDA. The department's 2013 budget outlay is for just under $941 billion, with provisions for 76,341 full–time–equivalent employees.

Under Congressional orders, HHS is required to produce a five–year strategic plan outlining its long–term goals and recent accomplishments. In its most recent plan, for fiscal years 2010–2015, the department has initiated a new policy of posting its strategic plan online, where it can be viewed by anyone. In this format, the plan is subject to constant review and revision that reflects changes that are likely to impact long–term goals. The most recent strategic plan consists of five major goals:

- Strengthen health care
- Advance scientific knowledge and innovation
- Advance the health, safety, and well–being of the American people
- Increase efficiency, transparency, and accountability of HHS programs
- Strengthen the nation's health and human services infrastructure and workforce

These very general goals are broken down into more specific objectives in each succeeding chapter of the strategic plan. For example, goal one is further defined as making healthcare coverage more affordable and extending health services to a larger portion of the American public; improving healthcare quality and patient safety; linking primary and preventative care to community **prevention** services; reducing the rate of healthcare costs; ensuring access to quality healthcare to **vulnerable populations**, and promoting the adoption of proven and useful healthcare technology. Appendix D of the report summarizes changes that have been made in goals, objectives, accomplishments, and other features of the plan since its original release in mid–2010.

Another major HHS initiative is a program called Healthy People, which originated in a 1979 Surgeon General's report of the same name. The report provided suggestions for federal involvement in programs to prevent disease and improve the general health of the American public. The initiative was reimagined and reformulated on a broader scale in 1990 as Healthy People 1990 and again as Healthy People 2000, Healthy People 2010, and, more recently, as Healthy People 2020. The most recent version of the program consists of 15 objectives and 42 topic areas, such as: adolescent health; **cancer**; chronic kidney disease; early and middle childhood; **food safety**; **genomics**; hearing and other sensory or communication disorders; lesbian, gay, bisexual, and transgender health; preparedness; sleep health; substance abuse; and vision.

Professional Publications

Each of the many divisions of HHS produces and distributes its own collection of books, articles, reports, newsletters, brochures, pamphlets, and other print and electronic publications. In addition, the department's web page at http://www.hhs.gov/news/reports/index.html provides a comprehensive guide to reports produced by all its divisions for the U.S. Congress and other governmental agencies. As an example of division offerings, the HHS Office of Adolescent Health offers (mostly free) publications on topics such as dating and sexual relationships; lesbian, gay, bisexual, and transgender issues; dating **violence**; youth violence; mental health disorders; access to health care; positive mental health skills; healthy eating; **immunization** and **vaccination**; chronic conditions; injuries; access to physical health services; teen pregnancy and childbearing; sexually transmitted infections; contraceptive and condom use; alcohol; tobacco; and licit and illicit drugs.

Resources

BOOKS

McKenzie, James F., R. R. Pinger, and Jerome Edward Kotecki. *An Introduction to Community Health*. Sudbury, MA: Jones and Bartlett Publishers, 2008.

PERIODICALS

Daulaire, N. "The Global Health Strategy of The Department Of Health And Human Services: Building On The Lessons Of PEPFAR." *Health Affairs*. 31. 7. (2012): 1573–77.

Radin, Beryl A. "When is a Health Department not a Health Department? The Case of the US Department of Health and Human Services." *Social Policy and Administration* 44. 2. (2010): 142–54.

WEBSITES

Department of Health and Human Services (HHS). USA.gov. http://www.usa.gov/Agencies/Federal/Executive/HHS.shtml (accessed October 10, 2012).

ORGANIZATIONS

U.S. Department of Health and Human Services (HHS), 200 Independence Ave., S.W., Washington, DC 20201, (877) 696-6775, http://wcdapps.hhs.gov/HHSFeedback/, http://www.hhs.gov/

David E. Newton, EdD

Diabetes mellitus

Definition

Diabetes mellitus is a condition in which the pancreas no longer produces enough insulin or cells stop responding to the insulin that is produced, so that glucose in the blood cannot be absorbed into the cells of the body. Symptoms include frequent urination, lethargy, excessive thirst, and hunger. Treatment can include changes in diet, oral medications, and daily injections of insulin, especially with type 1 diabetes.

Description

Diabetes mellitus is a chronic disease that causes serious health complications including renal (kidney) failure, **heart disease**, **stroke**, and blindness. Approximately 17 million Americans have diabetes. Unfortunately, as many as one-half are unaware they have it, and rates are expected to continue to increase due to the high prevalence of **obesity** in the United States.

Diabetes statistics for the United States

- 25.8 million Americans (8.3% of the U.S. population) have diabetes, with the estimate that 18.8 million are actually diagnosed, and seven million are walking around undiagnosed.
- An estimated 79 million American adults aged 20 years or older have prediabetes.
- Prediabetes is a condition in which individuals have blood glucose or A1c levels higher than normal but not high enough to be classified as diabetes. People with prediabetes have an increased risk of developing type 2 diabetes, heart disease, and stroke.
- People with prediabetes who lose weight and increase their physical activity can prevent or delay type 2 diabetes and in some cases return their blood glucose levels to normal.
- Among U.S. residents aged 65 years and older, 10.9 million, or 26.9%, had diabetes in 2010.
- About 215,000 people younger than 20 years had diabetes (type 1 or type 2) in the United States in 2010.
- About 1.9 million people aged 20 years or older were newly diagnosed with diabetes in 2010 in the United States.
- Diabetes is the leading cause of kidney failure, non-traumatic lower-limb amputations, and new cases of blindness among adults in the United States.
- Diabetes is a major cause of heart disease and stroke.
- Diabetes is the seventh leading cause of death in the United States.
- The risk for death among people with diabetes is about twice that of people of similar age but without diabetes.
- Medical expenses for people with diabetes are more than two times higher than for people without diabetes.
- Estimated cost of diabetes to the U.S. (direct medical costs and indirect, which includes disability, work loss, premature mortality): $174 billion dollars a year.

SOURCE: Centers for Disease Control and Prevention National Diabetes Fact Sheet 2011.

(Table by PreMediaGlobal. © 2013 Cengage Learning)

Background

Every cell in the human body needs energy in order to function. The body's primary energy source is glucose, a simple sugar resulting from the digestion of foods containing carbohydrates (sugars and starches). Glucose from the digested food circulates in the blood as a ready energy source for any cells that need it. Insulin is a hormone or chemical produced by cells in the pancreas, an organ located behind the stomach. Insulin binds to a receptor site on the outside of cell and acts like a key to open a doorway into the cell through which glucose can enter. Some of the glucose can be converted to concentrated energy sources like glycogen or fatty acids and saved for later use. When there is not enough insulin produced or when the doorway no longer recognizes the insulin key, glucose stays in the blood rather entering the cells.

The body will attempt to dilute the high level of glucose in the blood, a condition called hyperglycemia, by drawing **water** out of the cells and into the bloodstream in an effort to dilute the sugar and excrete it in the urine. It is not unusual for people with undiagnosed diabetes to be constantly thirsty, drink large quantities of water, and urinate frequently as their bodies try to get rid of the extra glucose. This creates high levels of glucose in the urine.

At the same time that the body is trying to get rid of glucose from the blood, the cells are starving for glucose and sending signals to the body to eat more food, thus making patients extremely hungry. To provide energy for the starving cells, the body also tries to convert fats and proteins to glucose. The breakdown of fats and proteins for energy causes acid compounds called ketones to form in the blood. Ketones also will be excreted in the urine. As ketones build up in the blood, a condition called ketoacidosis can occur. This condition can be life threatening if left untreated, leading to coma and death.

Types of diabetes mellitus

Type I diabetes, sometimes called juvenile diabetes, begins most commonly in childhood or adolescence. In this form of diabetes, the body produces little or no insulin. It is characterized by a sudden onset and occurs more frequently in populations descended from Northern European countries (Finland, Scotland, Scandinavia) than in those from Southern European countries, the Middle East, or Asia. In the United States, approximately three people in 1,000 develop Type I diabetes. This form also is called insulin-dependent diabetes because people who develop this type need to have daily injections of insulin.

Brittle diabetics are a subgroup of Type I where patients have frequent and rapid swings of blood sugar levels between hyperglycemia (a condition where there is too much glucose or sugar in the blood) and hypoglycemia (a condition where there are abnormally low levels of glucose or sugar in the blood). These patients may require several injections of different types of insulin during the day to keep the blood sugar level within a fairly normal range.

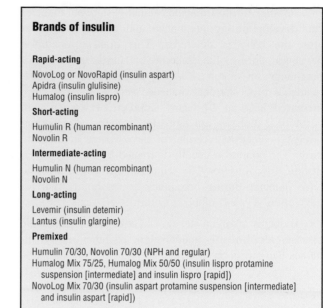

Brands of insulin

Rapid-acting

NovoLog or NovoRapid (insulin aspart)
Apidra (insulin glulisine)
Humalog (insulin lispro)

Short-acting

Humulin R (human recombinant)
Novolin R

Intermediate-acting

Humulin N (human recombinant)
Novolin N

Long-acting

Levemir (insulin detemir)
Lantus (insulin glargine)

Premixed

Humulin 70/30, Novolin 70/30 (NPH and regular)
Humalog Mix 75/25, Humalog Mix 50/50 (insulin lispro protamine suspension [intermediate] and insulin lispro [rapid])
NovoLog Mix 70/30 (insulin aspart protamine suspension [intermediate] and insulin aspart [rapid])

(Table by PreMediaGlobal. © 2013 Cengage Learning)

The more common form of diabetes, Type II, occurs in approximately 3–5% of Americans under 50 years of age, and increases to 10–15% in those over 50. More than 90% of the diabetics in the United States are Type II diabetics. Sometimes called age-onset or adult-onset diabetes, this form of diabetes occurs most often in people who are overweight and who do not exercise. It is also more common in people of Native American, Hispanic, and African-American descent. People who have migrated to Western cultures from East India, Japan, and Australian Aboriginal cultures also are more likely to develop Type II diabetes than those who remain in their original countries.

Type II is considered a milder form of diabetes because of its slow onset (sometimes developing over the course of several years) and because it usually can be controlled with diet and oral medication. The consequences of uncontrolled and untreated Type II diabetes, however, are the just as serious as those for Type I. This form is also called noninsulin-dependent diabetes, a term that is somewhat misleading. Many people with Type II diabetes can control the condition with diet and oral medications, however, insulin injections are sometimes necessary if treatment with diet and oral medication is not working.

Another form of diabetes called gestational diabetes can develop during pregnancy and generally resolves after the baby is delivered. This diabetic condition develops during the second or third trimester of pregnancy in about 2% of pregnancies. In 2004, incidence of gestational diabetes were reported to have increased 35% in 10 years. Children of women with gestational diabetes are more likely to be born prematurely, have hypoglycemia, or have severe jaundice at birth. The condition usually is treated by diet, however, insulin injections may be required. These women who have diabetes during pregnancy are at higher risk for developing Type II diabetes within 5–10 years.

Diabetes also can develop as a result of pancreatic disease, **alcoholism**, malnutrition, or other severe illnesses that stress the body.

Causes and symptoms

Causes

The causes of diabetes mellitus are unclear, however, there seem to be both hereditary (genetic factors passed on in families) and environmental factors involved. Research has shown that some people who develop diabetes have common genetic markers. In Type I diabetes, the immune system, the body's defense system against infection, is believed to be triggered by a virus or another microorganism that destroys cells in the pancreas that produce insulin. In Type II diabetes, age, obesity, and family history of diabetes play a role.

In Type II diabetes, the pancreas may produce enough insulin, however, cells have become resistant to the insulin produced and it may not work as effectively. Symptoms of Type II diabetes can begin so gradually that a person may not know that he or she has it. Early signs are lethargy, extreme thirst, and frequent urination. Other symptoms may include sudden weight loss, slow wound healing, urinary tract infections, gum disease, or blurred vision. It is not unusual for Type II diabetes to be detected while a patient is seeing a doctor about another health concern that is actually being caused by the yet undiagnosed diabetes.

Individuals who are at high risk of developing Type II diabetes mellitus include people who:

- are obese (more than 20% above their ideal body weight)
- have a relative with diabetes mellitus
- belong to a high-risk ethnic population (African-American, Native American, Hispanic, or Native Hawaiian)
- have been diagnosed with gestational diabetes or have delivered a baby weighing more than 9 lbs (4 kg)
- have high blood pressure (140/90 mmHg or above)
- have a high density lipoprotein cholesterol level less than or equal to 35 mg/dL and/or a triglyceride level greater than or equal to 250 mg/dL
- have had impaired glucose tolerance or impaired fasting glucose on previous testing

Several common medications can impair the body's use of insulin, causing a condition known as secondary diabetes. These medications include treatments for high blood pressure (furosemide, clonidine, and thiazide diuretics), drugs with hormonal activity (oral contraceptives, thyroid hormone, progestins, and glucocorticorids), and the anti-inflammation drug indomethacin. Several drugs that are used to treat mood disorders (such as anxiety and depression) also can impair glucose absorption. These drugs include haloperidol, lithium carbonate, phenothiazines, tricyclic antidepressants, and adrenergic agonists. Other medications that can cause diabetes symptoms include isoniazid, nicotinic acid, cimetidine, and heparin. A 2004 study found that low levels of the essential mineral chromium in the body may be linked to increased risk for diseases associated with insulin resistance.

Symptoms

Symptoms of diabetes can develop suddenly (over days or weeks) in previously healthy children or adolescents, or can develop gradually (over several years) in overweight adults over the age of 40. The classic symptoms include feeling tired and sick, frequent urination, excessive thirst, excessive hunger, and weight loss.

Ketoacidosis, a condition due to starvation or uncontrolled diabetes, is common in Type I diabetes. Ketones are acid compounds that form in the blood when the body breaks down fats and proteins. Symptoms include abdominal **pain**, vomiting, rapid breathing, extreme lethargy, and drowsiness. Patients with ketoacidosis will also have a sweet breath odor. Left untreated, this condition can lead to coma and death.

With Type II diabetes, the condition may not become evident until the patient presents for medical treatment for some other condition. A patient may have heart disease, chronic infections of the gums and urinary tract, blurred vision, numbness in the feet and legs, or slow-healing wounds. Women may experience genital itching.

Diagnosis

Diabetes is suspected based on symptoms. Urine tests and blood tests can be used to confirm a diagnose of diabetes based on the amount of glucose found. Urine can also detect ketones and protein in the urine that may help diagnose diabetes and assess how well the kidneys are functioning. These tests also can be used to monitor the disease once the patient is on a standardized diet, oral medications, or insulin.

Urine tests

Clinistix and Diastix are paper strips or dipsticks that change color when dipped in urine. The test strip is compared to a chart that shows the amount of glucose in the urine based on the change in color. The level of glucose in the urine lags behind the level of glucose in the blood. Testing the urine with a test stick, paper strip, or tablet that changes color when sugar is present is not as accurate as blood testing, however it can give a fast and simple reading.

Ketones in the urine can be detected using similar types of dipstick tests (Acetest or Ketostix). Ketoacidosis can be a life-threatening situation in Type I diabetics, so having a quick and simple test to detect ketones can assist in establishing a diagnosis sooner.

Another dipstick test can determine the presence of protein or albumin in the urine. Protein in the urine can indicate problems with kidney function and can be used to track the development of renal failure. A more sensitive test for urine protein uses radioactively tagged chemicals to detect microalbuminuria, small amounts of protein in the urine, that may not show up on dipstick tests.

Blood tests

FASTING GLUCOSE TEST. Blood is drawn from a vein in the patient's arm after a period at least eight hours when the patient has not eaten, usually in the morning before breakfast. The red blood cells are separated from the sample and the amount of glucose is measured in the remaining plasma. A plasma level of 7.8 mmol/L (200 mg/L) or greater can indicate diabetes. The fasting glucose test is usually repeated on another day to confirm the results.

POSTPRANDIAL GLUCOSE TEST. Blood is taken right after the patient has eaten a meal.

ORAL GLUCOSE TOLERANCE TEST. Blood samples are taken from a vein before and after a patient drinks a thick, sweet syrup of glucose and other sugars. In a non-diabetic, the level of glucose in the blood goes up immediately after the drink and then decreases gradually as insulin is used by the body to metabolize, or absorb, the sugar. In a diabetic, the glucose in the blood goes up and stays high after drinking the sweetened liquid. A plasma glucose level of 11.1 mmol/L (200 mg/dL) or higher at two hours after drinking the syrup and at one other point during the two-hour test period confirms the diagnosis of diabetes.

A diagnosis of diabetes is confirmed if there are symptoms of diabetes and a plasma glucose level of at least 11.1 mmol/L, a fasting plasma glucose level of at least 7.8 mmol/L; or a two-hour plasma glucose level of at least 11.1 mmol/L during an oral glucose tolerance test.

Home blood glucose monitoring kits are available so patients with diabetes can monitor their own levels. A small needle or lancet is used to prick the finger and a drop of blood is collected and analyzed by a monitoring device. Some patients may test their blood glucose levels several times during a day and use this information to adjust their doses of insulin.

Treatment

There is currently no cure for diabetes. The condition, however, can be managed so that patients can live a relatively normal life. Treatment of diabetes focuses on two goals: keeping blood glucose within normal range and preventing the development of long-term complications. Careful monitoring of diet, exercise, and blood glucose levels are as important as the use of insulin or oral medications in preventing complications of diabetes. Each year, the American Diabetes Association updates its standards of care for the management of diabetes. These standards help manage healthcare providers in the most recent recommendations for diagnosis and treatment of the disease.

Dietary changes

Diet and moderate exercise are the first treatments implemented in diabetes. For many Type II diabetics, weight loss may be an important goal in helping them to control their diabetes. A well-balanced, nutritious diet provides approximately 50–60% of calories from carbohydrates, approximately 10–20% of calories from protein, and less than 30% of calories from fat. The number of calories required by an individual depends on age, weight, and activity level. The calorie intake also needs to be distributed over the course of the entire day so surges of glucose entering the blood system are kept to a minimum.

Keeping track of the number of calories provided by different foods can become complicated, so patients usually are advised to consult a nutritionist or dietitian. An individualized, easy to manage diet plan can be set up for each patient. Both the American Diabetes Association and the Academy of Nutrition and Dietetics recommend diets based on the use of food exchange lists. Each food exchange contains a known amount of calories in the form of protein, fat, or carbohydrate. A patient's diet plan will consist of a certain number of exchanges from each food category (meat or protein, fruits, breads and starches, vegetables, and fats) to be eaten at meal times and as snacks. Patients have flexibility in choosing which foods they eat as long as they stick with the number of exchanges prescribed.

For many Type II diabetics, weight loss is an important factor in controlling their condition. The food exchange system, along with a plan of moderate exercise, can help them lose excess weight and improve their overall health.

Oral medications

Oral medications are available to lower blood glucose in Type II diabetics. In 1990, 23.4 outpatient prescriptions for oral antidiabetic agents were dispensed. By 2001, the number had increased to 91.8 million prescriptions. Oral antidiabetic agents accounted for more than $5 billion dollars in worldwide retail sales per year in the early twenty-first century and were the fastest-growing segment of diabetes drugs. The drugs first prescribed for Type II diabetes are in a class of compounds called sulfonylureas and include tolbutamide, tolazamide, acetohexamide, and chlorpropamide. Newer drugs in the same class are now available and include glyburide, glimeperide, and glipizide. How these drugs work is not well understood, however, they seem to stimulate cells of the pancreas to produce more insulin. New medications that are available to treat diabetes include metformin, acarbose, and troglitizone. The choice of medication depends in part on the individual patient profile. All drugs have side effects that may make them inappropriate for particular patients. Some for example, may stimulate weight gain or cause stomach irritation, so they may not be the best treatment for someone who is already overweight or who has stomach ulcers. Others, like metformin, have been shown to have positive effects such as reduced cardiovascular mortality, but but increased risk in other situations. While these medications are an important aspect of treatment for Type II diabetes, they are not a substitute for a well planned diet and moderate exercise. Oral medications have not been shown effective for Type I diabetes, in which the patient produces little or no insulin.

Constant advances are being made in development of new oral medications for persons with diabetes. In 2003, a drug called Metaglip combining glipizide and metformin was approved in a dingle tablet. Along with diet and exercise, the drug was used as initial therapy for Type 2 diabetes. Another drug approved by the U.S. Food and Drug Administration (FDA) combines metformin and rosiglitazone (Avandia), a medication that increases muscle cells' sensitivity to insulin. It is marketed under the name Avandamet. So many new drugs are under development that it is best to stay in touch with a physician for the latest information; physicians can find the best drug, diet and exercise program to fit an individual patient's need.

Insulin

Patients with Type I diabetes need daily injections of insulin to help their bodies use glucose. The amount and type of insulin required depends on the height, weight, age, food intake, and activity level of the individual diabetic patient. Some patients with Type II diabetes may need to use insulin injections if their diabetes cannot be controlled with diet, exercise, and oral medication. Injections are given subcutaneously, that is, just under the skin, using a small needle and syringe. Injection sites can be anywhere on the body where there is looser skin, including the upper arm, abdomen, or upper thigh.

Purified human insulin is most commonly used, however, insulin from beef and pork sources also are available. Insulin may be given as an injection of a single dose of one type of insulin once a day. Different types of insulin can be mixed and given in one dose or split into two or more doses during a day. Patients who require multiple injections over the course of a day may be able to use an insulin pump that administers small doses of insulin on demand. The small battery-operated pump is worn outside the body and is connected to a needle that is inserted into the abdomen. Pumps can be programmed to inject small doses of insulin at various times during the day, or the patient may be able to adjust the insulin doses to coincide with meals and exercise.

Regular insulin is fast-acting and starts to work within 15–30 minutes, with its peak glucose-lowering effect about two hours after it is injected. Its effects last for about four to six hours. NPH (neutral protamine Hagedorn) and Lente insulin are intermediate-acting, starting to work within one to three hours and lasting up to 18–26 hours. Ultra-lente is a long-acting form of insulin that starts to work within four to eight hours and lasts 28–36 hours.

Hypoglycemia, or low blood sugar, can be caused by too much insulin, too little food (or eating too late to coincide with the action of the insulin), alcohol consumption, or increased exercise. A patient with symptoms of hypoglycemia may be hungry, cranky, confused, and tired. The patient may become sweaty and shaky. Left untreated, the patient can lose consciousness or have a seizure. This condition is sometimes called an insulin reaction and should be treated by giving the patient something sweet to eat or drink like a candy, sugar cubes, juice, or another high sugar snack.

Surgery

Transplantation of a healthy pancreas into a diabetic patient is a successful treatment, however, this transplant is usually done only if a kidney transplant is performed at the same time. Although a pancreas transplant is possible, it is not clear if the potential benefits outweigh the risks of the surgery and drug therapy needed.

Alternative treatment

Since diabetes can be life-threatening if not properly managed, patients should not attempt to treat this condition without medical supervision. A variety of alternative therapies can be helpful in managing the symptoms of diabetes and supporting patients with the disease. Acupuncture can help relieve the pain associated with diabetic neuropathy by stimulation of certain points. A qualified practitioner should be consulted. Herbal remedies also may be helpful in managing diabetes. Although there is no herbal substitute for insulin, some herbs may help adjust blood sugar levels or manage other diabetic symptoms. Some options include:

- fenugreek (*Trigonella foenum-graecum*) has been shown in some studies to reduce blood insulin and glucose levels while also lowering cholesterol
- bilberry (*Vaccinium myrtillus*) may lower blood glucose levels, as well as helping to maintain healthy blood vessels
- garlic (*Allium sativum*) may lower blood sugar and cholesterol levels
- onions (*Allium cepa*) may help lower blood glucose levels by freeing insulin to metabolize them
- cayenne pepper (*Capsicum frutescens*) can help relieve pain in the peripheral nerves (a type of diabetic neuropathy)
- gingko (*Gingko biloba*) may maintain blood flow to the retina, helping to prevent diabetic retinopathy

Any therapy that lowers stress levels also can be useful in treating diabetes by helping to reduce insulin requirements. Among the alternative treatments that aim to lower stress are hypnotherapy, biofeedback, and meditation.

Prognosis

Uncontrolled diabetes is a leading cause of blindness, end-stage renal disease, and limb amputations. It also doubles the risks of heart disease and increases the risk of stroke. Eye problems including cataracts, glaucoma, and diabetic retinopathy also are more common in diabetics.

Diabetic peripheral neuropathy is a condition where nerve endings, particularly in the legs and feet, become less sensitive. Diabetic foot ulcers are a particular problem since the patient does not feel the pain of a blister, callous, or other minor injury. Poor blood circulation in the legs and feet contribute to delayed wound healing. The inability to sense pain along with the complications of delayed wound healing can result in minor injuries, blisters, or callouses becoming infected and difficult to treat. In cases of severe infection, the infected tissue begins to break down and rot away. The most serious consequence of this condition is the need for amputation of toes, feet, or legs due to severe infection.

Heart disease and kidney disease are common complications of diabetes. Long-term complications may include the need for kidney dialysis or a kidney transplant due to kidney failure.

Babies born to diabetic mothers have an increased risk of **birth defects** and distress at birth.

Prevention

Research continues on diabetes **prevention** and improved detection of those at risk for developing diabetes. While the onset of Type I diabetes is unpredictable, the risk of developing Type II diabetes can be reduced by maintaining ideal weight and exercising regularly. The physical and emotional stress of surgery, illness, pregnancy, and alcoholism can increase the risks of diabetes, so maintaining a healthy lifestyle is critical to preventing the onset of Type II diabetes and preventing further complications of the disease.

Resources

BOOKS

American Diabetes Association. *American Diabetes Association Complete Guide to Diabetes*. 5th ed. Alexandria, VA: American Diabetes Association, 2011.

PERIODICALS

Abbasi, A., et al. "Prediction Models for Risk of Developing Type 2 Diabetes: Systematic Literature Search and Independent External Validation Study." *BMJ* 18, no. 345 (September 18, 2012): e5900. http://dx.doi.org/10.1136/bmj.e5900 (accessed October 2, 2012).

American Diabetes Association. "Standards of Medical Care in Diabetes—2012." *Diabetes Care* 35, suppl. 1 (2012): S11–63.

Babbington, Gabrielle. "Metformin Tops Diabetes Trial." *Australian Doctor* (July 27, 2007): 3.

Buchanan, Thomas A., et al. "What is Gestational Diabetes?" *Diabetes Care* (July 2007): S105–S111.

Malik, Vasanti S., et al. "Sugar-Sweetened Beverages, Obesity, Type 2 Diabetes Mellitus, and Cardiovascular Disease Risk." *Circulation* 121 (2010):1356–64. http://dx.doi.org/10.1161/CIRCULATIONAHA.109.876185 (accessed October 2, 2012).

"Research: Lower Chromium Levels Linked to Increased Risk of Disease." *Diabetes Week* (March 29, 2004): 21.

"Standards of Medical Care for Patients with Diabetes Mellitus: American Diabetes Association." *Clinical Diabetes* (Winter 2003): 27.

WEBSITES

American Diabetes Association. "Diabetes Basics." http://www.diabetes.org/diabetes-basics (accessed September 9, 2012).

American Diabetes Association. "Low-Carb Diet for People with Diabetes." http://www.diabetes.org/news-research/research/access-diabetes-research/Ma-low-carb-diet.html (accessed October 3, 2012).

Centers for Disease Control and Prevention. "Diabetes Public Health Resource." http://www.cdc.gov/diabetes/# (accessed October 2, 2012).

Mayo Clinic staff. "Diabetes." MayoClinic.com. http://www.mayoclinic.com/health/diabetes/DS01121 (accessed October 2, 2012).

MedlinePlus. "Diabetes." U.S. National Library of Medicine, National Institutes of Health. http://www.nlm.nih.gov/medlineplus/diabetes.html (accessed October 2, 2012).

ORGANIZATIONS

Academy of Nutrition and Dietetics, 120 South Riverside Plz., Ste. 2000, Chicago, IL 60606-6995, (312) 899-0040, (800) 877-1600, amacmunn@eatright.org, http://www.eatright.org.

American Diabetes Association, 1701 North Beauregard St., Alexandria, VA 22311, (800) DIABETES (342-2383), askADA@diabetes.org, http://www.diabetes.org.

Canadian Diabetes Association, National Life Building, 1400–522 University Ave., Toronto, ON, Canada M5G 2R5, (800) 226-8464, info@diabetes.ca, http://www.diabetes.ca.

Centers for Disease Control and Prevention, 1600 Clifton Rd. NE, Atlanta, GA 30333, (800) CDC-INFO (232-4636), (888) 232-6348, cdcinfo@cdc.gov, http://www.cdc.gov.

Juvenile Diabetes Research Foundation International, 26 Broadway, 14th Fl., New York, NY 10004, (800) 533-CURE (2873), Fax: (212) 785-9595, info@jdrg.org, http://www.jdrf.org.

National Diabetes Education Program, One Diabetes Way, Bethesda, MD 20814-9692, (301) 496-3583, http://www.ndep.nih.gov.

National Diabetes Information Clearinghouse, 1 Information Way, Bethesda, MD 20892-3560, (800) 860-8747(866) 569-1162, Fax: (703) 738-4929, ndic@info.niddk.nih.gov, http://diabetes.niddk.nih.gov.

Altha Roberts Edgren
Teresa G. Odle

Dieticians *see* **Nutrition**

Diphtheria

Definition

Diphtheria is a potentially fatal, contagious disease that usually involves the nose, throat, and air passages, but may also infect the skin. Its most striking feature is the formation of a grayish membrane covering the tonsils and upper part of the throat.

Demographics

Before 1920 when the diphtheria toxoid was introduced, diphtheria was a major childhood killer, with 200,000 cases reported annually in the United States. In the twenty first century, diphtheria is rare and sporadic in the developed world because of widespread **immunization**. In countries that do not have routine immunization against this infection, periodic outbreaks occur. The largest recent outbreak occurred in the countries comprising the former Soviet Union and the Baltic States. From 1990–1995, 157,000 cases and 5,000 deaths were reported in this region, accounting for more than 80% of all diphtheria cases reported during those years. Other, smaller outbreaks have been reported in sub-Saharan Africa, India, and France. Like many other upper respiratory diseases, diphtheria is most likely to occur during the cold months. Individuals who have not been immunized may get diphtheria at any age; mortality rates are highest in those under five years or over 40 years of age.

Description

Diphtheria is spread most often by droplets from the coughing or sneezing of an infected person or carrier. The incubation period is two to seven days, with an average of three days. It is vital to seek medical help at once when diphtheria is suspected, because treatment requires emergency measures for adults as well as children.

Risk factors for developing diphtheria include:

- failure to immunize or incomplete immunization
- living in crowded, unhygienic conditions
- having a compromised immune system
- traveling to developing regions of the world where diphtheria is more common

Causes and symptoms

The symptoms of diphtheria are caused by toxins produced by the diphtheria bacillus, *Corynebacterium diphtheriae* (from the Greek for "rubber membrane"). In fact, toxin production is related to infections of the bacillus itself with a particular bacterial virus called a phage (from bacteriophage; a virus that infects bacteria). The infection destroys healthy tissue in the upper area of the throat around the tonsils, or in open wounds in the skin. Fluid from dying cells then coagulates to form the telltale gray or grayish-green membrane. Inside the membrane, the bacteria produce an exotoxin, which is a poisonous secretion that causes the life-threatening symptoms of diphtheria. The exotoxin is carried throughout the body in the bloodstream, destroying healthy tissue in other parts of the body.

The most serious complications caused by the exotoxin are inflammations of the heart muscle (myocarditis) and damage to the nervous system. The risk of serious complications is increased as the time between onset of symptoms and the administration of antitoxin increases and as the size of the membrane formed increases. Myocarditis may cause disturbances in the heart rhythm (arrhythmias) and may result in heart failure. Symptoms of nervous system involvement can include seeing double vision (diplopia), painful or difficult swallowing (dysphagia), and slurred speech or loss of voice, which are all indications of the exotoxin's effect on nerve functions. The exotoxin may also cause severe swelling in the neck ("bull neck").

The signs and symptoms of diphtheria vary according to the location of the infection.

Nasal

Nasal diphtheria produces few symptoms other than a watery or bloody discharge. On examination, there may be a small visible membrane in the nasal passages. Nasal infection rarely causes complications by itself, but it is a public health problem because it spreads the disease more rapidly than other forms of diphtheria.

Pharyngeal

Pharyngeal diphtheria gets its name from the pharynx, which is the part of the upper throat that connects the mouth and nasal passages with the voice box (larynx). This is the most common form of diphtheria, causing the characteristic grayish throat membrane. The membrane often bleeds if it is scraped or cut. It is important not to try to remove the membrane because the trauma may increase the body's absorption of the exotoxin. Other signs and symptoms of pharyngeal diphtheria include mild sore throat, fever of 101–102 °F (38.3–38.9 °C), a rapid pulse, and general body weakness.

Laryngeal

Laryngeal diphtheria, which involves the voice box or larynx, is the form most likely to produce serious complications. The fever is usually higher in this form of diphtheria (103–104 °F or 39.4–40 °C) and the patient is very weak. Patients may have a severe cough, have difficulty breathing, or lose their voice completely. The development of a "bull neck" indicates a high level of exotoxin in the bloodstream. Obstruction of the airway may result in difficulty breathing, respiratory compromise, and death.

KEY TERMS

Antitoxin—An antibody against an exotoxin, usually derived from horse serum.

Bacillus—A rod-shaped bacterium, such as the diphtheria bacterium.

Carrier—A person who may harbor an organism without symptoms and may transmit it to others.

Cutaneous—Located in the skin.

Diphtheria–tetanus–pertussis (DTP)—The standard preparation used to immunize children against diphtheria, tetanus, and whooping cough. A so-called "acellular pertussis" vaccine (aP) is usually used since its release in the mid-1990s in a combined vaccine known as DTaP.

Exotoxin—A poisonous secretion produced by bacilli which is carried in the bloodstream to other parts of the body.

Gram's stain—A dye staining technique used in laboratory tests to determine the presence and type of bacteria.

Loeffler's medium—A special substance used to grow diphtheria bacilli to confirm a diagnosis.

Myocarditis—Inflammation of the heart tissue.

Toxoid—A preparation made from inactivated exotoxin, used in immunization.

Skin

This form of diphtheria, which is sometimes called cutaneous diphtheria, accounts for about 33% of diphtheria cases. It is found chiefly among people with poor **hygiene**, and is more common in tropical climates. Any break in the skin can become infected with diphtheria. The infected tissue develops an ulcerated area and a diphtheria membrane may form over the wound but is not always present. The wound or ulcer is slow to heal and may be numb or insensitive when touched.

Diagnosis

Because diphtheria must be treated as quickly as possible, doctors usually make the diagnosis on the basis of the visible symptoms without waiting for test results.

Examination

In making the diagnosis, the doctor examines the patient's eyes, ears, nose, and throat in order to rule out other diseases that may cause fever and sore throat, such as infectious mononucleosis, a sinus infection, or strep throat. The most important single symptom that suggests diphtheria is the membrane. When a patient develops skin infections during an outbreak of diphtheria, the doctor will consider the possibility of cutaneous diphtheria and take a smear to confirm the diagnosis.

Tests

The diagnosis of diphtheria can be confirmed by the results of a culture obtained from the infected area. Material from the swab is put on a microscope slide and stained using a procedure called Gram's stain. The diphtheria bacillus is called Gram-positive because it holds the dye after the slide is rinsed with alcohol. Under the microscope, diphtheria bacilli look like beaded rod-shaped cells, grouped in patterns that resemble Chinese characters. Another laboratory test involves growing the diphtheria bacillus on a special material called Loeffler's medium.

Treatment

Diphtheria is a serious disease requiring hospital treatment in an intensive care unit if the patient has developed respiratory symptoms. Treatment includes a combination of medications and supportive care:

Antitoxin

The most important step is prompt administration of diphtheria antitoxin, without waiting for laboratory results. The antitoxin is made from horse serum and works by neutralizing any circulating exotoxin. The doctor must first test the patient for sensitivity to animal serum. Patients who are sensitive (about 10%) must be desensitized with diluted antitoxin, since the antitoxin is the only specific substance that will counteract diphtheria exotoxin. No other type if antitoxin is available for the treatment of diphtheria.

The dose of antitoxin ranges from 20,000–100,000 units, depending on the severity and length of time of symptoms occurring before treatment. Diphtheria antitoxin is usually given intravenously. It must be obtained from the United States **Centers for Disease Control and Prevention (CDC)** and may not be available in some parts of the world.

Antibiotics

Antibiotics are given to kill the bacteria, to prevent the spread of the disease, and to protect the patient from developing **pneumonia**. They are not a substitute for treatment with antitoxin. Both adults and children may be given penicillin, ampicillin, or erythromycin. Erythromycin appears to be more effective than penicillin in treating people who are carriers because of better penetration into the infected area.

Cutaneous diphtheria is usually treated by cleansing the wound thoroughly with soap and **water**, and giving the patient antibiotics for 10 days.

Supportive care

Diphtheria patients need bed rest with intensive nursing care, including extra fluids, oxygenation, and monitoring for possible heart problems, airway blockage, or involvement of the nervous system. Patients with laryngeal diphtheria are kept in a croup tent or high-humidity environment; they may also need throat suctioning or emergency surgery if their airway is blocked.

Patients recovering from diphtheria should rest at home for a minimum of two to three weeks, especially if they have heart complications. In addition, patients should be immunized against diphtheria after recovery, because having the disease does not always induce antitoxin formation and protect them from re-infection.

Prevention of complications

Diphtheria patients who develop myocarditis may be treated with oxygen and with medications to prevent irregular heart rhythms. An artificial pacemaker may be needed. Patients with difficulty swallowing can be fed through a tube inserted into the stomach through the nose. Patients who cannot breathe are usually put on mechanical respirators.

Public Health Response

Public health responders are generally not the first responders to suspected cases of diphtheria. Instead, they receive information about such cases from primary care physicians, emergency department personnel, and other healthcare workers. Public health workers then contact the infected person to obtain information about possible sources of the disease and contacts to whom the individual may have transmitted the diseases. **Vaccination** histories may also be collected to see if the individual may have been associated with others who have not been vaccinated. If necessary, public health workers provide information about the case to the state health department, other public health agencies, and other health organizations for whom such information may be useful in preventing the spread of the disease.

Prognosis

The prognosis depends on the size and location of the membrane and on early treatment with antitoxin; the longer the delay, the higher the death rate. The most vulnerable patients are children under age five and those who develop pneumonia or myocarditis. Death rates generally range from five to 10 percent and may reach as

QUESTIONS TO ASK YOUR DOCTOR

- Are there risks associated with the vaccination against diphtheria? If so, what are they?
- What reliable sources of information about the diphtheria inoculation program can you recommend?
- What should I do if I happen to miss one or more shots in the vaccination program for diphtheria?
- A number of children in my son's school have not been vaccinated against diphtheria. How does this fact affect my son's risk for contracting the disease?
- Why are some children excused from being vaccinated against diphtheria and still allowed to attend school?

high as 20% in young children and older adults. Nasal and cutaneous diphtheria are rarely fatal.

Prevention

Prevention of diphtheria has four aspects:

Immunization

Universal immunization is the most effective means of preventing diphtheria. The standard course of immunization for healthy children is three doses of DTaP (diphtheria-tetanus-acellular pertussis) preparation given between two months and six months of age, with booster doses given at 18 months and again between the ages of four and six years. At 12 years a booster shot is given. Adults should be immunized at 10-year intervals with Td (tetanus-diphtheria) toxoid. A toxoid is a bacterial toxin that is treated to make it harmless but still can induce immunity to the disease.

Isolation of patients

Diphtheria patients must be isolated for one to seven days or until two successive cultures show that they are no longer contagious (up to six weeks). Children placed in isolation are usually assigned a primary nurse for emotional support.

Identification and treatment of contacts

Because diphtheria is highly contagious and has a short incubation period, family members and other contacts of diphtheria patients must be watched for symptoms and tested to see if they are carriers. They are usually given antibiotics for seven days and a booster shot of diphtheria/tetanus toxoid.

Reporting cases to public health authorities

Reporting is necessary to track potential epidemics, to help doctors identify the specific strain of diphtheria, and to see if resistance to penicillin or erythromycin has developed.

Resources

BOOKS

Guilfoile, Patrick. *Diphtheria.* New York: Chelsea House, 2009.

Sears, Robert. *The Vaccine Book: Making The Right Decision for Your Child.* New York: Little, Brown, 2007.

OTHER

Diphtheria. Mayo Clinic. http://www.mayoclinic.com/health/diphtheria/DS00495 (accessed August 16, 2012).

Diphtheria. World Health Organization. http://www.who.int/topics/diphtheria/en (accessed August 16, 2012).

Diphtheria. MedlinPlus. http://www.nlm.nih.gov/medlineplus/diphtheria.html (accessed August 16, 2012).

Vaccines. Centers for Disease Control and Prevention. http://www.cdc.gov/vaccines (accessed August 16, 2012).

ORGANIZATIONS

Centers for Disease Control and Prevention (CDC), 1600 Clifton Rd., Atlanta, GA USA 30333, (404) 639–3534, (800) CDC-INFO (232-4636), (888) 232-6348, inquiry@cdc.gov, http://www.cdc.gov

World Health Organization (WHO), Avenue Appia 20, 1211 Geneva 27, Switzerland, +22 41 791 21 11, Fax: +22 41 791 31, info@who.int, http://www.who.int.

Rebecca J. Frey, PhD
Tish Davidson, A.M.

Disaster preparedness *see* **Emergency preparedness**

Distracted driving

Definition

Distracted driving is a term used to describe the operation of a motor vehicle while the driver's attention is occupied by factors other than those necessary for driving. This term is often used to discuss traffic accidents that result from distracted driving and is most frequently used when referring to the use of a cell phone—to send or receive phone calls or text messages—while driving.

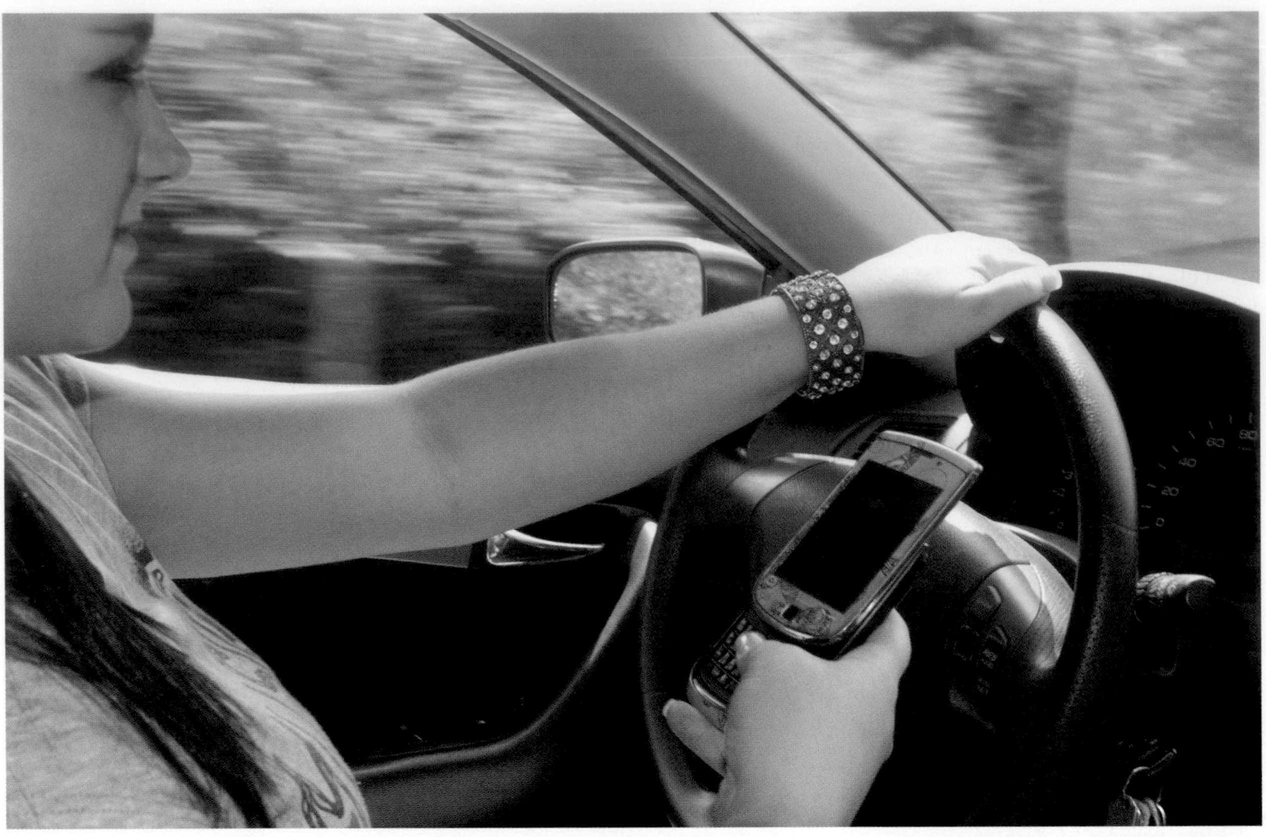

Teen girl texting while driving. *(CDC/Amanda Mills)*

Description

According to a survey by the National Highway Traffic Safety Administration (NHTSA), most participants were likely to use their phone or text, yet they also noted feeling unsafe in vehicles where the driver was texting. In many distracted driving surveys, participants report that they do not feel their own habits are dangerous, yet they agree to engaging in behaviors that they feel are dangerous in other drivers. The use of cell phones, though perhaps the most commonly discussed type of distracted driving is not the only example. There are three types of distracted driving:

- Visual—such as reading a book, newspaper, map, text message, or electronic billboard.
- Manual—such as eating or drinking, applying makeup, or smoking.
- Cognitive—such as talking on the phone or with other passengers.

Cell Phones and Driving

The cell phone was introduced in 1983 and cell phone usage has grown by 40% each year since. Studies suggest that driving performance and reaction time is impaired even with the use of a hands free cellular device and that distraction and limited driving performance with these devices is equal to that of drivers using handheld devices. Drivers operating any type of cell phone are more likely to experience inattention blindness—where they see objects and information in front of them but are delayed in processing and reacting to that information. This blindness applies equally to objects of small or great relevance to safe driving—such as a billboard or a pedestrian. Drivers operating a handheld or hands free cell phone could fail to recognize up to 50% of the information they would have recognized while not on the phone. Using a cell phone increases a driver's risk of collision four to six times over that of a driver not using a phone. Texting results in an estimated 35% reduction in reaction time while driving, and according to The Virginia Tech Transportation Institute (VTTI), drivers that text are 23 times more likely to be in an accident than drivers who do not text.

Not all distractions are equal, however. Studies show that it takes humans more brain power to create speech than it does to comprehend speech—so talking on a cell phone requires more brain power, and is therefore more likely to be a dangerous distraction than listening to a radio broadcast or audio book. Similarly, conversations that are taking place between the driver and other passengers are less likely to be a dangerous distraction because these conversations often follow the flow of traffic and other road conditions, and passengers may help the driver locate potential hazards in the road. Conversely, when the driver is speaking with someone via cell phone, that person is unaware of traffic conditions or potential hazards.

Teens and Distracted Driving

Motor vehicle accidents are the leading cause of death for people between 5 and 34 years of age, with the highest-risk group being teenagers and young adults aged 16 to 19. Though similar statistics around the world suggest that the dangers of young drivers are universal, fatality rates are higher in the United States than in Europe. Due to more efficient public transportation systems and more difficult driving tests, smaller percentages of teenagers obtain their drivers licenses in Europe, resulting in fewer automobile-related fatalities among those age groups. Additionally, in the United States, where the **population** is spread out over a bigger geographical area and a greater percentage of teenagers become licensed to drive, teenagers are more likely to be passengers in a vehicle with a novice teenage driver.

Multiple factors seem to contribute to the increase of car accidents among young drivers. One of these factors is that statistically, a teenage driver's risk of collision increases with each additional passenger in their vehicle. Additionally, young drivers are less likely to maintain appropriate focus on all necessary driving factors and are more likely to focus too long on any one object—either related or unrelated to operating their vehicle. Attention management while driving is a particular issue for young people with Attention Deficit Hyperactivity Disorder (ADHD) who experience much higher rates of driving distraction, accidents, and fatalities. Teens are also less experienced drivers and as such are generally less able to efficiently and safely drive while performing another visual task.

As a result of recent technological advances and the familiarity of most young people with these technologies, young drivers are more likely to operate various wireless devices while driving. According to the American Automobile Association (AAA), almost half of teens admit to texting while driving. Surveys also suggest that more than two-thirds of young drivers admit to talking on their cell phones while driving. These numbers imply that these behaviors are becoming a social norm, especially among young drivers.

Male occupants in a motor vehicle—particularly between the ages of 15 and 24—are two times more likely to die in a car accident than females. Male teenage drivers are more likely than female teenage drivers to engage in risky driving or make an illegal maneuver just before crashing. This likelihood increases for males when driving with passengers of either sex. Just prior to crashing, female teenage drivers are more likely to be engaged in at least one non-driving activity (not including passenger conversations). This likelihood increases for females when driving with male passengers. Female teenage drivers, however, rarely drive aggressively or make illegal maneuvers prior to a crash, regardless of whether or not they have passengers.

KEY TERMS

Graduated Drivers License (GDL)—A licensing program for young adults which requires them to complete a probationary period before obtaining a full license. This probationary period usually requires the novice driver to gain so many hours driving under the supervision of a licensed adult. The probationary period also limits the conditions under which a novice driver can drive, such as before a certain time of night, and without any additional passengers. GDLs have been shown to reduce the number of teenage driving accidents and fatalities.

Inattention Blindness—Commonly used when describing distracted driving, particularly while talking on a cell phone, this describes a driver's ability to see something but be delayed in recognizing or reacting to the information as a result of the cognitive distraction created by another activity.

Parent-Teen Driving Contracts—A contract drawn up and signed by a parent and prospective teenager driver, detailing the rules and responsibilities for the teenage driver. These contracts usually include what is considered safe driving behavior, prohibited or unsafe driving behaviors, and consequences for violating the contract. Such a contract helps the teenager feel more adult, while making the responsibilities of driving clear and carefully outlining what is expected of them. When using such a contract, it is important for parents to set the example by exhibiting the safe driving behaviors that they expect from their teenage driver.

Primary Enforcement—A law in which a police officer can pull over and ticket a driver for, without any other cause.

Risks

Studies show correlations in levels of impairment between driving while operating a cell phone and driving while under the influence of alcohol or marijuana. In support for its recommendation to ban the use of all cellular devices while driving, the National Transportation Safety Board (NTSB) cites a study originally performed by the University of Utah, showing that the degree of impairment experienced when using a cell phone is equal to the impairment of driving with a blood alcohol content (BAC) of .08, which is the national standard for driving under the influence.

Public Health

It is impossible to know the exact number of crashes, injuries, or fatalities attributed to distracted driving because not all drivers admit to these behaviors and many law enforcement teams do not record this type of information in accident reports. As a result, statics about the effects of distracted driving vary widely. The American Academy of Orthopedic Surgeons (AAOS) estimates that approximately 500,000 people are injured by distracted driving each year. The **Centers for Disease Control and Prevention (CDC)** suggest that total motor vehicle injuries (including those not attributed to distracted driving) could be as high as 3 million annually, with tens of thousands of annual fatalities in the United States alone. As of 2012, there are not concrete figures available to determine the public cost of distracted driving accidents, injuries, and fatalities. The CDC does estimate—citing a study by RB Naumann et al., which originally appeared in *Traffic Injury Prevention*—that in 2005, the lifetime costs of injuries and deaths as a result of motor vehicle accidents (not limited to distracted driving) was $70 billion. Some statistics put the percentage of accidents related to distracted driving as low as 11%, others as high as 90%, but wherever the actual number falls in that spectrum, the cost to the public in terms of injury, loss of life, and financial burden is great.

Solutions

Public Awareness

In June 2012, the U.S. Transportation Secretary announced the "Blueprint for Ending Distracted Driving." This initiative will:

- Help encourage the remaining 11 states without distracted driving laws to enact such legislation.
- Challenge the auto industry to develop new technologies and safety measures to combat distracted driving.
- Create new educational materials for drivers education professionals.

Provide actions for families, organizations, and lawmakers to create change nationwide.

Other organizations have established public educational programs and public service announcement to increase awareness about the dangers of distracted driving. An example of one such program is the "Decide to Drive" program created by the American Academy of Orthopedic Surgeons (AAOS) and the Orthopedic Trauma Association (OTA).

Legislation

In 2009, President Obama signed a mandate that banned federal employees from texting while driving. As of 2012, the federal government has banned the use of cell phones while driving for interstate truck and bus drivers. As of July 2012, ten states, the District of Columbia, Guam, and the Virgin Islands have prohibited all use of handheld cellular phones; 39 states, the District of Columbia, Guam, and the Virgin Islands have bans on text messaging for all drivers. The enforcement varies for these laws from state to state—some states have primary enforcement laws, which allow a police officer to pull a driver over for cell phone use even if the driver has committed no other traffic violation while other states require a traffic infraction in order for a driver to be cited for use of a cell phone. Some cities and other localities have made their own regulations, sometimes independent of existing or non-existing state legislation. According to the Governors Highway Safety Association (GHSA), some states including Florida, Louisiana, Nevada, Pennsylvania, and Oklahoma have laws in place which prevent individual localities within the state from creating their own distracted driving legislation.

Worker Safety

The Occupational Safety and Health Administration (OSHA) encourages employers to ban employees from texting while driving for work and to eliminate any company policies that may directly or indirectly encourage employees to text while driving for work. The OHSA also states that any employer with policies requiring an employee to text while driving is in violation of The Occupational Safety and Health Act of 1970, which requires employers to create a workplace free of known hazards. Workers who have questions or feel that their rights to a safe workplace are being jeopardized by company policies can contact the OSHA.

Prevention

Minimize Distractions

Though not all driving distractions can be avoided or controlled, drivers should take all precautions to minimize driving distractions. For example, before starting their engines, drivers can silence or turn off cell phones, preprogram GPS units, and properly secure children and pets within the vehicle. Drivers can also avoid eating and drinking on the road. For adults who drive with teenagers, it is especially important to set the example of safe driving and refrain from the use of a cell phone while driving.

Graduated Drivers Licenses

The use of Graduated Drivers License (GDL) programs in many states has led to reduced instances of teenage driving accidents. These programs provide more driving experience before the teenager is allowed to drive on their own, and minimize hazardous driving—often by limiting the hours in which a teenager can drive and the passengers that can be in the car. GDL programs also require the student to log driving hours under the supervision of a licensed adult.

Parent-Teen Driving Contracts

Parent-teen driving contracts are increasing in popularity and allow parents and young drivers to agree on acceptable driving behavior, rules, and consequences ahead of time. These consequences help teens to understand not only what is expected of them as a driver but the risks and responsibilities involved with driving, and help parents establish clear consequences for violating these expectations. It is important for parents and teens to be mutually involved in creating such a contract and parents must also be accountable for upholding the same driving standards that they expect to see in their teen drivers. In addition to establishing other safe driving patterns, parent-teen driving contracts can help parents open a dialogue about the dangers of distracted driving in particular.

Electronic Feedback Systems

Electronic Feedback Systems are another helpful tool in promoting safe driving habits and reducing distracted driving. These devices are often used by parents or insurance companies and help monitor driving performance by recording things like speed and hard braking. This data is used by some insurance companies to provide lower premiums to safe drivers and by parents to monitor their young drivers' driving habits.

Resources

BOOKS

"Adolescent Driving Behavior: A Developmental Challenge." *Encyclopedia of Adolescence.* Ed. B. Bradford Brown and Mitchell J. Prinstein. Vol. 1: Normative Processes in Development. London: Academic Press, 2011. 38-47. *Gale Virtual Reference Library.* Web. June 29, 2012.

Francescutti, Louis Hugo. "Cell Phone Use and Driving." *Encyclopedia of Lifestyle Medicine & Health.* Ed. James M. Rippe. Vol. 1. Thousand Oaks, CA: Sage Reference, 2012. 208-209. *Gale Virtual Reference Library.* Web. June 29, 2012.

"Parent-Teen Driving Contracts Deter Dangerous Driving Behaviors."*Teen Driving.* Ed. Linda Aksomitis. Detroit: Greenhaven Press, 2009. 64-72. Issues That Concern You. Web. June 29, 2012.

Roehler, Douglas R., David A. Sleet, and Ann M. Dellinger. "Preventing Traffic Injuries." *Encyclopedia of Lifestyle Medicine & Health.* Ed. James M. Rippe. Vol. 2. Thousand Oaks, CA: Sage Reference, 2012. 951-956. *Gale Virtual Reference Library.* Web. June 29, 2012.

Strayer, David L, and Joel M Cooper. "Cell Phones and Driver Distraction." *Encyclopedia of Perception.* E. Bruce Goldstein. Vol. 1. Thousand Oaks, CA: Sage Reference, 2010. 239-240. *Gale Virtual Reference Library.* Web. June 29, 2012.

Whitcomb, Dan. "Teens Ignore Laws to Curb Texting While Driving." *Risky Teen Behavior.* Ed. Heidi Watkins. Detroit: Greenhaven Press, 2012. 75-79. Issues That Concern You. *Gale Virtual Reference Library.* Web. June 29, 2012.

PERIODICALS

Currie, Donya. "Drivers unaware of risky behaviors." *The Nation's Health* July 2011: 7. *Health Reference Center Academic.* Web. June 29, 2012.

Curry, Allison E., et al. "Peer Passengers: How Do They Affect Teen Crashes?" *Journal of Adolescent Health* 50.6 (2012): 588+. *Health Reference Center Academic.* Web. June 29, 2012.

Issar, Neil M., et al. "Distracted driving: the emerging policy on cell phone use: lessons learned from drinking and driving are being applied." *AAOS Now* (2012): 24+. *Health Reference Center Academic.* Web. June 29, 2012.

Johnson, Teddi Dineley. "Distracted driving: stay focused when on the road." *The Nation's Health Feb.* 2012: 28. *Health Reference Center Academic.* Web. June 29, 2012.

Stanton, Terry. "Academy rolls out new public service messages: campaigns target overuse injuries, distracted driving, obesity, and lessons learned in wartime." *AAOS Now* (2012): 1+. *Health Reference Center Academic.* Web. June 29, 2012.

WEBSITES

Centers For Disease Control and Prevention "Distracted Driving" http://www.cdc.gov/Motorvehiclesafety/Distracted_Driving/ Accessed June 29, 2012.

Federal Communications Commission "Distracted Driving" http://www.fcc.gov/encyclopedia/distracted-driving Accessed June 29, 2012.

Federal Communications Commission "Distracted Driving Information Clearinghouse" http://www.fcc.gov/encyclopedia/distracted-driving-information-clearinghouse Accessed June 29, 2012.

Governors Highway Safety Administration "Cell Phone and Texting Laws" http://www.ghsa.org/html/stateinfo/laws/cellphone_laws.html Accessed June 29, 2012.

National Highway Traffic Safety Administration "Texting and Driving Prevention" http://www.stoptextsstopwrecks.org/#home Accessed June 29, 2012.

National Safety Council "Distracted Driving" http://www.nsc.org/safety_road/distracted_driving/pages/distracted_driving.aspx Accessed June 29, 2012.

Occupational Safety & Health Administration "Distracted Driving" http://www.osha.gov/distracted-driving/initiative.html Accessed June 29, 2012.

United States Government "Distraction.Gov" http://www.distraction.gov/ Accessed June 29, 2012.

ORGANIZATIONS

ONational Highway Traffic Safety Administration, 1200 New Jersey Avenue, SE, Washington, DC USA 20590, 1 (202) 366-9742, Fax: 1 (202) 366-6916, Lori.Millen@dot.gob, www.distraction.gov

Occupational Safety & Health Administration, 200 Constitution Avenue, Washington, DC USA 20210, 1 (800) 321-OSHA (6742), www.osha.gov

Andrea Nienstedt, MA

How domestic violence affects public health in the United States

- The cost of intimate partner violence exceeds $5.8 billion each year, $4.1 billion of which is for direct medical and mental health services.
- There are 16,800 homicides and $2.2 million (medically treated) injuries due to intimate partner violence annually, which costs $37 billion.
- In the United States, victims of intimate partner violence lose almost 8 million days of paid work a year because of the violence perpetrated against them.
- One in every four women will experience domestic violence in her lifetime.
- An estimated 1.3 million women are victims of physical assault by an intimate partner each year.
- 85% of domestic violence victims are women.
- Females who are 20–24 years of age are at the greatest risk of nonfatal intimate partner violence.
- Only approximately one-quarter of all physical assaults, one-fifth of all rapes, and one-half of all stalkings perpetuated against females by intimate partners are reported to the police.

SOURCE: National Coalition Against Domestic Violence (http://www.ncadv.org)

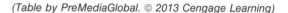

(Table by PreMediaGlobal. © 2013 Cengage Learning)

Domestic abuse

Definition

Domestic abuse is a form of coercion and assault against a family member or partner. It may include physical, psychological, sexual, verbal and economic tactics to gain control over the victim. Domestic abuse can further be classified as abuse of a spouse or domestic partner, child, or elder.

Description

In domestic abuse, the abuser seeks to dominate the other person, whether it is a spouse, child, or elderly family member. It is common for the abuser to regret the abuse, especially early on, and to promise not to do it in the future. Oftentimes, the abuser will blame a force such as **stress**, for causing the abuse. The three facets of domestic abuse are intimidation, humiliation, and physical injury.

The cycle of **violence** consists of these stages: abuse, guilt, excuses, normal behavior, fantasy and planning, and set-up. During the first phase, the abuser establishes control and power, but then feels guilty for being abusive. The abuser tries to rationalize the abuse by coming up with excuses for the behavior. Following this, there is a period during which the abuser takes action to keep the relationship intact; a sense of peace ensues. When this period has gone on for a time, the abuser thinks about how the partner has acted wrongly and deserves to be abused. In the final phase, the abuser orchestrates a scenario where the abuse can feel "justified" and the cycle starts over.

The American Academy of Experts in Traumatic Stress list the types of domestic abuse:

- Physical abuse—Inflicting physical harm via such violent acts as throwing, hitting, slapping, or using a weapon.
- Psychological abuse—Frightening the victim by making threats or using intimidation, destroying the partner's belongings, yelling, or acting violent by throwing an object in the sight of the victim.
- Sexual abuse—Forcing the partner to engage in sexual activity that may be undesired, not safe, or even degrading.
- Stalking (or cyberstalking)—Harassment or threats to the victim, either in person or on the Internet or via other forms of technology.
- Financial abuse—Not allowing the victim access to money, refusing to provide necessities such as food, clothing, or medicines, or not allowing the partner to gain financial independence through employment.
- Spiritual abuse—Manipulating the victim via religious or spiritual beliefs.

Demographics

Domestic abuse takes place throughout the world and is experienced by people of all socioeconomic levels, educational backgrounds, and religious beliefs. Domestic abuse occurs in heterosexual, as well as homosexual, relationships.

It is estimated that females represent 85–90% of domestic abuse victims. Women are especially vulnerable to abuse between the ages of 16 and 24. According to the National Library of Medicine, for women ages 15 to 44, domestic violence is the number one cause of injury.

There are 3.3 million reports of **child abuse** in the United States each year. These reports involve approximately 6 million children because one report may involve more than one child. Each day, five children die in the United States as a result of abuse.

Elder abuse, a form of domestic abuse, happens to approximately 2.1 million older people in the United States each year. Most of the time, elder abuse occurs at home, involving older persons who live alone or with a spouse, child, sibling, or other relative in a private home. Family members are usually the abusers.

Causes and symptoms

Causes

The root causes of domestic abuse are:

- Witnessing domestic abuse as a child
- Being victimized
- Experiencing violence in the school, community, or within a peer group
- Existing in a culture surrounded by violence in movies, video games, communities, and among cultures

Symptoms

Abusers may show certain characteristics early on in a relationship, prior to the abuse occurring or early in the process.

- Possessiveness—wants to monopolize the partner's time
- Jealousy—feels threatened if others pay attention to the partner
- Attempts to isolate—wants to keep partner shielded from others
- Very sensitive to comments—feelings hurt easily and perceives the partner is issuing insults
- Blames others—does not take responsibility for the abuse
- Pressures the partner—tells partner to do things "in the name of love"

A person who is being abused exhibits signs and symptoms that others can recognize, especially if the abuse is physical. If the abuse is psychological, it is often overlooked; however, there are also telltale signs of any abusive relationship.

- Fear—Fear of the partner who may humiliate, yell, or become physically abusive; seems overly anxious to please the partner
- Complacent—Agrees with the partners words and actions
- Overly communicative—Frequently must check-in with partner to report current location and activity
- Discuss partner's misgivings—Verbalizes partner's rage, jealousy, or possessiveness
- Visible injuries—Blames the injuries on accidents or wears long-sleeved clothing or dark glasses that seem inappropriate for the season (to hide injuries)
- Low self-esteem—Formerly confident individual seems to feel less self-worth
- Alterations in personality—Becomes withdrawn or less fun-loving
- Exhibits depression—May also seem anxious; may be suicidal

A person that is being abused should talk with a trusted friend, neighbor, relative, co-worker, or religious leader. Health professionals such as a physician, nurse, psychiatrist, or therapist can also provide support.

The National Domestic Hotline is available as well. Individuals in an abusive relationship may call the hotline at 1-800-799-SAFE (7233). If immediate danger is present, the victim should call 9-1-1.

Effects on Public Health

Domestic abuse can ultimately result in **behavioral health** issues such as anxiety, depression, panic attacks, posttraumatic stress disorder, or substance abuse. It can also lead to **suicide** attempts, episodes of psychosis, or homelessness.

Children who live in surroundings fraught with domestic abuse have the risk of developing behavioral health problems such as psychiatric disorders, academic difficulties, aggression, developmental issues, and low self-esteem.

Costs to society

According to the Child Welfare Information Gateway, an agency of the United States Department of Health and Human Resources, victims of domestic abuse lose about 8 million days of paid work a year, which is equal to 32,000 full-time jobs.

Partner rape, physical harm, and stalking cost more than $5.8 billion annually; approximately $4.1 billion covers direct medical and behavioral health services.

Children who are abused are at a 25% higher risk of becoming pregnant as teenagers. They are also less apt to

KEY TERM

Coercion—Use of force to threaten a person to do something against his or her will. In domestic abuse, the abuser uses coercion to gain control over the victim.

participate in safe sexual encounters, increasing their risk for **sexually transmitted diseases** (STDs).

Efforts and solutions

Before the 1970s, victims of rape or domestic abuse had no resources available to help them. Such matters were seen as private. A grass roots movement, often called the Battered Women's Movement, created programs in the community to help such victims.

Persons involved in the transformation to a society where help would be available to victims of domestic abuse are involved the goals of providing shelter for victims and their children, improving the criminal justice responses to these acts of violence and abuse, and heightening public awareness about domestic abuse.

The early grass roots efforts evolved into a wide range of resources for victims of domestic abuse. Among these resources are:

- Hotlines, which are available at the local, state, and national level
- Crisis counseling
- Shelters and safe houses, as well as services that provide housing and relocation
- Support groups
- Legal advocates
- Services for children
- Transportation
- Referrals to medical and behavioral health specialists

Resources

BOOKS

Neil Warner. *Signs of Emotional Abuse: Know about the War for Power and Control in Relationships.* Fort Lauderdale, FL: Creative Conflict Resolutions, Inc., 2012.

PERIODICALS

Payne, Darrell, and Linda Wermeling. "Domestic Violence and the Female Victim". *Journal of Multicultural, Gender and Minority Studies* 3, no. 1 (2009).

WEBSITES

Childhelp.org http://www.childhelp.org/pages/statistics (accessed September 29, 2012).

Child Welfare Information Gateway. U.S. Department of Health & Human Services. http://www.childwelfare.gov/pubs/usermanuals/domesticviolence/domesticviolencec.cfm (accessed September 29, 2012).

Domestic Violence. American Psychiatric Association. http://healthyminds.org/Main-Topic/Domestic-Violence.aspx (accessed September 28, 2012).

Domestic Violence and Abuse: Types, Signs, Symptoms, Causes, and Effects. http://www.aaets.org/article144.htm (accessed September 29, 2012).

Elder Abuse and Neglect: In Search of Solutions. http://www.apa.org/pi/aging/resources/guides/elder-abuse.aspx# (accessed September 29, 2012).

Helpguide.org. http://www.helpguide.org/mental/domestic_violence_abuse_types_signs_causes_effects.htm/Main-Topic/Domestic-Violence.aspx (accessed September 29, 2012).

U.S. National Library of Medicine. National Institutes of Health. http://vsearch.nlm.nih.gov/vivisimo/cgi-bin/query-meta?query=domestic+violence&v%3Aproject=nlm-main-website (accessed September 29, 2012).

ORGANIZATIONS

National Child Abuse Hotline, (800) 4-A-CHILD (422-4453), http://answers.usa.gov

National Council on Child Abuse & Family Violence, 1025 Connecticut Avenue NW, Suite 1000., Washington, DC 20036, www.nccafv.org

National Domestic Violence Hotline, (800) 799-SAFE (7233), http://answers.usa.gov.

Rhonda Cloos, RN

Domestic violence *see* **Domestic abuse**

Dracunculiasis infection

Definition

Dracunculiasis infection, also called guinea worm disease, occurs when the parasitic guinea worm *Dracunculus medinensis* resides within the body. Infection is not apparent until a pregnant female worm prepares to expel embryos. The infection is rarely fatal, but the latter stage is painful. The infection is also referred to as dracunculiasis, and less commonly as dracontiasis.

Description

To survive, guinea worms require three things: water during the embryo stage, an intermediate host during early maturation, and a human host during adulthood. In bodies of water, such as ponds, tiny, lobster-like water fleas in the genus *Cyclops* eat guinea worm embryos. Once ingested, the embryos mature into larvae.

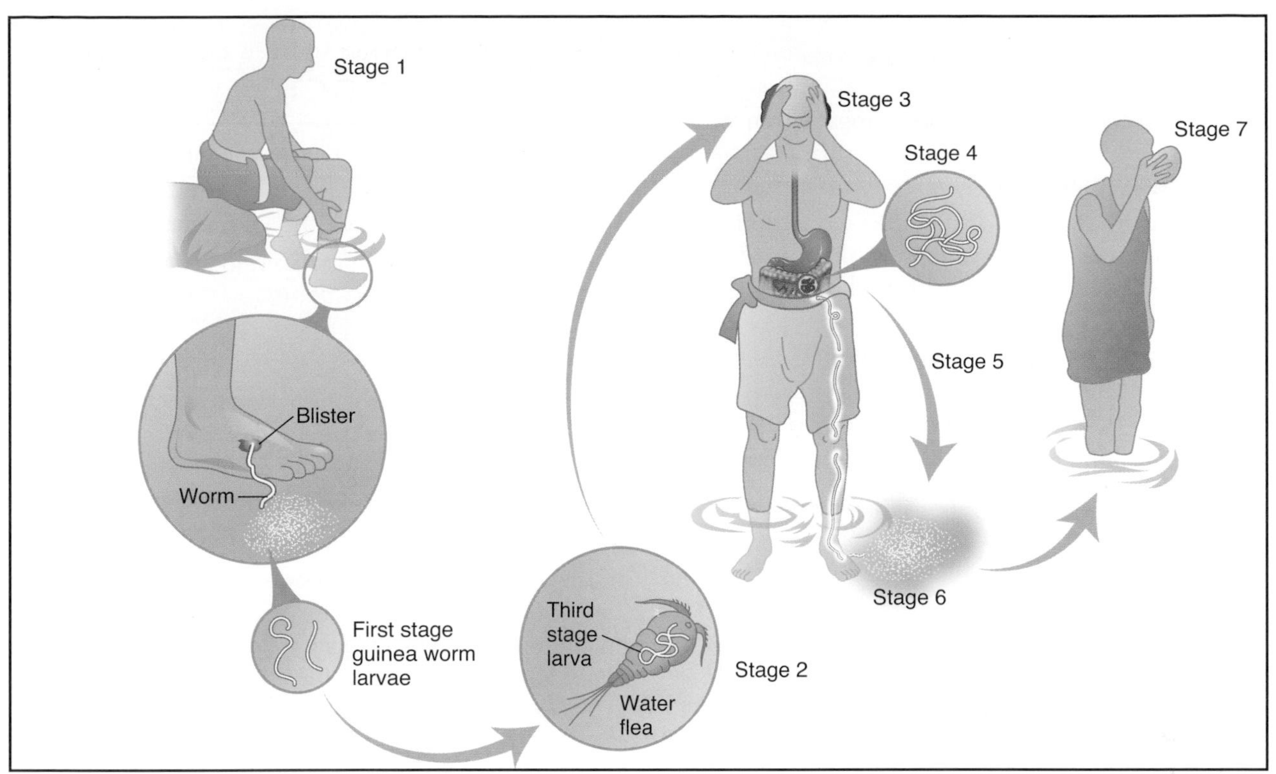

Stages of Dracunculiasis infection (Guinea Worm Disease). *(Illustration by Electronic Illustrators Group. © 2013 Cengage Learning)*

Humans become hosts by consuming water containing infected water fleas. Digestive juices in the stomach dissolve the fleas, which releases the guinea worm larvae. As they move into the intestine, the larvae burrow through the intestinal wall and into surrounding tissue. After three to four months, the worms mate. Males die soon after, but pregnant females continue to grow. As adults, each threadlike worm can be three feet long and harbor three million embryos. More than one guinea worm can infect a person at the same time.

About eight months later, the female prepares to expel mature embryos by migrating toward the skin surface. Until this point, most people are unaware that they are infected. Extreme **pain** occurs as the worm emerges from under the skin, often around the infected person's ankle. The pain is temporarily relieved by immersing the area in water, an act that contaminates the water and starts the cycle again.

Origins

Before the early 1980s, guinea worms infected as many as 10–15 million people annually in 20 countries of central Africa and parts of Asia. Following eradication efforts, the number of cases has declined dramatically. In 2011, the World Health Organization reported only 1,058 cases. The number of affected countries dropped, too, to just four: Chad, Ethiopia, Mali and South Sudan. Most of the 2011 cases were in South Sudan, which reported 1,028 cases. Ethiopia reported eight, Chad reported 10 and Mali reported 12 cases in 2011.

Causes and symptoms

CAUSES. *Dracunculus medinensis*, or guinea worm, causes infection.

SYMPTOMS. Symptoms are commonly absent until a pregnant worm prepares to expel embryos. At that time, it releases chemicals that create a blister on the skin, typically on the lower leg or foot, and then emerges through the skin at that point. Since more than one worm may infect the patient, several may emerge at approximately the same time. The emergence is accompanied by:

- blistering and ulceration of the skin
- burning, stabbing pain
- painful edema (swelling)
- intense itching
- Nausea.
- Vomiting.
- Dizziness.
- Diarrhea.

KEY TERMS

Guinea worm embryo—The guinea worm at its earliest life stage prior to or shortly after being expelled from an adult female worm.

Guinea worm larvae—The guinea worm during its middle life stage as it matures within a water flea. The larvae can only grow to adulthood within a human host.

Host—With regard to guinea worm infection, either the water flea or human from which the worm gets nourishment and shelter as it matures.

Secondary infection—An illness—typically caused by bacteria—that follows from a guinea worm infection.

The ulcers that result from the worm's emergence often develop bacterial infections. These infections can results in lingering inflammation and pain that may continue for several weeks, even months. If the worm ruptures inside the body, allergic reactions may also occur.

Diagnosis

Guinea worm infection is typically readily diagnosed by the presence of the characteristic blister that forms on the skin when the female worm is preparing to expel her embryos, or by the emergence of the worm itself.

Treatment

Most people infected with guinea worm rely on traditional medicine. Soaking the affected area in cool water encourages the worm to emerge through the skin. The worm is extracted by gently and gradually pulling the worm out, sometimes winding it around a small strip of wood. This removal process typically takes a least a week, and often several weeks. Surgical removal is possible, but rarely done in rural areas. Traditional treatment may include the application of herbs and oils, which may ease extraction and may help prevent secondary infections. Antibiotics can also reduce the risk of secondary infections.

Prognosis

Once the worm is completely removed, the wound heals in approximately two to four weeks. However, if a worm emerges from a sensitive area, such as the sole of a foot, or if several worms are involved, healing requires more time. Secondary infections may occur. Recovery is also complicated if the worm breaks during extraction. This can result in serious secondary infections and allergic reactions. Having one guinea worm infection does not confer immunity against future infections.

QUESTIONS TO ASK YOUR DOCTOR

- How do I take the pain medication?
- How long should I take the antibacterial medication following the worm removal?
- How should I store the pain medication and the antibacterial medication?

Prevention

Prevention of guinea worm infection is accomplished by disrupting transmission. Wells and other protected water sources are usually not contaminated with worm embryos. In open water sources, poisons may be used to kill water fleas. Otherwise, water must be boiled or filtered.

Effects on Public Health

Dracunculiasis has been an issue in developing countries, especially in tropical Africa. The intermediate host, the water flea, lives in stagnant water sources there—the same water sources with which residents have contact. As a result, it is a public-health issue because can spread to many thousands of people quickly.

Costs to Society

The sheer number of cases back in the 1980s, combined with the days or weeks of productivity lost due to the worm emergence or secondary infection, indicate that dracunculiasis was a drain of many millions of dollars from local economies. In addition, the infections are seasonal and usually occur during the height of agricultural season, when the demand for labor is great. A 1988 UNICEF study put the estimated annual loss in the rice-growing areas of three states in southern Nigeria at $20 million. Nigeria at the time was experiencing hundreds of thousands of cases. That has since changed. Nigeria went from more than 600,000 reported cases in 1988 to zero in 2009.

Efforts and Solutions

The World Health Organization, the U.S. Centers for Disease Control and Prevention, The Carter Center and UNICEF have been working together to eradicate dracunculiasis since the 1980s, and in 2011, WHO's World Health Assembly redoubled the efforts by calling on nations to establish surveillance programs to take various actions including: monitoring for cases of the infection; implementing containment measures in villages where the infection is found; ensuring safe drinking water; and educating its citizens about preventing dracunculiasis.

Since this eradication program has been in place, the number of cases of dracunculiasis has dropped precipitously: from millions a year to fewer than 1,100. As of 2011, only four remaining countries still experience cases of the infection.

Resources

PERIODICALS

Miri, Emmanuel S., et al. “Nigeria’s Triumph: Dracunculiasis Eradicated.” *American Journal of Tropical Medicine and Hygiene* 83, No. 2(2010): 215–225.

WEBSITES

“About Guinea Worm Disease. World Health Organization.” http://www.who.int/dracunculiasis/disease/en/. (accessed September 12, 2012).

“Dracunculiasis.” Centers for Disease Control and Prevention, Center for Global Health. http://www.dpd.cdc.gov/dpdx/HTML/Dracunculiasis. (accessed September 11, 2012).

“Dracunculiasis Epidemiology.” World Health Organization. http://www.who.int/dracunculiasis/epidemiology/en/. (accessed September 12, 2012).

“Guinea Worm Disease Frequently Asked Questions (FAQs).” Centers for Disease Control and Prevention (CDC). http://www.cdc.gov/parasites/guineaworm/gen_info/faqs.html. (accessed September 11, 2012).

“Guinea Worm Disease Eradication.” The Carter Center. http://www.cartercenter.org/health/guinea_worm/mini_site/index.html. (accessed September 11, 2012).

“Progress Toward Global Eradication of Dracunculiasis, January 2010–June 2011.” Centers for Disease Control and Prevention (CDC). http://www.cdc.gov/mmwr/preview/mmwrhtml/mm6042a2.htm?s_cid=mm6042a2_e&source=govdelivery. (accessed September 11, 2012).

“What Is Dracunculiasis?” BIO Ventures for Global Health. http://www.bvgh.org/Biopharmaceutical-Solutions/Global-Health-Primer/Diseases/cid/ViewDetails/ItemID/27.aspx. (accessed September 12, 2012).

ORGANIZATIONS

Centers for Disease Control and Prevention (CDC), 1600 Clifton Road, Atlanta, GA 30333, (800) 232-4636, cdcinfo@cdc.gov, http://www.cdc.gov.

The Carter Center, One Copenhill, 453 Freedom Parkway, Atlanta, GA 30307, (404) 420-5100, (800) 550-3560, carterweb@emory.edu, http://www.cartercenter.org/.

World Health Organization, Avenue Appia 20, 1211 Geneva 27, Switzerlandhttp://www.who.int/.

Julia Barrett
Leslie Mertz, Ph.D.

Drinking water

Definition

Drinking **water** comes from two sources, groundwater and surface water. Groundwater is brought up from under the earth by well pumps. Surface water is taken from sources open to the air such as lakes and streams. Many variables affect the quality of drinking water. Generally, surface water requires more treatment than groundwater. Water in public water systems can come from surface water, groundwater, or a combination of both. Groundwater is the source of water in wells and most private water systems. Bottled water can come from either source.

Description

Access to safe, clean drinking water is a major public health concern worldwide. The **World Health Organization (WHO)** estimated that in 2010, 780 million people lacked access to safe drinking water. Although the problem is most acute in the developing world, 120 million, or 15.4%, of these individuals lived in Europe. Good water quality is directly linked to the availability of effective **sanitation** systems. People who are least likely to have access to safe drinking water are those who live in rural areas, who live in **poverty**, and who live in a developing country.

Origins

Early civilizations including those of India, Egypt, and Greece experimented with ways to clarify water. Their main concern was to improve the look and taste of the water, as they did not yet understand that microscopic organisms in the water could cause disease. Early methods of water clarification included sand filtration, straining, and coagulation. As early as 1500 B.C. Egyptians added the chemical alum to water to improve its look and taste. These treatments improved water clarity and taste but did little to make drinking water safer.

By the 1700s, people were experimenting with other types of filters including those made of wool and charcoal. Nevertheless, slow sand filtration was the most common form of early water treatment. The first city water treatment plant was built in 1804 in Scotland, initiating the idea that all people should have access to clean, safe drinking water. More than 200 years later, that goal still has not been reached.

A massive **cholera** outbreak occurred in London in late August 1854. Within three days 127 people died. The death rate of those who became ill was about 12%. Before the outbreak was over, more than 600 people died. John Snow, a physician, mapped the locations where cholera cases occurred. From this map, he deduced that cholera was

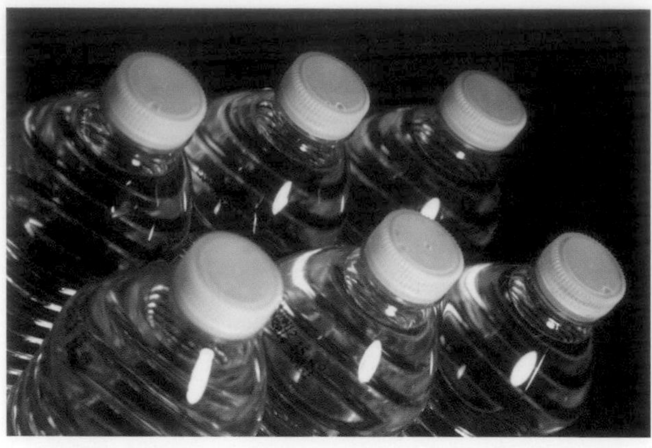

Six plastic bottles filled with spring drinking water. *(CDC/ Debora Cartagena)*

caused by contaminated water. He convinced the municipal authorities to disable a public pump in the Soho area of London where the number of cholera cases was highest. Almost immediately, the cholera outbreak subsided in that area. Snow's map showed that most cholera cases clustered around city water pumps, while very few cases of cholera occurred in buildings with private wells. From this, Snow as able to show that cholera was caused by contamination of the water. Snow's discovery was a major event in public health and helped shift the focus of water treatment from taste and clarity to controlling waterborne pathogens.

Through the 1970s, drinking water treatment focused on removing disease-causing organisms from the water supply. Many cities used sand filtration, supplemented beginning in the early 1900s by the addition of disinfectant agents such as chlorine and ozone. Jersey City, New Jersey, was the first American city to routinely add disinfectant to its municipal water supply.

In 1914, for the first time, the **United States Public Health Service** set national drinking water standards for the amount of bacteria permitted in water. These standards only applied to water that crossed state lines (such as water on trains and ships) and applied only to organisms that caused disease. The standards were not adopted by all communities until the 1940s. By 1962, federal standards regulated 28 substances in drinking water.

By the 1970s, concern increased about non-biological contaminants in water. Fertilizer and pesticide use had exploded, and runoff allowed these chemicals to enter lakes and streams and eventually the drinking-water supply. Other non-biological contaminants came from dumping chemicals used in manufacturing, materials used in construction such as lead pipes, and chemicals that leached out of containers such as cans and bottles.

The Safe Drinking Water Act, passed in 1974, required the United States **Environmental Protection Agency (EPA)** to develop guidelines for the treatment and monitoring of public water systems. In 1986, amendments to the act accelerated the regulation of contaminants, banned the future use of lead pipe, and required surface water from most sources to be filtered and disinfected. The amendments also provided for greater groundwater protection. Despite the improvement these regulations represent, the Act only covers public and private systems that serve a minimum of twenty-five people at least sixty days a year. As of 2010, there were more than 160,000 such water systems in the United States. Millions obtain their drinking water from privately owned wells that are not covered under the Act. The Act also does not apply to bottled water.

In the United States, the bottled water industry is not regulated by the **EPA** under the Safe Drinking Water Act or any other environmental law. Instead, the Food and Drug Administration (FDA) regulates bottled water under the Federal Food, Drug, and Cosmetic Act. Despite the image portrayed by advertising, studies indicate that bottled water is not any safer, in most cases, than tap water. Home water treatment units sometimes carry labels that claim they are EPA-approved, but these systems are not regulated either.

Effects on public health

The United States, Canada, and Western Europe have some of the safest drinking water supplies in the world. People in these areas can turn on the tap and feel confident that the water that comes out is safe to drink without additional treatment. Exceptions occur when **natural disasters** such as hurricanes, floods, or earthquakes cause the water supply to become contaminated with sewage. However, developed countries have well-established disaster relief response protocols to protect public health. These include warnings to temporarily not drink the water without boiling it first, providing disinfectant tablets for home use, and trucking in clean water for residents in areas where drinking water safety may be compromised.

In many parts of the world, however, the drinking water supply cannot be assumed safe. It may be contaminated with infectious agents (e.g., bacteria, viruses, **parasites**), toxic chemicals (e.g., pesticides, industrial chemicals), or radiological hazards. (e.g., naturally occurring radon or radioactive waste from nuclear power plants). According to **WHO**, two million people die each year from diarrhea caused by unsafe water. Most of these are children under age five. Many more, especially children, are permanently damaged by the presence of toxic chemicals or parasites in the water.

There is a direct relationship between adequate sanitation facilities and safe water. WHO estimates that at least 2.5 billion people in the developing world (more than one-third of the world's **population**) have no access to adequate sanitation. In many places, toilets are scarce and sewage and water treatment facilities are nonexistent. In 2012, UNICEF estimated that only 63% of the world's population had access to any type of improved sanitation. WHO estimates that improved water safety, sanitation, and **hygiene** have the potential to prevent 6.3% of all deaths worldwide.

Costs to society

The costs to society of contaminated drinking water are enormous. In addition to deaths caused by waterborne diseases, many children fail to reach their full mental and physical potential because of exposure to waterborne parasites and toxic chemicals during a time when their brains and bodies are developing rapidly. For example, 1.2 billion people in 57 countries suffer from **trachoma**, an infectious eye disease that causes blindness. Trachoma can be acquired by washing the face in contaminated water. In addition, areas without safe water, adequate sanitation, and other infrastructure are unlikely to attract development that will help pull the population out of poverty.

Efforts and solutions

WHO and UNICEF are the leaders in finding global solutions to the public health problems caused by unsafe drinking water. Both organizations celebrate World Water Day on March 22 each year. WHO sets global **millennium development goals** for improving water, sanitation, and hygiene. The organization works regionally on several levels. For example, WHO works in communities with unsafe water to promote water quality improvement in individual households. They educate people about the need for safe water and provide households with information about ways to improve water quality in their homes. The five most effective methods of water treatment that can be performed at the household level are **chlorination**, flocculent/disinfectant powder, solar disinfection, ceramic filtration, and slow sand filtration.

Another practice to improve water quality at the household level is safe water storage. Households are educated to store water in plastic, metal, or ceramic containers that provide barriers to recontamination. These containers are most effective when they have the following characteristics:

- are covered by a lid
- have a small opening that prevents people from putting their hands, cups, or other objects in the storage container
- have a spigot so that water can be removed without opening the container
- are cleaned regularly

UNICEF also works to achieve millennium development goals as it develops programs to help communities build sanitation and water systems. Between 1990 and 2012, UNICEF programs have given 2 billion people access to improved drinking water sources and 1.8 billion people access to improved sanitation. Water and sanitation improvement requires money. TAP is a program UNICEF developed to help fund its safe drinking-water programs. The TAP program encourages participating restaurants to ask their patrons to donate $1 for the tap water that they normally are served free of charge. Between 2007 and 2011, the TAP program raised $3 million.

Even though the drinking-water supply in the United States is clean and safe, the United States **Centers for Disease Control and Prevention (CDC)** works with WHO in the worldwide tracking of outbreaks of waterborne disease. It is, as of 2012, developing a National Well Data Repository, working with the National Park Service to assure the safety of water in parks and campgrounds, and providing on its website health information, including drinking-water safety, for travelers to other countries.

KEY TERMS

Cholera—An infection of the small intestine caused by a type of bacterium. The disease is spread by drinking water or eating seafood or other foods that have been contaminated with the feces of infected people. It occurs in parts of Asia, Africa, Latin America, India, and the Middle East. Symptoms include watery diarrhea and exhaustion and are often fatal to young children and the elderly.

Coagulation—In water treatment, this refers to adding a chemical to the water to cause particles in the water to clump so that they can be strained out.

Parasite—An organism that lives in or with another organism, called the host, in parasitism, a type of association characterized by the parasite obtaining benefits from the host, such as food, and the host being injured as a result.

Pathogen—Any disease-causing microorganism.

Resources

BOOKS

Salzman, James *Drinking Water: A History*. New York: Overlook Press, 2012

Spellman, Frank R. and Joanne E. Drinan. *The Drinking Water Handbook*. Boca Raton, FL: CRC Press, 2012.

WEBSITES

Centers for Disease Control and Prevention (CDC). "Drinking Water Quality." http://www.cdc.gov/healthywater/drinking (accessed September 13, 2012).

MedlinePlus. "Drinking Water." http://www.nlm.nih.gov/medlineplus/drinkingwater.html (accessed September 13, 2012).

United States Environmental Protection Agency (EPA). "Ground Water and Drinking Water." http://water.epa.gov/drink (accessed September 13. 2012).

World Health Organization. "Drinking Water." http://www.who.int/topics/drinking_water/en (accessed September 13, 2012).

ORGANIZATIONS

National Institute of Environmental Health Science, P.O. Box 12233, MD K3-16, Research Triangle Park, NC 27709, (919) 541-1919, Fax: (919) 541-4395, http://www.niehs.nih.gov.

United States Centers for Disease Control and Prevention (CDC), 1600 Clifton Road, Atlanta, GA 30333, (404) 639-3534, (800) CDC-INFO (800-232-4636); TTY: (888) 232-6348, inquiry@cdc.gov, http://www.cdc.gov.

United States Environmental Protection Agency, 1200 Pennsylvania Avenue, NW, Washington, DC 20460, (202) 272-0167; (202) 272-0165, http://water.epa.gov.

UNICEF Headquarters, 2 United Nations Plaza, New York, NY USA 10017, 1 (212) 326-7000, Fax: 1 (212) 887-7465, http://www.unicef.org.

World Health Organization, Avenue Appia 20, 1211 Geneva 27, Switzerland, +22 41 791 21 11, Fax: +22 41 791 31 11, info@who.int, http://www.who.int.

Tish Davidson, AM

Drug abuse *see* **Substance abuse and dependence**

Drug resistance

Definition

Drug resistance, also known as **antimicrobial resistance**, is the adaptation of a microbe to grow in the presence of chemicals that would normally kill it or limit its growth.

Description

Antimicrobial agents (**antibiotics**) and similar drugs are chemicals used in order to treat patients who have an **infectious disease**. Antimicrobial agents are developed to kill bacteria, **parasites**, and fungi in order to stop the growth and multiplication of the microbes making a person sick. Drug resistance occurs when an antimicrobial agent no longer has the desired effect, and the bacteria or other microbe continues to reproduce and cause continued illness.

Drug resistance occurs for several reasons. First, the resistance might be naturally occurring. Scientists tested a 2,000 year old bacterium found in a glacier and discovered that it was resistant against some types of antimicrobial agents, signifying that some resistance is naturally occurring. Natural resistance in microbes also develops because of selective pressure. Those strains that are resistant to particular antimicrobial agents are the same strains that go on to replicate, making those strains with drug resistant traits dominant.

Microbes may also become drug resistant due to mutations that take place. Microbes replicate every few hours, giving them the ability to adapt to their environment. During replication, a mutation may occur that gives resistance to certain drugs. The microbes with this mutation will then be more likely to continue to replicate, even after drug treatment has began. The result is a new drug resistant strain of bacteria.

A gene transfer can also cause a microbe to become drug resistant. In certain situations, microbes can get genes from each other, including genes that make them drug resistant and allow them to reproduce successfully even after drug treatment begins.

Microbes may become drug resistant because of human influences such as the inappropriate use of antimicrobial agents. An inadequate or incorrect diagnosis leading to the prescription of unneeded antimicrobials, can speed up the process of selective pressure and cause those microbes that have drug resistance qualities to become dominant. Some scientists believe that adding antibiotics to agricultural feed and the widespread overuse of antibiotic soaps and cleaners contributes to the increasing number of drug-resistant microbes. Because the scientific community has not reached consensus on this topic, research continues to better understand the effect antibiotics in feed and in household products can have on public health.

Together, all of these factors, in addition to the frequency and speed with which people travel around the world bringing with them foreign microbes, all lead to the increasing number of microbes being resistant to antimicrobial agents, both already in use and sometimes even before they have been released on the market.

Origins

Although since ancient times people had understood that something invisible to the eye could make them sick, ancient cultures were only able to try and reduce the likelihood of becoming ill, and had limited options to treat those who were infected. The ancient Egyptians, Chinese, and Indians of South American all used molds to treat infected wounds and skin rashes, but did not understand the reasoning behind this treatment that was often successful. The first real search to create antibiotics did not begin until the acceptance of the **germ theory** of disease.

Louis Pasteur, a researcher whose work supported the germ theory of disease, which states that diseases are caused by microbes, believed that microbes outside the body could get inside and make people sick. Before the germ theory of disease, people believed that life forms could come out of nowhere and begin to multiply on non-living matter. Through research and experimentation, Pasteur found that non-living matter placed in a sealed container could be kept indefinitely without growing anything. Only when the seal was broken would life forms begin to grow. It was this work, along with Robert Koch's discovery of **anthrax**, which led to both the field of immunology and the search for antibiotics.

The wide acceptance of the germ theory led scientists in the late 1800s to search for drugs that would kill disease-causing microbes. The first successful development of an antibiotic took place in the 1890s by two German physicians, Rudolf Emmerich and Oscar Low. Through their research, Emmerich and Low discovered that the microbes that caused one type of disease could be used as a cure for a different type of disease. By mixing the bacteria from infected wounds with other bacteria, they developed their own antibiotic known as pyocyanase. This new discovery was able to kill the bacteria strains causing diseases such as typhoid, **cholera**, and anthrax. Unfortunately, the resulting antibiotic did not always work as expected, sometimes hurting patients more than helping. For this reason, the work done by Emmerich and Low was later abandoned and research continued for a more reliable and better working antibiotic.

The first major breakthrough in the development of antibiotics came from the scientist Alexander Fleming. In 1928, while doing experiments in a hospital in London on **influenza**, Fleming noticed that a growth in his Petri dish had created a bacteria-free ring around it. Fleming named this **mold** he discovered penicillin. Although Fleming was the man who discovered penicillin, he did not develop it any further. Two men, Howard Florey and Ernst Chain, continued the development of penicillin, which enabled it to be developed into a drug to treat people. By the 1940s, the American drug industry was mass producing penicillin.

The development of antibiotics and other drugs that fought disease expanded rapidly after the discovery of penicillin. Gerhard J. P. Domagk worked for the company Bayer when he discovered Prontosil, a sulfonamide and the first synthetic drug effective against bacterial infections. Domagk won a Nobel prize in 1939 for his development of sulfonamides, or the class of synthetic drugs that fight some types of bacteria.

Since the 1940s, the number of antimicrobial agents on the market has continued to grow. Today, the knowledge about disease-causing microbes and the technology to fight them is greater than ever before.

KEY TERMS

Antimicrobial agents—A general term for drugs that kill or inhibit the growth of microbes.

Microbe—Any type of living organism made up of no cells, a single cell, or a cluster of cells. Bacteria, viruses, algae, eukaryotes, protozoa, and fungi are all common microbes.

Pathogen—Any disease-causing microbe.

Sulfonamides—A class of synthetic drugs used to prevent certain types of bacteria from reproducing.

However, with the increased use of antimicrobial agents comes increased resistance. The first case of antimicrobial resistance was discovered in 1947, only a few years after penicillin became mass produced. Some microbes that formerly had been killed using antibiotics now continue to reproduce and cause illness. As of 2011, about 70% of disease-causing bacteria found in hospitals is resistant to at least one of the common antibiotic agents used to treat it. This percentage reflects a large increase from even ten years earlier. Scientists and physicians track drug resistant microbes and are continuously developing new antibiotic agents in order to stay ahead of resistant strains. Antibiotic resistance is considered to be one of the world's most pressing health problems.

Effects on public health

Before the development of antimicrobial agents, infection due to microbes was a leading cause of death. Microbes such as bacteria, fungi, and parasites are still major killers in third world countries where the resources are limited. In the developed modern world, antimicrobial agents save millions of lives each year. The increased number of microbes resistant to the antibiotics on the market threaten the success of treatment and can lead to more time and money spent at the doctors, longer time spent on sick leave, or even death. Additionally, a major concern of physicians and scientists is the possibility of a drug-resistant strain spreading across cities, countries, and continents causing an epidemic.

Drug-resistant strains of diseases limit the number of options available to treat the sick. This forces researchers to continue developing new and often stronger antimicrobial agents, possibly with harmful side effects to those who are treated with them. Antimicrobial agents are currently the only way to treat bacterial infections successfully, making public health dependent on having a supply of successful antibiotics that can kill various types of bacteria. Some of the leading resistant pathogens in the community include

Mycobacterium tuberculosis, the cause of **tuberculosis**, *Escherichica coli* (commonly known as *E. coli*), and *Streptococcus pneumoniae*. These are only a few of the pathogens that threaten public health due to their resistance to drug treatments. Many bacteria found in hospitals, also threaten public health due to their resistance.

Researchers are specifically worried about the effect drug resistant pathogens have on children. Children have the highest rate of antibiotic use, meaning that if infections become drug resistant they will likely be sick longer, need more doctor visits, and in some cases, the illness may lead to death. Although drug resistance has been in existence since shortly after the mass production of antimicrobial agents, the problem has continued to grow. New drugs on the market are sometimes met with resistance before or as soon as they are released, making it important for physicians and researchers to be careful with how antimicrobial agent are used, including how long.

Costs to society

Drug resistance costs societies billions of dollars each year. Someone who is sick and first treated with an antibiotic that the strain of bacterium is resistant to, must follow up with additional visits to the doctor and additional, and often more expensive, prescriptions. Those who stay sick may find themselves with long hospital stays, taking time away from work, as well as increasing the cost to health insurance companies. Additionally, billions of dollars are spent on researching drug resistant microbes and doing research and development on variations of antimicrobial agents already on the market in order to find drugs that are more effective. Although there is no worldwide figure on the monetary cost drug resistance causes societies, in 2006, it was estimated that United States lost anywhere between $378 million to $18.6 billion because of the loss of effectiveness of outpatient antibiotic prescriptions. Another study from 2008, found that drug resistant infections in 188 people cost one healthcare institution between $13.35 and $18.75 million alone. This study only looked at a few patients out of the thousands affected by drug resistant infections each year.

Efforts and solutions

The threat drug resistance has on public health is understood by scientists, governments, and organizations. Especially since the early 2000s, much time, effort, and money has gone toward combating drug resistance. The U.S. Food and Drug Administration (FDA) is working against drug resistance by taking many steps, including increasing labeling regulations on drug prescriptions. This is being done in order to increase awareness about proper use of antimicrobial agents and encourage healthcare professionals to discuss proper drug use with their patients.

QUESTIONS TO ASK YOUR DOCTOR

- How can I know that the strain of infection I have is drug resistant?
- Is a drug-resistant disease more severe than a disease not drug resistant?
- What can I do to reduce the likelihood of more microbes becoming drug resistant?

Additionally, the FDA has partnered with the Center for Disease Control (**CDC**) to spread the message about proper antibiotic use in a campaign called, Germ Smart: Know When Antibiotics Work. The FDA and CDC hope to spread the message about how the public can play a role in preventing drug resistance through taking steps such as not skipping doses and taking the full course of drug prescriptions. The FDA also supports research and development of new antibiotics through guidance in developing clinical trials to evaluate new drugs. Additionally, the **World Health Organization (WHO)** is one of the main organizations supporting the surveillance and tracking of drug resistance around the world.

One of the main focuses on fighting drug resistance is the education of physicians and the public on the proper use of antibiotics. The CDC believes that there could be a 30% reduction in the number of prescriptions written for antibiotics in the United States without any negative effect on public health. This is mainly due to the misdiagnosis of virus-caused sicknesses, which cannot be treated using antibiotics, and the prescribing of medicine when not truly needed, which is prevalent in the United States.

Resources

BOOKS

Fong, I. W. and Karl Drlica*Antimicrobial Resistance and Implications for the 21st Century (Emerging Infectious Diseases of the 21st Century).*New York: Springer, 2008.

World Health Organization*The Evolving Threat of Antimicrobial Resistance: Options for Action.*Geneva: WHO, 2012.

PERIODICALS

Saga, Tomoo, Keizo Yamaguchi. "History of Antimicrobial Agents and Resistant Bacteria." *Japan Medical Association Journal*(2009) 52(2). http://112.140.39.164/english/journal/pdf/2009_02/103_108.pdf (accessed September 19, 2012).

WEBSITES

National Institute of Allergy and Infectious Diseases. "Antimicrobial (Drug) Resistance." http://www.niaid.nih.gov/topics/antimicrobialresistance/Pages/default.aspx (accessed September 19, 2012).

U.S. Food and Drug Administration. "Batter the Bug: Fighting Antibiotic Resistance." http://www.fda.gov/drugs/resourcesforyou/consumers/ucm143568.htm (accessed September 19, 2012).

World Health Organization. "Antimicrobial Resistance." http://www.who.int/drugresistance/en (accessed September 19, 2012).

ORGANIZATIONS

National Institute of Allergy and Infectious Diseases, 6610 Rockledge Drive, MSC 6612, Bethesda, MD 20892, (301) 496 5717, (866) 284 4107, Fax: (301) 402 3573, ocpostoffice@niaid.nih.gov, http://www.niaid.nih.gov.

United States Centers for Disease Control and Prevention (CDC), 1600 Clifton Road, Atlanta, GA 30333, (404) 639-3534, (800) 232-4636, inquiry@cdc.gov, http://www.cdc.gov.

United States Department of Human and Health Services, 200 Independence Avenue, S.W., Washington, DC 20201, (877) 696 6775, http://www.hhs.gov.

World Health Organization, Avenue Appia 20, Geneva 27, Switzerland 1211, 22 41 791 21 11, Fax: 22 41 791 31 11, info@who.int, http://www.who.int.

Tish Davidson, AM

Dysentery

Definition

Dysentery is a general term for a group of gastrointestinal disorders characterized by inflammation of the intestines, particularly the colon. Characteristic features include abdominal **pain** and cramps, straining at stool, and frequent passage of watery diarrhea or stools containing blood and mucus.

Description

Dysentery is a common but potentially serious disorder of the digestive tract that occurs throughout the world. It can be caused by a number of infectious agents ranging from viruses and bacteria to protozoa and parasitic worms; it may also result from chemical irritation of the intestines.

Dysentery is one of the oldest known gastrointestinal disorders. The English word dysentery comes from two Greek words meaning "ill" or "bad" and "intestine." Dysentery was described as early as the Peloponnesian War in the fifth century BC. Epidemics of dysentery were frequent occurrences aboard sailing vessels and in army camps, walled cities, and other places in the ancient world where large groups of people lived together in close quarters with poor **sanitation**. As late as the eighteenth and nineteenth centuries, sailors and soldiers were more likely to die from the "bloody flux" than from injuries received in battle. It was not until 1897 that a bacillus (rod-shaped bacterium) was identified as the cause of one major type of dysentery.

Risk factors

Poor sanitation, contaminated **water** supplies, and crowded living conditions are the greatest risk factors for developing dysentery. In the modern world, dysentery is most likely to affect people in less developed countries and travelers who visit these areas. According to the **Centers for Disease Control and Prevention (CDC)**, most cases of dysentery in the United States occur in immigrants from developing countries and in persons who live in inner-city housing with poor sanitation. Other groups of people at increased risk of contracting dysentery or developing severe symptoms are military personnel stationed in developing countries, frequent travelers, young children, especially those in day care centers, people in nursing homes, pregnant women, and men who have sex with other men.

Demographics

Dysentery is particularly common after **natural disasters** such as earthquakes, tsunamis, floods, or hurricanes where water supplies are contaminated, sewage treatment is disrupted, and people are forced to live crowded temporary shelters.

The **CDC** estimates that 450,000 cases of dysentery are caused by the various species of *Shigella* in the United States each year. The most common cause (about 85% of cases) in the United States is *S. sonnei*. Worldwide, *Shigella* are estimated to cause 165 million cases of dysentery and 1 million deaths annually. The most common species worldwide are *S. dysenteriae* and *S. boydii.*

Entamoeba histolytica, the cause of amebic dysentery, is found worldwide, but is most prevalent in developing countries where water and food are often contaminated with human feces and where, according to the CDC, as many as 50% of the population can be infected. Internationally, *E. histolytica* is second only to the organism that causes **malaria** as a protozoal cause of death. It is estimated to account for 40–50 million cases of dysentery each year and 40,000–100,000 deaths.

In the United States, amebic dysentery is uncommon. Most cases occur in recent immigrants from heavily infected areas or travelers returning from those areas. Between 1990 and 2007, only 134 deaths from amebic dysentery were reported in the United States.

Giardia lamblia is the most common parasite found in stool samples in the United States. It mainly causes dysentery in children under age three. Infection usually occurs through contaminated water. Most cases are reported in mountainous areas of the West. About 23,000 cases are reported to the CDC each year, although the infection rate is much higher.

G. lamblia is common worldwide in both tropical and temperate regions. It is estimated that 2–5% of the population in the developed world is infected. The rate is much higher in developing countries with a reported rate of more than 70% in Nepal.

There are about 3.5 million cases of viral dysentery in infants in the United States each year and about 23 million cases each year in adults. The CDC estimates that viruses are responsible for 9.2 million cases of dysentery related to food **poisoning** in the United States each year. The CDC reported that between 2009 and 2011, the number of cases of viral gastroenteritis caused by imported food rose sharply. About half the tainted food came from Asia, with imported fish as one of the most common sources of infection.

Worldwide, viral dysentery is the leading cause of infant death, accounting for 600,000–875,000 deaths per year.

Schistosomiasis is a widespread tropical disease. Although the disease is rare in the United States, travelers to countries where it is endemic may contract it. The **World Health Organization (WHO)** estimates that about 200 million people around the world carry the parasite in their bodies, with 20 million having severe disease.

Causes and symptoms

It should be noted that some doctors use the word "dysentery" to refer only to bacillary and amebic dysentery while others use the term in a broader sense. For example, some doctors speak of schistosomiasis, a disease caused by a parasitic worm, as bilharzial dysentery, while others refer to acute diarrhea caused by viruses as viral dysentery.

Causes

The most common types of dysentery and their causal agents are:

- Bacillary dysentery. Bacillary dysentery, also known as shigellosis, is caused by four species of the genus *Shigella*: *S. dysenteriae*, the most virulent species and the one most likely to cause epidemics; *S. sonnei*, the mildest species; *S. boydii*; and *S. flexneri*. *S. flexneri* is the species that causes Reiter's syndrome, a type of arthritis that develops as a late complication of shigellosis in the United States. The *Shigella* organisms cause the diarrhea and pain associated with dysentery by invading the tissues that line the colon and secreting an enterotoxin, or harmful protein that attacks the intestinal lining.
- Amebic dysentery. Amebic dysentery, also called intestinal amebiasis and amebic colitis, is caused by a protozoon, *Entamoeba histolytica*. *E. histolytica*, whose scientific name means "tissue-dissolving," is second only to the organism that causes malaria as a protozoal cause of death. *E. histolytica* usually enters the body during the cyst stage of its life cycle. The cysts may be found in food or water contaminated by human feces. Once in the digestive tract, the cysts break down, releasing an active form of the organism called a trophozoite. The trophozoites invade the tissues lining the intestine, where they are usually excreted in the patient's feces. They sometimes penetrate the lining itself and enter the bloodstream. If that happens, the trophozoites may be carried to the liver, lungs, or other organs. Involvement of the liver or other organs is sometimes called metastatic amebiasis.
- Balantidiasis, giardiasis, and cryptosporidiosis. These three intestinal infections are all caused by protozoa, *Balantidium coli*, *G. lamblia*, and *Cryptosporidium parvum* respectively. Although most people infected with these protozoa do not become severely ill, the disease agents may cause dysentery in children or immunocompromised individuals.
- Viral dysentery. Viral dysentery, sometimes called traveler's diarrhea or viral gastroenteritis, is caused by several families of viruses, including rotaviruses, caliciviruses, astroviruses, noroviruses, and adenoviruses. Whereas most cases of viral dysentery in infants are caused by rotaviruses, caliciviruses are the most common disease agents in adults. Noroviruses were responsible for about half of the outbreaks of dysentery on cruise ships reported to the CDC in the early 2000s.
- Dysentery caused by parasitic worms. Both whipworm (trichuriasis) and flatworm or fluke (schistosomiasis) infestations may produce the violent diarrhea and abdominal cramps associated with dysentery. Parasitic worm infection is uncommon in the developed world.

Symptoms

In addition to the characteristic bloody and/or watery diarrhea and abdominal cramps of dysentery, the various types have somewhat different symptom profiles:

- Bacillary dysentery. The symptoms of shigellosis may range from the classical bloody diarrhea and tenesmus characteristic of dysentery to the passage of non-bloody diarrhea that resembles the loose stools caused by other intestinal disorders. The high fever associated with shigellosis begins within one to three days after exposure to the organism. The patient may have pain in the rectum and abdominal cramping. The acute symptoms last for three to seven days, occasionally for as long as a month. Bacillary dysentery may lead to two potentially fatal complications outside the digestive tract: bacteremia (bacteria in the bloodstream), which is most likely to occur in malnourished children; and hemolytic uremic syndrome, a type of kidney failure that has a mortality rate above 50%.

- Amebic dysentery. Amebic dysentery often has a slow and gradual onset; most patients with amebiasis visit the doctor after several weeks of diarrhea and bloody stools. Fever is unusual with amebiasis unless the patient has developed a liver abscess as a complication of the infection. The most serious complication of amebic dysentery is fulminant or necrotizing colitis, which is a severe inflammation of the colon characterized by dehydration, severe abdominal pain, and the risk of perforation (rupture) of the colon.
- Dysentery caused by other protozoa. Dysentery associated with giardiasis begins about 1–3 weeks after infection with the organism. It is characterized by bloating and foul-smelling flatus, nausea and vomiting, headaches, and low-grade fever. These acute symptoms usually last three or four days. The symptoms of cryptosporidiosis are mild in most patients but are typically severe in patients with AIDS. Diarrhea usually starts between seven and 10 days after exposure to the organism and may be copious. The patient may have pain in the upper right abdomen, nausea, and vomiting, but fever is unusual.
- Viral dysentery. Viral dysentery has a relatively rapid onset; symptoms may begin within hours of infection. The patient may be severely dehydrated from the diarrhea but usually has only a low-grade fever. The diarrhea itself may be preceded by one to three days of nausea and vomiting. The patient's abdomen may be slightly tender but is not usually severely painful.
- Dysentery caused by parasitic worms. Patients with intestinal schistosomiasis typically have a gradual onset of symptoms. In addition to bloody diarrhea and abdominal pain, these patients usually have fatigue. An examination of the patient's colon will usually reveal areas of ulcerated tissue, which is the source of the bloody diarrhea.

Diagnosis

Patient history and physical examination

The physical examination in the primary care doctor's office will not usually allow the doctor to determine the specific parasite or other disease agent that is causing the bloody diarrhea and other symptoms of dysentery, although the presence or absence of fever may help to narrow the diagnostic possibilities. The patient's age and history are usually better sources of information. The doctor may ask about such matters as the household water supply and food preparation habits, recent contact with or employment in a nursing home or day care center, recent visits to tropical countries, and similar questions. The doctor will also need to know when the patient first noticed the symptoms.

The doctor will also evaluate the patient for signs of dehydration resulting from the loss of fluid through the intestines. Fatigue, drowsiness, dryness of the mucous membranes lining the mouth, low blood pressure, loss of normal skin tone, and rapid heartbeat (above 100 beats per minute) may indicate that the patient is dehydrated.

Laboratory tests

A stool sample is the most common laboratory test to determine the cause of dysentery. The patient should be asked to avoid using over-the-counter antacids or antidiarrheal medications until the sample has been collected, as these preparations can interfere with the test results. The organisms that cause cryptosporidiosis, bacillary dysentery, amebic dysentery, and giardiasis can be seen under the microscope, as can the eggs produced by parasitic worms. In some cases repeated stool samples, a sample of mucus from the intestinal lining obtained through a proctoscope, or a tissue sample from the patient's colon may be necessary to confirm the diagnosis. Antigen testing of a stool sample can be used to diagnose a **rotavirus** infection as well as parasitic worm **infestations**.

The doctor will usually order a blood test to evaluate the electrolyte levels in the patient's blood in order to assess the need for rehydration.

Imaging studies

Imaging studies (usually CT scans, x rays, or ultrasound) may be performed in patients with amebic dysentery to determine whether the lungs or liver have been affected. They may also be used to diagnose schistosomiasis, as the eggs produced by the worms will show up on ultrasound or MRI studies of the liver, intestinal wall, or bladder.

Treatment

Fluid replacement is given if the patient has shown signs of dehydration. The most common treatment is an oral rehydration fluid containing a precise amount of salt and a smaller amount of sugar to replace electrolytes as well as water lost through the intestines. Infalyte and Pedialyte are oral rehydration fluids formulated for the special replacement needs of infants and young children.

Medications are the primary form of treatment for dysentery:

- Bacillary dysentery. Dysentery caused by *Shigella* is usually treated with such antibiotics as trimethoprim-sulfamethoxazole (Bactrim, Septra), nalidixic acid (NegGram), or ciprofloxacin (Cipro, Ciloxan). Because the various species of *Shigella* are becoming resistant to these drugs, the doctor may prescribe one of the newer drugs. Patients with bacillary dysentery should not be given antidiarrheal medications, including loperamide (Imodium), paregoric, and diphenolate (Lomotil), because they may make the illness worse.
- Amebic dysentery. The most common drugs given for amebiasis are diloxanide furoate (Diloxide), iodoquinol (Diquinol, Yodoxin), and metronidazole (Flagyl). Metronidazole should not be given to pregnant women but paromomycin (Humatin) may be used instead. Patients with severe symptoms may be given emetine dihydrochloride or dehydroemetine, but these drugs should be stopped once the patient's symptoms are controlled.
- Dysentery caused by other protozoa. Balantidiasis, giardiasis, and cryptosporidiosis are treated with the same drugs as amebic dysentery; patients with giardiasis resistant to treatment may be given albendazole (Zentel) or furazolidone (Furoxone).
- Viral dysentery. The primary concern in treating viral dysentery, particularly in small children, is to prevent dehydration. Oral rehydration solution (ORS) developed by WHO or a commercial product such as Pedialyte is given as needed to keep the child hydrated. Antinausea and antidiarrhea medications should not be given to small children. Probiotics, including *Lactobacillus casei* and *Saccharomyces boulardii*, have been shown to reduce the duration and severity of viral diarrhea in small children by 30–70%.
- Dysentery caused by parasitic worms. Whipworm infestations are usually treated with anthelminthic medications, most commonly mebendazole (Vermox). Schistosomiasis may be treated with praziquantel (Biltricide), metrifonate (Trichlorfon), or oxamniquine, depending on the species causing the infestation.

Newer drugs that have been developed to treat dysentery include tinidazole (Tindamax, Fasigyn), an antiprotozoal drug approved by the Food and Drug Administration (FDA) in 2004 to treat giardiasis and **amebiasis** in adults and children over the age of three years. This drug should not be given to women in the first three months of pregnancy. Adults taking tinidazole should not drink alcoholic beverages while using it, or for three days after the end of treatment. Nitazoxanide (Alinia) is another new antiprotozoal medication that has the advantage of lacking the bitter taste of metronidazole and tinidazole.

Surgery

Surgery is rarely necessary in treating dysentery, but may be required in cases of fulminant colitis, particularly if the patient's colon has perforated. Patients with liver abscesses resulting from amebic dysentery may also require emergency surgery if the abscess ruptures. In some cases, exploratory surgery may be needed to determine whether severe abdominal pain is caused by schistosomiasis, amebic dysentery, or appendicitis.

Alternative treatments

There are a number of alternative treatments for dysentery, most of which are derived from plants used by healers for centuries. Because dysentery was known to ancient civilizations as well as modern societies, such alternative systems as traditional Chinese medicine (TCM) and Ayurvedic medicine developed treatments for it.

Ayurvedic medicine

Ayurvedic medicine recommends fruits and herbs, specifically cumin seed, bael fruit (*Aegle marmelos*, also known as Bengal quince), and arjuna (*Terminalia arjuna*) bark for the treatment of dysentery. Ayurvedic practitioners may also give the patient dietary supplements known as Isabbael, Lashunadi Bati, and Bhuwaneshar Ras. To rehydrate the body, adult patients may be given a combination of slippery elm water and barley to drink, at least a pint per day.

Traditional Chinese medicine

To treat dysentery, traditional Chinese doctors use astringent drugs, which are intended to constrict or tighten mucous membranes and other body tissues to slow down fluid loss. Myrobalan fruit (*Terminalia chebula*), nut galls (swellings produced on the leaves and stems of oak trees by the secretions of certain insects), and opium extracted from the opium poppy (*Papaver somniferum*) are the natural materials most commonly used. Paregoric, a water-based solution of morphine that is still used in the West to treat diarrhea, is derived from the opium poppy.

Other plant-based remedies

Researchers in Mexico reported in early 2005 that the roots of *Geranium mexicanum*, a plant that produces a sap traditionally used to treat coughs or diarrhea, contains compounds that are active against both *G. lamblia* and *E. histolytica*. Plant biologists in Africa are studying the effectiveness of African mistletoe (*Tapinanthus dodoneifolius*), a traditional remedy for dysentery among the Hausa and Fulani tribes of Nigeria.

Dietary supplements

The CDC reports that in many instances the administration of zinc at twice the recommended daily dietary allowance along with rehydration therapy and antibiotic therapy significantly shortens the duration and severity of dysentery in children.

Homeopathy

There are at least ten different homeopathic remedies used to treat diarrhea. Contemporary homeopaths distinguish between diarrhea that can be safely treated at home with such homeopathic remedies as *Podophyllum*, *Veratrum album*, *Bryonia*, and *Arsenicum*, and diarrhea that indicates dysentery and should be referred to a physician. Signs of dehydration (loss of normal skin texture, dry mouth, sunken eyes), severe abdominal pain, blood in the stool, and unrelieved vomiting are all indications that mainstream medical care is required.

Public health role and response

Public health measures to control the spread of dysentery include the following:

- Requiring doctors to report cases of disease caused by *Shigella*, *E. histolytica*, and other parasites that cause dysentery. Careful reporting allows the CDC and state public health agencies to investigate local outbreaks and plan prevention efforts.
- Posting advisories for travelers about outbreaks of dysentery and other health risks in foreign countries. The Travelers' Health section of the CDC website (http://wwwnc.cdc.gov/travel) is a good source of up-to date information.
- Instructing restaurant workers and other food handlers about proper methods of hand washing, food storage, and food preparation.
- Instructing workers in day care centers and nursing homes about the proper methods for changing and cleaning soiled diapers or bedding.
- Inspecting wells, other sources of drinking water, and swimming pools for evidence of fecal contamination.

Prognosis

Most adults in developed countries recover completely from an episode of dysentery. Children are at greater risk of becoming dehydrated, however; bacillary dysentery in particular can lead to a child's death from dehydration in as little as 12–24 hours.

- Bacillary dysentery. Most patients recover completely from shigellosis, although their bowel habits may not become completely normal for several months. About 3% of people infected by *S. flexneri* will develop Reiter's syndrome, which may lead to a chronic form of arthritis that is difficult to treat. Elderly patients or those with weakened immune systems sometimes develop secondary bacterial infections after an episode of shigellosis.

KEY TERMS

Anthelminthic (also spelled anthelmintic)—A type of drug or herbal preparation given to destroy parasitic worms or expel them from the body.

Bacillus—A rod-shaped bacterium. One common type of dysentery is known as bacillary dysentery because it is caused by a bacillus.

Endemic—Occurring naturally and consistently in a particular area.

Epidemic—An outbreak of disease where the number of cases exceeds the usual (endemic) or typical number of cases.

Enterotoxin—A type of harmful protein released by bacteria and other disease agents that affects the tissues lining the intestines.

Fulminant—Occurring or flaring up suddenly and with great severity. A potentially fatal complication of amebic dysentery is an inflammation of the colon known as fulminant colitis.

Probiotics—Food supplements containing live bacteria or other microbes intended to improve or restore the normal balance of microorganisms in the digestive tract.

Proctoscope—An instrument consisting of a thin tube with a light source, used to examine the inside of the rectum.

Protozoan (plural, protozoa)—A member of the simplest form of animal life, a one-celled organism. Amebic dysentery is caused by a protozoan.

Reiter's syndrome—A group of symptoms that includes arthritis, inflammation of the urethra, and conjunctivitis, and develops as a late complication of infection with *Shigella flexneri*. The syndrome was first described by a German doctor named Hans Reiter in 1918.

Tenesmus—Ineffective spasms of the rectum or bladder accompanied by the desire to evacuate the rectum or pass urine but without being able to do so. Tenesmus is a characteristic feature of bacillary dysentery.

Trophozoite—The active feeding stage of a protozoal parasite, as distinct from its encysted stage.

- Amebic dysentery. Most people in North America who become infected with *E. histolytica* do not become severely ill. Patients who develop a severe case of amebic dysentery, however, are at increased risk for such complications as fulminant colitis or liver abscess. About 0.5% of patients with amebic dysentery develop fulminant colitis, but almost half of these patients die. Between 2% and 7% of cases of amebic liver abscess result in rupture of the abscess with a high mortality rate. Men are 7–12 times more likely to develop a liver abscess than women. All patients diagnosed with amebic dysentery should have stool samples examined for relapse one, three, and six months after treatment with medications whether or not they have developed complications.
- Dysentery caused by other protozoa. Cryptosporidiosis may lead to respiratory infections or pancreatitis in patients with AIDS. The risk of these complications is reduced in AIDS patients who are receiving highly active antiretroviral therapy (HAART).
- Viral dysentery. Most people in North America recover completely without complications unless they become severely dehydrated. Viral dysentery in children in developing countries is a major cause of mortality.
- Dysentery caused by parasitic worms. Untreated whipworm infections can lead to loss of appetite, chronic diarrhea, and retarded growth in children. Untreated schistosomiasis can develop into a chronic intestinal disorder in which fibrous tissue, small growths, or strictures (abnormal narrowing) may form inside the intestine. Patients treated for schistosomiasis should have stool samples checked for the presence of worm eggs three and six months after the end of treatment.

Prevention

The disease agents that cause dysentery do not confer immunity against re-infection at a later date. There are no vaccines for bacillary dysentery or amebic dysentery; however, a vaccine against schistosomiasis is under investigation. An oral vaccine against rotavirus infections was developed for small children but was withdrawn in 2004 because it was associated with an increased risk of small-bowel disorders. Newer vaccines against rotaviruses and caliciviruses are being developed.

Personal precautions

Individuals can lower their risk of contracting dysentery by the following measures:

- Not allowing anyone in the household who has been diagnosed with amebic or bacillary dysentery to prepare food or pour water for others until their doctor confirms that they are no longer carrying the disease agent.
- Avoiding anal sex or oral-genital contacts.
- Washing the hands carefully with soap and water after using the bathroom, and supervising the hand washing of children in day care centers or those at home who are not completely toilet-trained.
- When traveling, drinking only boiled or treated water, and eating only cooked hot foods or fruits that can be peeled by the traveler.
- Not swimming in fresh water in areas known to have outbreaks of schistosomiasis.

QUESTIONS TO ASK YOUR DOCTOR

- I am planning to travel to an area where dysentery is common. Should I take any medications with me?
- How long should before the medication you gave me to slows/stops my diarrhea?
- Should I be aware of any side effects for the medication you gave me?
- How can I tell if my child is becoming dehydrated?
- Are there any likely long-term consequences from the type of infection causing my dysentery?

Resources

WEBSITES

Kroser, Joyann. “Shigellosis.” Medscape.com December 5, 2011. http://emedicine.medscape.com/article/182767-overview (accessed October 13, 2012).

Lacasse, Alexandre. “Amebiasis.” Medscape.com January 10, 2012. http://emedicine.medscape.com/article/212029-overview (accessed October 13, 2012).

Mukherjee, Sandeep. “Giardiasis.” Medscape.com June 29, 2011. http://emedicine.medscape.com/article/176718-overview (accessed October 13, 2012).

Tablang, Vincent F. “Viral Gastroenteritis.” Medscape.com March 19, 2012. http://emedicine.medscape.com/article/176515-overview (accessed October 13, 2012).

ORGANIZATIONS

Infectious Diseases Society of America (IDSA), 1300 Wilson Blvd., Ste. 300, Arlington, VA 22209, (703) 299-0200, Fax: (703) 299-0204, info@idsociety.org, http://www.idsociety.org

Centers for Disease Control and Prevention (CDC), 1600 Clifton Rd., Atlanta, GA 30333, (404) 639-3534, (800) CDC-INFO (800-232-4636), cdcinfo@cdc.gov, http://www.cdc.gov

World Health Organization, Avenue Appia 20, 1211 Geneva 27, Switzerland, 22 41 791 21 11, Fax: 22 41 791 31 11, info@who.int, http://www.who.int

Rebecca Frey, PhD
Tish Davidson, AM

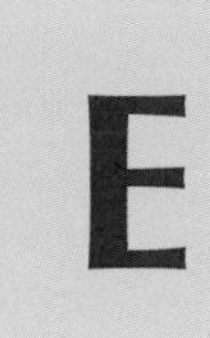

Eating disorders

Definition

Eating disorders (EDs) are psychiatric disorders that have diagnostic criteria based on psychologic, behavior, and physiologic characteristics that usually result in abnormal eating patterns that have a negative effect on health.

Demographics

According to the National Comorbidity Survey Replication study, reported lifetime prevalence rates for anorexia nervosa were 0.3% in men and 0.9% in women; for bulimia nervosa, 0.5% in men and 1.5% in women; and for binge eating disorder, 2% in men and 3.5% in women. In general, more women have eating disorders than men, and according to the National Eating Disorder Association, an estimated 10 million females in the United States have some form of eating disorder. The age at which a person develops an ED differs within conditions, with the greatest frequency of anorexia nervosa and bulimia nervosa occurring during adolescence, whereas binge eating disorder occurs well into adulthood. There are also clinical reports that show an increasing trend in EDs for middle-aged women. Longitudinal research has documented that 12% of adolescent girls aged 12 to 15 years, have experienced some form of ED. Anorexia athletica, muscle dysmorphic disorder, and orthorexia nervosa tend to be more common in men. Rumination, pica, and Prader-Willi syndrome affect men and women equally.

Anorexia nervosa begins primarily between the ages of 14 and 18 and affects mainly white girls. Bulimia usually develops slightly later in the late teens and early twenties. Binge eating disorder is a problem of middle age and affects blacks and whites equally. Prader-Willi syndrome begins in the toddler years. Not enough is known about the more newly classified disorders—such anorexia athletica, muscle dysmorphic disorder, and orthorexia nervosa—to determine when they are most likely to develop or which races or ethnic groups are most likely to be at risk.

Description

Eating disorders are largely psychological disorders. They develop when a person has an unrealistic attitude toward or abnormal perception of his or her body. This causes behaviors that lead to destructive eating patterns that have negative physical and emotional consequences. Individuals with eating disorders often hide their symptoms and resist seeking treatment. Depression, anxiety disorders, and other mental illnesses often are present in people who have eating disorders, although it is not clear whether these cause the eating disorder or are a result of it.

The two best-known eating disorders, anorexia nervosa and bulimia nervosa, have formal diagnostic criteria and are recognized as psychiatric disorders in the *Diagnostic and Statistical Manual for Mental Disorders*, fourth edition (*DSM-IV-TR*) published by the American Psychiatric Association (APA). Other eating disorders have recognized sets of symptoms, but have not been researched thoroughly enough to be considered separate psychiatric disorders as defined by the APA.

Well-known eating disorders

In North America and Europe, anorexia nervosa is the most publicized of all eating disorders. It gained widespread public attention with the rise of the ultra-thin fashion model. People who have anorexia nervosa are obsessed with body weight. They constantly monitor their food intake and starve themselves to become thin. No matter how much weight they lose, they continue to restrict their calorie intake in an effort to become ever thinner. Some people with anorexia overexercise or abuse drugs or herbal remedies that they believe will help them burn calories faster. A few purge their bodies of the few calories they do eat by abusing laxatives, enemas, and diuretics. In time, they reach a point where their health is seriously, and potentially fatally, impaired.

People with anorexia nervosa have an abnormal perception of their body. They genuinely believe that they are larger than they are, even if they are life-threateningly thin. People with anorexia may deny that they are too thin, or, if they admit they are thin, deny that their behavior is affecting their health. People with anorexia will lie to family, friends, and healthcare providers about how much they eat. Many vigorously resist treatment and accuse the people trying to cure them of wanting to make them fat. Anorexia nervosa is the most difficult eating disorder to recover from.

Bulimia nervosa is the only other eating disorder with specific diagnostic criteria defined by the (*DSM-IV-TR*). People with bulimia often consume unreasonably large amounts of food in a short time. Afterwards, they purge their body of calories. This is done most often by self-induced vomiting, often accompanied by laxative abuse. A subset of people with bulimia does not vomit after eating, but fast and exercise obsessively to burn calories. Both behaviors result in impaired health.

People with bulimia feel out of control when they are binge eating. Unlike people with anorexia, they recognize that their behavior is abnormal. Often they are ashamed and feel guilty about their behavior and will go to great lengths to hide their binge/purge cycles from their family and friends. People with bulimia are often of normal weight. Although their behavior results in negative health consequences, because they are less likely to be ultra-thin, these consequences are less likely to be life-threatening.

The APA does not formally recognize binge eating as an eating disorder. Binge eating is quite common, but it only rises to the level of a disorder when bingeing occurs at least twice a week for three months or more. People with binge eating disorder may eat thousands of calories in an hour or two. While they are eating, they feel out of control and may continue to eat long after they feel full. Unlike bulimia, people with binge eating disorder do not purge or exercise to get rid of the calories they have eaten. As a result, many people with binge eating disorder are obese, although not all obese people are binge eaters.

People with binge eating disorder may feel ashamed of their behavior and may try to hide it by eating in secret or hoarding food for future binges. After a binge, they usually feel guilty about their eating behavior. They might promise themselves that they will never binge again but are usually unable to keep this promise. Binge eating disorder often follow this seemingly endless cycle—rigorous dieting followed by an eating binge followed by guilt and rigorous dieting, followed by another eating binge. The main health consequences of binge eating are the development of obesity-related diseases such as type 2 diabetes, sleep apnea, **stroke**, and heart attack.

Lesser-known eating disorders

Quite a few eating problems are called disorders even though they do not have formal diagnostic criteria. They fall under the APA definition of eating disorders not otherwise specified. Many have only recently come to the attention of researchers and have been the subject of only a few small studies. Some have been known to the medical community for years but are rare.

Purge disorder is thought by some experts to be a separate disorder from bulimia. It is distinguished from bulimia by the fact that the individual maintains a normal or near normal weight despite purging by vomiting or laxative, enema, or diuretic abuse.

Anorexia athletica is a disorder of compulsive exercising. The individual places exercise above work, school, or relationships and defines his or her self-worth in terms of athletic performance. People with anorexia athletica also tend to be obsessed less with body weight than with maintaining an abnormally low percentage of body fat. This disorder is common among elite athletes.

Muscle dysmorphic disorder is the opposite of anorexia nervosa. Where people with anorexia believe that they are always overweight, people with muscle dysmorphic disorder believe that they are too small. This belief is maintained even when a person is clearly well-muscled. Abnormal eating patterns are less of a problem in people with muscle dysmorphic disorder than damage from compulsive exercising (even when injured) and the abuse of muscle-building drugs such as anabolic steroids.

Orthorexia nervosa is a term coined by Steven Bratman, a Colorado physician, to describe "a pathological fixation on eating 'proper,' 'pure,' or 'superior' foods." People with orthorexia allow their fixation with eating the correct amount of properly prepared healthy foods at the correct time of day to take over their lives. This obsession interferes with relationships and daily activities. For example, they may be unwilling to eat at restaurants or friends' homes because the food is impure or improperly prepared. The limitations they put on what they will eat can cause serious vitamin and mineral imbalances. Orthorectics are judgmental about what other people eat to the point where it interferes with personal relationships. They justify their fixation by claiming that their way of eating is healthy. Some experts believe orthorexia may be a variation of obsessive-compulsive disorder.

Rumination syndrome occurs when an individual, either voluntarily or involuntarily, regurgitates food almost immediately after swallowing it, chews it, and then either swallows it or spits it out. Regurgitation syndrome is the human equivalent of a cow chewing its cud. The behavior often lasts up to two hours after eating. It must continue for at least one month to be considered a disorder. Occasionally the behavior simply stops on its own, but it can last for years.

Pica is the eating of non-food substances by people developmentally past the stage where this is normal (usually around age two). Earth and clay are the most common non-foods eaten, although people have been known to eat hair, feces, lead, laundry starch, chalk, burnt matches, cigarette butts, light bulbs, and other equally bizarre non-foods. This disorder has been known to the medical community for years, and in some cultures (mainly tribes living in equatorial Africa) is considered normal. Pica is most common among people with mental retardation and developmental delays. It only rises to the level of a disorder when health complications require medical treatment.

Prader-Willi syndrome is a genetic defect that spontaneously arises in chromosome 15. It causes low muscle tone, short stature, incomplete sexual development, mental retardation, and an uncontrollable urge to eat. People with Prader-Willi syndrome never feel full. The only way to stop them from eating themselves to death is to keep them in environments where food is locked up and not available. Prader-Willi syndrome is a rare disease, and although it is caused by a genetic defect, tends not to run in families, but rather is an accident of development. Fewer than 15,000 people in the United States have Prader-Willi syndrome.

“Drunkorexia,” though not a medically recognized diagnosis, is the restriction of calories from food in order to consume greater amounts of alcohol without gaining weight. It is becoming increasingly common—a study conducted by professors at the University of Minnesota and published in the journal *Comprehensive Psychiatry* found that one in five students was substituting alcoholic beverages for meals. According to the U.S. **Centers for Disease Control and Prevention**, binge drinking is defined as having more than five drinks for men or four drinks for women in an short time frame. It is associated with a slew of adverse health effects, including higher risk of alcohol dependence, high blood pressure, stroke, **heart disease**, liver disease, neurological damage, sexual dysfunctions, injury (whether intentional or unintentional), and **sexually transmitted diseases** (due to lowered inhibitions while drunk). Replacing meals with alcohol can also place a person at risk of vitamin and nutrient deficiencies and malnutrition.

Causes and symptoms

Depression, low self-worth, and anxiety disorders are all common among people with eating disorders. Some disorders have obsessive-compulsive elements. The association between these psychiatric disorders and eating disorders is strong, but the cause and effect relationship is still unclear. Most specialists agree that eating disorders have multiple causes. There appears to be a genetic predisposition in some people toward developing an eating disorder. Biochemistry also seems to play a role. Neurotransmitters in the brain, such as serotonin, play a role in regulating appetite. Abnormalities in the amount of some neurotransmitters are thought to play a role in anorexia, bulimia, and binge eating disorder. Other disorders have not been studied enough to draw any conclusions.

Personality type can also put people at risk for developing an eating disorder. Low self-worth is common among people with eating disorders. Binge eaters and people with bulimia tend to have problems with impulse control and anger management. A tendency toward obsessive-compulsive behavior and black-or-white, all-or-nothing thinking also put people at higher risk.

Social and environmental factors also affect the development and maintenance of eating disorders and may trigger relapses during recovery. Relationship conflict, a disordered or unstructured home life, job or school **stress**, and transitional events such as moving or starting a new job are all potential triggers for some people to begin disordered eating behaviors. Dieting (nutritional and social stress) is the most common trigger of all. The United States in the early twenty-first century is a culture obsessed with thinness. The media constantly send the message through words and images that being not just thin, but ultra-thin, is fashionable and desirable. Magazines aimed mostly at women devote thousands of words every month to diet and exercise advice that creates a sense of dissatisfaction, unrealistic goals, and through air-brushing models to make them look thinner, many women develop a distorted body image.

Research has documented that comorbid illnesses and EDs tend to be diagnosed as a cluster of diagnoses; that is, patients with EDs often experience other psychiatric disorders. Axis I psychiatric disorders (including depression, anxiety, body dysmorphic disorder, or chemical dependency) and Axis II personality disorders (particularly borderline personality disorder) are frequently seen in the ED population. The breadth of these conditions increases the complexity of treatment and the skill required of the counselors and medical providers involved in the treatment.

Diagnosis

Diagnosis involves four components: a health history, a physical examination which will rule out hormone abnormalities that may result in loss of weight, laboratory tests, and a mental status evaluation that also assesses suicidal risk. Health histories tend to be unreliable, because many people with eating disorders lie about their eating behavior, purging habits, and medication abuse. Based on the health history and a physical examination of the patient, the physician will order appropriate laboratory tests. Mental status can be evaluated using several different scales. The goal is to get an accurate assessment of the individuals's physical condition and thinking in relationship to self-worth, body image, and food.

During the physical examination, other major medical complications may be diagnosed as well, such as cardiac arrhythmia, dehydration and eloctrolyte imbalances, delayed growth and development, endocrinological disturbances, gastrointestinal problems, oral health problems, osteopenia, osteoporosis, and protein/calorie malnutrition.

The mental health examination currently uses the *DSM-IV*, which provides diagnostic criteria for psychiatric disorders, including certain eating disorders. Expanded diagnostic criteria is under consideration for the fifth edition (*DSM-5*), expected to publish in 2013. The *DSM-IV* diagnostic criteria for anorexia nervosa includes an exaggerated drive for thinness, refusal to maintain a body weight above the standard minimum (e.g., 85% of expected weight), intense fear of becoming fat with self-worth based on weight or shape, and evidence of an endocrine disorder. The changes proposed for *DSM-5* include restricted energy intake relative to requirements (leading to a markedly low body weight), intense fear of gaining weight or becoming fat or persistent behavior to avoid weight gain, and considerable distress regarding one's weight or body shape.

KEY TERMS

Fast—A period of at least 24 hours in which a person eats nothing and drinks only water.

Type 2 diabetes—Sometimes called adult-onset diabetes, this disease prevents the body from properly using glucose (sugar).

Criteria in the *DSM-IV* for bulimia nervosa include overwhelming urges to overeat and inappropriate compensatory behaviors or purging that follow the binge episodes (e.g., vomiting, excessive exercise, alternating periods of starvation, and abuse of laxatives or drugs). Similar to anorexia nervosa, individuals with bulimia nervosa also display psychopathology, including a fear of being overweight. New criteria proposed for *DSM-5* include recurrent episodes of binge eating with a sense of a lack of control with inappropriate compensatory behavior, self-evaluation that is unduly influenced by body shape and weight, and the specification that the behaviors do not occur exclusively during episodes of anorexia nervosa.

The *DSM-IV* is somewhat vague when discussing eating disorders that are not specifically classified, merely noting that they tend to be compensatory behaviors distinguished by binge eating and a lack of self-control. Proposals for *DSM-5* include better definitions and diagnostic criteria for unspecified eating disorders, including binge eating disorder, purging disorder, and night-eating syndrome.

Treatment

Treatment depends on a collaborative approach by an interdisciplinary team of mental health, **nutrition**, and medical specialists. The degree to which the individual's health and mental status is impaired can direct what type of treatment plan is appropriate for the individual. People with EDs may need to be hospitalized or attend structured day programs for an extended period. Some people are also prescribed medication, but the mainstay of treatment is psychotherapy. An appropriate therapy is selected based on the type of eating disorder and the individual's psychological profile. Some of the common therapies used in treating eating disorders include:

- Cognitive behavior therapy (CBT) is designed to confront and then change the individual's thoughts and feelings about his or her body and behaviors toward food, but it does not address why those thoughts or feelings exist. Reasearch has shown that CBT is effective for those with binge eating behaviors by decreasing the frequency of binges through helping the person learn to normalize their thought patterns and find compensatory responses to binging. However, use of CBT with anorexia nervosa is compromised due to the addition of inborn disruptions in the person's neurotransmitter secretions, which places a limit on the extent to which CBT can assist in treatment.

- Psychodynamic therapy, also called psychoanalytic therapy, attempts to help the individual gain insight into the cause of the emotions that trigger their dysfunctional behavior. This therapy tends to be more long term than CBT.
- Interpersonal therapy is short-term therapy that helps the individual identify specific issues and problems in relationships. The individual may be asked to look back at his or her family history to try to recognize problem areas or stresses and work toward resolving them.
- Dialectical behavior therapy (DBT) consists of structured private and group sessions in which the therapist and patient(s) work at reducing behaviors that interfere with quality of life, finding alternate solutions to current problem situations, and learning to regulate emotions. In selected populations, some evidence suggests that DBT shows potential for decreasing binge eating and purging symptoms
- Family and couples therapy can be helpful in dealing with conflict or disorders that may be a factor in perpetuating the eating disorder. Family therapy is especially useful in helping parents with anorexia to avoid passing on their attitudes and behaviors to their children. Self-esteem and assertiveness training may also be helpful in some patients with EDs.

Drugs

As of 2012, there are no medications approved by the U.S. Food and Drug Administration (FDA) for the specific treatment of anorexia nervosa. Medications prescribed for those with anorexia nervosa focus on either reducing anxiety or alleviating mood symptoms to assist the person in eating. For the treatment of bulimia nervosa, the Food and Drug Administration has approved fluoxetine after (or in conjunction with) behavior therapy.

Nutrition/Dietetic concerns

Eating disorders result in malnutrition that can have life-threatening consequences. Death may be due to cardiac arrhythmia, acute cardiovascular failure, gastric hemorrhaging, or **suicide**. Nutrition inadequacies commonly seen in the eating disorder group are low energy intake (which can be as severe as eating fewer than 500 calories per day), protein intake that results in clinical signs of protein deficiency, insufficient dietary calcium intake, fluid and electrolyte imbalances, and an array of vitamin and mineral insufficiencies.

QUESTIONS TO ASK YOUR DOCTOR

- My child keeps saying he/she is fat and is unhappy with the way he/she looks. Is there someone in your office who can talk with her?
- My child seems to be avoiding eating or is only eating a limited amount of food. Is there a way to evaluate him/her for an eating disorder?
- Is my child's height and weight appropriate for his/her age?
- My daughter has not started her menstrual cycle. Is this normal?
- Can you recommend a family therapist?

Prognosis

Recovery from eating disorders can be a long, difficult process interrupted by relapses. About half of all people with anorexia. Up to 20% die of complications of the disorder. The recovery rate for people with bulimia is slightly higher. Binge eaters experience many relapses and may have trouble controlling their weight even if they stop bingeing. Not enough is known about the other eating disorders to determine recovery rates. All eating disorders have serious social and emotional consequences. All except rumination disorder have serious health consequences. The sooner a person with an eating disorder gets professional help, the better the chance of recovery.

Prevention

Prevention involves both preventing and relieving stresses and enlisting professional help as soon as abnormal eating patterns develop. Some things that may help prevent an eating disorder from developing are listed below:

- Parents should not obsess about their weight, appearance, and diet in front of their children.

- Parents should not put their child on a diet unless instructed to by a pediatrician.
- Do not tease people about their body shapes or compare them to others.
- Make it clear that family members are loved and accepted as they are.
- Try to eat meals together as a family whenever possible; avoid eating alone.
- Avoid using food for comfort in times of stress.
- Monitoring negative self-talk; practice positive self-talk
- Spend time doing something enjoyable every day
- Stay busy, but not overly busy; get enough sleep every night
- Become aware of the situations that are personal triggers for abnormal eating behaviors and look for ways to avoid or defuse them.
- Do not go on extreme diets.
- Be alert to signs of low self-worth, anxiety, depression, and drug or alcohol abuse. Seek help as soon as these signs appear.

Resources

BOOKS

Agras, W. Stewart. *Overcoming Eating Disorders: A Cognitive-Behavioral Therapy Approach for Bulimia Nervosa and Binge-Eating Disorder*. 2nd ed. New York: Oxford University Press, 2008.

Carleton, Pamela and Deborah Ashin.*Take Charge of Your Child's Eating Disorder: A Physician's Step-By-Step Guide to Defeating Anorexia and Bulimia*. New York: Marlowe & Co., 2007.

Heaton, Jeanne A. and Claudia J. Strauss. *Talking to Eating Disorders: Simple Ways to Support Someone Who Has Anorexia, Bulimia, Binge Eating or Body Image Issues*. New York: New American Library, 2005.

Kolodny, Nancy J. *The Beginner's Guide to Eating Disorders Recovery*. Carlsbad, CA: Gurze Books, 2004.

Liu, Aimee. *Gaining: The Truth About Life After Eating Disorders*. New York: Warner Books, 2007.

Messinger, Lisa, and Merle Goldberg. *My Thin Excuse: Understanding, Recognizing, and Overcoming Eating Disorders*. Garden City Park, NY: Square One Publishers, 2006.

Rubin, Jerome S., ed. *Eating Disorders and Weight Loss Research*. Hauppauge, NY: Nova Science Publishers, 2006.

Walsh, B. Timothy. *If Your Adolescent Has an Eating Disorder: An Essential Resource for Parents*. New York, NY: Oxford University Press, 2005.

PERIODICALS

Osborne, V. A., K. J. Sher, and R. P. Winograd. "Disordered Eating Patterns and Alcohol Misuse in College Students: Evidence for 'Drunkorexia?'" *Comprehensive Psychiatry* 52, no. 6 (2011): e12. http://dx.doi.org/10.1016/j.comppsych.2011.04.038 (accessed September 7, 2012).

Wilson, Jenny, et al. "Surfing for Thinness: A Pilot Study of Pro-Eating Disorder Web Site Usage in Adolescents With Eating Disorders." *Pediatrics* 118, no. 6 (December 2006): e1635–43. http://dx.doi.org/10.1542/peds.2006-1133 (accessed September 7, 2012).

WEBSITES

Anorexia Nervosa and Related Eating Disorders (ANRED). "Table of Contents." http://www.anred.com/toc.html (accessed September 7, 2012).

Centers for Disease Control and Prevention. "Fact Sheets: Binge Drinking." http://www.cdc.gov/alcohol/fact-sheets/binge-drinking.htm (accessed September 7, 2012).

Jennings, Ashley. "Drunkorexia: Alcohol Mixes With Eating Disorders." ABC News, October 21, 2010. http://abcnews.go.com/Health/drunkorexia-alcohol-mixes-eating-disorders/story?id=11936398 (accessed September 7, 2012).

MedlinePlus. "Eating Disorders." U.S. National Library of Medicine, National Institutes of Health. http://www.nlm.nih/gov/medlineplus/eatingdisorders.html (accessed September 7, 2012).

National Association of Anorexia Nervosa and Associated Disorders. "About Eating Disorders." http://www.anad.org/get-information/about-eating-disorders (accessed September 7, 2012).

Pearce, Tralee. "'Drunkorexia' a Growing Problem as Female Students Favour Booze over Food." *Globe and Mail*, October 19, 2011.

ORGANIZATIONS

American Psychological Association, 750 First St. NE, Washington, DC 20002-4242, (202) 336-5500, (800) 374-2721, http://www.apa.org.

National Association of Anorexia Nervosa & Associated Disorders, 800 E. Diehl Rd. #160, Naperville, IL 60563, (630) 577-1333 (630) 577-1330 (helpline), anadhelp@anad.org, http://www.anad.org.

National Eating Disorders Association, 165 West 46th Street, New York, NY 10036, (212) 575-6200, (800) 931-2237, info@NationalEatingDisorders.org, http://www.nationaleatingdisorders.org.

Tish Davidson, AM
Megan Porter, RD

Ebola hemorrhagic fever

Definition

Ebola, or Ebola hemorrhagic fever (HF), is a severe and often fatal viral disease that affects humans, chimpanzees, gorillas, and monkeys. The disease was first recognized in Africa in 1976. It is caused by a type of virus called the Ebola virus.

Description

In 1976, there were two simultaneous outbreaks of a mysterious fever, one in Nzara, Sudan, and the other in Yambuku, a village on the Ebola River in the Democratic Republic of Congo (DRC).

The Ebola virus belongs to a family of RNA viruses called the Filoviridae. Five subtypes or species of the virus have been identified: Ebola Zaire, Ebola Sudan, Ebola Ivory Coast, Ebola Bundibugyo, and Ebola-Reston. Of the five, only Ebola Reston does not appear to cause illness in humans, although the evidence is limited.

Origins

The origins and natural reservoirs of the Ebola virus are as yet unknown, although scientists believe that the virus is zoonotic, or animal-based, because of the nature of similar viruses and available evidence. The virus affects non-human primates, including chimpanzees, gorillas, and monkeys. However, researchers believe that they are accidental hosts, rather than natural reservoirs. Fruit bats, particularly *Hypsignathus monstrosus, Monycteris torquata,* and *Epomops franqueti,* may be possible natural hosts because of an overlap between the bats' natural ranges with the range of the virus. In addition, a species of fruit bat is the natural reservoir of the Marburg virus, another virus that causes hemorrhagic fever and the only other member of the family Filoviridae.

Demographics

According the **World Health Organization**, major outbreaks of Ebola HF have occurred only in African nations. Between 2000 and 2011, there were 11 major outbreaks, resulting in 1,202 cases and 734 deaths. Most cases occurred in Uganda and the DRC. During that period, 575 cases, resulting in 262 deaths, were recorded by the **WHO** in Uganda, while in the DRC, 545 cases resulted in 415 deaths, a 75 percent fatality rate. Overall since 2000, 61 percent of the people who have contracted Ebola have died. Another outbreak occurred in western Uganda in July and August, 2012.

Causes and Symptoms

Ebola HF is caused by a virus and as a result has symptoms similar to those of other viral diseases.

Causes

The cause of Ebola HF is the Ebola virus, one of the deadliest known viruses affecting humans. The U.S. **Centers for Disease Control and Prevention (CDC)** classifies the Ebola virus as a category A bioterrorism agent, along with **smallpox** and **anthrax**.

In 2011, researchers identified the means by which the Ebola virus enters a host cell. It depends on the protein Niemann-Pick C1 (NPC1), which is normally involved in the transport of cholesterol in and out of the cell. Researchers found that cells in which this protein did not function properly were resistant to infection by both the Ebola and the Marburg viruses. Although much remains to be learned, it is the first hopeful step toward learning how to control these deadly viruses.

The Ebola virus is passed to humans from infected animals. In Africa, these animals include chimpanzees, gorillas, porcupines, monkeys, fruit bats, and forest antelopes. The virus is present is the blood, secretions, organs, and other bodily fluids of these animals. Once infected, a human can transmit the virus through blood, secretions, bodily fluids, and organs; at burial ceremonies, mourners who have direct contact with the body of the dead person may contract the disease. The virus also remains active in semen for up to seven weeks after clinical recovery.

Healthcare workers have been infected with the Ebola virus when they have not followed infection-control procedures, such as not wearing gloves, goggles, or masks while treating infectious persons.

Ebola Reston, which appears to be less virulent, has caused infections in humans who work with monkeys and pigs that have the virus. It has caused severe outbreaks among macaque monkeys being raised in the Philippines; some of those monkeys were imported to the United States in 1989, 1990, and 1996 and to Italy in 1982.

Symptoms

The incubation period for the virus ranges from 2 to 21 days. Onset is abrupt and is characterized by fever, joint and muscle aches, headache, weakness and sore throat, soon followed by diarrhea, vomiting, and stomach **pain**. Red eyes, hiccups, rash, and internal and external bleeding may also occur.

Diagnosis

The disease can be difficult to diagnose because it can appear similar to **malaria**, **typhoid fever**, **cholera**, **leptospirosis**, **meningitis**, **hepatitis**, or other viral HFs.

Ebola Case Count and Location					
Year	**Ebola species**	**Country**	**No. of human cases**	**Reported no. (%) of deaths among cases**	**Situation**
1976	Ebola-Zaire	Zaire	318	280 (88%)	Occurred in Yambuku and surrounding area. Disease was spread by close personal contact and by use of contaminated needles and syringes in hospitals/clinics. This was the first recognition of the disease.
1976	Ebola-Sudan	Sudan	284	151 (53%)	Occurred in Nzara, Maridi and the surrounding area. Disease was spread mainly through close personal contact within hospitals. Many medical care personnel were infected.
1976	Ebola-Sudan	England	1	0 (0%)	Laboratory infection by accidental stick of contaminated needle.
1977	Ebola-Zaire	Zaire	1	1 (100%)	Noted retrospectively in the village of Tandala.
1979	Ebola-Sudan	Sudan	34	22 (65%)	Occurred in Nzara. Recurrent outbreak at the same site as the 1976 Sudan epidemic.
1989	Ebola-Reston	USA	0	0 (0%)	Ebola-Reston virus was introduced into quarantine facilities in Virginia and Pennsylvania by monkeys imported from the Philippines.
1990	Ebola-Reston	USA	4 (asymptomatic)	0 (0%)	Ebola was introduced once again into quarantine facilities in Virginia and Texas by monkeys imported from the Philippines. Four humans developed antibodies but did not get sick.
1989-1990	Ebola-Reston	Philippines	3 (asymptomatic)	0 (0%)	High mortality among cynomolgus macaques in a primate facility responsible for exporting animals in the USA. Three workers in the animal facility developed antibodies but did not get sick.
1992	Ebola-Reston	Italy	0	0 (0%)	Ebola-Reston was introduced into quarantine facilities in Sienna by monkeys imported from the same export facility in the Philippines that was involved in the episodes in the United States. No humans were infected.
1994	Ebola-Zaire	Gabon	52	31 (60%)	Occurred in Mékouka and other gold-mining camps deep in the rain forest. Initially thought to be yellow Fever; identified as Ebola hemorrhagic fever in 1995.
1994	Ebola-Ivory Coast	Ivory Coast	1	0 (0%)	Scientist became ill after conducting an autopsy on a wild chimpanzee in the Tai Forest. The patient was treated in Switzerland.
1995	Ebola-Zaire	Zaire	315	250 (81%)	Occurred in Kikwi and surrounding area. Traced to index case-patient who worked in forest adjoining the city. Epidemic spread through families and hospitals.
1996 (Jan-Apr)	Ebola-Zaire	Gabon	37	21 (57%)	Occurred in Mayibout area. A chimpanzee found dead in the forest was eaten by people hunting for food. Nineteen people who were involved in the butchery of the animal became ill; other cases occurred in family members.
1996 (Jul-Jan)	Ebola-Zaire	Gabon	60	45 (74%)	Occurred in Booué area with transport of patients to Libreville. Index case-patient was a hunter who lived in a forest camp. Disease was spread by close contact with infected persons. A dead chimpanzee found in the forest at the time was determined to be infected.
1996	Ebola-Zaire	South Africa	2	1 (50%)	A medical professional traveled from Gabon to Johannesburg, South Africa, after having treated Ebola virus-infected patients and thus having been exposed to the virus there. He was hospitalized, and a nurse who took care of him became infected and died.

(Illustration by Electronic Illustrators Group. © 2013 Cengage Learning)

Year	Ebola species	Country	No. of human cases	Reported no. (%) of deaths among cases	Situation
1996	Ebola-Reston	USA	0	0 (0%)	Ebola-Reston virus was introduced into a quarantine facility in Texas by monkeys imported from the Philippines. No human infections were identified.
1996	Ebola-Reston	Philippines	0	0 (0%)	Ebola-Reston virus was identified in a monkey export facility in the Philippines. No human infections were identified.
2000-2001	Ebola-Sudan	Uganda	425	224 (53%)	Occurred in Gulu, Masindi, and Mbarara districts of Uganda. The three most important risks associated with Ebola virus infection were attending funerals of Ebola hemorrhagic case-patients, having contact with case-patients in one's family, and providing medical care to Ebola case-patients without adequate personal protective measures.
2001-2001 (Oct'01 Mar'02)	Ebola-Zaire	Gabon	65	53 (82%)	Outbreak occurred over the border of Gabon and the Republic of the Congo.
2001-2002 (Oct'01 Mar'02)	Ebola-Zaire	Republic of the Congo	57	43 (75%)	Outbreak occurred over the border of Gabon and the Republic of the Congo. This was the first time Ebola hemorrhagic fever was reported in the Republic of the Congo.
2002-2003 (Dec'02 Apr'03)	Ebola-Zaire	Republic of the Congo	143	128 (89%)	Outbreak occurred in the districts of Mbomo and Kéllé in Cuvette Ouest Département.
2003 (Nov-Dec)	Ebola-Zaire	Republic of the Congo	35	29 (83%)	Outbreak occurred in Mbomo and Mbandza villages located in the Mbomo district, Cuvette Ouest Département
2004	Ebola-Sudan	Sudan	17	7 (41%)	Outbreak occurred in Yambio county of southern Sudan. This was concurrent with an outbreak of measles in the same area, and several suspected EHF cases were later reclassified as measles cases.
2007	Ebola-Zaire	Republic of the Congo	264	187 (71%)	Outbreak occurred in Kasai Occidental Province. The outbreak was declared over November 20. Last confirmed case on October 4 and last death on October 10.
Dec 2007 -Jan 2008	Ebola-Bundibugyo	Uganda	149	37 (25%)	Outbreak occurred in Bundibugyo District in Uganda. First reported occurrence of a new strain.
Nov 2008	Ebola-Reston	Philippines	6 (asymptomatic)	0 (0%)	First known occurrence of Ebola-Reston in pigs. Strain closely related to earlier strains. Six workers from the pig farm and slaughterhouse developed antibodies but did not become sick.
Dec 2008-Feb 2009	Ebola-Zaire	Democratic Republic of the Congo	32	15 (47%)	Outbreak occurred in the Mweka and Luebo health zones of the Province of Kasai Occidental.
May 2011	Ebola-Sudan	Uganda	1	1 (100%)	Single casein Luwero district, Uganda.
2012	Ebola-Sudan	Uganda	Ongoing	Ongoing	

(Illustration by Electronic Illustrators Group. © 2013 Cengage Learning)

If an Ebola infection is suspected, it can only be diagnosed definitively in the laboratory. Tests used to diagnose an Ebola infection are an antigen-capture enzyme-linked immunosorbent assay (ELISA) test, IGM ELISA, polymerase chain reaction assay, and virus isolation in cell culture within a few days of the appearance of the symptoms.

Treatment

There is no standard treatment for Ebola HF, nor is there any effective antiviral available. Patients are given supportive therapy, keeping their fluids and electrolytes in balance, monitoring their breathing and blood pressure, and treating any infections that may arise during the course of the illness.

Prevention

Because the natural reservoir of the virus is not known, there are few established **prevention** measures. For healthcare workers, the use of infection-control techniques, such as not reusing needles and completely sterilizing equipment, are important, as are the use of barrier garments such as gloves, gowns, and masks.

Those who work with victims of the virus must be cautious when handling the bodies of the dead to prevent direct contact with potentially infections fluids and tissues.

Efforts and Solutions

During the July and August 2012 outbreak in western Uganda, WHO provided expertise and support to healthcare workers and to those who had been thought to have the virus. Because their personal belongings had been buried or burned when they were suspected of being infected, people who tested negative would have been left with nothing. WHO provided a discharge package that included clothing, mattresses, and money to buy replacement goods to these people before they returned to their homes. WHO workers accompanied patients home and explained to fellow villagers that they had nothing to fear from the patient. The work of these social mobilization teams, including WHO staff, help educate people about the virus, reintegrate former patients, and rebuild community life.

KEY TERMS

virus—a parasitic microorganism that is smaller than a bacterium and has no independent metabolic activity. It is able to replicate only within a cell of a living plant or animal host.

zoonotic—a disease of animals that can be passed to humans.

Resources

PERIODICALS

Carette, J.E. et al. "Ebola virus entry requires the cholesterol transporter Niemann-Pick C1." *Nature* 477 340-343 (15 September 2011).

Whitehead Institute for Biomedical Research (2011, August 24). "Scientists identify point of entry for deadly Ebola virus." *Science Daily.* Accessed August 18, 2012. http://www.sciencedaily.com/releases/2011/08/110824131549.htm

WEBSITES

Centers for Disease Control and Prevention. "Ebola Hemorrhagic Fever Information Packet," accessed August 18, 2012, http://www.cdc.gov/ncidod/dvrd/spb/mnpages/dispages/Fact_Sheets/Ebola_Fact_Booklet.pdf

World Health Organization, "Ebola haemorrhagic fever," accessed August 18, 2012, http://www.who.int/mediacentre/factsheets/fs103/en

World Health Organization, "The journey home after having tested negative for Ebola," accessed August 23, 2012, http://www.who.int/features/2012/ebola/en/index.html

ORGANIZATIONS

Centers for Disease Control and Prevention, 1600 Clifton Road, Atlanta, GA USA 30333, (800) 232-4636, cdcinfo@cdc.gov, www.cdc.gov.

World Health Organization, Avenue Appia 20, 1211 Geneva 27, Switzerland 30333, 41 22 (791) 21 11, Fax: 41 22 (791) 21 11, www.who.int.

Fran Hodgkins

Economic and financial stress

Definition

Economic and financial **stress** is stress caused by a person's money or financial situation and is generally a reaction to the threat or worry of not having enough money to meet basic living needs. This perceived threat, known as a stressor, may result from an unanticipated situation or event that threatens a person's financial stability, or it may be experienced by those who have not yet been able to obtain financial stability.

Demographics

According to the American Psychological Association's *Stress in America* report, in 2011, 75% of Americans cited money as a source of stress. Additional stressors included the general economy (67%), work (70%), and relationships with spouse, children, friends, and others (58%). Overall, women were more likely to report that stress had an effect on their health than did men (88% compared to 78%). Among different age groups, adults aged 19–64 were more likely to name money as their top source of stress than seniors (65+), who cited health problems.

Description

Economic and financial stress may be arise from a number of circumstances, such as losing a job, moving, going to college, applying for a loan, incurring credit debt, having a child, or buying a house, to name a few. One of the potential factors in developing financial stress is a perceived sense of loss of control, especially when the circumstances surrounding financial stress are unpreventable or unforeseen. A person with a financial "safety net," who can maintain control of his or her life in the event of a layoff or loss of investments, for example, will experience relatively less stress and anxiety from the adverse event. Also, persons who consider their socioeconomic status to be based not only on financial resources but on other factors such as social connections and educational level may feel more optimistic when facing the threat of a financial disruption.

Most approaches to understanding stress emphasize that the cognitive evaluation of an event—that is, how a person thinks about the event—is what leads to the reaction of stress or no stress. After an adverse event, such as the loss of a job, the person evaluates the effects of the event and the amount of resources he or she has to deal with the adversity. If the strength of the resources—financial, social, and psychological—is greater than the strength of the adversity—reduced income—there is less stress. However, if the strength of the adversity is greater than the strength of the resources, there is greater stress. The amount of money a person needs is relative—as a person becomes accustomed to having less, the change in the standard of living starts to feel normal, and what is perceived as normal does not generally cause stress.

Relative deprivation

People tend to compare their circumstances with their peers. If a person perceives him- or herself to have less than friends or neighbors, the person may feel that his or her finances are inadequate. This is known as relative deprivation. Relative deprivation suggests that our evaluation of what is "normal" does not only rest on our own experience but is affected by the experience of others.

Learned helplessness

Another psychological effect of stress is learned helplessness. If rats in a cage receive an electric shock, they will move from the place of the shock to another part of the cage. However, if they receive a shock no matter where in the cage they go, they will lie down and accept the shock. When faced with a stressor, humans look for ways to deal with the threat, but if attempts all fail, learned helplessness—often in the form of depression—can develop. Anyone demonstrating the symptoms of agitation, lethargy, and depression in response to an aversive financial event may be experiencing economic and financial stress.

Finances and satisfaction with life

Money and financial stability do not necessarily equate with happiness. Satisfaction with life is considered a good resource against stress, although it may not prevent stress completely. A measure of satisfaction with life, as developed by psychologist Ed Diener, considers conditions such as having few regrets and achieving major goals. In the United States, for example, income has increased over the years, while measures of happiness have remained stable. Since the 1930s, the U.S. government has reported the average per-person income, and since the late 1950s, the National Opinion Research Center has asked participants in a survey study how happy they considered themselves. Although the buying power of individual Americans has steadily increased by nearly three times since 1957, the number of persons describing themselves as "very happy" has remained at close to 30%. If more money led to more happiness, the percentage of people rating themselves as "very happy" should have increased in relation to the increase in disposable income. Happiness is not connected directly with the amount of money one has, and among those who are meeting at least their basic needs (food, shelter), there is no correlation between the amount of income and satisfaction with life.

Risk factors

In general, anyone who misjudges his or her financial security is at risk for economic and financial stress. Those who either do not make financial goals or who strive for unrealistic financial goals are also at risk for economic and financial stress. Further, people who continuously live

Percentage of American adults (age 18+) experiencing debt stress, 2009–2011

HOW OFTEN DO YOU WORRY ABOUT THE TOTAL AMOUNT YOU (AND YOUR SPOUSE/PARTNER) OWE IN OVERALL DEBT?

	May/June 2009	November 2009	May 2010	November 2010	June 2011
All/most of the time	19%	23%	21%	20%	20%
All of the time	9%	11%	10%	9%	9%
Most of the time	10%	12%	11%	11%	11%
Some of the time	29%	27%	28%	25%	29%
Hardly ever/not at all	47%	45%	49%	52%	46%
Hardly ever	26%	20%	23%	23%	20%
Not at all	22%	25%	25%	29%	26%
No debt	5%	4%	2%	3%	5%
Don't know	*	*	*	*	*
Refused	*	*	*	*	1%
Total number of persons interviewed	**1,000**	**1,006**	**1,002**	**1,000**	**1,001**

HOW MUCH STRESS DOES THE TOTAL DEBT YOU CARRY CAUSE YOU (AND YOUR SPOUSE/PARTNER)?

	May/June 2009	November 2009	May 2010	November 2010	June 2011
Great deal/quite a bit of stress	17%	22%	20%	18%	16%
Great deal of stress	8%	12%	10%	7%	8%
Quite a bit of stress	9%	11%	10%	11%	8%
Some stress	29%	28%	26%	23%	31%
Not very much/no stress at all	54%	49%	53%	59%	53%
Not very much stress	28%	23%	25%	26%	23%
No stress at all	27%	26%	28%	33%	30%
Don't know	*	*	*	*	*
Refused	-	1%	*	*	1%
Total number of persons interviewed	**941**	**964**	**976**	**973**	**956**

SOURCE: GfK Roper Public Affairs & Corporate Communications, "A Telephone Survey of the American General Population (Ages 18+)," *The AP-GfK Poll*, June 2011.

(Table by PreMediaGlobal. © 2013 Cengage Learning)

beyond their means will eventually face the consequences that lead to economic and financial stress.

Causes and symptoms

It is a common perception that an aversive financial event is the cause of the economic and financial stress. However, the unpleasant event itself is not a stressor—it is the subjective evaluation of the event as a threat that makes it a stressor. As the stock market dips, a multimillionaire might lose more money in one day than most people make in a lifetime. Although unpleasant, this event is not a threat to the multimillionaire, who does not have to change his or her lifestyle or daily pattern.

The physiological effects of stress are the release of hormones usually reserved for reactions to physical danger. When faced with life-threatening situations, the body responds with a "fight-or-flight" reaction—the decision to fight the threat or run away. Natural selection developed "fight or flight" to increase survivability in the face of environmental threats to life. However, modern humans have been shown to react similarly to psychological and social threats. These physiological reactions over time can reduce the efficiency of the immune system. Symptoms of the "fight-or-flight" response include involuntary muscle contractions, increased heart rate, and trouble breathing.

Research shows that the physiological effects of stress are often manifested in specific, observable emotional reactions, such as irritability, anger, and depression. In the 2012 APA study, respondents reported experiencing the following emotions in response to increased stress:

- Irritability or anger (42% of respondents)
- Nervousness or anxiety (39%)
- Fatigue (37%)
- Depression or sadness (37%)
- Lack of interest, motivation or energy (35%)
- Headache (32%)
- Feeling as though one could cry (30%)
- Muscular tension (24%)
- Indigestion (24%)

Treatment

Economic and financial stress may be alleviated by finding a solution to the perceived problem. For instance, if the stressor is loss of a job, then searching for a new job may help reduce the stress. If the stressor is credit card debt, cutting up the credit cards to avoid accumulating further debt may help ease anxiety. If the stress persists and begins to interfere with activities of daily life, such as fulfilling familial responsibilities or socializing with friends, the person may wish to see a doctor or therapist to learn about other treatment options.

General treatments for stress

TRADITIONAL. Traditional psychotherapy focuses on the patient understanding his or her financial situation clearly. The humanistic approach to counseling encourages individuals to recognize their personal value, which may help counteract any feelings of diminished worth based on financial difficulties. Humanistic counseling often leads participants to more social interactions, which can shift their focus from a financial perspective to deriving pleasure from relationships.

DRUGS. Doctors do not usually prescribe drugs for treatment of commonplace stress brought on by financial difficulties. Some patients may use over-the-counter analgesics but should still discuss this option with their physician. If the stress becomes unmanageable, the doctor might prescribe an antianxiety medication.

ALTERNATIVE. Alternative stress management techniques are widely used and are easy for people to do at home. A person might keep a daily record of the onset of stress-related reactions, noting the exact time of the onset, whatever thoughts he or she might have had at the onset, and any events that prompted the onset. A therapist can then help the patient evaluate the record and identify any unknown stressors. If the patient recognizes that he or she is putting too much value into these stressors, including financial worries, then the stress reactions may be reduced.

Other alternative therapies include meditation, relaxation techniques, massage, yoga, exercise, aromatherapy, and more.

Home remedies

The best thing a person can do to treat financial stress is to organize his or her financial situation. Balancing the household budget is a great first step in regaining control of finances. The person should analyze his or her monthly spending and identify costs that are necessities (e.g., rent, food, bills) and those that are luxuries (e.g., dinners out, entertainment). By allotting a portion of income each month to cover all of the necessities, the person is able to see how much is left for luxuries, helping avoid unnecessary spending.

KEY TERMS

"Fight-or-flight" response—A function of the autonomic nervous system that prepares the brain to make an immediate decision to deal with a sudden threat.

Learned helplessness—The tendency to give up on solving a problem when efforts appear to bring no results.

Meditation—Technique of concentration for relaxing the mind and body.

Relative deprivation—The tendency to base one's criteria for normalcy on comparisons with neighbors and relatives.

"Satisfaction with Life"—Term coined by psychologist Ed Diener as a level of satisfaction determined by acceptance of the past, contentment with the present, and optimism for the future.

Socioeconomic status—Perceived status of an individual, family or community based on average income, education level, and social status.

Prevention

Though some circumstances surrounding economic and financial stress are not preventable, such as the state of the national economy or job layoffs, creating and following a budget can help to prevent some financial stress. Saving money, even a little bit at a time, can also help to prevent stress and may help to relieve stress when an unforeseen financial event does arise.

Resources

BOOKS

Perrewe, Pamela L., Jonathan Halbesleben, and Christopher C. Rosen, eds. *The Role of the Economic Crisis on Occupational Stress and Well Being*. Bingley, UK: Emerald Group Publishing, 2012.

Sasseville, Angela. *Families Under Financial Stress: Tools to Support Your Relationships and Your Continual Growth.* Concord, NH: Hummingbird Press, 2011.

PERIODICALS

Freshman, A. "Financial Disaster as a Risk Factor for Posttraumatic Stress Disorder: Internet Survey of Trauma in Victims of the Madoff Ponzi Scheme." *Health and Social Work* 37, 1. (2012): 39–48.

Uutela, Antti. "Economic Crisis and Mental Health." *Current Opinion in Psychiatry* 23, 2. (2010): 127–30.

Wahlbeck, Kristian, and David McDaid. "Actions to Alleviate the Mental Health Impact of the Economic Crisis." *World Psychiatry* 11, 3. (2012): 139–45.

WEBSITES

American Psychological Association. "Psychology Topics: Money." http://www.apa.org/topics/money/index.aspx (accessed October 18, 2012).

American Psychological Association. *Stress in America: Our Health at Risk*. Washington, DC: American Psychological Association, 2012. http://www.apa.org/news/press/releases/stress/2011/final-2011.pdf. Accessed on October 18, 2012.

Cox, Lauren. "Financial Stress: How Bad Can it Get?" ABC News. http://abcnews.go.com/Health/story?id=5867963&page=1#.TrMxY3LMqQw. Accessed on October 18, 2012.

Turner, Jo. "Coping with Financial Stress." University of Florida Extension, Institute of Food and Agricultural Sciences. http://miami-dade.ifas.ufl.edu/old/programs/efnep/publications/Coping-with-Financial-Stress.PDF. Accessed on October 18, 2012.

ORGANIZATIONS

American Institute of Stress, 124 Park Avenue, Yonkers, NY 10703, (914) 963-1200, stress125@optonline.net, http://www.stress.org.

American Psychological Association, 750 1st St. NE, Washington, DC 20002-4242, (202) 336-5500; TDD/TTY: (202) 336-6123, (800) 374-2721, http://www.apa.org.

National Institute of Mental Health, 6001 Executive Blvd., Rm. 8184, MSC 9663, Bethesda, MD 20892-9663, (301) 443-4513, (866) 615-6464, nimhinfo@nih.gov, http://www.nimh.nih.gov.

Ray F. Brogan, Ph.D.

Emergency health services

Definition

The term emergency health services refers to all those services and procedures put into service immedicately following a medical emergency, such as a heart attack or a traffic accident, up to and including a patient's appearance at the emergency department (ED) of a hospital or other medical facility. Emergency health services are also known by a number of other names, including emergency medical services (EMS), first aid squad, emergency squad, rescue squad, ambulance squad, ambulance service, ambulance corps, and life squad.

Purpose

The purpose of emergency health services (EHS) is to make available to a person who has suddenly and unexpectedly become ill or injured the very best medical care available as quickly as possible.

Description

The history of emergency health services dates to the end of the eighteenth century when Baron Dominique-Jean Larrey, chief physician in the French army, developed a system for moving injured soldiers from the battlefield to field hospitals. The first such services for civilians in the United States were put into place in Cincinnati in 1865 and in New York City in 1869. The modern EHS system is generally dated to the publication of a report by the Committee on Trauma and Committee on Shock of the National Research Council in 1966 that pointed out the inadequacies of the existing health care system for caring for emergency medical cases and made 29 recommendations for the establishment of a more efficient system for handling such emergencies. To a considerable extent, those recommendations have become the core of the modern emergency health system.

The core elements of an EHS are a toll–free telephone number (such as 911) that connects a caller with a central dispatch station and some type of ambulance staffed with individuals specially trained to deal with emergency medical problems. These individuals (usually called paramedics or emergency medical technicians [EMTs]) are trained in first aid and the treatment of medical emergencies such as trauma, heart attacks, strokes, and minor injuries. This team delivers injured or ill individuals to special centers called *emergency departments*, which have more extensive and more sophisticated equipment and personnel for treating a variety of health emergencies. Emergency departments were once called *emergency rooms*, with the name change reflecting the extended variety of technologies available for dealing with health emergencies.

Paramedics and EMTs are required to have the equivalent of college degree in some developed nations, such as Australia, South Africa, and the United Kingdom. Requirements are less severe in the United States, where some level of postsecondary education is required to obtain a license as an EMT or paramedic. All states do require licenses for the job, but specific requirements vary from state to state. Most states base their training requirements for EMTs and paramedics on the National Standard Curriculum for EMTs and paramedics, developed by the U.S. Department of

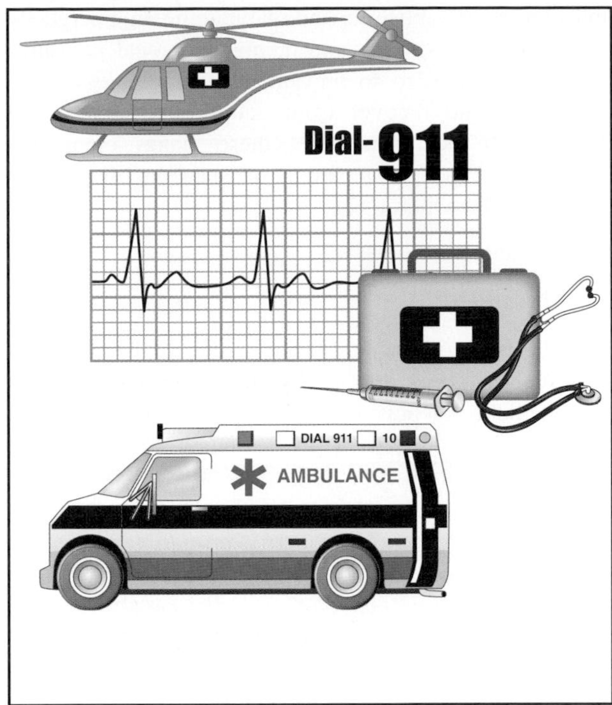

(Illustration by Electronic Illustrators Group. © 2013 Cengage Learning)

Transportation. Training programs tend to range in length from six months to two years. Some efforts are now underway to increase the professionalization of EMT and paramedic occupations, with a small number of colleges and universities offering bachelor degrees in the field. The University of Maryland, for example, offers both a bachelor's and a master's degree in emergency health management. These degrees allow a person not only to be involved in the traditional day–to–day work of an EMT or paramedic, but also to take administrative and supervisory responsibilities in emergency health programs. In addition, professional organizations have been formed to raise the level of skills and performance for EMTs and paramedics. One such organization is the National Association of Emergency Medical Technicians (NAEMT). Most EMTs and paramedics are now expected to have certificates from the National Registry of Emergency Medical Technicians, which offers classes and conducts examinations that lead to certification.

Professional Publications

The NAEMT publishes and distributes a wide variety of textbooks, workbooks, study guides, instructor manuals, field guides, DVDs, software, and other print and electronic materials dealing with emergency health issues. Included in this list are titles such as *Trauma Case Studies for the Paramedic, Exam Prep Paramedic, Paramedic Review Manual for National Certification, Atlas of Paramedic Skills, Street Scenarios, ALS Skills Review, Medical Case Studies for the Paramedic, Patient Assessment Handbook*, and *Drug Guide for Paramedics Pocket Reference*.

Resources

BOOKS

Batsie, Daniel A., Joseph J. Mistovich, and Daniel Limmer. *Topics for the Paramedic*. Boston: Brady, 2012.

DiPrima, Peter A. *Paramedic Survival Guide*. New York: McGraw-Hill Medical, 2012.

PERIODICALS

Ame, Jeremy T., et al. "The Core Content of Emergency Medical Services Medicine." *Prehospital Emergency Care*. 16. 3. (2012): 309–22.

Ragone, M. "Evolution or Revolution: EMS Industry Faces Difficult Changes." *JEMS: A Journal of Emergency Medical Services*. 37. 2. (2012): 34–9.

WEBSITES

EMSWorld. http://www.emsworld.com/ (accessed October 10, 2012).

JEMS Emergency Medical Services. http://www.jems.com/ (accessed October 10, 2012).

ORGANIZATIONS

National Association of Emergency Medical Technicians (NAEMT), PO Box 1400, Clinton, MS 39060–1400, (601) 924-7744, (800) 34-NAEMT, Fax: (601) 924-7325, info@naemt.org, http://www.naemt.org/.

David E. Newton, Ed.D.

Emergency preparedness

Definition

Emergency preparedness refers to precautions taken before an emergency or disaster to minimize the extent of damage and the impact on persons and property, as distinct from emergency response and recovery, which refer to measures taken after the event. Emergency preparedness may be considered the first phase of emergency management. It can be subdivided into two phases, mitigation and direct preparedness.

It is important to distinguish among emergencies, disasters, and catastrophes, even though the words are often used interchangeably in ordinary speech, because different types of planning and preparation are required to prevent or respond to these situations. The definitions used most often by emergency management professionals are as follows:

- Emergency: A localized unplanned event with the capacity to endanger life or property, disrupt business and other community activities, damage the environment, or threaten public safety, and which requires a comprehensive community-wide response. Examples of emergencies include such events as house fires, plane crashes, workplace or school shootings, and storms or other weather events that affect a relatively small area.
- Disaster: A large-scale event that differs from a local emergency in several respects: local organizations lose some of their capacity to respond; a greater degree of coordination among public- and private-sector organizations is needed; and standards of performance change (such as normal speed of response or standards of care). Examples of disasters include chemical spills or explosions; disease epidemics; dam or power plant failures; major floods, tornadoes, or forest fires; and large-scale terrorist attacks.
- Catastrophe: Catastrophes are distinguished from disasters in that most or all structures and functions are destroyed or interrupted simultaneously over a wide area; first responders and other personnel are themselves injured or affected by the event; and help from outside the affected area is not immediately available. Examples of catastrophes include major earthquakes followed by tsunamis, acts of warfare involving nuclear weapons, and disease pandemics.

Purpose

Public health organizations typically have well-thought-out and detailed plans for dealing with the everyday challenges they face in helping individuals and communities maintain a good health status and preventing disease and injury. They may be less well prepared to deal with disasters that arrive unexpectedly, produce a large number of casualities, disrupt the normal function of health agencies, and pose other unforeseen problems for a community. In such cases, large numbers of individuals may be placed at high risk for injury and disease, which a health agency's normal program is unprepared to deal with. Emergency preparedness programs are developed by health agencies to deal with these unexpected events.

Description

Emergency preparedness is a cycle of planning, training, and equipping first responders and volunteer emergency workers, stockpiling necessary equipment and supplies, establishing and maintaining an emergency communication system, and taking additional measures that may be needed to prevent, respond to, lessen the impact of, and recover from natural or human-made disasters. In actual practice, these stages or phases overlap; emergency preparedness is an ongoing set of activities rather than a final goal.

Mitigation

Mitigation is the first stage or phase of emergency preparedness. It is defined by the Federal Emergency Management Agency (FEMA) as "the effort to reduce loss of life and property by lessening the impact of disasters." It can also be defined as taking action in the present before a disaster occurs to prevent human and financial losses later. Mitigation is primarily undertaken at the community, state, or federal level in the United States.

Mitigation has four major aspects:

- Hazard identification. A hazard is defined as any agent or structure, whether biological, chemical, mechanical, or other, that is likely to cause harm to humans or the environment in the absence of protective measures. Hazards may be either natural or human-made; they include geographic features or weather patterns that increase the risk of natural disasters; methods of transportation (which are all inherently risky); unstable structures (weak dams or bridges, poorly designed buildings); waste dumps; chemical plants and oil refineries; biological disease agents or vectors; and others. Hazards are sometimes categorized as dormant (potentially dangerous but inactive at present) or active (the hazard is presently causing harm). Hazard identification is the process of detecting and evaluating the natural or human-made hazards present in the local community.
- Risk assessment. Risk assessment is the process of calculating the probability that a specific hazard will endanger the community and the extent of damage that is likely if the hazard becomes active. Risk is defined as the probability that exposure to a hazard will lead to a negative consequence (physical harm or death, property damage). A mathematical equation that is commonly used in risk assessment is as follows: Risk = Hazard x Dose (Exposure).
- Risk reduction. Risk reduction refers to strategies undertaken to lower the chance that a dormant hazard will become active, or to remove the hazard altogether. Risk reduction may include building codes, land use regulations, public health surveillance, measures to control air pollution, relocation of hazardous materials,

strengthening of bridges and dams, and similar measures.

- Insurance. FEMA provides insurance against flood damage at the state and community level. Individuals and homeowners may purchase insurance to protect themselves against financial loss in the event of illness, injury, or property damage.

Community emergency preparedness

FEMA identifies five stages in emergency preparedness at the community level following mitigation and risk assessment:

- Planning. Planning involves establishing procedures for operating during an emergency, including coordinating the activities of such different groups as firefighters, law enforcement, search and rescue personnel, emergency medical technicians, and the like. Planning also includes the identification of schools or other large buildings that could serve as emergency shelters. Another important part of planning is the establishment and maintenance of an effective emergency communication network. The Chemical Safety and Hazard Investigation Board (CSB) has repeatedly found that communication is one of the weakest aspects of many community emergency plans.
- Organizing and equipping. This stage involves the purchase and maintenance of emergency response equipment and the stockpiling of food, water, medicines, vaccines, batteries, generators, and other supplies that are usually required in emergencies.
- Training. Training involves providing first responders, civilian volunteers, military personnel, public health officials, and others with the information they need to respond effectively to different types of emergencies. The Centers for Disease Control and Prevention (CDC) classifies emergencies under six major categories: natural disasters and severe weather; bioterrorism; chemical emergencies; extreme heat and wildfires; mass casualty incidents (explosions, blasts, terrorist attacks); and radiation emergencies. Each of these requires specific understanding of the types of injuries most likely to result from the emergency, the possible scale of the emergency, and the most effective ways to coordinate responses to the emergency. There are training institutes at the national level for some groups of emergency workers, such as the National Fire Academy and the Emergency Management Institute.
- Exercising. Exercising refers to regularly scheduled events at the local and regional level in which first responders and civilian volunteers practice and rehearse lifesaving skills, search and rescue procedures, triage and trauma treatment, use of firefighting and other emergency equipment, and other skills that are needed in the event of an actual emergency. The goal is for these skills to become virtually automatic. Simulated accidents and emergencies are commonly included in these exercises.
- Evaluating and improving. This stage involves regular inspection of emergency equipment and facilities as well as evaluation of training programs and post-event critiquing of practice exercises.

In addition to first responders, civilian volunteers and military personnel may assist in responding to a community-level emergency. The Department of Homeland Security (DHS) has a Community Emergency Response Team (CERT) program that educates people about emergency preparedness for their local community and trains them in the specific skills needed to help survivors of an emergency. Training includes classroom instruction and simulation exercises; it covers fire safety, disaster medicine, terrorism, light search and rescue procedures, psychological issues in disasters, and team building and organization. More information about CERT is available at the link below.

Military personnel involved in emergency preparedness often include units of the National Guard as well as members of the various branches of the armed forces from nearby bases or installations. They may serve as instructors as well as participants in training exercises and CERT programs.

Household emergency preparedness

The American Red Cross and the **CDC** have joined together to provide a three-step program for emergency preparedness for households. A module detailing the three steps can be viewed at http://www.redcross.org/prepare/location/home-family. The three steps are:

- Get a kit. Sometimes called a 72-hour kit, the kit is a collection of food, water, and other supplies sufficient for survival for three days. FEMA recommends the following contents for the kit: one gallon of water per person per day for three days, nonperishable food items for each person for three days, a battery-powered or hand-crank radio and extra batteries, a flashlight for each person and extra batteries, a cell phone and charger, first aid kit, whistle, filter mask or cotton T-shirt for each person, moist towelettes, garbage bags and plastic ties, wrench or pliers, manual can opener, plastic sheeting and duct tape, important family documents, daily prescription medicine, emergency blankets, a map of the area, and special-needs items for infants, pets, and disabled family members.

- Make a plan. Planning includes discussing emergency plans with all family members on a regular basis, and assigning roles and responsibilities; setting up places to meet if the family is separated during an emergency; practicing evacuating (including traveling the evacuation route twice a year) if evacuation is necessary; setting up a safe room (a room that is tornado- or hurricane-proof) in the house if sheltering in place is necessary; and deciding on a contact person outside the area who can be notified in the event of an emergency.
- Be informed. This step includes familiarizing family members with local communications networks and procedures for notifying residents of an emergency; knowing the differences between various types of weather alerts and watches; finding out what (if any) hazards are present in the area; and ideally, having at least one member of the family trained in first aid and CPR.

The Red Cross and CDC offer additional information about emergency preparedness for vulnerable family members, such as the elderly, children, persons with disabilities, and pets.

Effects on public health

The effects of emergency preparedness on public health include closer coordination of local boards of public health and public health workers with emergency management experts and first responders. Increasing numbers of public health personnel participate in CERT programs and region-wide disaster simulations. Courses on emergency preparedness are offered in most schools of public health, and there are now several public health journals in the field, such as *Disaster Medicine and Public Health Preparedness*, published by the American Medical Association.

One important aspect of the relationship between public health and emergency preparedness is the matter of ethics. The health emergencies associated with disasters require triage and priority-setting and may require overriding the rights of individuals and property owners. Given the American tradition of respect for the individual, public health workers should take the ethical and social values of a community into account before approving coercive measures; identify the persons or groups most likely to bear the burdens of government use of power or coercion; and monitor the use of power when emergency plans must be carried out.

Efforts and solutions

Efforts and solutions in the field of public health include training programs and communications networks specific to the CDC and the Food and Drug Administration (FDA). The CDC website contains information regarding programs in disease surveillance, emergency preparedness for healthcare facilities, and training in risk communication and trauma management. The Health Alert Network (HAN) is a national program that provides emergency alerts, advisories, updates, and other public health-related information to state and local public health officers and epidemiologists.

The FDA's Center for Drug Evaluation and Research (CDER) assists public health workers in preparing medicines and vaccines against various forms of bioterrorism, **radiation** emergencies, and **emerging**

KEY TERMS

Emergency management—An overall term for organization and management procedures for critical events that includes response to, and recovery from, emergencies as well as emergency preparedness.

First responder—A generic term for the first medically trained responder to arrive at the scene of an emergency. First responders include police officers, firefighters, emergency medical technicians, and paramedics.

Hazard—In the context of emergency preparedness, a general term for any agent, whether biological, chemical, mechanical, or other, that is likely to cause harm to humans or the environment in the absence of protective measures.

Mitigation—A general term for attempts to prevent disasters or reduce their impact.

Pandemic—An epidemic of infectious disease that spreads over several continents or worldwide.

Risk—The probability that exposure to a hazard will have a negative consequence. There are mathematical equations and computer programs that can be used to calculate risk in specific situations.

Shelter in place—A phrase used to describe remaining indoors in a safe location during an emergency rather than evacuating the area.

Triage—A method for determining the priority of patient treatment during a disaster or mass casualty event according to the severity of the injuries.

Vector—In epidemiology, any person, animal, or microorganism that transmits a disease agent into another organism.

QUESTIONS TO ASK YOUR DOCTOR

- Have you ever participated in community meetings about emergency preparedness?
- Would you recommend participation in a CERT program? Is there one in our area?
- Are your own household and office prepared for an emergency?

diseases. The FDA also provides information about medication availability and safety during human-made and **natural disasters**, and coordinates responses to emergencies requiring large amounts of prescription medications or other regulated products.

Professional Publications

Many governmental, nongovernmental, and private health organizations have developed materials for use in preparing for and/or dealing with health emergencies. The **Centers for Disease Control and Prevention** is a particularly good example, with pamphlets, brochures, reports, and booklets on a number of emergency topics, such as *A Framework for Improving Cross-sector Coordination for Emergency Preparedness and Response: Action Steps for Public Health, Law Enforcement, the Judiciary, and Corrections*; *Public Health Preparedness: Mobilizing State by State: A CDC Report on the Public Health Emergency Preparedness Cooperative Agreement*; and *Public Health Preparedness: Strengthening the Nation's Emergency Response State by State: A Report on CDC–funded Preparedness and Response Activities in 50 States, 4 Cities, and 8 U.S. Insular Areas; A New Era of Preparedness*. Other governmental agencies, such as the **Environmental Protection Agency** and the Occupational Safety and Health Administration, also have similar resources.

Resources

BOOKS

Bernstein, Jonathan, with Bruce Bonafede. *Manager's Guide to Crisis Management*. New York: McGraw-Hill, 2011.

Creekmore, M.D. *31 Days to Survival: A Complete Plan for Emergency Preparedness*. Boulder, CO: Paladin Press, 2012.

Veenema, Tener Goodwin, ed. *Disaster Nursing and Emergency Preparedness for Chemical, Biological, and Radiological Terrorism and Other Hazards*, 3rd ed. New York: Springer, 2013.

Zhang, Derek C., ed. *Public Health Preparedness, Emergency Response and the CDC*. New York: Nova Science Publishers, 2011.

PERIODICALS

Centers for Disease Control and Prevention (CDC). "Household Preparedness for Public Health Emergencies—14 States, 2006–2010." *Morbidity and Mortality Weekly Report* 61 (September 14, 2012): 713–719.

Fernandez, E.R., et al. "Disaster Preparedness of Nationally Certified Emergency Medical Services Professionals." *Academic Emergency Medicine* 18 (April 2011): 403–412.

Gamboa-Maldonado, T., et al. "Building Capacity for Community Disaster Preparedness: A Call for Collaboration between Public Environmental Health and Emergency Preparedness and Response Programs." *Journal of Environmental Health* 75 (September 2012): 24–29.

Klima, D.A., et al. "Full-Scale Regional Exercises: Closing the Gaps in Disaster Preparedness." *Journal of Trauma and Acute Care Surgery* 73 (September 2012): 592–598.

Moore, M. "The Global Dimensions of Public Health Preparedness and Implications for U.S. Action." *American Journal of Public Health* 102 (June 2012): e1–e7.

Rambhia, K.J., et al. "A Survey of Hospitals to Determine the Prevalence and Characteristics of Healthcare Coalitions for Emergency Preparedness and Response." *Biosecurity and Bioterrorism* 10 (September 2012): 304–313.

Soomaroo, L., and V. Murray. "Weather and Environmental Hazards at Mass Gatherings." *PLoS Currents* (July 31, 2012): 4:e4fca9ee30afc4.

Vukotich, G., et al. "Prairie North: A Joint Civilian/Military Mass Casualty Exercise Highlights the Role of the National Guard in Community Disaster Response." *American Journal of Disaster Medicine* 7 (Winter 2012): 65–72.

WEBSITES

Are You Ready? An In-depth Guide to Citizen Preparedness. Federal Emergency Management Agency (FEMA). This is a 204-page manual regarding preparedness for most emergencies and disasters in PDF format. http://www.fema.gov/pdf/areyouready/areyouready_full.pdf (accessed October 11, 2012).

Community Emergency Response Team (CERT) Program. http://www.citizencorps.gov/cert/index.shtm (accessed October 12, 2012).

"Disaster Planning and Public Health." Hastings Center. This is an exploration of the ethical issues involved in public health responses to emergencies. http://www.thehastingscenter.org/Publications/BriefingBook/Detail.aspx?id=2160 (accessed October 13, 2012).

"Emergency Preparedness: Findings from CSB Accident Investigations." Engineering Failures: Case Studies in Engineering. This is a 21-minute video from the Chemical Safety and Hazard Investigation Board. http://engineeringfailures.org/?p=590 (accessed October 11, 2012).

"Emergency Preparedness and Response." Centers for Disease Control and Prevention (CDC). http://emergency.cdc.gov/ (accessed October 11, 2012),

"Emergency Preparedness and Response." Food and Drug Administration (FDA). http://www.fda.gov/Emergency-Preparedness/default.htm (accessed October 13, 2012).

"General Information for Disaster Preparedness and Response." Environmental Protection Agency (EPA).http://www.epa.gov/naturaldisasters/general.html (accessed October 9, 2012).

"Plan, Prepare, and Mitigate." Federal Emergency Management Agency (FEMA). https://www.fema.gov/plan-prepare-mitigate (accessed October 11, 2012).

"Plan and Prepare." American Red Cross. http://www.redcross.org/prepare (accessed October 12, 2012).

ORGANIZATIONS

American Red Cross, 2025 E Street, Washington, DC United States 20006, (202) 303-4498, (800) RED-CROSS (733-2767), http://www.redcross.org/.

Centers for Disease Control and Prevention (CDC), 1600 Clifton Road, Atlanta, GA United States 30333, (800) CDC-INFO (232-4636), http://www.cdc.gov/cdc-info/requestform.html, http://www.cdc.gov/.

Chemical Safety and Hazard Investigation Board (CSB), 2175 K Street NW, Washington, DC United States 20037, (202) 261-7600, Fax: (202) 261-7650, http://www.csb.gov/service/contact.aspx, http://www.csb.gov/.

Environmental Protection Agency (EPA), Ariel Rios Building, 1200 Pennsylvania Avenue, N.W., Washington, DC United States 20460, (202) 272-0167, http://www.epa.gov/.

Federal Emergency Management Agency (FEMA), 500 C Street SW, Washington, DC United States 20472, (202) 646-2500, (800) 621-3362, http://www.fema.gov/contact-us, http://www.fema.gov/.

Food and Drug Administration (FDA), 10903 New Hampshire Ave., Silver Spring, MD United States 20993-0002, (866) INFO-FDA (463-6332), http://www.fda.gov/default.htm.

National Institute of Environmental Health Sciences (NIEHS), P.O. Box 12233, MD K3-16, Research Triangle Park, NC United States 27709-2233, (919) 541-3345, Fax: (919) 541-4395, http://www.niehs.nih.gov/.

Rebecca J. Frey, Ph.D.

Emerging diseases

Definition

Emerging diseases, also known as emerging infectious diseases or EIDs, are defined by the National Institute of Allergy and Infectious Diseases (NIAID) as "outbreaks of previously unknown diseases or known diseases whose incidence in humans has significantly increased in the past two decades." The institute also defines reemerging diseases as "known diseases that have reappeared after a significant decline in incidence."

Description

NIAID classifies emerging diseases into three groups.

Group I: disease organisms newly recognized since 1990

Group I is the largest category of emerging diseases and pathogens. It includes:

- Acanthamebiasis. This is an inflammation of the brain (encephalitis) caused by an ameba belonging to the genus *Acanthamoeba*. It is a relatively rare disease in humans as of 2012 but has a survival rate of only 3%.
- Australian bat lyssavirus (ABLV). Lyssavirus is a disease agent closely related to the rabies virus. ABLV was first identified in Australia in 1996. It can be transmitted to humans directly from bats without an intermediate host but can be prevented and treated in the same way as rabies infection. There have been two known deaths from ABLV as of 2012.
- Atypical babesiosis. Babesiosis is a disease caused by a parasitic protozoon that ordinarily causes only mild fever and diarrhea in humans but is potentially fatal in persons with weakened immune systems. The disease is carried to humans through the bite of ticks living in the fur of the white-footed mouse.
- *Bartonella henselae*. *B. henselae* is the disease agent of cat-scratch fever, which usually causes swelling of the lymph nodes as well as fever in humans.
- Ehrlichiosis. Ehrlichiosis is a disease characterized by headache, muscle aches, and fatigue. It is caused by bacteria of the genus *Ehrlichia*, which are carried by mouse and deer ticks.
- *Encephalitozoon cuniculi* and *Encephalitozoon hellem*. These are two species of parasitic protozoa that cause an intestinal infection known as microsporidiosis in persons with weakened immune systems. Microsporidiosis is characterized by severe diarrhea and tissue wasting.
- *Enterocytozoon bieneusi*. *E. bieneusi* is another parasitic protozoon that was first discovered in an AIDS patient in France in 1985. In 1996, it was found that pigs are the largest animal reservoir of the parasite.
- *Helicobacter pylori*. *H. pylori* is a curved rod-shaped bacterium that was first discovered in 1982 and identified as the cause of gastric ulcers in humans—a stomach disorder that was not previously thought to have a microbial cause.
- Hendra virus. Hendra virus, sometimes referred to as equine morbillivirus, was first identified in Australia in 1994 when it cause the death of 13 horses and their

human trainer in Hendra, a suburb of Brisbane. Humans acquire the virus from close contact with horses. Four humans, including a veterinarian, have died of Hendra virus as of 2012.

- Hepatitis C and hepatitis E. These two forms of the hepatitis virus were discovered in 1989 and 1983, respectively. Hepatitis C exists only in humans and chimpanzees, while hepatitis E is commonly found in such animal reservoirs as pigs and deer.
- Human herpesvirus (HHV) 6 and HHV 8. Human herpesvirus 6 was first identified in 1986, with two subtypes, HHV-6A and HHV-6B. It is the cause of a childhood disease known as roseola infantum, characterized by fever and a reddish skin rash that lasts about two days. Human herpesvirus 8 is the virus associated with Kaposi's sarcoma, a skin cancer found in AIDS patients. HHV-8 was first identified in 1994.
- Lyme borreliosis. Lyme disease, also called Lyme borreliosis, was first diagnosed in Connecticut in 1978 although the disease agent, a bacterium belonging to the genus *Borrelia*, was not identified until 1981. Lyme disease is an emerging disease spread to humans by the bite of infected deer ticks.
- Parvovirus B19. Parvovirus B19 is a virus that causes a childhood disease called erythema infectiosum or slapped-cheek syndrome, so called because the affected person typically develops a bright red rash across the cheek area. It affects only humans. The virus may also cause chronic anemia in patients with AIDS.

Group II: reemerging disease organisms

Infectious diseases in this group include:

- Enterovirus 71. Enterovirus 71 is a virus that lives in the gut and is known to cause hand, foot and mouth disease (HFMD), a childhood infection characterized by fever, headache, and a red rash on the palms of the hands, soles of the feet, and the cheeks and area around the mouth. The virus is also capable, however, of causing severe and potentially fatal neurological disease in children.
- *Clostridium difficile*. *C. difficile* is a bacterium that lives in the human digestive tract; it can cause diarrhea and other intestinal disorders when the normal bacterial populations in the gut are wiped out by antibiotics.
- Mumps virus. Mumps virus infects only humans, where it causes a common childhood disease characterized by painful swelling of the salivary glands. It is vaccine-preventable, but has made a comeback in recent years due to opposition to compulsory vaccination on the part of some parents.
- Group A streptococci. Group A streptococci are a group of bacteria responsible for skin infections (erysipelas, impetigo), strep throat, septic arthritis, and pneumonia. Acute rheumatic fever is a potential complication of a respiratory infection caused by these bacteria.
- *Staphylococcus aureus*. *S. aureus* is a common cause of skin infections, food poisoning, and sinusitis. It is an increasing problem in hospitals worldwide because it has developed resistance to penicillin, methicillin, and other antibiotics.

Group III: disease agents with bioterrorism potential

NIAID subdivides these pathogens into three priority categories:

- Priority category A: Category A pathogens are the highest priority because they are easily transmitted from person to person; have high mortality rates; are likely to cause public panic and widespread social disruption; and require special actions for public health preparedness. They include the agents that cause anthrax, botulism, plague, tularemia (rabbit fever), dengue, smallpox, hantavirus infections, and the viral hemorrhagic fevers.
- Priority category B: Category B pathogens have a lower mortality rate than those in category A and are only moderately easy to disseminate. They include the agents that cause Q fever, West Nile fever, brucellosis, typhus, psittacosis (parrot fever), cholera, food poisoning (*Salmonella* and *Shigella* species), listeriosis, hepatitis A, toxoplasmosis, giardiasis, LaCrosse encephalitis, and Japanese encephalitis.
- Priority category C: Category C disease agents have the potential to be weaponized in the future because of their availability, ease of distribution, and potential for high mortality rates. They include the pathogens that cause multidrug-resistant tuberculosis, yellow fever, influenza, rabies, prion diseases (Creutzfeldt-Jakob disease and mad cow disease), SARS, and such emerging diseases as Nipah fever, a disease caused by a virus in the same family as Hendra virus.

Origins

In the 1960s, many epidemiologists thought that infectious diseases were on their way to being permanently controlled because of such medical advances as the discovery of **antibiotics** and the widespread use of pesticides in underdeveloped countries, which kill the mosquitoes that spread **malaria** and other insect-borne diseases. The appearance of previously unknown contagious diseases, including Legionnaires' disease in 1976 and a hantavirus outbreak in Korea in 1978, combined with a resurgence of such diseases as **tuberculosis** and malaria, led to a reexamination of the persistence of infectious diseases.

The specific phrase *emerging diseases* first appeared in the medical literature in 1971, but does not appear to have been widely used until the early 1990s, when an article by an epidemiologist working with the **World Health Organization (WHO)** titled "Surveillance and Control of Emerging Zoonoses" was published in the *World Health Statistics Quarterly*. *Emerging diseases* was originally applied to infectious diseases previously unknown in humans; later the term was extended to include diseases that have been diagnosed in humans for many years but have only recently been identified as caused by an infectious agent.

The number of EIDs that affect humans has quadrupled since 1960, largely because of human behavior, changing demographics, and changes in land use. Humans come into increasingly frequent contact with new disease organisms or become increasingly susceptible to known pathogens in the following ways:

- Overuse of antibiotics. The addition of antibiotics to animal feed to increase meat production as well as the overprescribing of antibiotics to humans (particularly for viral diseases, against which antibiotics are ineffective) has led to the development of resistant pathogens, allowing many diseases that were formerly treatable with drugs to make a comeback. These diseases include malaria, tuberculosis, foodborne infections, and nosocomial (hospital-acquired) infections.
- Frequent and increasingly rapid international travel. The introduction of jet airplanes for commercial travel in the 1950s speeded up not only international trade but also the spread of communicable diseases. SARS and AIDS are two emerging diseases that were spread worldwide by aircrews as well as travelers.
- Increased susceptibility to infection among some humans due to compromised immune systems. In addition to persons with AIDS and other diseases that weaken the immune system, persons taking immunosuppressant drugs to prevent rejection of a transplanted organ and those receiving chemotherapy for cancer are also susceptible to opportunistic infections.
- Opposition to vaccination programs. In Western countries, concern about the safety of vaccines—particularly the measles/mumps/rubella or MMR vaccine—led many parents to refuse vaccination for their children. The MMR vaccine controversy resulted from a 1998 paper published by a British medical researcher named Andrew Wakefield, who claimed that the vaccine caused autism and bowel disorders in some children. Although the paper was retracted in 2010, and Wakefield was subsequently charged with fraud, his 1998 article led to a sharp drop in the rate of vaccinations in the United Kingdom. There was a corresponding rise in the incidence of mumps and measles among British children, resulting in a number of deaths and permanent injuries.
- Changes in plant and animal habitats resulting from human interference with the natural environment—such as the widespread use of pesticides for disease control, deforestation in the tropics, and the expansion of human housing developments into previously intact temperate-zone forests. Lyme disease, for example, emerged as a human disease when the construction of new housing in central Connecticut chased away owls and other predators that kept the white-footed mouse population under control. When the mouse population multiplied fivefold, the infected deer ticks that live in the mouse's fur passed the bacteria that cause the disease to humans. Similarly, the Hendra virus emerged in Australia when infected fruit bats carrying the virus began to enter pastures and suburban back yards rather than remaining in the forests they previously inhabited. The movement of an EID from an animal reservoir to humans is known as spillover.
- Increased contact with exotic animals due to using them as food or keeping them as pets. The SARS virus is thought to have emerged into human communities in China, where the civet cats that carried the virus were used as meat. Similarly, there was an outbreak of monkeypox in the Midwestern United States in 2003 that was traced to an exotic animal dealer in Chicago who sold infected prairie dogs as pets.
- War and famine. People fleeing war zones or famine-stricken areas may carry emerging disease organisms with them to the countries where they seek refuge.
- Collapse of previously well-maintained systems of public health and hygiene. The recent political turmoil in Zimbabwe, for example, has led to the closure of hospitals, the emigration of most healthcare professionals, a rapid increase in the number of cases of HIV infection, and several outbreaks of cholera. The cholera epidemic has spread beyond Zimbabwe to Mozambique, Botswana, and Zambia as of 2012.
- Bioterrorism. The 2001 anthrax attacks that followed 9/11 in the United States offered a preview of the potential of weaponized disease organisms to cause widespread panic in the general public. Although only five people died (17 others were infected), thousands of fearful people requested prescriptions for ciprofloxacin (an antibiotic used to treat anthrax) from their doctors.

Demographics

One reason for concern about EIDs is their high death toll. Infectious diseases are the leading cause of death worldwide and the third highest cause of death in the United States. Most new emerging diseases—over 60%—are zoonoses; that is, they are transmitted to humans from animals. Of these zoonotic diseases, 70% originate in wildlife rather than domesticated animals or household pets.

An additional concern about EIDs is their capacity to interact with one another or with other diseases in ways that intensify the negative effects of each disease. The term *syndemic* has been coined to describe this type of disease combination. A syndemic differs from a comorbid condition in that it is possible for comorbid conditions to exist independently of each other even though the same patient has both disorders. An example of comorbidity would be a person who has both high blood pressure and arthritis. In a syndemic, by contrast, each illness worsens the virulence of the other. An example of a syndemic would be a patient who has both HIV and a herpesvirus infection; herpesvirus is known to speed the progression of HIV infection to full-blown **AIDS**. Syndemics associated with EIDs contribute significantly to the burden of disease worldwide.

Although some EIDs, such as Hendra virus, **SARS**, the hantaviruses, and acanthamebiasis are relatively uncommon as of 2012, the potential of others—particularly those caused by drug-resistant bacteria—to lead to epidemics or even pandemics affecting millions of people is of great concern to many epidemiologists. In addition, a bioterrorist attack involving any of the pathogens listed in NIAID's priority category A above has the potential to lead to open warfare between nations that would add to the death toll caused by the disease itself.

Efforts and solutions

Efforts to identify new EIDs and develop preventive measures against them include the following:

- Establishment of specialized research centers, programs, and publications to improve the identification and surveillance of new EIDs, and obtain a clearer understanding of their methods of transmission. The CDC has created a specialized center for research into EIDs, the National Center for Emerging and Zoonotic Infectious Diseases (NCEZID). NCEZID has a subsection called the Emerging Infections Programs or EIP. The EIP is a network of ten state health departments linked to schools of public health and clinical laboratories in their respective states. In addition, the CDC publishes a monthly specialized journal titled *Emerging Infectious Diseases*. The United States Army maintains the Armed Forces Health Surveillance Center in Silver Spring, Maryland, which focuses on EIDs of concern to military personnel stationed abroad, particularly those deployed in countries with tropical climates. Other recently established centers of research into EIDs include those at the University of California, Berkeley, and The Pennsylvania State University.
- Development of new vaccines, therapies, and diagnostic tests to detect and treat EIDs promptly and

KEY TERMS

Epidemic—An outbreak of a contagious disease that involves new cases of the disease in a specific human population during a given period substantially exceeding the number expected based on recent experience.

Incidence—The number of new cases of a specific disease within a specific time period within a specific population.

Opportunistic infection—An infection caused by pathogens that do not ordinarily cause disease in a healthy host but do produce disease in an immunocompromised person.

Pathogen—Any microorganism, virus, or other substance that causes disease in another organism.

Reservoir—In epidemiology, any species (including humans) that maintains a specific disease organism in nature.

Spillover—In epidemiology, the sporadic transmission of a disease agent from a reservoir species to a non-reservoir species.

Surveillance—In epidemiology, the monitoring and reporting of cases of contagious disease in order to establish patterns of its spread to prevent or minimize the development of epidemics and pandemics.

Syndemic—A combination of two or more diseases in a given population in which there is a positive biological interaction between the two diseases that intensifies their negative effects on health.

Virulence—The degree of a disease organism's ability to produce illness, as indicated by the mortality rate and/or the organism's ability to invade the host's tissues.

Zoonosis (plural, zoonoses)—Any disease that can be transmitted from animals to people or people to animals.

effectively. As of late 2012, there were 81 clinical trials registered with the National Institutes of Health to test the effectiveness of new vaccines, medications, and other treatments for EIDs ranging from hepatitis E and SARS to Group A streptococcal infections and West Nile virus.

- Setup and maintenance of international communication networks to monitor and report on EIDs. The International Society for Infectious Diseases (ISID) maintains a ProMED-mail system to facilitate international sharing of information and early warning about outbreaks of emerging and reemerging infectious diseases. ProMED stands for Program for Monitoring Emerging Diseases. More information about the system is available at the link below. The network currently links over 40,000 public health experts in 185 countries.
- Increasing cooperation among epidemiologists, veterinarians, and conservation biologists to better understand the emergence of new diseases from animal reservoirs, and the complexity of the interrelationships among humans, animals, geographic factors, and climate.

Resources

BOOKS

Beitz, Lisa A. *Emerging Infectious Diseases: A Guide to Diseases, Causative Agents, and Surveillance*. San Francisco, CA: Jossey-Bass, 2011.

Davis, Radford G., ed. *Animals, Diseases, and Human Health: Shaping Our Lives Now and in the Future*. Santa Barbara, CA: Praeger, 2011.

Kapur, G. Bobby, and Jeffrey P. Smith, eds. *Emergency Public Health: Preparedness and Response*. Sudbury, MA; Jones and Bartlett Learning, 2011.

Washer, Peter. *Emerging Infectious Diseases and Society*. New York: Palgrave Macmillan, 2010.

PERIODICALS

Burke, R.L., et al. "A Review of Zoonotic Disease Surveillance Supported by the Armed Forces Health Surveillance Center." *Zoonoses and Public Health* 59 (May 2012): 164–175.

Bush, L.M., and M.T. Perez. "The Anthrax Attacks 10 Years Later." *Annals of Internal Medicine* 156 (January 3, 2012) (1 Pt.1): 41–44.

Colpitts, T.M., et al. "West Nile Virus: Biology, Transmission, and Human Infection." *Clinical Microbiology Reviews* 25 (October 2012): 635–648.

Flaherty, D.K. "The Vaccine-Autism Connection: A Public Health Crisis Caused by Unethical Medical Practices and Fraudulent Science." *Annals of Pharmacotherapy* 45 (October 2011): 1302–1304.

Mahalingam, S., et al. "Hendra Virus: An Emerging Paramyxovirus in Australia." *Lancet Infectious Diseases* 12 (October 2012): 799–807.

Morris, J.G., Jr. "Cholera—Modern Pandemic Disease of Ancient Lineage." *Emerging Infectious Diseases* 17 (November 2011): 2099–2104.

Morse, S.S. "Public Health Surveillance and Infectious Disease Detection." *Biosecurity and Bioterrorism* 10 (March 2012): 6–16.

Reynolds, M.G., et al. "Spectrum of Infection and Risk Factors for Human Monkeypox, United States, 2003." *Emerging Infectious Diseases* 13 (September 2007): 1332–1339.

Singer, M. "Pathogen-Pathogen Interaction: A Syndemic Model of Complex Biosocial Processes in Disease." *Virulence* 1 (January-February 2010): 10–18.

WEBSITES

"About ProMED-mail." International Society for Infectious Diseases (ISID). http://www.isid.org/promedmail/promedmail.shtml (accessed October 29, 2012).

"Emerging and Re-emerging Infectious Diseases." National Institute of Allergy and Infectious Diseases (NIAID). http://www.niaid.nih.gov/topics/emerging/pages/default.aspx (accessed October 28, 2012).

"Emerging Diseases." Center for Infectious Disease Dynamics (CIDD). http://www.cidd.psu.edu/research/emerging-diseases (accessed October 30, 2012).

National Center for Emerging and Zoonotic Infectious Diseases (NCEZID), Centers for Disease Control and Prevention (CDC). http://www.cdc.gov/ncezid/index.html (accessed October 28, 2012).

ORGANIZATIONS

Armed Forces Health Surveillance Center (AFHSC), 11800 Tech Road, Suite 220, Silver Spring, MD United States 20904, (301) 319-3240, Fax: (301) 319-7620, AFHSC.Web@amedd.army.mil, http://www.afhsc.mil/home.

Center for Emerging and Neglected Diseases (CEND), University of California, Berkeley, 444A Li Ka Shing Center, Berkeley, CA United States 94720-3370, (510) 664-4867, cend@berkeley.edu, http://globalhealth.berkeley.edu/cend/index.html.

Center for Infectious Disease Dynamics (CIDD), The Pennsylvania State University, 208 Mueller Lab, University Park, PA United States 16802. http://www.cidd.psu.edu/contact-info, http://www.cidd.psu.edu/.

Centers for Disease Control and Prevention (CDC), Bacterial Diseases Branch, Foothills Campus, Fort Collins, CO United States 80521, (800) CDC-INFO (232-4636), cdcinfo@cdc.gov, http://www.cdc.gov/.

International Society for Infectious Diseases (ISID), 9 Babcock Street, 3rd Floor, Brookline, MA United States 02446, (617) 277-0551, Fax: (617) 278-9113, info@isid.org, http://www.isid.org/index.shtml.

National Institute of Allergy and Infectious Diseases (NIAID), 6610 Rockledge Drive, MSC 6612, Bethesda, MD United States 20892-6612, (301) 496-5717, (866) 284-4107, Fax: (301) 402-3573, ocpostoffice@niaid.nih.gov, http://www.niaid.nih.gov/Pages/default.aspx.

World Health Organization (WHO), Avenue Appia 20, Geneva, Switzerland 1211 Geneva 27, +41 22 791 21 11, Fax: +41 22 791 31 11, http://www.who.int/en/

Rebecca J. Frey, Ph.D.

Emphysema *see* **Smoking**

Encephalitis

Definition

Encephalitis is an inflammation of the brain, usually caused by a direct viral infection or a hypersensitivity reaction to a virus or foreign protein. Brain inflammation caused by a bacterial infection is sometimes called cerebritis. When both the brain and spinal cord are involved, the disorder is called encephalomyelitis. An inflammation of the brain's covering, or meninges, is called **meningitis**.

Description

Encephalitis is an inflammation of the brain. The inflammation is a reaction of the body's immune system to infection or invasion. During the inflammation, the brain's tissues become swollen. The combination of the infection and the immune reaction to it can cause headache and a fever, as well as more severe symptoms in some cases.

Approximately 2,000 cases of encephalitis are reported to the **Centers for Disease Control and Prevention (CDC)** each year. The viruses causing primary encephalitis can be epidemic or sporadic. The **polio** virus is an epidemic cause. Arthropod-borne viral (Arboviral) encephalitis is responsible for most epidemic viral encephalitis. Arboviral encephalitis has multiple causative agents, including St. Louis encephalitis (SLE), western equine encephalitis (WEE), Venezuelan equine encephalitis (VEE), eastern equine encephalitis (EEE), La Crosse virus, and other California serogroup viruses. The viruses live in animal hosts and mosquitoes that transmit the disease. The most common form of non-epidemic or sporadic encephalitis is caused by the **herpes** simplex virus, type 1 (HSV-1) and has a high rate of death. **Mumps** is another example of a sporadic cause.

Causes and symptoms

Causes

There are more than a dozen viruses that can cause encephalitis, spread by either human-to-human contact or animal bites. Encephalitis may occur with several common viral infections of childhood. Viruses and viral diseases that may cause encephalitis include:

- chickenpox
- measles
- mumps
- Epstein-Barr virus (EBV)
- cytomegalovirus infection
- HIV
- herpes simplex
- herpes zoster (shingles)
- herpes B
- polio
- rabies
- mosquito-borne viruses (arboviruses)

Primary encephalitis is caused by direct infection by the virus, while secondary encephalitis is due to a post-infectious immune reaction to viral infection elsewhere in the body. Secondary encephalitis may occur with **measles**, chickenpox, mumps, **rubella**, and EBV. In secondary encephalitis, symptoms usually begin five to 10 days after the onset of the disease itself and are related to the breakdown of the myelin sheath that covers nerve fibers.

In rare cases, encephalitis may follow **vaccination** against some of the viral diseases listed above. **Creutzfeldt-Jakob disease**, a very rare brain disorder caused by an infectious particle called a prion, may also cause encephalitis.

Mosquitoes spread viruses responsible for equine encephalitis (eastern and western types), St. Louis encephalitis, California encephalitis, and Japanese encephalitis. **Lyme disease**, spread by ticks, can cause encephalitis, as

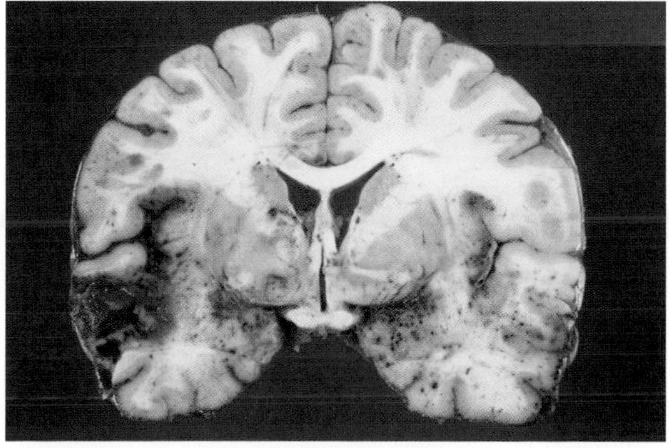

Coronal section of temporal lobe of a human brain showing effects of Encephalitis. *(Peter Berndt,M.D.,P.A.)*

can Colorado tick fever. **Rabies** is most often spread by animal bites from dogs, cats, mice, raccoons, squirrels, and bats and may cause encephalitis.

Equine encephalitis is carried by mosquitoes that do not normally bite humans but do bite horses and birds. It is occasionally picked up from these animals by mosquitoes that do bite humans. Japanese encephalitis and St. Louis encephalitis are also carried by mosquitoes. The risk of contracting a mosquito-borne virus is greatest in mid to late summer, when mosquitoes are most active, in those rural areas where these viruses are known to exist. Eastern equine encephalitis occurs in eastern and southeastern United States; western equine and California encephalitis occur throughout the West; and St. Louis encephalitis occurs throughout the country. Japanese encephalitis does not occur in the United States but is found throughout much of Asia. The viruses responsible for these diseases are classified as arboviruses, and these diseases are collectively called arbovirus encephalitis.

Herpes simplex encephalitis, the most common form of sporadic encephalitis in western countries, is a disease with significantly high mortality. It occurs in children and adults, and both sides of the brain are affected. It is theorized that brain infection is caused by the virus moving from a peripheral location to the brain via two nerves, the olfactory and the trigeminal (largest nerves in the skull).

Herpes simplex encephalitis is responsible for 10% of all encephalitis cases and is the main cause of sporadic, fatal encephalitis. In untreated patients, the rate of death is 70%, while the mortality is 15–20% in patients who have been treated with acyclovir. The symptoms of herpes simplex encephalitis are fever, rapidly disintegrating mental state, headache, and behavioral changes.

Symptoms

The symptoms of encephalitis range from very mild to very severe and may include:

- headache
- fever
- lethargy (sleepiness, decreased alertness, and fatigue)
- malaise
- nausea and vomiting
- visual disturbances
- tremor
- decreased consciousness (drowsiness, confusion, delirium, and unconsciousness)
- stiff neck
- seizures

Symptoms may progress rapidly, changing from mild to severe within several days or even several hours.

Diagnosis

Diagnosis of encephalitis includes careful questioning to determine possible exposure to viral sources. Tests that can help confirm the diagnosis and rule out other disorders include:

- Blood tests. These are to detect antibodies to viral antigens, and foreign proteins.
- Cerebrospinal fluid analysis (spinal tap). This detects viral antigens and provides culture specimens for the virus or bacteria that may be present in the cerebrospinal fluid.
- Electroencephalogram (EEG).
- CT and MRI scans.

A brain biopsy (surgical gathering of a small tissue sample) may be recommended in some cases where treatment to date has been ineffective, and the cause of the encephalitis is unclear. Definite diagnosis by biopsy may allow specific treatment that would otherwise be too risky.

Treatment

Choice of treatment for encephalitis will depend on the cause. Bacterial encephalitis is treated with **antibiotics**. Viral encephalitis is usually treated with antiviral drugs, including acyclovir, ganciclovir, foscarnet, ribovarin, and AZT. Viruses that respond to acyclovir include herpes simplex, the most common cause of sporadic (non-epidemic) encephalitis in the United States.

The symptoms of encephalitis may be treated with a number of different drugs. Corticosteroids, including prednisone and dexamethasone, are sometimes prescribed to reduce inflammation and brain swelling. Anticonvulsant drugs, including dilantin and phenytoin, are used to control seizures. Fever may be reduced with acetaminophen or other fever-reducing drugs.

A person with encephalitis must be monitored carefully, since symptoms may change rapidly. Blood tests may be required regularly to track levels of fluids and salts in the blood.

Prognosis

Encephalitis symptoms may last several weeks. Most cases of encephalitis are mild, and recovery is usually quick. Mild encephalitis usually leaves no residual neurological problems. Overall, approximately 10% of those with encephalitis die from their infections or complications such as secondary infection. Some forms of encephalitis have more severe courses, including herpes encephalitis, in which mortality is 15–20% with treatment, and 70–80% without. Antiviral treatment is ineffective for eastern equine encephalitis, and mortality is approximately 30%.

Permanent neurological consequences may follow recovery in some cases. Consequences may include personality changes, memory loss, language difficulties, seizures, and partial paralysis.

Prevention

Because encephalitis is due to infection, it may be prevented by avoiding the infection. Minimizing contact with others who have any of the viral illnesses listed above may reduce the chances of becoming infected. Most infections are spread by hand-to-hand or hand-to-mouth contact; frequent hand washing may reduce the likelihood of infection if contact cannot be avoided.

Mosquito-borne viruses may be avoided by preventing mosquito bites. Mosquitoes are most active at dawn and dusk and are most common in moist areas with standing **water**. Minimizing exposed skin and use of mosquito repellents on other areas can reduce the chances of being bitten.

Vaccines are available against some viruses, including polio, herpes B, Japanese encephalitis, and equine encephalitis. Rabies vaccine is available for animals; it is also given to people after exposure. Japanese encephalitis vaccine is recommended for those traveling to Asia and staying in affected rural areas during transmission season.

Costs to Society

In addition to the high fatality rates associated with encephalitis, there is a relatively high cost to public health associated with the condition. According to the **CDC**, the annual costs associated with encephalitis—including surveillance and vector control—are approximately $150 million. Though this cost may seem relatively low compared to the costs associated with other illnesses, it must be considered in relation to the number of cases, which is also much lower than many other nationally monitored illnesses. Assuming 2,000 cases per year (as reported by the CDC), the cost per case amounts to $75,000.

KEY TERMS

Cerebrospinal fluid analysis—An analysis that is important in diagnosing diseases of the central nervous system. The fluid within the spine will indicate the presence of viruses, bacteria, and blood. Infections such as encephalitis will be indicated by an increase of cell count and total protein in the fluid.

Computerized tomography (CT) Scan—A test to examine organs within the body and detect evidence of tumors, blood clots, and accumulation of fluids.

Electroencephalagram (EEG)—A chart of the brain waves picked up by the electrodes placed on the scalp. Changes in brain wave activity can be an indication of nervous system disorders.

Inflammation—A response from the immune system to an injury. The signs are redness, heat, swelling, and pain.

Magnetic resonance imaging (MRI)—MRI is diagnostic radiography using electromagnetic energy to create an image of the central nervous system (CNS), blood system, and musculoskeletal system.

Vaccine—A prepartation containing killed or weakened microorganisms used to build immunity against infection from that microorganism.

Virus—A very small organism that can only live within a cell. It is unable to reproduce outside that cell.

Resources

BOOKS

Carson–DeWitt, Rosalyn, and Rimas Lukas. "Encephalitis." *Infectious Diseases & Conditions.* Ed. H. Bradford Hawley. Vol. 1. Ipswich, MA: Salem Press, 2012. 367-369. Salem Health.

"Encephalitis." *Diseases, Disorders, and Injuries.* New York: Marshall Cavendish Reference, 2011. 107.

PERIODICALS

Rust, Robert S. "Human Arboviral Encephalitis." *Seminars in Pediatric Neurology* 19.3 (2012): 130+.

WEBSITES

Centers for Disease Control and Prevention. "Arboviral Encephalitis." http://www.cdc.gov/ncidod/dvbid/arbor/arbofact.htmAccessed November 12, 2012.

Medline Plus, National Institute of Health. "Encephalitis." http://www.nlm.nih.gov/medlineplus/encephalitis.html#cat22Accessed November 12, 2012.

ORGANIZATIONS

Centers for Disease Control and Prevention (CDC), 1600 Clifton Road, Atlanta, GA 30333, (800) 232-4636, cdcinfo@cdc.gov, http://www.cdc.gov.

Richard Robinson
Andrea Nienstedt, MA

Environmental disasters

Definition

Environmental disasters, also called environmental emergencies, are disasters caused to the natural environment by human activity—as distinct from **natural disasters**, which are calamities resulting from natural processes (e.g., weather events, geologic processes, asteroid strikes) The human activity resulting in an environmental disaster may be either intentional (acts of warfare, terrorism, or criminal behavior) or unintentional (e.g., engineering failures, industrial accidents). Environmental disasters may include loss of human, animal, or plant life; disruption of the ecosystem; or loss of biodiversity.

In some cases, an environmental disaster may be the end result of a chain of events in which a storm, earthquake, or other natural occurrence leads to the failure or collapse of a human-made structure; the Fukushima Daiichi disaster in 2011 is an example of this type of causal chain.

Description

Environmental disasters can be divided, for purposes of discussion, into several categories according to the nature of the event and/or its cause.

Nuclear accidents

Three Mile Island (1979). Three Mile Island was a partial nuclear meltdown that occurred at a power plant near Harrisburg, Pennsylvania. Although no one was killed or seriously injured in the incident, small amounts of radioactive gases and radioactive iodine were released. The investigation found that the emergency resulted from a combination of mechanical failures and human factors. Although Three Mile Island did not have any statistically significant short- or long-term effects on the physical health of the local population—including the incidence of cancer—it led to renewed concern about the safety of nuclear reactors.

Chernobyl explosion (1986). The Chernobyl reactor was part of a nuclear power plant located in Ukraine. Its explosion in 1986 is considered one of the two worst nuclear accidents in history, the other being the Fukushima Daiichi disaster of 2011. The reactor exploded during a systems test; the resulting fire discharged a plume of radioactive smoke that eventually covered most of Russia and Western Europe. About 60 people died at the time of the accident as a result of the explosion itself and acute **radiation poisoning**, all of them plant staff and emergency workers. An additional 4,000 deaths are expected to occur over the coming years as a result of the long-term effects of radiation poisoning. A total of 356,000 people were evacuated from the most heavily contaminated areas of Belarus, Ukraine, and Russia between 1986 and 2000, and resettled elsewhere.

Fukushima Daiichi disaster (2011). The Fukushima Daiichi disaster resulted from equipment failures and nuclear meltdown following an earthquake and tsunami that struck Japan on March 11, 2011. It is an instructive example of an environmental disaster resulting from the impact of a natural disaster on human-made structures and equipment. The tsunami that followed the earthquake flooded the rooms containing the plant's emergency generators, which stopped working, cutting off the flow of coolant **water** to the nuclear reactors, which then overheated. The earthquake and tsunami also kept workers from reaching the plant quickly enough to prevent or mitogate the disaster. While no deaths had been attributed directly to the accident as of 2012, people who were forced to evacuate their homes (about 1,760) are reported to have a high level of mental health issues.

Industrial toxins

Seveso (1976). The Seveso disaster was caused by the sudden release of large amounts of dioxin from a chemical manufacturing plant in a small town near Milan, Italy, as the result of a runway heat buildup and chemical reaction. Dioxin is a toxic substance that can contaminate soil as well as work its way up the food chain. About 3,300 animals were killed immediately, and others slaughtered to prevent the dioxin from entering the human food supply. The immediate effects on humans were chloracne and other skin inflammations, but long-term effects on the health of the affected local population are still being traced, as dioxin is a known carcinogen. A report published in 2011 found an increased incidence of **cancer** among the women of Seveso more than 30 years after the accident.

Love Canal (1978). The Love Canal disaster takes its name from a neighborhood in Niagara Falls, New York, named after a local politician who had proposed building a canal from the Niagara River to Lake Erie. A nearby chemical plant had used what was then empty land as a chemical disposal site from 1929 to 1953; it then then sealed the dump with a layer of red clay. Houses and a school were later built on the site. After a newly installed sewer line damaged the clay seal, residents began to notice strange odors and peculiar seepages in their back yards and basements. In 1978, the problems were traced to the waste dump, which was investigated and found to contain 22,000 tons of 248 different chemicals, including 130 pounds of dioxin. More than 900 families were relocated away from the neighborhood, and the dump was resealed. Effects on the inhabitants included a higher-than-normal rate of **birth defects**, damage to chromosomes, and mental health disorders.

Bhopal (1984). Considered the worst industrial disaster in world history, the Bhopal disaster occurred when a gas cloud containing 15 metric tons of methyl isocyanate (MIC) escaped from the Union Carbide pesticide factory near the town of Bhopal in India. About 4,000 people died instantly, with 15,000 more fatalities in the following years. As of 2012, about 100,000 people still suffer from chronic health disorders related to gas exposure, and the plant site itself contains thousands of tons of mercury and other toxic chemicals. The disaster was traced to poor maintenance of plant equipment, unsafe manufacturing processes, carelessness in regard to mandated safety procedures, and inadequate emergency plans and procedures. The disaster was made worse by the rapid recent growth in population of a slum neighborhood close to the plant.

Sandoz spill (1986). The Sandoz chemical spill resulted from a fire at the company's storehouse of agricultural chemicals near Basel, Switzerland, and subsequent attempts to extinguish the fire. Toxic chemicals were released into the atmosphere and eventually found their way into the Rhine River, turning its waters red. The chemicals led to a massive die-off of wildlife downstream from the plant. The cause of the fire was never established but has been attributed to sabotage by operatives from then-Communist East Germany; the destruction of the Sandoz plant was allegedly intended to divert attention from the disaster at Chernobyl six months earlier.

Oil spills

Exxon Valdez (1989). The *Exxon Valdez* was an oil tanker that ran aground on a reef in Prince William Sound in Alaska in March 1989. The resulting oil spill covered 1,300 miles of coastline and 12,000 square miles of ocean, and is estimated to have released 11 million gallons of oil (some estimates place the total closer to 25 million gallons. Until the *Deepwater Horizon* oil spill of 2010, the *Exxon Valdez* spill was the largest oil spill in terms of volume in United States waters. The accident was variously attributed to crew fatigue, inadequate training, and malfunctioning radar equipment. Although no human lives were lost, the impact on local animal life—particularly sea birds, otters, salmon, and whales—was devastating. As of 2012, the environment affected by the oil spill has still not completely recovered.

Deepwater Horizon (2010). In contrast to the *Exxon Valdez*, the *Deepwater Horizon* was not a tanker but a semi-submersible drilling unit located in the Gulf of Mexico about 40 miles off the Louisiana coast. It caught fire and exploded on April 20, 2010, killing 11 crew members and requiring the immediate evacuation of the 115 survivors. After the burning rig sank on April 22, oil began to seep from the damaged underwater well, eventually forming the largest oil spill ever recorded in U.S. waters—210 million gallons by the time the well was capped in September 2010. The coastlines of four states (Louisiana, Mississippi, Alabama, and Florida) were severely affected by the tar balls that washed up on the shore, damaging tourism as well as the fishing industry in the region. Effects on wildlife include strange genetic mutations that appeared among fish and shellfish in the Gulf in 2011 as well as evidence that small droplets of oil had entered the food chain by seeping under the shells of crabs and some shrimp species. The long-term effects of the *Deep Horizon* spill are still under investigation as of 2012.

Air pollution

Donora smog (1948). The Donora smog was an **air pollution** incident resulting from a temperature inversion, in which warmer air higher up in the atmosphere traps pollutants in colder air near the surface. Donora is a small town near Pittsburgh that had a zinc plant and a steel and wire factory that emitted large quantities of hydrogen fluoride, fluorine, and sulfur dioxide. A temperature inversion that lasted from October 27 to October 31, 1948, trapped these gases near the surface of the ground. The pollutants then mixed with damp fog to create a thick smog that killed 20 local residents and 800 animals, and sickened over 7,000 people in the town. Although the factories were shut down on October 31, the smog did not lift until the weather pattern changed. The disaster has been credited with sparking the clean-air movement in the United States, which led eventually to the establishment of the **Environmental Protection Agency**.

Great Smog of London (1952). The Great Smog of 1952 was a prolonged episode of air pollution that lasted from December 1952 to March 1953. The smog resulted from a combination of unusually cold weather resulting in increased use of low-quality coal to heat homes and businesses; a temperature inversion coupled with light winds that did not disperse pollutants in the air; and the need for most Londoners to travel by automobile or bus, which added to the atmospheric pollution. The concentration of particulates in the air was 56 times greater than normal levels. It is thought that as many as 12,000 people died in 1952 and 1953 from bronchitis and other respiratory disorders caused by the smog. The Great

Smog brought about the passage of the United Kingdom's Clean Air Act of 1956.

Food chain contamination

Minamata/Niigata disease (1956, 1965). Minamata disease is a neurological disorder caused by mercury poisoning due to bioaccumulation. The disorder is characterized by inability to walk normally (ataxia), general weakness, and damage to hearing, vision, and speech. Long-term effects included elevated blood pressure and **heart disease**. In severe cases, the victims become psychotic, lapse into coma, and die. It was first identified in humans in the Japanese city of Minamata in 1956; residents had noticed from 1950 onward that their cats would sometimes go into convulsions and die. They referred to the strange phenomenon as "dancing cat fever." When the disorder appeared in humans, researchers eventually found that it was the end result of methylmercury wastes that had been dumped into the local river from 1932 onward by a chemical factory. Over the years following, shellfish and fish in Minamata Bay accumulated mercury in their tissues. Residents living near the bay—and their cats—were gradually poisoned by the mercury they took in through their fish-heavy diet. By 2001, almost 1,800 people had died from Minamata disease. A second outbreak of poisoning from bioaccumulated mercury in the local fish occurred in Niigata in 1965.

Bovine spongiform encephalopathy (BSE; also known as mad cow disease; 1986). BSE is a transmissible prion disease that can be passed from animal to animal through consumption of contaminated tissues. It is thought that the epidemic of BSE that decimated British cattle in 1987 resulted from supplementing their normal grass-based diet with protein supplements made from animal byproducts obtained from sick animals. By 1987, about 165 people had sickened and died from a neurological disease with similar symptoms to BSE that is now called variant **Creutzfeldt-Jakob disease** or vCJD. The evidence indicates that most of those diagnosed in the 1980s with vCJD had eaten tainted beef from infected cows. An estimated 400,000 cattle infected with BSE had entered the European food chain in the 1980s.

Acts of warfare

Chemical warfare (1915 and following). Poisonous gases intended to kill or disable soldiers were first used during World War I (1914–1918), beginning with the German use of chlorine gas at Ypres in 1915. Phosgene and mustard gas were later used by the Allies as well as the Central Powers. The Italian dictator Benito Mussolini used mustard gas during the invasion of Ethiopia in 1935, and the Japanese used it during the invasion of China in 1938. Scientists in Nazi Germany in the 1930s discovered two nerve gases, Sarin and Tabun, but neither agent was used during World War II (1939–1945). Sarin would later be used by Iraq in the war between Iraq and Iran in the 1980s. Sarin is a nerve gas which is lethal even in small quantities. The long-term aftereffects of chemical warfare include not only chronic physical and mental illnesses among veterans but also unexploded World War I gas shells that still turn up on the battlefields of Western Europe.

Biological warfare (1930s and following). Although interest in the use of various disease agents in warfare was stimulated by the discovery of the **germ theory** of disease in the 1880s, the only known use of bioweapons in warfare was the Japanese war with China between 1937 and 1945. About 580,000 Chinese civilians are thought to have died as a result of the Japanese distribution of foodstuffs carrying the agents of bubonic **plague** and **cholera**. During the Cold War (1947–1991), the United Kingdom, the United States, and the Soviet Union experimented with the weaponization of **anthrax**, botulinum toxin, and **brucellosis**, but these agents were never used.

Nuclear warfare (1945). The effects of the atomic bombs dropped on Hiroshima and Nagasaki in August 1945 include immediate death tolls of 245,000 (in both cities); about 21,000 survivors have been diagnosed with illnesses caused by exposure to radiation in the years since. These two nuclear bombs are the only such devices used in warfare as of 2012.

Kuwaiti oil fires (1991). The Kuwaiti oil fires were deliberately set by Iraqi military forces during the Gulf War to prevent oil wells from being captured by Coalition forces. About 600 wells were set ablaze, leading to widespread pollution of the soil and air. It took 11 months to put out the last of the fires because the Iraqis had placed land mines around the wells to prevent the entrance of firefighting crews. The smoke from the fires caused smoke-filled skies and carbon fallout across Bahrain and Saudi Arabia throughout 1991.

Engineering and planning failures

Chinese anti-sparrow campaign (1958–1962). The Chinese anti-sparrow campaign was a misguided government intervention that was part of Mao Zedong's Great Leap Forward. The Chinese Communist government began in 1958 to encourage the population to trap, kill, and prevent the reproduction of sparrows on the grounds that the birds ate grain that could be used to feed people instead. By 1960, however, it was discovered that the birds were actually useful because they ate insects as well as grains. The near-eradication of the sparrows led to a rapid increase in the locust population; the hungry insects devouring of the 1960 rice harvest contributed to the Great Chinese **Famine**, in which nearly 30 million people died of hunger.

Guadalajara sewer explosions (1992). The 1992 explosions in Guadalajara, Mexico, were caused by the poor design and placement of zinc-coated water pipes too close to an underground steel gasoline pipeline. The humid climate of the city facilitated a chemical reaction between the zinc and the steel that caused the gasoline pipeline to corrode and leak gasoline into the city water supply and the sewer system. Residents complained of a smell of gasoline on April 19, but no action was taken. On April 22, a series of ten explosions in the sewer system destroyed five miles of streets, killed 252 people, and injured another 500.

Baia Mare (2000). The Baia Mare cyanide disaster occurred in Romania and neighboring countries in Eastern Europe in January 2000 when a dam constructed by a gold mining company failed following heavy snowfall. The ruptured dam released over 300,000 cubic feet of water contaminated by cyanide used in gold processing operations. The cyanide-contaminated water spilled over farmland and eventually reached the Tisza River and then the Danube. The cyanide contaminated **drinking water** in Hungary and Serbia as well as Romania, and killed fish and wildlife along the course of the Tisza. Five weeks after the failure of the Baia Mare dam, another nearby dam burst, releasing such heavy metals as zinc, copper, and lead into the Tisza. As of 2012, the fisheries along the Danube and Tisza Rivers have still not fully recovered from the disaster.

Criminal behavior

Forest and brush fires (1980 and following). According to the U.S. Forest Service, between a quarter and a third of all forest fires in the United States since 1980 have been set by arsonists, accounting for the burning of over a million acres of land each year. Many of the firesetters suffer from a disorder of impulse control known as pyromania, but others have been linked to Al Qaeda since the summer of 2011. Forest fires not only kill wildlife and destroy homes and businesses, but also lead to human deaths, some resulting from heart attacks as well as fire-related injuries. Forest fires also release large amounts of carbon and soot into the air, causing or increasing the severity of respiratory and cardiovascular disorders. The February 2009 bushfires in Australia known as "Black Saturday" resulted in part from arson; they cost the lives of 173 people as well as burning 1.1 million acres of land.

KEY TERMS

Bioaccumulation—The absorption and buildup of a toxic substance within the tissues of an organism. Bioaccumulation can move up the food chain when one animal feeds on another contaminated by the toxin and is in turn consumed by a larger predator.

Biodiversity—The extent of the variety of life forms within a given ecosystem. Biodiversity is an important measurement of the health of an ecosystem.

Carcinogen—A chemical or other agent that is known to cause cancer.

Chloracne—A skin eruption of blackheads, cysts, and acne-like pustules, most often caused by exposure to toxic chemicals.

Dioxin—The name of a family of highly toxic chlorinated chemicals that are known carcinogens as well as environmental pollutants.

Prion—An infectious agent consisting of a protein in a misfolded form. The term is derived from a combination of the words *protein* and *infection*.

Pyromania—A disorder of impulse control in which a person sets fires either for gratification or to relieve tension. About 90% of persons diagnosed with pyromania are males.

Temperature inversion—A weather condition in which cooler air near the ground has a layer of warmer air above it, in contrast to the normal pattern of air temperature decreasing steadily with altitude. Temperature inversions have been implicated in several instances of smog-related disasters.

Bioterrorism (2001 anthrax attacks). The 2001 anthrax attacks consisted of a series of letters containing anthrax spores mailed to various media offices and politicians in the United States between September 18 and October 9, 2001, right after 9/11. At least 22 people were infected with anthrax from the letters; five of them died. The suspected perpetrator was identified as Bruce Ivins, a research scientist who committed **suicide** in 2008. Although the anthrax letters did not cause extensive loss of life, they demonstrated the capacity of bioterrorism to affect a large area, as those infected lived in different locations ranging from Florida to Connecticut. In addition, decontamination of post offices and other buildings exposed to the letters took over 26 months to complete, cost millions of dollars, and required the use of chlorine dioxide, a disinfectant gas that requires careful handling as it can contaminate drinking water. In sum, the anthrax letters were a painful reminder not only of the dangerous potential of bioterrorism but also of the difficulty of preventing environmental disasters caused by the intentional acts of disturbed human beings.

Demographics

Statistics regarding loss of life and other effects on human and animal health were included in the preceding descriptions when they were available.

Prevention

The many different types of environmental disasters; their relationship to natural weather patterns and storms; and the dependence of modern society on complex construction and manufacturing processes, equipment, and techniques make it unlikely that environmental disasters can ever be completely prevented. On the other hand, humans have the ability to learn from environmental disasters; many of the events described in this entry have led to improved understanding of the human factors (e.g., fatigue, inadequate training, poor interpersonal relationships within an organization) that contribute to such disasters as well as the engineering and equipment failures. The virtual disappearance of smog-related disasters since the 1950s is an example of human ability to respond effectively to environmental disasters once the cause(s) are understood.

Effects on public health

The effects of environmental disasters on public health range from skin disorders, digestive problems, and upper respiratory complaints to an increased incidence of cancer, birth defects, and fatal neurological syndromes. The specific diseases and disorders depend on the nature of the disaster, the chemical agents (if any) involved, the timeline of the disaster, and the size of the population affected. One finding that appears to be common to almost all environmental disasters is a significant increase in mental health disorders (particularly depression and anxiety disorders) in the human witnesses, first responders, and survivors of such disasters. Public health workers are increasingly aware of the need for mental health treatment as well as medical assistance in the days and weeks following an environmental disaster.

Efforts and solutions

An emerging trend among public health experts is to coordinate more closely with disaster management and **emergency preparedness** organizations. Environmental disasters often present unusual and unexpected challenges to mental as well as physical well-being that are very different from the situations commonly encountered by local boards of public health. In addition, environmental disasters often require some "detective work" in identifying the cause(s) as well as the extent of the problem before health issues can be effectively addressed.

In addition to working more closely with disaster management experts, public health experts are also increasingly aware of the need for more long-term research into the aftereffects of environmental disasters. Although the immediate loss of human and animal life can be measured fairly quickly, the long-term effects on health may take decades to appear. Disasters involving chemical and nuclear explosions and contamination of the food chain appear to be especially likely to produce measurable harm over long periods of time.

QUESTIONS TO ASK YOUR DOCTOR

- Have you ever treated immediate survivors of an environmental disaster?
- Have you ever treated a patient whose illness turned out to be a long-term consequence of an environmental disaster?
- What is your opinion of preventive measures against environmental disasters?

Resources

BOOKS

Duke, Shirley. *Environmental Disasters*. Vero Beach, FL: Rourke Publishing, 2012.

Hernan, Robert Emmet. *This Borrowed Earth: Lessons from the Fifteen Worst Environmental Disasters around the World*. New York: Palgrave Macmillan, 2010.

Hunting, Katharine L., and Brenda L. Gleason. *Essential Case Studies in Public Health: Putting Public Health into Practice*. Sudbury, MA: Jones and Bartlett Learning, 2012.

Jenks, Andrew L. *Perils of Progress: Environmental Disasters in the Twentieth Century*. Boston, MA: Prentice Hall, 2011.

Vallero, Daniel, and Trevor Letcher. *Unraveling Environmental Disasters*. Waltham, MA: Elsevier, 2012.

PERIODICALS

Atlas, R.M., and T.C. Hazen. "Oil Biodegradation and Bioremediation: A Tale of the Two Worst Spills in U.S. History." *Environmental Science and Technology* 45 (August 15, 2011): 6709–6715.

Austin, A.A. "Reproductive Outcomes among Former Love Canal Residents, Niagara Falls, New York." *Environmental Research* 111 (July 2011): 693–701.

Buttke, D., et al. "Community Assessment for Public Health Emergency Response (CASPER) One Year Following the Gulf Coast Oil Spill: Alabama and Mississippi, 2011." *Prehospital and Disaster Medicine* September 25, 2012: 1–7 [E-pub ahead of print].

Gamboa-Maldonado, T., et al. "Building Capacity for Community Disaster Preparedness: A Call for Collaboration between Public Environmental Health and Emergency Preparedness and Response Programs." *Journal of Environmental Health* 75 (September 2012): 24–29.

Goyal, N., et al. "Thyroid Cancer Characteristics in the Population Surrounding Three Mile Island." *Laryngoscope* 122 (June 2012): 1415–1421.

Helfand, W.H., et al. "Donora, Pennsylvania: An Environmental Disaster of the Twentieth Century." *American Journal of Public Health* 91 (April 2001): 553.

Inoue, S., et al. "Short-Term Effect of Severe Exposure to Methylmercury on Atherosclerotic Heart disease and Hypertension Mortality in Minamata." *Science of the Total Environment* 417 (February 15, 2012): 291–293.

Ivanov, V.K. et al. "Formation of Potential Radiation Risk Groups to Render Timely Targeted Medical Care: Lessons of Chernobyl." *Radiation Protection Dosimetry* 151 (April 2012): 666–670.

Sheehan, H.E. "The Bhopal Gas Disaster: Focus on Community Health and Environmental Effects." *Indian Journal of Medical Ethics* 8 (April-June 2011): 95–96.

Warner, M., et al. "Dioxin Exposure and Cancer Risk in the Seveso Women's Health Study." *Environmental Health Perspectives* 119 (December 2011): 1700–1705.

WEBSITES

"Disaster Types and Topics." Disaster Information Management Resource Center, National Library of Medicine. http://sis.nlm.nih.gov/dimrc/disasters.html (accessed October 9, 2012).

"Emergency Response." National Institute of Environmental Health Sciences (NIEHS). http://www.niehs.nih.gov/health/topics/population/response/index.cfm (accessed October 8, 2012).

Engineering Failures: Case Studies in Engineering. http://engineeringfailures.org/ (accessed October 8, 2012).

"FAQs and Fact Sheets." National Toxicology Program (NTP). http://ntp.niehs.nih.gov/index.cfm?objectid=EF1E5313-F1F6-975E-73B55D30B2966A5A (accessed October 8, 2012).

"General Information for Disaster Preparedness and Response." Environmental Protection Agency (EPA).http://www.epa.gov/naturaldisasters/general.html (accessed October 9, 2012).

ORGANIZATIONS

Association of Occupational and Environmental Clinics (AOEC), 1010 Vermont Ave., NW #513, Washington, DC United States 20005, (202) 347-4976, (888) 347-AOEC, Fax: (202) 347-4950, aoec@aoec.org, http://www.aoec.org/.

Environmental Protection Agency (EPA), Ariel Rios Building, 1200 Pennsylvania Avenue, N.W., Washington, DC United States 20460, (202) 272-0167, http://www.epa.gov/.

National Institute of Environmental Health Sciences (NIEHS), P.O. Box 12233, MD K3-16, Research Triangle Park, NC United States 27709-2233, (919) 541-3345, Fax: (919) 541-4395, http://www.niehs.nih.gov/.

National Toxicology Program (NTP), P.O. Box 12233, MD K2-05, Research Triangle Park, NC United States 27709, (919) 541-3419, http://ntp.niehs.nih.gov/.

Rebecca J. Frey, Ph.D.

Environmental health

Definition

Environmental health is that field of public health that relates to all health issues that may arise in connection with the natural or human-made environments. The **World Health Organization (WHO)** defines environmental health as all of those "physical, chemical and biological factors external to a person, and all the related factors impacting behaviours."

Purpose

The purpose of environmental health is to use the principles of public health and environmental science to prevent and control contaminants in the natural and artificial environment, thus providing a safer and healthier milieu within which humans may live and work.

Description

The modern science of environmental health dates to the work of Sir Edwin Chadwick in the last quarter of the nineteenth century. Chadwick was a social reformer who studied living conditions in England's urban areas and concluded that filthy environmental conditions were major contributors to the generally poor health of residents of the area. His 1842 report to the English Parliament on *The Sanitary Condition of the Labouring Population* is generally considered to have been a "wake up" call to the government about the risks posed by environmental factors to the health of the average English citizen. In 1884, Chadwick founded the Association of Public Sanitary Inspectors, which survives today as the Chartered Institute of Environmental Health. Other nations have a much shorter history of formal acknowledgment of the health risks posed by environmental factors. In the United States, for example, the National

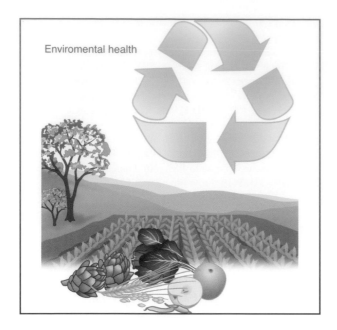

(Illustration by Electronic Illustrators Group. © 2013 Cengage Learning)

Center for Environmental Health (NCEH) of the **Centers for Disease Control and Prevention (CDC)** was created only in 1980. The NCEH today is the primary federal agency with responsibility for environmental health issues.

The field of environmental health is often divided into three major subdisciplines:

- Environmental epidemiology studies the effects of exposure to environmental hazards on human health. Such studies are always observational and retrospective in nature because it is unethical to design or conduct experiments in which humans are intentionally exposed to agents that can cause them harm. A typical epidemiological study might attempt to measure, for example, the number of cases of cancer in a community located adjacent to a petroleum refinery compared to the number of cases in a community distant from such a source of pollution.
- Exposure science is somewhat similar to environmental epidemiology in that it involves studies in the field of the ways in which environmental factors can affect human health. The science is based on the fact that virtually all humans are constantly being exposed to agents that might have harmful effects on their health, but those effects differ significantly from person to person and from agent to agent. The exposure scientist works in the everyday environment of the average person, attempting to determine the range of health effects that can be expected from a range of exposure to such agents.
- Toxicology, on the other hand, relies on experiments conducted on nonhuman animals, such as rats and mice, to determine directly how environmental agents affect the health of those animals. The results of such studies are then commonly extrapolated to human health, with the understanding that human and nonhuman biology, while similar, are not identical in their response to environmental factors. One type of toxicological study might expose a population of rats to low levels of carbon monoxide over extended periods of time and then determine the effects of this exposure on their health. Assumptions about comparable exposure of humans to the same levels of carbon monoxide might then be made.

The field of environmental health covers a very wide range of subjects, as indicated by the topics of fact sheets published by **WHO** in the discipline. They include:

- Mercury and health
- Waste from healthcare activities
- Indoor air pollution and health
- Air quality and health
- Electromagnetic fields and public health: mobile phones
- Environmental and occupational cancers
- Elimination of asbestos-related diseases
- Dioxins and their effects on human health
- Climate change and health
- Sunbeds, tanning, and UV exposure
- Radon and cancer
- Base stations and wireless technologies
- Static electricity and magnetic fields
- Electromagnetic hypersensitivity
- Legionellosis
- Depleted uranium

Other topics of interest to environmental health workers that might be included in this list are:

- Health effects of tattoos and other forms of body art
- Second-hand smoke
- Food safety
- Airborne and waterborne diseases
- Lead poisoning
- Land use policies
- Noise pollution
- Drinking water quality
- Vector control

The number and range of topics listed here provide a sense of the scope of environmental health issues in today's world. A large array of resources are available

KEY TERMS

Environmental epidemiology—The study of the effects of exposure to environmental hazards on human health.

Exposure science—The study of the ways in which environmental factors can affect human health.

Toxicology—The study of the direct effects of substances on the health of experimental animals.

for both professional and laypersons in the field, including peer-reviewed journals such as *Environmental Health, Journal of Environmental Health, Environmental Health Perspectives, Journal of Toxicology and Environmental Health, Journal of Clinical Epidemiology, International Journal of Hygiene and Environmental Health, Environmental Research, International Journal of Occupational and Environmental Health, Environmental Health Insights, Toxicology Mechanisms and Methods*, and *Journal of Exposure Science and Environmental Epidemiology*. The U.S. National Library of Medicine (NLM) also maintains two resources of potential benefit and interest to the general public on environmental health issues, TOXNET and TOXMAP. TOXNET is a searachable resource that provides access to more than a dozen databases with information on environmental health issues in the United States, such as the Hazardous Substances Data Bank (HSDB), Toxicology Literature Online (TOXLINE), Developmental and Reproductive Toxicology Database (DART), and Genetic Toxicology Data Base (GENETOX). TOXNET can be accessed at http://toxnet.nlm.nih.gov/. NLM also maintains TOXMAP, which is a searchable database of all sites listed in the Environmental Protection Agency's Toxic Release Inventory (TRI) and the Superfund National Priorities List (NPL). TOXMAP is available online at http://toxmap.nlm.nih.gov/toxmap/main/index.jsp.

QUESTIONS TO ASK YOUR DOCTOR

- What are the three most important environmental health issues about which members of our community should be concerned?
- What kinds of studies have been or are being conducted in our community on the effects of environmental factors on human health?
- Are there any Superfund or toxic waste sites in or near our community and, if so, what is being done about having them cleaned up?
- How often do you see patients with illnesses that can be attributed to environmental factors?
- What resources in our community are available to individuals who have been exposed to potential environmental hazards?

Resources

BOOKS

Friis, Robert H. *The Praeger Handbook of Environmental Health*. Santa Barbara, CA: Praeger, 2012.

Spellman, Frank R., and Revonna M. Bieber. *Environmental Health and Science Desk Reference*. Lanham, MD: Government Institutes, 2012.

Theodore, Louis, and R. Ryan Dupont. *Environmental Health and Hazard Risk Assessment: Principles and Calculations*. Boca Raton, FL: CRC Press, 2012.

PERIODICALS

Greenberg, Michael, and Lauren Babcock-Dunning. "Worrying About Terrorism and Other Acute Environmental Health Hazard Events." *American Journal of Public Health* 102. 4. (2012): 651–56.

Lioy, Paul, et al. "Letter to the Editor: Defining Exposure Science."*Journal of Exposure Analysis and Environmental Epidemiology*. 15 (2005): 463.

Pohjola, M.V., et al. "State of the Art in Benefit-risk Analysis: Environmental Health." *Food and Chemical Toxicology* 50. 1. (2012): 40–55

"The 2011 Japanese Earthquake: An Overview of Environmental Health Impacts." *Journal of Environmental Health* 74. 6 (2012): 42–51.

WEBSITES

Center for Environmental Health. http://www.ceh.org/. Accessed on September 13, 2012.

Environmental Health Coalition. http://www.environmental-health.org/index.php/en/. Accessed on September 13, 2012.

Environmental Health. Medline Plus. http://www.nlm.nih.gov/medlineplus/environmentalhealth.html. Accessed on September 13, 2012.

Environmental Health News. http://www.environmentalhealthnews.org/. Accessed on September 13, 2012.

ORGANIZATIONS

National Center for Environmental Health, Centers for Disease Control and Prevention, 1600 Clifton Rd., N.E., Atlanta, GA USA 30333, 1 (800) 232-4636, cdcinfo@cdc.gov, www.cdc.gov/nceh/.

David E. Newton, Ed.D.

Environmental Protection Agency (EPA)

Definition

The U.S. Environmental Protection Agency (EPA) is the primary federal agency responsible for protecting human health and the natural environment.

Purpose

The EPA's statement of purposes lists seven specific objectives:

- protecting Americans from threats to their health and to the environment;
- reducing environmental risks based on the best available scientific information;
- enforcing federal laws dealing with human health and the environmental in a fair and balanced way;
- carrying out federal policy in a balanced way that gives due consideration to all aspects of American society;
- ensuring that all parts of American society have equal access to accurate information about health and environmental issues;
- working to make ecosystems diverse, sustainable, and economically productive; and
- playing a leadership role in addressing global environmental issues.

Description

The Environmental Protection Agency was created on July 9, 1970, under President Richard M. Nixon's Reorganization Plan #3. That plan brought together a number of agencies from various parts of the federal government into a single new department, the EPA. Among the agencies transferred to the new EPA were the Federal Water Quality Administration from the Department of the Interior; the National **Air Pollution** Control Administration, Bureau of Solid Waste Management, Bureau of Water **Hygiene**, and Bureau of Radiological Health from the Department of Health, Education, and Welfare; certain agencies dealing with pesticides from the Food and Drug Administration and the Department of Agriculture; and the regulation of nuclear materials from the Atomic Energy Commission. That mix of responsibilities is reflected in the organization of the department today. In addition to a number of administrative offices (such as the Office of the Inspector General and the Office of the General Counsel), the major divisions of the EPA are:

- Office of Air and Radiation;
- Office of Chemical Safety and Pollution Prevention;
- Office of Environmental Information;
- Office of Research and Development;
- Office of Solid Waste and Emergency Response;
- Office of Water.

These offices are responsible for administering and carrying out the provisions of the full arsenal of U.S. environmental laws, including such legislation as the Clean Air Act and all of its amendments; the Clean Water Act and Water Quality Act; the Toxic Substances Control Act; the Safe **Drinking Water** Act and its amendments; the Federal Insecticide, Fungicide, and Rodenticide Act; the Food Quality Protection Act; the Endangered Species Protection Act; the Solid Waste Disposal Act; the Comprehensive Environmental Response, Compensation, and Liability Act ("Superfund"); the Nuclear Waste Repository Act; and the Hazardous and Solid Wastes Amendments Act. In order to carry out this ambitious program, the EPA employs about 17,400 men and women (as of 2011) with a budget at the time of $8.682 billion. In addition to its headquarters in Washington, the EPA maintains ten regional offices around the country that include the 50 states, the District of Columbia, and eight U.S. territories in the Atlantic and Pacific Oceans. In addition to its regional offices (each of which has its own affiliated research laboratory), the EPA sponsors a number of research centers that focus on specific topics of environmental and health interest, including the National Center for Computational Toxicology in Research Triangle Park, North Carolina; National Center for Environmental Assessment in Arlington, Virginia, Cincinnati, Ohio, and Research Triangle Park; National Center for Environmental Research in Washington, D.C.; National Exposure Research Laboratory in Durham, North Carolina; National Health and Environmental Effects Research Laboratory in Research Triangle Park, Gulf Breeze, Florida, Duluth, Minnesota, Corvallis Oregon, and Narragansett, Rhode Island; National Homeland Security Research Center in Cincinnati; and National Risk Management Research Laboratory in Cincinnati; Durham; Ada, Oklahoma; and Edison, New Jersey.

The EPA website is an invaluable resource on laws and regulations dealing with every conceivable aspect of human health and environmental issues and the repository of extensive scientific data on such issues. It also provides extensive scientific information on a wide range of health and environmental topics, which it currently classifies under nine major topics: air; climate change; emergencies; green living; health and safety; land and cleanup; pesticides, chemicals, and toxics; waste; and water.

Professional Publications

The EPA publishes a number of newsletters pertaining to health and environmental issues, such as *Enforcement Alert*, *Fish Advisories Newsletter*, *Go Green!*,

Pipeline, *Small Flows Quarterly*, *Technology News and Trends*, *Tribal Air*, *Tribal Waste Journal*, *Volunteer Monitoring*, and *Water Talk*. These publications range in complexity from technical journals intended for experts in the field to general publications of interest to the public as a whole. The EPA also publishes many thousands of technical reports concerning every aspect of its health and environment mission. Many of these publications are available from the EPA directly, while others can be ordered through one or more of the regional offices or specialized offices listed above. For a complete list of publications from all sources, see the EPA web page at http://www.epa.gov/epahome/publications.htm#tech.

Resources

BOOKS

Cooper, Terry F., and Clark D. Morgan. *The Environmental Protection Agency "regulation train": Proposals and Controversies*. Hauppauge, NY: Nova Science Publishers, 2012.

Roberts, Ashley B. *The EPA and the Clean Air Act: Authority and Regulation Issues*. New York: Nova Science Publishers, 2011.

PERIODICALS

Cline, K. "Negotiating the Superfund: Are Environmental Protection Agency Regional Officials Willing to Bargain with States?" *Social Science Journal* 47. 1. (2010): 106–20.

Payne-Sturges, Devon. "Humanizing Science at the US Environmental Protection Agency." *American Journal of Public Health* 101. S1. (2011): S8–S12.

WEBSITES

How the EPA Works. How Stuff Works. http://people.howstuffworks.com/epa1.htm. (Accessed September 11, 2012).

Interference at the EPA. Union of Concerned Scientists. http://www.ucsusa.org/assets/documents/scientific_integrity/interference-at the-epa.pdf. (Accessed September 11, 2012).

ORGANIZATIONS

Environmental Protection Agency (EPA), Ariel Rios Building, 1200 Pennsylvania Ave., N.W., Washington, DC 20460, 1 (202) 272–0167, http://publicaccess.supportportal.com/ics/support/ticketnewwizard.asp?style=classic, http://www.epa.gov/.

David E. Newton, Ed.D.

Environmental toxins

Definition

Environmental toxins are chemicals found in the air, soil, **water**, food, or buildings, that are harmful to humans. They include a wide range of natural as well as synthetic compounds that damage human health. Some scientists prefer the term *toxicant* for toxic chemicals produced by human activity, to differentiate them from toxins produced by disease organisms, plants, and marine or land animals.

Purpose

Some environmental toxins are byproducts of such natural processes as the decay of animal wastes and plant matter or the release of volcanic gases during an eruption. Some environmental toxins are found in poisonous plants or animals. Some, like lead, mercury, arsenic, and plutonium, are elements that occur naturally in the Earth's crust and may cause harm to humans accidentally. Others are byproducts of manufacturing processes that were not intended to cause deliberate harm to people or the environment.

Some environmental toxins are designed to cause harm or are purposely consumed by humans for other reasons:

- Pesticides and weed killers (herbicides). These products are used in parts of Asia and Africa to commit suicide as well as to rid crops or buildings of pests.
- Disinfectants and sanitizing agents.
- Chemicals used in warfare. These include nerve gases (Sarin and VX); suffocating agents (phosgene); and vesicants or blister-causing agents (nitrogen mustard and sulfur mustard). These agents could also be used by terrorists.
- Alcohol, tobacco, and drugs of abuse. These include wood alcohol and other toxic alcohols not ordinarily intended for consumption as well as aerosol propellants and organic solvents used by adolescent "glue sniffers."
- Chemicals used for crowd or riot control. These include tear gas, mace, and similar chemicals.

Demographics

It is difficult to estimate how many people are harmed each year by environmental toxins either worldwide or in specific countries, and how severe is the damage to health. There are a number of reasons for this difficulty:

- Most environmental toxins have not been studied frequently enough or have not been produced long enough to allow researchers to gauge their long-term effects on health. Of the more than 80,000 chemicals that have been developed, used, and released into the environment since the end of World War II, only a few (such as asbestos, lead, and vinyl chloride) have been studied closely over many years.

- Environmental toxins rarely occur in isolation. Most people are exposed to mixtures of chemicals in their environments. Scientists have not yet mapped all of the potential interactions among them. Some toxins counteract each other, while some have an additive or multiplicative effect. One example is the combination of tobacco smoking and asbestos exposure. In combination with each other, these two toxins increase the risk of lung cancer 25-fold—a risk much higher than the sum of the risks of the toxic substances taken separately.
- Using human subjects for experiments using toxic substances is unethical. Much of the available information about the health effects of environmental toxins therefore comes from animal studies, case studies of accidental exposures to toxins, industrial disasters, or long-term workplace exposures.
- It can also be difficult to measure the effects of exposure to environmental contaminants because people frequently move to new geographical locations or change occupations.
- The toxicity of environmental toxins varies considerably, ranging from substances that have negligible effects on people unless touched, swallowed, or inhaled in large amounts, to substances that are potentially deadly even in small quantities.
- The health effects of exposure to environmental toxins depend on a number of factors, including length of time of exposure; frequency of exposure; age at exposure (before birth; childhood, adolescence, adulthood); route of exposure (inhalation, skin contact, ingestion); and differences in individual susceptibility, including genetic factors.

Precautions

Precautions for dealing with environmental toxins are highly specific to the substance involved. The Agency for Toxic Substances and Disease Registry (ATSDR) has public health statements (PHSs) written for the general public on its website at http://www.atsdr.cdc.gov/PHS/Index.asp for over 180 different natural and synthetic toxins. Each PHS answers the following questions:

- What is [name of chemical]?
- What happens to it when it enters the environment?
- How might I be exposed to it?
- How can it enter and leave my body?
- How can it affect my health?
- Is there a medical test to determine whether I have been exposed to it?
- What recommendations have been made to protect human health?

Description

Natural environmental toxins

Some toxins occur naturally:

- Volcanic gases. About 3% of all deaths resulting from volcanic eruptions are caused by suffocation or damage to the lungs from the acids, sulfur, ash, and other compounds in volcanic gases.
- Biotoxins. Biotoxins is the term for toxic substances produced by living organisms. They have two primary purposes: predation (catching or killing prey) and defense. Biotoxins include hemotoxins (toxins that destroy red blood cells); neurotoxins (toxins that attack the nervous system); and necrotoxins (toxins that destroy cells and cause the death of tissue). Biotoxins vary greatly in chemical composition and the mechanisms by which they are delivered to animals or humans.
- Biogases. Biogases are gases produced by the anaerobic decay of organic matter. Methane is the most common biogas. Sources of biogases include swamps, landfills, marshes, animal manure, and sewage sludge.

Synthetic toxicants

Synthetic toxicants are chemicals made by humans or produced as byproducts of human smelting, refining, and manufacturing processes. The **Centers for Disease Control and Prevention (CDC)** divides these toxicants into the following categories:

- Vesicants. Vesicants are chemicals that cause blistering of the skin and mucous membranes. They include mustard gas, nitrogen mustard, and sulfur mustard.
- Long-acting blood anticoagulants. These chemicals are typically used in mouse and rat poisons. Super warfarin is the most commonly used chemical in this category.
- Blood agents. These toxic chemicals are absorbed directly into the blood. They include carbon monoxide, cyanide, and arsine, a colorless gas made from arsenic.
- Choking and pulmonary agents. These are chemicals that irritate the eyes and respiratory tract, causing severe irritation and swelling. They include chlorine, ammonia, phosgene (a poison gas used in World War I), and elemental white, or yellow phosphorus.
- Caustics. These are substances that burn or corrode people's skin, eyes, and mucus membranes (lining of the nose, mouth, throat, and lungs) on contact. They include strong acids (hydrochloric acid, sulfuric acid) and alkalis (lye [caustic soda] and potassium hydroxide).

- Metals. Poisonous metallic substances include lead, mercury, barium, thallium, and arsenic.
- Incapacitating agents. There are drugs that make people unable to think clearly or that cause an altered state of consciousness or even loss of consciousness. They include fentanyl and other opioids, and BZ (benzilic acid), used to make some hallucinogenic drugs.
- Organic solvents. These chemicals dissolve fats and oils in living tissue, resulting in tissue damage. The most common of these is benzene, formerly used as a gasoline additive and in dry cleaning. Benzene is produced in small amounts by volcanoes and forest fires as well as by human industrial processes.
- Nerve agents. These prevent the nervous system from functioning properly. They include Sarin, Tabun, VX, and Soman.
- Toxic alcohols. Toxic alcohols include ethylene glycol, used to make antifreeze; methanol (wood alcohol); and isopropyl alcohol (rubbing alcohol). Note that ethanol (beverage alcohol) is also toxic in large amounts and can lead to death.
- Vomiting agents. The most common is adamsite, which has been used for riot control.

Specific environmental health hazards

The National Institute of **Environmental Health** Sciences (NIEHS) considers the following substances or categories of substances to be particularly harmful as of 2012:

- Dioxins. Dioxins are chemicals formed by burning, ranging from forest fires to backyard trash burning and incineration of industrial wastes. They are also formed by paper pulp bleaching and herbicide production. People take in dioxins mostly by eating food contaminated with them. Dioxins accumulate in the fatty tissues of the body; they can lead to a skin disorder known as chloracne and to an increased risk of cancer.
- Endocrine disruptors. Endocrine disruptors are a class of chemicals that affect the body's endocrine system, leading to various disorders in reproduction, growth and development, the nervous system, and the immune system. Endocrine disruptors include dioxins, some pharmaceuticals, pesticides, and some chemicals used to make plastic bottles, metal food cans, cosmetics, household detergents, pesticides, and flame-retardant materials.
- Ozone. Ozone is a reactive form of oxygen found naturally in the upper atmosphere. It is also produced in the lower atmosphere by the interaction of automobile exhaust and factory emissions with sunlight. High concentrations of ozone in urban areas can lead to respiratory distress in persons with asthma and other chronic lung diseases.
- Lead. Lead is one of the best-studied environmental toxins. Found naturally in the earth's crust, lead has been used by humans for millennia to make cosmetics, ceramic glazes, pewter cups and plates, batteries, pipes, house paints, and many other items. Extreme forms of lead poisoning are marked by lack of muscular coordination, convulsions, and coma; however, much lower lead levels have been associated with measurable changes in children's mental development and behavior. Chronic lead exposure in adults can lead to high blood pressure, infertility, cataracts, nerve disorders, muscle and joint pains, and problems with memory or concentration.
- Molds. Molds are fungi that occur naturally in shady, damp, or moist areas outdoors, where they help to break down plant and animal matter. Indoors, molds can grow around pipes and plumbing fixtures, in damp basements, or in any location that supplies them with oxygen, moisture, and organic matter. When molds are disturbed, they release spores that can irritate the skin, eyes, nasal passages, and throat. People with chronic respiratory illnesses may have difficulty breathing after exposure to mold spores, and people with weakened immune systems are at increased risk of lung infections.
- Mercury. Like lead, mercury is found naturally in the earth's crust. It is used to make thermometers, barometers, and fluorescent light bulbs. It is also discharged into the air by volcanic eruptions and by waste incinerators. Mercury released into the air is eventually taken up by microscopic organisms in the sea and enters the food chain when fish consume these organisms and store the mercury in their own tissues. Humans can be exposed to mercury in the form of elemental mercury or through eating large quantities of fish. Mercury poisoning includes such symptoms as difficulty walking, "pins and needles" sensations, muscle weakness, skin rashes, mood changes, memory loss, and difficulties with vision, hearing, or speech.
- Pesticides. Pesticides include a wide variety of compounds intended to destroy unwanted plants, animals, or microorganisms. They include herbicides, fungicides, disinfectants for use in hospitals and similar facilities, insecticides, and chemicals to kill rats and mice. Researchers do not yet have a clear understanding of all the possible health effects of these substances nor the concentrations of them that are needed to become dangerous, but preliminary studies of farmers indicate that pesticides can cause a variety of neurological symptoms, including chronic headaches, dizziness, insomnia, fatigue, and hand tremors.
- Bisphenol A. Bisphenol A is used in the production of a wide variety of plastics. It is used to make packaging

material for foods and drinks, compact discs, impact-resistant safety equipment, medical devices, lacquers to coat metal products, and some types of dental sealants and composites. Considerable disagreement exists over possible health effects on humans of bisphenol A, although some evidence suggests that it may be responsible for prenatal damage to the neurological system.

- Radon. Radon is a colorless, odorless, radioactive gas formed during the decay of uranium and thorium in the soil and the air. It occurs commonly in basements, floors, walls, and other enclosed areas in homes and other buildings. The U.S. Environmental Protection Agency (EPA) estimates that about 21,000 deaths from lung cancer annually are attributable to radon exposure.

Readers who wish to find out more about the known or suspected health effects of specific toxicants or who wish information about the associations between specific diseases and toxic chemicals may find the database compiled by the Collaborative on Health and the Environment (CHE) helpful. The database is searchable for over 180 different diseases or conditions and can be searched for toxicant or disease category. It can be found at http://www.healthandenvironment.org/tddb.

Origins

As has already been noted, some environmental toxins are the result of natural processes or substances that have been present since the formation of the planet's crust and the beginnings of plant and animal life. The human contribution to environmental toxicants appears to have begun with the mining and smelting of metals in the Bronze Age (about 3000 B.C.). Measurable residues of pollution taken from glacier ice core samples have been dated as far back as 500 B.C.. The earliest-known references to environmental contamination occur in Arab medical treatises written between the ninth and thirteenth centuries A.D.

Preparation

Preparation for exposure to environmental toxins varies widely, depending on the nature of the toxin or contaminant. Some can be simply avoided; some may require special handling, while others may require various types of protective equipment. Detailed information about specific chemicals can be obtained from the ATSDR or local public health officials.

Aftercare

People do not always need to take special measures after exposure to some environmental toxins, particularly if the substance is of low toxicity and the exposure has been brief. In the case of severe exposure or a chemical accident, advice about personal aftercare and treatment of contaminated clothing can be found on the **CDC** website at http://emergency.cdc.gov/planning/personalcleaningfacts.asp.

Results

The results of cleaning up environmental toxins depends on the nature of the contamination and its

KEY TERMS

Anaerobic—Occurring or growing in the absence of oxygen.

Biogas—Gas produced by the decay of organic matter in the absence of oxygen. Sources of biogas include sewage, manure, landfills, swamps, marshes, and animal manure.

Biomonitoring—The direct measurement of people's exposure to toxic substances in the environment through analysis of blood and urine samples.

Biotoxin—Any toxin produced by a living organism.

Brownfield—A term used to describe previously used or underused commercial or industrial buildings that are contaminated by sufficiently low levels of pollutants that they can be reused after being cleaned up.

Chelation therapy—The use of such chemicals as BAL (British Anti-Lewisite) or EDTA in conventional medicine to treat heavy metal poisoning. Some practitioners of alternative medicine use these chemicals to remove toxins in general from the body or to treat autism and heart disease.

Colonic hydrotherapy—In alternative medicine, the use of enemas to cleanse the lower bowel in the belief that this process removes toxic wastes from the body.

Endocrine disruptors—Chemicals that interfere with the production or activity of hormones produced by the body's endocrine glands. These glands include the pancreas, pituitary, thyroid, adrenals, and male and female reproductive glands.

Toxicant—Any toxic chemical produced by human activity, as distinct from natural toxins.

Toxicity—The degree to which a substance is able to harm a human or other organism exposed to it.

Vesicant—The scientific name for a toxic chemical that causes blistering of the skin, mucous membranes, and respiratory tract.

QUESTIONS TO ASK YOUR DOCTOR

- Are any of my health problems related to environmental toxins, in your opinion?
- What treatments are available?
- What can I do about environmental toxins in my home or workplace?
- What precautions should I take regarding the use of household chemicals?

location. In some cases, unused buildings or factories in urban areas with low levels of environmental toxins can be reused after cleaning, decontamination, or demolition. These buildings or the areas of their location are known as brownfields or brownfield land.

Health care team roles

Health care team roles include public health surveillance and biomonitoring of people in workplaces, factories, other buildings, landfills, and the like; research into the short- and long-term health effects of natural and synthetic toxins and toxicants; research into better methods of pollution **prevention** and environmental cleanup; and treatment of individuals who develop physical illnesses or mental disorders as a result of exposure to environmental toxins.

Alternatives

Some forms of **alternative medicine** claim to be able to improve health by removing environmental toxins from the human body. These systems and approaches include traditional Chinese medicine (TCM), Ayurveda (the traditional medical system of India), lemon juice and other detoxification diets, chelation therapy, colonic hydrotherapy, the use of laxatives to cleanse the colon, juice fasts, water diets, polarity therapy, or herbal cleansing.

Research & general acceptance

There are a growing number of clinical trials investigating the effects of environmental toxins on human health. As of early 2010, there were 156 studies of lead **poisoning** under way, 4 of asbestos, 10 of cadmium poisoning, 3 of mercury toxicity, 4 of endocrine disruptors, 47 of pesticide exposure, 24 of susceptibility to high ozone levels, 23 of mold-related illnesses, 522 of tobacco, 2 of inhalant abuse, and 19 of alcohol toxicity.

As of 2012, there was no evidence that detoxification diets, Chinese herbal medicines, colonic hydrotherapy or laxative use, fasting, or any other form of alternative medicine is effective in removing environmental toxins from the body.

Caregiver concerns

Caregiver concerns include checking the house and surrounding environment for possible sources of contamination; having the house professionally inspected for **mold**, lead paint, asbestos, or other toxic substances often found in buildings; taking necessary precautions in the use and storage of cleaning products; and keeping the house free of tobacco products and smoke. These precautions are particularly important if the person being cared for has **asthma**, bronchitis, or another chronic respiratory disorder.

Resources

BOOKS

Friis, Robert H. *Essentials of Environmental Health*, 2nd ed. Sudbury, MA: Jones & Bartlett Learning, 2010.

Frumkin, Howard, ed. *Environmental Health: From Global to Local*, 2nd ed. New York: Jossey-Bass, 2010.

Maczulak, Anne. *Pollution: Treating Environmental Toxins*. New York: Facts On File, 2010.

PERIODICALS

Chatham-Stephens, Kevin M., et al. "First, Do No Harm: Children's Environmental Health in Schools." *American Educator* 35, 4. (2012): 22–31.

Rourigny, P.D., and C. Hall. "Diagnosis and Management of Environmental Thoracic Emergencies." *Emergency Clinics of North America* 30, 2. (2012): 501–28.

Roy, J.R., S. Chakraborty, and T. R. Chakraborty. "Estrogen-like Endocrine Disrupting Chemicals Affecting Puberty in Humans—A Review." *Medical Science Monitoring* 15, 6. (2009): RA137–45.

Salama, Mohamed, and Oscar Arias-Carri'n. "Natural Toxins Implicated in the Development of Parkinson's Disease." *Therapeutic Advances in Neurological Disorders* 4, 6. (2011): 361–73.

WEBSITES

"Chemical Contaminants and Human Disease: A Summary of Evidence." Collaborative on Health and the Environment. http://guamagentorange.info/yahoo_site_admin/assets/docs/CHE_Toxicants_and_Disease_Database.160121218.pdf. Accessed on October 20, 2012.

"Environmental Toxins/Hazardous Materials." Environmental Protection Agency. http://www.cdc.gov/nceh/ehs/topics/toxins.htm. Accessed on October 20, 2012.

"National Report on Human Exposure to Environmental Chemicals." Centers for Disease Control and Prevention. http://www.cdc.gov/exposurereport/index.html. Accessed on October 20, 2012.

"Top 10 Most Common Environmental Toxins." Canada.com http://www.canada.com/vancouversun/news/story.html?id=57586947-9466-4fcf-bb1b-2c464dd19e5c. Accessed on October 20, 2012.

"Toxic Substances Portal." Agency for Toxic Substances and Disease Registry. http://www.atsdr.cdc.gov/substances/index.asp. Accessed on October 20, 2012.

ORGANIZATIONS

Agency for Toxic Substances and Disease Registry (ATSDR), 4770 Buford Hwy. NE, Atlanta, GA 30341, 800-232-4636, cdcinfo@cdc.gov, http://www.atsdr.cdc.gov/.

Centers for Disease Control and Prevention (CDC), 1600 Clifton Rd., Atlanta, GA 30333, 800-232-4636, cdcinfo@cdc.gov, http://www.cdc.gov.

Collaborative on Health and the Environment (CHE), P.O. Box 316, Bolinas, CA 94924, 415-868-0970, Fax: 415-868-2230, info@HealthandEnvironment.org, http://www.healthandenvironment.org/index.php.

Environmental Protection Agency (EPA), Ariel Rios Building, 1200 Pennsylvania Ave., NW, Washington, DC 20460, 202-272-0167, http://www.epa.gov/epahome/comments.htm, http://www.epa.gov/.

National Institute of Environmental Health Sciences (NIEHS), 111 T.W. Alexander Dr., Research Triangle Park, NC 27709, 919-541-3345, Fax: 919-541-4395, webcenter@niehs.nih.gov, http://www.niehs.nih.gov/.

National Toxicology Program (NTP), P.O. Box 12233, MD K2-03, Research Triangle Park, NC 27709, 919-541-0530, http://ntp.niehs.nih.gov/index.cfm?objectid=720166E6-BDB7-CEBA-F0032407A834B400, http://ntp.niehs.nih.gov/.

U.S. Food and Drug Administration (FDA), 10903 New Hampshire Ave., Silver Spring, MD 20993, 888-463-6332, http://www.fda.gov/AboutFDA/ContactFDA/default.htm, http://www.fda.gov/.

World Health Organization (WHO), Avenue Appia 20, 1211 Geneva 27, Switzerland, + 41 22 791 21 11, Fax: + 41 22 791 31 11, info@who.int, http://www.who.int/en/.

Rebecca J. Frey, Ph.D.
David E. Newton, Ed.D.

Epidemic *see* **Epidemiology**

Epidemiology

Definition

Epidemiology is the branch of medicine and public health that deals with the study of factors associated with either communicable or noncommunicable diseases which affect the health of populations rather than individuals. A more formal definition is that given by the **World Health Organization (WHO)**: "the study of the distribution and determinants of health-related states or events (including disease), and the application of this study to the control of diseases and other health problems." Epidemiologists gather and analyze data about the occurrence or spread of disease and communicate their findings to policy makers and the general public. They are also commonly tasked with managing or planning public health programs, monitoring their progress, and seeking ways to improve the programs.

There are two main approaches to epidemiology: descriptive and analytical. Descriptive epidemiologists study and report on the distribution, occurrence, and patterns of diseases. For example, it is known that the incidence of Alzheimer's disease increases with age. A descriptive epidemiologist would draw up a table with different age categories and note the corresponding incidence rates for Alzheimer's in each age group. By contrast, analytical epidemiologists use statistics to evaluate the impact of different factors on the occurrence of a disease. To use Alzheimer's disease again as an example, an analytical epidemiologist might look at factors thought to affect a person's risk of developing Alzheimer's, such as diet, exercise, or mental stimulation, and use statistics to determine whether in fact these factors play a part in the development of the disease along with increasing age.

Applied epidemiology refers to the use of both descriptive and analytical approaches to epidemiology in practice-based settings, which may be state or local government public health agencies, pharmaceutical firms, international agencies, or hospitals and other healthcare institutions. Applied epidemiology includes investigations of outbreaks and epidemics of infectious diseases, disease surveillance, and studies of such chronic diseases as diabetes and heart disorders.

Description

History

Epidemiology as the study of the origin and spread of diseases goes back to ancient Greece, to Hippocrates (c. 460–370 B.C.), the so-called father of Western medicine. Hippocrates attempted to trace the sources of the contagious diseases known to him, and coined the term *epidemic* for diseases that spread rapidly throughout a **population**. The earliest writer who recognized the importance of clean **water**, avoidance of environmental contaminants, and frequent bathing to lower the risk of disease was the Roman military engineer Vitruvius (c. 80–15 B.C.), who noted that the use of lead for water pipes was dangerous to health, and recommended ceramic pipes instead. Vitruvius was responsible for overseeing the cleanliness of Julius Caesar's army camps as well as guaranteeing a safe and adequate water supply.

During the Renaissance, an Italian physician named Girolamo Fracastoro (1478–1553) published a book in 1543 titled *De contagione et contagiosis morbis* ("On Contagion and Communicable Diseases"), in which he theorized that infectious diseases were spread by "spores" that were too small to see but were nonetheless alive. Like Vitruvius, Fracastoro recommended personal cleanliness and environmental **hygiene** to prevent outbreaks of disease.

Modern epidemiology began with John Snow (1813–1858), an English physician who traced the source of an outbreak of **cholera** in London in 1854 to a public water pump whose water was contaminated by sewage. Although Snow's work was not widely accepted until some years after his death, the establishment of the **germ theory** of disease by Louis Pasteur (1822–1895) and Robert Koch (1843–1910) helped to confirm the importance of Snow's work and establish epidemiology as a branch of preventive medicine. In the twentieth century, such physicians as Ronald Ross (1857–1932), a British doctor who won the 1902 Nobel Prize in Medicine for his work on **malaria**, and Anderson Gray McKendrick (1876–1943), a Scottish doctor who worked with Ross in India, pioneered the application of mathematical models to analytical epidemiology. McKendrick in particular was a gifted mathematician who published a noteworthy set of papers from 1927 onward on a general theory of disease transmission.

Specialties within epidemiology

As of 2012, several specialties have developed within the wider field of epidemiology:

- Disease etiology. Disease etiology is the branch of epidemiology that traces a disease outbreak or emerging disease to its source or cause.
- Investigation of disease outbreaks. Epidemiologists who specialize in this branch of epidemiology are called field epidemiologists. Field epidemiology is a branch of applied epidemiology intended to solve public health problems of an urgent or emergency nature, particularly outbreaks or epidemics in underdeveloped countries. Both the CDC and WHO offer training programs in field epidemiology.
- Disease surveillance and screening. Surveillance is another form of applied epidemiology; it involves collecting case reports of reportable (notifiable) diseases in order to predict, monitor, and reduce the harm caused by outbreaks or epidemics of viral or bacterial diseases. The CDC maintains a countrywide surveillance system in the United States known as the National Notifiable Diseases Surveillance System or NNDSS.
- Biomonitoring. Biomonitoring is the study and assessment of chemicals in the environment, measured by the amounts of these substances that actually enter the human body and can be detected in blood or urine samples. Epidemiologists who specialize in biomonitoring often work in the fields of environmental or occupational health. The Centers for Disease Control and Prevention (CDC) has established a National Biomonitoring Program (NBP) that collects data on more than 450 different chemicals that can be found in human body fluids.
- Comparison of management or treatment options. Sometimes known as pharmacoepidemiologists, specialists in this field conduct clinical studies to compare the safety and effectiveness of a new drug or treatment for a specific disease with the safety and efficacy of current treatment options.
- Forensic epidemiology. Forensic epidemiologists investigate incidents of bioterrorism and other aspects of disease related to law enforcement and the criminal justice system. There has been increasing interest in forensic epidemiology in the United States since the anthrax attacks of 2001, with a growing number of schools of public health offering courses in this field.
- Veterinary epidemiology. Veterinary epidemiology is the study of disease transmission and outbreaks in animal populations. It utilizes the same observational methods, data collection, and statistical analyses as human epidemiology. Some schools of veterinary medicine in the United States have specialized departments of veterinary epidemiology.

Work settings

Epidemiologists work in a variety of different public health, academic, laboratory, and other settings:

- Federal, state, and local government: 54%. Most epidemiologists who work in government agencies are applied epidemiologists; the most common area of concern is infectious diseases. Other areas of special interest include bioterrorism and emergency management; maternal and child health; chronic diseases; environmental health; injuries and accidents; occupational health; substance abuse; animal health; and oral health.
- State, local, and private hospitals: 13%. Hospital-based epidemiologists typically collect and analyze patient data—including observations, interviews with patients, staff surveys, and samples of blood or other bodily fluids—to find the causes of diseases or other health problems in the population served by the hospital.
- Colleges, universities, graduate, and professional schools: 9%. Most epidemiologists who teach at the

university or professional school level are research epidemiologists.

- Scientific research and clinical trials: 7%. Clinical trial design and conduct is a growing field within epidemiology; there are 1547 clinical trials registered with the National Institutes of Health (NIH) as of 2012 that involve epidemiological studies of diseases ranging from lymphoma and pancreatic cancer to HIV infection and nosocomial (hospital-acquired) infections.
- Pharmaceutical companies: 5%. Epidemiologists who work in pharmaceutical companies are usually pharmacoepidemiologists who hold the Pharm.D. degree or have obtained other specialized training in pharmacology. They study infectious or chronic diseases whose outcome may be affected by a medication or biologic agent.

According to the U.S. Bureau of Labor Statistics (BLS), the average annual salary for an epidemiologist as of 2012 is about $65,000. Most full-time epidemiologists work regular hours; the exception is field epidemiologists during an epidemic or other public health crisis, who may asked to work irregular hours to conduct interviews and gather data.

Undergraduate education

Very few colleges and universities in North America offer undergraduate majors in epidemiology as such; the basic requirement for employment in the field is a master's degree, and preferably a doctorate. To prepare for a career in epidemiology, an undergraduate should have a strong background in mathematics as well as the biological sciences and other premedical courses. Admission to most departments of epidemiology and schools of public health in the United States is highly competitive as of 2012.

Advanced education and training

Students with appropriate undergraduate preparation and performance may apply for a master's degree program with an emphasis in epidemiology, most often a master of public health (M.P.H.) or a master of science (M.Sc.) degree. As of 2012, there are 82 universities in the United States and 10 in Canada that offer degree programs in epidemiology; some have separate schools of epidemiology and public health while others have divisions or departments of epidemiology and preventive medicine within their schools of medicine, health sciences, or **veterinary medicine**. Students interested in research or academic positions in the field usually obtain doctorates, usually a Ph.D. (doctor of philosophy) or Dr. P.H. (doctor of public health) degree. Some medical schools offer joint M.D./M.P.H. degree programs, which allow students to qualify as medical practitioners as well as epidemiologists. In addition, some persons who already hold the M.D., D.O. (doctor of osteopathy), or D.V.M. (doctor of veterinary medicine) degree may obtain an additional master's or doctoral degree in public health in order to qualify as epidemiologists.

Coursework in epidemiology places a heavy emphasis on competence in mathematics as well as the biological sciences and public health. Classes include statistical methods, causal analysis, and survey design. Advanced courses offer instruction in multiple regression, medical informatics, reviews of previous biomedical research, and practical applications of medical data. Epidemiologists must be skilled in both qualitative research (observations of patients or research subjects and interviews with them) and quantitative methods (survey methods and analysis of the data collected). In addition, epidemiologists must be able to communicate health information clearly and accurately in written reports and oral presentations, whether they are speaking to other health professionals and policy makers, or addressing the general public.

Advanced training in applied epidemiology began in the United States in 1951, when the **CDC** instituted a two-year postgraduate program for epidemiologists known as the Epidemic Intelligence Service or EIS. The program is open to physicians, veterinarians, those with a Ph.D. in epidemiology, and other health professionals who have completed an M.P.H. degree. The Rollins School of Public Health at Emory University in Atlanta offers an applied epidemiology track within its M.P.H. program that is coordinated with the CDC's EIS.

Epidemiologists may also seek advanced training in psychology and the social sciences to better understand the human factors in the spread of disease; engineering to specialize in **occupational health** or assess the degree of people's exposure to contaminants in the environment; pharmacology in order to work in drug development; or law to specialize in forensic epidemiology or advocate for changes in public policy.

Future outlook

There are about 5,000 people in the United States employed as epidemiologists as of 2012. Employment in the field is expected to increase by 24% by 2020, particularly in state and local government public **health departments**. The reason for the increase is renewed interest in disease **prevention**, **emergency preparedness** related to bioterrorism, and monitoring of emerging and reemerging diseases. As of 2012, a number of states are reporting a shortage of applied epidemiologists.

KEY TERMS

Biomonitoring—A method for detecting the presence and amount of environmental chemicals in the human body, usually obtained from blood or urine samples. It is a more accurate measure of the effects of chemical exposure on human health than simply measuring the levels of chemicals in soil, air, water, or food.

Epidemic—An outbreak of a contagious disease that involves new cases of the disease in a specific human population during a given period substantially exceeding the number expected based on recent experience.

Etiology—The cause or origin of a disease; also, the scientific study of disease causation.

Forensic—Pertaining to matters of interest in a court of law.

Incidence—The number of new cases of a specific disease within a specific time period within a specific population.

Reportable disease—Any disease that is required by law to be reported to government authorities or to such organizations as the CDC or WHO. Reportable diseases are also called notifiable diseases.

Surveillance—In epidemiology, the monitoring and reporting of cases of contagious disease in order to establish patterns of its spread to prevent or minimize the development of epidemics and pandemics.

Resources

BOOKS

Gerstman, B. Burt. *Epidemiology Kept Simple: An Introduction to Traditional and Modern Epidemiology*, 3rd ed. Chichester, UK: John Wiley and Sons, 2013.

Gregg, Michael. *Field Epidemiology*, 3rd ed. New York: Oxford University Press, 2008.

Macera, Caroline A., Richard A. Shaffer, and Peggy M. Shaffer. *Introduction to Epidemiology: Distribution and Determinants of Disease in Humans*. Clifton, NY: Delmar Cengage Learning, 2012.

Merrill, Ray M. *Introduction to Epidemiology*, 6th ed. Burlington, MA: Jones and Bartlett Learning, 2013.

Thrusfield, Michael V. *Veterinary Epidemiology*, 3rd ed. Ames, IA: Blackwell, 2005.

PERIODICALS

Becker, K.M., et al. "Field Epidemiology and Laboratory Training Programs in West Africa as a Model for Sustainable Partnerships in Animal and Human Health." *Journal of the American Veterinary Medical Association* 241 (September 1, 2012): 572–579.

Boulton, M.L., et al. "Assessment of Epidemiology Capacity in State Health Departments, 2001–2006." *Journal of Public Health Management and Practice* 15 (July-August 2009): 328–336.

Burns, C.J., and G.M. Swaen. "Review of 2,4-Dichlorophenoxyacetic Acid (2,4-D) Biomonitoring and Epidemiology." *Critical Reviews in Toxicology* 42 (October 2012): 768–786.

Carter-Pokras, O.D., et al. "Epidemiology, Policy, and Racial/Ethnic Minority Health Disparities." *Annals of Epidemiology* 22 (June 2012): 446–455.

Centers for Disease Control and Prevention (CDC). "Surveillance for Foodborne Disease Outbreaks—United States, 2008." *Morbidity and Mortality Weekly Report* 60 (September 9, 2011): 1197–1202.

Haas, J. "Commentary: Epidemiology and the Pharmaceutical Industry: An Inside Perspective." *International Journal of Epidemiology* 37 (February 2008): 53–55.

Kinyua, J., and T.A. Anderson. "Temporal Analysis of the Cocaine Metabolite Benzoylecgonine in Wastewater to Estimate Community Drug Use." *Journal of Forensic Sciences* 57 (September 2012): 1349–1353.

Koplan, J.P., and W.H. Foege. "Introduction: The Centers for Disease Control and Prevention's Epi-Aids—A Fond Recollection." *American Journal of Epidemiology* 174 (December 1, 2011): Suppl. 11: S1–S3.

Miguel, A., et al. "Frequency of Adverse Drug Reactions in Hospitalized Patients: A Systematic Review and Meta-analysis." *Pharmacoepidemiology and Drug Safety* 21 (November 2012): 1139–1154.

WEBSITES

"Biomonitoring: Making a Difference." Centers for Disease Control and Prevention (CDC). http://www.cdc.gov/biomonitoring/biomonitoring_presentation.html (accessed November 4, 2012).

"Epidemic Intelligence Service (EIS)." Centers for Disease Control and Prevention (CDC). http://www.cdc.gov/eis/index.html (accessed November 3, 2012).

"Epidemiology." Association of Schools of Public Health (ASPH). This is a list of core competencies expected of a person with an M.P.H. degree. http://www.asph.org/document.cfm?page=704 (accessed November 3, 2012).

"Forensic Epidemiology." Johns Hopkins Bloomberg School of Public Health. http://www.jhsph.edu/research/centers-and-institutes/johns-hopkins-center-for-public-health-prepared ness/training/forensicepi.html (accessed November 4, 2012).

"Member Schools." Association of Schools of Public Health (ASPH). http://www.asph.org/document.cfm?page=200 (accessed October 4, 2012).

"National Notifiable Diseases Surveillance System (NNDSS)." Centers for Disease Control and Prevention (CDC). http://wwwn.cdc.gov/nndss/ (accessed November 3, 2012).

"What Is Epidemiology?" University of Alabama at Birmingham (UAB) School of Public Health. http://www.soph

.uab.edu/epi/academics/studenthandbook/what (accessed November 3, 2012).

WWW Virtual Library: Medicine and Health: Epidemiology. This is a website that lists the various agencies worldwide that hire epidemiologists as well as lists of schools and universities in various countries that offer degree programs in epidemiology.http://www.epibiostat.ucsf.edu/epidem/epidem.html (accessed November 4, 2012).

ORGANIZATIONS

American College of Epidemiology (ACE), 1500 Sunday Drive, Suite 102, Raleigh, NC United States 27607, (919) 861-5573, Fax: (919) 787-4916, info@acepidemiology.org, http://acepidemiology.org/.

American Public Health Association (APHA), 800 I Street, NW, Washington, DC United States 20001-3710, (202) 777-APHA, Fax: (202) 777-2534, http://apha.org/.

Association of Schools of Public Health (ASPH), 1900 M Street NW, Suite 710, Washington, DC United States 20036, (202) 296-1099, Fax: (202) 296-1252, info@asph.org, http://www.asph.org/.

Council on Education for Public Health (CEPH), 1010 Wayne Avenue, Suite 220, Silver Spring, MD United States 20910, (202) 789-1060, Fax: (202) 789-1895, http://www.ceph.org/.

Council of State and Territorial Epidemiologists (CSTE), 2872 Woodcock Blvd. Suite 303, Atlanta, GA United States 30341, (770) 458-3811, Fax: (770) 458-8516 , http://www.cste.org/dnn/.

World Health Organization (WHO), Avenue Appia 20, Geneva, Switzerland 1211 Geneva 27, +41 22 791 21 11, Fax: +41 22 791 31 11, http://www.who.int/en/.

Rebecca J. Frey, Ph.D.

Epstein-Barr virus

Definition

Epstein-Barr virus, or EBV, is the name given to a member of the herpesvirus family that is associated with a variety of illnesses—from infectious mononucleosis (IM) and multiple sclerosis to nasopharyngeal **cancer** and Burkitt's lymphoma. EBV is also known as human herpesvirus 4 or HHV-4. It is named for Anthony Epstein and Yvonne Barr, who identified the virus in 1964 in tissue samples sent to them from Uganda by Denis Burkitt (1911–1993), for whom Burkitt's lymphoma was named.

Demographics

EBV occurs in nearly all regions of the world, and is considered among the most common infectious viruses known to humankind. It is likely as of 2012 that its genetic diversity is greater than was thought when it was first identified. In the United States, the **Centers for Disease Control and Prevention (CDC)** estimates that 95% of adult Americans between the ages of 35 and 40 years have been infected with EBV, but it is less prevalent in children and teenagers. This pattern of infecting adults more than children persists throughout other prosperous Western countries, but does not hold true in underdeveloped regions such as Africa and Asia. In Africa, most children have been infected by EBV by the age of three years.

About 10% of cancers of the stomach are associated with EBV. The reason for this association is not known as of 2012.

Nasopharyngeal cancer is uncommon in the West but more prevalent in the Far East. It affects three times as many men as women, and usually occurs in adults between the ages of 40 and 50 years. This type of cancer is diagnosed in fewer than one in every 100,000 Caucasians but in 10–53 persons per 100,000 in mainland China, Taiwan, Hong Kong, and Malaysia. It also occurs more frequently in Eskimos in Greenland and Alaska, and in Tunisians, with about 20 cases per 100,000 people per year. The prevalence rate for adults of Asian descent in the United States is 3–4.2 cases per 100,000 persons per year. Nasopharyngeal cancer accounts for fewer than 1% of malignancies in children. It affects one in every 100,000 children in North America and Europe each year, but between 8 and 25 of every 100,000 children in Asia.

Description

Herpesviruses have long been known. The name actually comes from the Greek adjective *herpestes*, which means creeping. Many herpesvirus species appear to establish a lifelong presence in the human body, remaining dormant for long periods and becoming active for some, often inexplicable, reason. EBV is only one of several members of the Herpesvirus family that have similar traits. Others include varicella zoster virus—the cause of both chickenpox and shingles—and the **herpes** simplex virus responsible for both cold sores and genital herpes. EBV is usually transmitted through saliva but not blood, and is not normally an airborne infection.

Individuals with EBV infections typically show some elevation in the white blood cell count and a noticeable increase in lymphocytes—white blood cells associated with the immune response of the body. IM is a time-limited infection that usually lasts from one to two months. Symptoms include fever, malaise, sore throat, swollen glands and (sometimes) swollen spleen and/or liver.

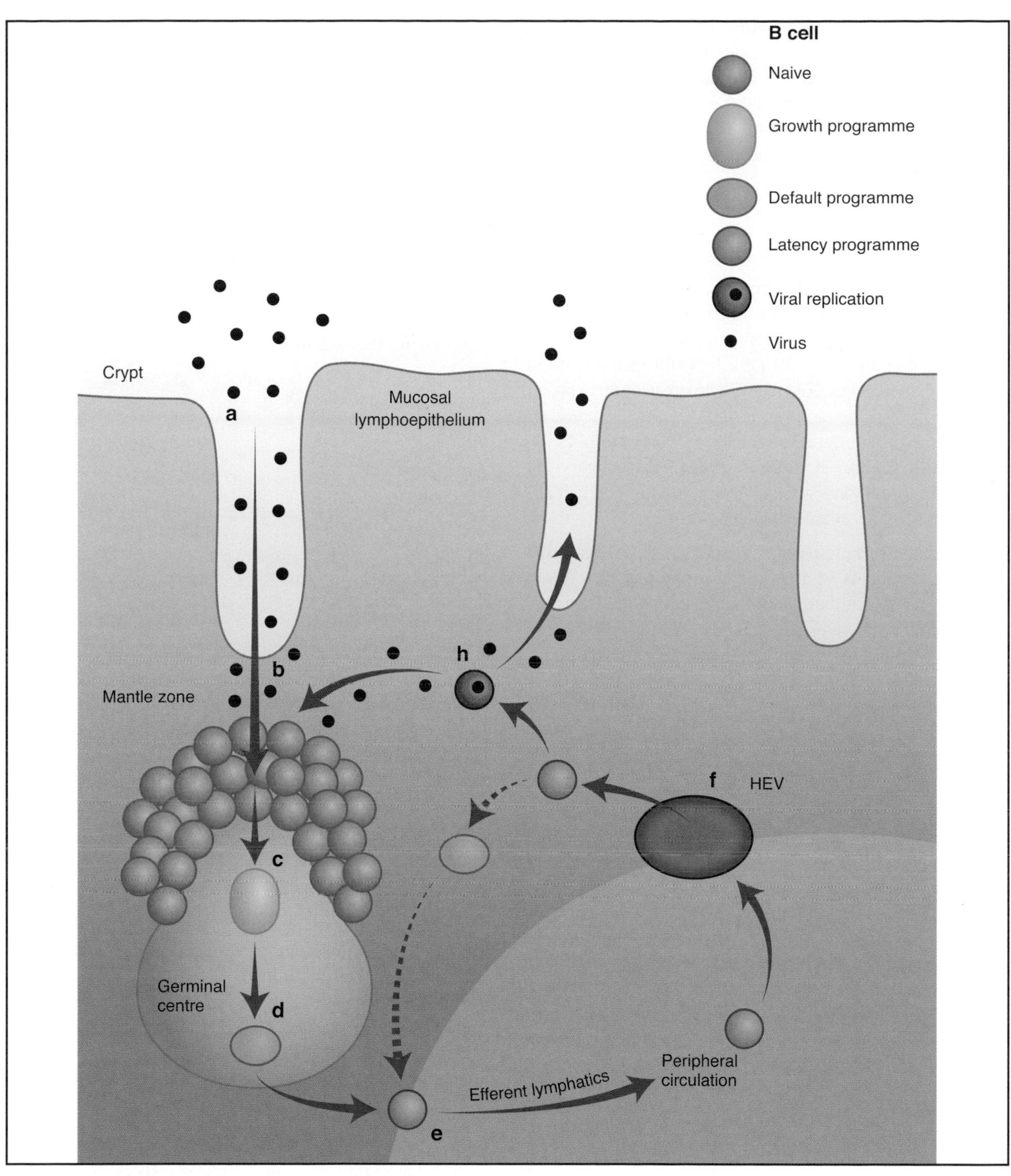

Epstein-Barr virus. *(Illustration by Electronic Illustrators Group. © 2013 Cengage Learning)*

EBV infections that lead to Burkitt's lymphoma in Africa typically affect the jaw and mouth area, while the (very rare) incidences of Burkitt's lymphoma found in developed countries are more apt to manifest tumors in the abdominal region, most commonly in the intestines, kidneys, or ovaries.

Causes and symptoms

EBV and mononucleosis

EBV is normally transmitted by contact with the saliva of an infected person; it is not ordinarily transmitted through the air. The virus takes about 4 to

6 weeks to incubate, and thus infected persons can spread the disease to others over a period of several weeks. After entering the patient's mouth and upper throat, the virus infects B cells, which are a type of white blood cell produced in the bone marrow. The infected B cells are then carried into the lymphatic system, where they affect the liver and spleen and cause the lymph nodes to swell and enlarge. The infected B cells are also responsible for the fever, swelling of the tonsils, and sore throat that characterize mononucleosis.

Most people who become infected with EBV do not have any symptoms, however. In children, EBV infection is usually asymptomatic; when it does cause symptoms, they are difficult to distinguish from routine mild childhood infections. Teenagers who were not exposed to EBV in childhood have a 35% to 50% chance of developing infectious mononucleosis (IM) from EBV. The most common symptoms of IM in teenagers are fever, sore throat, and swollen lymph glands. The patient may also have an enlarged spleen and liver.

After the symptoms of mononucleosis go away, the EBV virus remains in a few cells in the patient's throat tissues or blood for the rest of the person's life. The virus occasionally reactivates and may appear in samples of the person's saliva, but it does not cause new symptoms of illness. EBV infection does not cause any problems during pregnancy, such as miscarriages or **birth defects**.

EBV and cancer

EBV has been linked to IM in the Western world for decades. It has also become associated consistently with nasopharyngeal cancers in Asia (especially China) and Burkitt's lymphoma in Africa and Papua New Guinea. According to the **CDC**, EBV is not the sole cause of these two malignancies but does play an important role in the development of both cancers. The mechanism that allows Epstein-Barr virus to at least help in producing such diverse illnesses in diverse regions of the world has been the subject of increasing research and scrutiny. One theory regarding the higher rate of nasopharyngeal cancer in Asia is that EBV interacts with chemicals called nitrosamines, used in the preparation of salted fish and other preserved foods popular in the region, to trigger changes in cells that lead to cancer.

It is known that EBV is one of the herpesviruses that remain in the human body for life. Under certain, still not-understood conditions, it alters white blood cells normally associated with the immune system, changing the B cells (white blood cells normally associated with making antibodies) and causing them to reproduce uncontrollably. EBV can bind to these white blood cells to produce a solid mass made up of B cells—called Burkitt's lymphoma—or to the mucous membranes of the mouth and nose and cause nasopharyngeal cancer. Since Burkitt's lymphoma typically occurs in people living in moist, tropical climates, the same regions where people usually contract **malaria**, some doctors speculate that the immune system is altered by its response to malaria. When EBV infection occurs, the altered immune system reacts by producing a tumor.

KEY TERMS

B cell—A type of white blood cell produced in the bone marrow that makes antibodies against viruses.

Lymphocyte—Any of a group of white blood cells of crucial importance to the immune system's production of a tailor-made defense against specific invading organisms.

Lymphoma—A group of cancers in which the cells of tissue usually found in the lymph nodes or spleen multiply abnormally.

Malaria—A serious disease prevalent in the tropics. It is caused by parasites and produces severe fever and sometimes complications affecting the kidneys, liver, brain, and blood. It is spread by the Anopheles mosquito and can be fatal.

Nasopharyngeal—Referring to the passage connecting the nasal cavity behind the nose to the top of the throat behind the soft palate.

Special concerns

Though studies about the hereditary tendency of abnormal cell development after EBV infection are incomplete, researchers have found it to be associated with abnormalities on multiple human chromosomes, including chromosomes 1, 2, 3, 4, 5, 6, 8, 9, 11, 13, 14, 15, 16, 17, 22, and the X chromosome.

Diagnosis

The diagnosis of mononucleosis caused by EBV is usually based on the results of blood tests combined with the doctor's examination of the patient's throat and neck. The doctor will also tap on or feel the patient's abdomen to see whether the liver and spleen have become enlarged.

A patient infected by EBV will have an increased number of white blood cells in the blood sample, an increased number of abnormal white blood cells, and antibodies to the Epstein-Barr virus. These antibodies can be detected by a test called the monospot test, which gives results within a day but may not be accurate during the first week of the patient's illness. Another type of blood test for EBV antibodies takes longer to perform but gives more accurate results within the first week of symptoms.

Treatment

Traditional

Drugs

Because EBV infections are viral in origin, **antibiotics** are ineffective against them. Much research is geared toward the development of a vaccines effective against both the virus and cancer.

Treatment for mononucleosis caused by EBV consists of self-care at home until the symptoms go away. Patients should rest in bed if possible and drink plenty of fluids. Nonaspirin **pain** relievers like Advil or Tylenol can be taken to bring down the fever and relieve muscle aches and pains. Throat lozenges or gargling with warm salt water may help ease the discomfort of a sore throat.

Because mononucleosis can affect the spleen, patients should avoid vigorous exercise or contact sports for at least one month after the onset of symptoms or until the spleen returns to its normal size. This precaution will lower the risk of rupture of the spleen.

With regard to cancers associated with EBV, such anticancer drugs as cyclophosphamide or **radiation** therapy have been shown to be effective against Burkitt's lymphoma in four out of five cases.

Alternative treatment/therapy

The goal of alternative treatment is to lower the white blood cell count to normal levels. Treatment often includes such nutritional supplements as flaxseed oil or shark cartilage, vitamins—including **vitamins** C and K, and mineral supplements containing magnesium and potassium. Well-conducted randomized clinical trials have not yet been conducted to prove the efficacy of these therapies.

Public Health Response

Epstein-Barr infections are not generally a reportable disease, so public **health departments** are not necessarily involved in the collection of data, treatment, or **epidemiology** of the disease and related conditions. However, public health agencies are always good sources of information about any disease and can serve as useful references both for health and medical professionals, as well as for the general public.

QUESTIONS TO ASK YOUR DOCTOR

- Are there precautions I should take to protect my child for becoming infected with Epstein-Barr virus?
- What are the risks of Epstein-Barr disease for my elderly parents?
- Are there characteristics symptoms by which EBV disease can be recognized?
- Are there parts of the world to which I might travel where I should be especially concerned about encountering EBV disease?
- With what other infections is EBV disease sometimes confused, and how serious is the risk of misdiagnosis for the condition?

Prognosis

Mononucleosis caused by EBV rarely leads to serious complications. In most patients, the fever goes down in about 10 days, but fatigue may last for several weeks or months. Some people do not feel normal again for about three months. A patient who feels sick longer than 4 months, however, should go back to the doctor to see whether they have another disease or disorder in addition to mononucleosis. In some cases, the patient is diagnosed with chronic fatigue syndrome or CFS. The Epstein-Barr virus does not cause CFS; however, it appears to make some patients with mononucleosis more susceptible to developing chronic fatigue syndrome.

The prognosis for nasopharyngeal cancer associated with EBV in adults is poor, because about 60% of these cancers have already metastasized to other regions of the head and neck by the time diagnosis is made. The prognosis for this type of cancer in children is also relatively poor. The survival rates for children treated only with radiation therapy are about 45%. When chemotherapy and radiation therapy are used together, long-term survival rates range from 55% to 80%.

Prevention

As of 2012, there is no vaccine that can prevent mononucleosis caused by EBV. In addition, the fact that many people can be infected with the virus and transmit it to others without having symptoms of the disease means that mononucleosis is almost impossible to prevent. The best precautionary measure is for patients who have been diagnosed with mono to avoid kissing or other close personal contact with others, and to wash their drinking glasses, food dishes, and eating utensils separately from those of other family members or friends for several days after the fever goes down. It is not necessary for people with mono to be completely isolated from other people, however.

Because the Epstein-Barr virus remains in the body after the symptoms of mononucleosis go away, people who have had IM should not donate blood for at least 6 months after their symptoms started.

Resources

BOOKS

Gluckman, Toma R. *Herpesviridae Viral Structure, Life Cycle, and Infections*. New York: Nova Science Publishers, 2009.

Krueger, Hans, et al. *HPV and Other Infectious Agents in Cancer: Opportunities for Prevention and Public Health*. New York: Oxford University Press, 2010.

Tao, H.E., ed. *DNA Tumor Viruses*. New York: Nova Science Publishers, 2009.

PERIODICALS

Agliari, E., et al. "Can Persistent Epstein-Barr Virus Infection Induce Chronic Fatigue Syndrome as a Pavlov Reflex of the Immune Response?" *Journal of Biological Dynamics* 6, 2. (2012): 740–62.

Bagert, B.A. "Epstein-Barr Virus in Multiple Sclerosis." *Current Neurology and Neuroscience Reports* 9, 5. (2009): 405–410.

Boysen, T., et al. "EBV-associated Gastric Carcinoma in High- and Low-incidence Areas for Nasopharyngeal Carcinoma." *British Journal of Cancer* 101, 3. (2009): 530–33.

Chang, C.M., et al. "The Extent of Genetic Diversity of Epstein-Barr Virus and its Geographic and Disease Patterns: A Need for Reappraisal." *Virus Research* 143, 2. (2009): 209–21.

Leruez-Ville M., et al. "Blood Epstein-Barr Virus DNA Load and Risk of Progression to AIDS-related Systemic B Lymphoma." *HIV Medicine* 13, 8. (2012): 479–87.

OTHER

Epstein-Barr Virus and Infectious Mononucleosis. Centers for Disease Control and Prevention. http://www.cdc.gov/ncidod/diseases/ebv.htm (accessed August 16, 2012).

Lin, Ho-Sheng, and Willard E. Fee, Jr. *Malignant Nasopharyngeal Tumors.* eMedicine. http://emedicine.medscape.com/article/848163-overview (accessed August 16, 2012).

National Library of Medicine Tutorial. http://www.nlm.nih.gov/medlineplus/tutorials/epsteinbarrvirusmono/htm/index.htm (accessed August 16, 2012).

Paulino, Arnold C., and Stephan A. Grupp. *Nasopharyngeal Cancer.* eMedicine. http://emedicine.medscape.com/article/988165-overview (accessed August 16, 2012).

Virology Down Under. http://www.uq.edu.au/vdu/VDUEBV.htm (accessed August 16, 2012).

ORGANIZATIONS

Centers for Disease Control and Prevention (CDC), 1600 Clifton Rd., Atlanta, GA USA 30333, 1 (404) 639–3534, 800 CDC–INFO (800–232–4636). TTY: (888) 232–6348, inquiry@cdc.gov, http://www.cdc.gov.

Joan Schonbeck, RN
Rebecca J. Frey, Ph.D.

Escherichia coli

Definition

Escherichia coli (*E. coli*) is a gram-negative, rod-shaped bacterium. It is one of several types of bacteria that normally inhabit the lower intestine of humans and other warm-blooded animals (commensal organisms). Some strains of the bacterium are harmless, but other strains of *E. coli* are capable of causing disease under certain conditions when the immune system is compromised, or disease may result from an environmental exposure to the organism. The *E. coli* bacterium has been responsible for product recalls, along with food **poisoning** in humans, due to **food contamination**.

Description

E. coli bacteria may give rise to infections in wounds, the urinary tract, biliary tract, and abdominal cavity (peritonitis). This organism may cause septicemia, neonatal **meningitis**, infantile gastroenteritis, tourist diarrhea, and hemorrhagic diarrhea. An *E. coli* infection may also arise due to environmental exposure. Infections with this type of bacteria pose a serious threat to public health with outbreaks arising from food and **water** contaminated with human or animal feces or sewage. This type of bacteria has been used as a biological indicator for safety of **drinking water** since the 1890s. Exposure may occur during hospitalization, resulting in **pneumonia** in immunocompromised patients or those on a ventilator.

Origins

German pediatrician Theodor Escherich (1857–1911) first discovered this bacterium in 1885, in the feces of healthy individuals. Escherich named the bacterium species *Bacterium coli*. It was renamed *Bacillus coli* in 1895, following invalidation to the genus *Bacterium*,

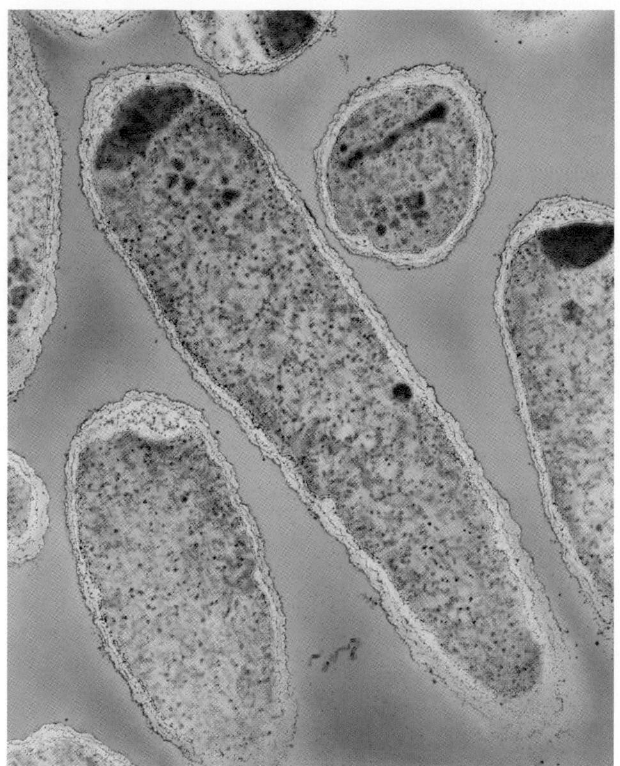

Color transmission electron micrograph of Escherichia coli O157:H7 bacteria, cause of foodborn illness. *(K. Lounatmaa / Science Source/Photo Researchers, Inc.)*

and changed again to its current species name after the new genus *Escherichia* was created.

Effects on public health

E. coli can multiply in recreational waters, such as ponds, lakes, and other swimming areas, which can cause health officials to warn the public that it has exceeded a permissible level in such waters. Such warnings may eventually lead to the closing of these areas. Levels of *E. coli* in drinking water are also regulated by government officials, through the Safe Drinking Water Act. Municipalities often issue a boil order for all water used for cooking, drinking, and other uses when levels of the bacterium have been exceeded in the water supply.

Demographics

Neonatal meningitis caused by *E. coli* is associated with a mortality rate of 8%. The organism is the leading cause of urinary tract infections in men and women. The bacterium also causes approximately 30% to 45% of traveler's diarrhea in people traveling to Mexico. The U.S. **Centers for Disease Control and Prevention (CDC)** found that 1,034 foodborne disease outbreaks were reported in 2008, with 23,000 people getting sick, over 1,200 being hospitalized, and 22 dying. *Salmonella* was the most frequent reason for these problems, at 62%, but *E. coli* made up 17% of the cases, and the norovirus 7%. As of June 20, 2012, the **CDC** reports that 18 people have been infected with the strain of Shiga toxin-producing *Escherichia coli* O145 infection, with the first report on April 15, 2012. Four people had hospitalized, and one death had been reported in Louisiana, with nine states reporting outbreaks: Alabama (2), California (1), Florida (1), Georgia (5), Kentucky (1), Louisiana (5), Maryland (1), Tennessee (1), and Virginia (1). The CDC makes the following general statement: "Germs such as norovirus, *Salmonella*, and *E. coli* cause thousands of illnesses and deaths in the United States each year. Hospitalizations resulting from foodborne disease outbreaks have increased in recent years but can be prevented if people follow proper food-handling practices."

Causes and symptoms

The causes and symptoms of *E. coli* are described below.

Causes

An *E. coli* infection is caused when one comes into contact with water or food that has been contaminated with feces or into direct contact with the feces of humans or animals.

Symptoms

The symptoms of infection and resulting complications are dependent upon the strain of *E. coli* and the site of infection. These bacteria produce toxins that have a wide range of effects. Symptoms caused by some *E. coli* infections range from mild to severe, bloody diarrhea, acute abdominal **pain**, vomiting, and fever. Gastrointestinal complications that can cause *E. coli* infections include irritable bowel syndrome (IBS), ischemic colitis, appendicitis, perforation of the large bowel, and, in some instances, gangrene, in the colon. Other known *E. coli*-causing infections include chronic renal failure, pancreatitis, and **diabetes mellitus**. Neurological symptoms such as drowsiness, seizure, and coma may occur. In infants, *E. coli* infections are present in cases of infantile gastroenteritis and neonatal meningitis.

Strains of *E. coli* that produce diarrhea were initially distinguished by their O (somatic) antigens found on the bacterial surface. Although there is an overlap in characteristics among strains, they may be classified into four main groups: enterohemorrahagic (0157), enteropathogenic (055,0111), enterotoxigenic (06,078), and enteroinvasive (0124,0164).

E.coli O157 (VTEC)

The O157:H7 strain is the member of the group most often associated with a particularly severe form of diarrhea. (The O indicates the somatic antigen, while the H denotes the flagellar antigen, both of which are found on the cell surface of the bacteria.) The bacterium was discovered in 1977, and first reports of infections followed in 1982. *E. coli* O157:H7, as researchers frequently refer to it, causes bloody diarrhea in many infected patients. It accounts for about 2% of all cases of diarrhea in the Western Hemisphere, and at least one-third of cases of hemorrhagic colitis, or about 20,000 cases per year.

E. coli O157:H7 is also the most common cause of unique syndromes, known as hemolytic-uremic syndrome (HUS) and thrombocytopenic purpura (TTP), which cause kidney failure, hemolytic anemia, and thrombocytopenia. Infection with this strain of bacteria often subsides without further complications. However, about 5% of people who are infected develop HUS/TTP. This infection also accounts for the majority of episodes of HUS, especially in children.

This strain of bacteria produces a potent toxin called verotoxin, named for the toxin's ability to kill green monkey kidney or "vero" cells. Bacteria that produce verotoxin are referred to as "verotoxin-producing" *E. coli* (VTEC). The numbers of bacteria that are necessary to reproduce infectious levels of bacteria are quite small, estimated at 10–100 viable bacteria. These toxins are lethal for intestinal cells and those that line vessels (endothelial cells), inhibiting protein synthesis and causing cell death. Scientists contend that the damage to blood vessels results in the formation of clots, which eventually leads to HUS. HUS/TTP is a serious, often fatal, syndrome that has other causes besides *E. coli* O157:H7; it is characterized by the breaking up of red blood cells (hemolysis) and kidney failure (uremia). The syndrome occurs most often in the very young and very old.

E. coli O157:H7 is commonly found in cattle and poultry, and outbreaks of disease have been associated with cattle and bovine products. There have been reports of contamination from unpasteurized apple juice, hamburger meat, radish sprouts, lettuce, and potatoes, as well as other food sources. Environmental contamination may occur in water drained from cattle pastures or water containing human sewage used for drinking or swimming. Human-to-human transmission, through contact with fecal matter, has also been identified in daycare centers.

After an incubation period of three to four days on average, watery diarrhea begins, which rapidly progresses to bloody diarrhea in many cases. Nausea, vomiting, and low-grade fever are frequently present. Gastrointestinal symptoms last about one week, and recovery is often spontaneous. Symptomatic infection may occur in about 10% of infected individuals. About 5–10% of individuals, usually at the extremes of age, develop HUS/TTP and, ultimately, kidney failure. Patients taking **antibiotics** or medications for gastric acidity may also be at risk. Neurological symptoms can occur as part of HUS/TTP and consist of seizures, paralysis, and coma. Rectal prolapse may be a complication, and in some cases, colitis, appendicitis, perforation of the large bowel, and gangrene in the bowel. Systemically, the most prevalent complications of *E. coli* 157 infections are HUS and TTP.

E. coli non-O157 (VTEC)

These strains of *E. coli* produce verotoxin but are strains other than O157. There have been as many as 100 different types implicated in the development of disease. Strain OH111 was found to be involved in outbreaks in Australia, Japan, and Italy. The O128, O103, and O55 groups have also been implicated in diarrhea outbreaks. In Britain, cases of infantile gastroenteritis in maternity hospitals and neonatal units have been attributed to the *E. coli*) non-0157 group. Many of these organisms have been identified in cattle.

Enterotoxigenic *E. coli*

Two toxins may be produced by this group, the heat-labile enterotoxin (LT) that can produce enteritis in infants, and a heat-stable enterotoxin (ST), the action of which has yet to be determined.

Enteroinvasive *E. coli*

Some strains of the enteroinvasive *E. coli* have been involved in the development of gastroenteritis in infants. These organisms do not produce an enterotoxin. The cells of the intestine are affected, with the development of symptoms that are typical of a shigellae infection.

Diagnosis

Diagnosis of a specific type of infection is dependent upon the characteristics of the particular strain of the organism.

E. coli O157:H7 (HUS)

This particular strain of *E. coli* is suspected when bloody diarrhea, bloody stools, lack of fever, elevated leukocyte count, and abdominal tenderness are present. Stool cultures are used to tentatively identify the bacteria. Unfortunately, cultures are often negative or inconclusive if done after 48 hours of symptoms. Further tests are usually needed for confirmation of infection. This may include a full blood count, blood film, and tests to determine urea, electrolyte, and LDH (lactate dehydrogenase) levels. Damaged red blood cells and elevated levels of creatinine, urea, and LDH with a drop in platelet count may indicate that HUS will develop. Immunomagnetic separation is used for diagnosis as well.

E. coli non-O157 (VTEC)

Diagnosis is often difficult for these types of bacteria, but production of enterohemolysin (Ehly) is used as an indicator. Other diagnostic tests are used to detect verotoxins, including ELISA (enzyme-linked immunosorbent assays), colony immunoblotting, and DNA-based tests.

E. coli 0157 STEC

Methods for detection of this type of bacteria are under development, including culture growth media selective for this organism. Immunomagnetic separation and specific ELISA, latex agglutination tests, colony immunoblot assays, and other immunological-based detection methods are being explored.

Prevention

Thorough cooking of all meat and poultry products and adhering to proper food preparation are the most effective ways to avoid infection. More studies are needed to determine the appropriate safety margins for killing these bacteria. Food-irradiation methods are also being developed to sanitize food. The enforcement of regulations for meat production and water are critical. Steam **pasteurization** is used in the United States and is being explored in other countries. Vaccinations to *E. coli* 0157 are under development, as are medications aimed at limiting the effects of the verotoxin.

Prevention of *E. coli* gastroenteritis in infants is best achieved by breastfeeding. Breast milk contains antibodies that combat the infection. For bottle-fed infants, care should be taken in the preparation of the milk and bottles. Good **hygiene** of the umbilical cord area is important. Keeping this area clean and dry may reduce infection.

Treatment

The treatment of *E. coli* may involve the use of proven medical countermeasures, however, others are more controversial.

Traditional

Uncomplicated cases of the *E. coli* O157:H7 infection clear up within ten days. It is not certain that antibiotics are helpful in treating *E. coli* O157:H7. Antimicrobials that may be administered include doxycycline (Vibramycin), trimethoprim/sulfamethoxazole (Bactrim DS, Septra), fluoroquinolones (Cipro), and rifaximin (Xifaxan, RedActiv, Flonorm). Dehydration resulting from diarrhea must be treated with either Oral Rehydration Solution (ORS) or intravenous fluids. Anti-motility agents that decrease the intestines' ability to contract should not be used in any patient with bloody diarrhea. Treatment of HUS, if it develops, involves correction of clotting factors, plasma exchange, and kidney dialysis. Blood transfusions may be required. Treatment methods for other *E. coli* infections are similar.

Drugs

Antibiotics are often used in the treatment of *E. coli* infections, but their role is controversial. Some antibiotics may enhance the development of HUS/TTP, depending upon their action, as well as the use of anti-diarrhea medications that should be avoided. Treatment with third-generation cephalosporin antibiotics, such as ceftriaxone (Rocephin), is indicated for neonatal meningitis.

Antibiotic therapy may be complicated by the presence of antibiotic resistant organisms. These organisms appear to have been increasing since the late 1990s and are resistant to the penicillins and cephalosporins as well as to the fluoroquinolones and gentamicin, which in the past were reserved to treat only the most serious of infections.

Prognosis

In most cases of O157:H7, symptoms last for about a week, and recovery is often spontaneous. Ten percent of individuals with *E. coli* O157:H7 infection develop HUS; 5% of those die of the disease. Some who recover from HUS are left with a degree of kidney damage and possibly irritable bowel syndrome. Additionally, there is a possibility of chronic *E. coli* infection.

Infants who develop *E. coli* infections may be permanently affected. Gastroenteritis may leave the child with lactose intolerance. Neonates who develop meningitis from *E. coli* strains have a high morbidity and mortality rate. Some may develop neurological and developmental dysfunction.

Precautions

The CDC recommends the following to minimize the chances of contracting an *E. coli* infection:

- Thoroughly wash hands, cutting boards, utensils, and countertops.

KEY TERMS

Antigen—A substance, usually a protein, that causes the formation of an antibody and reacts specifically with that antibody.

Anti-motility medications—Medications such as loperamide (Imodium), dephenoxylate (Lomotil), or medications containing Codeine or narcotics that decrease the ability of the intestine to contract. This can worsen the condition of a patient with dysentery or colitis.

Colitis—Inflammation of the colon or large intestine, usually causing diarrhea that may be bloody.

Food-irradiation methods—A process using radiant energy to kill microorganisms in food, to extend the amount of time in which food can be sold and eaten safely.

Oral Rehydration Solution (ORS)—A liquid preparation developed by the World Health Organization that can decrease fluid loss in persons with diarrhea. Originally developed to be prepared with materials available in the home, commercial preparations have recently come into use.

Urea—Chemical formed during the body's metabolism of nitrogen and normally excreted by the kidney. Urea levels rise in the blood when kidney failure occurs.

- Keep raw meat, poultry, and seafood separate from other foods.
- Use a food thermometer to ensure that foods are cooked to a safe internal temperature: 145°F (63°C) for whole meats (allowing an additional three minutes before carving or consuming the meat), 160°F (71°C) for ground meats, and 165°F (74°C) for all poultry.
- Keep the refrigerator at a temperature below 40°F (4.4°C), and refrigerate food that will spoil.
- Report suspected illness from food to the local health department.
- Do not prepare food for others if you have diarrhea or have been vomiting.
- Be careful when preparing food for children, pregnant women, those in poor health, and older adults.

Risks

The Mayo Clinic states that *E. coli* can be contracted by anyone. However, some people are more susceptible to the infection and are more likely to develop serious

QUESTIONS TO ASK YOUR DOCTOR

- How soon do symptoms of *E. coli* infection develop?
- How is *E. coli* infection diagnosed?
- How long is an infected person infectious to others?
- Should an infected person be excluded from work or school?
- Where can I learn more information?

problems than are others. These risk factors include age, weakened immune systems, and eating certain types of foods. A further description is:

- Young children and older adults are at higher risk of experiencing sickness caused by *E. coli* and more-serious complications from the infection.
- People who have weakened immune systems, such as from acquired immune deficiency syndrome (AIDS) or drugs to treat cancer or to prevent the rejection of organ transplants, are more likely to have symptoms from ingesting *E. coli*.
- Foods that put a person at greater risk for contracting *E. coli* include undercooked hamburger; unpasteurized milk, apple juice or cider; and soft cheeses made from raw milk.

Resources

BOOKS

Manning, Shannon D. editor. *Escherichia Coli Infections*. Philadelphia: Chelsea House, 2010.

Rogers, Morgan C., and Nancy D. Peterson. *E. Coli Infections: Causes, Treatment, and Prevention*. Hauppauge, NY: Nova Science, 2011.

Zimmer, Carl. *Microcosm: E. Coli and the New Science of Life*. New York: Pantheon Books, 2008.

WEBSITES

E. Coli (Escherichia coli). Centers for Disease Control and Prevention. (July 17, 2012). http://www.cdc.gov/ecoli/ (accessed August 8, 2012).

E. Coli Infection. WebMD. (June 14, 2010). http://www.webmd.com/a-to-z-guides/e-coli-infection-topic-overview (accessed August 8, 2012).

E. Coli. Mayo Clinic. (July 28, 2011). http://www.mayoclinic.com/health/e-coli/DS01007 (accessed August 8, 2012).

Foodborne Disease Outbreaks Are Deadly Serious—What You Can Do to Avoid Them. Centers for Disease Control and Prevention. (September 15, 2011). http://www.cdc.gov/features/dsFoodborneOutbreaks/ (accessed August 8, 2012).

Multistate Outbreak of Shiga Toxin-producing Escherichia coli O145 Infections (Final Update). Centers for Disease Control and Prevention. (July 20, 2012). http://www.cdc.gov/ecoli/2012/O145-06-12/index.html (accessed August 8, 2012).

ORGANIZATIONS

American Medical Association, 515 N. State St., Chicago, IL U.S.A. 60654, (800) 621-8335, http://www.ama-assn.org/.

Centers for Disease Control and Prevention, 1600 Clifton Rd., Atlanta, GA U.S.A. 30333, (800) 232-4636, cdcinfo@cdc.gov, http://www.cdc.gov/.

Environmental Protection Agency, 1200 Pennsylvania Ave., N.W. (Ariel Rios Building), Washington, D.C. U.S.A. 20460, 1 (202) 272-0167, http://www.epa.gov/.

National Center for Emerging and Zoonotic Infectious Diseases, Centers for Disease Control and Prevention, 1600 Clifton Rd., Atlanta, GA U.S.A. 30333, (800) 232-4635, cdcinfo@cdc.gov, http://www.cdc.gov/ncezid/.

National Institute of Allergy and Infectious Diseases (NIAID Office of Communications and Government Relations), 6610 Rockledge Dr., MSC 6612, Bethesda, MD U.S.A. 20892-6612, 1 (301) 496-5717, Fax: 1 (301) 402-3573, (866) 284-4107, ocpostoffice@niaid.nih.gov, http://www.niaid.nih.gov.

Jill Granger, MS
David Kaminstein, MD
Melinda Granger Oberleitner, RN, DNS, APRN, CNS
William A. Atkins, BB, BS, MBA

Essential medicines

Definition

The **World Health Organization** defines *essential medicines* as "those drugs that satisfy the health care needs of the majority of the **population**; they should therefore be available at all times in adequate amounts and in appropriate dosage forms, at a price the community can afford."

Description

Healthcare providers in the modern world are faced with the daunting challenge of selecting among the vast number of drugs currently available those that are most appropriate for the health issues they face in their own specific geographical setting. Those decisions are especially difficult in low-income areas where money is often not available for purchasing the wide variety of drugs one might wish to have available for the best possible health care of people in the region. In an effort to help solve this problem, the **World Health Organization (WHO)** produced its first list of essential medicines in 1977. That list consisted of 208 medicines thought to constitute a bare minimum for healthcare providers in most settings. Since that time, **WHO** has updated and revised its list of essential medicines, with the most recent version, the 17th edition, having been released in 2011. That newest list contained 368 pharmaceuticals. The essential medicine list (EML) is prepared by the WHO Expert Committee on Selection and Use of Medicines, which had begun working on the 18th edition of the list in March 2011.

The EML was never considered to be a "one size fits all" scheme for all nations but, rather, a list of suggestions from which individual nations can pick and choose to select a formulary that is best suited to their own specific needs and capabilities. As of 2012, 150 nations, almost all of which are developing nations, had created their own national essential medicines list based on WHO recommendations. The United States, Canada, and most European nations are not among those to have developed national essential medicines lists, largely because financing of medications is not a critical issue in those nations.

The WHO EML actually consists of three distinct lists, the first of which, the core list, consists of the safest, most cost-effective, and efficacious medicines needed to treat basic, priority health conditions. The second list, the complementary list, contains medications recommended for priority conditions that required specialized treatment, such as specialized diagnostic procedures or specialized medical care. The third list is a special list for children's medicine, the *WHO Model List of Essential Medicines for Children*. The third edition of that list was published in 2011 and contains 270 items.

The WHO EML classifies drugs according to their therapeutic action into the following categories:

- anaesthetics
- analgesics, antipyretics, non-steroidal anti-inflammatory medicines (NSAIMs), medicines used to treat gout and disease modifying agents in rheumatoid disorders (DMARDs)
- antiallergics and medicines used in anaphylaxis
- antidotes and other substances used in poisonings
- anticonvulsants and antiepileptics
- anti-infective medicines (by far the largest category in the list)
- antimigraine medicines
- antineoplastic, immunosuppressives and medicines used in palliative care

- antiparinsonian medicines
- medicines affecting the blood
- blood products and plasma substitutes
- cardiovascular medicines
- dermatological medicines (topical)
- diagnostic agents
- disinfectants and antiseptics
- diuretics
- gastrointestinal medicines
- hormones, other endocrine medicines and contraceptives
- immunologicals
- muscle relaxants (peripherally acting) and cholinesterase inhibitors
- opththamological preparations
- oxytocics and antioxytocics
- peritoneal dialysis solution
- medicines for mental and behavioral disorders
- medicines acting on the respiratory tract
- solutions correcting water, electrolyte and acid-base disturbances
- vitamins and minerals
- specific medicines for neonatal care

Some examples of the hundreds of drugs listed on the three WHO essential medicine lists are the following medications:

- aciclovir
- ascorbic acid
- barium sulfate
- condoms
- diaphragms
- glucose with sodium chloride
- hepatitis A and hepatitis B vaccines
- lidocaine
- measles vaccine
- phenobarbitol
- misoprostol

WHO has pointed to a number of advantages in having a list of essential medicines for use by individual nations. First, such a list helps nations decide how best to spend their limited healthcare funds by selecting drugs that are safe and efficacious, as well as relatively inexpensive. The vast majority of drugs on the EML are available in generic form and, thus, available at the lowest possible price. An international list also facilitates the sale and distribution of drugs between countries with the least amount of confusion and misunderstanding. The expert advice that has gone into the creation of EML also tends to ensure that healthcare authorities in all countries know that they are getting the best possible recommendations for dealing with their own health issues. This advice also ensures that nations will be able to purchase, store, and distribute drugs in the most efficient manner possible.

KEY TERMS

Essential medicines—Drugs that satisfy the health care needs of the majority of the population; they should therefore be available at all times in adequate amounts and in appropriate dosage forms, at a price the community can afford.

Formulary—A book containing a list of pharmaceutical substances along with their formulas, uses, and methods of preparation.

Demographics

WHO conducts surveys of member nations from time to time to determine the extent to which selected medicines on the EML are available in public and private healthcare agencies. As might be expected, availability varies widely over time and countries. For example, the availability of selected generic medicines in Yemen in 2006 varied from 5% percent in public agencies to 90% percent in private agencies. In surveys conducted in 2007 and 2008, some nations showed ranges similar to that of Yemen, and others, very different ranges, as follows:

- Bolivia: 31.9%; 86.7% (2008)
- Ecuador: 41.7%; 71.7% (2008)
- Nicaragua: 50.0%; 87.1% (2008)
- Sao Tome and Principe: 56.3%; 22.2% (2008)
- Congo: 21.2%; 31.3% (2007)
- Democratic Republic of the Congo: 55.6%; 65.4% (2007)
- Iran: 96.7%; 96.7% (2007)
- Oman: 96.7%; 70.3% (2007)
- Ukaine: 100.0%; 90.0% (2007)

A 2012 report by the United Nations Global Parternship for Development attempted to provide a very general, overall view of the success of the WHO essential medicine program. It concluded that worldwide, as of the end of 2011, essential medicines were available in 51.8% of all public healthcare facilities and 68.5% of all private healthcare facilities. It further noted that the price of these medicines in public facilities was 2.6 times that of the established international reference price and 5 times that in private healthcare facilities.

Resources

BOOKS

Pogge, Thomas, Matthew Rimmer, and Kim Rubenstein, eds. *Incentives for Global Public Health: Patent Law and Access to Essential Medicines*. Cambridge, UK: Cambridge University Press, 2010.

The Selection and Use of Essential Medicines, 17th ed. Geneva: World Health Organization, 2011.

PERIODICALS

Cottingham, J., and M. Berer. "Access to Essential Medicines for Sexual and Reproductive Health Care: The Role of the Pharmaceutical Industry and International Regulation." *Reproductive Health Matters* 19, 38. (2011): 69–84.

Gilson, A.M., et al. "Ensuring Patient Access to Essential Medicines while Minimizing Harmful Use: A Revised World Health Organization Tool to Improve National Drug Control Policy." *Journal of Pain and Palliative Care Pharmacotherpy* 25, 3. (2011): 246–51.

Nunan, M., and T. Duke. "Effectiveness of Pharmacy Interventions in Improving Availability of Essential Medicines at the Primary Healthcare Level." *Tropical Medicine and International Health* 16, 5. (2011): 647–58.

WEBSITES

"Access Campaign." Doctors without Borders. http://www.msfaccess.org/. Accessed on October 1, 2012.

"Essential Medicines." World Health Organization. http://www.who.int/topics/essential_medicines/en/. Accessed on October 1, 2012.

"UAEM: Universities Allied for Essential Medicines." http://essentialmedicine.org/. Accessed on October 1, 2012.

"WHO Model List of Essential Medicines." World Health Organization. http://whqlibdoc.who.int/hq/2011/a95053_eng.pdf. Accessed on October 1, 2012.

ORGANIZATIONS

World Health Organization (WHO), Avenue Appia 20, 1211 Geneva 27, Switzerland, +41 22 791 21 11, Fax: +41 22 791 31 11, http://www.who.int/about/contact_form/en/index.html, http://www.who.int/en/.

David E. Newton, Ed.D.

Ethics and legal issues of public health

Definition

The policies and practices that make up public health do not exist in a vacuum. Rather, they interact with many other aspects of society, including its ethical and legal principles. Out of that interaction arise a number of issues about the proper role of each element in the system: public law, the legal system, and ethical guidelines.

Purpose

The purposes of discussions over the proper relationship of public health, the law, and ethical principles is to clarify the appropriate actions of each of the three elements in dealing with problems that limit a society's achieving the best possible health conditions for its citizens.

Description

The objectives, policies, and practices of public health programs have evolved dramatically over the past two centuries. In the late nineteenth century, public health was generally viewed as a somewhat limited, if essential, set of practices that helped prevent the spread of disease within a **population**. As scientists began to develop a better understanding of the nature of infectious diseases and the way they are spread throughout a community, it became obvious that government had a reasonable obligation to become involved in certain types of actions with the potential for reducing epidemics and the spread of many common diseases. One of the earliest of these actions occurred in 1854 when physician John Snow hypothesized that a **cholera** epidemic in London was being spread through common use of a contaminated well in the city's Broad Street. When the Board of Guardians of St. James parish removed the pump handle, the epidemic was resolved. As an example of the very limited reach of public health efforts at the time, however, it should be noted that the pump handle was replaced as soon as the disease retreated from the area.

Over time, governments began to accept as a legitimate and reasonable part of their activities whatever actions might be necessary to eliminate the proximate causes of disease, injury, and other health problems in a community. By the early twentieth century, cities, counties, and states operated a number of services designed to head off disease and protect the health of constituents, services such as the construction of sanitary sewage systems, **water** purification plants, the regular collection and disposal of garbage, and the draining of swamps and other pools of standing water, where insect vectors bred. As the causative agents of infectious diseases were discovered, and vaccinations developed against those agents, governments also began to make required immunizations a part of their regular activities.

To a considerable extent, then, the first century of public health was characterized by scientific and medical decisions about the most effective ways to prevent disease and ensure the general health of individuals. Critics always existed who felt that governmental and public health agencies had no right to impose their views and their policies on individual citizens, but the vast majority of people were glad for the efforts that removed the causes of disease from their daily lives. That situation began to change as the twentieth century progressed, however. Over time, public health authorities began to have a somewhat more expansive view of their role in society. They began to think more broadly of the host of ways in which the quality of a person's life was diminished by social, economic, environmental, and other factors. For example, in the 1950s, researchers discovered that the addition of very small amounts of fluoride to the public water supply produced a significant decrease in the number of dental caries (cavities) among children and adults in the region. To some individuals, the idea of adding a bit of a relatively harmless chemical to the water to reduce society's most serious dental problem seemed like a reasonable effort to undertake. Other individuals had very different views, suggesting that fluoridation of water was going one step too far for public health agencies. Individual families could very well take responsibility for their own dental care, they argued. Besides, no one was going to die from having bad teeth. The time had arrived, then, when increasing numbers of ordinary citizens were asking how far public health agencies should go in ensuring their health.

The expansion of the public health mission in many parts of the world reflected a growing appreciation by experts in the field that many of the most serious health problems people face do not exist in a vacuum. People become ill and die for a number of reasons that, at first glance, seem have little or nothing to do with health. But research continued to show that social, economic, political, and other problems such as race, ethnicity, economic status, and educational background were critical factors in the development of disease and other health problems. Study after study showed that lower-income minorities in urban areas were consistently at higher risk not only for disease, but also for accidents and generally poorer health than were their better-off, non-minority neighbors. Most public health officials began to conclude that a society's health problems could not be resolved with dealing with more fundamental problems of income, education, social standing, and other factors.

As a consequence, public health programs began to expand into areas that would never have fit that definition a century earlier. For example, by the end of the twentieth century, many public health experts had concluded that the problem of firearms injuries in deaths in many countries could best be dealt with as a public health problem, in which deaths by gunshot wounds could be thought of as an epidemic, not so different from a cholera epidemic. Public health agencies began to call on legislatures to pass laws that supported their view on gunshot accidents, automobile accidents, falls in the home, exposure to ultraviolet **radiation** in tanning parlors, and a host of other newly defined "public health problems." In 2011, for example, the mayor of New York City decided that soft drinks were contributing to the problem of **obesity** among the city's citizens and proposed a ban on sugary drinks of more than 16 ounces.

The increasing view of topics appropriate to the field of public health has had some practical effects on the size of both the profession itself and the governmental bureaucracy that has grown up to enforce legislative decisions, write rules and regulations, educate the public about new public health practices, and, in general, support the public health profession itself. Perhaps not surprisingly, a growing number of individuals have begun to ask what limits there are to the activities of the field of public health. It sometimes seems as if every aspect of human life might be a legitimate target of public health concern, ranging from the foods one eats to the number of hours one exercises to the hours of sunlight to which one should be exposed. As a consequence, individuals and groups have begun to push back against what they view as unreasonable expansion of public health activities into areas where they do not belong. For example, prohibitions on **smoking** have expanded significantly over the past few decades in a number of countries around the world. In some places in the United States, smoking in a public park or on a public beach is prohibited. A few governmental agencies have even discussed the possibility of prohibiting people from smoking in their own residences. Some individuals ask whether such regulations are a step too far.

One of the most fundamental issues that arise as public health agencies expand their view of their responsibilities is the point at which public health programs conflict with individual rights. The right of individuals to make their own decisions as to how they will live their own lives is an essential cornerstone of democratic societies. People may sometimes make decisions that harm themselves—they may choose not to wear a seat belt when they drive, for example—but perhaps that is a decision that each person should make on his or her own. Citizens of New York City would almost certainly be healthier if they were to drink smaller quantities of sugary drinks, as the mayor suggests. But does it really fall within the purview of the government and public health agencies to insist by law that individuals follow diets prescribed by experts in the field? The question that now arises more and more often is the point at which governmental health regulations and public health policies and practices impinge on individual rights.

There probably are certain public health activities on which almost everyone can agree. **Chlorination** of public water supplies is probably a virtually unanimously popular public health program. The practice has saved countless numbers of human lives over the past century. But can the same be said for fluoridation of water supplies? Critics of that practice argue that individual citizens have the means to achieve the same health results as fluoridation by taking actions such as following a well-designed program of **dental health**, using fluoridated toothpaste, and making regular visits to the dentist. Should anyone who prefers not to ingest fluorides in the public water supply (for whatever reason) actually be required to do so?

The ultimate ethical and legal challenge for the public health profession, then, is to find a reasonable balance between the rights and needs of society as a whole and those of individuals. On the one hand, public health authorities and governmental officials are justified in acknowledging the array of social, political, economic, environmental, and other factors that influence the health status of diverse groups of citizens in a society. And they are justified in wanting to develop programs that will improve the status of all citizens in such a way as to guarantee them healthier, safer lives. On the other hand, the development of public health policies and programs must also take into consideration the rights that individuals in a democracy have to make fundamental decisions about their own lives, even when such decisions may ultimately result in a less healthy, less safe life for themselves.

Until recently, there has been no widely accepted, specific code of ethics to which public health practitioners could turn for guidance in making some of the most difficult decisions with which they are faced on an almost daily basis. Individual agencies and practitioners had to make ethical decisions about their policies and actions based on their own training, experience, and sense of responsibility to the community and the individuals of whom it was composed. That situation began to change in the early 2000s when members of the graduating class of the Public Health Leadership Institute undertook the task of developing such a code. After extensive discussion and review, that code was published in 2002. The code consists of two parts, one of which is a statement of values and beliefs underlying the code in three areas: health, community, and bases for action. The heart of the code is a statement of Principles of the Ethical Practice of Public Health. The 12 principles that make up that statement are as follows:

- Public health should address principally the fundamental causes of disease and requirements for health, aiming to prevent adverse health outcomes.

KEY TERM

Ethics—A set of principles of correct conduct that help individuals and groups decide the moral action to take in a specific situation.

- Public health should achieve community health in a way that respects the rights of individuals in the community.
- Public health policies, programs, and priorities should be developed and evaluated through processes that ensure an opportunity for input from community members.
- Public health should advocate for, or work for the empowerment of, disenfranchised community members, ensuring that the basic resources and conditions necessary for health are accessible to all people in the community.
- Public health should seek the information needed to implement effective policies and programs that protect and promote health.
- Public health institutions should provide communities with the information they have that is needed for decisions on policies or programs and should obtain the community's consent for their implementation.
- Public health institutions should act in a timely manner on the information they have within the resources and the mandate given to them by the public.
- Public health programs and policies should incorporate a variety of approaches that anticipate and respect diverse values, beliefs, and cultures in the community.
- Public health programs and policies should be implemented in a manner that most enhances the physical and social environment.
- Public health institutions should protect the confidentiality of information that can bring harm to an individual or community if made public. Exceptions must be justified on the basis of the high likelihood of significant harm to the individual or others.
- Public health institutions should ensure the professional competence of their employees.
- Public health institutions and their employees should engage in collaborations and affiliations in ways that build the public's trust and the institution's effectiveness.

The 12 Ethical Principles have been widely praised within the public health profession, as well as by legal experts and ethicists. Not everyone is convinced that the ethical code provides adequate assistance for individuals faced with specific, concrete dilemmas, but publication of the code has moved the discussion of legal and ethical issues in public health to a new level.

Resources

BOOKS

Coughlin, Steven S. *Case Studies in Public Health Ethics*, 2nd ed. New York: American Public Health Association, 2011.

Dawson, Angus, ed. *Public Health Ethics: Key Concepts and Issues in Policy and Practice*. Cambridge, UK: Cambridge University Press, 2011.

Freeman, Michael. *The Ethics of Public Health*. Surrey, UK: Ashgate, 2011.

Gosten, Lawrence O. *Public Health Law and Ethics: A Reader*, 2nd ed. Berkeley: University of California Press, 2011.

PERIODICALS

Lee, L.M. "Public Health Ethics Theory: Review and Path to Convergence." *Journal of Law, Medicine, and Ethics* 40, 1. (2012): 85–98.

Lee, L.M., et al. "Ethical Justification for Conducting Public Health Surveillance without Patient Consent." *American Journal of Public Health* 102, 1. (2012): 38–44.

Pierce, M.W., et al. "Testing Public Health Ethics: Why the CDC's HIV Screening Recommendations May Violate the Least Infringement Principle." *Journal of Law, Medicine, and Ethics* 39, 2. (2011): 263–71.

Roberts, Marc J., and Michael R. Reich. "Ethical Analysis in Public Health." *Lancet* 359, 9311. (2002): 1055–9.

WEBSITES

Gostin, Lawrence O. "Mapping the Issues: Public Health, Law and Ethics." Georgetown Law Faculty Publications and Other Works. Paper 374. http://scholarship.law.georgetown.edu/cgi/viewcontent.cgi?article=1373&context=facpub. Accessed on October 13, 2012.

Jennings, Bruce, et al. "Ethics and Public Health: Model Curriculum." http://www.asph.org/UserFiles/EthicsCurriculum.pdf. Accessed on October 13, 2012.

"Public Health: Ethical Issues." Nuffield Council on Bioethics. http://www.nuffieldbioethics.org/sites/default/files/Public%20health%20-%20ethical%20issues.pdf. Accessed on October 13, 2012.

"Public Health - Legal and Ethical Issues." Pediatrics Ethics Consortium. http://www.pediatricethics.org/index.php?option=com_content&view=article&id=171&Itemid=61. Accessed on October 13, 2012.

ORGANIZATIONS

American Public Health Association (APHA), 800 I St., N.W., Washington, D.C. USA 20001–3710, 1 (202) 777-APHA, Fax: 1 (202) 777-2534, comments@apha.org, http://www.apha.org/.

David E. Newton, Ed.D.

Evidence-based policy

Definition

Evidence-based policy in the area of health care is public policy based on rigorously defined scientific evidence. It can also be defined as an extension of the concept of evidence-based medicine to all areas of public policy and planning. *Policy,* as such, is a broad term that includes budget priorities and guidelines published by agencies or professional organizations outside federal, state, or local governments, as well as government legislation, regulations, and judicial decisions.

Within the specific field of public health, evidence-based programs or policies have the following characteristics:

- The best and most up-to-date peer-reviewed evidence is used to guide decision making.
- There is a systematic use and application of data and information systems.
- Information from the behavioral sciences (psychology and neuroscience) is used in program planning.
- The group or community that will be affected by the policy is involved in planning and decision making.
- The outcomes of the policy are analyzed and evaluated.
- The results are published and distributed to all stakeholders and others involved in decision making.

Description

Types of evidence

Evidence-based policy making requires an understanding of the different types of evidence gathered by researchers and the various levels of quality involved. The basic distinction in medical and public health research is between quantitative and qualitative evidence. Quantitative evidence is based on numerical data derived from large population samples that can be analyzed by statistical methods and expressed as percentages or other numerical values. Quantitative data can be obtained from scientific information found in peer-reviewed journals, data from public health surveillance systems, or evaluations of individual programs or policies. Some researchers think that the best quantitative evidence comes from systematic reviews like those collected in the Cochrane Library (described in more detail below).

Qualitative evidence, by contrast, is derived from personal interviews, participant observation, or conducting focus groups; it does not involve numerical calculations or mathematical models but rather in-depth interviews with individuals. Qualitative evidence is considered less rigorous than quantitative evidence but is often highly effective in providing a narrative outline or specific examples when researchers in the health sciences need to explain quantitative findings to policy makers in government or the general public.

The overall quality of evidence, whether quantitative or qualitative, can be measured by several different criteria:

- Number of observations: multiple observations are preferable to only one observation.
- Type of research: Randomized controlled studies are considered to be more rigorous than isolated case reports or anecdotes.
- Publication: Studies published in peer-reviewed journals are considered more significant than so-called gray literature (unpublished government reports, conference proceedings, technical reports, and other printed materials that may be relevant to public health but are difficult to access).
- Novelty: New findings are considered less reliable than findings that confirm the results of previous studies.
- Subject type: Studies using animal subjects are considered less significant in the field of public health than studies using human subjects.
- Comparison to other studies: Studies that situate themselves in the context of the existing body of knowledge on the subject are considered better evidence than those that do not attempt to relate their results to previous work.
- Hypothesis testing: Studies intended to test a hypothesis are regarded as providing stronger evidence than those that do not relate their findings to a hypothesis.

Aspects of public health policy

Evidence-based policies in public health can be described under three headings:

PROCESS. Process refers to taking into account the complexities involved in public **health policy** making. One of these factors is that many policy makers outside the health professions do not always understand the ways in which scientific evidence is collected and evaluated, or the reasons for judging some studies to be better guides to policy than others. Moreover, policy makers often have different criteria for decision making, such as election cycles, competing sources of information, public opinion, or relationships with special interests. On the other side, many public health researchers do not think through the consequences of their research for policy making. As a result, there is often limited personal contact between researchers and clinical practitioners in the health professions on the one hand and legislators, judges, and others involved in politics on the other.

Policy making is a complicated process that typically involves numerous interactions between the different stakeholders involved; it is not a simple linear movement from point A to point B, so to speak. One analyst has described three stages or phases that increase the likelihood that a policy will be adopted: 1) defining the issue or problem as worthy of government involvement; 2) defining alternative policy measures that may be taken to address the problem; and 3) recognizing the factors outside as well as inside government that affect policy-making. In other words, public health policy must be politically and administratively feasible as well as based on the best available scientific evidence. Factors that can affect policy making range from the mood of the general public and the involvement of organized political groups to turnover within the government and the need to compromise or bargain with some stakeholders. In general, evidence-based policies that introduce gradual or incremental changes are more likely to succeed than those that take an all-or-nothing approach.

CONTENT. The content of evidence-based public health policy is derived from systematic reviews and qualitative as well as quantitative research, as described above. It incorporates findings from many different disciplines, including **epidemiology**, biostatistics, library science, psychology and other behavioral sciences, health care management, and policy development. One approach that has been taken in recent years is to look for and analyze the use of evidence-based materials or elements within existing or proposed policies. An example of this approach is the finding that the Institute of Medicine's (IOM) 2005 study of the relationship between trans fats in food and **heart disease** resulted in state or county regulations as early as 2008—a relatively brief time span between publication of the IOM study and policy formulation and introduction.

OUTCOMES. Sound evidence-based policy requires documentation of the results (outcomes) of recently implemented interventions or programs. Policy evaluations may make use of both quantitative and qualitative methods to assess the outcome of the policy's adoption and implementation. Outcome measurements typically result in modifications of the new policy in a repeated cycle of feedback, collection of updated scientific evidence, and improvement of the policy or program. In short, evidence-based policies in public health involve ongoing evaluation and fine-tuning; they are not once-and-done accomplishments.

Origins

Evidence-based policy in medicine in general and public health in particular began with the work of Archie (Archibald) Cochrane (1909–1988), a Scottish physician and epidemiologist whose service as a medical officer in prisoner-of-war camps during World War II led him to conclude that many of the interventions he had been trained to use—particularly treatments for tuberculosis—were not based on scientific evidence. He later stated in his autobiography, "I knew that there was no real evidence that anything we had to offer had any effect on **tuberculosis**, and I was afraid that I shortened the lives of some of my friends by unnecessary intervention." Cochrane spent the remainder of his career urging physicians to use the best available scientific evidence as the basis for clinical practice. In 1960 he was appointed a professor of medicine, and in 1969 he became the director of a new epidemiology research unit in Cardiff, Wales. His most influential book, *Effectiveness and Efficiency: Random Reflections on Health Services*, was published in 1972.

Cochrane was an early proponent of randomized controlled trials (RCTs) as the benchmark for scientific evidence in medicine. His work led to the Cochrane Library, a collection of databases of systematic reviews and meta-analyses that summarize and interpret the results of medical research—particularly the results of well-conducted clinical trials. The Library, which is available by subscription, is maintained by the Cochrane Collaboration, an international nonprofit organization. Subscription to the Cochrane Library is free in many countries.

Evidence-based practice

The influence of Cochrane's work first appeared in the form of evidence-based medical practice or EBP. EBP is one form of translational science, a new discipline concerned with applying research findings to real-life situations at the level of **community health** as well as the bedside of the individual patient. EBP has been defined as "the integration of clinical expertise, patient values, and the best research evidence into the decision making process for patient care." This integration involves a multi-step process that requires a doctor to search the medical literature for relevant scientific evidence as well as interact with the patient. The steps in the process can be summarized as the five A's:

- Assess the patient. Good care of the patient usually involves recognizing the patient's clinical problem or question. For example, the doctor may find that the patient's blood pressure is higher than normal. This observation may indicate that the patient has some kind of underlying disorder.
- Ask the question. This step involves formulating a clinical question involved in the patient's case. In this case, the doctor will ask why the patient's blood pressure is elevated.
- Acquire the evidence. The physician must select the appropriate medical literature or other resources and conduct a search. To continue the example, the doctor will search for journal articles or other resources for the latest findings about the differential diagnosis of high blood pressure.
- Appraise the evidence. The physician must carefully evaluate the evidence for its scientific validity and its clinical applicability to the patient in question.
- Apply the findings. This step represents the effective translation of clinical research to real-life patient care. It involves integrating the evidence collected from the literature with the physician's training and clinical experience along with the patient's preferences and values, and then talking with the patient. In this case, the doctor will discuss the high blood pressure reading with the patient. He or she might suggest modification of the patient's lifestyle, followed by a retest of the blood pressure, a different type of diagnostic test, referral to a specialist, or some other next step. The doctor will base the conversation on his or her knowledge of the individual patient as well as his or her evaluation of the most recent medical research.The final step in EBP is the physician's self-evaluation after the discussion with the patient.

Evidence-based public health

EBP was modified in some respects when it was introduced into public health for one obvious reason: public health policies and interventions are based on, and in turn affect, populations rather than individuals. The population-based aspect of public health in turn requires healthcare professionals in the field to interact with community groups, policy makers, and other stakeholders rather than individual patients. The process underlying the formulation and introduction of evidence-based public health (EBPH) policies and interventions can be outlined in six steps:

- Identify public health priorities, and define the relevant issue. The priorities may be disease-specific, or they may be derived from consumer concerns, legislative priorities, state or local needs, or preventive issues.
- Collect quantitative data related to the specific population, its location, and the expected outcomes.
- Develop program or policy options and select the appropriate evidence-based approach and performance measures.
- Choose an appropriate evaluation strategy; then implement the program or other intervention.
- Measure the program's effects, and evaluate its processes and outcomes.
- Publish the findings and results.

KEY TERMS

Gray literature—A term used by librarians to refer to written material that is not published commercially or is not generally accessible to the public. Gray literature includes such material as conference proceedings, working papers, technical reports, and the like.

Intervention—In public health, any plan, policy, or activity intended to encourage behaviors conducive to good health or discourage behaviors harmful to health. Interventions may include treatments, prevention strategies, screening programs, diagnostic tests, different health care settings, and educational materials or programs.

Meta-analysis—A method of contrasting and combining results from different studies in order to identify patterns among study results, sources of disagreement among those results, or other significant relationships among the various studies.

Participant observation—A type of qualitative research in which the observer or researcher becomes involved with a specific group of individuals, such as a religious congregation, extended family, or other small group over an extended period of time, and participates in the life of the group as well as making direct observations of the group members.

Qualitative research—An approach to research that focuses on human behavior and the reasons for it; it is usually based on social interactions, words, or images rather than numbers and statistics. Qualitative research typically uses a small study sample, and the information obtained is regarded as limited to that sample rather than applicable to the general population.

Quantitative research—A quantifiable approach to research in which raw data are collected and turned into usable information by mathematical computation. Quantitative research uses statistics to make generalizations or predictions about a population larger than the study sample.

Randomized controlled trial (RCT)—A study in which subjects are allocated at random to receive one of several clinical interventions.

Stakeholder—Any person, group, organization, or other entity who affects or can be affected by an organization's actions or policies.

Systematic review—A summary of the medical literature that uses explicit methods to perform a comprehensive literature search and critical appraisal of individual studies, and also uses appropriate statistical techniques to combine these valid studies.

Translational science—A term used in the health sciences to describe the transfer and application of laboratory science to bedside clinical practice or population-based public health interventions.

Effects on public health

Evidence-based policy is an increasingly important topic within the field of public health. Students as well as professionals already in the field should acquaint themselves with the basic principles and methods of EBPH.

Resources

The current interest in evidence-based policy has resulted in the creation of a number of training programs for persons with an M.P.H. degree or work experience in public health. One such training program has been established at the **Prevention** Research Center in St. Louis (PRC-StL), which offers a four-day on-site course that has trained over 1,300 persons since it was started in 1997. The **CDC** also funds 36 other prevention research centers (PRCs) across the United States that offer programs in preventive medicine and public health research. A map of all 37 currently funded PRCs and contact information for each center is available at http://www.cdc.gov/prc/center-descriptions/index.htm.

In addition to on-site training programs, there are numerous online resources for students or professionals in public health interested in evidence-based policy. These resources range from free online training modules, some of which are listed below, to such databases as the Cochrane Library, CDC surveillance systems, guides to gray literature, and access to legislative information that allows researchers to track the progress of policy initiatives and legislation.

Benefits of evidence-based policies

The benefits of evidence-based policies in the field of public health include:

- Meeting the requirements of federal and state agencies for funding public health programs. Government requirements that proposed programs be evidence-based are becoming increasingly rigorous as of 2012.
- Access to more accurate information about the feasibility of public health policies.
- Increased likelihood of implementing effective and successful programs and interventions.
- Greater workforce productivity.
- More efficient use of limited public and private funding and other resources.

Resources

BOOKS

Brownson, Ross C., et al. *Evidence-based Public Health*, 2nd ed. New York: Oxford University Press, 2011.

Fink, Arlene G.*Evidence-Based Public Health Practice*. Thousand Oaks, CA: Sage Publications, 2013.

Hunting, Katherine L, and Brenda L. Gleason. *Essential Case Studies in Public Health: Putting Public Health into Practice*. Sudbury, MA: Jones and Bartlett Learning, 2012.

Killoran, Amanda, and Michael P. Kelly. *Evidence-based Public Health: Effectiveness and Efficiency*. New York: Oxford University Press, 2010.

PERIODICALS

Brownson, R.C., et al. "Evidence-Based Public Health: A Fundamental Concept for Public Health Practice." *Annual Review of Public Health* 30 (2009): 175–201.

Brownson, R.C., et al. "Understanding Evidence-based Public Health Policy." *American Journal of Public Health* 99 (September 2009): 1576–1583.

Cilenti, D., et al. "Information-Seeking Behaviors and Other Factors Contributing to Successful Implementation of Evidence-Based Practices in Local Health Departments." *Journal of Public Health Management and Practice* 18 (November 2012): 571–576.

Jacobs, J.A., et al. "Tools for Implementing an Evidence-Based Approach in Public Health Practice." *Preventing Chronic Disease* 9 (2012): 110324.

Kansagra, S.M., and T.A. Farley. "Public Health Research: Lost in Translation or Speaking the Wrong Language?" *American Journal of Public Health* 101 (December 2011): 2203–2206.

Mirvis, D.M. "From Research to Public Policy: An Essential Extension of the Translation Research Agenda." *Clinical and Translational Science* 2 (October 2009): 379–381.

WEBSITES

"EBPH Training Course Information." Prevention Research Center in St. Louis (PRC-StL). The nine modules in the course can be opened separately in PowerPoint format. http://prcstl.wustl.edu/EBPH/Pages/Evidence-Based PublicHealthCourse.aspx (accessed November 7, 2012).

"Evidence-Based Public Health." Prevention Research Center in St. Louis (PRC-StL). http://prcstl.wustl.edu/EBPH/Pages/default.aspx (accessed November 7, 2012).

"Evidence-based Public Health Online Course." University of Illinois at Chicago Institute for Health Research and Policy. http://ebph.ihrp.uic.edu/ (accessed November 7, 2012).

"Understanding Evidence-Based Healthcare: A Foundation for Action." United States Cochrane Center. This is a free online course that requires registration. http://us.cochrane.org/understanding-evidence-based-healthcare-foundation-action (accessed November 8, 2012).

ORGANIZATIONS

Agency for Healthcare Research and Quality (AHRQ), 540 Gaither Road, Suite 2000, Rockville, MD United States 20850, (301) 427-1104, http://www.ahrq.gov/.

Center for Evidence-Based Policy, Oregon Health and Science University, 3455 SW US Veterans Hospital Road, Mail-stop SN-4N, Portland, OR United States 97239-2941, (503) 494-2182, Fax: (503) 494-3807, centerebp@ohsu.edu, http://www.ohsu.edu/xd/research/centers-institutes/evidence-based-policy-center/index.cfm/.

Coalition for Evidence-Based Policy, 1725 I Street, NW, Suite 300, Washington, DC United States 20006, (202) 349-1130, Fax: (202) 349-3915, jbaron@coalition4evidence.org, http://coalition4evidence.org/wordpress/.

Cochrane Collaboration, United States Cochrane Center, Center for Clinical Trials, Johns Hopkins Bloomberg School of Public Health, 615 N. Wolfe Street, Mail RM W5010, Baltimore, MD United States 21205, (410) 502-4419, Fax: (410) 502-4621, uscc@jhsph.edu, http://www.cochrane.org/United States home page: http://us.cochrane.org/.

Prevention Research Center in St. Louis (PRC-StL), Washington University, 660 S. Euclid Ave., Campus Box 8109, Saint Louis, MO United States 63110, (314) 362-9643, prcstl@wustl.edu, http://prcstl.wustl.edu/Pages/default.aspx.

Rebecca J. Frey, Ph.D.

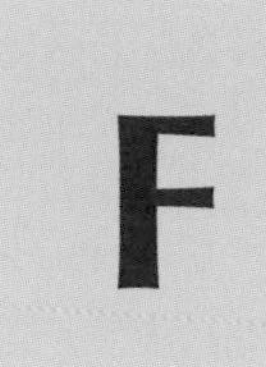

Famine

Definition

A famine is an extreme and widespread scarcity of food that affects the general **population** of a large area, such as a particular country or geographic region. It is typically accompanied or followed by starvation, epidemics of contagious disease, political instability, and increased mortality. Famines may result from natural causes, human practices, or policies, or a combination of these. The English word *famine* is derived from *fames*, the Latin word for hunger.

Description

Famines have been a recurrent form of disaster throughout human history. The earliest recorded famine affected ancient Egypt around 2200 B.C. Another severe famine struck ancient Rome in the fifth century B.C. Famines were frequent in Western Europe, Russia, India, Africa, Mexico, Central and South America, China, Japan, and southeastern Asia from the fifth century A.D. up through the nineteenth century. Improvements in agricultural science, farm equipment, irrigation techniques, weather forecasting, and other technological advances that followed the Industrial Revolution lowered the frequency and severity of famines in the developed countries, with the exception of wars. Periodic famines continue to affect large portions of sub-Saharan Africa, Central America, Bangladesh, and North Korea as of 2012.

Famines are complex disasters in that they may cause as well as result from disease, political conflict, and poor agricultural practices. The complicated interconnections of natural and human factors involved in famines is one reason why famine **prevention** and relief are difficult even in the twenty-first century; and why famines so often have severe consequences for public health. Up until 1981 famines were usually understood as resulting from a simple lack of available food; this theory is known as the food availability decline (FAD) hypothesis. More recently, however, public health experts have learned that famines can result from difficulties in food distribution as well as food availability. The destruction of roads, railroads, and other means of transportation during a war is one example of a situation in which famine can develop in one part of a country even though there is ample food in other areas.

Demographics

Famines are a major cause of mortality in the present as well as the past; some major famines, such as the famine that struck Russia in 1601, the Deccan famine of India in 1630, and the French famine of 1693 are estimated to have killed 2 million people each. The four famines that affected China between 1810 and 1849 cost 45 million lives. The North Korean famine of 1996 is estimated to have killed between 600,000 and 3.5 million people. The only major countries that have never been affected by large-scale famines are Australia, Canada, New Zealand, and the United States.

As of 2012, the geographic region most consistently affected by famine is sub-Saharan Africa, with Asia also affected by chronic famines. Countries with food emergencies declared by the United Nations since 2005 include Niger, Chad, Darfur, Ethiopia, South Sudan, Zimbabwe, Somalia, Kenya, Djibouti, and the Horn of Africa. Worldwide, the UN estimates that as of 2012 several hundred million people suffer from chronic food shortages if not outright famine.

Although all segments of a population are affected by famine, those most vulnerable are the very young, the very old, and people with chronic diseases. Interestingly, in all recorded famines, mortality is higher among adult males than adult females. It is thought that the higher survival rate among women is due to women's lower daily caloric needs compared to the requirements of an adult male, and women's higher percentage of stored body fat.

Causes

Famines may be caused by **natural disasters**, human policies and actions, or both.

Natural causes

Natural causes of famine include animal and microscopic pests as well as weather- and soil-related problems, any of which can lead to crop failure.

WEATHER, CLIMATE, AND NATURAL DISASTERS. Weather- and climate-related causes of famine include periodic droughts, floods, earthquakes and tsunamis, hurricanes and typhoons, and tornadoes. The famine that affected what is now the southwestern United States occurred in the thirteenth century, when the Anasazi peoples of the Four Corners region were forced to leave the area because of repeated crop failures due to drought.

Another natural cause of famine is volcanic eruptions, which lead to famine by releasing aerosols and dust into the atmosphere and blocking the sunlight needed for plants to grow. The famine of 1740–1741 in Europe followed an unusually cold winter that is thought to have been caused by volcanic dust. In addition to destroying crops directly, storms and floods lead to famine by contributing to soil erosion or contamination. Natural disasters of any kind may also lead to famine by killing or displacing farmers and agricultural workers.

A recurrent weather pattern that has been implicated in famines in countries bordering the southern Pacific Ocean is the El Niño-Southern Oscillation or ENSO. This weather pattern, which recurs every three to seven years, is characterized by alternating wetter-than-usual and drier-than-usual conditions. Severe famines in 1876 (India, China, Brazil), 1896 (China), and 1902 (India) have all been described as ENSO famines.

SOIL EROSION AND EXHAUSTION. The loss of topsoil through erosion by wind or **water**, or the depletion of minerals in soil that are necessary for crops (particularly nitrogen, phosphorus, and potassium) is a common cause of famine in Africa. Erosion of the soil is a frequent consequence of deforestation, while the loss of minerals in the soil is the result of poor agricultural practices. An additional complication is the cost of fertilizer; many African farmers are so poor that they cannot afford to purchase fertilizer to protect the mineral content of the soil.

PESTS. Famine may result from **fungal infections** of food crops or animal pests that compete with humans for the crops. The Great Irish Famine of 1847–1852 resulted from the destruction of the potato crop by a water **mold**, *Phytophthora infestans*. Wheat rust is a disease caused by fungi belonging to the genus *Puccinia* that has led to major losses of wheat, barley, and rye crops in Africa, Asia, and Latin America as of 2012. Animal pests that have destroyed crops across large areas include locusts, rats, and mice.

Human causes

Human causes of famine include intentional acts of war and genocide as well as unintentional behaviors that affect food supplies or food distribution.

POPULATION IMBALANCE. A frequent cause of famine is an imbalance between the supply of available food and the number of people who need food. In some cases famine results from simple overpopulation, but in others, it may result from the loss of farmers and agricultural workers due to war or migration. In the second type of situation, there are not enough healthy adults to cultivate and harvest crops on the available land relative to the number of people left behind who still need food.

AGRICULTURAL PRACTICES AND TECHNIQUES. Poor agricultural practices are associated with the loss of topsoil through erosion and the depletion of mineral nutrients in the soil. In many parts of Africa, farmers no longer allow some of their land to lie fallow for a year or two between crops in order to restore its mineral content but instead raise crops on the same plot year after year without fertilizer until the soil is completely exhausted. In addition, they typically raise the same kind of food crop in successive years rather than practicing crop rotation.

The role of deforestation in leading to soil erosion has already been mentioned. Deforestation itself results from a practice known as slash-and-burn agriculture, which refers to the cutting and burning of forest trees in order to create new fields. After the soil in the new fields has been depleted, the farmer repeats the process in another forested area. There are an estimated 250 million farmers around the world who practice slash-and-burn agriculture as of 2012.

WAR AND POLITICAL UNREST. War and political unrest are major causes of famine in that they interrupt the distribution of available food as well as directly destroying crops and other food supplies. The weapons of modern warfare can crush, burn, or chemically contaminate large areas of cultivated land; destruction on this scale was not possible before the mid-nineteenth century. In addition, an occupying army may deliberately take food from the civilian population to feed its own troops; the German occupiers of the Netherlands caused a massive famine in the winter of 1944–1945 to punish the Dutch for their refusal to help the Nazi war effort. About 22,000 people died during the "hunger winter," particularly elderly men.

Another wartime practice that can lead to famine is a scorched-earth policy, in which an invading army destroys the fields and crops of the civilian population in order to lower its morale. The best-known American example of scorched earth comes from the Civil War: Sherman's march from Atlanta to Savannah, Georgia, in the fall of 1864, in which Union troops destroyed Confederate railroads and killed livestock as well as burning crops along their path. In other instances of scorched earth practices, the civilian population in the path of an invader may destroy its own crops and food supply in order to deprive the invading army of easily obtained food. This type of scorched earth policy goes back to the first century BC, when the Gallic tribes in what is now France and Belgium burned large parts of the countryside to try to starve the Roman legions led by Julius Caesar.

GOVERNMENT POLICY. Misguided government policies can lead to famine. The most disastrous example is China's so-called Great Leap Forward in 1958–1962. Mao Zedong attempted to turn China from an agricultural to an industrial power in a very brief period of time; the government seized food supplies, melted down farm tools for the metal they contained, and deprived the peasants of enough food to continue their work of growing crops. The famine that resulted killed between 35 and 45 million people; it is considered the greatest peacetime disaster in human history.

Governments may also bring about the deliberate starvation of a segment of their population as an act of genocide. Examples of genocidal famines include the 1915 starvation of the Armenians by Ottoman Turkey and the 1932 famine in Ukraine resulting from Josef Stalin's intention to punish the Ukrainians for their opposition to his regime. The Ukrainian famine is estimated to have cost 7.5 million lives.

Effects on public health

Famines have a number of damaging effects on public health, ranging from increased mortality and population displacement to environmental damage and destruction.

- Increased mortality. Increased mortality in famine-stricken areas may result directly from malnutrition or starvation, or indirectly from epidemics of communicable or vaccine-preventable diseases. The diseases that most often accompany famines are the diarrheal diseases, particularly cholera; malaria; tuberculosis; other respiratory infections; and measles.
- Contamination or loss of water supplies.
- Population displacement and migration. Famines commonly drive people in the area affected by the famine to move elsewhere, often bringing communicable disease with them. They may also cause stress on the food supply or food distribution in their new area, possibly leading to political conflict. Last, the loss of population in the affected area may hinder recovery after the cause of the famine is resolved. For example, the Great Irish Famine of the 1840s led to mass emigration to Australia, the United States, and Canada. As late as 1970, the population of Ireland was only half of what it had been before the famine.
- Long-term chronic health problems. Studies of children conceived during the Dutch famine of 1944–1945 have shown that they have higher-than-average rates of obesity, diabetes, and cardiovascular disease as adults. They are also more prone to depression and other mood disorders. One particularly interesting finding is that these people were not only shorter and smaller than average at birth, but that their own children are smaller than average. This finding suggests that famine may have multigenerational genetic effects.

Efforts and solutions

Famine prevention

Famine prevention in the twenty-first century begins with attempts to measure problems with food availability and distribution in a distressed area before a full-blown famine develops. The first scale to measure the severity of famine was devised by the British in India in the 1880s, and had three levels: near-scarcity of food; scarcity; and famine. The most widely used scale as of 2012 is the Integrated Food Security Phase Classification or IPC scale. Originally devised by the UN to evaluate the 1992 famine in Somalia, the IPC defines five levels of food insecurity:

- Generally food-secure: over 80% of households can meet their nutritional needs without resorting to destructive coping strategies (theft, rioting, or liquidation of household assets).
- Borderline food-insecure: at least 20% of households have difficulty meeting nutritional needs and cannot fully protect their livelihood.
- Acute food crisis: More than 20% of households can meet their needs for food only by liquidating their assets. Levels of malnutrition are higher than normal.
- Humanitarian emergency: More than 20% of households have extreme gaps in food consumption, leading to very high levels of malnutrition and higher-than-normal mortality.
- Famine: More than 20% of households have a complete lack of food and other basic needs; levels of severe

malnutrition have risen above 30%, and mortality exceeds 2/10,000 per day.

The United States Agency for International Development (USAID) has set up the Famine Early Warning System Network or FEWS NET to monitor climatic and agricultural conditions as well as food supplies around the world.

Other measures taken to prevent famine include the provision of seeds for high-yielding crops such as those developed by the so-called Green Revolution of the 1970s; donations of fertilizer and pesticides to prevent soil depletion and crop failure due to insects and rodents; improved maintenance of irrigation canals and other water supplies for crops; improved maintenance of roads and railroads to ensure adequate food distribution; and public health measures to prevent disease through **immunization** and clean **drinking water** campaigns.

Famine relief

Famine relief relied in the past on direct donations of food from the developed countries to famine-stricken areas. As of 2012, however, the World Food Programme (WFP) and other humanitarian organizations have found that giving cash or cash vouchers to the hungry is a more effective way to counter famine in countries where food is available but costly. Direct delivery of food is still carried out in drought-stricken areas and locations where people live long distances from food markets.

Other measures to relieve famine include delivery of fortified or nutrient-rich foods, such as spirulina and a peanut butter-based food called Plumpy'nut that is manufactured by a French company called Nutriset. Both spirulina and Plumpy'nut have the advantages of being easily digested by malnourished people; do not require refrigeration; and do not need to be mixed with scarce drinking water. Famished people affected by **cholera** or other diarrheal diseases are treated with oral rehydration solution (ORS), zinc supplements, vitamin A, and **antibiotics**.

Future concerns

Most public health experts as well as other policy makers expect famine to be an ongoing problem throughout the twenty-first century. Particular concerns include diminishing water supplies worldwide; the fact that 40% of the world's cultivated land is presently considered seriously degraded; an epidemic of wheat rust that has spread from Africa to Asia as of 2012; and the side effects of fertilizers and pesticides on the environment. Some experts predict massive starvation as early as 2050 unless the world population is rapidly reduced.

KEY TERMS

Crop rotation—The practice of growing a series of different crops with different water and nutrient requirements in the same plot of land in successive seasons. Crop rotation helps to restore nutrients to the soil and reduces the likelihood of crop failure due to plant diseases or pests.

El Niño-Southern Oscillation (ENSO)—A recurrent weather pattern across the tropical Pacific characterized by alternating wetter-than-normal and drier-than-normal conditions in large portions of Africa, eastern Asia, and South America.

Food insecurity—A limited or uncertain ability to obtain nutritionally adequate and safe foods in socially acceptable ways.

Green Revolution—A series of agricultural research and development programs from the 1940s through the 1970s that included the development of high-yielding food crops, expansion of irrigation, and distribution of seeds and fertilizers in India and other countries with recurrent famines.

Scorched earth—A military strategy that includes confiscating or destroying the civilian food supply as well as destroying other resources that might be useful to the enemy.

Slash-and-burn—An agricultural practice that involves the cutting and burning of trees in a forested area to create new fields. It quickly results in soil depletion followed by soil erosion.

Spirulina—A nutritional supplement made from two species of blue-green algae belonging to the genus *Arthrospira*.

Resources

BOOKS

Behnassi, Mohamed, Sidney Draggan, and Sanni Yaya, eds. *Global Food Insecurity: Rethinking Agricultural and Rural Development Paradigm and Policy*. New York: Springer, 2011.

Dando, William A., ed. *Food and Famine in the 21st Century*. Santa Varbara, CA: ABC-CLIO, 2012.

Dikötter, Frank. *Mao's Great Famine: The History of China's Most Devastating Catastrophe, 1958–1962*. New York: Walker and Co., 2010.

Ó Gráda, Cormac. *Famine: A Short History*. Princeton, NJ: Princeton University Press, 2009.

PERIODICALS

Castillo, D.C., et al. "Inconsistent Access to Food and Cardiometabolic Disease: The Effect of Food Insecurity."

Current Cardiovascular Risk Reports 5 (June 2012): 245–250.

D'Alessandro, S. "Modernization, Weather Variability, and Vulnerability to Famine." *Oxford Economic Papers* 63 (April 2011): 625–647.

Gilbert, N. "African Agriculture: Dirt Poor." *Nature* 483 (March 28, 2012): 525–527.

McMichael, A.J. "Insights from Past Millennia into Climatic Impacts on Human Health and Survival." *Proceedings of the National Academy of Sciences of the United States of America* 109 (March 27, 2012): 4730–4737.

Nackers, F., et al. "Effectiveness of Ready-to-use Therapeutic Food [Plumpy'nut] Compared to a Corn/soy-blend-based Pre-mix for the Treatment of Childhood Moderate Acute Malnutrition in Niger." *Journal of Tropical Pediatrics* 56 (December 2010): 407–413.

van Abeelen, A.F., et al. "Survival Effects of Prenatal Famine Exposure." *American Journal of Clinical Nutrition* 95 (January 2012): 179–183.

WEBSITES

Famine Early Warning System Network (FEWS NET). FEWS NET is a network funded by USAID that monitors climatic and food security issues in underdeveloped parts of the world in order to provide timely warning about hunger and other early signs of famine. http://www.fews.net/Pages/default.aspx?l=en (accessed October 5, 2012).

ORGANIZATIONS

Centers for Disease Control and Prevention (CDC), 1600 Clifton Road, Atlanta, GA United States 30333, (800) CDC-INFO (232-4636), http://www.cdc.gov/cdc-info/requestform.html, http://www.cdc.gov/.

United States Agency for International Development (USAID), Office of the Administrator, Ronald Reagan Building, 1300 Pennsylvania Avenue, N.W., Washington, DC United States 20523, (202) 712-4810, Fax: (202) 216-3524, http://www.usaid.gov/comment, http://www.usaid.gov/.

World Food Programme (WFP), Via C. G. Viola 68, Parco dei Medici, Rome, Italy 00148, +39 06 65131, Fax: +39 06 6590632, http://www.wfp.org/contact, http://www.wfp.org/.

World Health Organization (WHO), Avenue Appia 20, Geneva, Switzerland 1211 Geneva 27, +41 22 791 21 11, Fax: +41 22 791 31 11, http://www.who.int/en/.

Rebecca J. Frey, Ph.D.

Federally qualified health centers

Definition

Federally qualified health centers (FQHCs) are community-based health centers that provide primary health, dental, behavioral, and mental care to uninsured, underinsured, and underserved populations in the United States.

Purpose

The purpose of FQHCs is to provide comprehensive basic health and medical care to citizens and non-citizens who would not otherwise have access to such services.

Description

Federally Qualified Health Centers were created under terms of the Omnibus Budget Reconciliation Act of 1989. The concept on which they are based evolved out of earlier programs, the Community and Migrant Health Center programs, originally enacted in the 1960s and 1970s to provide comprehensive health and medical care to populations who otherwise had no access to such services. The primary difference between FQHCs and their predecessors is that the former fall under the Medicare and Medicaid programs, which the Community and Migrant Health Center programs did not. The activities of the FQHCs were consolidated with those of a number of federal health and medical programs in the Health Center Consolidation Act of 1996, commonly referred to as Section 330, as that is its location in the current Public Health Service Act.

FGHCs fall into four major categories:

- Community Health Centers, which are designated sites for providing basic health and medical care to medically underserved areas (MUA) or populations (MUP), categories that are described in federal law;
- Migrant Health Centers, whose primary purpose is the health and medical care of documented and undocumented migrants and seasonal agricultural workers;
- Health Care for the Homeless Programs, whose function it is to provide health and medical care and substance abuse care and counseling for the homeless and their families; and
- Public Housing Primary Care Programs, facilities that are sited within or adjacent to public housing projects, for which they are typically the sole or primary healthcare provider.

Two additional categories of facilities are classified along with FQHCs: FQHC Look Alikes (FQHCLA) and Indian Health Service FQHCs. Both categories have the same general objectives as FQHCs, but differ in other respects. For example, FQHCLAs do not receive funding from the so-called 330 grants paid to regular FQHCs. Indian Health Service FQHCs also have some of their own provisions established under with the Indian Self-Determination Act of 1975 or the Indian Health Care Improvement Act of 1976.

FQHCs are supported financially by the federal government in a number of ways, most important of which is a start-up grant of as much as $650,000. Centers then continue to operate with other 330 grants for ongoing operational expenses. Centers are also reimbursed for actual patient care from the Medicare fund on a cost-based reimbursement schedule. The federal government also provides medical malpractice coverage to all FQHCs through the Federal Tort Claims Act, makes available purchase of prescription drugs through the federal 340B Drug Pricing Program, offers access to the Vaccine for Children Program, and makes available volunteers from the National Health Service Corps. As part of the Affordable Care Act of 2010, the federal government will begin reimbursing FQHCs in 2014 on a Prospective Payment System (PPS) basis, in which payments are determined by a standard developed through the analysis of previous payments for particular types of services. In addition to these financial benefits, FQHCs are also eligible for a number of other grant and loan programs offered by the federal government.

Federal funding for FQHCLAs is similar to that for FQHCs with one major exception: the former meet all of the same requirements as do FQHCs, but they are not eligible for 330 grants.

Both FQHCs and FQHCLAs are administered by a board of directors, of whom at least 51% must be clients of the facilities who are representative of the community that is being served by the clinic. Clinic facilities must be available to all members of a community, but a sliding fee must also be established that requires that those who are able to make some payment towards their care do, in fact, do so. In any case, neither an FQHC nor FQHCLA may be a profit-making facility.

FQHCs and FQHCLAs provide a wide array of primary care services in the areas of health and medical serivces, dental services, mental health and substance abuse services, transportation services necessary for adequate patient care, and hospital and specialty care. Examples of the specific services available at a typical FQHC or FQHCLA include

- Nutritional assessment and referral
- Children's eye and ear examination
- Well child care
- Immunization
- Family planning services
- Physical examination
- Blood pressure measurement
- Cholesterol screening
- Hearing screening
- Vision screening
- Tuberculosis testing
- Risk assessment and counseling
- Preventive health education
- Prenatal and post-partum care
- Thyroid function test
- Breast examination.

To carry out their extensive missions, FQHCs and FQHCLAs typically provide a wide variety of staff, including general physicians and medical specialists, nurse practitioners, physician assistants, various levels of nurses, clinical social workers, clinical psychologists, certified nurse midwives, dentists, dental technicians, and mental health counselors.

KEY TERMS

Primary health care—A level of health care that is necessary for an individual to maintain good health that normally involves preventive education and treatment and early diagnosis and treatment of possible health and medical problems.

Prospective Payment System (PPS)—A method of making medical payments based on a standard developed through the analysis of previous payments for particular types of services.

Underserved population—A group of individuals who receive fewer services than would normally be considered necessary for a normal lifestyle.

Demographics

The most recent data available (2010) indicate that there were 1,124 FQHCs in the 50 states, the District of Columbia, and Puerto Rico. The largest number of centers were in California, with 118 FQHCs, and the fewest in Nevada, with two. In 2010, the program served an estimated 20 million clients, 62% of whom belonged to some ethnic minority (primarily Hispanic). More than a third (38%) of all clients were uninsured, 72% lived at or below the 100% **poverty** level ($22,314 for a family of four in 2010), and 93% lived at or below 200% of the poverty level.

Resources

BOOKS

California HealthCare Foundation. *The Clinic's Tale: Chasing FQHC Status Not for the Faint-hearted.* Sacramento, CA: California HealthCare Foundation, 2012.

Travers, Karen L. *Comparison of the Rural Health Clinic and Federally Qualified Health Center Programs.* Washington, DC: U.S. Department of Health and Human Services, Health Resources and Services Administration, [2006].

PERIODICALS

Feder, J.L. "Innovation Profile: Restructuring Care in a Federally Qualified Health Center to Better Meet Patients' Needs." *Health Affairs* 30, 3. (2011): 419–21.

Omojasola, Anthony, et al. "Federally Qualified Health Center Patients and Generic Drug Discount Programs." *Journal of Health Care for the Poor and Underserved* 23, 1. (2012): 358–66.

Sefton, M., et al. "A Journey to Become a Federally Qualified Health Center." *Journal of the American Academy of Nurse Practitioners* 23, 7. (2011): 346–50.

Sieber, W.J., et al. "Establishing the Collaborative Care Research Network (CCRN): A Description of Initial Participating Sites." *Families, Systems & Health* 30, 3. (2012): 210–23.

WEBSITES

"Comparison of the Rural Health Clinic and Federally Qualified Health Center Programs." U.S. Department of Health and Human Services. http://www.ask.hrsa.gov/downloads/fqhc-rhccomparison.pdf. Accessed on October 21, 2012.

"Enhancing the Capacity of Community Health Centers to Achieve High Performance: Findings from the 2009 Commonwealth Fund National Survey of Federally Qualified Health Centers." The Commonwealth Fund. http://www.commonwealthfund.org/Publications/Fund-Reports/2010/May/Enhancing-the-Capacity-of-Community-Health-Centers-to-Achieve-High-Performance.aspx?page=all. Accessed on October 21, 2012.

"Federally Qualified Health Center." Department of Health and Human Services. http://www.cms.gov/Outreach-and-Education/Medicare-Learning-Network-MLN/MLN Products/downloads/fqhcfactsheet.pdf. Accessed on October 21, 2012.

"Federally Qualified Health Centers." Rural Assistance Center. http://www.raconline.org/topics/clinics/fqhc.php. Accessed on October 21, 2012.

ORGANIZATIONS

Centers for Medicare & Medicaid Services, 7500 Security Blvd., Baltimore, MD 21244, 1 (410) 786–3000, (877) 267–2323, https://www.cms.gov/.

David E. Newton, Ed.D.

Female genital mutilation

Definition

Female genital mutilation (FGM)—also called "female genital cutting" (FGC) or "female circumcision"—is the cutting or partial or total removal of the external female genitalia. The **World Health Organization** states that FGM "includes procedures that intentionally alter or cause injury to the female genital organs for non-medical reasons." It is performed for cultural or other non–medical reasons, most often on girls between the ages of four and ten years, but may be performed as young as a few days after being born, to as late as the age of puberty (up to 15 years). Sometimes it is performed at ages even older.

Description

FGM includes a wide range of procedures. They are divided generally into four groups:

- Clitoridectomy: partial or total removal of the clitoris and, in very rare cases, only the prepuce.
- Excision: partial or total removal of the clitoris and the labia minora, with or without excision of the labia majora.
- Infibulation: narrowing of the vaginal opening through the creation of a covering seal. The seal is formed by cutting and repositioning the inner, or outer, labia, with or without removal of the clitoris.
- Other: all other harmful procedures to the female genitalia for non-medical purposes (for example, cauterizing, incising, piercing, pricking, and scraping the genital area).

The simplest form of FGM involves a small cut to the clitoris or labial tissue. A Sunna circumcision removes the prepuce—a fold of skin that covers the clitoris—and/or the tip of the clitoris. A clitoridectomy is the removal of the entire clitoris and some or all of the surrounding tissue. Clitoridectomies account for approximately 80% of FGMs. The extreme form of genital mutilation is excision and infibulation, in which the clitoris and all of the surrounding tissues of the external genitalia are cut away, and the remaining skin is sewn together, leaving only a small opening for the passage of urine and menstrual blood. This sewing shut of the vagina is designed to ensure virginity until marriage. Infibulation accounts for approximately 15% of FGM procedures.

FGM is usually performed in the home or some other non–medical setting. It is often performed by a family member or a local "circumciser," using scissors, knives, razor blades, or other instruments that have not necessarily been sterilized. However, in Egypt up to 90% of FGMs are now performed by medical professionals.

With increased immigration to Western countries from regions where female circumcision is common, the practice has come to the attention of health professionals in the United States, Canada, Europe, and Australia. Some families return to their native countries to have their daughters circumcised. In an effort to integrate old customs with modern medical care, some immigrant families have requested that Western physicians perform the procedure. This can place doctors in the difficult position of trying to be sensitive to cultural traditions and choosing between performing female circumcision in a medical facility under anesthesia and sanitary conditions, or refusing, knowing that the FGM may be performed without medical supervision. In 2010, the American Academy of Pediatrics, in a controversial change of policy, suggested that U.S. doctors be allowed to perform a ceremonial pinprick on girls to prevent them from being sent abroad for FGM.

Origins

FGM has been practiced before the first century A.D. Decorations surrounding ancient Egyptian mummies indicate the practice of genital mutilation. Historians have found references to FGM by ancient Greek historian Herodotus (c. 484 B.C.–425 B.C.), who claimed that the Ethiopians, Hittites, and Phoenicians practiced female circumcision in the fifth century B.C. Other ancient reports document the practice by peoples in the tropical regions of Africa, the Philippines, the Upper Amazon River, and in Australia. It also was practiced among the early Arabs and Romans. As recent as the 1950s, clitoridectomy was practiced in the United States and Western Europe to treat such so-called problems in women as epilepsy, hysteria, lesbianism, masturbation, melancholia, mental disorders, and nymphomania.

Demographics

The **World Health Organization (WHO)** estimates that about 140 million girls and women worldwide have undergone some form of FGM, with as many as three million girls at risk for the procedure each year. The **WHO** estimates that in Africa, alone, an estimated 92 million girls who are 10 years old and older have undergone FGM. The procedure is a deeply rooted cultural tradition in some 28 African countries and a few Middle Eastern and Asian nations. Although it is illegal in many countries, including 18 African nations, enforcement is minimal. In the United States, it is illegal to perform FGM on anyone under age 18. The WHO states that FGM is a violation of the **human rights** of girls and women. The organization makes the following statement: "FGM is recognized internationally as a violation of the human rights of girls and women. It reflects deep-rooted inequality between the sexes, and constitutes an extreme form of discrimination against women. It is nearly always carried out on minors and is a violation of the rights of children. The practice also violates a person's rights to health, security and physical integrity, the right to be free from torture and cruel, inhuman or degrading treatment, and the right to life when the procedure results in death."

Nearly half of all women who have been genitally mutilated live in Egypt or Ethiopia, although the rates of FGM in Egypt and some other countries appear to be on the decline. FGM is practiced to a lesser degree in Indonesia, India, and Pakistan. The countries in which the highest percentages of females are subjected to FGM are as follows. (Where two percentages are given, the lower percentage refers to girls aged 15–19, and the higher percentage is for women aged 35–39, suggesting that the practice is on the decline):

- Guinea: 99%
- Somalia: 97–99%
- Djibouti: 98%
- Egypt: 81–96%
- Eritrea: 95%
- Mali: 94%
- Sierra Leone: 90%
- Ethiopia: 62–81%
- Gambia: 80%
- Côte d'Ivoire: 28–44%
- Kenya: 15–35%

FGM is practiced by people of all educational levels and social classes and various religions, including Christians, Muslims, and animists (who believe in the existence of non-human spiritual beings). In some countries, it is more common in rural areas, and in other countries, it is more prevalent in cities.

Although FGM is most often performed on girls before they reach puberty, it is practiced on women of all ages, from infancy through adulthood. The usual age for FGM varies with the country and region within a country. Sometimes it is performed just before a woman marries or during her first pregnancy. In Egypt, about 90% of girls are cut between the ages of four and 12 years. In Yemen, more than 75% of girls are cut during the first two weeks of life. In Burkina Faso, Côte d'Ivoire, Egypt, Kenya, and Mali, the age for FGM is decreasing, perhaps because younger children are less able to resist or because in countries where it is illegal, the practice is more easily concealed with younger girls.

Purpose

The World Health Organization states that FGM "has no health benefits for girls and women."

Causes and symptoms

The causes of female genital mutilation are mixed, while the symptoms vary widely, depending on the type of mutilation performed.

Causes

The causes of female genital mutilation include a mix of cultural, religious, and social factors within families and communities. FGM is practiced for the following reasons:

- It is usually an integral part of community tradition; social pressure to conform to what others do, and have been doing, is a strong motivation to perpetuate the practice.
- Most parents believe that genital cutting protects—rather than harms—their daughters.
- In some cultures, FGM is considered a necessary rite of passage for girls, may even mark their introduction to sexual activity, and is a way to prepare girls for adulthood and marriage.
- Although it represents social and cultural control of female sexuality, some cultures believe that FGM actually empowers women by protecting their family's reputation and ensuring that they will marry.
- Female circumcision is believed to protect a girl's virginity and prevent unwed pregnancy, which could bring shame upon the family.
- In some cultures, uncircumcised females are considered to be dirty or unmarriageable and may be treated poorly; the practice is associated with femininity and modesty, which include the idea that girls are clean and beautiful after removal of body parts that are considered male or unclean.
- In some societies, it is believed to quell female sexual desire.
- Some people believe that their religion requires female circumcision. Most people who advocate FGM state that the practice has religious support, although no religious scripts advocate it.
- Some people believe in superstitions—that the clitoris will continue to grow if it is not removed or that external genitalia are unclean and can kill an infant during birth.

Symptoms

The symptoms of FGM depend on the degree of cutting, the cleanliness of the instruments, and the health of the female at the time of the procedure. FGM is usually performed without anesthesia and almost always causes bleeding and **pain**. The pain is usually most severe on the following day, when the patient first urinates onto the wound.

Diagnosis

Diagnosis and treatment of FGM requires the care of culturally sensitive gynecologists and women's health-care specialists who are familiar with the different types of FGM and their complications.

Prevention

Many national and international medical organizations—including the American Medical Association, Canadian medical associations, and the World Health Organization (WHO)—oppose the practice of female genital mutilation. The United Nations considers FGM to be a violation of human rights, and several African and Asian nations have called for an end to the practice. The WHO has undertaken a number of projects aimed at decreasing the incidence of FGM. These include:

- publicizing a statement that addresses the regional status of FGM and encourages the development of national policies against the practice
- training community workers to oppose FGM
- developing educational materials about FGM for community healthcare workers
- providing alternative job training for circumcisers

Specifically, in 1997, the WHO issued a joint statement with the United Nations Children's Fund (UNICEF), and the United Nations **Population** Fund (UNFPA) made a stand against the practice of FGM. The statement was strengthened in 2008, adding support to increase the advocacy for the abandonment of FGM. During this time, the WHO focused its efforts to eliminate female genital mutilation with the following actions:

- advocacy: developing publications and advocacy tools for international, regional, and local efforts to end FGM within a generation
- research: generating knowledge about the causes and consequences of FGM, along with ways to eliminate it, and ways to care for those who have experienced it
- guidance for health systems: develop training materials and guidelines for health professionals to help them treat and counsel women who have undergone FGM

In 2010, the WHO published its *Global Strategy to Stop Health Care Providers from Performing Female Genital Mutilation*, which was supported by several international organizations, such as the United Nations.

Other approaches to halting the practice of FGM include:

- community meetings, discussions, theater productions, and songs

- educational programs conducted by respected local women
- work by Islamic and other religious leaders to change the perception that FGM is required by religion
- substitution of other coming-of-age rituals for girls
- laws prohibiting FGM except as the free choice of an adult woman

Treatment

Treatment for symptoms caused by female genital mutation includes tradition methods that have been used for generations, along with the use of drugs.

Traditional

A girl or young woman who has recently had FGM may require supportive care to control bleeding. Treatment may be necessary for any complications. Women who have undergone FGM may require specialized gynecologic, obstetric, and reproductive care by knowledgeable practitioners.

In the United States, female immigrants with FGM often undergo defibulation or reconstructive surgery to reverse or repair their genitalia. Some surgical procedures that were originally developed for sex-change operations have been adapted for treating women with FGM. These techniques may involve cutting away scar tissue and skin to expose whatever remains of the clitoris, as well as more extensive reconstruction.

Drugs

Females who have recently undergone FGM may require **antibiotics** to prevent infection.

Prognosis

FGM can adversely affect a woman's quality of life, particularly with regard to sexual enjoyment and childbirth. It is associated with postpartum hemorrhage, episiotomy, extended hospital stays, stillbirth, infant resuscitation, and infant and maternal death. Circumcised pregnant women sometimes must deliver by Caesarian section.

Risks

The immediate risks of FGM include:

- physical and/or psychological trauma
- hemorrhage (excessive bleeding)
- severe pain, shock
- open sores in the genital region
- injury to nearby genital tissue

KEY TERMS

Circumcision—A procedure, usually with religious or cultural significance, in which the prepuce—the skin covering the tip of the male penis or the female clitoris, is cut away.

Clitoridectomy—A procedure in which the clitoris and possibly some of the surrounding labial tissue at the opening of the vagina is removed.

Clitoris—The small erectile organ at the front of the female vulva that is the site of female sexual pleasure.

Infibulation—A procedure that closes the labia majora to prevent sexual intercourse, leaving only a small opening for the passage of urine and menstrual blood.

Labia majora—The outer fatty folds of the vulva; sometimes also called the "lips" surrounding the vagina.

Prepuce—The fold of tissue covering the clitoris in females and the tip of the penis in males.

Vulva—The external female genital organs, including the labia majora, labia minora, clitoris, and vestibule of the vagina.

- infection, including abscesses, fever, sepsis (blood infection), shock, tetanus, or gangrene
- infertility
- death due to excessive blood loss or infection

Long–term complications usually occur with the more severe forms of FGM and include:

- scarring
- urination problems, such as urine retention; recurrent bladder and urinary tract infections
- chronic urinary tract infections
- cysts and abscesses
- incontinence
- pelvic and back pain
- painful menstruation
- very painful sexual intercourse due to scarring of most of the vagina
- lack of sexual pleasure
- inability to undergo normal gynecological exams and procedures
- increased risk for sexually transmitted infections (STIs), including HIV/AIDS, both from contaminated instruments and also because the damaged tissues are more

QUESTIONS TO ASK YOUR DOCTOR

- Where do I learn more about female genital mutilation?
- How can I help to prevent FGM from happening in the future?
- Does FGM still occur in the United States?
- What organizations help women with FGM?

likely to tear during sex, facilitating the transmission of infectious agents

- infertility rates as high as 25–30%, usually related to vaginal scarring that makes sexual intercourse difficult
- childbirth complications, including prolonged labor, tearing, heavy bleeding, and infection, along with newborn deaths
- psychological symptoms similar to post–traumatic stress syndrome (PTSD), including anxiety, depression, and sleep abnormalities, although these conditions are rare

Results

Female genital mutilation can leave lasting psychological marks on women. Immediate behavioral disturbances in children can be caused by the loss of trust and confidence in caregivers. In the longer term, women may have feelings of anxiety, depression, and frigidity. Sexual dysfunction may also be the cause of marital problems and divorce.

Resources

BOOKS

French, Kathy. *Sexual Health.* Ames, IA: Blackwell, 2009.

Levin, Tobe, and Augustine H. Asaah. *Empathy and Rage: Female Genital Mutilation in African Literature.* Boulder, CO: Lynne Rienner Publishers, 2009.

Mottin-Sylla, Marie-Helene, and Joelle Palmieri. *Confronting Female Genital Mutilation: The Role of Youth and ICTs in Changing Africa.* Gardners Books, 2011.

World Health Organization, United Nations Population Fund, Key Centre for Women's Health in Society. *Mental Health Aspects of Women's Reproductive Health: A Global Review of the Literature.* Geneva: World Health Organization, 2009.

Zabus, Chantal J. *Fearful Symmetries: Essays and Testimonies About Excision and Circumcision.* New York: Rodopi, 2008.

PERIODICALS

Adam, Taghreed, et al. "Estimating the Obstetric Costs of Female Genital Mutilation in Six African Countries." *Bulletin of the World Health Organization* 88, no. 4 (April 2010): 281–288.

Auge, Karen. "'I Want to Be Like Everyone Else.'" *Denver Post* (March 7, 2010): A1.

Belluck, Pam. "Group Backs Ritual 'Nick' as Female Circumcision Option." *New York Times* May 7, 2010: A16.

di Giovanni, Janine. "From Torture to Triumph." *Harper's Bazaar* no. 3579 (February 2010): 115.

"Ritual Genital Cutting of Female Minors." *Pediatrics* 125, no. 5 (May 2010): 1088.

WEBSITES

Female Genital Mutilation. World Health Organization. (February 2012). http://www.who.int/mediacentre/factsheets/fs241/en/ (accessed August 10, 2012).

Feldman–Jacobs, Charlotte, and Donna Clifton. *Female Genital Mutilation/Cutting: Data and Trends Update 2010.* Population Reference Bureau. (2010). http://www.prb.org/Publications/Datasheets/2010/fgm2010.aspx (accessed August 10, 2012).

Feldman–Jacobs, Charlotte, and Donna Clifton. *Female Genital Cutting Fact Sheet.* WomenHealth.gov, Department of Health and Human Services. (December 15, 2009). http://womenshealth.gov/publications/our-publications/fact-sheet/female-genital-cutting.cfm (accessed August 10, 2012).

ORGANIZATIONS

African Women's Health Center, Brigham and Women's Hospital, 75 Francis St., Boston, MA U.S.A. 02115, 1 (617) 732-5500, http://www.brighamandwomens.org/Departments_and_Services/obgyn/services/africanwomenscenter/default.aspx.

Center for Reproductive Rights, 120 Wall St., New York, NY 10005, 1 (917) 637-3600, Fax: (917) 637-3666, http://reproductiverights.org/.

Office on Women's Health, U.S. Department of Health and Human Services, 200 Independence Ave., S.W., Washington, D.C. U.S.A. 20201, 1 (917) 637-3600, http://www.womenshealth.gov/.

World Health Organization, Avenue Appia 20, Geneva, Switzerland 1211 27, 41 22 791-2111, Fax: 41 22 791-3111, cdcinfo@cdc.gov, http://www.who.int/en/.

Altha Roberts Edgren
Margaret Alic, Ph.D.
William A. Atkins, BB, BS, MBA

Fetal alcohol syndrome

Definition

Fetal alcohol syndrome (FAS) is a pattern of **birth defects**, learning, and behavioral problems affecting individuals whose mothers drank alcohol during pregnancy. FAS is the most severe of a range of disorders represented by the term fetal alcohol spectrum disorder (FASD).

Demographics

The occurrence of FAS/FASD is independent of the race, ethnicity, or gender of the individual. Individuals from different genetic backgrounds exposed to similar amounts of alcohol during pregnancy may show different symptoms of FAS. The reported rates of FAS vary widely among different populations studied, depending on the degree of alcohol use within the population and the monitoring methods used. Studies by the U.S. **Centers for Disease Control and Prevention (CDC)** show that, as of 2012, FAS occurs in 0.2 to 1.5 per 1,000 live births in different areas of the United States. FASDs are believed to occur approximately three times as often as FAS.

Description

FAS/FASD is caused by exposure of a developing fetus to alcohol. FASD is used to describe individuals with some, but not all, of the features of FAS. Other terms used to describe specific types of FASD are alcohol-related neurodevelopmental disorder (ARND) and alcohol-related birth defects (ARBD).

FAS is the most common preventable cause of mental retardation. This condition was first recognized and reported in the medical literature in 1968 in France and in 1973 in the United States. Alcohol is a teratogen, the term used for any drug, chemical, maternal disease, or other environmental exposure that can cause birth defects or functional impairment in a developing fetus. Some features of FAS that may be present at birth include low birth weight, prematurity, and microcephaly. Characteristic facial features may be present at birth or may become more obvious over time. Signs of brain damage include delays in development, behavioral abnormalities, and mental retardation, but affected individuals exhibit a wide range of abilities and disabilities.

FAS is a lifelong condition. It is not curable and has serious long-term consequences. Learning, behavioral, and emotional problems are common in adolescents and adults with FAS/FASD. The costs of FAS to the American economy were estimated most recently to be $321 million annually.

Risk factors

The only risk factor for a child to develop FAS is the consumption of alcohol by a women who is pregnant. There is no known amount of alcohol use that is safe during pregnancy, nor is there a particular stage of pregnancy during which alcohol use is safe.

Causes and symptoms

The only cause of FAS is maternal use of alcohol during pregnancy. FAS is not a genetic or inherited disorder. Alcohol consumed by the mother freely crosses the placenta and damages the developing fetus. Alcohol use by the father cannot cause FAS. Not all offspring who are exposed to alcohol during pregnancy have signs or symptoms of FAS; individuals of different genetic backgrounds may be more or less susceptible to the damage that alcohol can cause. The amount of alcohol, stage of development of the fetus, and pattern of alcohol use create the range of symptoms that encompass FASD.

Classic features of FAS include short stature, low birth weight, poor weight gain, microcephaly, and a characteristic pattern of abnormal facial features. These facial features in infants and children may include small eye openings (measured from inner corner to outer corner), epicanthal folds (folds of tissue at the inner corner of the eye), small or short nose, low or flat nasal bridge, smooth or poorly developed philtrum (the area of the upper lip above the colored part of the lip and below the nose), thin upper lip, and small chin. Some of these features are nonspecific, meaning they can occur in other conditions, or be appropriate for age, racial, or family background.

Other major and minor birth defects that have been reported to occur in conjunction with FAS/FASD include cleft palate, congenital heart defects, strabismus, **hearing loss**, defects of the spine and joints, alteration of the hand creases, small fingernails, and toenails. Since FAS was first described in infants and children, the diagnosis is sometimes more difficult to recognize in older adolescents and adults. Short stature and microcephaly remain common features, but weight may normalize, and the individual may actually become overweight for his/her height. The chin and nose grow proportionately more than the middle part of the face, and dental crowding may become a problem. The small eye openings and the appearance of the upper lip and philtrum may continue to be characteristic. Pubertal changes typically occur at the normal time.

Newborns with FAS may have difficulty nursing due to a poor sucking response, have irregular sleep-wake cycles, decreased or increased muscle tone, seizures or tremors. Delays in achieving developmental milestones such as rolling over, crawling, walking, and talking may become apparent in infancy. Behavior and learning difficulties typical in the preschool or early school years include poor attention span, hyperactivity, poor motor skills, and slow language development. Attention deficit-hyperactivity disorder (ADHD) is often associated with FASD. Learning disabilities or mental retardation may be diagnosed during this time.

During middle-school and high-school years, the behavioral difficulties and learning difficulties can be significant. Memory problems, poor judgment, difficulties with daily living skills, difficulties with abstract reasoning skills, and poor social skills are often apparent by this time. It is important to note that animal and human studies have shown that neurologic and behavioral abnormalities can be present without characteristic facial features. These individuals may not be identified as having FAS but may fulfill criteria for alcohol-related neurodevelopmental disorder (ARND).

FASD continues to affect individuals into adulthood. One study looked at FAS adults and found that about 95% had mental health problems, 82% lacked the ability to live independently, 70% had problems staying employed, 60% had been in trouble with the law, and 50% of men and 70% of women were alcohol or drug abusers.

Another long-term study found that the average IQ of the group of adolescents and adults with FAS in the study was 68 (70 is lower limit of the normal range). However, the range of IQ was quite large, ranging from a low of 20 (severely retarded) to a high of 105 (normal). Academic abilities and social skills were also below normal levels. The average achievement levels for reading, spelling, and arithmetic were fourth grade, third grade, and second grade, respectively. The Vineland Adaptive Behavior Scale was used to measure adaptive functioning in these individuals. The composite score for this group showed functioning at the level of a seven-year-old. Daily living skills were at a level of nine years, and social skills were at the level of a six-year-old.

KEY TERMS

Cleft plate—A congenital malformation in which there is an abnormal opening in the roof of the mouth that allows the nasal passages and the mouth to be improperly connected.

IQ—Abbreviation for intelligence quotient, the comparison of an individual's mental age to his/her true or chronological age multiplied by 100.

Microcephaly—An abnormally small head.

Miscarriage—Spontaneous pregnancy loss.

Placenta—The organ responsible for oxygen and nutrition exchange between a pregnant mother and her developing baby.

Strabismus—An improper muscle balance of the ocular, muscles resulting in crossed or divergent eyes.

Teratogen—Any drug, chemical, maternal disease, or exposure that can cause physical or functional defects in an exposed embryo or fetus.

Diagnosis

In 1996, the U.S. Institute of Medicine suggested a five-level system to describe the birth defects, learning problems, and behavioral difficulties in offspring of women who drank alcohol during pregnancy. This system contains criteria including confirmation of maternal alcohol exposure, characteristic facial features, growth problems, learning and behavioral problems, and birth defects known to be associated with prenatal alcohol exposure.

FAS is a clinical diagnosis, which means that there is no blood, x ray or psychological test that can be performed to confirm the suspected diagnosis. The diagnosis is made based on the history of maternal alcohol use, and detailed physical examination for the characteristic major and minor birth defects and characteristic facial features. It is often helpful to examine siblings and parents of an individual suspected of having FAS, either in person or by photographs, to determine whether findings on the examination might be familial, of if other siblings may also be affected. Sometimes, genetic tests are performed to rule out other conditions that may present with developmental delay or birth defects. Individuals with developmental delay, birth defects, or other unusual features are often referred to a clinical geneticist, developmental pediatrician, or neurologist for evaluation and diagnosis of FAS. Psychoeducational testing to determine IQ and/or the presence of learning disabilities may also be part of the evaluation process.

Treatment

There is no cure for FAS. The disorder is irreversible. Nothing can change the physical features or brain damage associated with maternal alcohol use during the pregnancy. Children should have psychoeducational evaluation to help plan appropriate educational interventions. Common associated diagnoses such ADHD, depression, or anxiety can be recognized and treated. The disabilities that present during childhood persist into adult life. However, some of the behavioral problems mentioned above may be avoided or lessened by early and correct diagnosis, better understanding of the life-long complications of FAS, and intervention. The goal of treatment is to help the individual affected by FAS become as independent and successful in school, employment, and social relationships as possible.

Public Health Response

Fetal alcohol syndrome is not a condition that can be spread throughout a community by contact among people

QUESTIONS TO ASK YOUR DOCTOR

- I drank alcohol before I knew I was pregnant. How might this affect my baby?
- How soon can you evaluate the degree to which my baby has been affected by my use of alcohol?
- I am a heavy drinker. Can you refer me to a program to help me control my drinking while I am pregnant?
- My baby was born with FAS. What kind of social services are available to our family?

who have the condition. So, many typical public health practices may not be invoked in dealing with FAS. A considerable effort has been exerted by public health workers, however, to prevent the condition by providing information and education for women and their families about the risks posed by drinking alcohol during pregnancy. In addition, the U.S. Substance Abuse and Mental Health Services Administration's (SAMHSA), Center for Substance Abuse **Prevention** (CSAP) has created the Partnership to Prevent Fetal Alcohol Syndrome Disorders (PFASD), a program that encourages pregnant women and their significant others to become aware of the problems of alcohol consumption during pregnancy and to avoid producing children at risk for the condition.

Prognosis

The prognosis for FAS/FASD depends on the severity of birth defects and the brain damage present at birth. Miscarriage, stillbirth, or death in the first few weeks of life may be outcomes in very severe cases. Generally individuals with FAS have a long list of mental health problems and associated social difficulties: alcohol and drug problems, inappropriate sexual behavior, problems with employment, trouble with the law, inability to live independently, and often confinement in prison, drug or alcohol treatment centers, or psychiatric institutions.

Some of the factors that have been found to reduce the risk of learning and behavioral disabilities in FAS individuals include diagnosis before the age of six years, stable and nurturing home environments, never having experienced personal **violence**, and referral and eligibility for disability services. Some physical birth defects associated with FAS are treatable with surgery. The long-term data help in understanding the difficulties that individuals with FAS encounter throughout their lifetime and can help families, caregivers, and professionals provide the care, supervision, education and treatment geared toward their special needs.

Prevention

FAS and FASD are completely preventable by avoiding all use of alcohol while pregnant. Prevention efforts include public education efforts aimed at the entire population, not just women of child bearing age, appropriate treatment for women with high-risk drinking habits, and increased recognition and knowledge about FAS/FASD by professionals, parents, and caregivers.

Resources

BOOKS

Alters, Sandra. *Fetal Alcohol Disorders*. San Diego, CA: ReferencePoint Press, 2012.

Blackburn, Carolyn, Barry Carpenter, and Jo Egerton. *Educating Children and Young People with Fetal Alcohol Spectrum Disorders: Constructing Personalised Pathways to Learning*. New York: Routledge, 2012.

Golden, Janet. *Message in a Bottle: The Making of Fetal Alcohol Syndrome*. Cambridge, MA: Harvard University Press, 2006.

Kulp, Jodie. *The Best I Can Be: Living with Fetal Alcohol Syndrome—Effects*. Brooklyn Park, MN: Better Endings New Beginnings, 2006.

Lawryk, Liz. *Finding Perspective: Raising Successful Children Affected by Fetal Alcohol Spectrum Disorders*. Bragg Creek, AB (Canada): OBD Triage Institute, 2005.

Soby, Jeanette M. *Prenatal Exposure to Drugs/Alcohol: Characteristics and Educational Implications of Fetal Alcohol Syndrome and Cocaine/Polydrug Effects,* 2nd ed. Springfield, IL: Charles C Thomas, 2006.

PERIODICALS

Alex, K., and R. Feldmann. "Children and Adolescents with Fetal Alcohol Syndrome (FAS): Better Social and Emotional Integration After Early Diagnosis." *Klinische Padiatrie* 224, 2. (2012): 66-71.

Kully-Martens, K., et al. "A Review of Social Skills Deficits in Individuals with Fetal Alcohol Spectrum Disorders and Prenatal Alcohol Exposure: Profiles, Mechanisms, and Interventions." *Alcoholism, Clinical and Experimental Research* 36, 4. (2012): 568-76.

OTHER

Chambers, Christine and Keith Vaux. *Fetal Alcohol Syndrome*. http://emedicine.medscape.com/article/974016-overview (accessed August 17, 2012).

Fetal Alcohol Spectrum Disorders (FASDs). United States Centers for Disease Control and Prevention. http://www.cdc.gov/ncbddd/fasd/index.html (accessed August 17, 2012).

Fetal Alcohol Syndrome. Medline Plus. http://www.nlm.nih.gov/medlineplus/fetalalcoholsyndrome.html (accessed August 17, 2012).

ORGANIZATIONS

Fetal Alcohol Spectrum Disorders Center for Excellence, 2101 Gaither Road., Suite 600, Rockville, MD 20850, (866) STOP-FAS (786-7327), http://fasdcenter.samhsa.gov.

Fetal Alcohol Syndrome (FAS) World Canada, 250 Scarborough Golf Club Rd., Toronto, Canada M1J 3G8, (416) 264-8000, Fax: (416) 264-8222, info@fasworld.com, http://www.fasworld.com.

March of Dimes Foundation, 1275 Mamaroneck Avenue, White Plains, NY 10605, (914) 997-4488, askus@marchofdimes.com, http://www.marchofdimes.com.

National Institute on Alcohol Abuse and Alcoholism (NIAAA), 5635 Fishers Lane, MSC 9304, Bethesda, MD 20892-9304, (301) 443-3860, http://www.niaaa.nih.gov.

National Organization on Fetal Alcohol Syndrome (NOFAS), 900 17th St., NW, Suite 910, Washington, DC 20006, (202) 785-4585, (800) 66-NOFAS, Fax: (202) 466-6456, http://www.nofas.org.

Laurie Heron Seaver, M.D.
Tish Davidson, A.M.

Filariasis

Definition

Filiariasis is the name for a group of tropical diseases caused by various thread-like parasitic round worms (nematodes) and their larvae. The larvae transmit the disease to humans through a mosquito bite. Filariasis is characterized by fever, chills, headache, and skin lesions in the early stages and, if untreated, can progress to include gross enlargement of the limbs and genitalia in a condition called elephantiasis.

Description

Approximately 170 million people in the tropical and subtropical areas of Southeast Asia, South America, Africa, and the islands of the Pacific are affected by this debilitating parasitic disease. While filariasis is rarely fatal, it is the second leading cause of permanent and long-term disability in the world. The **World Health Organization (WHO)** has named filariasis one of only six "potentially eradicable" infectious diseases and has embarked upon a 20-year campaign to eradicate the disease.

In all cases, a mosquito first bites an infected individual then bites another uninfected individual, transferring some of the worm larvae to the new host. Once within the body, the larvae migrate to a particular part of the body and mature to adult worms. Filariasis is classified into three distinct types according to the part of the body that becomes infected: lymphatic filariasis affects the circulatory system that moves tissue fluid and immune cells (lymphatic system); subcutaneous filariasis infects the areas beneath the skin and whites of the eye; and serous cavity filariasis infects body cavities but does not cause disease. Several different types of worms can be responsible for each type of filariasis, but the most common species include the following: *Wucheria bancrofti, Brugia malayi* (lymphatic filariasis), *Onchocerca volvulus, Loa loa, Mansonella streptocerca, Dracunculus medinensis* (subcutaneous filariasis), *Mansonella pustans*, and *Mansonella ozzardi* (serous cavity filariasis).

The two most common types of the disease are Bancroftian and Malayan filariasis, both forms of lymphatic filariasis. The Bancroftian variety is found throughout Africa, southern and southeastern Asia, the Pacific islands, and the tropical and subtropical regions of South America and the Caribbean. Malayan filariasis occurs only in southern and southeastern Asia. Filariasis is occasionally found in the United States, especially among immigrants from the Caribbean and Pacific islands.

A larva matures into an adult worm within six months to one year and can live between four and six years. Each female worm can produce millions of larvae, and these larvae appear in the bloodstream only at night, when they may be transmitted, via an insect bite, to another host. A single bite is usually not enough to acquire an infection; therefore, short-term travelers are usually safe. A series of multiple bites over a period of time is required to establish an infection. As a result, those individuals who are regularly active outdoors at night and those who spend more time in remote jungle areas are at an increased risk of contracting the filariasis infection.

Causes and symptoms

In cases of lymphatic filariasis, the most common form of the disease, the disease is caused by the adult worms actually living in the lymphatic vessels near the lymph nodes, where they distort the vessels and cause local inflammation. In advanced stages, the worms can actually obstruct the vessels, causing the surrounding tissue to become enlarged. In Bancroftian filariasis, the legs and genitals are most often involved, while the Malayan variety affects the legs below the knees. Repeated episodes of inflammation lead to blockages of the lymphatic system, especially in the genitals and legs. This causes the affected area to become grossly enlarged, with thickened, coarse skin, leading to a condition called elephantiasis.

In conjunctiva filariasis, the worms' larvae migrate to the eye and can sometimes be seen moving beneath the skin or beneath the white part of the eye (conjunctiva). If untreated, this disease can cause a type of blindness known as onchocerciasis.

Symptoms vary, depending on what type of parasitic worm has caused the infection, but all infections usually begin with chills, headache, and fever between three months and one year after the insect bite. Swelling, redness, and **pain** may also occur in the arms, legs, or scrotum. Areas of pus (abscesses) may appear as a result of dying worms or a secondary bacterial infection.

Diagnosis

The disease is diagnosed by taking a patient history, performing a physical examination, and by screening blood specimens for specific proteins produced by the immune system in response to this infection (antibodies). Early diagnosis may be difficult because, in the first stages, the disease mimics other bacterial skin infections. To make an accurate diagnosis, the physician looks for a pattern of inflammation and signs of lymphatic obstruction, together with the patient's possible exposure to filariasis in an area where filariasis is common. The larvae (microfilariae) can also be found in the blood, but because mosquitoes, which spread the disease, are active at night, the larvae are usually found in the blood only between about 10 p.m. and 2 a.m.

KEY TERMS

Abscess—An area of inflamed and injured body tissue that fills with pus.

Antibody—A specific protein produced by the immune system in response to a specific foreign protein or particle called an antigen.

Conjunctiva—The mucous membrane that lines the inside of the eyelid and the exposed surface of the eyeball.

Elephantiasis—A condition characterized by the gross enlargement of limbs and/or the genitalia that is also accompanied by a hardening and stretching of the overlying skin. Often a result of an obstruction in the lymphatic system caused by infection with a filarial worm.

Encephalitis—Inflammation of the brain.

Lymphatic system—The circulatory system that drains and circulates fluid containing nutrients, waste products, and immune cells, from between cells, organs, and other tissue spaces.

Microfilariae—The larvae and infective form of filarial worms.

Nematode—Round worms.

Subcutaneous—The area directly beneath the skin.

Public Health Response

An effective public health response to filariasis involves a number of steps, the first of which is often a surveillance program to determine characteristics such as how many individuals in a community are infected, how they became infected, and what the mechanism(s) of spread within the community is. This step is likely to include an element of testing suspected carriers of the disease, since such individuals may be asymptomatic for the infection. A program of treatment for infected individuals may also be necessary in which attention is paid not only to health and medical issues, but also, social, interpersonal, economic, and other issues associated with the spread of the disease. Preventative steps to control spread of the disease may also be necessary, often including intensive educational programs to help individuals understand the steps they can take to avoid infection and spread of the disease.

Treatment

Ivermectin, albendazole, and diethylcarbamazine are used to treat a filariasis infection by eliminating the larvae, impairing the adult worms' ability to reproduce, and actually killing adult worms. Unfortunately, much of the tissue damage may not be reversible. The medication is started at low doses to prevent reactions caused by large numbers of dying **parasites**.

While effective, the medications can cause severe side effects in up to 70% of patients as a result either of the drug itself or the massive death of parasites in the blood. Diethylcarbamazine, for example, can cause severe allergic reactions and the formation of pus-filled sores (abscesses). These side effects can be controlled using antihistamines and anti-inflammatory drugs (corticosteroids). Rarely, treatment with diethylcarbamazine in someone with very high levels of parasite infection may lead to a fatal inflammation of the brain (**encephalitis**). In these cases, the fever is followed by headache and confusion, then stupor and coma caused when massive numbers of larvae and parasites die. Other common drug reactions include dizziness, weakness, and nausea.

Symptoms caused by the death of the parasites include fever, headache, muscle pain, abdominal pain, nausea and vomiting, weakness, dizziness, lethargy, and

QUESTIONS TO ASK YOUR DOCTOR

- How can I find out if I am likely to be at risk for filariasis in an area to which I am traveling?
- What precautions and preventative measures can I take to reduce my risk of becoming infected with filariasis?
- Are there symptoms of a filariasis infection with which I should become familiar?
- Can you recommend a print or online resource where I can learn more about filariasis infections?

asthma. Reactions usually begin within two days of starting treatment and may last between two and four days.

No treatment can reverse elephantiasis. Surgery may be used to remove surplus tissue and provide a way to drain the fluid around the damaged lymphatic vessels. Surgery may also be used to ease massive enlargement of the scrotum. Elephantiasis of the legs can also be helped by elevating the legs and providing support with elastic bandages.

Prognosis

The outlook is good in early or mild cases, especially if the patient can avoid being infected again. The disease is rarely fatal, and with continued **WHO** medical intervention, even gross elephantiasis is now becoming rare.

Prevention

The best method of preventing filariasis is to avoid repeated bites by the mosquitoes that carry the disease. Some methods of preventing insect bites include the following:

- limiting outdoor activities at night, particularly in rural or jungle areas
- wearing long sleeves and pants, and avoiding dark-colored clothing that attracts mosquitoes
- avoiding perfumes and colognes
- treating one or two sets of clothing ahead of time with permethrin (Duramon, Permanone).
- wearing DEET insect repellent or, especially for children, trying citronella or lemon eucalyptus, to repel insects
- if sleeping in an open area or in a room with poor screens, use a bed net to avoid being bitten while asleep
- using air conditioning; the cooler air makes insects less active.

In addition, filariasis can be controlled in highly infested areas by taking ivermectin preventatively before being bitten. Currently, there is no vaccine available, but scientists are working on a preventative vaccine at this time.

Resources

OTHER

Lymphatic Filariasis Support Center. http://www.filariasis.us/ (accessed August 17, 2012).

Parasites – Lymphatic Filariasis. Centers for Disease Control and Prevention. http://www.cdc.gov/parasites/lymphatic-filariasis/ (accessed August 17, 2012).

Global Alliance to Eliminate Lymphatic Filariasis. http://www.filariasis.org/ (accessed August 17, 2012).

ORGANIZATIONS

Centers for Disease Control and Prevention. 1600 Clifton Rd., NE, Atlanta, GA 30333. (800) CDC-INFO (800 232-4636) or (404) 639-3534. cdcinfo@cdc.gov. www.cdc.gov.

Carol A. Turkington

Food additives

Definition

The U.S. Food and Drug Administration (FDA) defines food additives as "any substance, the intended use of which results or may reasonably be expected to result, directly or indirectly, in its becoming a component or otherwise affecting the characteristics of any food." In other words, an additive is any substance that is added to food.

Purpose

Direct additives are those that are intentionally added to foods for a specific purpose, such as coloring. Indirect additives are those to which the food is exposed during processing, packaging, or storing. Preservatives are additives that inhibit the growth of bacteria, yeasts, and molds in foods.

Description

Additives and preservatives have been used in foods for centuries. When meats are smoked to preserve them, compounds such as butylated hydroxyanisole (BHA) and butyl gallate are formed and provide both antioxidant and bacteriostatic effects. Salt has also been used as a preservative for centuries. Salt lowers the water activity of meats and other foods and inhibits bacterial growth.

Food additives

Types of ingredients	What they do	Examples of uses	Names found on product labels
Preservatives	Prevent food spoilage from bacteria, molds, fungi, or yeast (antimicrobials); slow or prevent changes in color, flavor, or texture and delay rancidity (antioxidants); maintain freshness	Fruit sauces and jellies, beverages, baked goods, cured meats, oils and margarines, cereals, dressings, snack foods, fruits and vegetables	Ascorbic acid, citric acid, sodium benzoate, calcium propionate, sodium erythorbate, sodium nitrite, calcium sorbate, potassium sorbate, BHA, BHT, EDTA, tocopherols (Vitamin E)
Sweeteners	Add sweetness with or without the extra calories	Beverages, baked goods, confections, table-top sugar, substitutes, many processed foods	Sucrose (sugar), glucose, fructose, sorbitol, mannitol, corn syrup, high fructose corn syrup, saccharin, aspartame, sucralose, acesulfame potassium (acesulfame-K), neotame
Color additives	Offset color loss due to exposure to light, air, temperature extremes, moisture, and storage conditions; correct natural variations in color; enhance colors that occur naturally; provide color to colorless and "fun" foods	Many processed foods (candies, snack foods, margarine, cheese, soft drinks, jams/jellies, gelatins, pudding and pie fillings)	FD&C Blue Nos. 1 and 2, FD&C Green No. 3, FD&C Red Nos. 3 and 40, FD&C Yellow Nos. 5 and 6, Orange B, Citrus Red No. 2, annatto extract, beta-carotene, grape skin extract, cochineal extract or carmine, paprika oleoresin, caramel color, fruit and vegetable juices, saffron (Note: Exempt color additives are not required to be declared by name on labels but may be declared simply as colorings or color added)
Flavors and spices	Add specific flavors (natural and synthetic)	Pudding and pie fillings, gelatin dessert mixes, cake mixes, salad dressings, candies, soft drinks, ice cream, BBQ sauce	Natural flavoring, artificial flavor, and spices
Flavor enhancers	Enhance flavors already present in foods (without providing their own separate flavor)	Many processed foods	Monosodium glutamate (MSG), hydrolyzed soy protein, autolyzed yeast extract, disodium guanylate or inosinate
Fat replacers (and components of formulations used to replace fats)	Provide expected texture in reduced-fat foods	Baked goods, dressings, frozen desserts, confections, cake and dessert mixes, dairy products	Olestra, cellulose gel, carrageenan, polydextrose, modified food starch, microparticulated egg white protein, guar gum, xanthan gum, whey protein concentrate

[continued]

Excess water in foods can enhance the growth of bacteria, yeast, and fungi. Pickling, which involves the addition of acids, such as vinegar, increases the acidity (lowers the pH) of foods to levels that slow bacterial growth. Some herbs and spices, such as curry, cinnamon, and chili pepper, also contain antioxidants and may provide bactericidal effects.

Uses of additives and preservatives in foods

Additives and preservatives are used to maintain product consistency and quality, improve or maintain nutritional value, maintain palatability and wholesomeness, provide leavening, control pH, enhance flavor, or provide color. Classes of food additives include:

- Antimicrobial agents prevent spoilage of food by mold or microorganisms. These include not only vinegar and salt but also compounds such as calcium propionate and sorbic acid, which are used in products such as baked goods, salad dressings, cheeses, margarines, and pickled foods.
- Antioxidants prevent rancidity in foods containing fats, and damage to foods caused by oxygen. Examples of antioxidants include vitamin C, vitamin E, BHA, BHT (butylated hydroxytolene), and propyl gallate.
- Artificial colors are intended to make food more appealing and to provide certain foods with coloring more indicative of their flavor (e.g., red for cherry, green for lime).
- Artificial flavors and flavor enhancers are the largest class of additives and function to make food taste better or to give them a specific taste. Examples are salt, sugar, and vanilla, which are used to complement the flavor of certain foods. Synthetic flavoring agents, such

Types of ingredients	What they do	Examples of uses	Names found on product labels
Nutrients	Replace vitamins and minerals lost in processing (enrichment), add nutrients that may be lacking in the diet (fortification)	Flour, breads, cereals, rice, macaroni, margarine, salt, milk, fruit beverages, energy bars, Instant breakfast drinks	Thiamine hydrochloride, riboflavin (Vitamin B2), niacin, niacinamide, folate or folic acid, beta carotene, potassium iodide, iron or ferrous sulfate, alpha tocopherols, ascorbic acid, Vitamin D, amino acids (L-tryptophan, L-lysine, L-leucine, L-methionine)
Emulsifiers	Allow smooth mixing of ingredients, prevent separation, keep emulsified products stable, reduce stickiness, control crystallization, keep ingredients dispersed, help products dissolve more easily	Salad dressings, peanut butter, chocolate, margarine, frozen desserts	Soy lecithin, mono- and diglycerides, egg yolks, polysorbates, sorbitan monostearate
Stabilizers and thickeners, binders, texturizers	Produce uniform texture, improve texture	Frozen desserts, dairy products, cakes, pudding and gelatin mixes, dressings, jams and jellies, sauces	Gelatin, pectin, guar gum, carrageenan, xanthan gum, whey
pH Control agents and acidulants	Control acidity and alkalinity, prevent spoilage	Beverages, frozen desserts, chocolate, low-acid canned foods, baking powder	Lactic acid, citric acid, ammonium hydroxide, sodium carbonate
Leavening agents	Promote rising of baked goods	Breads and other baked goods	Baking soda, monocalcium phosphate, calcium carbonate
Anti-caking agents	Keep powdered foods from clumping, prevent moisture absorption	Salt, baking powder, confectioner's sugar	Calcium silicate, iron ammonium citrate, silicon dioxide
Humectants	Retain moisture	Shredded coconut, marshmallows, soft candies, confections	Glycerin, sorbitol
Yeast nutrients	Promote growth of yeast	Breads and other baked goods	Calcium sulfate, ammonium phosphate
Dough strengtheners and conditioners	Produce more stable dough	Breads and other baked goods	Ammonium sulfate, azodicarbonamide, L-cysteine
Firming agents	Maintain crispness and firmness	Processed fruits and vegetables	Calcium chloride, calcium lactate
Enzyme preparations	Modify proteins, polysaccharides, and fats	Cheese, dairy products, meat	Enzymes, lactase, papain, rennet, chymosin
Gases	Serve as propellant, aerate, or create carbonation	Oil cooking spray, whipped cream, carbonated beverages	Carbon dioxide, nitrous oxide

SOURCE: Center for Food Safety and Applied Nutrition, Food and Drug Administration, U.S. Department of Health and Human Services.

(Table by PreMediaGlobal. © 2013 Cengage Learning)

as benzaldehyde for cherry or almond flavor, may be used to simulate natural flavors. Flavor enhancers, such as monosodium glutamate (MSG), intensify the flavor of other compounds in a food.

- Bleaching agents, such as peroxides, are used to whiten foods, such as wheat flour and cheese.
- Chelating agents are used to prevent discoloration, flavor changes, and rancidity that might occur during the processing of foods. Examples include citric acid, malic acid, and tartaric acid.
- Nutrient additives include vitamins and minerals and are added to foods during enrichment or fortification. For example, milk is fortified with vitamin D, and rice is enriched with thiamin, riboflavin, and niacin.
- Thickening and stabilizing agents function to alter the texture of a food. Examples include the emulsifier lecithin, which keeps oil and vinegar blended in salad dressings, and carrageen, which is used as a thickener in ice creams and low-calorie jellies.

Regulating safety of food additives and preservatives

Based on the 1958 Food Additives Amendment to the Federal Food, Drug, and Cosmetic (FD&C) Act of 1938, the FDA must approve the use of all additives. Manufacturers bear the responsibility of proving that additives are safe for their intended uses. The Food Additives Amendment excluded additives and preservatives deemed safe for consumption before 1958, such as salt, sugar, spices, **vitamins**, vinegar, and monosodium glutamate. These substances are considered "generally recognized as safe" (GRAS) and may be used in any food, although the FDA may remove additives from the GRAS list if safety concerns arise. The 1960 Color Additives Amendment to the FD&C Act required the FDA to approve synthetic coloring agents used in foods, drugs, cosmetics, and certain medical devices. The Delaney Clause, which was included in both the Food Additives Amendment and Color Additives Amendment, prohibited approval of any additive that had been found to cause **cancer** in humans or animals. However, in 1996, the Delaney Clause was modified, and the commissioner of the FDA was charged with assessing the risk from consumption of additives that may cause cancer and making a determination as to the use of those additives.

In the United States, food additives and preservatives play an important role in ensuring that the food supply remains the safest and most abundant in the world. Despite consumer concerns about use of food additives and preservatives, there is very little scientific evidence that they are harmful at the levels at which they are used.

In Europe, food additives and preservatives are evaluated by the European Commission's Scientific Committee on Food. Regulations in the European Union countries are similar to those in the United States. The Food and Agricultural Organization (FAO) of the United Nations and the **World Health Organization (WHO)** Expert Committee on Food Additives work together to evaluate the safety of food additives, as well as contaminants, naturally occurring toxicants, and residues of veterinary drugs in foods. Acceptable Daily Intakes (ADIs) are established on the basis of toxicology and other information.

Precautions

Food additives can induce a wide range of adverse reactions in sensitive individuals. A prevalence of 0.03% to 0.23% is estimated. Before any substance can be added to food, the **Food Safety** and Inspection Service (FSIS) of the U.S. Department of Agriculture (USDA) share responsibility with the FDA to ensure the safety of food additives used in meat, poultry, and egg products. Initially, all additives are evaluated for safety by FDA.

Safe is defined by Congress as "reasonable certainty that no harm will result from use" of an additive in the food supply. Substances that are found to be harmful to either people or animals may be allowed as an additive, but only at the level of 1/100th of the amount that is considered harmful. This margin of safety is intended as a protection for the consumer by limiting the intake of dangerous substances. For example, some people are allergic to certain food additives, and their reaction can be mild or very severe when consumed.

Interactions

Nitrites are controversial additives. When used in combination with salt, nitrites serve as antimicrobials and add flavor and color to meats. However, nitrite salts can react with certain amines in food to produce nitrosamines, many of which are known carcinogens. Food manufacturers must show that nitrosamines will not form in harmful amounts, or will be prevented from forming, in their products.

KEY TERMS

Bacteria—Single-celled organisms without nuclei, some of which are infectious.

Bactericidal—A state that prevents growth of bacteria.

Bacteriostatic—A substance that kills bacteria.

Carcinogen—A cancer-causing substance.

Enrichment—The addition of vitamins and minerals to improve the nutritional content of a food.

Fermentation—A reaction performed by yeast or bacteria to make alcohol.

Fortification—The addition of vitamins and minerals to improve the nutritional content of a food.

Leavening—Yeast or other agents used for rising bread.

Microorganisms—Bacteria and protists; single-celled organisms.

The flavoring enhancer MSG is another controversial food additive. MSG is made commercially from a natural fermentation process using starch and sugar. Despite anecdotal reports of MSG triggering headaches or exacerbating **asthma**, the Joint Expert Committee on Food Additives of the FAO, **WHO**, the European Commission's Scientific Committee for Food, the American Medical Association, and the National Academy of Sciences have all affirmed the safety of MSG at normal consumption levels.

Another controversial additive is ammonia, which is present in very small amounts in a number of foods, including ground beef and cheese. Ammonium hydroxide has been considered GRAS by the FDA since 1974, but many consumers are unaware of its presence in foods. If a substance is used during processing and is not considered to be part of the product, it is not required to be listed as an ingredient on the label.

Complications

There are numerous difficulties that may be encountered by the FDA in assessing potential harm that may come from food additives. These are due to the inadequacies and complications of animal models and the variability of human exposure and reporting of adverse reactions. Typically, testing for food additive toxicity is designed so that the additive is administered to an animal model for the life of that animal in a range of doses, of which the highest dose is much greater than that expected to occur during the course of human exposure. It is also too complicated to predict all of the possible interactions or reactions that can occur with any given food additive, such as from the packaging, the heating or cooling process, other additions to the food, or consumption of the food.

The FDA continually monitors the safety of all food additives as new scientific evidence becomes available. For example, use of erythrosine (FD&C Red No. 3) in cosmetics and externally applied drugs was banned in 1990 after it was implicated in the development of thyroid tumors in male rats. However, the cancer risk associated with FD&C Red No. 3 is about 1 in 100,000 over a 70-year lifetime, and its use in some foods, such as candies and maraschino cherries, is still allowed. Tartrazine (FD&C Yellow No. 5) has been found to cause dermatological reactions ranging from itching to hives in a small **population** subgroup. Given the mild nature of the reaction, however, it still may be used in foods. In 2012, consumer groups, such as the Center for Science in the Public Interest (CSPI), were seeking a ban on caramel coloring used in soft drinks (4-methylimidazole) due to its potential risk as a carcinogen. However, this claim was based on study of mice, and re-evaluations of the additive by the European Food Safety Authority did not find any risk to humans.

Resources

BOOKS

Minich, Deanna. *An A–Z Guide to Food Additives: Never Eat What You Can't Pronounce.* San Francisco: Conari Press, 2012.

Taub-Dix, Bonnie. *Read it Before You Eat it: How to Decode Food Labels and Make the Healthiest Choice Every Time.* New York: Penguin Group, 2010.

Smith, Jim, Hong-Shum, Lily. *A Consumer's Food Additive Data Book.* 2nd ed. Wiley-Blackwell, 2011.

WEBSITES

European Commission, Directorate General for Health and Consumers. "Food Additives." http://ec.europa.eu/food/food/fAEF/additives/index_en.htm (accessed July 9, 2012).

Food Safety and Inspection Service. "Additives in Meat and Poultry Products." U.S. Department of Agriculture. http://www.fsis.usda.gov/Fact%5FSheets/Additives_in_Meat_&_Poultry_Products/index.asp (accessed July 9, 2012).

Geller, Martinne. "Ammonia Used in Many Foods, not Just 'Pink Slime.'" MSNBC.com. http://www.msnbc.msn.com/id/46958231/ns/health-diet_and_nutrition (accessed July 9, 2012).

International Food Information Council Foundation. "Questions and Answers about Caramel Coloring and 4-methylimidazole (4-MEI or 4-MI)." FoodInsight.org. http://www.foodinsight.org/Resources/Detail.aspx?topic=Questions_and_Answers_about_4_MEI (accessed July 9, 2012).

International Food Information Council Foundation. "The Rigorous Road to Food Ingredient Approval." FoodInsight.org. http://www.foodinsight.org/Newsletter/Detail.aspx?topic=The_Rigorous_Road_to_Food_Ingredient_Approval (accessed July 9, 2012).

Lembert, Phil. "The 5 Things You Need to Know About Deli Meats." TODAY Food, MSNBC.com. http://today.msnbc.msn.com/id/16361276/ns/today-food/t/things-you-need-know-about-deli-meats (accessed July 9, 2012).

U.S. Food and Drug Administration. "Color Additives." http://www.fda.gov/ForIndustry/ColorAdditives/default.htm (accessed July 9, 2012).

U.S. Food and Drug Administration. "Food Additives." http://www.fda.gov/food/foodingredientspackaging/foodadditives/default.htm (accessed July 9, 2011).

U.S. Food and Drug Administration. "Generally Recognized as Safe (GRAS)." http://www.fda.gov/Food/FoodIngredientsPackaging/GenerallyRecognizedasSafeGRAS/default.htm (accessed July 9, 2012).

ORGANIZATIONS

Center for Food Safety and Applied Nutrition (CFSAN), U.S. Food and Drug Administration, 5100 Paint Branch Pkwy., College Park, MD 20740, (888) SAFEFOOD (723-3366), consumer@fda.gov, http://www.fda.gov/Food/default.htm.

European Commission, Directorate General for Health and Consumers, B-1049, Brussels, Belgium, 011 32 (2) 299-11-11, http://ec.europa.eu/dgs/health_consumer/index_en.htm.

Food and Nutrition Information Center, National Agricultural Library, 10301 Baltimore Ave., Rm. 105, Beltsville, MD 20705, (301) 504-5414, Fax: (301) 504-6409, fnic@ars.usda.gov, http://fnic.nal.usda.gov.

Food Safety and Inspection Service (FSIS), U.S. Department of Agriculture (USDA) , 1400 Independence Ave. SW, Washington, DC 20250-3700, (888) 674-6854 (USDA Meat and Poultry Consumer Hotline), MPHotline.fsis@usda.gov, http://www.fsis.usda.gov.

Food Allergy and Anaphylaxis Network (FAAN), 11781 Lee Jackson Hwy., Ste. 160, Fairfax, VA 22033, (800) 929-4040, Fax: (703) 691-2713, faan@foodallergy.org, http://www.foodallergy.org.

Institute of Food Technologies, 525 W. Van Buren, Ste. 1000, Chicago, IL 60607, (312) 782-8424, Fax: (312) 792-8348, info@ift.org, http://www.ift.org.

International Food Information Council Foundation, 1100 Connecticut Ave., NW Ste. 430, Washington, DC 20036, (202) 296-6540, info@foodinsight.org, http://www.foodinsight.org.

U.S. Food and Drug Administration (FDA), 10903 New Hampshire Ave., Silver Spring, MD 20993, (888) 463-6332, http://www.fda.gov.

M. Elizabeth Kunkel
Tish Davidson, AM
Megan Porter, RD

Food contamination

Definition

Food contamination occurs when potentially harmful substances render food unsafe for consumption. Microorganisms—viruses, bacteria, and other parasites—are the most common food contaminants. Naturally occurring or manmade chemicals can also contaminate food.

Demographics

Although widespread contamination is relatively rare in the United States, food contamination remains a serious public health concern throughout the world. In 2011, the U.S. **Centers for Disease Control and Prevention (CDC)** reported that about 48 million Americans—one in six—suffer the effects of food contamination every year, accounting for 128,000 hospitalizations and 3,000 deaths annually.

While disease-causing microorganisms are by far the most common contaminants in food, naturally occurring toxins sometimes contaminate shellfish and other organisms. Food can also be contaminated with heavy metals, manmade chemicals such as pesticides and herbicides, and radioactive iodine and cesium from nuclear accidents, such as the 2011 Fukushima Daiichi nuclear power plant disaster in Japan.

Although most food contamination is unintentional, sometimes contaminants are introduced as a means of "stretching" or extending the life of a product. Bioterrorism experts worry that disease-causing organisms or toxic chemicals could be intentionally introduced into food or **water** supplies to cause mass contamination. Scientists also worry that climate change may increase the risk of contamination of crops and seafood from biotoxins, pathogenic microbes, pesticides, and other chemicals.

Description

Of the more than 250 identified foodborne diseases, most are caused by pathogenic microorganisms. For example, the U.S. Food and Drug Administration (FDA) estimates that 90% of purchased raw poultry carries some disease-causing bacteria. Most pathogenic food contaminants originate from animal or human feces, and food contamination is directly responsible for many infectious digestive diseases.

In the United States, most food contamination is caused by one of eight pathogens:

- Noroviruses are responsible for 58% of illnesses and 11% of deaths from identified food contaminants. Unlike other foodborne pathogens, noroviruses are spread primarily by infected people, especially food-service workers. Noroviruses have been responsible for major outbreaks of foodborne illness on cruise ships and in nursing homes.
- *Salmonella* spp. are widespread intestinal bacteria that cause salmonellosis, a major cause of illness and death from food contamination.
- *Clostridium perfringens* is found throughout the environment, including human and animal intestines, and is common on raw meat and poultry.
- *Campylobacter* spp. are the most commonly identified cause of diarrheal illness worldwide. The bacteria live in the intestines of healthy birds and are found in most raw poultry. Undercooked chicken, foods contaminated with juices from raw chicken, and cross-contamination between raw and cooked foods are the most common sources of infection.
- *Staphylococcus aureus* is a bacterium in dust, air, and sewage. It is spread primarily through unsanitary food handling and can contaminate almost any food.
- *Toxoplasma gondii* is a single-celled parasite that causes toxoplasmosis, a potentially fatal condition that can result from consuming contaminated water or undercooked meat.
- *Escherichia coli* is a common, normally harmless bacterium in the human gut. However, some Shiga toxin-producing *E. coli* (STEC) strains, especially strain O157:H7, can cause severe food poisoning. O157:H7 is most often found in undercooked hamburger but has also contaminated produce and unpasteurized juice.
- *Listeria monocytogenes*, a ubiquitous bacterium in soil, groundwater, plants, and animals, can contaminate food and cause listeriosis. Listeriosis appears to be on the increase in the United States—in 2011, at least 29 people died, and at least 139 people across 28 states were sickened from eating contaminated cantaloupe that was traced to unsanitary conditions and poor handling at a single Colorado farm.

Other pathogenic food contaminants are serious problems worldwide:

- *Clostridium botulinum* is a rare bacterium that can contaminate food with a deadly paralytic nerve toxin called botulinum. Botulism is associated with improperly canned food, especially home-canned products, smoked fish, and honey.
- *Shigella* is a bacterial family that is a common cause of diarrhea in developing countries.
- *Vibrio cholera* is a fecal bacterial contaminant of food and water that is endemic in many parts of the world and causes deadly cholera outbreaks.

- *Vibrio vulnificus* and *Vibrio parahemolyticus* are ocean bacteria that can contaminate filter-feeding shellfish such as oysters.
- *Yersinia enterocolitica* is a bacterium that can contaminate water, raw milk, and meat.
- Rotavirus is a major cause of diarrhea and death in infants and children.
- Hepatitis A virus can contaminate food.
- *Giardia lamblia* and *Cryptosporidium parvum* are intestinal parasites that contaminate water.
- *Entamoeba histolytica* is a parasite transmitted by contaminated water that causes amoebic dysentery and is prevalent in developing nations.
- *Cyclospora cayetanensis* is an emerging foodborne parasite.
- *Trichinella spiralis*, contracted from undercooked pork and wild game, is an intestinal roundworm that invades human muscle.
- *Taenia* spp. are parasitic tapeworms contracted from beef and pork.

Seafood contamination

Seafood can be contaminated in various ways, including via agricultural and other runoff, sewage, natural toxins, mercury, and chemical pollutants in water and the food chain. Filter-feeding shellfish, such as oysters, clams, scallops, and mussels, can accumulate toxins. Scombroid is caused by chemicals produced by bacteria in fish that are not refrigerated or frozen immediately.

Toxins associated with algal blooms called red and brown tides can accumulate in fish and shellfish:

- Ciguatera fish poisoning is caused by ciguatoxin or maitotoxin produced by various algal species.
- Paralytic shellfish poisoning (PSP) is caused by saxitoxins from several different red tide dinoflagellates.
- Neurotoxic shellfish poisoning is caused by brevetoxins from *Karenia brevis*, a dinoflagellate that accumulates in oysters, mussels, and clams.
- Amnesic shellfish poisoning is caused by domoic acid from *Pseudonitzschia* spp. of diatoms.

Causes and symptoms

Causes

Food can be contaminated at any point in the production chain—in the field, through animal feed, in the slaughterhouse or processing plant, during transport, in markets and restaurants, or in the home kitchen. Sources include:

- application of illegal or higher-than-approved pesticides or herbicides to crops
- waste disposal on agricultural land
- bacteria on growing fruits and vegetables
- molds and their toxic products that develop in grains during growth, harvesting, or storage
- during processing, improper handling of raw materials, contaminated water, inadequate or improper disinfection, equipment malfunctions, inadequate temperatures, rodent or insect infestations, or contamination with poisons used to control pests
- during transportation and storage, improper temperatures, inappropriate use of fumigants, inadequate sanitization of food-carrying tanker trucks, or contamination with insects or rodent droppings
- in stores and restaurants, improper temperatures, cross-contamination between raw and cooked foods, improper disinfection of food-preparation surfaces, transmission by infected food handlers, or improper hand washing by food handlers
- in the home, unhygienic food handling, food left at room temperature, inadequate cooking, cross-contamination between raw and cooked foods, or failure to properly reheat leftovers

Although any food can be contaminated, raw or undercooked meat, poultry, eggs, fish, and raw (unpasteurized) milk are the most common. Processed foods that pool ingredients from multiple sources are particularly prone to contamination. Washing raw fruits and vegetables reduces but does not eliminate contaminants. Improperly canned foods, luncheon and deli meats, soft cheeses, and any products containing raw eggs are subject to contamination. A few bacteria in alfalfa or bean seeds can multiply to contaminate an entire batch of sprouts. Refrigeration or freezing generally prevents bacteria from multiplying. However, *L. monocytogenes* and *Y. enterocolitica* can grow and multiply at refrigerator temperatures. High levels of salt, sugar, or acid prevent bacteria from growing in preserved foods, and thorough cooking kills pathogenic microorganisms.

Symptoms

Although symptoms of food contamination depend on the type, abdominal **pain** and cramps, diarrhea, nausea, and vomiting are most common. After ingesting contaminated food, there is usually a delay before symptoms develop. However, symptoms of chemical food **poisoning** often appear very quickly, usually beginning with a tingling in the mouth, then in the arms and legs, followed by dizziness and possibly difficulty breathing. Symptoms of poisoning from manmade toxic chemicals that have accidentally contaminated food may

KEY TERMS

Botulism—A life-threatening paralytic illness from food contaminated with botulinum toxin from the bacterium *Clostridium botulinum*.

Campylobacter—A genus of bacteria that is found in almost all raw poultry.

Clostridium perfringens—A bacterium that is a common food contaminant.

Dehydration—The abnormal depletion of body fluids, as from vomiting and diarrhea.

Electrolytes—Ions—such as sodium, potassium, calcium, magnesium, chloride, phosphate, bicarbonate, and sulfate—that are dissolved in bodily fluids such as blood and regulate or affect most metabolic processes.

Gastroenteritis—Inflammation of the lining of the stomach and intestines.

Hemolytic uremic syndrome (HUS)—Kidney failure, usually in infants and young children, that can be caused by food contaminated with bacteria such as STEC or *Shigella*.

Listeriosis—Illness caused by food contaminated with the bacterium *Listeria monocytogenes*.

Norovirus—Norwalk virus; a large family of RNA viruses that are the most common cause of illness from contaminated food.

Parasite—An organism that survives by living with, on, or in another organism, usually to the detriment of the host.

Pathogen—A causative agent of disease, such as a bacteria, virus, or parasite.

Salmonellosis—Severe diarrhea caused by food contaminated with bacteria of the genus *Salmonella*.

Shiga toxin-producing *E. coli* (STEC)—Strains of the common, normally harmless, intestinal bacterium *Escherichia coli* that can contaminate food with Shiga toxin; *E. coli* O157:H7 is the most commonly identified STEC in North America.

spp.—Species.

Staphylococcus aureus—Staph; a bacterium that can contaminate food.

Toxoplasma gondii—A very common parasite that is a leading cause of death from food contamination; although it infects large numbers of people, *T. gondii* is usually dangerous only in immunocompromised patients and newly infected pregnant women.

develop rapidly or slowly and vary with the type of chemical and degree of exposure.

Treatment

Most illnesses caused by contaminated foods are mild and resolve on their own within one or a few days. Diarrhea and vomiting can cause dehydration if more fluids and salts (electrolytes) are lost than are taken in; oral medications, such as Ceralyte, Pedialyte, or Oralyte, can be used to replace fluid losses. An electrolyte replacement fluid can be made at home with one teaspoon of salt and four teaspoons of sugar per quart of water. Severe dehydration may require hospitalization and intravenous fluids. Drugs are sometimes prescribed to stop persistent vomiting. Over-the-counter medications to stop or slow diarrhea, such as Kaopectate, Pepto-Bismol, or Imodium, may provide some relief. **Antibiotics** are not usually required.

Botulism, shellfish poisoning, and **chemical poisoning** are medical emergencies. Botulism requires hospitalization, often in an intensive care unit. Adults are given botulism antitoxin if it can be administered within 72 hours of the appearance of symptoms. Patients may require mechanical ventilation to assist breathing, as well as intravenous feeding until the paralysis passes.

Prognosis

Most illnesses resulting from food contamination resolve quickly without complications. However, contaminated food can cause serious and potentially life-threatening complications, especially for the very young, the elderly, pregnant women and their unborn babies, and anyone with a weakened immune system. It is estimated that 2%–3% of acute illnesses from food contamination lead to secondary long-term illnesses and complications that may affect any part of the body, such as the joints, nervous system, kidneys, or heart. **Listeriosis** can be serious or even fatal in newborns, the elderly, and the immunocompromised and can cause miscarriage, stillbirth, or premature birth if contracted during pregnancy. *Campylobacter* infection can cause Guillain-Barré syndrome. STEC can cause hemolytic uremic syndrome (HUS), the most common cause of acute kidney failure in children. In the elderly, food contamination can even cause gastroenteritis-induced death.

Chemical food contamination is more likely to cause serious long-term health problems than the various forms of microbial contamination. Toxins in fish can cause permanent liver damage. Pesticides and other chemical contaminants can cause liver damage, kidney failure, and nervous system complications.

Prevention

Avoiding food contamination requires vigilance at every level of the food-production process. Growers must use only approved pesticides and herbicides at no higher than recommended levels. Processors must use clean sources of water, regularly disinfect machinery, and use only safe pesticides around food. Canning requires high temperatures and pressure. Irradiation of meat and other foods destroys contaminating microbes. Bacterial toxins vary in their heat sensitivity. For example, although botulinum is completely inactivated by boiling, staphylococcal toxin is not.

Most food contamination is preventable, since the **CDC** estimates that about 97% of all poisonings from contaminated food result from improper food handling, such as undercooking or poor refrigeration. Simple precautions in restaurants, cafeterias, and home kitchens include:

- washing hands thoroughly with soap and water before, during, and after preparing food, and after using the bathroom or changing diapers
- preventing cross-contamination of foods by keeping hands, utensils, and food-preparation surfaces clean
- keeping raw foods, especially meat, poultry, fish, and shellfish, separated from ready-to-eat foods, such as fruits and vegetables
- washing all fruits and vegetables thoroughly before and after peeling
- discarding the outer leaves of lettuce and cabbage
- keeping foods above 140°F (60°C) or below 40°F (4°C)
- cooking food thoroughly to an internal temperature of 160°F (78°C), which kills most bacteria, viruses, and parasites
- cooking egg yolks until firm
- never placing cooked food on plates or surfaces that held raw food
- refrigerating or freezing perishable foods within two hours of purchasing or preparing them
- avoiding thawing and refreezing food
- defrosting food in the refrigerator, in cold water, or in a microwave and cooking immediately

QUESTIONS TO ASK YOUR DOCTOR

- What are the best ways to avoid food contamination?
- Are there specific foods that I should avoid because of possible contamination?
- Should I avoid luncheon meats and fish during pregnancy?
- What type of oral rehydration fluid do you recommend for diarrhea and vomiting?
- Does illness from food contamination require medical attention?

- discarding any food or leftovers that have been at room temperature for more than two hours (or more than one hour in hot weather)
- dividing large quantities of food into shallow containers to cool faster
- avoiding any suspect foods, such as raw meat, fish, and milk or unpasteurized juice and cider

As a general safety rule, "when in doubt, throw it out."

Parental concerns

Breastfeeding is the best way to protect infants from food contamination. Baby formula should never be left at room temperature, and baby bottles must be kept clean and disinfected.

Infants and young children are particularly susceptible to dehydration from food contamination–induced diarrhea and vomiting, since they can lose water and electrolytes very quickly. Small sips of oral rehydration solution should be given to children as soon as vomiting or diarrhea begins. A physician should be consulted before giving antidiarrheal medicines to children.

Resources

BOOKS

Hewitt, Ben. *Making Supper Safe: One Man's Quest to Learn the Truth about Food Safety*. New York: Rodale, 2011.

Hwang, Andy, and Lihan Huang, eds. *Ready-to-Eat Foods: Microbial Concerns and Control Measures*. Boca Raton, FL: CRC, 2010.

Perrett, Heli. *The Safe Food Handbook: How to Make Smart Choices About Risky Food*. New York: Experiment, 2011.

PERIODICALS

"Don't Let Food Poisoning Spoil Your Picnic." *U.S. News & World Report* (May 2011). http://health.usnews.com/health-news/diet-fitness/diet/articles/2011/05/28/dont-let-food-poisoning-spoil-your-picnic (accessed July 9, 2012)

Dwoskin, Elizabeth. "Your Food Has Been Touched by Multitudes." *Bloomberg Businessweek*, August 29, 2011. http://www.businessweek.com/magazine/your-food-has-been-touched-by-multitudes-08252011.html (accessed July 9, 2012).

Kowalski, Kathiann. "How Safe is Your Food?" *Current Health Kids* 34, no. 7 (March 2011): 16–19.

Landro, Laura. "The Informed Patient: Food Illness and the Kitchen—Salmonella Infections Rose Last Year; Home Cooks Fail to Act Safely, Studies Say." *Wall Street Journal*, June 14, 2011, D3. http://online.wsj.com/article/SB10001424052702304665904576383582242952932.html (accessed July 9, 2012).

Lowenstein, Kate. "Not Safe to Eat." *Health* 25, no. 8 (October 2011): 86.

Park, Alice. "How to Stop the Superbugs." *Time*, June 20, 2011. http://www.time.com/time/magazine/article/0,9171,2076723,00.html (accessed July 9, 2012).

Rosenthal, Elisabeth. "My Salad, My Health." *New York Times*, June 12, 2011, WK3.

Tarshis, Lauren. "Delicious or DEADLY?" *Scholastic Scope* 60, no. 7 (January 9, 2012): 4–9.

"Tips for Safer Food." *Consumer Reports on Health* 23, no. 8 (August 2011): 8.

WEBSITES

American Academy of Family Physicians. "Food Poisoning." FamilyDoctor.org. http://familydoctor.org/familydoctor/en/diseases-conditions/food-poisoning.html (accessed July 9, 2012).

Centers for Disease Control and Prevention. "Questions and Answers About Foodborne Illness." National Center for Emerging and Zoonotic Infectious Diseases. http://www.cdc.gov/foodsafety/facts.html (accessed July 9, 2012).

Gammara, Roberto M."Food Poisoning." Medscape Reference. http://emedicine.medscape.com/article/175569-overview (accessed July 9, 2012).

Mahon, Barbara. "Preventing Foodborne Illnesses." Centers for Disease Control and Prevention, Podcasts at CDC. April 15, 2010. http://www2c.cdc.gov/podcasts/player.asp?f=1266133 (accessed July 9, 2012).

MedlinePlus. "Foodborne Illness." http://www.nlm.nih.gov/medlineplus/foodborneillness.html (accessed July 9, 2012).

ORGANIZATIONS

National Agriculture Compliance Assistance Center, U.S. Environmental Protection Agency, 901 North 5th St., Kansas City, KS 66101, (888) 663-2155, Fax: (913) 551-7270, agcenter@epa.gov, http://www.epa.gov/agriculture.

Partnership for Food Safety Education, 2345 Crystal Dr., Ste. 800, Arlington, VA 22202, (202) 220-0651, Fax: (202) 220-0873, info@fightbac.org, http://www.fightbac.org.

U.S. Centers for Disease Control and Prevention, 1600 Clifton Rd., Atlanta, GA 30333, (800) CDC-INFO (232-4636), cdcinfo@cdc.gov, http://www.cdc.gov.

U.S. Department of Agriculture, 1400 Independence Ave. SW, Washington, DC 20250, (202) 720-2791, http://www.usda.gov/wps/portal/usdahome.

U.S. Food and Drug Administration, 10903 New Hampshire Ave., Silver Spring, MD 20993-0002, (888) INFO-FDA (463-6332), http://www.fda.gov.

Monique Laberge, Ph.D.
Margaret Alic, Ph.D.

Food fortification

Definition

Food fortification is the intentional act of adding **vitamins** and essential trace elements, also known as micronutrients, to foodstuffs.

Description

Food fortification is the deliberate addition of essential micronutrients to foods and drinks. This includes the addition of vitamins, essential minerals, fatty acids, amino acids, and proteins. Although similar, food enrichment is different from food fortification because only micronutrients lost in production are added during food enrichment, and both micronutrients lost during production and micronutrients never present may be added during food fortification. Examples of commonly fortified foods include milk, fortified with vitamin D; orange juice, fortified with vitamin C;, and salt, fortified with iodine.

Purpose

The purpose of fortifying foods is to add micronutrients into the diets of people who may not obtain the recommended amount of **nutrition** from their everyday eating habits. The practice of fortifying food started around the same time that nutritional deficiency diseases began to be identified and tracked. Over two billion people worldwide experience micronutrient deficiencies. Beginning in 1992, a joint Food and Agriculture Organization of the United Nations (FAO) and World Health Organization (WHO) conference gained the agreement of 159 countries to support food fortification as a way to combat micronutrient deficiencies worldwide. Common justification for food fortification includes replacing nutrients lost during production, combating nutritional deficiency diseases, ensuring that food eaten as a substitute (i.e., soy milk instead of cow's milk) is equivalent to the original food, and to ensure that special dietary foods (i.e., gluten-free foods) have appropriate nutritional content.

Origins

Food fortification has a relatively short history in the United States and around the world. In 1924, the United States began a voluntary program to add iodine to salt. This addition was a result of recommendations by many prominent organizations including the **American Public Health Association**, the American Medical Association, and the Council on Foods and Nutrition. It was seen as a way to decrease the number of goiter cases in the United States. In 1933, milk began to be fortified with vitamin D through irradiating the milk and feeding milk cows irradiated yeast. This practice was replaced in the 1940s by the addition of concentrated vitamin D directly to milk. This practice has continued in the United States. As of 2012, milk and salt were still two of the most commonly consumed fortified foods.

Organizations in the United States recommended additional food fortification practices in the 1930s and 1940s, when deficiency disease syndromes were first identified. These included adding the micronutrients riboflavin, iron, thiamin, and niacin to flour. In 1941, the Food and Drug Administration (FDA) developed requirements that fortified flour must be labeled as enriched. The labeling of fortified and enriched foods remains an FDA regulation.

Bread began to be enriched in 1941 out of concern for the poor nutritional health of men enlisted during World War II. By the middle of 1942, 75% of white bread in the United States was being fortified. This was accomplished only through the voluntary participation of bakery associations. Although fortification was never made mandatory by the FDA, and as of 2012 still was not, individual states were allowed to pass their own state legislation on the matter. In 1952, 26 states had laws making the enrichment of flour and bread mandatory. That same year, the FDA developed new regulations regarding the standards that must be met by fortified flour and bread in order to be labeled as enriched. State laws requiring mandatory fortification of flour and bread were ended by passage of the National Labeling Education Act of 1990.

In 1962, the FDA proposed limits in food fortification and developed a list of 12 essential micronutrients allowed to be used and developed suitable amounts of fortification. An additional 11 micronutrients were listed as essential micronutrients but unsuitable for fortification. The FDA tried to strengthen the regulation of food fortification in 1966, by proposing a limit of food fortification to only eight classes for foodstuffs, but the legislation never passed.

KEY TERMS

Amino acids—Complex molecules that form proteins. There are 20 different common types of amino acids that join to form proteins. A diet must include a minimum number of amino acids to keep a person healthy.

Fatty acids—Complex molecules found in fats and oils. Essential fatty acids are fatty acids that the body needs but cannot synthesize. Essential fatty acids are made by plants and must be present in the diet to maintain health.

Micronutrient—A substance needed in small amounts to allow for normal growth and development. Common examples of micronutrients include vitamins, such as vitamin C and vitamin D, and minerals, such as iron and zinc.

Non-staple foods—Food that is not a dominant portion of a population's standard diet. Examples for the United States include carbonated beverages, snack foods, and chocolate.

Over the years, additional foods beyond salt, flour, and bread have begun to be enriched or fortified. Many of these were non-staple foods. Between 2006 and 2008, the number of foods fortified with omega-3 fatty acids increased by 68%. Although the FDA is very involved in food fortification standards, the FDA has, for the most part, only released policies and not legal regulations. Some of these policies include the idea that it is not appropriate to fortify meat, poultry, fish, fresh produce, or candy. Additionally, food fortification should be only used to correct a dietary insufficiency that has been recognized by the scientific community or to replace micronutrients lost in production. Although recommended, these policies have not been enacted into laws.

In 1980, the U.S. Department of Agriculture's Food Safety and Inspection Service (FSIS) adopted the food fortification policies set forth by the FDA. Although the same policy is used, the FSIS has made some of its own exceptions, such as allowing certain meats to be fortified.

Effects on public health

The consensus among researchers and physicians is that for the most part, fortified foods benefit public health. Between 1998, when the FDA made the addition of folic acid to enriched grains mandatory, and 2004, the number of babies born with neural-tube deficits (which result from folic acid deficiency early in pregnancy) went down by 25%. The **Centers for Disease Control and Prevention (CDC)** believes that this drop was at least partially due to the FDA's regulation. This is just one example of how fortified food has reduced the inidence of health problems caused by nutrient deficiencies.

Food fortification, many physicians say, is similar to taking a multi-vitamin. At times, food fortification can be even more beneficial than a multi-vitamin because many essential micronutrients are digested better when taken with food instead of alone. In other cases, a multi-vitamin may be more beneficial than only relying on fortified and enriched foods because the amount of micronutrients in each type of fortified food can be difficult to monitor accurately.

Although consuming fortified food benefits public health, fortified food does not always have as many health benefits as whole foods, such as whole grain breads. Additionally, many unhealthy foods such as fortified snack food and sodas can be found on the market. Fortification does not overcome or offset the high sugar and fat content in these foods. Some researchers worry that people may eat a diet higher in fat than they normally would because they focus on the fact that these unhealthy foods are fortified with healthy nutrients.

Another problem some people worry about is that high concentrations of micronutrients can cause health problems, just as insufficient concentrations of micronutrients can. This worry, however, is minimal, and regulations by governmental organizations, such as the FDA in the United States, limit the likelihood of someone getting too much of a particular micronutrient from fortified foods. Even with the large number of fortified foods available to consumers, many people still do not have enough micronutrients in their diet. According to a 2009 study, three in four Americans do not consume the recommended daily allowance of minerals and nutrients.

Outside of developed nations, food fortification allows people with access to limited amounts and types of food to get additional micronutrients. Vitamin and mineral deficiencies are responsible for reducing work capacity, disability, and death throughout the underdeveloped world. Although food fortification is not common in most of these countries, organizations work to get fortified food or powdered vitamins, which allow people to fortify their own food, into communities in need.

Costs and benefits to society

Although the costs and benefits of food fortification are hard to measure directly, studies show that the benefits of food fortification far outweigh the costs to society. Food fortification has reduced the number of cases of many nutrient-deficient syndromes. One study estimated that in the developing world, salt fortification costs about USD $0.5 billion annually in comparison to the $35.7 billion that could be potentially spent on a widespread iodine deficiency. Another study estimated that the median potential benefit of iron fortification in the developing world is 6:1, when focusing on physical benefits, and as high as 36:1 when taking into account cognitive benefits. These benefits, especially when considering the costs of healthcare, productivity, and the general health of a society, can be substantial. The main cost food fortification has to society is the increase in price in some foods that are fortified compared to the same food that is not fortified.

QUESTIONS TO ASK YOUR DOCTOR

- Can I maintain a healthy diet even if I avoid all enriched or fortified foods?
- Is it better for me to eat whole grain bread or enriched white bread?
- Should I take extra vitamin supplements above eating vitamin-fortified foods?
- Can enriched foods harm me when I am pregnant?

Efforts and solutions

Food fortification has been found to play an important role in the health of a society, however, many efforts are focused on educating the public about food fortification and how to eat a healthy diet without relying only on fortified foods. Fortified food cannot solve all micronutrient problems in either the developed or the developing world. Many organizations are working to increase the availability of fortified food programs to undeveloped nations that suffer from widespread nutritional deficiencies. Other organizations and governmental agencies are working to determine the best way to regulate food fortification and to determine which fortifications are important to public health and which are unneeded or could possibly do more harm than good.

Resources

BOOKS

Allen, L., et al. *Guidelines on Food Fortification with Micronutrients.* Geneva: WHO, 2006.

Committee on Use of Dietary Reference Intakes in Nutrition Labeling. *Guiding Principles for Nutrition Labeling and Fortification.* Washington, DC: National Academic Press, 2003.

WEBSITES

FAO Agriculture and Consumer Protection. "Food Fortification Technology." http://www.fao.org/docrep/w2840e/w2840e03.htm (accessed September 20, 2012).

International Food Information Council Foundation. "Food Fortification in Today' World." http://www.foodinsight.org/Newsletter/Detail.aspx?topic=Food_Fortification_in_Today_s_World (accessed September 20, 2012).

Reistad-Long, Sara. "Fortified Food: How Healthy Are They?" http://online.wsj.com/article/SB124267976477131801.html (accessed September 20, 2012).

ORGANIZATIONS

Food and Agriculture Organization of the United Nations (FAO Headquarters), Viale delle Terme di Caracalla, Rome, Italy 00153, 39 06 570 53625, Fax: 39 06 5705 3699, AGN-Director@fao.org (Nutrition and Consumer Protection), http://www.fao.org.

United States Department of Agriculture Food Safety and Inspection Service, 1400 Independence Ave., S.W., Washington, DC 20250, (402) 344 5000, (800) 233 3935, Fax: (402) 344 5005, http://www.fsis.usda.gov.

United States Food and Drug Administration (FDA), 10903 New Hampshire Avenue, Silver Spring, MD 20993, (888) INFO-FDA (463-6332), http://www.fda.gov.

World Health Organization, Avenue Appia 20, Geneva 27, Switzerland 1211, 22 41 791 21 11, Fax: 22 41 791 31 11, info@who.int, http://www.who.int.

Tish Davidson, AM

Food safety

Definition

Food safety involves protecting food from all contamination—including pathogenic organisms, chemicals, toxins, and physical contaminants—at all stages of the food-production chain. This includes farming through harvesting or slaughtering, processing, packaging, distribution, retail sales, and meal preparation.

Purpose

The food supply in the United States is probably the safest in the world, and serious breaches of food safety are relatively rare. Nevertheless, the U.S. **Centers for Disease Control and Prevention (CDC)** reported in 2011 that about 48 million Americans—one in six—suffer from foodborne illness (food **poisoning**) every year. Internationally, **food contamination** and large scale food recalls appear to be on the rise. The 2011 Fukushima Daiichi nuclear power plant disaster in Japan raised fears of radiation-contaminated food. Bioterrorism experts worry that disease-causing organisms or toxic chemicals could be intentionally introduced into food or **water** supplies causing mass contamination. Scientists worry that climate change may increase the risk of contamination from pesticides and other chemicals, biotoxins, and pathogenic microbes. Various groups question the safety of food derived from genetically modified organisms (GMOs).

Although food safety includes preventing the contamination of crops with unsafe levels of pesticides and herbicides and avoiding poisonous mushrooms, mercury-contaminated fish, and shellfish contaminated with algal toxins, most illnesses resulting from food contamination are caused by pathogenic organisms—bacteria, viruses, and **parasites**. Although foodborne illnesses can be very unpleasant, they are usually mild and short-lived. However, they can cause serious complications and even death, particularly among the very young, the very old, pregnant women and their unborn children, and people with weakened or compromised immune systems. Foods that are tainted with natural toxins, synthetic chemicals, or physical contaminants can also cause serious or fatal illnesses.

Description

In the United States, the vast majority of food poisonings of known origin are caused by one of eight pathogens:

- noroviruses, a large group of viruses that are responsible for the majority of food poisonings of known origin, including major outbreaks on cruise ships and in nursing homes, and that, unlike most other food pathogens, appear to be spread primarily by infected food-service workers
- *Salmonella* spp., widespread intestinal bacteria that cause salmonellosis
- *Clostridium perfringens*, common bacteria found throughout the environment, including in human and animal intestines
- *Campylobacter* spp., bacteria present in most raw poultry and the most commonly identified cause of diarrheal illness worldwide
- *Staphylococcus aureus*, a bacterium in dust, air, and sewage that can contaminate almost any food
- *Toxoplasma gondii*, a parasite that can cause life-threatening illness
- certain strains of the normally harmless, human-gut bacterium *Escherichia coli*, called Shiga toxin-producing *E. coli* (STEC)
- *Listeria monocytogenes*, a bacterium that is ubiquitous in soil, groundwater, plants, and animals and that causes listeriosis

Safe food storage limits

Category	Food	Refrigerator (40 °F or below)	Freezer (0 °F or below)
Salads	Egg, chicken, ham, tuna, and macaroni salads	3–5 days	Does not freeze well
Hot dogs	Opened package	1 week	1–2 months
	Unopened package	2 weeks	1–2 months
Luncheon meat	Opened package or deli sliced	3–5 days	1–2 months
	Unopened package	2 weeks	1–2 months
Bacon and sausage	Bacon	7 days	1 month
	Sausage, raw, from chicken, turkey, pork, beef	1–2 days	1–2 months
Ground meats	Hamburger, ground beef, turkey, veal, pork, lamb, and mixtures of them	1–2 days	3–4 months
Fresh beef, veal, lamb and pork	Steaks	3–5 days	6–12 months
	Chops	3–5 days	4–6 months
	Roasts	3–5 days	4–12 months
Fresh poultry	Chicken or turkey, whole	1–2 days	1 year
	Chicken or turkey, pieces	1–2 days	9 months
Soups and stews	Vegetable or meat added	3–4 days	2–3 months
Leftovers	Cooked meat or poultry	3–4 days	2–6 months
	Chicken nuggets or patties	3–4 days	1–3 months
	Pizza	3–4 days	1–2 months

SOURCE: U.S. Department of Health and Human Services, FoodSafety.gov.

(Table by PreMediaGlobal. © 2013 Cengage Learning)

Contaminants that jeopardize food safety change over time, requiring constant surveillance. Improved food safety techniques—including milk **pasteurization**, safer canning methods, and water treatment—have helped overcome diseases, such as **typhoid fever**, **tuberculosis**, and **cholera** in the developed world. However, other foodborne diseases, such as **listeriosis**, appear to be on the rise. In 2011, at least 29 people died and at least 139 people across 28 states were sickened from eating cantaloupe contaminated with *L. monocytogenes*, which was traced to unsanitary conditions and poor handling at a single farm. There have been major recalls of ground beef, lettuce, and spinach contaminated with STEC. Strain O157:H7 is the most commonly identified STEC in the United States. There have also been nationwide recalls of peanut butter contaminated with **salmonella**.

Media reports of contaminated foods, frequent product recalls, and U.S. government initiatives have raised public awareness of food-safety issues. However, globalization of the food supply, industrial farming, concentrated animal feeding operations (CAFOs), and centralized slaughterhouses and processing facilities that pool ingredients from hundreds or thousands of plants and animals have made monitoring food safety very difficult.

The U.S. Food and Drug Administration's (FDA) Food Safety Modernization Act (FSMA) of 2011 was the most sweeping overhaul of food-safety laws in more than 70 years. It aimed to establish a comprehensive, prevention-based system of farm-to-table food safety. As of 2012, however, there were still more than a dozen federal agencies in charge of various aspects of food safety. For example, in the 2011 State of the Union address, President Barack Obama pointed out that the Interior Department is responsible for salmon while they are in fresh water, but once they hit saltwater, the Commerce Department takes over. The Food Safety and Inspection Service (FSIS) of the Department of Agriculture (USDA) is responsible for meat, poultry, and processed egg products that are produced in federally inspected facilities, while the FDA is responsible for the safety of most other foods. The **Environmental Protection Agency (EPA)** is in charge of pesticides and other toxic chemicals used in food production.

The FDA can request the recall of about 80% of foods consumed domestically, as well as contaminated animal feed. Additives and substances that contact food, such as packaging, must be approved by the FDA as safe. However, other food ingredients, including some that have been used for many years, do not require FDA approval. The FDA also regulates food irradiation that helps protect against disease-causing bacteria and delays spoilage. Irradiated foods include spices, red meat, poultry, some shellfish, and fresh iceberg lettuce and spinach.

Despite government regulation, almost all food safety testing is performed by the food companies themselves. This means that the responsibility of ensuring food is safe to eat falls upon food manufacturers and producers, as well as consumers. Cleanliness, food separation, and proper cooling and cooking are key to food safety.

Cutting boards and food safety

- **Type of boards**
  Choose either wood or a nonporous surface cutting board such as plastic, marble, glass, or pyroceramic. Nonporous surfaces are easier to clean than wood.
- **Avoid cross-contamination**
  Use one cutting board for fresh produce and bread and a separate one for raw meat, poultry, and seafood. This will prevent bacteria on a cutting board that is used for raw meat, poultry, or seafood from contaminating a food that requires no further cooking.
- **Cleaning cutting boards**
  To keep all cutting boards clean, wash them with hot, soapy water after each use; then rinse with clear water and air dry or pat dry with clean paper towels. Nonporous acrylic, plastic, or glass boards and solid wood boards can be washed in a dishwasher (laminated boards may crack and split).
  Both wooden and plastic cutting boards can be sanitized with a solution of 1 tablespoon of unscented, liquid chlorine bleach per gallon of water. Flood the surface with the bleach solution and allow it to stand for several minutes. Rinse with clear water and air dry or pat dry with clean paper towels.
- **Replace worn cutting boards**
  All plastic and wooden cutting boards wear out over time. Once cutting boards become excessively worn or develop hard-to-clean grooves, they should be discarded.

SOURCE: Food Safety and Inspections Service, U.S. Department of Agriculture

(Table by PreMediaGlobal. © 2013 Cengage Learning)

Cleanliness

Frequent hand washing before, during, and after preparing and eating food is a central tenet of food safety. Hand washing is especially important after handling raw meat, poultry, eggs, and seafood. Hands should be rubbed together with soap under warm, running water for at least 20 seconds (two choruses of "Happy Birthday"). Soap should be rubbed between fingers, down to the wrists, and into fingernails. Paper towels should be used for drying, since cloths spread microbes.

Fresh fruits and vegetables should be washed under running water and scrubbed with a clean brush or with both hands just before cooking or eating. They should be washed both before and after peeling to prevent salmonellosis. Outside leaves of lettuce and cabbage should be discarded. Produce that is not eaten immediately should be dried with a clean cloth or disposable towel, since surface moisture can promote microbial growth. Raw meat and poultry should not be washed, because washing increases the danger of cross-contaminating surfaces.

Cutting boards, utensils, dishes, appliances, kitchen bins, and countertops should be carefully cleaned regularly with hot, soapy water. Dishtowels should be washed in hot water. Sponges should be disinfected in a chlorine bleach solution and replaced frequently. Two minutes in the microwave will kill harmful bacteria in wet sponges. Smelly sponges, cloths, utensils, or surfaces suggest microbial growth and require proper cleaning or disposal.

Food separation

Juices from raw meat, poultry, seafood, and eggs should never come in contact with uncooked, ready-to-eat foods, such as fruits and vegetables. Such foods should remain separated in the grocery cart, in bags, and in the refrigerator with their juices contained.

Cutting boards are a common source of cross-contamination. One cutting board should be set aside for raw meat, poultry, and seafood, and another for cutting vegetables, breads, and other ready-to-eat foods. Boards can be appropriately labeled or colored (e.g., green for vegetables). The meat board should be washed thoroughly with hot, soapy water or in a dishwasher immediately after use. Old cutting boards, especially wooden boards with cracks, crevices, and knife scars, should be discarded. Cross-contamination of cooked foods can occur when plates or surfaces that held raw meat, poultry, or seafood are reused for cooked food.

Cooling

Cold temperatures slow or halt bacterial growth. Although refrigerating leftovers might seem obvious, among the most common calls fielded by the USDA Meat and Poultry Hotline are from college students asking whether it is safe to eat pizza that sat out overnight (it's not). Refrigerators should be kept at 40°F (4°C) or below and freezers at 0°F (-18°C). A refrigerator thermometer can ensure the correct temperature. Raw meat, poultry, eggs, seafood, cut fruits and vegetables, and leftovers should not be left at room temperature for more than two hours or one hour at temperatures above 90°F (32°C). Refrigerators should be cleaned out often, since too much food can prevent cold air from circulating properly.

Foods are generally labeled with refrigeration/freezing instructions and expiration dates. Most foods are safe in the refrigerator for at least three to four days. Exceptions include stuffing, some cooked patties, gravies, and broths, which should only be kept for one to two days. Raw meats should be marinated in the refrigerator rather than at room temperature. Frozen foods should be defrosted in the refrigerator. Food defrosted in warm water or a microwave should be cooked immediately.

Cooking

Uncooked or undercooked meat, poultry, eggs, and egg products are potentially unsafe. Only a good meat thermometer—not the color of the meat or its juices—can determine whether meat is adequately cooked. The thermometer should be placed in the thickest portion of meat or poultry pieces, away from bone, fat, and gristle, and at the center of casseroles and egg dishes. Appropriate minimum temperatures include:

- hamburger patties and meatballs, 160°F (71°C)
- roasts and steaks, 165°F (74°C)
- chicken and turkey, 180°F (82°C)
- fish, 140°F (60°C)
- egg dishes and casseroles, 160°F (71°C)

Cold and hot spots must be avoided when cooking in a microwave. Stirring halfway through cooking evenly distributes the heat and ensures consistent temperature. Leftovers should be heated to at least 165°F (74°C). Leftover sauces, soups, and gravy should be brought to a boil.

Precautions

The most important food safety rule may be "When in doubt, throw it out." Although spoiled foods often have an unpleasant taste or smell, some people, especially the elderly, may have difficulty telling whether food has gone bad by smell alone. Further, bacterial growth does not necessarily result in a bad taste or smell or discoloration. Dating foods when first refrigerated can help prevent the consumption of outdated items.

Consumers should be aware of updated food safety information and food recalls. Reports of suspect food should be made to the store where the food was purchased, to the manufacturer, or to the FDA or FSIS, depending on the type of food. Any identifying information on the packaging should be noted.

Complications

Ignorance of or disregard for food safety can lead to foodborne illness. Outbreaks of foodborne illness are common in restaurants, cafeterias, nursing homes, prisons, and family and community gatherings where large numbers of people are fed "from the same pot." Contaminated food usually causes diarrhea and often causes nausea, vomiting, abdominal cramps, and fever, which can pose significant health risks for infants, the elderly, and those with special medical conditions. Even moderate diarrhea and vomiting pose a risk for dehydration, especially in infants and young children. Although symptoms of food poisoning often occur soon after eating contaminated food, symptoms may not be apparent for up to a week.

KEY TERMS

Botulism—Life-threatening paralytic illness from contaminated food caused by the botulinum toxin from the bacterium *Clostridium botulinum*.

Campylobacter—A genus of bacteria that is found in almost all raw poultry and that can contaminate food and cause illness.

Concentrated animal feeding operation (CAFO)—An agricultural operation in which animals are raised in confined situations, with animals, feed, manure, urine, dead animals, and production operations concentrated in a small area.

Dehydration—The abnormal depletion of body fluids, as from vomiting and diarrhea.

Food Safety and Inspection Service (FSIS)—The public health agency within the U.S. Department of Agriculture that is responsible for the safety of meat, poultry, and egg products.

Genetically modified (GM or GMO) foods—Food or ingredients derived from genetically modified organisms.

Listeriosis—Illness caused by food contaminated with the bacterium *Listeria monocytogenes*.

Norovirus—Norwalk virus; a large family of RNA viruses that are the most common cause of illness from contaminated food.

Parasite—An organism that survives by living with, on, or in another organism, usually to the detriment of the host.

Pathogen—A causative agent of disease, such as a bacteria, virus, or parasite.

Salmonellosis—Food poisoning caused by bacteria of the genus *Salmonella*, which usually leads to severe diarrhea and may be transmitted to a fetus.

Shiga toxin-producing *E. coli* (STEC)—Strains of the common, normally harmless, intestinal bacterium *Escherichia coli* that contaminate food with Shiga toxin; *E. coli* O157:H7 is the most commonly identified STEC in North America.

Parental concerns

Pregnant women and their unborn babies, infants, and young children are particularly vulnerable to the effects of contaminated food. Thus, awareness of food safety, good food-hygiene practices, and possibly the avoidance of "high-risk" foods are especially important for pregnant women, parents, and caregivers. Vigilant

QUESTIONS TO ASK YOUR DOCTOR

- What are the most important ways to keep my family's food safe?
- Are there specific foods that I should avoid because of possible contamination?
- Should lunch meats and fish be avoided during pregnancy?
- At what point does an illness from food contamination require medical attention?

food safety is particularly important when young children attend summer picnics, cookouts, and outdoor buffets.

Breast-feeding is the best food-safety practice for babies. Breast milk and infant formula must be carefully stored. Mixed formula should be kept in the refrigerator for no more than 24 hours. Expired formula and any formula or breast milk left in the bottle after feeding should be discarded. Bottles can become contaminated with salmonella within two hours at room temperature. Infants under one year should never be given food containing honey, even if it is cooked, since honey can contain spores of *Clostridium botulinum*, the bacterium that produces the deadly paralytic toxin that causes botulism. Although the toxin is destroyed by boiling, the spores are not.

Baby food containers should always be checked to ensure that they have been well sealed and that the food has not reached its expiration date. Leftover food that has been contaminated with the spoon used to feed a baby should be discarded or moved to a dish that the same child will eat from again.

Resources

BOOKS

Bartos, Judeen, ed. *Food Safety*. Detroit: Greenhaven, 2011.

Benedict, Jeff. *Poisoned: The True Story of the Deadly E. coli Outbreak that Changed the Way Americans Eat*. Buena Vista, VA: Inspire, Mariner Media, 2011.

Hewitt, Ben. *Making Supper Safe: One Man's Quest to Learn the Truth about Food Safety*. New York: Rodale, 2011.

Juneja, Vijay K., and John Nikolaos Sofos. *Pathogens and Toxins in Foods: Challenges and Interventions*. Washington, DC: American Society for Microbiology, 2010.

Moby, and Miyun Park, eds. *Gristle: From Factory Farms to Food Safety (Thinking Twice About the Meat We Eat)*. New York: New Press, 2010.

Nestle, Marion. *Safe Food: The Politics of Food Safety*. Berkeley: University of California, 2010.

O'Reilly, James T. *A Consumer's Guide to Food Regulation & Safety*. New York: Oceana, 2010.

Paarlberg, Robert L. *Food Politics: What Everyone Needs to Know*. New York: Oxford University, 2010.

Wallace, Robert B., and Maria Oria. *Enhancing Food Safety: The Role of the Food and Drug Administration*. Washington, DC: National Academies, 2010.

PERIODICALS

Kowalski, Kathiann. "How Safe is Your Food?" *Current Health Kids* 34, no. 7 (March 2011): 16–19.

Palmer, Sharon. "8 Food Safety Myths Busted." *Environmental Nutrition* 34, no. 8 (August 2011): 2.

Roan, Shari, and Eryn Brown. "Q&A; Radiation and Food Safety." *Los Angeles Times*, March 22, 2011, A5.

Stacey, Michelle. "A Good Egg." *Prevention*, May 2011, 124–33.

Voelker, Rebecca. "FDA Tries to Catch Up on Food Safety." *Journal of the American Medical Association* 303, no. 18 (May 12, 2010): 1797.

WEBSITES

Food Safety and Inspection Service. "Food Safety Education." U.S. Department of Agriculture. http://www.fsis.usda.gov/Food_Safety_Education/index.asp (accessed August 19, 2012).

FoodSafety.gov. U.S. Department of Health & Human Services. http://www.foodsafety.gov (accessed August 19, 2012).

Partnership for Food Safety Education. "Safe Food Handling." http://www.fightbac.org/safe-food-handling (accessed August 19, 2012).

U.S. Centers for Disease Control and Prevention. "Food Safety at CDC." http://www.cdc.gov/foodsafety (accessed August 19, 2012).

U.S. Food and Drug Administration. "Food Safety." http://www.fda.gov/Food/FoodSafety/default.htm (accessed August 19, 2012).

U.S. Food and Drug Administration. "The New FDA Food Safety Modernization Act (FSMA)." http://www.fda.gov/food/foodsafety/fsma/default.htm (accessed August 19, 2012).

U.S. Food Safety and Inspection Service. "USDA Meat and Poultry Hotline." Food Safety Education. http://www.fsis.usda.gov/education/usda_meat_&_poultry_hotline/index.asp (accessed August 19, 2012).

ORGANIZATIONS

Academy of Nutrition and Dietetics, 120 South Riverside Plz., Ste. 2000, Chicago, IL 60606-6995, (312) 899-0040, (800) 877-1600, amacmunn@eatright.org, http://www.eatright.org.

Center for Food Safety, 660 Pennsylvania Ave. SE, Ste. 302, Washington, DC 20003, (202) 547-9359, Fax: (202) 547-9429, office@centerforfoodsafety.org, http://www.centerforfoodsafety.org.

Food Safety and Inspection Service (FSIS), U.S. Department of Agriculture (USDA), 1400 Independence Ave. SW, Washington, DC 20250-3700, (888) 674-6854 (USDA Meat and Poultry Consumer Hotline), MPHotline.fsis@usda.gov, http://www.fsis.usda.gov.

National Agriculture Center, U.S. Environmental Protection Agency, 901 N 5th St., Kansas City, KS 66101, (888) 663-2155, Fax: (913) 551-7270, agcenter@epa.gov, http://www.epa.gov/agriculture/agctr.html.

Partnership for Food Safety Education, 2345 Crystal Dr., Ste. 800, Arlington, VA 22202, (202) 220-0651, Fax: (202) 220-0873, info@fightbac.org, http://www.fightbac.org.

U.S. Centers for Disease Control and Prevention, 1600 Clifton Rd., Atlanta, GA 30333, (800) 232-4636, cdcinfor@cdc.gov, http://www.cdc.gov.

U.S. Food and Drug Administration, 10903 New Hampshire Ave., Silver Spring, MD 20993, (888) 463-6332, http://www.fda.gov/Safety/Recalls/default.htm.

Teresa G. Odle
Margaret Alic, Ph.D.

Fungal infections

Definition

A fungal infection is an infection caused by a member of the Kingdom Fungi. Fungi are eukaryotic organisms that are structurally similar to plants, but functionally similar to animals. They include a number of common and well-known organisms, such as molds, mildew, yeasts, and mushrooms.

Description

Fungi are ubiquitous in the environment. They occur in the air and the soil, on plants, and in **water**. Fungi become part of the human body primarily in one of two ways: by being inhaled from the air or by having fungi or their spores land on the outer surface of the body. Once resident on or in the body, fungi may reproduce and cause a fungal infection, such as ringworm, athlete's foot, jock itch, or systemic diseases, such as aspergillosis, blastomycosis, candidosis, coccidioidomycosis, cryptococcosis, histoplasmosis, mucormycosis, pneumocystis **pneumonia**, and sporotrichosis. Most of these infections are relatively harmless, although they can become life-threatening for certain populations, such as the elderly and those with compromised immune systems.

Causes and Symptoms

In general, fungal infections can be classified as superficial or systemic. Superficial infections are those that occur when fungi settle on the outer surface of the body and colonize there. Systemic infections are those that are caused by fungi that enter the body and colonize the respiratory system or some other part of the body.

Demographics

Few data are available on the incidence and prevalence of superficial fungal infections, although most experts agree that such diseases are very common in the general population. It is probably safe to say that the vast majority of people in all cultures have at one time or another contracted one or more forms of such disease. Such is not the case with systemic infections, however, which tend to afflict only very small numbers of the general, otherwise healthy, population. For non-reportable diseases, such as aspergillosis and blastomycosis, one must rely on estimates based on informal studies. For these two diseases, that estimate was about one to two cases per 100,000 persons. More reliable data are available for reportable conditions, such as coccidioidomycosis. In 2010, the U.S. **Centers for Disease Control and Prevention (CDC)** reported that there were about 16,000 cases of the infection in the United States, almost all of which were reported from two states, Arizona and California. For other fungal infections, data are not available even though a disease itself may be reportable. For example, the **CDC** estimates that as many as 80% of all individuals who live in regions where histoplasmosis is common carry antibodies to the fungus. They also estimate that anywhere from 10 to 25% of immune-compromised patients with HIV infection have active cases of histoplasmosis infection, although no specific data are available to support that estimate.

Causes

One of the two most common causes of superficial fungal infections is a group of organisms classified as tineal fungi. The term *tinea* refers in general to any skin disease caused by a fungus. Some of the most common tineal organisms and the diseases they cause are

- Tinea cruris: Jock itch
- Tinea pedis: Athlete's foot
- Tinea capitis: Ringworm
- Tinea barbae: Infection of the hair follicles
- Tinea faciei: Infection of the face
- Tinea unguium: Infection of the fingernails and toenails

The most common cause of all fungal infections is a member of the genus *Candida*, especially the species *C. albicans*. Scientists estimate that about four-fifths of all humans harbor *C. albicans* on or in their bodies, especially in the mouth and gastrointestinal system. Normally, these fungi live with their human hosts in a symbiotic relationships in which they cause no harm to the human. In some circumstances, the fungus may cause a mild disease known as candidiasis, or thrush, that appears most commonly in the mouth or the genital region (oral thrush or vaginitis, for example). Although unpleasant and uncomfortable, most cases of candidiasis are relatively benign and often resolve without treatment. For a number of reasons, however, they can also become more serious and may even be life-threatening for some infected individuals.

A number of other fungi cause other types of systemic infections, including

- Members of the genus *Aspergillus*, especially *A. fumigatus,* cause a group of respiratory disorders known as allergic bronchopulmonary aspergillosis, pulmonary aspergilloma, and invasive aspergillosis.
- The fungi *Coccidioides immitis* and *C. posadasii* are primarily responsible for the disease known as coccidioidomycosis, also called valley fever. California fever, desert rheumatism, or San Joaquin Valley fever.
- *Cryptococcus neoformans* and *C. gattii* are the causative agents for cryptococcosis, an infection of the respiratory system that may spread throughout the body.
- *Histoplasma capsulatum* is responsible for the disease known as histoplasmosis. Since the fungus often lives in caves, the disease is also called cave or caver's disease or spelunker's lung. Other common names are Darling's disease, Ohio Valley disease (for one of the regions in which it is most common), and reticuloendotheliosis. If allowed to spread throughout the body, the disease can be fatal.
- The fungus *Paracoccidioides brasiliensis* is responsible for the disease known as paracoccidioidomycosis, which is also known as Brazilian blastomycosis, South American blastomycosis, Lutz-Splendore-de Almeida disease, and paracoccidioidal granuloma. The disease occurs primarily in the respiratory system.

Symptoms

The signs and symptoms of superficial fungal infections are generally similar and include cracking, flaking, peeling skin that usually is very itchy and/or burning, causing considerable discomfort. The skin may also becme red, with the formation of blisters. In the case of ringworm, the fungus produces a flat, circular, raised, red sore that gives the disease one part of its name ("ring"), although no "worm" is involved in the infection. Candida infections are characterized by a painful, reddish rash at the site of the infection, often accomplanied by small, pimple-like bumps that are very itchy and/or painful. The bumps may ooze a white or yellowish fluid.

KEY TERMS

Compromised—Lacking adequate resistance to disease.

Eukaryote—A single-cell or multicellular organism with a clearly defined nucleus.

Fungicide—A substance capable of killing or stopping the growth of fungi.

Incidence—The number of new cases of a disease in some given time period, such as one year.

Prevalence—The total number of cases of a disease at any one time in a region.

Spore—A small, one-cell reproductive body produced by an organism, such as a fungus.

Symbiotic—Having to do with a close physical association between individuals of two different species.

Systemic—Relating to the complete body of an organism.

The symptoms of systemic infections tend to differ somewhat from condition to condition. Since most tend to begin in the respiratory system, however, they also have certain common features, such as coughing, low-grade fever, chest **pain**, and difficulty in breathing. Indications of more advanced stages of these disease depend on the involvement of other body systems. In the case of aspergillosis, for example, advance of the disease may be accompanied by a higher fever, chills, shock, and delirium. Progress of the disease may also result in liver and kidney failure and, in a relatively short period of time, death may occur.

Diagnosis

Diagnosis of superficial fungal infections is usually based on visual and/or microscopic examination of the patient's skin. Physical features of the infections are so characteristic that they generally leave little doubt as to the existence of a fungal infection, although the specific agent responsible for the infection might not be identified. Such identification is not necessary, because the chemicals used to treat the infection are equally effective with any of the possible agents responsible for the condition.

Diagnosis for systemic fungal infections generally requires a fungal culture or urine, blood, or other test. In a fungal culture, a physician takes a sample of blood, sputum, or some other body fluid and cultures the material over an extended period of antigens to any fungus are present in the body. Imaging tests may be used also to determine whether a fungus has spread to other parts of the body beyond the respiratory system and, if so, what other systems may be involved with what types of complications.

Treatment

The first level of treatment for superficial fungal infections includes a number of over-the-counter (OTC) products that can be obtained without a prescription. These include products that include the fungicides miconazole (Micatin), tolnaftate (Tinactin) or clotrimazole (Lotramin). These products may take a matter of weeks before the fungus is completely killed. If an OTC product is not effective in treating the infection, a stronger prescription medication may be necessary. Among the products available are ointments and creams that are used directly on the infection (ketoconazole [Nizoral], ciclopirox [Penlac; Loprox] or selenium sulfide) or oral medications such as fluconazole (Diflucan), itraconazole (Sporanox), or ketoconazole (Nizoral). Oral medications should be used with caution as they may have severe hepatic effects that are far more serious than the fungal infection itself.

A number of antifungal medications are available for treating systemic fungal infections. These include voriconazole (Vfend), itraconazole (Sporanox), lipid amphotericin formulations, caspofungin (Cancidas), micafungin (Mycamine), and posaconazole (Noxafil).

Prevention

The prevalence of fungi in a variety of settings that one might visit on a regular basis make it difficult to entirely avoid fungal infections. However, a number of steps can be taken to reduce that risk, most based on the concept that fungi grow and reproduce best in damp, warm settings. Locker room floors, for example, are an almost ideal environment for the growth of fungi. Individuals who have already had one fungal infection may be prone to acquire a second such infection, so some of the following preventive measures are of particular value:

- Avoid walking barefoot in locker rooms, bathrooms, gyms, and other areas that are likely to remain damp and are used by many individuals.
- Make sure your footwear fits properly, and replace footwear when it becomes worn out. Never share footwear with other people.
- Use a light dusting of antifungal powder if sensitive to fungal infections.
- In any case, keep your feet clean, cool, and dry to the extent possible when wearing socks and shoes.
- Showering with an anti-dandruff shampoo, such as Selsun Blue (selenium sulfide), can be used to protect the groin area against infection.
- Keep toenails and fingernails short and neatly groomed.
- Wear loose clothing to prevent the development of fungal infections on the body.
- Avoid contact with anyone known to be infected with any type of superficial fungal infection.
- Do not share personal items with other individuals, such as combs, brushes, or sports gear.
- Avoid contact with animals who appear to have fungal infections, such as those with bald spots on their body.

People with compromised immune systems may need to take special precautions to avoid contracting more dangerous systemic infections. One approach is to avoid, wherever possible, going to an area where a specific type of fungal infection is known to be more common. Generally speaking, one should also avoid coming into contact with soil where fungi may be present, and it may be necessary upon occasion to wear a face mask or filter if the risk of encountering fungi is known to be high. In any case, aggressive hand washing and other hygienic procedures are always important.

Prognosis

Most cases of superficial fungal infections can be cured with OTC medications at the very least, or prescription medications if OTC products do not work. Systemic infections may present more of a problem, although they are also susceptible to most treatments or likely to resolve on their own, even without treatment. Patients with compromised immune systems or others who may be at greater risk pose a very different problem. In such cases, prognosis for recovery significantly depends on a person's overall general health and the stage at which the infection is diagnosed. In the most serious cases, spread of fungi throughout the body may overwhelm the body's immune system, ultimately resulting in death.

Public Health Concerns

Fungal infections are becoming an issue of increasing concern among public health agencies primarily for three reasons. First, the HIV/AIDS epidemic that has swept through the United States (and the rest of the world) since the 1980s has vastly increased the number of individuals with weakened immune systems. These individuals are at significantly greater risk for infections such as aspergillosis and cryptococcosis then is the general population. Second, fungal infections have become a vastly more important source of hospital infections over the past few decades. Today, infections caused by *C. albicans* are the

QUESTIONS TO ASK YOUR DOCTOR

- The fungal infection on my feet has lasted for a long time. Is it likely to develop into a more serious medical problem?
- My job requires me to spend a great deal of time in remote desert regions of Arizona. Am I at risk for any particular fungal infection in this region?
- Are there special precautionary steps I should take to avoid fungal infections in our region of the country?
- What risks do I face from fungal infections during my forthcoming stay in the hospital?
- What are the risks my chidren will face in pre-school and kindergarten for fungal infections? What steps should I take to reduce those risks?
- What steps can I take to reduce the risks my children are likely to encounter for fungal infections at high school?

primary cause of hospital-associated infections in the United States. Third, a number of fungal infections endemic to certain regions of the United States are becoming increasingly common as community-acquired infections. Primary among these diseases are blastomycosis in the eastern states, cryptococcus along the Pacific coast, and coccidioidomycosis in the Southwestern states.

Efforts and Solutions

In the United States, the Mycotic Diseases Branch of the CDC has undertaken an aggressive program to learn more about fungal infections and to develop programs for bringing these diseases under better control. Some of the activities involved in this effort include:

- following up on outbreaks of a disease with epidemiologic studies of the region involved
- monitoring long-term trends of disease patterns for each type of infection
- developing, evaluating, and promoting guidelines and strategies for dealing with each type of infection
- conducting laboratory research to learn more about the etiology, epidemiology, and transmission of each infection
- improving the physical capabilities of laboratories for the study and treatment of fungal infections.

Resources

BOOKS

Kauffmann, Carol A. *Essentials of Clinical Mycology*. New York: Springer, 2011.

Larone, Davise H. *Medically Important Fungi: A Guide to Identification*. Washington, DC: ASM Press, 2011.

Sax, Paul E., Calvin J. Cohen, and Daniel R. Kuritzkes. *HIV essentials*. Burlington, MA: Jones & Bartlett Learning, 2012.

Wertheim, Heiman F.L., Peter Horby, and John P. Woodall. *Atlas of Human Infectious Diseases*. Hoboken, NJ: John Wiley & Sons, 2012.

PERIODICALS

Barron, Michelle A. "Medical Mycology for the Hospital Epidemiologist." *Current Fungal Infection Reports* 6, 1. (2012): 74–80.

Baskova, L., and V. Buchta. "Laboratory Diagnostics of Invasive Fungal Infections: An Overview with Emphasis on Molecular Approach." *Folia Microbiologica* 57, 5. (2012): 421–30.

Lionakis, Michail S. "Genetic Susceptibility to Fungal Infections in Humans." *Current Fungal Infection Reports* 6, 1. (2012): 11–22.

Repetto, E.C., C.G. Giacomazzi, and F. Castelli. "Hospital-related Outbreaks Due to Rare Fungal Pathogens: A Review of the Literature from 1990 to June 2011." *European Journal of Clinical Microbiology & Infectious Diseases* 31, 11. (2012): 2897–904.

WEBSITES

"Fungal Diseases." Centers for Disease Control and Prevention. http://www.cdc.gov/fungal/. Accessed October 30, 2012.

"Fungal Infections." Better Medicine. http://www.localhealth.com/article/fungal-infections. Accessed October 30, 2012.

"Fungal Infections of the Skin." WebMD. http://www.webmd.com/skin-problems-and-treatments/guide/fungal-infections-skin. Accessed October 30, 2012.

"How A Benign Fungus Can Become Life-Threatening." Science Daily. http://www.sciencedaily.com/releases/2007/10/071004165553.htm. Accessed October 30, 2012.

ORGANIZATIONS

Centers for Disease Control and Prevention, 1600 Clifton Rd., N.E., Atlanta, GA USA 30333, 1 (800) 232–4636, cdcinfo@cdc.gov., www.cdc.gov.

David E. Newton, Ed.D.

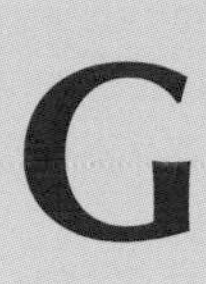

Genetic testing and counseling

Definition

A genetic test seeks to identify changes in a person's chromosomes, genes, or proteins, that are associated with inherited disorders. Genetic testing is performed to determine whether a person has, or will develop, a certain disease or could pass a disease to his or her offspring. Genetic tests also determine whether couples are at a higher risk than the general population for having a child affected with a genetic disorder. Genetic testing is often followed by genetic counseling, which is a communication process by which personal genetic risk information is translated into practical information for families. Genetic counselors are commonly health care professionals with specialized training and experience in the areas of medical genetics and counseling. They work as members of a health care team, providing individuals and families with information on the nature, inheritance, and implications of genetic disorders to help them make informed medical and personal decisions.

Purpose

Some families or ethnic groups have a higher incidence of a certain disease than does the population as a whole. For example, individuals from Eastern European, Ashkenazi Jewish descent are at higher risk for carrying genes for rare conditions that occur much less frequently in populations from other parts of the world. Before having a child, a couple from such a family or ethnic group may want to know whether their child would be at risk of having that disease. Genetic testing for this purpose is called genetic screening.

During pregnancy, a baby's cells can be studied for certain genetic disorders or chromosomal problems such as Down syndrome. Chromosome testing is most commonly offered when the mother is 35 years or older at the time of delivery. When there is a family medical history of a genetic disease or there are individuals in a family affected with developmental and physical delays, genetic testing may also be offered during pregnancy. Genetic testing during pregnancy is called prenatal diagnosis.

Prior to becoming pregnant, couples who are having difficulty conceiving a child or who have suffered multiple miscarriages may be tested to see whether a genetic cause can be identified.

A genetic disease may be diagnosed at birth by doing a physical evaluation of the baby and observing characteristics of the disorder. Genetic testing can help to confirm the diagnosis made by the physical evaluation. In addition, genetic testing is used routinely on all newborns to screen for certain genetic diseases that can affect a newborn baby's health shortly after birth.

There are several genetic diseases and conditions in which the symptoms do not occur until adulthood. One such example is Huntington's disease. This is a serious disorder affecting the way in which individuals walk, talk, and function on a daily basis. Genetic testing may be able to determine whether someone at risk for the disease will in fact develop the disease.

Some genetic defects may make a person more susceptible to certain types of **cancer**. Testing for these defects can help predict a person's risk. Other types of genetic tests help diagnose and predict and monitor the course of certain kinds of cancer, particularly leukemia and lymphoma.

Following a genetic test, an individual or couple may be offered genetic counseling to better understand the results and implications of the test. Specifically, the process of genetic counseling supports families by:

- Helping them understand information about birth defects or genetic disorders. This includes explaining patterns of inheritance, recurrence risks, natural history of diseases, and genetic testing options.

- Providing nondirective supportive counseling regarding emotional issues related to a diagnosis or testing options.
- Helping individuals or families make decisions that they are comfortable with, based on their personal ethical and religious standards.
- Connecting families with appropriate resources, such as support groups or specific types of medical clinics, locally and nationally.

As of 2012, 25 universities in the United States and three universities in Canada were offering genetic counseling study programs that had been approved by the American Board of Genetic Counseling (ABGC). Most genetic counseling programs are two-year programs that include course work, clinical rotations, and an independent research project. Most applicants enter the field from a variety of disciplines, including biology, genetics, psychology, and nursing.

Description

Gene tests

Gene tests look for signs of a disease by examining DNA taken from a person's blood, body fluids, or tissues. The tests can look for large changes, such as a gene that has a section missing or added, or small changes, such as a missing, added, or altered chemical base within the DNA strand. Other important changes can be genes with too many copies, genes that are too active, genes that are turned off, or those that are lost entirely.

Various techniques are used for gene tests. Direct DNA sequencing examines the direct base pair sequence of a gene for specific gene mutations. Some genes contain more than 100,000 bases; a mutation of any base can make the gene nonfunctional and cause disease. The more mutations possible, the less likely it is for a test to detect all of them. This test is usually done on white blood cells from a person's blood but can also be performed on other tissues. There are different ways in which to perform direct DNA mutation analysis. When the specific genetic mutation is known, it is possible to perform a complete analysis of the genetic code, also called direct sequencing. There are several different lab techniques used to test for a direct mutation. One common approach begins by using chemicals to separate DNA from the rest of the cell. Next, the two strands of DNA are separated by heating. Special enzymes (called restriction enzymes) are added to the single strands of DNA, where they act like scissors and cut the strands in specific places. The DNA fragments are then sorted by size through a process called electrophoresis. A special piece of DNA, called a probe, is added to the fragments. The probe is designed to bind to specific mutated portions of the gene. When bound to the probe, the mutated portions appear on x-ray film with a distinct banding pattern.

Another gene test technique is indirect DNA testing. Family linkage studies are done to study a disease when the exact type and location of the genetic alteration is not known, but the general location on the chromosome has been identified. These studies are possible when a chromosome marker has been found associated with a disease. Chromosomes contain certain regions that vary in appearance among individuals. These regions are called polymorphisms and do not cause a genetic disease to occur. If a polymorphism is always present in family members with the same genetic disease, and absent in family members without the disease, it is likely that the gene responsible for the disease is near that polymorphism. The gene mutation can be indirectly detected in family members by looking for the polymorphism.

To look for the polymorphism, DNA is isolated from cells in the same way it is for direct DNA mutation analysis. A probe is added that will detect the large polymorphism on the chromosome. When bound to the probe, this region will appear on x-ray film with a distinct banding pattern. The pattern of banding of a person being tested for the disease is compared to the pattern from a family member affected by the disease.

Linkage studies have disadvantages not found in direct DNA mutation analysis. These studies require multiple family members to participate in the testing. If key family members choose not to participate, the incomplete family history may make testing other members useless. The indirect method of detecting a mutated gene also brings more opportunity for error.

Chromosome tests

Various genetic syndromes are caused by structural chromosome abnormalities. To analyze a person's chromosomes, his or her cells are allowed to grow and multiply in the laboratory until they reach a certain stage of growth. The length of growing time varies with the type of cells. Cells from blood and bone marrow take one to two days; fetal cells from amniotic fluid take 7–10 days.

When the cells are ready, they are placed on a microscope slide using a technique to make them burst open, spreading their chromosomes. The slides are stained: the stain creates a banding pattern unique to each chromosome. Under a microscope, the chromosomes are counted, identified, and analyzed based on their size, shape, and stained appearance.

Types of chromosome tests include the karyotype test and the FISH (fluorescent in situ hybridization) test.

In a karyotype test, the chromosomes are counted, and a photograph is taken of the chromosomes from one or more cells as seen through the microscope. Then the chromosomes are cut out and arranged side-by-side with their partner in ascending numerical order, from largest to smallest. The karyotype is done either manually or by using a computer attached to the microscope. The FISH test identifies specific regions on chromosomes using fluorescent DNA probes. FISH analysis can find small pieces of chromosomes that are missing or have extra copies and that can be missed by the karyotype test.

Biochemical tests

Genes contain instructions for making proteins, and abnormal protein levels can be indicative of a genetic disorder. Biochemical tests look at the level of key proteins. This level can identify genes that are not working normally. These tests are typically used for newborn screening. For example, this screening can detect infants who have metabolic conditions such as phenylketonuria (PKU).

Applications of genetic testing

Newborn screening

In the United States, genetic testing is used most often for newborn screening, a major public health program that can find disorders in newborns that have long-term health effects. Newborn screening tests infant blood samples for abnormal or missing gene products. Every year, millions of newborn babies have their blood samples tested for potentially serious genetic diseases. As of 2012, all 50 states and the District of Columbia required newborn screening for eight conditions, including two endocrine deficiencies, three blood-related disorders, cystic fibrosis, and two enzyme deficiency disorders. Thirty-four states and the District also required a test for hearing problems; the remaining 14 states offered that test as an option. A new technology called tandem mass spectrometry allows screening of up to 30 other metabolic disorders.

Carrier testing

An individual who has a gene associated with a disease but never exhibits any symptoms of the disease is called a carrier. A carrier is a person who is not affected by the mutated gene he or she possesses, but can pass the gene to an offspring. Genetic tests have been developed that tell prospective parents whether they are carriers of certain diseases. If one or both parents are a carrier, the risk of passing the disease to a child can be predicted.

To predict the risk, it is necessary to know if the gene in question is autosomal or sex–linked. If the gene is carried on any of chromosomes 1–22, the resulting disease is called an autosomal disease. If the gene is carried on the X or Y chromosome, it is called a sex-linked disease.

Sex-linked diseases, such as the bleeding condition hemophilia, are usually carried on the X chromosome. A woman who carries a disease–associated gene on one of her X chromosomes has a 50% chance of passing that gene to her son. A son who inherits that gene will develop the disease because he does not have another normal copy of the gene on a second X chromosome to compensate for the abnormal copy. A daughter who inherits the disease-associated gene from her mother will be at risk for having a son affected with the disease.

The risk of passing an autosomal disease to a child depends on whether the gene is dominant or recessive. A prospective parent carrying a dominant gene has a 50% chance of passing the gene to a child. A child needs to receive only one copy of the mutated gene to be affected by the disease.

If the gene is recessive, a child needs to receive two copies of the mutated gene, one from each parent, to be affected by the disease. When both parents are carriers, their child has a 25% chance of inheriting two copies of the mutated gene and being affected by the disease; a 50% chance of inheriting one copy of the mutated gene, and being a carrier of the disease but not affected; and a 25% chance of inheriting two normal genes. When only one parent is a carrier, a child has a 50% chance of inheriting one mutated gene and being an unaffected carrier of the disease, and a 50% chance of inheriting two normal genes.

Cystic fibrosis is a disease that affects the lungs and pancreas and is discovered in early childhood. It is the most common autosomal recessive genetic disease found in the Caucasian population: one in 25 people of Northern European ancestry is a carrier of a mutated cystic fibrosis gene. The gene, located on chromosome 7, was identified in 1989.

The gene mutation for cystic fibrosis is detected by a direct DNA test. Over 600 mutations of the cystic fibrosis gene have been found; each of these mutations causes the same disease. Tests are available for the most common mutations. Tests that check for the 86 of the most common mutations in the Caucasian population will detect 90% of carriers for cystic fibrosis. (The percentage of mutations detected varies according to the individual's ethnic background). If a person tests negative, it is likely, but not guaranteed, that he or she does not have the gene. Both parents must be carriers of the gene to have a child with cystic fibrosis.

Tay–Sachs disease, also autosomal recessive, affects children primarily of Ashkenazi Jewish descent. Children with this disease usually die between the ages of two and five. This disease was previously detected by looking for a missing enzyme. The mutated gene has now been identified and can be detected using direct DNA mutation analysis.

Presymptomatic testing

Not all genetic diseases show their effect immediately at birth or early in childhood. Although the gene mutation is present at birth, some diseases do not appear until adulthood. If a specific mutated gene responsible for a late-onset disease has been identified, a person from an affected family can be tested before symptoms appear.

Huntington disease is one example of a late-onset autosomal dominant disease. Its symptoms of mental confusion and abnormal body movements do not appear until middle to late adulthood. The chromosome location of the gene responsible for Huntington chorea was located in 1983 after studying the DNA from a large Venezuelan family affected by the disease. Ten years later, the gene was identified. A test is now available to detect the presence of the expanded base pair sequence responsible for causing the disease. The presence of this expanded sequence means the person will develop the disease.

Another late-onset disease, Alzheimer's, does not have as well-understood a genetic cause as Huntington disease. The specific genetic cause of Alzheimer disease is not as clear. Although many cases appear to be inherited in an autosomal dominant pattern, many cases exist as single incidents in a family. Like Huntington, symptoms of mental deterioration first appear in adulthood. Genetic research has found an association between this disease and genes on four different chromosomes. The validity of looking for these genes in a person without symptoms or without family history of the disease is still being studied.

CANCER SUSCEPTIBILITY TESTING. Cancer can result from an inherited (germline) mutated gene or a gene that mutated sometime during a person's lifetime (acquired mutation). Some genes, called tumor suppressor genes, produce proteins that protect the body from cancer. If one of these genes develops a mutation, it is unable to produce the protective protein. If the second copy of the gene is normal, its action may be sufficient to continue production, but if that gene later also develops a mutation, the person is vulnerable to cancer. Other genes, called oncogenes, are involved in the normal growth of cells. A mutation in an oncogene can cause too much growth, which is the beginning of cancer.

Direct DNA tests are currently available to look for gene mutations identified and linked to several kinds of cancer. People with a family history of these cancers are those most likely to be tested. If one of these mutated genes is found, the person is more susceptible to developing the cancer. The likelihood that the person will develop the cancer, even with the mutated gene, is not always known because other genetic and environmental factors are also involved in the development of cancer.

Cancer susceptibility tests are most useful when a positive test result can be followed with clear treatment options. In families with familial polyposis of the colon, testing a child for a mutated APC gene can reveal whether the child needs frequent monitoring for the disease. In families with potentially fatal familial medullary thyroid cancer or multiple endocrine neoplasia type 2, finding a mutated RET gene in a child provides the opportunity for that child to have preventive removal of the thyroid gland. In the same way, MSH1 and MSH2 mutations can reveal which members in an affected family are vulnerable to familiar colorectal cancer and would benefit from aggressive monitoring.

In 1994, a mutation linked to early-onset familial breast and ovarian cancer was identified. BRCA1 is located on chromosome 17. Women with a mutated form of this gene have an increased risk of developing breast and ovarian cancer. A second related gene, BRCA2, was later discovered. Located on chromosome 13, it also carries increased risk of breast and ovarian cancer. Although both genes are rare in the general population, they are slightly more common in women of Ashkenazi Jewish descent.

When a woman is found to have a mutation in one of these genes, the likelihood that she will develop breast or ovarian cancer increases, but not to 100%. Other genetic and environmental factors influence the outcome.

Testing for these genes is most valuable in families where a mutation has already been found. BRCA1 and BRCA2 are large genes; BRCA1 includes 100,000 bases. More than 120 mutations to this gene have been discovered, but a mutation could occur in any of the bases. Studies show tests for these genes may miss 30% of existing mutations. The rate of missed mutations, the unknown disease likelihood in spite of a positive result, and the lack of a clear preventive response to a positive result make the value of this test for the general population uncertain.

Prenatal and postnatal chromosome analysis

Chromosome analysis is performed on fetal cells primarily when the mother is age 35 or older at the time of delivery, has experienced multiple miscarriages, or reports a family history of a genetic abnormality.

Prenatal testing is done on the fetal cells from a chorionic villus sampling (from the baby's developing placenta) at 10–12 weeks or from the amniotic fluid (the fluid surrounding the baby) at 16–18 weeks of pregnancy. Cells from amniotic fluid grow for 7–10 days before they are ready to be analyzed. Chorionic villi cells have the potential to grow faster and can be analyzed sooner.

Chromosome analysis using blood cells is done on a child who is born with, or later develops, signs of mental retardation or physical malformation. In the older child, chromosome analysis may be done to investigate developmental delays.

Extra or missing chromosomes cause mental and physical abnormalities. A child born with an extra chromosome 21 (trisomy 21) has Down syndrome. An extra chromosome 13 or 18 also produces well-known syndromes. A missing X chromosome causes Turner syndrome, and an extra X in a male causes Klinefelter syndrome. Other abnormalities are caused by extra or missing pieces of chromosomes. Fragile X syndrome is a sex-linked disease that causes mental retardation in males.

Chromosomal material may also be rearranged, such as the end of chromosome 1 moving to the end of chromosome 3. This is called a chromosomal translocation. If no material is added or deleted in the exchange, the person might not be affected. Such an exchange, however, can cause **infertility** or abnormalities if passed to children.

Evaluation of a man and woman's infertility or repeated miscarriages will include blood studies of both to check for a chromosome translocation. Many chromosome abnormalities are incompatible with life; babies with these abnormalities often miscarrry during the first trimester. Cells from a baby that died before birth can be studied to look for chromosome abnormalities that may have caused the death.

Diagnostic testing

This type of genetic testing is used to confirm a diagnosis when a person has signs or symptoms of a genetic disease. The genetic test used depends on the disease for which a person is tested. For example, if a patient has physical features indicative of Down syndrome, a chromosomal test is used. To test for Duchenne muscular dystrophy, a gene test is done to look for missing sections in the dystrophin gene.

Chromosome tests are also used to diagnose certain cancers, particularly leukemia and lymphoma, which are associated with changes in chromosomes: extra or missing complete chromosomes, extra or missing portions of chromosomes, or exchanges of material (translocations) between chromosomes. Studies show that the locations of the chromosome breaks are at locations of tumor-suppressor genes or oncogenes.

Chromosome analysis on cells from blood, bone marrow, or solid tumor helps diagnose certain kinds of leukemia and lymphoma and often helps predict how well the person will respond to treatment. After treatment has begun, periodic monitoring of these chromosome changes in the blood and bone marrow gives the physician information as to the effectiveness of the treatment.

A well-known chromosome rearrangement is found in chronic myelogenous leukemia. This leukemia is associated with an exchange of material between chromosomes 9 and 22. The resulting smaller chromosome 22 is called the Philadelphia chromosome.

Pharmacogenetic testing

Among the latest types of genetic testing is pharmacogenetic testing. This test examines a person's genes to gain information on how drugs would be broken down by the body. Pharmacogenetic testing aims to design drug treatments that are specific to each person. For example, a test used in patients who have chronic myelogenous leukemia can show which patients would benefit from a medicine called Gleevac (Imatinib). Another test looks at a liver enzyme called cytochrome P450, which breaks down certain types of drugs. Gene mutations can affect the ability of the body to break down certain drugs, and people with a less active form of P450 might be taking excessive levels of a drug. Pharmacogenetic testing seeks to help patients obtain the right amount of a medication.

Precautions

Because genetic testing is not always accurate, and because there are privacy concerns for the individual receiving a genetic test, genetic counseling should always be performed prior to genetic testing. Genetic counseling is also commonly offered after a test has been performed.

Prenatal genetic counseling

There are several different reasons why a person or couple may seek prenatal genetic counseling. If a woman is age 35 or older and pregnant, there is an increased chance that the fetus may have a change in the number of chromosomes present. Changes in chromosome number may lead to mental retardation and **birth defects**. Down syndrome is the most common change in chromosome number that occurs more often in the fetuses of older women. Couples may seek prenatal genetic counseling because of abnormal results of screening tests performed during pregnancy. A blood test called the alpha fetal protein (AFP) test is offered to all pregnant women. This blood test screens for Down syndrome, open spine defects (spina bifida), and another type of mental retardation caused by a change in chromosome number called trisomy 18. When this test is abnormal, further tests are offered to obtain more information about the chance of these conditions in the fetus. Another reason that people seek prenatal genetic counseling is a family history of birth defects or inherited diseases. In some cases, blood tests on the parents may be available to indicate whether their children would be at risk of being affected. Genetic counselors assess risk in each case, help patients understand their risks, and explore how patients feel about, or cope with, these risks.

Prenatal tests that are offered during genetic counseling include level II ultrasounds, maternal serum AFP screening, chorionic villus sampling (CVS), and amniocentesis. Level II ultrasound is a detailed ultrasound surveying fetal anatomy for birth defects. Ultrasound is limited to detection of structural changes in anatomy and cannot detect changes in chromosome number. The maternal serum AFP screening is used to indicate whether a pregnant woman has a higher or lower chance of certain birth defects. This test can only change the chances for a birth defect. The screening cannot diagnose a birth defect. CVS is a way of learning how many chromosomes are present in a fetus. A small piece of placental tissue is obtained for these studies during the tenth to twelfth weeks of pregnancy. Amniocentesis is also a way of learning how many chromosomes are present in a fetus. Amniotic fluid is obtained for these studies, usually between 16 and 18 weeks of pregnancy. There is a small risk for miscarriage with both of these tests. Genetic counseling regarding these procedures involves the careful explanation of benefits and limitations of each testing option. The counselor also tries to explore how patients feel about prenatal testing and the impact of such testing on the pregnancy. Genetic counselors are supportive of any decision a patient makes about whether to have prenatal tests performed.

Pediatric genetic counseling

Families or pediatricians seek genetic counseling when a child has features of an inherited condition. Any child who is born with more than one birth defect, mental retardation, or dysmorphic features has an increased chance of having a genetic syndrome. One common type of mental retardation in males for which genetic testing is available is fragile X syndrome. Genetic testing is also available for many other childhood illnesses, such as hemophilia and muscular dystrophy. Genetic counselors work with medical geneticists to determine if a genetic syndrome is present. This process includes a careful examination of family history, medical history of the child, review of pertinent medical records in the family, a physical examination of the child, and sometimes blood work or other diagnostic tests. If a diagnosis is made, then the medical geneticist and genetic counselor review what is known about the inheritance of the condition, the natural history of the condition, treatment options, further examinations that may be needed for health problems common in the diagnosed syndrome, and resources for helping the family. The genetic counselor also helps the family adjust to the diagnosis by emotional support and counseling. Many families are devastated by receiving a diagnosis, learning of the likely outcome for the child, and the loss of the hoped-for healthy child. There would also be a discussion about recurrence risks in the family and who else in the family may be at risk.

Adult genetic counseling

Adults seek genetic counseling when a person in the family decides to be tested for a known genetic condition in the family, when an adult begins exhibiting symptoms of an inherited condition, or when there is a new diagnosis of someone with an adult onset disorder in the family. In addition, sometimes the birth of a child with obvious features of a genetic disease leads to diagnosis of a parent who is affected more mildly. Genetic counseling for adults may lead to the consideration of presymptomatic genetic testing. Testing a person to determine whether they will be symptomatic for a condition before the symptoms occur is an area of controversy. Huntington disease is an example of a genetic disease for which presymptomatic testing is available. It is a neurological disease resulting in dementia. Onset of the condition is between 30 to 50 years of age. Huntington disease is inherited in an autosomal dominant pattern. If a person has a parent with the disease, his or her risk of being affected is 50%. Would presymptomatic testing relieve or create anxiety? Would a person benefit from removal of doubt about being affected? Would knowing help a person with life planning? Genetic counselors help patients sort through their feelings about such testing and whether the results would be helpful to them.

Cancer genetic counseling

A family history of early-onset breast, ovarian, or colon cancer in multiple generations of a family is a common reason why a person would seek a genetic counselor who works with cancer patients. While most cancer is not inherited, there are some families in which a dominant gene is present and causing the disease. The genetic counselor can discuss with a patient the chance that the cancer in the family is related to a dominantly inherited gene. The counselor can also discuss the option of testing for the breast and ovarian cancer genes, BRCA1 and BRCA2. In some cases, the person seeking testing has already had cancer. Therefore, presymptomatic testing is also an issue in cancer genetics. Emotional support is important for these patients as they have often lost close relatives from cancer and are fearful of their own risks. For families in which a dominant form of cancer is detected through genetic testing, a plan for increased surveillance for the disease can be made.

Pedigree

In all types of genetic counseling, one important aspect of the genetic counseling session is information gathering about family and medical history. Information gathering is performed by drawing a chart called a pedigree. A pedigree is made of symbols and lines that represent the family history. To accurately assess the risk of inherited diseases, information about three generations of the family, including health status and/or cause of death, is usually needed. If the family history is complicated, information from more distant relatives may be helpful, and medical records may be requested for any family members who have had a genetic disorder. Through an examination of the family history, a counselor may be able to discuss the probability of future occurrence of genetic disorders.

ETHNICITY. In taking a family history, a genetic counselor asks for the patient's ethnicity or ancestral origin. There are some ethnic groups that have a higher chance of being carriers of specific genetic diseases. For instance, the chance that an African American is a carrier of a gene for sickle cell disease is one in ten individuals. People of Jewish ancestry are more likely to be carriers of several conditions, including Tay–Sachs disease, Canavan disease, and cystic fibrosis. People of Mediterranean ancestry are more likely to be carriers of a type of anemia called thalassemia. Genetic counselors discuss inheritance patterns of these diseases, carrier risks, and genetic screening or testing options.

CONSANGUNITY. Another question a genetic counselor asks in taking a family history is if the couple is related to one another by blood. The practice of marrying or having children with relatives is infrequent in the United States, but is more common in some countries. When two people are related by blood, there is an increased chance for their children to be affected with conditions inherited in a recessive pattern. In recessive inheritance, each parent of a child affected with a disease carries a single gene for the disease. The child gets two copies, one from each parent, and is affected. People who have a common ancestor are more likely than unrelated people to be carriers of genes for the same recessively inherited genes. Depending on family history and ethnic background, blood tests can be offered to couples to get more information about the chance for these conditions to occur.

EXPOSURES DURING PREGNANCY. During prenatal genetic counseling, the counselor will ask about pregnancy history. If the patient has taken a medication or has had a harmful exposure (like **radiation**), the genetic counselor can discuss the possibility of harmful effects. Ultrasound is often a useful tool to look for some affects of exposures.

Ethical issues in genetic counseling

Prenatal diagnosis of anomalies or chromosomal abnormalities leads to a decision about whether a couple wishes to continue a pregnancy. Some couples chose to continue a pregnancy. Prenatal counseling gives them additional time to prepare emotionally for the birth of the child and to gather resources. Others choose not to continue a pregnancy in which problems have been diagnosed. These couples have unique emotional needs. Often the child is very much a desired addition to the family, and parents are devastated that the child is not healthy. Presymptomatic testing for adult onset disorders and cancer raise difficult issues regarding the need to know and the reality of dealing with abnormal results before symptoms. The National Society of Genetic Counselors (NSGC) has established a Code of Ethics to guide genetic counselors in caring for patients. The NSGC Code of Ethics, last updated in 2006, is based on four ethical principles:

- Beneficience is the promotion of personal well-being in others. The genetic counselor is an advocate for the patient.
- Nonmaleficience is the idea of doing no harm to a patient.
- Autonomy is recognizing the value of the individual, the person's abilities, and their point of view. Important aspects of autonomy include truthfulness with patients, respecting confidentiality, and practicing informed consent.
- Justice is providing equal care for all, freedom of choice, and a high quality of care.

Perhaps the main ethical principle of genetic counseling is the attempt to provide nondirective counseling. This requires a patient-centered approach by providing care focused on the thoughts and feelings of the patient. Five percent of the Human Genome Project budget is assigned to research involving the best way to address ethical issues that arise as new genetic tests become available. Genetic counselors can help patients navigate through the unfamiliar territory of genetic testing.

Preparation

Most tests for genetic diseases of children and adults are done on blood. To collect the 5–10 mL of blood needed, a health care worker draws blood from a vein in the inner elbow region. Collection of the sample takes only a few minutes.

Prenatal testing is done either on amniotic fluid or a chorionic villus sampling. To collect amniotic fluid, a physician performs a procedure called amniocentesis. An ultrasound is done to find the baby's position and an area filled with amniotic fluid. The physician inserts a needle through the woman's skin and the wall of her uterus and withdraws 5–10 mL of amniotic fluid. Placental tissue for a chorionic villus sampling is taken through the cervix. Each procedure takes approximately 30 minutes.

Bone marrow is used for chromosome analysis in a person with leukemia or lymphoma. The person is given local anesthesia. Then the physician inserts a needle through the skin and into the bone (usually the sternum or hip bone). One–half to 2 mL of bone marrow is withdrawn. This procedure takes approximately 30 minutes.

Aftercare

After blood collection, the person can feel discomfort or bruising at the puncture site or may become dizzy or faint. Pressure to the puncture site until the bleeding stops reduces bruising. Warm packs to the puncture site relieve discomfort.

The chorionic villus sampling, amniocentesis, and bone marrow procedures are all done under a physician's supervision. The person is asked to rest after the procedure and is watched for weakness and signs of bleeding.

Risks

Collection of amniotic fluid and chorionic villus sampling have the risk of miscarriage, infection, and bleeding; the risks are higher for the chorionic villus sampling. Because of the potential risks for miscarriage—0.5% following the amniocentesis and 1% following the chorionic villus sampling procedure—both of these prenatal tests are offered to couples, but not required. A woman should tell her physician immediately if she has cramping, bleeding, fluid loss, an increased temperature, or a change in the baby's movement following either of these procedures.

KEY TERMS

Autosomal disease—A disease caused by a gene mutation located on a chromosome other than a sex chromosome.

Carrier—An individual who possesses a genetic mutation associated with a recessive disorder, but who usually does not display symptoms of that disease. Carriers can pass the mutation on to their offspring.

Consangunity—Relation to a common ancestor; blood relative.

Dominant inheritance—A pattern of inheritance in which a trait or disease is conferred by one gene or allele. A parent with a disorder caused by a dominant allele has a 50% chance of passing the trait for disease to their offspring.

Karyotype—A photomicrograph (picture taken through a microscope) of a person's 46 chromosomes, lined up in 23 pairs, that is used to identify some types of genetic disorders.

Oncogene—A gene that causes normal cell growth, but if mutated or expressed at high levels, encourages normal cells to change into cancerous cells.

Recessive inheritance—A pattern of inheritance where both parents carry the gene responsible for a trait or disease (although they seldom show symptoms). Their offspring will have a 25% chance of having the trait or disease. Recessive inheritance is also responsible for disorders such as hemophilia, where the mother carries the affected gene on the X chromosome and passes it to her son.

Sex-linked genetic disorder—A disease or disorder caused by a gene mutation located on the X (female) or Y (male) chromosome.

Translocation—The rearrangement or exchange of segments of chromosomes that does not alter the total number of chromosomes, but sometimes results in a genetic disorder or disease.

After bone marrow collection, the puncture site may become tender, and the person's temperature may rise. These are signs of a possible infection.

Genetic testing involves other nonphysical risks. Many people fear the possible loss of privacy about personal health information. Other family members may be affected by the results of a person's genetic test. Privacy of the person tested and the family members affected is a consideration when deciding to have a test and to share the results.

A positive result carries a psychological burden, especially if the test indicates the person will develop a disease later in life, such as Huntington's chorea. The news that a person may be susceptible to a specific kind of cancer, while it may encourage positive preventive measures, may also negatively shadow many decisions and activities.

A genetic test result may also be inconclusive, meaning that no definitive result can be given to the individual or family. This may cause the individual to feel more anxious and frustrated and to experience psychological difficulties.

Prior to undergoing genetic testing, individuals need to learn from the genetic counselor the likelihood that the test could miss a mutation or abnormality.

Results

A normal result for chromosome analysis is 46, XX or 46, XY. This means there are 46 chromosomes (including two X chromosomes for a female or one X and one Y for a male) with no structural abnormalities. A normal result for a direct DNA mutation analysis or linkage study includes no gene mutations found.

There can be some benefits from genetic testing when the individual tested is not found to carry a genetic mutation. Those who learn with great certainty they are no longer at risk for a genetic disease may choose not to undergo prophylactic therapies and may feel relieved and less anxious.

An abnormal chromosome analysis report will include the total number of chromosomes and will identify the abnormality found. Tests for gene mutations will report the mutations found.

There are many ethical issues to consider with an abnormal prenatal test result. Many of the diseases tested for during a pregnancy cannot be treated or cured. In addition, some diseases tested for during pregnancy may have a late onset of symptoms or have minimal effects on the affected individual.

Before making decisions based on an abnormal test result, the person should meet again with a genetic counselor to fully understand the meaning of the results and learn what options are available based on the test result and what are the risks and benefits of each of those options.

Resources

BOOKS

Arribas-Ayllon, Michael, Srikant Sarangi, and Angus Clarke. *Genetic Testing: Accounts of Autonomy, Responsibility, and Blame*. London; New York: Routledge, 2011.

Parker, Michael. *Ethical Problems and Genetics Practice*. New York: Cambridge University Press, 2012.

Pfleiderer, Georg, Manuel Battegay, and Klaus Lindpaintner. *Knowing One's Medical Fate in Advance: Challenges for Diagnosis and Treatment, Philosophy, Ethics and Religion*. Basel: Karger, 2012.

Schneider, Katherine A. *Counseling about Cancer: Strategies for Genetic Counseling*. Hoboken, NJ: Wiley-Blackwell, 2012.

Stern, Alexandra. *Telling Genes: The Story of Genetic Counseling in America*. Baltimore: Johns Hopkins University Press, 2012.

Wiggins, Jennifer, and Anna Middleton. *Getting the Message Across: Communication with Diverse Populations in Clinical Genetics*. Oxford: Oxford University Press, 2013.

PERIODICALS

Caga-anan, E.C., et al. "Testing Children for Adult-onset Genetic Diseases." *Pediatrics* 129, 1. (2012): 163–7.

Cassa, C.A., et al. "Disclosing Pathogenic Genetic Variants to Research Participants: Quantifying an Emerging Ethical Responsibility." *Genome Research* 22, 3. (2012): 421–8.

Caulfield, Timothy, and Amy L. McGuire. "Direct-to-Consumer Genetic Testing: Perceptions, Problems, and Policy Responses." *Annual Review of Medicine* 63, 1. (2012): 23–33.

Hickeron, C.L., et al. "Did You Find That out in Time?: New Life Trajectories of Parents Who Choose to Continue a Pregnancy Where a Genetic Disorder Is Diagnosed or Likely." *American Journal of Medical Genetics.* 158A, 2. (2012): 373–83.

Kaphingst, K.A., et al. "Patients Understanding of and Responses to Multiplex Genetic Susceptibility Test Results." *Genetics in Medicine* 14, 7. (2012): 681–87.

Riley, Bronson D., et al. "Essential Elements of Genetic Cancer Risk Assessment, Counseling, and Testing: Updated Recommendations of the National Society of Genetic Counselors." *Journal of Genetic Counseling* 21, 2. (2012): 151–61.

OTHER

"Genetic Counseling." Human Gene Project Information. http://www.ornl.gov/sci/techresources/Human_Genome/medicine/genecounseling.shtml. Accessed on October 31, 2012.

"Genetic Counseling." March of Dimes http://www.marchofdimes.com/pregnancy/trying_geneticcounseling.html. Accessed on October 31, 2012.

"Gene Testing." Human Genome Project Information. http://www.ornl.gov/sci/techresources/Human_Genome/medicine/genetest.shtml. Accessed on October 31, 2012.

"Genetic Testing." Medline Plus. http://www.nlm.nih.gov/medlineplus/genetictesting.html. Accessed on October 31, 2012.

"Genetic Testing: What You Need to Know." American Cancer Society. http://www.cancer.org/cancer/cancercauses/geneticsandcancer/genetictesting/genetic-testing-what-you-need-to-know-toc. Accessed on October 31, 2012.

Murry, Mary M. "Prenatal Genetic Screening: Is It Right for You?" Mayo Clinic. http://www.mayoclinic.com/health/prenatal-genetic-screening/MY01966. Accessed on October 31, 2012.

"Newborn Screening." Centers for Disease Control and Prevention. http://www.cdc.gov/ncbddd/pediatricgenetics/newborn_screening.html. Accessed on October 31, 2012.

ORGANIZATIONS

EuroGentest, Gasthuisberg O&N, Herestraat 49, Box 602, Leuven, Belgium 3000, (+32)16 345860, Fax: (+32) 16 34599, http://www.eurogentest.org

March of Dimes Foundation, 1275 Mamaroneck Ave., White Plains, NY 10605, (914) 428–7100, (888) MODIMES (663–4637), Fax: (914) 428–8203, askus@marchofdimes.com, http://www.marchofdimes.com

National Office of Public Health Genomics, 1600 Clifton Rd., Atlanta, GA 30333, (770) 488–8510, (888) MODIMES (663–4637), Fax: (770) 488–8355, genetics@cdc.gov, http://www.cdc.gov/genomics

National Society of Genetic Counselors, 401 N. Michigan Ave., Chicago, IL 60611, (312) 321–6834, Fax: (312) 673–6972, nsgc@nsgc.org, http://www.nsgc.org.

Katherine S. Hunt, MS
Brenda W. Lerner

Genetically modified food

Definition

Genetically modified foods (GMFs) are substances for human or animal consumption that have been altered by the insertion of a gene from a different species of plant or other organism in order to produce a desired characteristic or trait. GMFs are also referred to as bioengineered foods, genetically modified organisms (GMOs), or transgenetic foods.

Description

All people have deoxyribonucleic acid (DNA) in their cells. DNA is where the information needed to produce and sustain life is stored. DNA is made up of strands of nucleic acids that are grouped to form individual genes. Genes contain information about how to synthesize particular proteins. The proteins synthesized lead to individual characteristics, such as hair and eye color in humans.

Plants also contain DNA, as do almost all other living things. When scientists genetically modify a plant, they take a gene from another plant or another organism, such as a bacterium, and insert it into the original plant or trade it for a gene in the original plant. Trading of genes is called transposing.

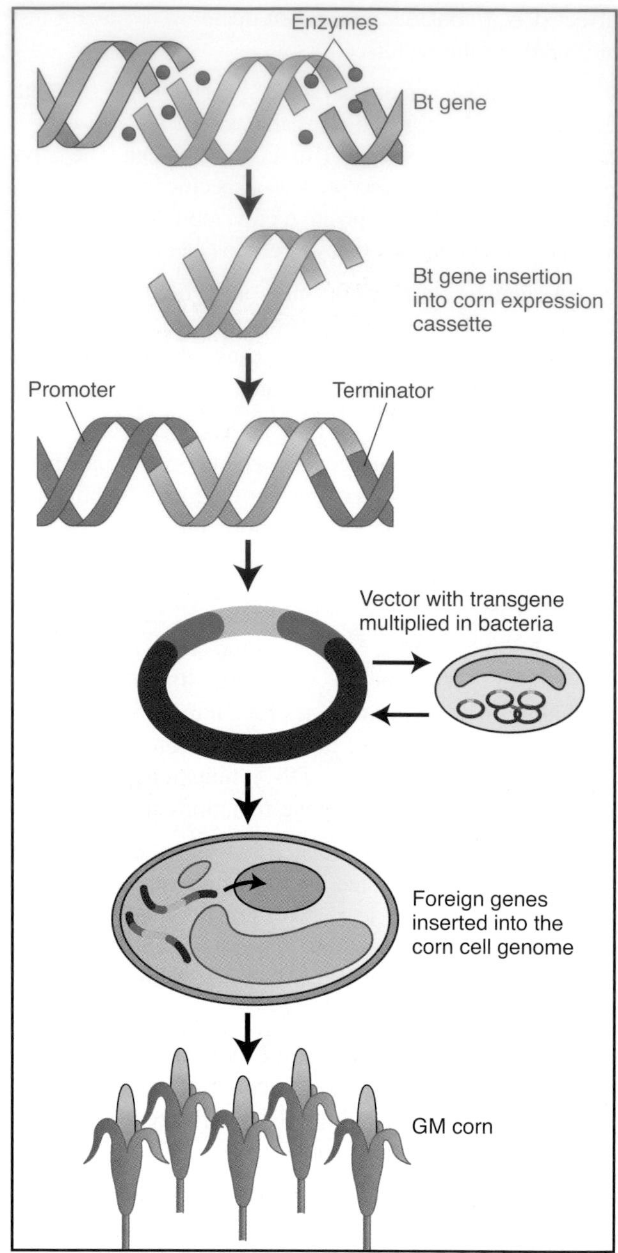

Gentically modified corn process. *(Illustration by Electronic Illustrators Group. © 2013 Cengage Learning)*

Origins

From the beginning of agriculture, people have tried breed better plants and animals. But not until the work of Gregor Mendel in the nineteenth century did people begin to understand how traits were passed from one generation to the next. Mendel did research on pea plants and discovered that traits were passed from one generation to the next in a way that could be predicted. Peas had a much simpler inheritance pattern than most organisms, so even with this knowledge it was very difficult for scientists to produce plants with the exact traits they wanted. Plants with the desired trait had to be crossbred, and then plants from the resulting generation that had the desired traits had to be selected and crossbred again and again. It takes many generations of plants to produce offspring that regularly have the desired trait. The tangelo, a cross between the tangerine and the grapefruit, was developed this way, as was the nectarine, which is a selectively bred peach.

In the 1980s, scientists learned how to successfully insert and transpose genes. In 1994, the first GMF introduced to the consumer market in the United States was the Flavr Savr tomato. This tomato was bioengineered to ripen more slowly and to remain on the vine longer so that it would be available to consumers later in the year than other tomatoes. Today, instead of crossbreeding plants repeatedly to get a new variety with the traits or characteristics they desire, scientists search for a gene in another organism that will produce the desired characteristics and then insert it into the DNA of the original plant. Often two or three different genes are inserted, sometimes each from different plants or animals.

Purpose

The purpose of genetic modification is to create plants that are in some way superior to the plant breeds currently being used. Some genetically modified plants are engineered to resist specific insects, diseases, or herbicide applications. Crops that are modified to be herbicide tolerant can thrive when an herbicide that would normally kill them is sprayed on fields to control weeds. This gives farmers a greater choice of herbicides to use. According the USDA, in 2012, 93% of the acreage planted in soybeans in the United States was genetically modified to be herbicide tolerant.

Some genetic modifications introduce a gene that creates insect disease resistance. For example, introducing a gene from *Bacillus thuringiensis*, a bacterium found in soil, makes corn (maize) resistant to corn rootworm. This means that these plants are more likely to grow big and stay healthy. Because nonorganic farming uses insecticides to protect plants, selecting plants that are genetically modified to be pest resistant allow farmers to use fewer chemical pesticides. This is good for the environment, as well as possibly less costly for the farmer, and may provide less expensive products for consumers. According to the United States Department of Agriculture (USDA), in 2012, 73% of the acreage of corn planted in the United States was genetically modified to be insect resistant and/or herbicide tolerant.

Other plants are genetically modified to increase their nutrient content or to add **vitamins** that are not usually found in the plant. A variety of rice, sometimes called "golden rice," that includes beta-carotene has been developed through genetic modification. Beta-carotene is a provitamin to vitamin A, which means that the body can use it to produce vitamin A. Rice is a staple of the diet of many Asians, and because rice does not normally contain vitamin A, many people in Asia are deficient in vitamin A. This deficiency is thought to have resulted in blindness in a quarter of a million children in southeast Asia alone. If the new strain of rice that contains beta-carotene is introduced to the area, it could help to eliminate vitamin A deficiency and significantly reduce the incidence of childhood blindness.

In addition to producing heartier crops, genetic modification is used to improve the taste of crops. Other genetic modifications introduce traits that help crops get to consumers in better condition or to have longer periods of freshness. Some plants are genetically modified to withstand drought or cold to increase the range in which they can be grown. Others have been altered to withstand high levels of salt in the soil.

Regulation

In the United States, genetically modified foods are regulated and monitored by three different government agencies: the Food and Drug Administration (FDA), the Department of Agriculture (USDA) and the **Environmental Protection Agency (EPA)**. This has given rise to some confusion about regulatory roles. The FDA is responsible for regulating nutrient content and production of genetically modified foods. The USDA oversees the safety and completeness of test fields used by bioengineering companies to test their new plants. The **EPA** regulates any genetically modified foods plants that contain pesticide-related genes and determines the effects genetically modified plants may have on the environment.

Major companies that produce genetically modified seed include Monsanto, Dow Chemical, and Syngenta. Before companies can put a genetically modified food on the market, they need to prove that it is safe for consumers. The food is evaluated for

- toxicity and direct health effects
- tendency to cause allergic reactions in humans
- the kinds of proteins synthesized by the new gene(s)
- the stability of the inserted gene(s)
- nutritional effects caused by genetic modification
- any unintended effects from gene insertion

The European Union (EU) regulates genetically modified organisms through an application procedure that combines a single approval for GMO cultivation, use in human foods, and use in animal feeds. The European Food Safety Authority (EFSA) is responsible for risk assessment of GMF crops. The EFSA report is then evaluated by at least two more commissions and committees before approval can be granted.

In Australia, the Office of the Gene Technology Regulator (OGTR) is responsible for overseeing all genetically modified organisms and genetically modified products. GMFs must undergo a safety assessment by Food Standards Australia New Zealand (FSANZ), a government agency, before they can be sold in Australia or New Zealand.

One major difference between the regulation of GMFs in the United States and the EU is in labeling requirements. In the United States, labeling of GMFs is voluntary, and the decision to label a food as genetically modified is left up to individual companies. This, however, may change in the future. A proposition (citizen-originated law) was be put to a vote in November 2012 that required all GMFs to be labeled as such if sold in the state of California. The law did not pass, which points to the efforts being derailed for the immediate future, and may well indicate the direction the United States will take in the labeling of GMFs. In the EU, labeling of GMFs is mandatory. Other differences between the EU and the US involve tracking GMFs through the production process to prevent unintended contamination.

Research and general acceptance

The appropriateness of GMFs is a hotly debated topic. GMFs are much more widely accepted in the United States than in Europe. Initially, multiple member states in the EU banned all genetically modified products. As of 2012, although there is no longer a blanket ban on GMFs in the EU, there is still much skepticism about their safety. In the United States, the **Centers for Disease Control and Prevention (CDC)** have declared GMFs to be safe for consumption. Research as of 2012 has generally supported this assessment, although some studies have suggested that long-term consumption of GMFs may increase the risk of developing **cancer**. The **CDC** does not assess environmental risks caused by GMOs.

The arguments in favor of genetically modified plants and foods include the following:

- Improved pest and disease resistance will increase crop yield, especially in the developing world.
- Increased drought, cold, and salinity tolerance will expand the range in which crops can be grown, especially in the developing world.
- Increased yields may drive down food prices.
- Plants may be genetically engineered to be more nutritious.
- Non-food plants may be genetically modified to help clean the environment by removing heavy metal pollutants.

The arguments against genetically modified plants and foods include the following:

- Genetic modification may cause plants to produce allergens, causing allergic reactions in people who would not normally be allergic to the food.
- Genetic modification may accelerate the development of drug resistant organisms, especially antibiotic resistant bacteria.
- The inserted genes may not be stable over generations of plants and may mutate in ways that harm human health or the environment.
- Genetically modified plants may crossbreed with other non-target plants and transfer genes in ways that are harmful or allow the development of plants with undesirable qualities that are difficult to control.
- Although many generations of farm animals have eaten GMFs without apparent harm, there is no way to know the long-term effects on humans.

As of 2012, the majority of scientific research appears to indicate that GMFs brought to market so far are safe. However, there is substantial concern in the United States that the process for regulating new GMOs and GMFs is not strict enough, is divided among too many agencies, and needs to be streamlined and tightened to ensure that future GMFs are safe and beneficial.

Despite scientific findings, acceptance of GMFs is low in much of Europe. In the United States, several studies have reported that consumers are aware that GMFs exist, but are not aware of how pervasive they are. For example, many consumers do not know that most

KEY TERMS

Allergen—A foreign substance that causes an allergic reaction in some sensitive people but not in most others.

Provitamin—A substance that the body can convert into a vitamin.

QUESTIONS TO ASK YOUR DOCTOR

- Are GMFs of special concern during pregnancy for me or my young children?
- Could my allergic reaction be caused by a GMF?
- Could GMFs interact with any of the medications I am taking?

foods in the United States that contain canola oil or corn products, including corn-based sweeteners, contain genetically modified ingredients. If labeling of GMFs becomes required in the United States, increased awareness of the pervasive nature of GM ingredients may cause pushback against GMFs.

Resources

BOOKS

Forman, Lillian E. *Genetically Modified Foods*. Edina, MN: ABDO Pub., 2010.

Rees, Andy *Genetically Modified Food: A Short Guide for the Confused*. Ann Arbor, MI: Pluto Press, 2006.

WEBSITES

European Union. "Food and Feed (GMO)." http://europa.eu/legislation_summaries/agriculture/food/l21154_en.htm (accessed September 20, 2012).

National Academy of Sciences. "Technology to Feed the World." http://www.nationalacademies.org/webextra/crops (accessed September 18, 2012)

WebMD. "Are Biotech Foods Safe to Eat?." http://www.webmd.com/food-recipes/features/are-biotech-foods-safe-to-eat (accessed September 18, 2012).

Whitman, Deborah B. "Genetically Modified Foods: Harmful or Helpful?." CSA Discovery Guide http://www.csa.com/discoveryguides/gmfood/overview.php (accessed September 18, 2012)

World Health Organization. "Questions on Genetically Modified Foods." http://www.who.int/foodsafety/publications/biotech/20questions/en (accessed September 18, 2012).

ORGANIZATIONS

United States Department of Agriculture, 1400 Independence Avenue, S.W., Room 1180, Washington, DC 20250, (202) 720-2791, http://www.usda.gov

United States Food and Drug Administration (FDA), 10903 New Hampshire Avenue, Silver Spring, MD 20993, (888) INFO-FDA (463-6332), http://www.fda.gov

World Health Organization, Avenue Appia 20, 1211 Geneva 27, Switzerland, +22 41 791 21 11, Fax: +22 41 791 31 11, info@who.int, http://www.who.int.

Tish Davidson, AM

Genomics

Definition

Genomics is the study of a genome, the complete collection of genes present in an organism. It includes the determination of the DNA sequence within a genome, a map of all genes present, a study of the way in which individual genes are turned on and off, the way in which genes direct the production of proteins in an organism, and the way in which genes interact with each other. Some researchers now find it useful to subdivide the general field of genomics into four discrete categories:

- Genome mapping and sequencing, which involves locating the position of genes on a chromosome and the precise sequence of base pairs within each gene
- Structural genomics, which attempts to determine the relationship between genes and the complete set of proteins for which they code in an organism
- Functional genomics, which is an effort to discover the relationship between genes and phenotypical characteristics
- Comparative genomics, in which the genomes of different species or different individuals are compared to each other.

Purpose

In one regard, the primary purpose of genomics is to discover the structure and function of all genes present in an organism. In a more comprehensive view of the goal of genomics, researchers David J. Lockhart and Elizabeth A. Winzeler explained in a 2000 paper that the purpose of genomics is "to understand biology not simply to identify its component parts." By this comment, Lockhart and Winzeler meant that it is not sufficient simply to discover the arrangement of base pairs in the DNA molecules that make up genes. It is also necessary then to determine how these arrangements explain how genes actually perform the functions they do, how the proteins they produce assemble into cells, how cells assemble into organisms, what causes cells and organisms to malfunction producing disease and causing death, and similar elements of the process called "life."

Description

Although the term *genomics* was coined as early as 1920 by the German botanist Hans Winkler (long before DNA was discovered), the first breakthrough in the field of that name did not occur until 1975, when Robert W. Holley determined the sequence of nucleotides in the RNA of the MS2 bacteriophage. The next major step in the growth of genomics occurred almost a decade later

KEY TERMS

Base pair—A pair of two nitrogen bases, such as adenine and thymine or guanine and cytosine.

DNA—The abbreviation for deoxyribonucleic acid, the molecule in which genetic information is stored.

Gene mapping—The process of determining the location of genes (or DNA segments) on a chromosome.

Genome—The complete set of genetic information in an organism.

Genomics—The study of an organism's complete genome.

Sequencing—The process of discovering the sequence of amino acids in a protein or nucleotides in a DNA molecule.

when researchers at the Chiron Corporation determined the entire sequence of the HIV-1 virus in 1984. It was another decade later, in 1995, when researchers at the Institute for Genomic Research (IGR) reported the complete genomic structure for the *Haemophilus influenzae* bacterium, the first free-living organism to have its genome sequenced. The genome consisted of 1,830,140 base pairs in a singular circular chromosome with 1,740 protein-coding genes, 58 genes coding for transfer RNA molecules and 18 genes for other RNA molecules. A year later, the complete genome for the important bacterium *Escherichia coli* was announced, and two years later, the complete genome for the first multicellular organism, the nematode (roundworm) *Caenorhabditis elegans* was also reported. By the end of the twentieth century, techniques for sequencing genomes had vastly improved, and the genomes of more and more organisms were being announced. Finally, in 2001, the first reports of a complete human genome were announced by a joint team of researchers from the Human Genome Project (HGP) and IGR. As of 2012, 180 species had had their genomes completely sequenced. The complete list of all proteins and all forms of living organisms, however, is much larger. According to the National Center for Biotechnology Information, the total number of discrete organisms for which complete genomes were available as of July 11, 2012, was 17,605. The number of completely sequenced proteins was much larger, more than 1.6 million.

The earliest DNA sequencing projects focused on determining a complete genome for certain species, such as *H. influenzae* and *E. coli*. Relatively small differences in the genomes of two individuals within the same species were not very important at that point. Determining the genomes of humans, on the other hand, requires attention to such intraspecies differences because of the information they provide about individual characteristics, such as the tendency to develop a noncommunicable disease. In fact, one researcher has suggested that genomics may provide an equivalent to the **germ theory** for noninfectious diseases. The point is that by recognizing the genomic differences between individuals who are and are not at risk for diseases such as diabetes, **cancer**, and cardiac disease, it may be possible to develop preventive technologies (similar to **vaccination** for infectious diseases) that will help prevent those diseases. As of 2012, 69 individuals had had their individual genomes sequenced. They include such well known individuals as Craig Venter, one of the pioneers in gene sequencing; James Watson, codiscoverer of the structure of the DNA molecule and formerly head of the Human Genome Project; and Steve Jobs, founder of Apple, Inc.; as well as less-well-known individuals, including members of the Han Chinese and Nigerian Yoruban populations; and a few individuals selected because of their medical condition (one being a patient with leukemia).

Effects on Public Health

Most researchers now believe that genomics has the potential for producing profound developments in the field of public health. As noted above, that belief is based on the assumption that detailed knowledge of an individual's genetic makeup should provide invaluable information as to how to prevent and/or treat many, if not all, noninfectious (and, perhaps, infectious) diseases. For example, imagine researchers finding out that certain individuals have a specific type of genome that one might describe as "leukemia-prone." And suppose that that type of genome tends to be found most commonly in a specific population, such as Korean residents of urban American cities. Then public health officials can bring to bear the full force of their knowledge, skills, and technologies on the susceptible population with the aim of reducing the risk of developing the disease among members of that population.

A 2011 study by the Center for Public Health and Community Genomics and Genetic Alliance found a number of ways in which public health agencies were making use of genomics, such as:

- The Michigan Neonatal Bank has blood samples dating to 1984 that can be analyzed to better understand health disparities among various populations in the state.

- The Michigan Department of Community Health has used genomic data to develop a better understanding of young adults at risk for sudden cardiac death and to counsel such individuals and their parents about possible preventive behaviors.
- The Hawaii Department of Health employs four full time genetic counselors to work with at risk individuals with potential medical problems identified by genomics research.
- Public health departments in four states (Michigan, Minnesota, Oregon, and Utah) have developed programs that integrate family history and surveillance data into chronic disease prevention programs.
- A number of academic institutions and public health departments have initiated research programs to determine the interaction of genetic background with environmental factors in the development of chronic noncommunicable diseases and differences observed in this pattern among varying populations.
- The U.S. Office of Minority Health has recently issued new standards for linguistically and culturally appropriate services, one of which calls for providers to maintain a demographic profile based in part on genomic research that can be used in developing prevention programs.
- The Midwest Latino Health Research, Training and Policy Center employees multilingual staff who train public health workers in the region to better understand and make use of information provided by genomics research on at-risk populations.
- The U.S. Institute of Medicine Roundtable on Translating Genomic-Based Research for Health is developing detailed plans for making use of increasingly common whole genome sequencing studies into clinical applications for individual consumers.
- Some repositories of biological materials, such as the Mayo Clinic and the Marshfield Clinic, are developing methods for integrating genomic information about populations and individuals into medical records that can be used for management recommendations for patients who fit certain profiles.
- A number of institutions of higher education, such as the University of Michigan and the University of Washington, are integrating courses on the genetic basis of disease into their regular public health programs.
- A number of public health agencies have developed educational programs for the general public about the applications of genomics research for specific medical disorders. An example is the Asthma Genomic Community Consultation held in Seattle, Washington, in 2005.

In many respects, the public health aspects of genomics are still in their earliest days, with agencies still trying to decide the best way in which to make use of the abundance of new information. A 2011 study by European researchers found, for example, that public health authorities in the Netherlands, the United Kingdom, and Germany were taking very different approaches to the use of new genetic knowledge about the diagnosis and treatment of familial hypercholesterolaemia (FH), a predisposing factor for coronary **heart disease**. In the Netherlands, an infant screening program aims to identify two specific gene mutations that genomics research has shown to be associated with FH. In the United Kingdom, the genomic research is a subsidiary factor, with diagnosis based primarily on phenotypic characteristics. In Germany, diagnosis is left to individual physicians who may or may not use available genomic data in their decisions.

QUESTIONS TO ASK YOUR DOCTOR

- Can you explain how information obtained about certain groups of people applies to health issues for me as an individual?
- If my child is screened for a disease at a young age, what protection is there to prevent that information from becoming generally available?
- Suppose that I belong to a population at risk for a particular genetic disorder, discovered by genomic research. How can that information be used specifically to improve my future health prospects?
- Can you explain how genomics information can or cannot be used in the treatment of breast cancer?

Resources

BOOKS

Kumbar, Dhavendra, ed. *Genomics and Health in the Developing World*. Oxford: Oxford University Press, 2012.

Mikail, Claudia N. *Public Health Genomics: The Essentials* San Francisco: Jossey-Bass, 2008.

Nelson, Karen E., and Barbara Jones-Nelson. *Genomics Applications for the Developing World*. New York: Springer, 2012.

Rosenberg, Leon, and Diane Drobnis Rosenberg. *Human Genes and Genomes: Science, Health, Society*. Burlington, VT: Elsevier Science, 2012.

PERIODICALS

Khoury, Muin J., et al. "Beyond Base Pairs to Bedside: A Population Perspective on How Genomics Can Improve

Health." *American Journal of Public Health* 102. 1. (2012): 34–37.

Lockhart, David J., and Elizabeth A. Winzeler. "Genomics, Gene Expression, and DNA Arrays." *Nature*. 405. 6788. (2000): 827–36.

McGrath, B. B. "Advancing the Post-genomic Era Agenda: Contributions from Public Health." *Public Health Genomics* 15. 3–4. (2012): 125–31.

Williams, M. S. "The Public Health Genomics Translation Gap: What We Don't Have and Why It Matters." *Public Health Genomics* 15. 3–4. (2012): 132–38.

Zimmern, R. L., and M. J. Khoury. "The Impact of Genomics on Public Health Practice: The Case for Change." *Public Health Genomics* 15. 3–4. (2012): 118–24.

WEBSITES

Priorities for Public Health Genomics. Center for Public Health and Community Genomics and Genetic Alliance. http://genomicsforum.org/files/geno_report_WEB_w_RFI_1122rev.pdf. Accessed on September 12, 2012.

Public Health Genomics European Network. http://www.phgen.eu/typo3/index.php. Accessed on September 12, 2012.

What Is Public Health Genomics? A Day in the Invisible Life of Public Health Genomics. Centers for Disease Control and Prevention. http://blogs.cdc.gov/genomics/2011/06/02/what-is-public-health-genomics-a-day-in-the-invisible-life-of-public-health-genomics/. Accessed on September 12, 2012.

ORGANIZATIONS

Office of Public Health Genomics, Centers for Disease Control and Prevention, 1600 Clifton Rd., N.E., MS E61, Atlanta, GA USA 30333, 1 (404) 498–0001, genomics@cdc.gov, http://www.cdc.gov/genomics/.

David E. Newton, Ed.D.

Germ theory

Definition

The germ theory states that microorganisms are the cause of certain diseases.

Description

Prior to the mid-nineteenth century, a number of theories were proposed for the existence of infectious diseases such as **malaria**, **tuberculosis**, and **diphtheria**. Many people believed that such diseases were caused by superhuman forces, such as gods and spirits. Diseases might appear, according to this theory, as punishment for the sins of individuals or communities. Relief from disease under this theory came about only as the result of prayer, sacrifice, and ritual observances. Another theory attributed the spread of disease to **miasma**, a poisonous vapor produced by decaying matter. This theory led to a number of public health practices that actually reduced the risk of **infectious disease** by removing garbage, cleaning streets, purifying **water**, and removing other possible sources of the supposed disease-causing miasma. Perhaps the most common explanation for disease in the early modern period was the humoral theory, which posited the existence in the human body of four types of fluids, or *humors*. The four humors were thought to be black bile, yellow or red bile, blood, and phlegm. Each of these humors was thought to be associated with a specific psychological trait, such as melancholy or a phlegmatic disposition (from whence the term came). According to this theory, illness was caused by an imbalance among the humors and could be cured by finding a way to restore the proper balance of humors. One such approach was bleeding, in which a practitioner withdrew some quantity of a person's blood.

The idea that microscopic organisms might have a role in human disease has a very old history. In the first century BCE, for example, the Roman scholar Marcus Terentius Varro speculated that "minute creatures live that cannot be discerned with the eye and they enter the body through the mouth and nostrils and cause serious diseases." He had, however, no concrete evidence for this theory. Still, the notion that disease could be transferred from one person to another by a nonhuman agent persisted through the centuries. In the eleventh century CE, for example, the Arab philosopher Avicenna described the transmission of disease from one person to another by means of the guinea worm which, although not a microorganism, still operated in the same way as would a germ.

A crucial breakthrough in the evolution of the germ theory came in about 1674 when the Dutch tradesman and lensmaker Anton van Leeuwenhoek invented a microscope which allowed him to observe organisms that were otherwise invisible to the human eye. For the first time, possible living microscopic agents capable of transmitting disease had been identified. And within a few years, such a theory was first put forth by French physician Nicolas Andry de Bois-Regard, who suggested that microscopic "worms" like those seen by van Leeuwenhoek were responsible for certain infectious diseases such as **smallpox**.

Over the next 150 years, evidence began to accumulate for a theory similar to that put forth by Andry that at least some diseases are caused by microscopic organisms. Much of that evidence came from the clinical experience of medical practitioners. In the 1840s, for example, the Austro-Hugarian physician Ignaz Semmelweiss was able to dramatically reduce the rates of puerperal fever among women who had just delivered babies when (which, at first, was not very often) he could convince physicians simply to wash their hands more often, a result that suggested the transfer of some infectious organisms from hands to patient. Other evidence came from the new science of public health. In one of the most famous of these events, the English physician John Snow was able to show in 1854 that an outbreak of **cholera** in London was related to the use of water from a single well and not, as most physicians at the time believed, because of the spread of miasma in the area. When access to water from the infected well was denied to people, cholera cases rapidly dropped, suggesting that something in the well water had been causing the disease.

Most historians of science assign credit for final development of the germ theory to two men, the French chemist Louis Pasteur and the German bacteriologist Robert Koch. Pasteur came to his understanding of disease through his research on the spoilage of beer, wine, and milk. He found that the cause of these changes were microorganisms that multiplied rapidly as the liquids *went bad*. He obtained the same result in his studies of the decay of meat and concluded that microorganisms similar to those that cause spoilage might also cause disease. This hypothesis was finally confirmed in the 1870s when he was able to prove unequivocally that a specific microorganism, the bacterium *Bacillus anthracis*, was responsible for the disease **anthrax**.

Over the next two decades, Koch also developed a number of procedures for isolating, growing, and studying disease-causing microorganisms. For example, he developed techniques for staining microorganisms in order to see and study them more clearly. In 1884, he also published the first version of what were to become known as Koch's postulates, a set of rules for establishing a causal relationship between a microorganism and a disease. Those postulates, as revised in 1890, are as follows:

- The microorganisms must be found in all organisms that have a disease, but in no healthy organism.
- It must be possible to isolate the microorganisms for a diseases organism and to culture that microorganism successfully.
- The cultured microorganisms must be capable of causing the given disease in an otherwise healthy organism.
- It must be possible to isolate and culture the microorganisms from the newly infected organisms, and they must be identical to the original microorganism.

By the time Koch died in 1910, he and his associates and colleagues had identified the causative microorganisms for a number of major infectious diseases, such as **typhus** (1880), tuberculosis (1882), cholera (1883), **tetanus** (1884), gangarene (1892), and **plague** (1894).

Effects on Public Health

The impact of the germ theory on the growth of public health can hardly be overemphasized. Indeed, the origin of the modern public health movement can be traced to the recognition that many infectious diseases are caused by microorganisms that are easily spread among humans and between humans and nonhuman animals by environmental conditions that encourage the growth of those microorganisms. Among the most significant documents in the early history of public health was a report issued in 1842 by English social reformer Edwin Chadwick, *The Sanitary Condition of the Labouring Population*. In that report, Chadwick pointed out that the unsanitary conditions in which the British urban **population** lived were primarily responsible for the high rates of morbidity and mortality they experienced. Without yet understanding the role of microorganisms in this problem, Chadwick nonetheless published drawings of the abundance of tiny organisms present in the water, ground, and air or urban areas which, Chadwick seemed certain, were associated with the unhealthy lifestyle of those he studied. He concluded his report with the observation that "the removal of noxious physical circumstances [that he had described in his report], and the promotion of civic, household, and personal cleanliness, are necessary to the improvement of the moral condition of the population," certainly a clarion call for the beginnings of a new science of public health. Six years later, Chadwick saw the first fruits of his efforts in passage of England's first public health law, the Public Health Act of 1848. Once health authorities began to understand and adopt the germ theory, they then had a concrete tool for addressing the unhealthy conditions that Chadwick had identified. They knew, for example, that not only was purification of water a crucial goal of public health, but that killing disease-causing agents in water (as with **chlorination**) was a concrete and specific way of achieving that objective.

Today, many of the concrete activities of a public health program reflect in one way or another the role of microorganisms in causing disease. Whether it be educational programs designed to increase **handwashing** among the general public; improving programs for the storage and removal of garbage and trash; developing and implementing programs of **vaccination**; maintaining adequate water purification facilities; or designing and implementing efforts to reduce diseases such as HIV/AIDS and sexually transmitted infections, many public health programs implicitly or explicitly acknowledge the importance of the germ theory in public **health policy**.

KEY TERMS

causative agent—An organism that causes a disease.

germ—A common term for a microorganism that causes disease.

humor—A theoretical liquid contained in the human body once thought to be responsible for ill health.

miasma—A theoretical agent in the air that causes disease and is produced by the decay of dead organisms.

microorganism—An organism so small that it can be seen only by a microscope, such as a bacterium or virus.

Resources

BOOKS

Gaynes, Robert P. *Germ Theory: Medical Pioneers in Infectious Diseases* Washington, DC: ASM Press, 2011.

Lee, R. Alton. *From Snake Oil to Medicine: Pioneering Public Health*. Westport, CT: Praeger Publishers, 2007.

Magner, Lois N. *A History of Infectious Diseases and the Microbial World*. Westport, CT: Praeger, 2009.

PERIODICALS

Barnard, F. A. P. "The Germ Theory of Disease and its Relation to Hygiene." *Public Health Papers and Reports*. 1. (1873): 70–87.

Fry, Donald E. "Prions: Reassessment of the Germ Theory of Disease." *Journal of the American College of Surgeons* 211. 4. (2010): 546–52.

Rutecki, G. "A Revised Timeline for Biological Agents: Revisiting the Early Years of the Germ Theory of Disease." *Medical Hypotheses* 68. 1. (2007): 222–26.

Tomes, Nancy J., and John Harley Warner. "Introduction to Special Issue on Rethinking the Reception of the Germ Theory of Disease: Comparative Perspectives." *Journal of the History of Medicine and Allied Sciences*. 52. 1. (1997): 7–16.

WEBSITES

Germ Theory. Harvard University Library. http://ocp.hul.harvard.edu/contagion/germtheory.html. Accessed on September 12, 2012.

Hooper, Judith. "A New Germ Theory." The Atlantic Online. http://www.theatlantic.com/past/docs/issues/99feb/germs.htm. Accessed on September 12, 2012.

ORGANIZATIONS

Centers for Disease Control and Prevention, 1600 Clifton Rd., N.E., Atlanta, GA USA 30333, 1 (800) 232–4636, cdcinfo@cdc.gov., www.cdc.gov.

David E. Newton, Ed.D.

Global public health

Definition

Global public health is that field of study that focuses on public health issues that are international in scope.

Purpose

The purposes of global public health programs are to conduct research on worldwide health problems, develop potential solutions for those problems, disseminate information and technologies relating to these solutions, and reduce disparities among various populations in the pursuit of healthy peoples around the world.

Description

The origin of global public health concerns can be traced to the years immediately following the end of World War II, which saw the creation of the United Nations and a number of other international agencies. Foremost of those international health agencies was the **World Health Organization (WHO)**, created on April 7, 1948, to deal with health problems both within individual nations and across international boundaries. **WHO** has been a leader in global health issues ever since, although a number of international, regional, and national health organizations, universities, and nonprofit organizations have also become active in the field. As an example, a number of universities in the United States now offer undergraduate and graduate degrees in the field of global public health, including the University of North Carolina's Gillings School of Global Public Health, the Center for Global Public Health at the University of California at Berkeley, the University of California at San Diego Division of Global Public Health, and the Global Health Program at the University of Michigan School of Public Health.

The field of global public health includes a very wide array of topics of concern at the local, state, and national levels, as well as the international level.

Women's health

One of the most universal issues in the field of global public health is the lower status of women in most parts of the world. This lower status has led to a reduced interest and attention to the health of women, both in general and in regard to uniquely female issues, such as contraception, family planning, pregnancy, and childbirth. Virtually all global public health programs, then, allocate significant resources to study the social, economic, and medical roots of **women's health** problems and the ways these factors can be changed to provide better health care to individuals regardless of gender. These efforts also include programs for helping women better understand their own potential and develop methods for empowering their efforts in controlling their own health options. Developing a better understanding of the causes of **violence** to women and ways to combat this problem is an essential element of global public health programs. Addressing the disparity between health care for women and men involves better training and education for men and for governmental and private agencies that provide health care in a community.

Infectious diseases

While great strides have been made in the control of infectious diseases in developed nations, the same cannot be said for developing nations. Diseases such as **malaria**, HIV/AIDS, African trypanosomiasis (sleeping sickness), **cholera**, and **hepatitis** are responsible for millions of deaths annually throughout Africa, Asia, and parts of South and Central America. Efforts by global public health agencies are often aimed at bringing to the developing world the same levels of **prevention** and treatment for these diseases as are currently available in the developed world.

Double burden of diseases

Some regions of the world are dealing with what has been called the double burden of disease, that is, facing deaths and disabilities from both infectious and non-infectious (degenerative) diseases. In many parts of the developed world, for example, nations are still dealing with unacceptable rates of **infectious disease** among their poorest citizens, while also having to face the challenge of caring for older citizens who develop diseases such as **cancer**, cardiovascular disease, **obesity**, diabetes, and chronic pulmonary disease that are linked to lifestyle and dietary choices as well as problems that emerge from environmental issues. Global public health agencies are looking for ways that nations and regions can develop multifaceted programs that recognize and address this wide range of health challenges.

Biostatistics and epidemiology

A key element involved in addressing any global public health problem involves collecting data related to the source and distribution of the problem. In the case of an infectious disease epidemic, for example, the most fundamental questions are those that can be answered by **epidemiology**: Where was the disease first seen, how was it first identified, what were the signs and symptoms that characterized the disease, and how did it spread through the **population**? Answering these questions involves the collection of quantitative data—biostatistics—as well as qualitative observations. Biostatistics involves the collection of data, analysis of those data, interpretation of their results, and the development of policies and practices based on the results of that interpretation.

Finances and economics

Economic issues are an inherent part of public health problems worldwide. Indeed, many such problems exist or survive simply because governmental agencies lack the financial resources to manage them successfully. In the case of infectious diseases, for example, drugs may be available for use in the prevention and treatment of many conditions, but individuals and health agencies in many parts of the world may not have the financial resources to purchase and distribute those drugs. Health problems are not restricted to science and technology, then, but usually also involve economics.

Politics

A similar argument can be made for political factors when a nation may have the economic and technical resources to address a health problem, but for one reason or another, lacks the political will to do so. As a recent example, the government of Pakistan suspended the **vaccination** of children because a physician associated with health agencies providing immunizations was involved in the uncovering and ultimate death of Osama bin Laden in 2011. That decision placed in jeopardy the nation's efforts to eradicate **polio** from the country.

Education programs

Two other related but critical elements of virtually all global public health programs are education and changes in behavior. No matter the specific health problem, getting people to understand the causes of that problem and the changes in behavior needed to solve it are fundamental. Whether the issue is HIV/AIDS, sexually transmitted infections, firearm violence, violence against women, binge drinking, seatbelt use, or any other public health topic, progress probably cannot be made without programs to educate individuals at risk for the particular harmful behavior. Reducing the rate of HIV infections, for example, ultimately depends almost entirely on individuals' understanding the ways in which the virus is spread and the changes in sexual habits needed to reduce the risk of transmission.

Global climate change

An issue of growing concern worldwide is global climate change and the effects it may have on health problems. As regions become warmer or cooler, patterns of infectious disease are almost certainly likely to change in ways that have no regard for national boundaries. In addition, climate change is likely to result in the movement of populations across national boundaries, carrying with them endemic diseases to regions where such conditions have traditionally been absent. As an extreme example, some small island nations have already begun exploring the possibility of having to move their entire populations to other parts of the world, creating at least the potential for bringing with them their unique health problems. One challenge of global public health programs, then, is identifying populations who are at risk for new health problems and ways of dealing with those problems.

Nutrition

One irony of global public health issues is that some of the most developed countries of the world are struggling with problems related to obesity, the excessive intake of calories by citizens, while most developing countries are addressing some level of poor **nutrition**, an inadequate supply of healthy foods for the majority of their populations. The fundamental nutritional problem facing the world is not a lack of food, but an inability to create a fair and equitable distribution of food throughout the world. This situation has forced public health agencies in developed nations to establish programs educating people about the need to control caloric intake and obtain adequate levels of exercise to maintain a healthy body weight and public health agencies in developing countries to find ways of providing their populations with better access to adequate amounts of healthful foods.

Food safety

A relatively new global public health problem involves the spread of disease through the distribution of contaminated foods across international boundaries. Today, food distribution has become an international industry, with foods grown in one part of the world routinely being shipped hundreds or thousands of miles away to other parts of the world. WHO estimates that three-quarters of all new infectious diseases in the world have arisen from pathogens that started in animals and animal products and then were carried to human populations in other parts of the globe. Such foodborne diseases are thought to be responsible for the vast majority of the more than 1.5 million deaths among children in the world each year.

KEY TERMS

Biostatistics—The branch of statistics that focuses on the collection and analysis of biological and medical data.

Bioterrorism—The intentional use of pathogens to cause illness in large population groups or to cause fear of such harm.

Double burden of disease—The situation in which a country or region has to simultaneously address problems posed by both infectious and non-infectious (degenerative) diseases.

Empowerment—The act of investing individuals with an understanding of their own potential and their own self-worth, while simultaneously providing them with the tools by which to achive their maximum personal potential.

Epidemiology—The study of the distribution of diseases in large groups of people.

Pathogen—An organism that causes disease.

Potable—Safe for drinking.

Bioterrorism

The risks posed by bioterrorism to the world's population have been recognized for more than four decades. In 1970, WHO published a manual recommending ways in which nations could prepare for and respond to bioterrorist attacks, a manual that was updated in 2002. The manual noted that an attack using pathogens such as those responsible for **anthrax**, **measles**, cholera, malaria, or HIV can be met by essentially the same technologies and methods used against these diseases in everyday public health programs. However, preparing for such attacks adds new dimensions that are not part of the usual public health agenda. With the increasing level of terrorist attacks in the past decade, preparing for bioterrorist events throughout multinational regions is increasingly important.

Water supplies and safety

One problem facing people in many parts of the world is simply a shortage of potable **water**. According to some estimates, the women of the world spend more than 200 million hours on an average day simply collecting the water needed for drinking, washing, and cooking for their families. A second water problem is **sanitation**. Much of the water that is readily available for human use is contaminated. As a result, waterborne diseases are among the most serious of all public health problems in the world. WHO estimates that every 20 seconds, a child somewhere in the world dies because of waterborne diseases. The shortage of safe water supplies affects about one in nine humans alive today, a total of about 780 million people worldwide. Without access to potable water, almost any public health program is doomed to failure.

Refugee health

People are constantly moving across international boundaries for a variety of reasons. When war or civil unrest breaks out in one country, for example, many inhabitants of that country are like to seek refuge in a neighboring nation. Also, many people voluntarily leave their native land in order to seek better lives in some other nation. Migrants can be an important global public health problem when they bring diseases from their native countries into their new homes, perhaps introducing health issues previously unknown in the latter nation. Host nations for refugees must be concerned not only with the health of the men, women, and children moving into the country, but also the public health of the native residents of that nation.

Resources

BOOKS

Beaglehole, Robert, and Ruth Bonita, eds. *Global Public Health: A New Era*, 2nd ed. New York: Oxford University Press, 2009.

Gaist, Paul A., ed. *Igniting the Power of Community: The Role of CBOs and NGOs in Global Public Health*. New York: Springer 2009.

Garrett, Laurie. *Betrayal of Trust: The Collapse of Global Public Health*. New York: Hyperion Books, 2011.

Weir, Lorna, and Eric Mykhalovskiy. *Global Public Health Vigilance: Creating a World on Alert*. London: Routledge, 2010.

PERIODICALS

Fried, L. P., et al. "Global Public Health Leadership for the Twenty-First Century: Towards Improved Health of All Populations." *Global Public Health* 7, Suppl. 1. (2012): S5–S15.

Hill, D. R., R. M. Ainsworth, and U. Partap. "Teaching Global Public Health in the Undergraduate Liberal Arts: A Survey of 50 Colleges." *American Journal of Tropical Medicine and Hygiene* 87, 1. (2012): 11–15.

Kohl, H. W., 3rd, et al. "The Pandemic of Physical Inactivity: Global Action for Public Health." *Lancet* 380, 9838. (2012): 294–305.

Morse, S. S. "Public Health Surveillance and Infectious Disease Detection." *Biosecurity and Bioterrorism* 10, 1. (2012): 6–16.

WEBSITES

"Global Health." Centers for Disease Control and Prevention. http://www.cdc.gov/globalhealth/. Accessed on October 6, 2012.

"Global Health Issues. Global Issues."http://www.globalissues.org/article/588/global-health-overview. Accessed on October 6, 2012.

"Global Health Topics." U.S. Department of Health and Human Services. http://www.globalhealth.gov/. Accessed on October 6, 2012.

"Global Public Health." McKinsey & Company. http://mckinseyonsociety.com/topics/global-public-health/. Accessed on October 6, 2012.

ORGANIZATIONS

World Health Organization (WHO), Avenue Appia 20, 1211 Geneva 27, Switzerland, +41 22 791 21 11, Fax: +41 22 791 31 11, http://www.who.int/about/contact_form/en/index.html, http://www.who.int/en/.

David E. Newton, Ed.D.

Grief counseling *see* **Community Mental health**

Guinea worm *see* **Dracunculiasis infection**

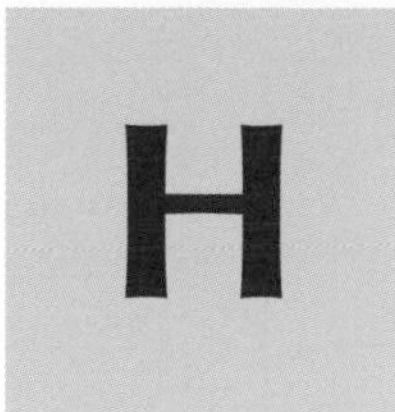

H1N1 influenza A

Definition

Pandemic 2009 H1N1 **influenza**, initially termed a swine flu, is an infectious respiratory disease caused by a subtype of the influenza A virus first identified in April 2009. It is also denoted as the A (H1N1) virus. The virus and associated influenza spread rapidly around the world, and on June 11, 2009, **World Health Organization (WHO)** officials declared H1N1 influenza to be a global pandemic, the first new pandemic of the twenty-first century.

Demographics

Because the 2009 H1N1 influenza virus was a novel (not previously identified) virus, and because the virus and associated flu became subjects of intense research, information about the virus accumulated rapidly. As of July 2009, the **WHO** offices reported over 94,000 laboratory-confirmed cases of 2009 H1N1 influenza in 135 countries. At least 700 deaths had been attributed to the novel virus, and WHO officials characterized the 2009 H1N1 flu as the fastest spreading pandemic on record.

Despite high initial estimates, by June 24, 2009, Mexico had reported 7,847 confirmed cases and 115 laboratory-confirmed deaths. The United States reported 21,449 confirmed cases and 87 deaths, and Canada reported 6,457 cases and 15 deaths. Deaths were also reported in Columbia, Costa Rica, Dominican Republic, Guatemala, the Philippines, and the United Kingdom. The spread of the virus into the Southern Hemisphere was evidenced by Australia's reporting of 2,857 cases, including two deaths; Argentina's reporting of 1,213 cases, including seven deaths; and Chile's reporting of 4,315 cases, including four deaths. As with all reports related to a developing outbreak, daily reports of cases and deaths were simply considered by experts to be a snapshot of data; both the number of countries reporting and cases confirmed were expected to increase until the pandemic subsided. In July 2009, with the pandemic well established in both the Northern and Southern Hemispheres, WHO officials stopped accumulating individual case counts in favor of concentrating on pandemic flu mitigation strategies such as vaccine and antiviral medication development and delivery. In developing countries with established outbreaks, data were difficult to collect and prone to error. Counting individual cases was also difficult because many were mild and went unreported.

Newswires were often filled with unverified reports and even the time difference between offices reporting laboratory-confirmed results could seemingly swing figures rapidly. In addition, there was often a delay or backlog in such reporting. Uncertainties in the number of cases and confirmed deaths created a degree of uncertainty in assessments of the lethality of the virus and course of the outbreak. As of August 2009, there was no evidence that the H1N1 pandemic would be more lethal on a case-by-case basis than a typical seasonal flu. However, pandemic flu viruses often cause significant global deaths because so many more people are infected than in normal influenza seasons.

Common seasonal influenza (the type for which vaccinations are offered each year) normally accounts for about 200,000 hospitalizations and 36,000 deaths annually in the United States. Globally, WHO officials estimate that between 300,000 and 500,000 people die from flu complications each year. Although people of all ages can contract influenza, young children and the elderly, along with those with compromised immune systems (e.g., **cancer** patients or those with HIV/AIDS) are most at risk during a normal seasonal flu. Most deaths are caused by **pneumonia**, a common complication of seasonal flu. During the initial outbreak of 2009 H1N1 flu in Mexico, reports indicated that otherwise healthy adults aged 20 to 44 years were dying of the disease in higher than expected numbers. By the end of July 2009, in the United States, approximately 50 percent of the

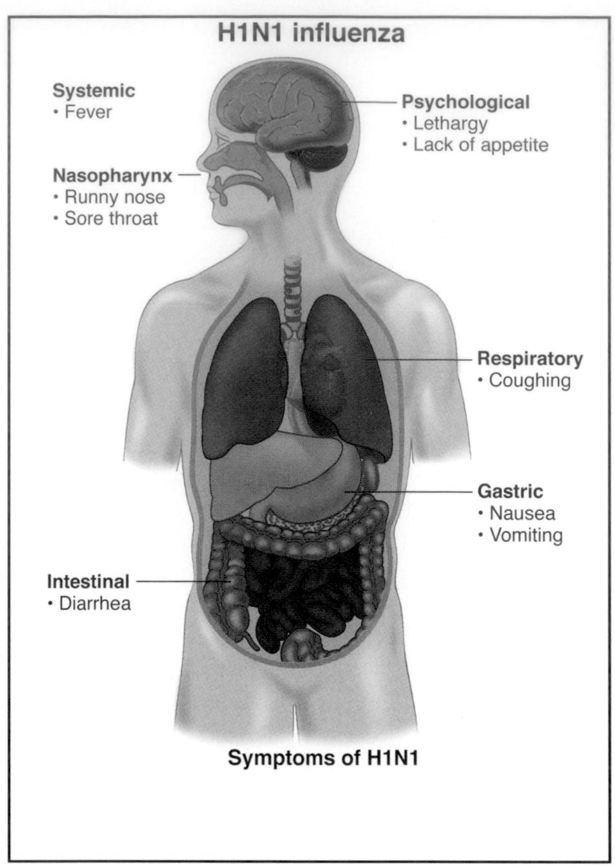

(Illustration by Electronic Illustrators Group. © 2013 Cengage Learning)

reported cases of pandemic H1N1 flu occurred in young people from five to 24 years of age, and the highest rate of hospitalization was among infants and young children under four years of age. Although there is no definitive cause, the pattern of illness differs from normal seasonal flu, which usually results in a greater number of cases in the elderly. A report published in the medical journal *The Lancet* showed that early in the pandemic, pregnant women were four times as likely as other people who contract swine flu to require hospitalization. The physiological reasons remain under study.

Description

In April 2009, scientists at the U.S. **Centers for Disease Control and Prevention (CDC)** and at a research laboratory in Winnipeg, Canada, confirmed that a new strain of influenza was causing illness in humans. Genetic analysis showed that although the H1N1 virus is a novel genetic reassortment of genes of swine, human, and avian origin, the majority of the H1N1 genome is traceable and comparable to other viruses that cause seasonal influenza.

It remained a subject of intense research as to when and where the 2009 H1N1 flu virus may have entered the human population. Although the first cases erupted in Mexico and the United States in March and April 2009, this did not mean that that the genetic reassortment of the virus took place in Mexico or the United States or that the virus entered the human population in either country.

The 2009 H1N1 influenza virus was initially classified as a swine flu because it contains swine flu genes. This means only that the virus passed through swine at some point in its evolution. When and where the virus passed through swine was a subject of continued investigation. Although probable, it was not a certainty that the virus was most recently transmitted from swine to humans. Based on preliminary genetic analysis, experts conjectured such a transfer might have taken place in late 2008. As of June 12, 2009, however, none of the cases encountered in the 2009 H1N1 flu outbreak could be definitively traced to contact with pigs. In fact, the first confirmed outbreak of H1N1 recorded in swine was on a Canadian farm. Experts strongly suspected that a human farm worker who had traveled from Mexico infected the swine.

H1N1 strains of influenza are common in pigs, and swine flu viruses can be transmitted from pigs to humans who are in close contact with infected animals. However, before the 2009 H1N1 outbreak, documented transmission of recent swine flu viruses from person to person was extremely limited and had not resulted in documented outbreaks of human disease.

What made health experts in 2009 so concerned about the new H1N1 virus was its being a novel virus of unknown lethality that had gained the ability to efficiently pass from person to person (human transmission). Because 2009 H1N1 flu was new, humans had no immunity to it. As a result, the resources of the WHO, the **CDC**, state public **health departments**, and various international organizations charged with protecting public health were mobilized to attempt to mitigate a worldwide influenza pandemic.

Understanding the influenza virus

Viruses are simple organisms consisting of a protein matrix containing genetic information. They are so small that they can be seen only with an electron microscope. Because they are metabolically inert outside a host cell, viruses cannot reproduce on their own. They are **parasites** and must enter a host cell and take over the host cell's resources in order to make millions of new virus particles.

Influenza is caused by a hardy group of viruses belonging to the Orthomyxoviridae family. There are three types of influenza viruses: types A, B, and C. Type A influenza virus is the most threatening to humans. The type B virus is stable, changing little from year to year, and can be effectively controlled through **vaccination**. Type C influenza viruses cause only mild illness in humans. The type A virus, however, easily changes, or mutates, into new strains or subtypes. Each strain contains slightly different genetic information. Because of this difference, no single vaccine is completely effective against all type A viruses, and whenever a new strain arises, as in the case of the 2009 H1N1, the body's immune system treats the virus as a completely new antigen.

How new strains develop

Humans are not the only animals vulnerable to influenza A infections. Different strains of influenza A cause disease in other animals, including wild birds, chickens, ducks, and turkeys (collectively called avian or bird flu), in addition to pigs, horses, ferrets, whales, seals, and dogs. Pigs and birds are the critical species in the development of new flu strains that can infect humans. Wild birds serve as a reservoir for the influenza A viruses; some strain of **avian flu** is always present in the wild bird population. Birds shed live virus in their droppings (feces), and because many species of birds migrate long distances, they can infect large areas. Pigs carry their own strains of influenza A, but they also can become infected with avian influenza if they are exposed to infected bird droppings or contaminated **water**. If a pig simultaneously becomes infected with a strain of swine influenza and a strain of avian influenza, when the virus reproduces, genetic information can be exchanged so that new strains of influenza A develop that incorporate some genetic material from the avian virus and some genetic material from the swine virus.

Most new strains of influenza that result from a recombination or reassortment of avian and swine flu viruses do not survive, cannot infect humans, or die out quickly. Occasionally, however, a strain develops that can infect humans and that has the ability to pass from pig to human and from person to person. Because the virus is new to humans, the body has few defenses against it, and the vaccines included in seasonal flu shots are ineffective against it. When a new strain of flu arises that can pass easily from person to person, it has the potential to cause a pandemic, rapidly infecting and sometimes killing millions of people across the world.

Influenza pandemics have occurred during thousands of years of recorded history. The worst influenza pandemic in modern history occurred in 1918–1919 and killed an estimated 20 to 40 million people. In 1957, another pandemic known as the asian flu killed about 70,000 Americans. This was followed by the pandemic Hong Kong flu in 1968. Then in 1976, Americans experienced a swine flu scare. During February 1976, several recruits at the Army Fort Dix in New Jersey developed unusually severe flu symptoms. When samples from some of the sick men were sent to the CDC for analysis, four samples showed a previously unknown flu virus that appeared to be similar to the virus that caused the 1918–1919 pandemic. After one soldier died of flu, the United States began a $135 million emergency **immunization** program. However, the 1976 virus proved to be much less dangerous than the 1918 virus. In the end, the 1976 swine flu never spread beyond Fort Dix. About 500 people became sick and only one person died.

People who were most likely to become infected with the 2009 H1N1 influenza were those who had close contact with someone who was infected. The incubation period was uncertain, although it was most likely less than seven days. The disease was passed to others through infected droplets that were spread by coughing, sneezing, kissing, and close physical contact. The virus could also spread indirectly. Tests of other viral strains typically show that Type A viruses can live up to two hours on hard surfaces such as door knobs, telephones, or children's toys. This means that an infected person can leave the flu virus on objects where it can be picked up by another person who then touches his or her own mouth, nose, or eyes and becomes infected. People are contagious for about one day before symptoms appear. Adults remain contagious for about seven days after they begin to show symptoms; children can remain contagious for up to ten days.

Causes and symptoms

The 2009 H1N1 flu was caused by a newly identified strain of influenza virus. Genetic tests established that H1N1 strains encountered before that were consistent (nearing 99% genetic matches among viruses examined from patient samples taken from six countries). Of particular interest to **infectious disease** research were the genes that control hemagglutinin (H), neuraminidase (N), two surface proteins with subtypes that are numbered, hence H1N1 flu or H5N1 avian flu virus, genes that control the nucleoprotein, the surrounding matrix, and three key polymerase enzymes (designated PA, PB1, and PB2) that the virus must have to reproduce. Genetically, the 2009 H1N1 presented a mixed background, with these key genes derived from human, swine, and avian sources (a triple reassortment). The hemagglutinin [H] produced was equidistant to the swine flu sequences found in North America, Europe, and Asia. The neuraminidase and matrix genes sequences were close to genes found in swine flu strains found in

KEY TERMS

Incubation period—The time between when an individual becomes infected with a disease-causing agent and when symptoms begin to appear.

Pandemic—The occurrence of a disease that in a short time infects a large percentage of the population over a wide geographical area.

Parasite—An organism that lives in or with another organism, called the host, in parasitism, a type of association characterized by the parasite obtaining benefits from the host, such as food, and the host being injured as a result.

Asia. Early evidence indicated similarities to influenza strains where the PB1 gene is of human origin and the PA and PB2 genes are from avian sources.

Symptoms of 2009 H1N1 flu were similar to the symptoms of seasonal influenza. These included fever, cough, sore throat, runny nose, body aches, headaches, chills, loss of appetite, and exhaustion. Some people experienced nausea, vomiting, and diarrhea. Although most cases of 2009 H1N1 flu were mild to moderate, complications such as severe pneumonia could result in respiratory failure and death. Neurological complications, including seizures, were also linked to 2009 H1N1 flu in children. The case fatality rate was only 0.03% compared with more than 2.5% in the Spanish flu epidemic of 1918–1919. Worldwide there may have been between 14,000 and 18,000 deaths from the H1N1 flu during the 2009 pandemic.

Diagnosis

Normally influenza is diagnosed on the basis of symptoms and the health care provider's knowledge of whether influenza is prevalent in the local area. An influenza test can be performed in the doctor's office that is about 75% accurate. However, this test cannot distinguish between strains of influenza A and, therefore, was not useful in determining if the patient had H1N1 (2009). To make this determination, a mucus sample had to be sent to a laboratory capable of rapid PCR analysis. Prior to May 1, 2009, only two laboratories in North America, the CDC laboratories in Atlanta and Canadian research laboratories in Winnipeg, were capable of definitively diagnosing the 2009 H1N1 flu. However, PCR machines were installed in labs in Mexico that allowed rapid definitive diagnosis.

Tests

The most accurate test for influenza is done by taking a mucus sample from the throat of an infected person. Because of the time delay involved in testing, knowing the strain of flu does not provide much help to the patient, but this information helps the CDC and WHO understand how and where flu is spreading. During an influenza pandemic, physicians often forgo laboratory confirmation of influenza, relying on signs and symptoms for diagnosis. In the United Kingdom, persons with flu symptoms are given access to antiviral drugs after answering questions that indicate an influenza diagnosis on a government-sponsored public health website. This saves physician resources for handling severe or emergent cases, provides quick access to treatment, and helps the person with symptoms to stay home, thereby reducing the pool of infected persons in public available to infect others.

Treatment

Supportive treatment for H1N1 (2009) appears to be the same as for all influenza viruses and included drinking plenty of fluids, extended bed rest, and use of acetaminophen to treat aches and fever. 2009 H1N1 influenza A virus also responded to two antiviral drugs, oseltamivir (Tamiflu) and zanamivir (Relenza). These drugs do not prevent or cure flu, but if taken within 48 hours of the start of symptoms, they reduce the severity and duration of the disease. In late April 2009, the U.S. government released stockpiled supplies of these antiviral drugs to combat 2009 H1N1 flu. Initial tests showed that 2009 H1N1 was resistant to two other antiviral drugs, amantadine (Symmetrel, Symadine), and rimantadine (Flumandine), making these drugs ineffective. **Antibiotics** also were ineffective against all viruses, including H1N1, but could be used to treat bacterial complications of influenza, such as pneumonia.

In late June 2009, public health officials in Denmark reported the first case of 2009 A/H1N1 influenza that was resistant to oseltamivir. Although some cases of resistance normally occurred and developed with seasonal influenzas, any emergence of Tamiflu-resistant 2009 A/H1N1 influenza virus put public health officials on alert for appearance of the resistant virus elsewhere. Isolated cases of Tamiflu-resistant 2009 H1N1 were identified in Japan, Hong Kong (Special Administrative Region of China), and Canada. Thus far, the Tamiflu-resistant viral influenza remained treatable with zanamivir (Relenza), the other antiviral drug usually effective against the A/H1N1 virus.

Alternative treatment

No scientific testing exists to validate any claim of effectiveness of any alternative medical treatments specific to H1N1 flu. Although claims of effectiveness (and/or potential harm) for any alternative medical treatment should be carefully scrutinized for supporting scientific evidence, there are a number of alternative treatments commonly used to support relief of symptoms. Because there is no scientifically validated antiviral treatment, if flu is suspected, persons should consult a physician to determine if they are in need of antiviral medicines.

Alternative practitioners recommend herbal teas to soothe the throat and allegedly boost the immune system. Other herbal treatments recommended by alternative practitioners for seasonal flu routinely include the following:

- Ginger (*Zingiber officinalis*) to reduce fever and pain, settle the stomach, and suppress cough.
- Echinacea (*Echinacea purpurea* or *angustifolia*) to reduce flu symptoms, including sore throat, chills, sweating, fatigue, weakness, body aches, and headaches.
- Cordyceps (*Cordyceps sinensis*) to modulate and allegedly boost the immune system and improve respiration.
- Eucalyptus (*Eucalyptus globulus*) or peppermint (*Mentha piperita*) essential oils added to a steam vaporizer to help clear chest and nasal congestion.

Prognosis

Because 2009 H1N1 was a new strain of influenza, it was difficult to predict the course of the disease. Generally cases were mild, but as with all flu, cases could be life-threatening if complications develop. Underlying health conditions might be worsened by the disease, and pneumonia, a common and sometimes fatal complication of seasonal flu, might develop.

Prevention

The best ways to prevent H1N1 (2009) infection are the following:

- Wash hands well and often. Hands should be washed with soap and warm water to above the wrists for 15–20 seconds or about the time it takes to sing the happy birthday song slowly. If soap and water are not available, use an alcohol-based hand sanitizer.
- Cover the mouth when coughing.
- Dispose of used tissues in a covered container.
- Avoid touching the nose, mouth, and eyes.
- Stay home if flu symptoms appear.
- Avoid crowded places such as movie theaters.

Note that surgical masks are unlikely to protect against the influenza virus but are effective in reducing dissemination of droplets that can contain viral particles.

QUESTIONS TO ASK YOUR DOCTOR

- How can I know if I have H1N1 (2009) influenza A?
- Should I begin taking oseltamivir (Tamiflu) or zanamivir (Relenza)?
- Should other members of my household be tested for H1N1 (2009)?
- What are some warning signs that my flu is getting worse?
- When should I contact a doctor or go to the emergency room?

In addition, antiviral medications do not prevent influenza; they simply help shorten the intensity and duration of the illness.

Vaccination

The first H1N1-specific vaccine was anticipated by late September or early October 2009. World public health officials recommended prioritizing vaccine recipients according to individual risk, as well as to ensure the greatest benefit for overall public health. Pregnant women and people caring for infants, children, young people under 25 years of age, and persons with underlying health conditions such as **asthma** or diabetes were recommended to receive priority vaccination against pandemic 2009 H1N1 influenza. In addition, healthcare workers were suggested to be among the first immunized in order to keep hospitals, doctors' offices, and other critical healthcare infrastructure functional during the pandemic flu.

Public health officials acknowledged that even under the best scenarios, production of the H1N1 vaccine was expected to fall far short of global demand. As of 2009 production rates, 900 million doses of the new H1N1 vaccine could be produced each year (as two doses are required per person, enough to vaccinate 450 million people). The vaccine is produced in only a handful of countries and there were concerns these countries, along with wealthier nations, would obtain the vast majority of vaccine produced. The shortages might also hinder WHO efforts to secure donations of vaccine or agreements that will enable poorer countries to purchase vaccine at a lower price.

Resources

BOOKS

Friis, Robert H. *Essentials of Environmental Health*. 2nd ed. Sudbury, MA: Jones & Bartlett, 2012.

Shors, Teri. *Understanding Viruses*. Sudbury, MA: Jones and Bartlett, 2009.

WEBSITES

"2009 HINI (Swine Flu) and You." Centers for Disease Control and Prevention. http://www.cdc.gov/h1n1flu/qa.htm (accessed November 1, 2012).

"Influenza." National Geographic Society. http://science.nationalgeographic.com/science/health-and-human-body/human-diseases/influenza-article.html (accessed November 1, 2012).

ORGANIZATIONS

Centers for Disease Control and Prevention, 1600 Clifton Rd., Atlanta, GA 30333, (800) 232-4636, cdcinfor@cdc.gov, http://www.cdc.gov

World Health Organization, Avenue Appia 20, 1211 Geneva 27, Switzerland, +22 41 791 21 11, Fax: +22 41 791 31 11, info@who.int, http://www.who.int.

Brenda Wilmoth Lerner
Tish Davidson, AM

Haemophilus influenzae type b

Definition

Sometimes called H. influenzae type B or Hib, Haemophilus **influenza** type B is a fairly common bacterium found all over the world and in most healthy human beings. In spite of the bacterium's name, it does not cause influenza.

Description

Haemophilus influenzae was first described in 1892 by Richard Johannes Pfeiffer (1858–1945). For many years, H. influenzae was mistakenly believed to cause the flu—this misunderstanding was corrected in 1933. H. influenzae are typically oval-shaped organisms with a cell wall consisting of two membranes separated by a plasma membrane.

Though H. influenzae is a relatively common organism, it is especially harmful to infants and small children. If the bacterium spreads to the lungs or into the bloodstream, it can cause serious illnesses—including **pneumonia**, **meningitis**, sepsis, epiglottitis, or death. The illnesses resulting from a Hib infection are relatively common and usually not life-threatening for adults. These illnesses include pneumonia, bronchitis, sinusitis, and some types of ear infections. These same illnesses when caused by a Hib infection can prove highly fatal, however, to children, particularly those who are very young. Children are often infected by individuals who are not aware they are carrying the bacteria.

The bacterium is not harmful to children if it stays on their skin or in their nose. H. influenzae is dangerous when it is spread into the lungs or blood stream. In the United States and other developed countries with standardized inoculation, Hib infections and their subsequent illnesses have dropped drastically. For instance, epiglottitis is primarily associated with Hib. Since the introduction of the Hib vaccine, cases of epiglottitis have almost disappeared in the United States.

Individuals who become seriously infected with H. influenzae and survive are likely to suffer serious long-term health consequences such as mental retardation, deafness, or other permanent disabilities.

Vaccination is a problem in some developed countries that do not have standardized vaccination programs or where vaccinations are not frequently utilized. However, undeveloped nations suffer H. influenzae infections and deaths because of insufficient information and funding. Hib can be difficult to diagnose, and often causes death without being identified. Additionally, the Hib vaccine is relatively costly—approximately seven times more than the cost of vaccines against **measles**, **polio**, **tuberculosis**, **diphtheria**, **tetanus**, and pertussis combined.

Demographics

Approximately 80% of those who develop H. influenzae infections are children younger than five years of age.

Children from 6–12 months of age are at the greatest risk for contracting meningitis from an H. influenzae infection.

Children over the age of two are at the greatest risk for epiglottitis caused by an H. influenzae infection.

Before the introduction of the H. influenzae vaccine in the 1980s, there were roughly 20,000 invasive (serious) cases of Hib and 1,000 deaths per year in the United States alone.

The standardization of an H. influenzae vaccination in developed countries has reduced the rate of infection by about 95%.

Rates of H. influenzae infection and subsequent infant deaths are still relatively high in developed countries with low vaccination rates. The **World Health Organization (WHO)** estimates that in the poorest countries, children's vaccination rates are as low as 8% and that in many developed countries, it is still less than 50%.

The **WHO** estimates that H. influenzae infections are responsible for roughly three million serious illnesses and 386,000 deaths per year.

Symptoms

An H. influenzae infection can present with various symptoms—the most common symptoms are those of illnesses related to Hib. These infections often involve the respiratory tract and include sinusitis, bronchitis, pneumonia, and otitis media. Symptoms associated with these illnesses include sneezing, coughing, and **pain**. Symptoms of other related illnesses such as meningitis may be more severe.

Diagnosis

Since H. influenzae is a bacterium, a culture is used to definitively diagnose the infection. This process requires a sample from the patient, which is then added to a growth medium in a laboratory and subsequently studied under a microscope.

Prevention

The Haemophilus influenza type B vaccination was first introduced in 1985. The vaccination was added to the schedule of recommended pediatric immunizations in 1989. Proof that a child has received the vaccinations on this list is usually required before the child can be enrolled in school or day care. The vaccine is usually administered to children at 2, 4, 6, and 12–15 months of age. Children under six weeks of age should not be vaccinated and children who are seriously ill should not be vaccinated until they recover from the original illness. The **Centers for Disease Control and Prevention (CDC)** defines "seriously ill" in this case as any illness more severe than a cold.

Both the **CDC** and the WHO suggest that all infants receive a vaccination against H. influenzae infection. Serious side effects to the vaccination, though rare, can occur. The most common reaction is inflammation near the injection site, often accompanied by a fever. These symptoms may not develop for up to 24 hours and may linger for two or three days. Any more serious side effects, including a high fever, breathing difficulties, or heart palpitations should receive immediate medical treatment.

Treatment

A long and intensive course of **antibiotics** is used to treat H. influenzae infections. Hib tends to resist more common and inexpensive antibiotics.

As of 2012, Danish research suggests that treating H. influenzae infections with cefuroxime/aminopenicillin antibiotics is preferable to treatment with benzylpenicillins because it reduces mortality.

KEY TERMS

Sepsis—an infection of the blood that can be caused by a number of organisms, including H. influenzae.

Epiglottitis—an infection of the epiglottis that causes inflammation and can lead to an obstructed airway and inability to breathe. Epiglottitis can be caused by H. influenzae.

Vaccination—the process of intentionally injecting a person with a vaccine—a small amount of a potentially harmful disease, bacteria, or virus. This injection allows the individual's immune system to develop an appropriate response to the agent, thereby allowing the individual's immune system to fight off the agent in the future.

Effects on public health

The effects of H. influenzae on the public health in the United States have largely disappeared as a result of widespread inoculation against the infection. As long as the vaccination is administered on the recommended schedule, H. influenzae should remain a minimal threat in the United States and other developed nations. The international health community, through organizations like the WHO, continues work to standardize the Hib vaccination worldwide, especially in underdeveloped and developing nations.

Efforts and solutions

The presence and standard use of the H. influenzae vaccine in the United States and other developed nations requires little other public health effort to combat the infection, since it is not usually seriously dangerous to adults.

The CDC and the WHO have developed a "Rapid Assessment Tool" that helps countries estimate the numbers of H. influenzae infections by studying available public records such as instances of pneumonia and detailed mortality rates. This method has already proven successful in many regions, though to a lesser degree in Eastern Europe and Asia. The WHO is working on adjusting this tool to improve its efficacy in more areas of the world, including Eastern Europe and Asia.

As of 2012, conjugate vaccines are available—vaccines that serve to protect individuals against multiple illnesses. This development has the potential to make inoculation easier in undeveloped countries, and help to reduce the cost.

Resources

BOOKS

Birkhauser, Jennifer. "Hib Vaccine." *Infection Diseases & Conditions.* Ed. H. Bradford Hawley. Vol. 2. Ipswich, MA: Salem Press, 2012.

Hoyle, Brian. "Haemophilus Influenzae." *Infectious Diseases: In Context.* Ed. Brenda Wilmoth Lerner and K. Lee Lerner. Vol. 1. Detroit: Gale, 2008.

Krapp, Kristine, and Tish Davidson. "Hib Vaccine." *The Gale Encyclopedia of Children's Health: Infancy through Adolescence.* Ed. Jacqueline L. Longe. 2nd ed. Vol. 2. Detroit: Gale, 2011.

Knight, Jeffrey A. "Haemophilus Influenzae Infection." *Infectious Diseases & Conditions.* Ed. H. Bradford Hawley. Vol. 2. Ipswich, MA: Salem Press, 2012.

PERIODICALS

Beurret, Michel, Ahd Hamidi, and Hans Kreeftenberg. "Development and technology transfer of Haemophilus influenzae type b conjugate vaccines for developing countires." *Vaccine* 30.33 (2012):4897.

Ostergaard, Christian, and Sara Thonnings. "Treatment of Haemophilus bacteremia with benzylpenicillin is associated with increased (30–day) mortality." *BMC Infectious Diseases* 12 (2012): 153.

WEBSITES

Medline Plus "Hib—vaccine." http://www.nlm.nih.gov/medlineplus/ency/article/002023.htm Accessed September 20, 2012.

CDC "Haemophilus Influenzae Type b (Hib) Vaccine." http://www.cdc.gov/vaccines/pubs/vis/downloads/vis-hib.pdf Accessed September 20, 2012.

WHO "Haemophilus Influenzae Type b (Hib) Vaccine." http://www.who.int/mediacentre/factsheets/fs294/en/index.html Accessed September 20, 2012.

ORGANIZATIONS

Centers for Disease Control and Prevention, 1600 Clifton Road, Atlanta, GA USA 30333, (800) 232-4636, inquiry@cdc.gov, www.cdc.gov.

Andrea Nienstedt, MA

Hand-foot-and-mouth disease

Definition

Hand-foot-and-mouth disease is an infection of young children in which characteristic fluid–filled blisters appear on the hands, feet, and inside the mouth.

Demographics

Hand-foot-and-mouth disease is very common among young children and often occurs in clusters of children who are in daycare together.

An outbreak of hand-foot-and-mouth disease occurred in Singapore in 2000, with more than 1,000 diagnosed cases, all in children, resulting in four deaths. Asmaller outbreak occurred in Malaysia in 2000. In 1998, a serious outbreak of enterovirus 71 in Taiwan resulted in more than one million cases of hand-foot-and-mouth disease. Of these, there were 405 severe cases and 78 deaths, 71 of which were children younger than five years of age.

Hand-foot-and-mouth should not be confused with foot and mouth disease, which infects cattle but is extremely rare in humans. An outbreak of foot and mouth disease swept through Great Britain and into other parts of Europe and South America in 2001.

Description

Coxsackie viruses, the viruses that cause hand-foot-and-mouth disease, belong to a family of viruses called enteroviruses. These viruses live in the gastrointestinal tract and are therefore present in feces. They can be spread easily from one person to another when poor **hygiene** allows the virus within the feces to be passed from person to person. After exposure to the virus, development of symptoms takes only four to six days. Hand–foot–and–mouth disease can occur year–round, although the largest number of cases are in summer and fall months.

Causes and symptoms

Hand-foot-and-mouth disease is very common among young children and often occurs in clusters of

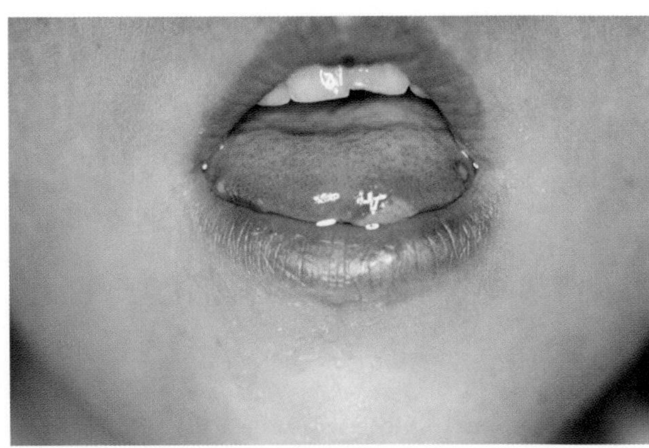

Hand-foot-and-mouth disease (HFMD) is a comon viral infection that afflicts infants and children. This image reveals the blisters that erupt on the mouth, and are usually accompanied by fever and skin rashes. *(Photo Researchers/Gettyimages.com)*

KEY TERMS

Enteroviruses—Viruses that live in the gastrointestinal tract. Coxsackie viruses, viruses that cause hand-foot-and-mouth disease, are an enterovirus.

Vesicle—A bump on the skin filled with fluid.

children who are in daycare together. It is spread when poor hand–washing after a diaper change or contact with saliva (drool) allows the virus to be passed from one child to another.

Within about four to six days of acquiring the virus, an infected child may develop a relatively low–grade fever, ranging from 99–102°F (37–38.9°C). Other symptoms include fatigue, loss of energy, decreased appetite, and a sore sensation in the mouth that may interfere with feeding. After one to two days, fluid–filled bumps (vesicles) appear on the inside of the mouth, along the surface of the tongue, on the roof of the mouth, and on the insides of the cheeks. These are tiny blisters, about three to seven millimeters in diameter. Eventually, they may appear on the palms of the hands and on the soles of the feet. Occasionally, these vesicles may occur in the diaper region.

The vesicles in the mouth cause the majority of discomfort, and the child may refuse to eat or drink due to **pain**. This phase usually lasts for an average of a week. As long as the bumps have clear fluid within them, the disease is at its most contagious. The fluid within the vesicles contains large quantities of the causative viruses. Extra care should be taken to avoid contact with this fluid.

Diagnosis

Diagnosis is made by most practitioners solely on the basis of the unique appearance of blisters of the mouth, hands, and feet in a child not appearing very ill.

Treatment

There are no treatments available to cure or decrease the duration of the disease. Medications like acetaminophen or ibuprofen may be helpful for decreasing pain, and allowing the child to eat and drink. It is important to try to encourage the child to take in adequate amounts of fluids, in the form of ice chips or popsicles if other foods or liquids are too uncomfortable.

Public Health Response

Hand-foot-and-mouth disease is a condition for which public health practices have a number of useful applications. The first step in public health procedures usually involves the identification of an area in which the disease occurs; the number, type, and other characteristics of those individuals infected with the virus; and provision of the needed equipment and personnel skills needed to test for the virus and for treatment of those infected with the disease. Of special importance to public health workers is the need to develop programs of education for individuals living within an area where hand, foot, and mouth disease is prevalent to prevent to the extent possible spread of the disease. The procedures required for such an instructional program are those that, in any case, are essential to the spread of other infectious diseases, focusing on the need for good hygiene to the extent possible. Educational programs should focus not only on children themselves, the most likely victims of the disease, but also parents, teachers, and local health workers.

QUESTIONS TO ASK YOUR DOCTOR

- Are there regions in the United States where my family is likely to encounter hand-foot-and-mouth disease?
- What precautions should our family take in traveling overseas to reduce the risk of becoming infected with hand-foot-and-mouth disease?
- What long-term health problems may be associated with a case of hand-foot-and-mouth disease?
- Is there any biological connection between hand-foot-and-mouth and foot-and-mouth diseases? If so, what is that connection?

Alternative treatment

There are no effective alternative treatments for hand-foot-and-mouth disease.

Prognosis

The prognosis for a child with hand-foot-and-mouth disease is excellent. The child is usually completely better within about a week of the start of the illness.

Prevention

Prevention involves careful attention to hygiene. Thorough, consistent hand–washing practices and discouraging the sharing of clothes, towels, and stuffed toys are all helpful. The virus continues to be passed in the feces for several weeks after infection, so good hygiene should be practiced long after all signs of infection have passed.

Resources

BOOKS

Morag, Abraham, and Pearay L. Ogra. "Viral Infections." In Behrman, Richard, ed. *Nelson Textbook of Pediatrics,* 19th ed. Philadelphia: W.B. Saunders Co., 2011.

PERIODICALS

Lee T.C., et al. "Diseases Caused by Enterovirus 71 Infection." *The Pediatric Infectious Disease Journal.* 28, 10 (2009): 904–10.

Ooi M.H., et al. "Identification and Validation of Clinical Predictors for the Risk of Neurological Involvement in Children with Hand, Foot, and Mouth Disease in Sarawak." *BMC Infectious Diseases.* 9 (2009): 3.

OTHER

Hand, Foot, and Mouth Disease. Centers for Disease Control and Prevention. http://www.cdc.gov/hand-foot-mouth/index.html (accessed August 17, 2012).

Hadn-foot-and-mouth Disease. Mayo Clinic. http://www.mayoclinic.com/health/hand-foot-and-mouth-disease/DS00599/ (accessed August 17, 2012).

Rosalyn Carson–DeWitt, MD
Ken R. Wells
Karl Finley

Handwashing

Definition

In health and medicine, handwashing is a procedure that reduces the risk of spreading disease between two individuals. Handwashing is an essential component of standard precaution procedures, a set of minimum infection **prevention** practices used in all types of patient care, regardless of suspected or confirmed infection status of the patient, in any setting where healthcare is delivered.

Description

The term *handwashing* suggests a familiar practice common to almost any household in which a person uses soap and water to cleanse the hands of dirt and other materials. In health and medicine, however, the term has a much broader and more specific meaning. One of the most common methods by which disease is transmitted is the transfer of microbes from a patient or a contaminated surface to a health worker and back to a patient again. Public health authorities have developed a number of procedures for reducing the risk of infection by this process. One set of procedures is described as some form of *handwashing*, in which some type of antiseptic agent, such as plain or antiseptic soap and water, is used to cleanse the hands, after which they are dried with some form of towel. A second set of procedures is known as *handrubbing*, in which some type of antiseptic material without the use of water or a drying material is used. By far the most common antiseptic used for this purpose is an alcoholic preparation. Alcohol-based hand rubs are a more efficient antimicrobial material than are either plain soap or antibacterial soap, and they also tend to be gentler on the hands than are soaps of any kind. Handwash and handrub procedures for surgical purposes tend to be somewhat stronger and more persistent than are those used for routine hospital or other forms of health or medical procedures.

Handwashing and handrubbing materials come in a variety of formats. The traditional soap and water handwash, for example, can be accomplished with a solid or liquid soap with or without an added antiseptic agent with water, followed by drying with a cloth. A variety of substances can be added to plain soap to provide antiseptic action, including various kinds of alcohol, chlorhexidine gluconate (CHG), derivatives of chlorine, iodine, chloroxylenol (PCMX), quaternary ammonium compounds, and triclosan. Alcohol-based handrubs can be provided in liquid, gel, or foam form, which are usually all self-drying. Antiseptic handwipes are fabric or paper which contain an antiseptic material dissolved in an alcohol-base which evaporates rapidly after use.

The role of handwashing in surgical procedures is especially important, and the **World Health Organization (WHO)** has developed a very detailed methodology for the practice consisting of 17 discrete and clearly-defined steps. That procedure begins with the collection of about 5 mL of alcohol-based handrub from a dispenser in the left hand while manipulating the dispenser lever with the right elbow, dipping the fingertips of the right hand in the handrub being held in the left hand, smearing the handrub on the right forearm up to the elbow . . . and so on to the final steps, which include rubbing the thumb of the left hand by rotating it in the palm of the right hand, and vice versa. (The complete procedure is described at http://whqlibdoc.who.int/publications/2009/9789241597906_eng.pdf, pp. 59-60.)

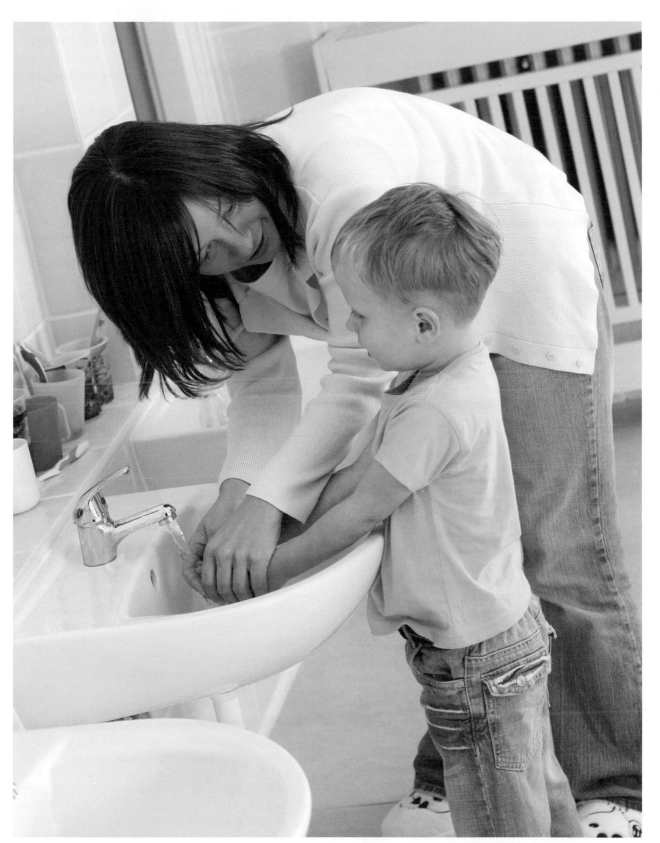

Teacher helping a preshooler with the proper techniques of hand washing. *(matka_Wariatka/Shutterstock.com)*

Origins

Although the risk of transfering pathogens from healthcare workers to patients is well known today, such has not always been the case. In fact, the realization that healthcare workers can be a serious health threat to their patients dates only to the middle of the nineteenth century, when Hungarian physician Ignaz Semmelweiss became convinced that the high rate of puerperal fever among new mothers was the result of physician behavior. Specifically, it was not uncommon at the time for physicians in a hospital to move from one patient to the next without washing one's hands. If a prior patient was contaminated with pathogens, which was almost always the case, the physician then served as the vector through which those pathogens were carried to the next patient, often an expectant mother. Efforts by Semmelweiss to change physician practice in the hospitals for which he was responsible were largely a failure at first (and Semmelweiss himself was eventually commited to an asylum), but his ideas proved true in the end, and handwashing today is an unquestionable and essential part of all responsible healthcare practice.

Sick people and healthcare facilities such as hospitals are, almost by definition, hotbeds of disease. Pathogens are present on many parts of a patient's body and on virtually every part of the surrounding environment, including pillows, sheets, tables, chairs, and medical equipment used to treat a patient. A healthcare worker simply cannot avoid coming into contact with those pathogens and collecting them on her or his skin. Without handwashing as an intermediary step between touching one patient and the next, the healthcare worker is almost certain to transmit at least some of those pathogens to the second patient. Studies of handwashing practices in hospitals and other care facilities have found that doctors, nurses, and other healthcare workers have literally dozens of opportunities for handwashing during every shift at work. The extent to which they take advantage of those opportunities, however, varies greatly, depending on a number of factors. In a number of studies of adherence to handwashing opportunities, researchers have found that healthcare workers take advantage of such opportunities anywhere from 5 to 89 percent of the time, with the overall average of 38.7 percent adherence. These results suggest that even when healthcare workers understand the importance of handwashing procedures, they do not always take advantage of the opportunities to follow up on the practice.

A number of factors affect adherence to handwashing protocols, such as:

- one's status within the profession (doctors may feel less motivated to follow handwashing protocols than nurses)
- duration of contact with a patient (shorter times with a patient may lead to a reduced use of handwashing)
- degree of risk posed by patients (handwashing after interaction with an HIV patient is more likely than contact with someone who has back pain)
- patient-to-nurse ratio (the more patients one sees, the less time one may have to do handwashes)
- availability of handwashing sinks (the less available equipment is, the less likely workers may use handwashing)
- higher demand for patient attention (the more time one spends with patients, the less time one may have for handwashing)
- increased practice of glove use (workers may believe—incorrectly—that by using gloves they should not have to handwash as often)
- lack of institutional guidelines (if the institution does not seem to care, maybe healthcare workers won't care either)
- personal doubts about the value of handwashing (some workers may not be convinced that handwashing is really all that important, and so may ignore the practice to some extent)

Interestingly enough, cultural and religious beliefs may have a strong influence on the extent to which healthcare workers adhere to recommended handwashing practices. That is, some religions and cultures place a high value on hand cleanliness in the everyday world, so that such practices within the healthcare world are not an unusual concept. The Muslim religion, for example, teaches that one should wash one's hands many times a day: five times before prayers, before and after every meal, after using the toilet, after touching a dog or shoes, and after anything that has been soiled. Other religions, such as Christianity, do not have such severe admonitions about everyday handwashing, so the health and medical practice presents a new level of adherence. On the other hand, the use of alcohol rubs is generally thought to be prohibited by the Muslim religion, so that healthcare workers in Islamic nations must develop acceptable alternatives to some recommended health and medical handcare practices.

Costs to society

A substantial amount of research is now available about the costs to societies of diseases that result from healthcare-worker-transmitted disease. Authorities now estimate that, at any moment in time, about 1.4 million patients worldwide are under care from healthcare-associated infections (HCAI). In developed countries, HCAI infections may account for anywhere from 5 to 15 percent of all hospitalized patients and for 9 to 37 percent of all intensive care unit patients. In Europe, an estimated 50,000 people die every year as a result of HCAI infections, and such

KEY TERMS

Antiseptic agent—Any substance that inactivates microorganisms or inhibits their growth on living tissues.

Antiseptic handrubbing—Cleaning the hands with any antiseptic agent that does not require the use of water or a drying cloth.

Antiseptic handwashing—Washing the hands with soap and water, or other detergents containing an antiseptic agent.

Hand cleansing—Any act or set of acts performed to remove dirt, microbes, and other materials from the hands.

Standard precaution procedures—A set of minimum infection prevention practices used in all types of patient care, regardless of suspected or confirmed infection status of the patient, in any setting where healthcare is delivered.

Surgical hand antisepsis—An antiseptic handwash or handrub in preparation for surgery that follows a carefully prescribed sequence of steps. Also known as surgical hand preparation or presurgical hand preparation.

infections are a contributing factor in an additional 135,000 deaths per year. The latest data for the United States (2002) showed 1.7 million individuals with HCAI infections and 99,000 deaths, producing an estimated economic impact on the nation of $6.5 billion in 2004. In the United States, the most common type of HCAI case reported was urinary tract infection, accounting for 36% of all HCAI infections, followed by surgical site infections (20%), and bloodstream infections and **pneumonia** (both 11%).

Data for HCAI infections in developing countries are generally not as readily available as they are for developed countries. The few reliable studies that have been done suggest infection rates from HCAI in the 15 to 25 percent range for hospitals and other healthcare facilities. Contributing factors in these countries include understaffing, poor **hygiene** and **sanitation** in general, lack or shortage of basic medicines and equipment, and inadequate structures and overcrowding of facilities.

Efforts and solutions

The irony that healthcare workers and facilities are a major source of health and medical problems around the world has not been lost on the public health community. Aggressive programs have been developed to better inform healthcare workers and policymakers about the importance of handwashing in protecting patients and the general **population**. The **World Health Organization** has developed a recommended training and education program for healthcare workers on the topic of handwashing. The program consists of four major elements:

- Morbidity, mortality, and economic costs associated with healthcare-associated infections.
- Transmission of pathogens, including routes of transmission and consequences for both the patient and healthcare workers.
- Strategies for the prevention of pathogen transmission, including standard precautions, hand hygiene, and care-associated precautions.
- Indications for hand hygiene, including the concept of a health-care area and patient zone, the principle of "my five moments for hand hygiene," and hand hygiene agents and procedures.

Resources

BOOKS

Graupp, Patrick, and Martha Purrier. *Getting to Standard Work in Health Care: Using TWI to Create a Foundation for Quality Care.* London: Productivity Press, 2012.

Rothrock, Jane C. *Alexander's Care of the Patient in Surgery*, 14th ed. St. Louis: Mosby, 2010.

PERIODICALS

Kendall, A., et al. "Point-of-care Hand Hygiene: Preventing Infection behind the Curtain." *American Journal of Infection Control.* 40, 4, Suppl 1 (2012): S3–10.

Landers, T., et al. "Patient-centered Hand Hygiene: The Next Step in Infection Prevention." *American Journal of Infection Control.* 40, 4, Suppl 1. (2012): S11–17.

Vindigni, S. M., P. L. Riley, and M. Jhung. "Systematic Review: Handwashing Behaviour in Low- to Middle-income Countries: Outcome Measures and Behaviour Maintenance." *Tropical Medicine and International Health.* 16, 4. (2011): 466–77.

WEBSITES

"Hand Hygiene in Healthcare Settings." Centers for Disease Control and Prevention. http://www.cdc.gov/handhygiene/. Accessed on September 26, 2012.

"Improved Hand Hygiene to Prevent Health Care-Associated Infections." The Joint Commission. http://www.ccforpatientsafety.org/common/pdfs/fpdf/presskit/PS-Solution9.pdf. Accessed on September 26, 2012.

"WHO Guidelines on Hand Hygiene in Health Care." World Health Organization. http://whqlibdoc.who.int/publications/2009/9789241597906_eng.pdf. Accessed on September 26, 2012.

ORGANIZATIONS

World Health Organization (WHO), 20 Avenue Appia, 1211, Geneva 27, Switzerland, +41 22 791 4140, http://www.who.int/about/contacthq/en/index.html, http://www.who.int.

David E. Newton, Ed.D.

Hantavirus infections

Definition

Hantavirus infection is caused by a group of viruses that can infect humans with two serious illnesses: hemorrhagic fever with renal syndrome (HFRS), and hantavirus pulmonary syndrome (HPS).

Description

Hantaviruses are found without causing symptoms within various species of rodents and are passed to humans by exposure to the urine, feces, or saliva of those infected rodents. Ten different hantaviruses have been identified as important in humans. Each is found in specific geographic regions and therefore is spread by different rodent carriers. Further, each type of virus causes a slightly different form of illness in its human hosts:

- Hantaan virus is carried by the striped field mouse and exists in Korea, China, Eastern Russia, and the Balkans. Hantaan virus causes a severe form of HFRS.
- Puumula virus is carried by bank voles and exists in Scandinavia, western Russia, and Europe. Puumula virus causes a milder form of HFRS, usually termed *nephropathia epidemica*.
- Seoul virus is carried by a type of rat called the Norway rat and exists worldwide, but causes disease almost exclusively in Asia. Seoul virus causes a form of HFRS that is slightly milder than that caused by Hantaan virus, but results in liver complications.
- Prospect Hill virus is carried by meadow voles and exists in the United States, but has not been found to cause human disease.
- Sin Nombre virus, the most predominant strain in the United States, is carried by the deer mouse. This virus was responsible for severe cases of HPS that occurred in the southwestern United States in 1993.
- Black Creek Canal virus has been found in Florida. It is predominantly carried by cotton rats.
- New York virus strain has been documented in New York. The vectors for this virus seem to be deer mice and white-footed mice.
- Bayou virus has been reported in Louisiana and Texas and is carried by the marsh rice rat.
- Blue River virus has been found in Indiana and Oklahoma and seems to be associated with the white-footed mouse.
- Monongahela virus, discovered in 2000, has been found in Pennsylvania and is transmitted by the white-footed mouse.

At least 30 additional species of hantavirus have been identified, most with little or no known effect on human health.

Causes and symptoms

Hemorrhagic fever with renal syndrome (HFRS)

Hantaviruses that produce forms of HFRS cause a classic group of symptoms, including fever, malfunction of the kidneys, and low platelet count. Because platelets are blood cells important in proper clotting, low numbers of circulating platelets can result in spontaneous bleeding, or hemorrhage.

Patients with HFRS have **pain** in the head, abdomen, and lower back and may report bloodshot eyes and blurry vision. Tiny pinpoint hemorrhages, called petechiae, may appear on the upper body and the soft palate in the mouth. The patient's face, chest, abdomen, and back often appear flushed and red, as if sunburned.

After about five days, the patient may have a sudden drop in blood pressure; often it drops low enough to cause the clinical syndrome called shock. Shock is a state in which blood circulation throughout the body is insufficient to deliver proper quantities of oxygen. Lengthy shock can result in permanent damage to the body's organs, particularly the brain, which is very sensitive to oxygen deprivation.

Around day eight of HFRS, kidney involvement results in multiple derangements of the body chemistry. Simultaneously, the hemorrhagic features of the illness begin to cause spontaneous bleeding, as demonstrated by bloody urine, bloody vomit, and in very serious cases, brain hemorrhages with resulting changes in consciousness.

Day 11 often brings further chemical derangements, with associated confusion, hallucinations, seizures, and lung complications. Those who survive this final phase usually begin to turn the corner toward recovery at this time, although recovery takes approximately six weeks.

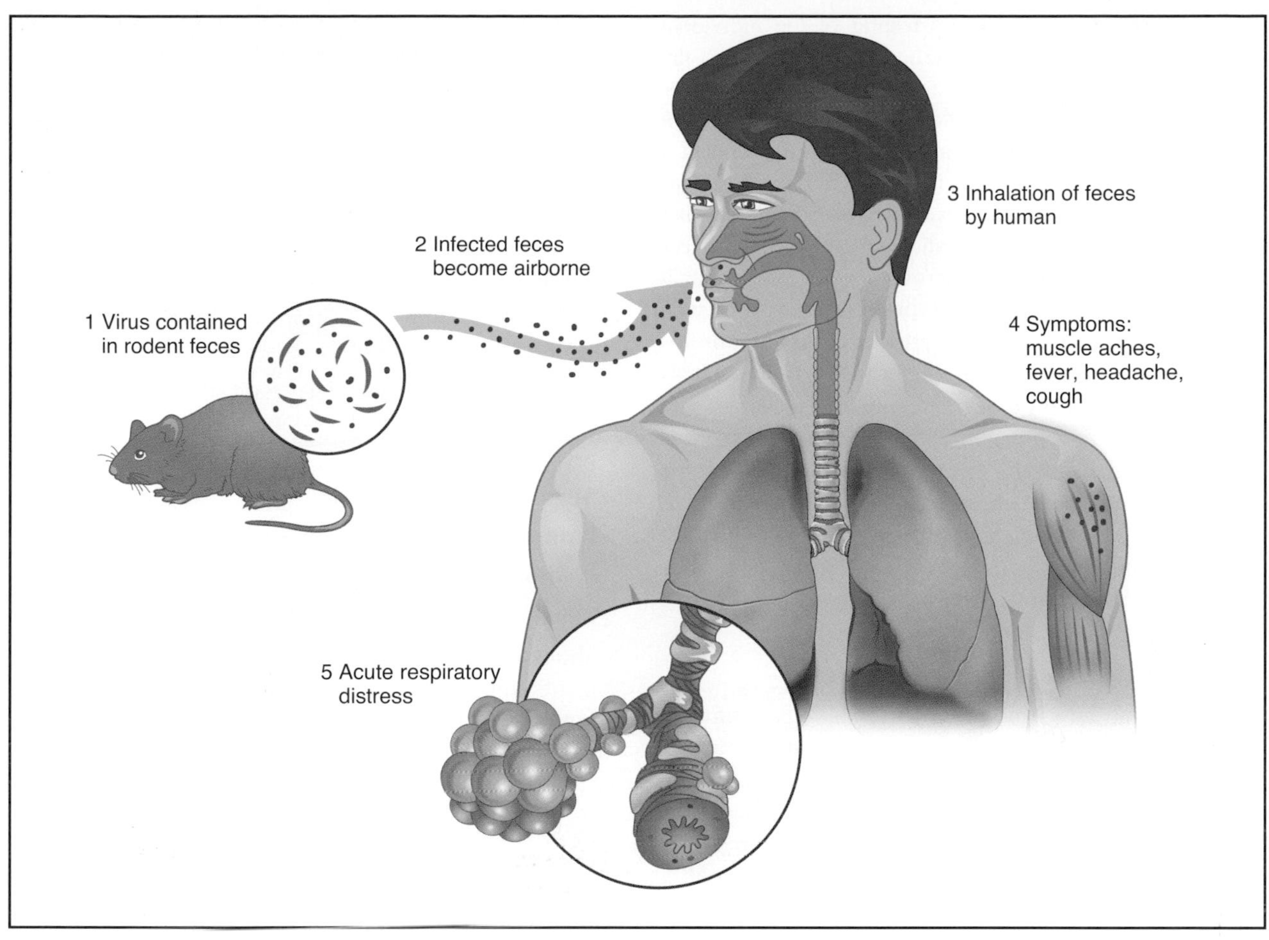

Hanta virus transmission *(Illustration by Electronic Illustrators Group. © 2013 Cengage Learning)*

Hantavirus pulmonary syndrome (HPS)

HPS develops in four stages. They are:

- The incubation period. This lasts from one to five weeks from exposure. Here, the patient may exhibit no symptoms.
- The prodrome, or warning signs, stage. Symptoms begin with a fever, muscle aches, headache, dizziness, abdominal pain, and stomach upset. Sometimes there is vomiting and diarrhea.
- The cardiopulmonary stage. The patient slips into this stage rapidly, sometimes within a day or two of initial symptoms, sometimes as long as 10 days later. There is a drop in blood pressure, shock, and leaking of the blood vessels of the lungs, which results in fluid accumulation in the lungs, and subsequent shortness of breath. The fluid accumulation can be so rapid and so severe as to put the patient in respiratory failure within only a few hours. Some patients experience severe abdominal tenderness.
- The convalescent stage. If the patient survives the respiratory complications of the previous stage, there is a rapid recovery, usually within a day or two. However, abnormal liver and lung functioning may persist for six months.

Diagnosis

Serologic techniques help diagnose a hantavirus infection. The patient's blood is drawn, and the ELISA (enzyme-linked immunosorbent assay) is done in a laboratory to identify the presence of specific immune substances (antibodies), which an individual's body would only produce in response to the hantavirus.

It is difficult to demonstrate the actual virus in human tissue or to grow cultures of the virus within the laboratory, so the majority of diagnostic tests use indirect means to demonstrate the presence of the virus.

Public health response

The first stage in the public health response to a reported hantavirus infection is likely to be confirmation of the existence of the disease by testing of the individual involved. In many cases it may be necessary to send the sample collected from a victim to the U.S. **Centers for Disease Control and Prevention (CDC)** for confirmation of diagnosis. A public health agency may then conduct a survey to determine the source from which the disease was obtained and the way it may have been spread among other community members. Identification of a hantavirus infection should intensify and improve existing educational programs about the disease and its **prevention** or, if no such program exists, one should be initiated. A program of this kind normally includes not only information to individuals who may be at risk for the disease, but also materials with which a prevention program can be conducted, such as cleaning materials, rat and mouse traps, and the like. Some forms of hantavirus, such as hantavirus pulmonary syndrome, are reportable diseases, so data for infected individuals must be sent to the National Notifiable Diseases Surveillance System at the **CDC**.

Treatment

Treatment of hantavirus infections is primarily supportive because there are no agents available to kill the viruses and interrupt the infection. Broad-spectrum **antibiotics** are given until the diagnosis is confirmed. Supportive care consists of providing treatment in response to the patient's symptoms. Because both HFRS and HPS progress so rapidly, patients must be closely monitored so that treatment may be started at the first sign of a particular problem. Low blood pressure is treated with medications. Blood transfusions are given for both hemorrhage and shock states. Hemodialysis is used in kidney failure. (Hemodialysis involves mechanically cleansing the blood outside of the body, to replace the kidney's normal function of removing various toxins form the blood.) Rapid respiratory assistance is critical, often requiring intubation.

The anti-viral agent ribavirin has been approved for use in early treatment of hantavirus infections.

Prognosis

The diseases caused by hantaviruses are extraordinarily lethal. About 6–15% of people who contract HFRS have died. Almost half of all people who contract HPS will die. This gives HPS one of the highest fatality rates of any acute viral disease. It is essential that people living in areas where the hantaviruses exist seek quick medical treatment should they begin to develop an illness that might be due to a hantavirus.

Prevention

As of late 2012, there are no immunizations currently available against any of the hantaviruses. Developments in genetic science are expected to help researchers work on a possible **vaccination** and therapy for several versions of hantavirus, including the Sin Nombre virus that causes HPS. With further work, a gene-based vaccine could become available in the future. However, the only known forms of hantavirus prevention involve rodent control within the community and within individual households. The following is a list of preventive measures:

- Avoiding areas known to be infested by rodents is essential.
- Keeping a clean home and keeping food in rodent-proof containers.
- Disposing of garbage and emptying pet food dishes at night.
- Setting rodent traps around baseboards and in tight places.
- Disposing of dead animals with gloves and disinfecting the area with bleach.
- Using rodenticide as necessary.
- Sealing any entry holes 0.25 inch wide or wider around foundations with screen, cement, or metal flashing.
- Clearing brush and junk from house foundations.
- Putting metal flashing around house foundations.
- Elevating hay, woodpiles, and refuse containers.
- Airing out all sealed outbuildings or cabins 30 minutes before cleaning for the season.

KEY TERMS

Hemodialysis—A method of mechanically cleansing the blood outside of the body, in order to remove various substances that would normally be cleared by the kidneys. Hemodialysis is used when an individual is in relative, or complete, kidney failure.

Hemorrhagic—A condition resulting in massive, difficult-to-control bleeding.

Petechiae—Pinpoint size red spots caused by hemorrhaging under the skin.

Platelets—Circulating blood cells that are crucial to the mechanism of clotting.

Prodrome—Early symptoms or warning signs

Pulmonary—Referring to the lungs.

Renal—Referring to the kidneys.

Shock—A state in which blood circulation is insufficient to deliver adequate oxygen to vital organs.

QUESTIONS TO ASK YOUR DOCTOR

- What public health resources are available in our community for additional information about hantavirus infections?
- Which forms of hantavirus are known to occur in our area of the country?
- What new developments can you tell me about with regard to treatment or prevention of hantavirus infections?

- When camping, avoiding sleeping on the bare ground. It is advised to sleep on a cot or in a tent with a floor.

Resources

BOOKS

Beltz, Lisa A. *Emerging Infectious Diseases: A Guide to Diseases, Causative Agents, and Surveillance*. San Francisco: Jossey-Bass, 2011.

Fong, I.W., and Ken Alibek. *New and Evolving Infections of the 21st Century*. New York: Springer, 2007.

PERIODICALS

Schmaljohn, C. "Vaccines for Hantaviruses." *Vaccine* 27, Supp. 4. (2012): D61–D64.

Clement, J., et al. "A Unifying Hypothesis and a Single Name for a Complex Globally Emerging Infection: Hantavirus Disease." *European Journal of Clinical Microbiology & Infectious Diseases* 31, 1. (2012): 1–5.

OTHER

Hantavirus. Centers for Disease Control and Prevention. http://www.cdc.gov/hantavirus/ (accessed August 18, 2012).

Hantavirus. PubMed Health. http://www.ncbi.nlm.nih.gov/pubmedhealth/PMH0002358/ (accessed August 18, 2012).

Janie F. Franz
Teresa G. Odle

Health commissioners

Definition

A health commissioner is the chief administrative officer for a public or private health agency, such as a city or county health department. The health commissioner is appointed by and reports to a board of directors or some other governing board. It is her or his responsibility, in general, to carry out the health policies set by that governing board.

Purpose

The health commissioner is the person in a health agency who is the intermediary between the governing board, which sets policies for the organization, and the staff of the agency, which ultimately carries out those policies.

Description

A health commissioner may have a range of responsibilities, depending on the size and purpose of the organization he or she leads. Those responsibilities might include:

- Appointing and supervising managers, department heads, and other midlevel managers who are to report to the health commissioner.
- Preparing financial budgets for the agency for which he or she is responsible.
- Preparing reports on programs, activities, accomplishments, and other functions of the health agency.
- Defining the responsibilities and chain of command for offices, divisions, personnel, and other agency employees.
- Assuming overall responsibility for the functioning of the agency, which may involve solving problems that arise from within the agency.
- Representing the agency to the general public as spokesperson for the agency's mission and activities.
- Negotiating contracts with other companies and agencies that supply personnel, services, or materials for the agency's operations.
- Representing the agency before legislative, regulatory, administrative, and other governmental agencies to which the health agency is responsible.
- Having ultimate responsibility for research and development functions that take place within the agency.
- Reviewing legislative, regulatory, adiministrative and other governmental rules and regulations that may apply to the health agency, determining how those rules and regulations will affect the agency, and designing mechanisms by which they can be carried out.
- Working with the governing board to determine long–range policies and practices for the agency.
- Demonstrating the type of leadership for the agency that will encourage employees to understand and carry out the goals and mission of the agency.
- Acting as the negotiating office between and among stakeholders within the agency, including between employees and between employees and nonemployees.
- Working to develop harmonious cooperation among employees to accomplish agency objectives.

- Developing methods for forecasting future trends within the industry and for the specific agency for which she or he is responsible.

The job requirements for health commissioner vary considerably depending on the type of agency, the geographic location, and other factors. Generally speaking, most agencies prefer to have medical doctors in the position of health commissioner, although some accept other degrees, such as higher degrees in nursing, law degrees, a master of public health or master of business administration, or some comparable degree. Degrees in ancillary fields, such as **veterinary medicine**, dentistry, podiatry, or chiropractic may also be acceptable in some cases. Applicants for the position of health commissioner may also be required to have experience in the same or related fields before being considered for a post, and they may be required to have earned a certificate of advanced training in health sciences management. An example of such a certificate is one given in the field of National Incident Management, issued by the U.S. Federal Emergency Management Administration (FEMA). Most applicants for the position of health commissioner are also expected to display a rather extensive list of management and interpersonal skills, such as the ability to analyze quantitative and qualitative data; to ensure that local policies and practices are consistent with local, state, and national laws and regulations; to communicate effectively in verbal and written communications with superiors, subordinates, lawmakers, and the general public; to recognize and understand how to appreciate and deal with individuals from a variety of cultural backgrounds; to develop and carry out mechanisms that recognize and make use of the skills and talents of all stakeholders engaged in the specific public health agency involved, and to have command of the science and technology of public health as a discipline and to know how to apply that knowledge to local problems and issues.

Professional publications

Lacking a specific professional organization of their own, health commissioners tend to rely on publications available to them from other professional organizations to which they might belong, such as the **Association of State and Territorial Health Officers (ASTHO)** or the National Association of **Community Health** Centers (NACHC). **ASTHO**, for example, provides books, pamphlets, brochures, and other print materials on topics such as state and local public health, at-risk populations, health equity, health reform, public health funding, state public health issues, substance abuse, workforce issues, and **environmental health**.

Resources

BOOKS

Fallon, L. Fleming, and Eric J. Zgodzinski. *Essentials of Public Health Management*. Sudbury, MA: Jones and Bartlett Publishers, 2005.

Stahl, Michael J. *Encyclopedia of Health Care Management*. Thousand Oaks, CA: Sage Publications, 2004.

PERIODICALS

Sigmond, Robert. "Community-Based Health Organizations." *Health Promotion Practice* 7. 2. (2006): 157–58

Thompson, Amy, et al. "Public Policy Involvement by Health Commissioners." *Journal of Community Health* 34. 4. (2009): 239–45

WEBSITES

Career: Health Commissioner. MyMajors. http://www.mymajors.com/careers-and-jobs/Health-Commissioner (accessed October 12, 2012).

Health Officer Medical Director. Santa Barbara County Human Resources Department. http://www.jobaps.com/sbc/specs/CSPEC3933.asp (accessed October 12, 2012).

ORGANIZATIONS

Association of State and Territorial Health Officers (ASTHO), 2231 Crystal Dr., Suite 450, Arlington, VA 22202, (202) 371-9090, Fax: (571) 527-3189, http://www.astho.org/

National Association of Community Health Centers (NACHC), 7501 Wisconsin, Ave., Suite 1100W, Bethesda, MD 20814, (301) 347-0400, http://www.nachc.com/contact-us.cfm, http://www.nachc.com/.

David E. Newton, EdD

Health departments

Definition

A health department is a division of a larger governmental agency, such as a city, county, or state, with general responsibility for matters relating to public health.

Purpose

The purpose of a health department is to promote the general health of all individuals subsumed within the entity covered by the department. For public health departments, this statement applies to all of the men, women, and children who live within a specific geographical region, such as a city, county, or state. For private health departments, it applies to the individuals employed within a particular work setting, such as an office, department, or company. One of the major aspects of such a function is preventing disease and injury among individuals within the entity, as well as promoting a general understanding of the elements of a healthful lifestyle and ways in which those elements can be incorporated in the workplace and/or one's daily life.

Description

The National Association of County and City Health Officials (**NACCHO**) has developed a self-assessment tool for health departments that allows them to evaluate their proficiencies in a number of areas that are generally considered to be part of the work of a health department. Some of those areas are the following:

- The health department staff collects data from the community about its health status and practices, collates and analyzes those data, retains them as permanent records, and uses those data to develop policies and practices for the department's use in the future. Staff members search for trends in health patterns in the community or the company that can be used to formulate new and revised policies and practices.
- It makes use of its own expertise to develop community health surveys on a regular basis of no less than every five years and shares the data collected from such surveys with other organizations and agencies within the community who can make use of this information.
- It possesses and makes use of skills needed to investigate outbreaks of infectious diseases, environmental hazards, or other public health issues that may arise in the community.
- It takes actions that may be necessary to reduce the risk of such outbreaks and environmental hazards by educating the public about conditions that may lead to the outbreak of disease or that may lead to environmental threats to the community.
- It makes use of knowledge, skills, personnel, materials, and other resources from other health agencies to achieve its objectives of reducing the threat of disease outbreak, the rise of environmental hazards, or other public health problems. At the same time, staff members share their own knowledge and skills with other agencies and companies.
- It is familiar with resources available for dealing with natural or manmade disasters, by knowing how to implement programs such as the National Incident Management System for bioterrorist attacks or other unexpected emergencies. Staff members are expected to participate in training exercises and other activities that are part of such preparedness programs.
- It is skilled in or has access to individuals who are familiar with and have the equipment to carry out essential laboratory analyses that may be related to public health issues, such as the identification of causative agents in disease outbreaks.
- It develops and implements public education programs that will include information and activities that teach people about ways of avoiding infectious diseases, maintaining healthy lifestyles, preparing for natural and manmade emergencies, and being aware of information and material resources available to deal with public health issues.
- It recognizes the special needs of various populations, such as the poor, homeless, nonspeakers of English, immigrants, or others for whom adequate health care may be less accessible than it is to the general population.
- It develops and implements programs for individuals and groups within the general population who have special health problems, such as those who are diabetic or obese, those who are HIV positive, or those who have substance abuse problems.
- It works with the general public and other stakeholders to develop long-term health policies and practices that are appropriate for the community or the company.
- It acts as a resource to governmental policymaking and regulatory agencies about public health issues within a community or a company.
- It carries out enforcement activities specific to national, state, and local laws and regulations dealing with public health issues.
- It serves as a link between individuals with special housing needs, such as those requiring hospice care, and facilities in the community that can meet those needs.
- It recruits, trains, and assesses the staff for the health department.
- It makes sure that the health department staff has the physical and informational resources needed to carry out their duties in the department.
- It plans and carries out regular reviews of the accomplishments and activities of the department in terms of the agency's or company's long-term goals and mission.

This list of health department activities varies from agency to agency and does not apply in every detail to every agency. It is suggestive, however, of the types of responsibilities of most health departments.

Professional publications

The professional body most closely associated with the work of health departments is the National Association of County & City Health Officers (NACCHO), which provides a limited number of print and electronic resources for its members and for the general public. The most important of these resources is the bimonthly *Journal of Public Health Management and Practice*, which publishes peer–reviewed articles on topics such as

emergency preparedness; bioterrorism; **infectious disease** surveillance; **environmental health**; **community health assessment**; and chronic disease **prevention** and health promotion. Another useful publication is the *Achieving Healthier Communities through MAPP* handbook, developed for the **Mobilizing for Action through Planning and Partnerships** program. Two other publications developed for use with the **MAPP** program are the MAPP Field Guide and the MAPP Brochure, which provide additional information about the program and its implementation in health departments and other public health facilities.

Resources

BOOKS

Fallon, L. Fleming, and Eric J. Zgodzinski. *Essentials of Public Health Management*. Sudbury, MA: Jones and Bartlett Publishers, 2005.

Schneider, Mary-Jane. *Introduction to Public Health*, 2nd ed. Sudbury, MA: Jones and Bartlett, 2006.

Stahl, Michael J. *Encyclopedia of Health Care Management*. Thousand Oaks, CA: Sage Publications, 2004.

PERIODICALS

Novick, L. F. "Local Health Departments: Time of Challenge and Change." *Journal of Public Health Management and Practice* 18. 2. (2012): 103–105

Stanbury, M., et al. "Functions of Environmental Epidemiology and Surveillance in State Health Departments." *Journal of Public Health Management and Practice* 18. 5. (2012): 453–460.

WEBSITES

Local Health Departments in the USA. Health Guide USA. http://www.healthguideusa.org/local_health_departments.htm (accessed October 13, 2012).

Public Health Resources: State Health Departments. Centers for Disease Control and Prevention. http://www.cdc.gov/mmwr/international/relres.html (accessed October 13, 2012).

ORGANIZATIONS

National Association of County and City Health Officials (NACCHO), 1100 17th St., N.W., 17th floor, Washington, DC 20036, (202) 783-5550, Fax: (202) 783-1583, info@naccho.org, www.naccho.org/

David E. Newton, EdD

Health education

Definition

One of the most commonly quoted definitions of health education comes from a 1998 publication by the **World Health Organization**, which describes it as "consciously constructed opportunities for learning involving some form of communication designed to improve **health literacy**, including improving knowledge, and developing life skills which are conducive to individual and community health." Since the field of health itself is large and complex, health education is often subdivided into smaller categories, such as physical health, sexual health, mental health, emotional health, **environmental health**, and social health.

Purpose

The purpose of health education is to provide individuals and communities with the knowledge, skills, and attitudes they need to make the best choices possible to ensure that they will experience a safe, healthy, and productive life.

Description

In some respects, health education has probably always been part of the human community, with parents and those with special skills in medicine teaching younger members of the group the best practices for staying alive and healthy. Health education as we know it, however, dates only to the late nineteenth and early twentieth century in most developed countries. It was during this period that researchers began to discover the causes of infectious diseases, which are the primary threat to the health of most individuals in a society. The first understanding of the principles of public health also began to appear during this period, with researchers discovering the ways in which polluted air and **water** contributed to the outbreak of disease and ill health in communities. The key breakthrough in health education in the United States occurred in 1915 with the publication of a report by William Welch and Wickliffe Rose, sponsored by the Rockefeller Foundation, outlining a program for health education in the United States. That report called for a program that focused on teaching about infectious diseases, was located in university programs, relied heavily on research, and was independent of existing medical schools. The first institution along these lines, the Johns Hopkins School of **Hygiene** and Public Health, opened a year later, in 1916. Over the next two decades, nine more such institutions were established, with an emphasis on teaching the practical aspects of health, such as **public health administration**, public health nursing, vital statistics, disease control, and **community health** services and field programs. Growth in health education at the university level soon slowed, however, and did not become a national priority until 1957 when the U.S. Congress passed the Hill-Rhodes bill, which provided federal funding for the establishment of university health education courses, programs, and degrees. As of 2013, there were 50 fully accredited and seven non-accredited schools of public health in the United States.

Health education is a required part of the curriculum in 40 U.S. states. In addition, many individual school systems voluntarily offer such classes in the remaining 10 states. Some form of health education is often offered at every grade level from kindergarten through grade 12, with individual school systems generally offering programs designed to meet their own needs and expectations. Generally speaking, such courses tend to cover subjects such as the human body; infectious diseases and disease **prevention**; physical fitness; alcohol, tobacco, and drug abuse; sexually transmitted infections; emotional health and self image; misconceptions and myths about health; sexuality and sexual relationships; pregnancy, contraception, and famiy planning; environmental health; community and public health; and careers in the health sciences, such as medicine, nursing, public health, and other related occupations. Under the best circumstances health education courses are taught by individuals specially trained in the field, although teachers are also often recruited from other fields, such as biology, general science, or physical education.

National guidelines for primary and secondary level health education courses were first issued in 1995 under the auspices of the U.S. Department of Education. A set of eight standards make up the guidelines, with performance indicators indicated for each grade level, pre-kindergarten through grade two; grades 3 through 5; 6 through 8; and 9 through 12. The eight standards deal with the following general topics:

1. promotion of health and disease prevention
2. the influence of family, peers, culture, media, technology, and other factors on health behaviors
3. information products and services available for the enhancement of health
4. the use of interpersonal communication skills for the enhancement of health and avoidance of disease
5. the use of decision-making skills in enhancing personal and community health
6. learning how to set goals to improve personal and community health
7. putting into practice the skills needed to improve health and avoid disease
8. learning how to advocate for personal, family, and community health

The so-called performance indicators used in the standards consist of observable behaviors by which one can determine whether and to what extent an individual has progressed towards each of the standards. For example, a performance indicator for standard 4 at the youngest grade level consists of a child's ability to "demonstrate ways to tell a trusted adult if threatened or harmed." A performance indicator at the highest grade level for standard 3 is to "determine when professional health services may be required."

Health educators work in a wide variety of settings in addition to primary and secondary schools and colleges and universities. They also find employment in health care facilities, public **health departments**, nonprofit organizations, and private businesses. Among their responsibilities in these settings are the following:

- teaching patients about ways of handling their health problems, such as necessary treatments they may need to carry out
- arranging for testing and screenings for patients
- working with medical staff to improve the interaction between providers and patients
- organize and operate specialized programs on disease prevention and other public health issues
- provide administrative support by writing grant requests and maintaining contact with outside agencies
- design and execute programs focusing on specific health issues of concern to a community or a business, such as obesity or smoking
- conduct assessments and evaluations of health needs in a community, school, business, or other setting
- serve as members on and as liaisons to other health organizations at the local, regional, state, and national level.

Most schools and agencies require that health educators have at least a bachelor's degree in health education, with a master's degree often being preferred. Many institutions also require that a candidate become a Certified Health Education Specialist (CHES), a title earned from the National Commission for Health Education Credentialing, Inc. The certificate is awarded to individuals who have passed a specialized test and remains valid as long as a person takes an additional 75 hours of approved course work in each of the following five years.

Professional publications

Resources

BOOKS

Glanz, Karen, Barbara K. Rimer, and K. Viswanath. *Health Behavior and Health Education: Theory, Research, and Practice*, 4th ed. Hoboken, NJ: John Wiley & Sons, Inc., 2011.

Gilbert, Glen G., Robin G. Sawyer, and Beth McNeill. *Health Education: Creating Strategies for School and Community*

Health, 3rd ed. Sudbury, MA: Jones and Bartlett Publishers, 2011.

Meeks, Linda Brower, Philip Heit, and Randy M. Page. *Comprehensive School Health Education: Totally Awesome Strategies for Teaching Health*, 8th ed. New York, NY: McGraw-Hill, 2012.

PERIODICALS

Hisanaga, N. "Occupational Safety and Health Education in Schools." *Industrial Health* 50. 4. (2012): 251–52.

Sanderson, K. "Health Education in Schools: Strengths and Weaknesses in Relation to Long–term Behaviour Development." *Perspectives in Public Health* 132. 1. (2012): 19–20.

WEBSITES

Health Education. World Health Organization. http://www.who.int/topics/health_education/en/ (accessed October 13, 2012).

What Is Health Education? http://www.cnheo.org/PDF%20files/health_ed.pdf (accessed October 13, 2012).

ORGANIZATIONS

Society for Public Health Education (SOPHE), 10 G St., N.W., Suite 605, Washington, DC 20002, (202) 408-9804, Fax: (202) 408-9815, info@sophe.org, www.sophe.org.

David E. Newton, EdD

Health inspectors

Definition

Health inspectors are public employees who visit and assess a wide range of facilities to help ensure good public health practices in a community. Such facilities may include restaurants, public schools, day care facilities, nursing homes, swimming pools, public housing units, wells, public and private **water** and sewage systems, correctional institutions, campgrounds, beauty salons, tattoo parlors, and other facilities.

Purpose

The job of health inspectors is to ensure that facilities being examined meet standards established by local health authorities for providing safe and healthful conditions to their customers and clients. Most inspectors also work with owners and managers of such establishments to help them understand the need for such standards and the way their establishment can come into compliance when they are not doing so. Inspectors may examine a whole range of materials and procedures at an establishment, ranging from **handwashing**, dishwashing, and food storage procedures to the cleanliness and safety of chemicals and equipment used in the establishment's operation.

Description

Most individuals probably associate the job of health inspector with public facilities, such as restaurants and stores, where they check to make sure that food, water, air, and the general environment are maintained in a safe and healthy way to prevent physical injury and the spread of disease to customers. But food inspectors may carry out these tasks in any setting to which the public is exposed and where they may be at risk for unhealthful practices. Health inspectors use local, state, and federal laws and standards for the basis of their inspections, but they also apply their own knowledge of health to aid facilities in meeting the required standards. In addition to the investigation of facilities that serve the public, health inspectors may carry out a number of other jobs, such as ensuring that bars, restaurants, and other public facilities observe all laws and regulations about **smoking**; following up on bite victims for possible spread of infectious diseases; collecting and studying dead animals that may be carrying infectious agents; and assisting in determining the source of infectious diseases, such as **dengue fever** and West Nile fever. Many health inspectors also regard public education and health issues as a major part of their job.

Individuals who work as health inspectors are generally required to have at least a bachelor's degree with a major in biology, chemistry, food sciences, or some related degree. Such individuals may also be required to earn a specialized certificate related to the topic of health inspection, such as a certificate issued by the American Board of Industrial **Hygiene** or the National **Environmental Health** Association. Health inspectors work both for governmental agencies, such as a city or county health department, or for consulting firms, who supply health inspectors to governmental and nongovernmental agencies and companies on a contract basis.

Professional publications

There is no national professional organization of health inspectors, although people in the field may join any one of a number of other related organizations, such as the National Environmental Health Association (NEHA) or the American Industrial Hygiene Association (AIHA). The relevant professional group in Canada is the Canadian Institute of Public Health Inspectors (CIPHI). The CIPHI publishes the *Environmental Health Review*, which is available as part of a membership in the organization. The NEHA publishes the *Journal of Environmental Health*, along with other publications that may be of interest and value to health inspectors, such as *Food Alert! The Ultimate Sourcebook for Food Safety, Food Hygiene, Microbiology, and HAACP*; *Food Regulation: Laws, Science, Policy, and Practice*; *Food Safety Fundamentals*; *Food Safety: Theory and Practice*, and *Guide to Food Laws and Regulations*.

Resources

BOOKS

Newbold, Paul, et al. *Restaurant Inspection Frequency and Food Safety Compliance*. White Rock, BC: Canadian Institute of Public Health Inspectors and D2C3 Enterprises Incorporated, 2008.

Tulchinsky, Theodore H., and Elena Varavikova. *The New Public Health*. Amsterdam; Boston: Elsevier/Academic Press, 2009.

PERIODICALS

Newbold, K. B., et al. "Restaurant Inspection Frequency and Food Safety Compliance." *Journal of Environmental Health* 71, 4 (2008): 56–61.

Pham, Mai T., et al. "A Qualitative Exploration of the Perceptions and Information Needs of Public Health Inspectors Responsible for Food Safety." *BMC Public Health* 10 (2010): 345.

WEBSITES

Become an Environmental Health Inspector: Education and Career Roadmap. Education-Portal.com. http://education-portal.com/articles/Become_an_Environmental_Health_Inspector_Education_and_Career_Roadmap.html (accessed October 11, 2012).

Public Health Inspectors Do More than You Think. Leeds, Grenville, & Lanark District. http://www.healthunit.org/jobs/careers/phi_description.htm (accessed October 11, 2012).

ORGANIZATIONS

National Environmental Health Association (NEHA), 720 S. Colorado Blvd., Suite 1000-N, Denver, CO 80246, (303) 756-9090, (866) 956-2258, Fax: (303) 691-9490, staff@neha.org, www.neha.org

David E. Newton, EdD

Health literacy

Definition

The term *health literacy* describes a relatively new concept in the field of public health, the ability of consumers to adequately understand written and spoken instructions as to how best to maintain a healthy lifestyle. According to a report on health literacy prepared by the National Network of Libraries of Medicine, one generally accepted definition of the term is "the degree to which individuals have the capacity to obtain, process, and understand basic health information and services needed to make appropriate health decisions."

Purpose

The need for improved health literacy has grown in the United States and elsewhere because of two factors, one of which is the increasing complexity of health and medical information available to professionals and the general public. The other factor is the increasing number of individuals throughout the world who do not speak a national language, such as the large number of Americans for whom English is not their first language.

Demographics

Estimating the extent of health literacy in the United States is difficult because researchers may use somewhat different definitions for the term. Some studies have shown, however, that as many as half of people interviewed on the topic appear to lack sufficient health literacy to function at acceptable levels. Some of the specific data that have been reported include the following:

- The health of as many as 90 million Americans may be at risk because of low health literacy.
- One in five Americans reads at grade 5 level or below, and the average American reads at about grade 8 level; yet health instructions are usually written at grade 10 reading level.
- Half of all Hispanics, 40 percent of all African-Americans, and a third of all Asians have literacy problems that may affect their ability to read and understand health information.
- More than two-thirds of Americans over the age of 60 have marginal or deficient health literacy skills.
- Anywhere from a quarter to three-fifths of hospital patients are unable to understand medication directions given to them by hospital staff.

Five groups of individuals appear to be especially vulnerable to poor health literacy. They are: minority populations, immigrants, and low-income groups, all of whom tend to have poor educational backgrounds and/or poor English language skills; the elderly, who often experience cognitive decline as they age; and people with chronic physical and health problems, who may also experience some deterioration of their cognitive abilities.

Description

The modern health literacy movement owes its beginnings to two groups of professionals. One group consists of health and medical providers and educators who deal on a day-to-day basis with individuals to whom they have to explain fundamental principles of good health practices. In many cases, these individuals simply do not have the language skills needed to fully comprehend the instructions provided to them. The second group of professionals consists of adult education providers and teachers of English as a second language who often receive feedback from their clients about an inability to maintain the best health practices because they do not understand linguistically or conceptually the suggestions made to them by health and medical professionals.

For more than two decades, research findings have been accumulating about the effects of poor health literacy on a person's overall health status. The 1992 Adult Literacy Survey conducted by the National Center for Education Statistics of the U.S. Department of Education, for example, was one of the first studies to show that low health literacy was directly related to poor health status. A 1999 study by the American Medical Association confirmed these findings, concluding that poor health literacy is "a stronger predictor of a person's health than age, income, employment status, education level, and race." Other research focusing on specific health conditions, such as **cancer**, diabetes, and **asthma**, have reported similar results. A 1998 health literacy study among asthmatics found, for example, that less than a third of patients described as having low health literacy scores understood that they should see a physician even when they were asymptomatic, compared to 90 percent of high literacy patients who did understand that concept. In the same study, more than half of low literacy patients went to an emergency department when they had an asthma attack, compared to about a third of high literacy patients who did so. Based on studies such as these, there no longer appears to be any question that less well people understand the basic principles of good health care, and are likely todevelop an unsatisfactory health status.

Health literacy involves a number of more specific skills, such as:

- Simply being able to read in the language provided the directions for performing a health task, such as taking a medication according to a schedule provided.
- Understanding the meaning of test results.
- Knowing where to look for additional health information on a given topic.
- Having the mathematical skills needed to calculate correct doses of medication.
- Understanding the risks and benefits of various health actions and decisions.
- Knowing how to judge the relative accuracy and value of information on specific health choices or procedures.
- Understanding how to operate a computer to obtain or evaluate health information.
- Being able to express oneself clearly to a health professional in order to explain one's health status.
- Being able to articulate questions about health status, health options, and potential health outcomes.

Costs to society

Lack of health literacy skills also has economic impacts on both individuals and the society overall. According to a 2012 estimate, the additional health care costs in the United States resulting from poor health literacy skills amounted to about $73 billion, of which an estimated $30 billion can be attributed to people who are defined as functionally illiterate about health matters and $43 billion to those who are marginally illiterate in the topic. Of these totals, the federal government pays just over half of all the estimated expenses, with 39 percent coming from Medicare billings and 14 percent from the Medicaid program.

Efforts and solutions

The crisis in health literacy has created new challenges for the public health profession, as much as it has for individuals with health literacy problems. Some of the demands placed on public health workers are not new, but they are receiving greater emphasis in light of health literacy needs. For example, public health agencies need to be increasingly conscious of the need for recognizing poor language skills among immigrants, minority groups, the elderly, and other especially vulnerable populations for poor health literacy skills. They also need to recognize how gaps in cultural backgrounds can exacerbate the development of poor health literacy skills and require the development of programs that can address those gaps. Public health workers also may need to acknowledge the widening gap in scientific background between people in health and medical fields and the average citizen, which requires a greater emphasis on more extensive training for the general public in the science and technology of modern health and medicine.

QUESTIONS TO ASK YOUR DOCTOR

- My neighbors do not speak English at all. To whom can I refer them for advice on a health problem they are experiencing?
- My elderly mother has trouble remaining on the prescribed regimen for her medications. What can I do to help her with this problem?
- I always understand what the doctor tells me when I am in her office, but then get confused when I try to remember her instructions afterwards. What can I do to make sure I'm following the essential health advice she has given me?

In recognition of these challenges, a number of governmental and nongovernmental agencies and organizations have developed programs specializing in health literacy over the past two decades. The U.S. Department of Health and Human Services, for example, now has a free online course on health literacy designed for healthcare professionals. The course consists of five lessons that takes about five hours to complete. It can be taken for credit or not, depending on the format one chooses. Among professional organizations, the American Medical Association has perhaps the oldest health literacy program in the nation, begun in 1998. It provides toolkits, safety monographs, safety tip cards, reports, and other resources for use in health literacy improvement programs. The Canadian Public Health Association has a similar program called National Literacy and Health Program, designed to promote awareness among public health professionals about the issue. A number of educational institutions have also instituted health literacy programs. The Harvard University School of Public Health, for example, has a Health Literacy Studies division, which conducts research on ways to reduce deficiencies in health literacy among **vulnerable populations**. The division produces reports on its research and pursues the implementation of these research findings in real-world public health settings. A similar program is available at the University of New England's Health Literacy Center in Biddeford, Maine. Private industry is also involved in the health literacy movement. The Pfizer drug company, for example, sponsors a program known as Clear Health Communication, designed to help consumers develop a better understanding of ways in which to interpret and make use of medical and health information.

Resources

BOOKS

Gillis, Doris, Deborah Begoray, and Gillian Rowlands. *Health Literacy in Context: International Perspectives.* New York: Nova Science Publishers, 2012.

Hewitt, Maria Elizabeth, ed. *Improving Health Literacy within a State: Workshop Summary.* Washington, DC: National Academies Press, 2011.

Kars, Marge, Lynda Baker, and Feleta L. Wilson. *The Medical Library Association Guide to Health Literacy.* New York: Neal-Schuman Publishers, 2008.

Marks, Ray. *Health Literacy and School-based Health Education.* Bingley, UK: Emerald Press, 2012.

PERIODICALS

Freedman, A. M., et al. "Better Learning Through Instructional Science: A Health Literacy Case Study in 'How to Teach So Learners Can Learn'." *Health Promotion Practice* 13. 5. (2012): 648–56.

Paakkari, Leena, and Olli Paakkari. "Health Literacy as a Learning Outcome in Schools." *Health Education* 112. 2. (2012): 133–52.

Rudd, Rima E. "Health Literacy Skills of U.S. Adults." *American Journal of Health Behavior* 31. Suppl 1. (2007): S8–18.

Xie, Bo. "Improving Older Adults' E-health Literacy through Computer Training Using NIH Online Resources." *Library & Information Science Research* 34. 1. (2012): 63–71.

WEBSITES

Health Literacy. Health.gov. http://www.health.gov/communication/literacy/. Accessed on September 14, 2012.

Health Literacy. Medline Plus. http://www.nlm.nih.gov/medlineplus/healthliteracy.html. Accessed on September 14, 2012.

Health Literacy: Accurate, Accessible and Actionable Health Information for All. Centers for Disease Control and Prevention. http://www.cdc.gov/healthliteracy/. Accessed on September 14, 2012.

ORGANIZATIONS

Ask Me 3, National Patient Safety Foundation (NPSF), 268 Summer Street, 6th floor, Boston, MA USA 02210, 1 (617) 391–9900, Fax: 1 (617) 391–9999, http://www.npsf.org/contact-us/, http://www.npsf.org/for-healthcare-professionals/programs/ask-me-3/.

David E. Newton, Ed.D.

Health policy

Definition

The **World Health Organization (WHO)** defines health policy as those "decisions, plans, and actions that are undertaken to achieve specific health care goals within a society."

Purpose

The purpose of a health policy is to express an agency's vision of the future with respect to health care, outlining specific objectives for both the short and long term. It allows stakeholders to understand what the health priorities of an agency or organization are and how various individuals and organizations are involved in the actions of the healthcare organization.

Description

In principle, the term *health policy* can apply to the long-term goals and mission of any healthcare agency or organization, although in practice it is most often used for the vision of states, nations, or even the international community as a whole. Perhaps the most common expression of the concept is in the area of personal healthcare policy, the determination by a state or nation as to how the health and wellbeing of individuals is to be managed. In some nations, for economic, political, historical, or other reasons, health care is regarded as an individual's private concern. When a medical needs arises, it is up to the individual to decide whether or not to see a medical professional, which professional to visit, and how to pay for those services. In other nations, a decision has been made that health care is the right of all citizens and that it is the duty of the national government to arrange for adequate care for all citizens, whether they can pay for it personally or not. Indeed, the view of the United Nations' Universal Declaration of **Human Rights** takes this position, noting that "everyone has the right to a standard of living adequate for the health and well-being of himself and of his family," even in circumstances of old age, disability, sickness, or other circumstances beyond his or her control.

In the twenty-first century, virtually every developed nation in the world has adopted a health policy that reflects this view, agreeing to provide medical care that one needs whether or not a person can afford to pay for that care, a so-called "universal health care" approach. The one major exception to that rule is the United States, which remains committed to the proposition that individual citizens should have the right to make many, most, or all of their own healthcare decisions, even if it means that they must pay all or some of their own healthcare costs. Indeed, one of the most vigorous political debates in the United States in the second decade of the twenty-first century is centered on this question, with opposing forces arguing for a more government-centered program reflected in the 2010 Affordable Care Act, or a more decentralized program reflected in a variety of other healthcare options. Most experts believe that the current U.S. health policy is unsustainable in the long run because the financial costs of the existing system are greater than the federal government and individual citizens will be able to pay for in coming decades.

The term *health policy* is also used in a number of other contexts, usually in dealing with specific healthcare issues, such as **aging**, various specific diseases, disparities in access, systems of healthcare delivery, economics of health care, governmental programs (such as Medicare and Medicaid), mental health, prescription drugs, quality of care, tobacco and alcohol consumption, and health research. In each case the elements of a health policy are similar, with the need for decisions as to which aspects of a problem should receive priority, on what information decisions about the program should be made, what educational tools can be developed, how the program will be paid for, what individuals and organizations will be involved in the program, and how the results of the program will be assessed.

Professional publications

In addition to a host of books, reports, articles, and websites on the topic of health policy, a number of journals are devoted exclusively or primarily to this topic, including *Health Policy* (Elsevier), *Journal of Public Health Policy* (Palgrave), *Health Affairs* (Project HOPE), *Health Policy and Planning* (Oxford Press), *Journal of Health Politics, Policy and Law* (Duke University Press), *Journal of Health Economics* (Elsevier), *American Journal of Public Health* (**American Public Health Association**), *World Health Report* (**World Health Organization**), and *Milbank Quarterly* (Milbank Memorial Fund). Also, more than two dozen national organizations have a major interest in health policy issues and publish books, reports, articles, newsletters, and other materials on the topic. These organizations include the Alliance for Health Reform, Institute for Health Policy Solutions, the American Pharmaceutical Association, the American Association of Health Plans, the Center for Health Care Strategies, the Healthcare Leadership Council, and the Henry J. Kaiser Family Foundation.

Resources

BOOKS

Alaszewski, Andy, and Patrick Brown. *Making Health Policy: A Critical Introduction*. Cambridge, UK: Polity, 2012.

Bodenheimer, Thomas, and Kevin Grumbach. *Understanding Health Policy: A Clinical Approach*. New York: McGraw-Hill Medical, 2009.

Exworthy, Mark, et al., eds. *Shaping Health Policy: Case Study Methods and Analysis*. Chicago: Policy Press, 2012.

Ho, Lok–Sang. *Health Policy and the Public Interest.* London; New York: Routledge, 2011.

PERIODICALS

Field, P., R. Gauld, and M. Lawrence. "Evidence–informed Health Policy—The Crucial Role of Advocacy." *International Journal of Clinical Practice* 66. 4. (2012): 337–41

Goldberg, Daniel S. "Against the Very Idea of the Politicization of Public Health Policy." *American Journal of Public Health* 102. 1. (2012): 44–49

WEBSITES

Health Policy. World Health Organization. http://www.who.int/topics/health_policy/en/ (accessed October 13, 2012).

National Health Policy. http://www.nhpf.org/ (accessed October 13, 2012).

ORGANIZATIONS

Institute for Health Policy Solutions, 1444 "Eye" St., N.W., Suite 900, Washington, DC 20005, (202) 789-1491, Fax: 789-1879, pshrestha@ihps.org, http://www.ihps.org/.

David E. Newton, EdD

Healthy Cities

Definition

Healthy Cities is a term used to describe a particular type of **health policy** aimed at improving the health of individuals who live and work in urban areas. The concept is also known by a number of other names, such as Healthy City, Healthy Communities, Healthy Community, and, in Spanish-speaking regions of the world, *Municipios saludables*.

Purpose

Healthy Cities is based on the presumption that life in an urban area presents health issues not necessarily faced by individuals who live in more rural areas and that governments should develop policies and practices that meet these special needs and provide inhabitants of cities with the best possible health environment and experience.

Description

Healthy Cities is a relatively old concept, whose origin can be traced to a Health of Towns Association formed in Great Britain in 1844. The motivation for that association was a report written by Edwin Chadwick, the son of a successful businessman and social activist. The report documented the generally poor and unhealthful living conditions in which most townspeople lived at the time and recommended a number of actions to improve these conditions. The modern Healthy Cities movement is often dated to the creation of a meeting held in Toronto in 1984 called Healthy Toronto 2000, whose goal it was to achieve a higher standard of healthful living for that city in the time period mentioned. The Healthy City movement soon earned greater recognition when it was picked up by the **World Health Organization (WHO)** in 1986, which adopted it as the basis for its new Healthy Cities and Villages program in that year. That program initially focused on the improvement of urban health within the European Union, but has since grown to become a worldwide movement. **WHO** has defined a Health City as one that "is continually creating and improving those physical and social environments and expanding those community resources which enable people to mutually support each other in performing all the functions of life and in developing to their maximum potential."

The fundamental principle that underlies the Healthy City movement is that inequalities in social conditions, such as access to adequate health care, are not morally justified and that governmental agencies have a moral responsibility to do whatever they can to eliminate such inequalities. Thus, while Healthy Cities is focused on health issues, it is fundamentally also a philosophy of the way governments should organize and operate to deliver health resources to everyone in an urban area who needs them. The development of a Healthy City involves a number of fundamental commitments, the first of which is the explicit commitment of governmental leaders to the philosophical and operational principles on which the concept is based. The city government must then make such organizational changes as may be necessary to provide a mechanism by which this commitment can be put into practice. The city must also develop a plan of action to which the community as a whole can become committed and specific action themes must be adopted through which the overall program can be carried out. Finally, specific methods for developing networks of stakeholders that provide mechanisms of cooperation must be developed.

The WHO Healthy Cities program is currently in Phase V of its development. As of 2012, there were 90 cities that had been certified as members of the WHO European Healthy Cities Network and an additional 1,400 cities and towns enrolled in 30 national Healthy Cities programs in Europe. A review of the program's accomplishments to date and an outline of its goals and programs for Phase V (2009–2013) was adopted at Zagreb in 2009 and is available online at http://www.euro.who.int/__data/assets/pdf_file/0015/101076/E92343.pdf. The Healthy Cities movement has found

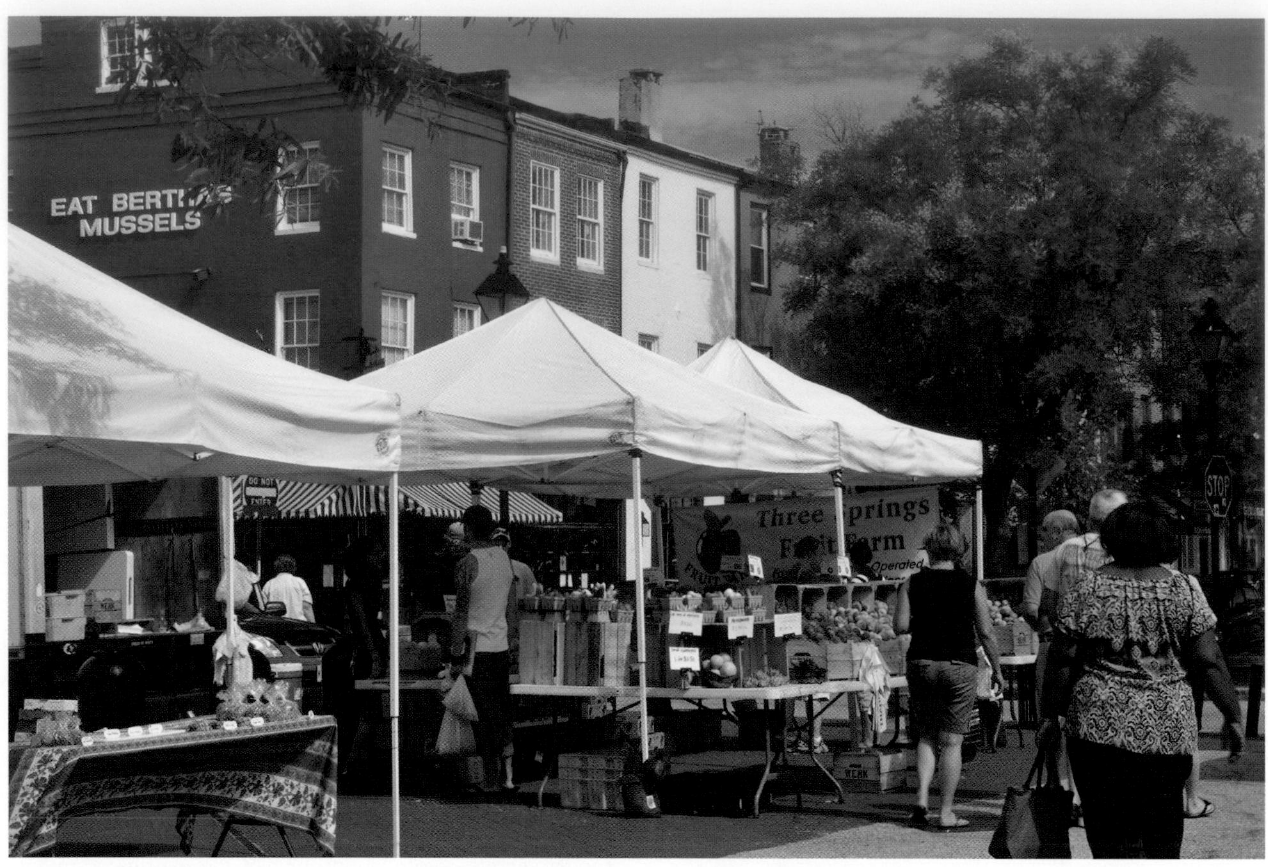

Fell's Point Farmers Market in Baltimore is an example of a community embracing and promoting fresh produce. *(© iStockphoto.com/Aimin Tang)*

most of its success in developed nations, particularly within the European Union and, to a lesser extent, in North America. The failure of the movement to take hold in developing nations seems a result of many factors, such as the lack of necessary governmental structures in less developed areas, the failure of the Healthy Cities model to take into consideration basic issues of **poverty** and **violence**, the polarization of social and economic classes, the very low baseline of existing health care in most developing nations, the inability to transfer successful European models to less developed nations, and the relative lack of concern about health matters in developing nations compared to that in developed nations.

The Healthy Cities movement in the United States appears to have taken a somewhat different direction from that in Europe. According to the Healthy Communities Institute, there were more than 1,000 cities in the United States that had undertaken Healthy City projects, although such projects often appeared to be less comprehensive than those in Europe. A U.S. program somewhat similar to the Healthy Cities movement is called Healthy People. The program grew out of a report issued by the Surgeon General in 1979, which provided suggestions for federal involvement in programs to prevent disease and improve the general health of the American public. The initiative was revised and reformulated on a broader scale in 1990 as Healthy People 1990, and again as Healthy People 2000, Healthy People 2010, and, more recently, as Healthy People 2020. The most recent version of the program consists of 15 objectives and 42 topic areas, such as: adolescent health; **cancer**; chronic kidney disease; early and middle childhood; **food safety**; **genomics**; hearing and other sensory or communication disorders; lesbian, gay, bisexual, and transgender health; preparedness; sleep health; substance abuse; and vision.

In recent years, increasing attention has been paid to the role of transportation systems in the consideration of urban health problems. Transportation systems affect human health in a number of ways, ranging from the deaths and injuries caused by vehicular accidents, to the air and **water** pollutants released by cars, trucks, buses, trains, and other modes of motorized transportation. Human health can also be affected by the very materials of which roads and streets are made (such as tar and asphalt). Many individuals responsible for urban policy decisions are now recognizing that the choices a community makes vis-à-vis its transportation system have direct and vital influences on the health of individuals living and working in an urban area. A recent document dealing with this issue is the report *The Transportation Prescription*, produced by a consortium consisting of The **Prevention** Institute, Convergence Partnership, and Policy Link. The thesis of the report is that, for as long as urban areas have existed, modes of transportation have contributed to a host of health problems experienced by city dwellers, but that transportation systems can now be reimagined not only to reduce their negative impacts, but also to actually contribute to the improvement of the health and safety of city dwellers.

Professional publications

Information about the Healthy Cities movement is available from a variety of sources, one of the most important of which is WHO. Its 2012 booklet *Healthy Cities Tackle the Social Determinants of Inequities in Health: A Framework for Action* lays out the fundamental philosophy of the movement, provides some historical background, and describes the essential elements of the modern Healthy Cities program. The WHO website also contains essential historical documents about the movement, including the Ottawa Charter for Health Promotion, which is sometimes described as the founding document for the Healthy Cities movement. Information about the U.S. Healthy People movement is available from the U.S. **Department of Health and Human Services** on its website at HealthyPeople.gov (http://www.healthypeople.gov/2020/default.aspx). *The Transportation Prescription* is available online at http://www.convergencepartnership.org/atf/cf/%7B245a9b44-6dcd-4abd-a392-ae583809e350%7D/TRANSPORTATIONRX.PDF.

Resources

BOOKS

Kushner, James A. *Healthy Cities: The Intersection of Urban Planning, Law and Health*. Durham, NC: Carolina Academic Press, 2007.

Otgaar, Alexander H. J., Jeroen Klijs, and Leo van den Berg. *Towards Healthy Cities: Comparing Conditions for Change*. Farnham, UK; Burlington, VT: Ashgate Publishing Company, 2011.

PERIODICALS

Barten, Francoise. "Toward Healthy Cities. People, Places, the Politics of Urban Planning and Power." *Journal of Urban Health* 88. 2. (2011): 376–77

Leeuw, Evelyne. "Do Healthy Cities Work? A Logic of Method for Assessing Impact and Outcome of Healthy Cities." *Journal of Urban Health* 89. 2. (2012): 217–31.

WEBSITES

An Introduction to Healthy Cities and Communities. Healthy Cities/Healthy Communities. http://www.well.com/~bbear/hc_articles.html (accessed October 10, 2012).

Shaping Cities for Health: Complexity and the Planning of Urban Environments in the 21st Century. The Lancet. http://www.thelancet.com/commissions/healthy-cities (accessed October 10, 2012).

ORGANIZATIONS

Alliance for Healthy Cities, Kanda–surugadai 2–1–19–1112, Chiyoda–ku, Tokyo, Japan 101–0062, +81 3 5577 6780, Fax: +81 3 5577 6780, alliance.ith@tmd.ac.jp, http://www.alliance-healthycities.com/

World Health Organization (WHO). Regional Office for Europe, Scherfigsvej 8, DK-2100 Copenhagen, Denmark, +45 39 17 17 17, infohcp@euro.who.int, http://www.euro.who.int/en/what-we-do/health-topics/environment-and-health/urban-health/activities/healthy-cities.

David E. Newton, EdD

Healthy Lives, Healthy People

Definition

Healthy Lives, Healthy People is the name of a new approach to public health adopted in the United Kingdom in 2010. It transfers responsibilities for many public health activities from the national government to Local Authorities, administrative bodies responsible for policy and programs at the town, city, county, or other local area.

Purpose

The purpose of Healthy Lives, Healthy People is to transfer decision-making and programs for public health from large, national bureaucratic organization at a significant distance from ordinary people to local governments with whom they have much closer contact. In addition, local authorities are to be provided with so-called ring-fenced financing for their public health programs that protects funds from being used for purposes other than those for which they are intended (public health programs).

Demographics

All residents of the United Kingdom are to be covered by the Healthy Lives, Healthy People program.

Description

Healthy Lives, Healthy People evolved out of a study conducted by a committee of health experts chaired by Sir Michael Marmot, professor of **epidemiology** and public health at University College London. The committee was created in 2008 by Prime Minister at that time Gordon Brown in light of troubling statistics about the health of British citizens. Studies had shown that the British were the most obese people in Europe; the nation was losing 80,000 people a year to smoking-related diseases; 1.6 million people had been diagnosed as alcohol dependent; and a half million new cases of sexually transmitted infections were being reported annually. The committee's charge was to study the basis for these statistics and to suggest programs by which they could be reduced. The committee was also charged with investigating the nature of health inequalities in the United Kingdom, the reasons for these inequalities, and the steps that should be taken to reduce or eliminate those inequalities. The committee issued its final report, Fair Society, Healthy Lives, in February 2010. It became the basis of a white paper issued on November 30, 2010 entitled "Healthy Lives, Healthy People."

As with most reports of its kind, "Healthy Lives, Healthy People" is a long and detailed analysis of the causes of, and possible solutions for, Great Britain's current health crisis. Two main features of the report stand out, however. First, the emphasis in health care shifts from treatment to **prevention**. The Marmot report repeatedly noted the importance of dealing with health problems before they develop, not after they occur. Thus, the report emphasized greater need for: prenatal care, health programs for pregnant women and newborn children, in-school **health education**, on-the-job health programs, and greater attention to the health needs of elderly citizens. The goal of this part of the report was to prevent health problems, such as **obesity** and **smoking**, from developing in the first place, reducing health problems and health costs.

The second major feature of the white paper was a shift in focus of health treatment from the national to the local level. The Marmot report had emphasized that health issues, and preventative programs in particular, can best be dealt with by caregivers who are in physically close connection to their clients. There are certainly circumstances in which the national government may and should take actions to reduce a health issue—as when they pass laws prohibiting the use of certain types of drugs—but most health problems can best be handled by local health officers, physicians, nurses, health educators, and other health workers.

To accomplish this goal, the white paper announced the creation of a new national health authority, Public Health England. Rather than assuming a whole new set of health care responsibilities, Public Health England was designed to be primarily an enabling agency, providing funding and assistance to local governmental bodies (called Local Authorities). It then falls to the Local Authorities to design and implement programs in keeping with the spirit of Healthy Lives, Healthy People that are most appropriate to their own settings. To ensure that programs are actually designed and operate according to this philosophy, the white paper announced so-called "ring-fenced" financing to Local Authorities. Ring-fencing means that the funds allocated to Local Authorities are guaranteed to be used for local health activities entirely, and are not available for any other purposes, no matter how closely related to health care those activities may appear to be.

A crucial feature of Healthy Lives, Healthy People is to improve the health care available to poor people. Over the years, the spread in the quality of health care between classes has grown until it reached its maximum level in the first decade of the twenty-first century. Healthy Lives, Healthy People attempts to reverse that trend by focusing on the four R's of the program: **R**each out and reach across, an attempt to make contact with the people who need health care the most; **R**epresentative, allowing communities to develop the health care program that they need, not what national government provides for everyone; **R**igorous, making use of the best available scientific information about causes and treatments; and **R**esilient, involving the development of programs appropriate for both current and future health needs.

Results

Healthy Lives, Healthy People is a new program that had just begun implementation in 2011. No assessment of its eventual success in meeting the goals set out in the Marmot report of the white paper is possible. What can be said is that the national government clearly understands it has a responsibility to keep the general public informed about the goals and programmatic features of Healthy Lives, Healthy People, and to ensure that citizens have an opportunity to make their own ideas about the program known. After issuing the white paper in November 2010, the Department of Health organized or cooperated in more than 60 listening exercises, and supported many more such exercises of the type. In total, it received more than 2,100 responses to ideas proposed in the white paper. As a consequence of these feedback events, the Department of Health issued in July 2011 a report entitled "Healthy Lives, Healthy People: Update and Forward," summarizing the most important issues raised in the listening exercises and written responses and outlining the ways in which the government anticipated responding to these concerns. The July 2011 report concluded with a section describing the next steps to be taken in the transition to the new Healthy Lives, Healthy People program, and a tentative timetable for those changes. It also provided a summary of progress on certain key health issues.

KEY TERMS

Department of Health (UK)—The national agency responsible for public health, adult social care, and the National Health Service.

Local Authority—In the United Kingdom, administrative bodies responsible for policy and programs at the town, city, county, or other local area. The term has somewhat different meanings in England, Wales, Scotland, and Northern Ireland.

Public Health England—A new agency in the United Kingdom created to carry out the provisions of the white paper, "Healthy Lives, Healthy People." It is currently within the bureaucratic structure of the Department of Health.

Ring-fenced financing—Financing for a particular project that is protected from use for any purpose than that for which it was specifically designated.

Resources

WEBSITES

Secretary of State for Health. "Healthy Lives, Healthy People: Our Strategy for Public Health in England." http://www.dh.gov.uk/prod_consum_dh/groups/dh_digitalassets/documents/digitalasset/dh_127424.pdf (accessed November 23, 2011).

Secretary of State for Health. "Healthy Lives, Healthy People: Update and Way Forward." http://www.dh.gov.uk/prod_consum_dh/groups/dh_digitalassets/documents/digital asset/dh_128333.pdf (accessed November 23, 2011).

ORGANIZATIONS

Department of Health (UK), Customer Service Centre, Richmond House, 79 Whitehall, London, England SW1A 2NS, 020 7210 4850, Fax: 020 7210 5952, http://www.info.doh.gov.uk/contactus.nsf/memo?openform, http://www.dh.gov.uk/en

David E. Newton, AB, MA EdD

Hearing loss

Definition

Hearing loss is impairment of the ability to apprehend sound. The impairment may be in any degree. Such impairment occurs primarily due to natural causes (heredity) and environmental factors (e.g., extended exposure to loud sounds). Secondary factors of hearing loss include obstructions within the ear canal, primarily ear wax, but sometimes other natural or foreign materials.

Description

Sound can be measured accurately. The term "decibel" (dB) refers to an amount of energy moving sound from its source to one's ears or to a microphone. For instance, a whisper is equivalent to about 30 dB, and a washing machine is around 70 dB, and both fall well within the range that will not produce hearing loss. On the other hand, heavy traffic and a hair dryer each produce about 85–90 dB, which is within the range that is considered risky for producing a loss of hearing. Even worse, a jet taking off and a shotgun blast each produce 140–165 dB, which is within the range that can cause considerable degradation to one's hearing.

The ear has three main parts: the external ear, the middle ear, and the inner ear. The external ear includes the pinna, which is the part that is visible on the outside of the head, and the ear canal. The pinna guide sound waves into the ear canal. The sound waves travel down to the eardrum, which is the boundary between the external ear and the middle ear. The middle ear transmits those vibrations to the three tiny bones, called the ossicles, which lie within it. These bones move in response, thereby changing the sound waves into mechanical waves. These mechanical waves are relayed to the inner ear and a snail-shaped bony structure called the cochlea. The cochlea contains two different fluids—endolymph and perilymph—and the sensory receptor Organ of Corti, which holds the nerve receptors, or "hair cells," that ultimately send the nerve signals to the brain for processing into hearing. In summary, the hearing process is divided into five steps:

- air conduction through the external ear to the ear drum
- bone conduction through the middle ear to the inner ear
- water conduction to the Organ of Corti
- nerve conduction into the brain
- interpretation by the brain

Hearing can be interrupted (i.e., hearing loss can result) in several ways at each of the five steps.

Demographics

Generally, some hearing loss occurs gradually as humans age. According to the National Institutes of Health, about one out of three older Americans between the ages of 65 and 74 years has hearing loss. Over the age of 75 years, hearing loss occurs in 47% of people in the United States.

Although it is more common among older individuals, hearing loss can happen to any person regardless of age. The NIH reports that about 17% of American adults, or 36 million, say that they have some degree of hearing loss. It is more common among men than women.

Causes and symptoms

Causes

The external ear canal can be blocked with ear wax, foreign objects, infection, and tumors. Wax build-up can cause hearing loss in people of any age. Overgrowth of the bone, a condition that occurs when the ear canal has been flushed with cold water repeatedly for years, can also narrow the passageway, making blockage and infection more likely. This condition occurs often in Northern Californian surfers and is therefore called "surfer's ear."

The eardrum is so thin a physician can see through it into the middle ear. Sharp objects, pressure from an infection in the middle ear, or even a firm cuffing or slapping of the ear, can rupture it. It is also susceptible to pressure changes during scuba diving.

Several conditions can diminish the mobility of the ossicles in the middle ear. Otitis media (an infection in the middle ear) occurs when fluid cannot escape into the throat because of blockage of the eustachian tube. The fluid then accumulates—whether it is pus or just mucus—and this dampens the motion of the ossicles. A disease called otosclerosis scars and limits the motion of the small conducting bones in the middle ear and may cause deafness.

Sensory hearing loss may also occur. This refers to damage to the Organ of Corti and the acoustic nerve. Prolonged exposure to loud noise is the leading cause of sensory hearing loss. Causes include exposure to loud music and occupational noise. This is known as noise-induced hearing loss (NIHL). A third of people over 65 years of age have presbycusis—sensory hearing loss due to **aging**. Both NIHL and presbycusis are primarily high-frequency losses. In most languages, the high-frequency sounds define speech, so these people cannot easily make out spoken words, especially when it is accompanied by background noise.

Brain infections such as like **meningitis**, drugs such as the aminoglycoside **antibiotics** (streptomycin, gentamycin, kanamycin, tobramycin), and Meniere's disease also cause permanent sensory hearing loss. Meniere's disease combines attacks of hearing loss with attacks of vertigo. The symptoms may occur together or separately. High doses of salicylates such as aspirin and quinine can cause a temporary high-frequency loss. Prolonged high doses can lead to permanent deafness. A hereditary form of sensory deafness and a congenital form occur, and these are most often caused by **rubella** (German **measles**).

Sudden hearing loss—at least 30dB in less than three days—is most commonly caused by cochleitis, a mysterious viral infection.

The final category of hearing loss is neural. Damage to the acoustic nerve and the parts of the brain that perform hearing are the most likely to produce permanent hearing loss. Strokes, multiple sclerosis, and acoustic neuromas are all possible causes of neural hearing loss.

Hearing can also be diminished by extra sounds generated by the ear, most of them from the same kinds of disorders that cause diminished hearing. These sounds are referred to as tinnitus and can be ringing, blowing, clicking, or anything else that no one but the patient hears.

Symptoms

The general symptoms of hearing loss include:

- unclear (muffled) voices and noises
- difficulty with the understanding of spoken words, especially when background noises are present, resulting in requests for people to talk slowly or more distinctly
- inability to participate in conversations

Diagnosis

An examination of the ears and nose, combined with simple hearing tests done in the physician's office, can detect many common causes of hearing loss. An audiogram often concludes the evaluation, and often produces a diagnosis. If the defect is in the brain or the acoustic nerve, further neurological testing and imaging will be required.

The audiogram has many uses in diagnosing hearing deficits. The pattern of hearing loss across the audible frequencies gives clues to the cause. Several alterations in the testing procedure can give additional information. For example, speech is perceived differently than pure tones. Adequate perception of sound, combined with inability to recognize words, points to a brain problem rather than a sensory or conductive deficit. Loudness perception is distorted by disease in certain areas but not in others. Acoustic neuromas often distort the perception of loudness.

Treatment

Conductive hearing loss can almost always be restored to some degree, if not completely. Some examples are:

- Matter in the ear canal can be easily removed with a dramatic improvement in hearing.
- Surfer's ear gradually regresses if cold water is avoided or a special ear plug is used. In advanced cases, surgeons can grind away the excess bone.
- Middle ear infection with fluid may be treated with medications. If they do not work, surgical drainage of the ear is accomplished through the ear drum, which heals completely after treatment.
- Tiny skin grafts can repair traumatically damaged ear drums.

- Surgical repair of otosclerosis is accomplished by substituting tiny artificial parts for the original ossicles.

Sensory and neural hearing loss, on the other hand, cannot readily be cured. Since the loss is not often complete, however, hearing aids can fill the deficit.

In-the-ear hearing aids can boost the volume of sound by up to 70 dB. (Normal speech is about 60 dB.) Physicians will perform tests and recommend proper hearing aids, which, depending on the type of hearing loss, may include devices that can be surgically implanted in the cochlea.

Tinnitus can sometimes be relieved by adding white noise (like the sound of wind or waves crashing on the shore) to the environment.

Prognosis

The prognosis for reducing or eliminating hearing loss varies widely. Whether hearing loss can be solved is generally dependent on the cause. Conductive hearing loss is usually curable, but sensory hearing loss is more complicated to treat and is usually not curable. People can regain a majority of their hearing with the use of hearing aids.

Prevention

Prompt treatment and attentive follow-up of middle ear infections in children will prevent this cause of conductive hearing loss. Control of infectious childhood diseases, such as measles, has greatly reduced sensory hearing loss as a complication of epidemic diseases. Laws that require protection from loud noise in the workplace have achieved substantial reduction in noise-induced hearing loss. Surfers should use the right kind of ear plugs, and all persons should avoid prolonged exposure to loud noises, including music.

Effects on public health

Depending on its extent, hearing loss can be isolating. People with hearing loss may find it difficult to hold conversations with friends and family, and may begin to withdraw. At the same time, older individuals who have hearing loss may appear to be confused or obstinate because of their inability to decipher speech, and family members may become frustrated and begin to ignore them. This compounds the isolation that many older individuals feel as a result of the hearing loss.

This hearing loss can affect job performance. For drivers, hearing loss may cause them to miss sirens, horn honks, and other warning sounds. Individuals with hearing loss might not be able to comprehend important information from a healthcare professional; they might not hear smoke alarms or other alert sounds in the home; and they might be oblivious to people knocking at the door or ringing the doorbell.

KEY TERMS

Decibel—A unit of the intensity of sound, a measure of loudness.

Meniere's disease—The combination of vertigo and decreased hearing caused by abnormalities in the inner ear.

Multiple sclerosis—A progressive disease of brain and nerve tissue.

Otosclerosis—A disease that scars and limits the motion of the small conducting bones in the middle ear.

Stroke—Sudden loss of blood supply to part of the brain.

Costs to society

As the **population** ages, the number of people who have hearing loss will increase. Although many would benefit from hearing aids, they are expensive and often not covered by insurance. A pair of hearing aids may run $2,000–$6,000. This expense precludes many individuals from regaining the ability to understand the spoken word, to engage in conversations, and to participate fully in society. According to a 2011 study in *Hearing Journal*, most people with a hearing impairment have a mild-to-moderate loss, and of that number, more than 90% do not get hearing aids. The study notes that about half of those with hearing loss report that financial cost is the reason they do not get hearing aids.

Efforts and solutions

Decreased hearing is such a common problem that legions of organizations have arisen to provide assistance. Special language training, both in lip reading and signing, special schools, and special camps for children are all available in most regions of the United States. In addition to hearing aids, which are always improving, many assistive devices are available. These include telephone-amplification systems, television-listening devices, and visual alerts to accompany important sounds, such as smoke alarm sirens or ringing doorbells.

Research on cochlear implants is continuing, and many people with severe hearing loss are finding them beneficial.

Resources

BOOKS

Luxford, William M., M.D., M. Jennifer Derebery, M.D., and Karen I. Berliner Ph.D. The Complete Idiot's Guide to Hearing Loss. New York: Alpha, 2010.

Cole, Elizabeth, Ed.D., and Carol Flexer Ph.D. Children with Hearing Loss: Developing Listening and Talking, Birth to Six. Second edition. San Diego, CA: Plural Publishing, 2010.

PERIODICALS

Ramachandran, Virginia Au.D.; Brad A. Stach, Ph.D.; and Erika Becker. Reducing hearing aid cost does not influence device acquisition for milder hearing loss, but eliminating it does. *Hearing Journal* 64, no. 5 (May 2011): pp. 10–18.

WEBSITES

MedlinePlus "Hearing Disorders and Deafness." U.S. National Library of Medicine, National Institutes of Health. http://www.nlm.nih.gov/medlineplus/hearingdisordersanddeafness.html (accessed November 8, 2012).

"Hearing Loss." American Speech-Language-Hearing Association. http://www.asha.org/public/hearing/Hearing-Loss/ (accessed November 8, 2012).

"Hearing Loss." National Institute on Aging, National Institutes of Health. http://www.nia.nih.gov/health/publication/hearing-loss (accessed November 8, 2012).

"Hearing Loss in Children: What Should You Know?" U.S. Centers for Disease Control and Prevention. http://www.cdc.gov/ncbddd/hearingloss/index.html (accessed November 8, 2012).

"What Is Hearing Loss?" NIH SeniorHealth, National Institutes of Health (NIH). http://nihseniorhealth.gov/index.html (accessed November 8, 2012).

ORGANIZATIONS

Alexander Graham Bell Association for the Deaf and Hard of Hearing, 3417 Volta Place NW, Washington, DC 20007, (202) 337-5220, http://nc.agbell.org/

Better Hearing Institute, 1444 I Street NW; Suite 700, Washington, DC 20005, (202) 449-1100, mail@betterhearing.org, http://www.betterhearing.org/

Center for Hearing and Communications, 50 Broadway, Sixth Floor, New York City, NY 10004, (917) 305-7700, http://www.chchearing.org/

Central Institute for the Deaf, 825 South Taylor Avenue, St. Louis, MO 63110, (314) 977-0132, (877) 444-4574, http://www.cid.edu/home.aspx

Hearing Loss Association of America, 7910 Woodmont Avenue, Suite 1200, Bethesda, MD 20814, (301) 657-2248, http://www.hearingloss.org/

National Association of the Deaf, 8630 Fenton Street, Suite 820, Silver Spring, MD 20910, (301) 587-1788, http://www.nad.org/

The Sight & Hearing Association, 1246 University Avenue West, Suite 226, St. Paul, MN 55104-4125, (651) 645-2546, (800) 992-0424, mail@sightandhearing.org, http://www.sightandhearing.org/

World Recreation Association of the Deaf, Post Office Box 3211, Quartz Hill, CA 93586, (661) 952-7752, http://www.wrad.org/.

J. Ricker Polsdorfer, M.D.
Leslie Mertz, Ph.D.

Heart disease

Definition

Heart disease is a group of conditions affecting the structure and functions of the heart. The four primary conditions that make up heart disease are coronary artery disease, heart attack, congenital heart disease, and rheumatic heart disease. Other diseases include angina (chest **pain**) and arrhythmia (irregular heartbeat).

Description

The heart is a muscle that gets energy from blood carrying oxygen and nutrients. Having a constant supply of blood keeps the heart working properly. Most people think of heart disease as one condition. However, heart disease is a group of conditions affecting the structure and functions of the heart and has many root causes. Coronary artery disease (CAD) is the most common of these conditions and occurs when blood vessels in the heart become blocked or narrowed. This blockage limits the flow of blood through the coronary arteries, the major arteries supplying oxygen-rich blood to the heart. The coronary arteries expand when the heart is working harder and needs more oxygen. If the arteries are unable to expand, the heart is deprived of oxygen (myocardial ischemia). When the blockage is limited, chest pain or pressure called angina may occur. When the blockage cuts off the blood flow, the result is heart attack (myocardial infarction or heart muscle death).

A normal heart is a strong muscular pump. It weighs between 200 and 425 grams (7–15 ounces) and is a little larger than the size of an adult fist. During an average lifetime, the human heart will beat more than 2.5 billion times. The average heart beats about 100,000 times each day and pumps about 7,200 liters (1,900 gallons) of blood. The heart sits between the lungs in the middle of the chest, behind and slightly to the left of the breastbone. A double-layered membrane called the pericardium surrounds the heart like a sac. Blood loaded with oxygen comes from the lungs and enters the heart. To function, the heart needs a continuous supply of oxygen and nutrients, which it gets from the blood that is pumped through the coronary arteries. The heart and circulatory system make up the cardiovascular system. The heart pumps blood to the organs, tissues, and cells of the body, delivering oxygen and nutrients to every cell and removing carbon dioxide and waste products made by those cells. Oxygen-rich blood is carried from the heart to the rest of the body through a complex network of arteries, arterioles, and capillaries. Oxygen-poor blood is carried back to the heart through veins.

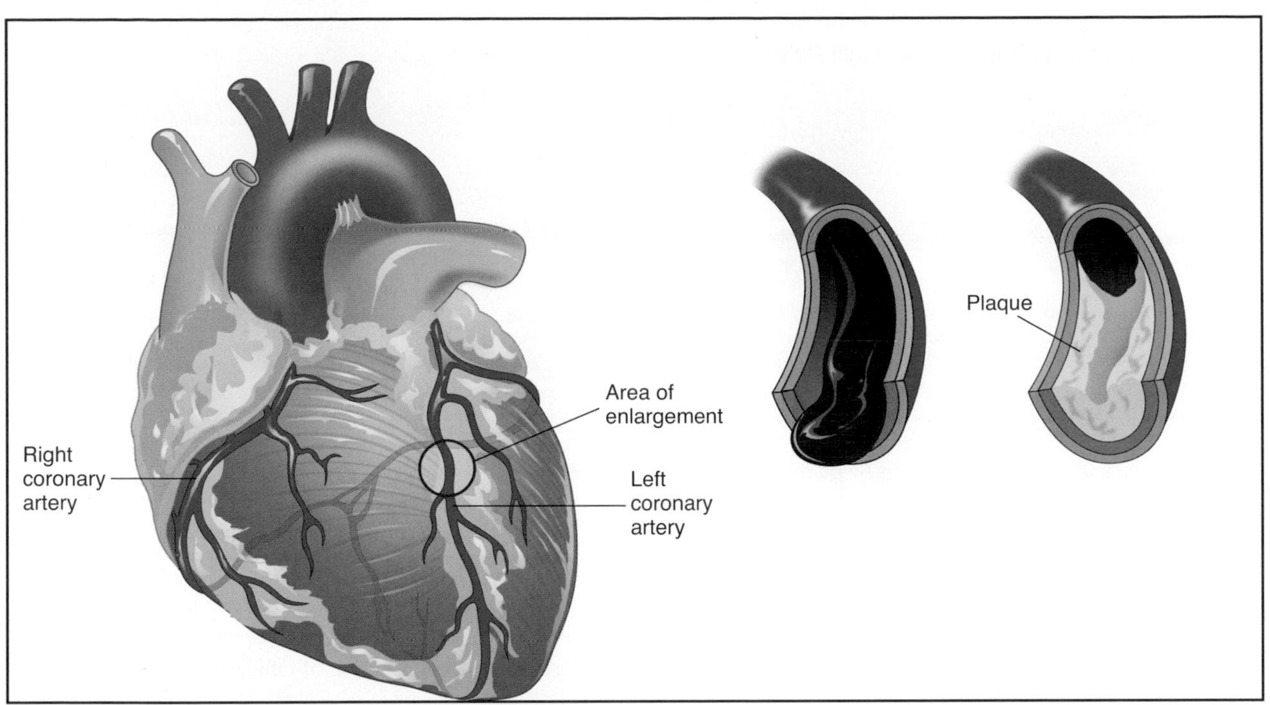

Coronary artery disease. *(Illustration by Electronic Illustrators Group. © 2013 Cengage Learning)*

Coronary artery disease

Healthy coronary arteries are open, elastic, smooth, and slick. The artery walls are flexible and expand to let more blood through when the heart needs to work harder. The disease process is thought to begin with an injury to the linings and walls of the arteries. This injury makes them susceptible to atherosclerosis and production of blood clots (thrombosis).

Coronary artery disease (CAD) is a condition in which plaque builds up inside the coronary arteries. These arteries supply the heart muscle with oxygen-rich blood. Plaque is made up of fat, cholesterol, calcium, and other substances found in the blood. When plaque builds up in the arteries, the condition is called atherosclerosis, commonly called hardening of the arteries. Plaque narrows the arteries and reduces blood flow to the heart. It also makes it more likely that blood clots will form in arteries. Blood clots can partially or completely block blood flow. When coronary arteries are narrowed or blocked, oxygen-rich blood cannot reach the heart. This can cause angina or a heart attack. Angina is chest pain or discomfort that occurs when not enough oxygen-rich blood is flowing to an area of the heart. Angina may feel like pressure or squeezing in the chest. The pain also may occur in the shoulders, arms, neck, jaw, or back. A heart attack occurs when blood flow to an area of the heart is completely blocked. This prevents oxygen-rich blood from reaching that area of the heart and causes it to die. Without quick treatment, a heart attack can lead to serious problems and even death. Over time, CAD can weaken the heart and lead to heart failure and arrhythmias. Heart failure is a condition in which the heart cannot pump enough blood throughout the body. Arrhythmias are irregularities with the speed or rhythm of the heartbeat.

Heart attack (myocardial infarction)

A heart attack (myocardial infarction) occurs when the blood supply to the heart is slowed or stopped because of a blockage. Atherosclerosis, the narrowing of coronary arteries due to plaque buildup, causes more than 90% of heart attacks. A heart attack may also occur when a coronary artery temporarily contracts or goes into a severe spasm, effectively shutting off the flow of blood to the heart. The length of time the blood supply is cut off determines the amount of damage to the heart.

Congenital heart disease

Congenital means existing at birth. A congenital heart defect happens when the heart or the blood vessels near the heart do not develop normally before birth. Congenital heart defects are present in about 1% of live births and are the most frequent congenital malformations in newborns. In most cases, researchers do not know the reason they happen. Some causes include viral infections, certain conditions such as Down Syndrome,

Prevalence of heart disease in the United States[1]

	African American		Caucasian	
	Females	Males	Females	Males
Coronary heart disease	8.8%	7.8%	6.9%	9.4%
Heart attack	2.9%	3.6%	2.6%	5.1%
Angina pectoris	5.4%	4.0%	4.5%	4.7%
Total cardiovascular disease	**46.9%**	**44.6%**	**34.4%**	**38.1%**

[1]All statistics are from 2006, the most recent year for which data was available.

SOURCE: American Heart Association, *Heart Disease and Stroke Statistics—2010 Update*. Available online at: http://www.americanheart.org (accessed September 23, 2010).

(Table by PreMediaGlobal. Reproduced by permission of Gale, a part of Cengage Learning.)

and drug abuse during pregnancy, especially of alcohol, cocaine, and methamphetamines.

Rheumatic heart disease

Rheumatic heart disease describes a group of acute (short-term) and chronic (long-term) heart disorders that can occur as a result of rheumatic fever. One common result of rheumatic fever is heart valve damage. Due to the control of rheumatic fever in the United States and most developed countries, it is relatively rare in these regions but is still a significant heart disease in parts of Africa, Asia, and South America. Rheumatic fever is an inflammatory disease that may affect many connective tissues of the body, especially those of the heart, joints, brain or skin. It usually starts out as a strep throat (streptococcal) infection. Anyone can get acute rheumatic fever, but it usually occurs in children between the ages of 5 and 15 years. About 60% of people with rheumatic fever develop some degree of subsequent heart disease.

Demographics

Heart disease is the leading cause of death in the United States, and it is a major cause of disability. About 600,000 people die of heart disease in the United States each year, about 25% of all U.S. deaths. Statistics from the **Centers for Disease Control and Prevention (CDC)** report that coronary heart disease is the principal type of heart disease, reponsible for about 385,000 deaths each year, or about 65% of all cases of heart disease. In 2012, cardiovascular disease killed more than 17 million people worldwide, almost one-third of all deaths globally, according to the **World Health Organization (WHO)**. Experts estimate that, by 2020, heart disease and **stroke** will become the leading causes of both death and disability worldwide, with the number of fatalities projected to increase to over 20 million a year and by 2030 to over 24 million a year. Men are slightly more likely to develop heart disease than women. An increasing number of women are experiencing heart disease but they are under-diagnosed. For both sexes, the risk of heart disease increases with age. According to the most recent data available (2008), heart disease is the leading cause of death among whites (25.1% of all deaths), African Americans (24.5% of all deaths), and Hispanics (20.8% of all deaths), and the second leading cause of death, after **cancer**, among Asians or Pacific Islanders (23.2% of all deaths) and American Indians or Alaskan Natives (18.0% of all deaths). In 2010, heart disease was responsible for 3% of all deaths among the age group 1 to 24 years, 12% of all deaths among 25- to 44-year-olds, 21% of all deaths among 45- to 64-year-olds, and 27% of all those over the age of 65.

Causes and symptoms

Coronary artery disease

Over many years, plaque builds up on artery walls. Plaque is a sticky, yellow substance made of fatty substances like cholesterol, as well as calcium and waste products from cells. It narrows and clogs the arteries, slowing the flow of blood. The process is called atherosclerosis. Atherosclerosis is a slow, progressive condition that may begin as early as childhood and occur anywhere in the body, but it usually affects large and medium sized arteries. Atherosclerotic plaques often form blood clots that can also block the coronary arteries (coronary thrombosis). Sometimes plaque in an artery can rupture. The body's repair system in turn creates a blood clot to heal the wound. The clot, however, can block the artery, leading to a heart attack or stroke.

Congenital defects and muscle spasms of arteries or heart muscles also block blood flow. Some research indicates that infection from organisms such as chlamydia bacteria may be responsible for some cases of heart disease.

Early warning signs may include fatigue, pain, and dizziness, as well as the symptoms associated with angina: a squeezing, suffocating, or burning feeling in the chest that tends to start in the center of the chest but may move to the arm, neck, back, throat, or jaw. Women are more likely to experience atypical symptoms, such as vague chest discomfort.

Heart attack (myocardial infarction)

A heart attack occurs when the blood supply to the heart is partially or completely blocked. Symptoms include pain in the chest, neck, jaw, shoulder, arms or back, sudden discomfort or pain (especially in the chest) that does not go away, difficulty breathing, nausea, sweating, and anxiety.

Congenital heart disease

Congenital heart disease is caused by a defect in the heart at birth. The most common symptoms of congenital heart defects are a heart murmur, a bluish tint to the skin, lips, or fingernails, fast breathing, shortness of breath, and fatigue, especially during exercise or **physical activity**.

Rheumatic heart disease

It may take several years after an episode of rheumatic fever for valve damage to develop or symptoms to appear. **Antibiotics** can prevent streptococcal infection from developing into rheumatic fever. Any child with a persistent sore throat should have a throat culture to check for strep infection. Penicillin or another antibiotic will usually prevent strep throat from developing into rheumatic fever. Symptoms of heart valve problems, which are often the result of rheumatic heart disease, can include chest pain, excessive fatigue, heart palpitations (when the heart flutters or misses beats), a thumping sensation in the chest, shortness of breath, and swollen ankles, wrists or stomach.

Major risk factors

A number of major contributing risk factors increase the chance of developing heart disease. Some of these can be changed and some cannot. The greater the number of risk factors, the greater the chance of developing heart disease. Major risk factors significantly increase the chance of developing heart disease. These include:

- Heredity. People whose parents have heart disease are more likely to develop it. African Americans are also at increased risk because they experience a high rate of severe hypertension.
- Gender. Men are more likely to have heart attacks than women and to have them at a younger age. Above the age of 60, however, women have heart disease at a rate equal to that of men.
- Age. Men who are 45 years of age and older and women who are 55 years of age and older are more likely to have heart disease. Occasionally, heart disease may strike men or women in their 30s. People more than 65 years old are more likely to die from a heart attack. Older women are twice as likely as older men to die within a few weeks of a heart attack.
- Smoking. Smoking increases both the chance of developing heart disease and the chance of dying from it. Smokers are more than twice as likely as non-smokers to have a heart attack and are two to four times more likely die from it.
- High cholesterol levels. Dietary sources of cholesterol are meat, dairy food, eggs, and other animal-fat products. Cholesterol is also produced by the body. Age, body fat, diet, exercise, heredity, and sex affect one's blood cholesterol. For typical, healthy patients, the American Heart Association recommends a total blood cholesterol below 200 mg/dL, which puts the person at a comparatively low risk for coronary heart disease. For these individuals, a total cholesterol level of 200–239 mg/dL is considered borderline high-risk, and a level of 240 mg/dL or above is considered high risk and doubles the risk for coronary heart disease. Persons with such risk factors as elevated low-density lipoprotein (LDL cholesterol, or "bad" cholesterol) levels, low high-density lipoprotein (HDL or "good" cholesterol) levels, or high triglyceride levels should consult with their doctor about what their target cholesterol level should be.
- High blood pressure. High blood pressure makes the heart work harder and weakens it over time. It increases the risk of heart attack, stroke, kidney failure, and congestive heart failure. A blood pressure of 140 over 90 or above is considered high. The risk of heart attack or stroke is raised several times for people with high blood pressure combined with obesity, smoking, high cholesterol levels, or diabetes. Nearly one-third of American adults have high blood pressure.
- Lack of physical activity. Lack of exercise increases the risk of heart disease. Even modest physical activity, such as walking, is beneficial if done regularly.
- Diabetes mellitus. The risk of developing heart disease is seriously increased for diabetics. About two-thirds of people who have type I or type II diabetes die as the result of a heart attack or stroke.

Contributing risk factors

Contributing risk factors have been linked to heart disease. These include:

- Obesity. Excess weight increases the strain on the heart and increases the risk of developing heart disease even if no other risk factors are present. Obesity increases blood pressure and blood cholesterol and can lead to diabetes.

- Hormone replacement therapy (HRT). Even though physicians once believed that HRT could help prevent heart disease in women, the Women's Health Initiative (WHI) released information in 2002 and 2003 showing that use of combined hormones (estrogen and progestin) is harmful in women who already have coronary artery disease. As of 2012, experts no longer recommend the use of HRT as protection against heart disease.
- Stress and anger. Some scientists believe that poorly managed stress and anger can contribute to the development of heart disease and increase the blood's tendency to form clots (thrombosis). Stress increases the heart rate and blood pressure and can injure the lining of the arteries.
- Chest pain (angina). Angina is the main symptom of coronary heart disease, but it is not always present. Other symptoms include shortness of breath, chest heaviness, tightness, pain, a burning sensation, squeezing, or pressure either behind the breastbone or in the left arm, neck, or jaws. According to the American Heart Association, 64 percent of women and 50 percent of men who died suddenly of heart disease had no previous symptoms of the disease.

Diagnosis

Diagnosis begins with a doctor's review of the medical history, discussion of symptoms, listening to the heart, and performing basic screening tests. These tests measure blood lipid levels, blood pressure, fasting blood-glucose levels, weight, and other indicators. Other diagnostic tests include resting and exercise electrocardiograms, echocardiography, radionuclide scans, and coronary angiography. The treadmill exercise (stress) test is an appropriate screening test for those with high risk factors even though they feel well.

Angiogram

Coronary angiography is considered the most accurate method for making a diagnosis of heart disease, but it is also the most invasive. This test involves taking x-ray pictures of the coronary arteries and the vessels that supply blood to the heart. During coronary angiography, the patient is awake but sedated. The cardiologist inserts a catheter into a blood vessel and guides it into the heart. A contrast dye (a radiopaque substance that is visible on x-ray) is injected into the catheter, and x-rays are taken. This dye makes the blood vessels visible when an x-ray is taken of them. Angiography allows doctors to clearly see how blood flows into the heart. This helps them to pinpoint problems with the coronary arteries. Angiography may be recommended for patients with angina or those with suspected coronary artery disease. The test gives doctors valuable information on the condition of the coronary arteries, such as atherosclerosis, regurgitation (blood flowing backward through the heart valves), or pooling of blood in a chamber because of a valve malfunction. Coronary angiography is performed in a cardiac catheterization laboratory in either an outpatient or an inpatient surgery unit.

Radionuclide angiography enables physicians to see the blood flow of the coronary arteries. Nuclear scans are performed by injecting a small amount of radiopharmaceutical, such as thallium, into the bloodstream. As the patient lies on a table, a camera that detects gamma rays to produce an image of the radioactive material passes over the patient and records pictures of the heart. Radionuclide angiography is usually performed in a hospital's nuclear medicine department. The **radiation** exposure is about the same as that in a chest x-ray.

Echocardiogram

An echocardiogram uses sound waves (ultrasound) to create a picture of the heart. The recorded waves show the shape, texture, and movement of the heart valves, as well as the size of the heart chambers and how well they are working. A technician applies gel to a hand-held transducer and then presses it against the patient's chest. The heart's sound waves are converted into an image that can be displayed on a monitor. An echocardiogram may be done to determine whether a stroke was caused by a heart condition and can also help determine whether there is a risk of blood clots forming in the heart. It may also be recommended if the patient is experiencing abnormal heart sounds, shortness of breath, palpitations, or angina or has a history of stroke. It is very useful in diagnosing heart valve problems. It does not reveal the coronary arteries themselves but can detect abnormalities in the heart wall caused by heart disease. Typically performed in a doctor's office or outpatient facility, the test takes 30 to 60 minutes.

Electrocardiogram

An electrocardiogram (ECG or EKG) is a test that checks how the heart is functioning by measuring the electrical activity of the heart. Electrodes are placed on the patient's chest, arms, and legs. They send impulses of the heart's activity through an oscilloscope (a monitor) to a recorder that traces them on paper. With each heartbeat, an electrical impulse (wave) travels through the heart. This wave causes the muscle to squeeze and pump blood from the heart. By measuring how long the electrical wave takes to pass through the heart, a cardiologist can determine whether the electrical activity is normal, fast, or irregular. The cardiologist may also be able to determine whether the heart is enlarged or overworked. It may be recommended if the patient is experiencing arrhythmia, palpitations, dizziness, excessive fatigue, or angina. An ECG is used to:

- Detect abnormal heart rhythms that may have caused blood clots to form.
- Detect heart problems, including a recent or ongoing heart attack, abnormal heart rhythms (arrhythmias), coronary artery blockage, areas of damaged heart muscle (from a prior heart attack), enlargement of the heart, and inflammation of the sac surrounding the heart (pericarditis).
- Detect non-heart conditions such as electrolyte imbalances and lung diseases.
- Monitor recovery from a heart attack, progression of heart disease, or the effectiveness of certain heart medications or a pacemaker.
- Rule out hidden heart disease in patients about to undergo surgery.

Exercise stress test

This test measures how the heart and blood vessels respond to exertion when the patient is exercising on a treadmill or a stationary bike. It can be performed in a physician's office or outpatient facility.

Treatment

Heart disease can be treated many ways. The choice of treatment depends on the patient and the severity of the disease. Treatments include lifestyle changes, drug therapy, and coronary artery bypass surgery. These, however, are not a cure. Heart disease is a chronic disease requiring lifelong care.

Medications

People with moderate heart disease may gain adequate control through lifestyle changes and drug therapy. Drugs such as nitrates, beta-blockers, and calcium channel blockers relieve chest pain and complications of heart disease, but they cannot clear blocked arteries. Nitrates improve blood flow to the heart, and beta-blockers reduce the amount of oxygen required by the heart during stress. Calcium channel blockers help keep the arteries open and reduce blood pressure. Aspirin helps prevent blood clots from forming on plaques, reducing the likelihood of a heart attack and stroke. Cholesterol-lowering medications are also indicated in many cases.

ANTIPLATELETS. Antiplatelets help prevent dangerous blood clots from forming. They may be used to reduce the risk of clot-induced heart attack or stroke, which is called preventive or prophylactic treatment. One of the most common antiplatelets is aspirin. Ticlopidine (Ticlid) may be prescribed to stroke survivors or those who are at high risk of stroke, particularly if they are not able to take aspirin. Clopidogrel (Plavix) is an antiplatelet drug that is effective in preventing strokes and heart attacks and is often prescribed for patients who receive a coronary stent. Dipyridmalole (Persantine) may also be given with other antiplatelet or anticoagulant medications. It can also be given by injection during tests on the heart.

ACE INHIBITORS. Angiotensin converting enzyme (ACE) inhibitors are usually given to people with high blood pressure, congestive heart failure, or a high likelihood of developing coronary artery disease. They may also be given after a heart attack to prevent more complications and to people living with congestive heart failure. They help control blood pressure to make it easier for the heart to pump. ACE inhibitors may also make people with CAD feel less tired and short of breath, reduce the time they spend in a hospital, and help them live longer. ACE inhibitors have been shown to reduce the risk of heart attack, stroke, and death in people with a history of coronary artery disease. Since ACE inhibitors are used to control and prevent conditions of the heart, they are usually prescribed for the long term.

BETA-BLOCKERS. Beta-blockers are used to treat high blood pressure, congestive heart failure, abnormal heart rhythms, and chest pain. They are sometimes used to prevent future heart attacks in someone who has had a heart attack and to treat tremors caused by an overactive thyroid, as well as anxiety or migraines. Beta-blocker is short for beta-adrenergic blocking drugs. Beta-blockers block the responses from the beta nerve receptors. This slows the heart rate and lowers blood pressure to reduce the workload on the heart.

CALCIUM CHANNEL BLOCKERS. Calcium channel blockers, sometimes called calcium channel antagonists, are used to control high blood pressure, chest pain caused by coronary artery disease, and irregular heartbeats. Calcium channel blockers are often taken in combination with beta-blockers or diuretics to help reduce blood pressure. Calcium channel blockers are vasodilators, which means they widen (dilate) blood vessels, letting blood flow through more easily. By relaxing blood vessels, the blood pressure drops, and the heart does not have to work as hard.

NITRATES. Nitrates are vasodilators and can be used to prevent chest pain, limit the number of angina attacks, relieve the pain of a current attack, or treat the symptoms of congestive heart failure. Nitroglycerin is a type of nitrate.

Medical procedures

ANGIOPLASTY WITH STENT. Percutaneous Coronary Intervention (PCI), commonly called angioplasty with a stent, is a non-surgical procedure that uses a catheter (a thin flexible tube) to place a small structure called a stent (a small tubular structure made of stainless steel or plastic) to open up blood vessels in the heart that have been narrowed by plaque buildup. PCI improves blood flow, thus decreasing heart-related chest pain, making the patient feel better and increasing his or her ability to be physically active. During the procedure, a catheter is inserted into the blood vessels either in the groin or in the arm. Using a special type of x-ray called fluoroscopy, the catheter is threaded through the blood vessels into the heart where the coronary artery is narrowed. When the tip is in place, a balloon tip covered with a stent is inflated. The balloon tip compresses the plaque and expands the stent. Once the plaque is compressed, and the stent is in place, the balloon is deflated and withdrawn. The stent stays in the artery, holding it open. The doctor may use a coated stent or a bare metal stent. A coated stent has medicine on its outside that slows the regrowth of the artery wall and blocking the stent. If a coated stent is used, the patient will need to take Plavix for at least two years, perhaps for life.

CORONARY ARTERY BYPASS SURGERY. Coronary artery bypass surgery improves the blood flow to the heart muscle. It is commonly referred to as bypass surgery or Coronary Artery Bypass Graft (CABG, pronounced like cabbage) surgery. Bypass surgery is performed to improve blood flow problems to the heart muscle caused by the buildup of plaque in the coronary arteries. The surgery involves using a piece of blood vessel (artery, vein) taken from elsewhere in the body to create a detour or bypass around the blocked portion of the coronary artery. By improving blood flow, bypass surgery may decrease heart-related chest pain, making patients feel better and increasing their ability for physical activity.

In coronary artery bypass surgery, a piece of a healthy blood vessel from the patient's leg, arm, or chest will be removed to be used as the bypass. Unless a patient is undergoing one of the newer procedures (minimally invasive bypass or off-pump or beating-heart surgery), the heart is stopped so the surgeons can work on it. A machine called the heart-lung machine will take over the work of the heart and lungs while the surgeon is operating on the heart. The section of healthy blood vessel is attached above and below the blocked artery. When the heart is restarted, blood flow is diverted through the bypass around the narrowed portion of the diseased artery. Depending upon the number of blockages, one to five bypasses may be created.

COUNTER PULSATION. Another medical procedure that can help with CAD is counter pulsation. In this procedure, inflatable cuffs are placed on the legs and lower abdomen. When the heart relaxes, the cuffs inflate and push blood into the blood vessels of the heart. This procedure is repeated over a few days, and it stimulates improved blood flow to the heart. Counter pulsation can not be done in people with dilated aortas or severe peripheral vascular disease.

Heart attack (myocardial infarction)

A person who is experiencing or believes they may be experiencing a heart attack should seek immediate emergency help. In the United States, call or have someone else call 911 and request paramedics or emergency medical technicians (EMTs). Most fire departments in the United States and Canada have paramedics and/or EMTs. Doctors also recommend that at the first sign of a heart attack, the patient chew and swallow an adult (325 mg) aspirin, which can help improve blood flow to the heart. Only aspirin can improve blood flow; no other pain medications, such as acetaminophen (Tylenol) or ibuprofen (Advil), will work. Until medical help arrives, the patient should sit or lie down. If the patient is on the drug nitroglycerine, they should take a normal dose. Following a heart attack, patients may be put on nitrates, ACE inhibitors, beta-blockers, and antiplatelets (all described under coronary artery disease medications). Other drugs used include thrombolytic drugs, used to dissolve blood clots that are blocking the coronary arteries, and anticoagulants, used to thin the blood and prevent clots from forming in the arteries. Surgical treatments include angioplasty and coronary bypass (both described under coronary artery disease medical procedures).

Congenital heart disease

The heart defects of congenital heart disease are treated with several medications, including ACE inhibitors, beta-blockers, diuretics, and digoxin. Diuretics act on the kidneys to produce more urine and remove excess salt and water from the body. By decreasing water and salt, diuretics lower blood pressure and help reduce the workload on the heart. This may make it easier for the heart to pump, improve shortness of breath, reduce swelling and bloating, reduce the time spent in a hospital, and help patients live longer. Digoxin helps the heart pump more strongly and slows down the heart rate to improve its pumping action.

In many cases, the strain to the heart requires procedures that either fix holes between the chambers, replace valves, or repair or reconnect major blood vessels. In severe cases, heart transplant surgery may be needed. Several other surgical procedures can be used to repair and correct congenital heart defects:

- Cardiac catheterization is often used to repair simple holes in the heart. A catheter (thin tube) is inserted into a blood vessel in the groin or arm and guided to the heart so that a surgeon can insert a plug inside the hole to repair it.
- Angioplasty is used to repair defective cardiac valves that can be either too narrow or leaky. A tiny balloon is guided to the heart inside a catheter (a thin tube). When the balloon is inflated, it can stretch the opening of a narrowed heart valve and restore normal blood flow. It is removed once blood flow returns.

Rheumatic heart disease

If heart damage from rheumatic fever is identified in childhood or young adulthood, daily antibiotics may be required until the age of 25 or 30 to help prevent recurrence of rheumatic fever and avoid the development of infective bacterial endocarditis, an infection of the heart valves or lining of the heart. Additional treatment will depend on the type of heart damage. Surgery may be required to repair or replace damaged heart valves. In rare cases, heart transplant surgery may be recommended.

Other treatment options

Herbal-medicine practitioners recommend a variety of remedies that may have a beneficial effect on heart disease. They may suggest garlic (*Allium sativum*), myrrh (*Commiphora molmol*), and oats (*Avena sativa*) to help reduce cholesterol, and hawthorn (*Crataegus* spp.), linden (*Tilia europaea*), and yarrow (*Achillea millefolium*) to control high blood pressure, a risk factor for heart disease. Tea, especially green tea (*Camellia sinensis*), is high in antioxidants, and studies have shown that it may have a preventive effect against atherosclerosis. Coenzyme Q10 has been shown to be beneficial for patients with congestive heart failure. Taurine, an amino acid found in meat and fish proteins, has also been suggested as a way to treat heart arrhythmia.

Some alternative-medicine practitioners believe that yoga and other bodywork, massage, relaxation, aromatherapy, and music therapies may also help prevent heart disease and stop, or even reverse, the progression of atherosclerosis. Vitamin and mineral supplements that are believed to reduce, reverse, or protect against heart disease include B-complex **vitamins**, calcium, chromium, magnesium, L-carnitine, zinc, and the antioxidant vitamins C and E. Notably, a study in 2004 showed a relationship between high doses of supplemental vitamin C and reduced coronary heart disease but found little risk reduction with supplemental vitamin E.

Traditional Chinese medicine (TCM) may recommend herbal remedies, massage, acupuncture, and dietary modification. A healthy diet (including cold-water fish as a source of essential fatty acids) and exercise are important components of both alternative and conventional **prevention** and treatment strategies.

Nutrition and diet concerns

A healthy diet includes a variety of foods that are low in fat, especially saturated fat; low in cholesterol; and high in fiber. It includes plenty of fruits and vegetables and limits salt. According to the American Heart Association, fats should comprise no more than 25 to 35 percent of total daily calories and should total less than 7 percent saturated fats, less than 1 percent trans fats, and the remainder as monounsaturated and polyunsaturated fats from such sources as nuts, seeds, fish, and vegetable oils. Cholesterol intake should be limited to 300 mg per day for the average person. Those individuals who have coronary heart disease or who have an LDL cholesterol level of 100 mg/dL or more should lower their daily cholesterol intake to less than 200 mg per day. Eating cold-water fish or taking comparable omega-3 polyunsaturated fatty acid supplements can help prevent cardiac death. The American Heart Association advocates eating fish (particularly fatty fish) at least twice a week. It also recommends adding soybeans (including tofu), canola, walnut, flaxseed, and other oils to the diet because these contain alpha-linolenic acid that can transform into omega-3 fatty acid in the body. The association also notes that individuals consult with their doctor before taking omega-3 fatty acid supplements in excess of 3 grams per day because of the potential for bleeding.

Cholesterol, a waxy substance containing fats, is found in foods such as meat, dairy, eggs, and other animal products. It is also produced in the liver. Soluble fiber can help lower cholesterol. Dietary cholesterol should be below 300 milligrams per day. Many popular lipid-lowering drugs can reduce LDL cholesterol by an average of 25 to 30 percent or more when used with a low-fat, low-cholesterol diet.

Antioxidants are chemical compounds in plant foods. When people eat antioxidant-rich foods, they may improve the function of the arteries and prevent arterial plaque formation and reduce their risk of cancer. Colorful vegetables and fruits are sources of antioxidants and are rich in fiber, vitamins, and minerals. They are low in calories and nearly fat-free. Vitamin C and beta-carotene, found in many fruits and vegetables, keep LDL-cholesterol from turning into a form that damages coronary arteries. Whole grains, especially whole oats and oat bran, reduce cholesterol.

Excess **sodium** can increase the risk of high blood pressure. Many processed foods contain large amounts of sodium. Daily intake should be limited to about 2,300 milligrams, about the amount in a teaspoon of salt.

New reports on diet and heart disease have answered some questions, but others remain unclear. While one study concludes that four servings per day of fruit and vegetables are associated with a slight drop in risk of heart disease, eight or more servings per day can produce a significant drop in risk. Another study showed that consuming legumes at least four times per week lowered risk of heart disease from 11 percent to 22 percent, compared with consuming legumes less than once a week. Research on antioxidants continues to produce mixed findings, with some reports showing that vitamins E, C, and other antioxidants can help prevent heart disease, and other studies showing they have no effect. Although scientists and medical professionals had not reached a consensus about the benefits of antioxidants as of 2012, the American Heart Association reported that up to 30 percent of Americans take antioxidant supplements. As of 2012, however, the association did not recommend supplements. Instead, it advised a diet containing a variety of nutrient-rich foods, including fruits, vegetables, whole grains, and nuts.

The MyPlate nutritional guide developed by the Center for **Nutrition** Policy and Promotion, an organization of the U.S. Department of Agriculture, provides easy-to-follow guidelines for daily heart-healthy eating.

Exercising regularly

Regular aerobic exercise can lower blood pressure, help control weight, and increase HDL (good) cholesterol. It also may keep the blood vessels more flexible. The American Heart Association recommends moderate-to-vigorous intensity aerobic activity (50 to 85 percent of the maximum heart rate) for 150 minutes every week. Those 150 minutes can be divided into five 30-minute sessions per week, or any other system that a person prefers, as long as a total of 150 minutes is achieved each week. Aerobic exercise—activities such as walking, jogging, and cycling—use the large muscle groups and forces the body to use oxygen more efficiently. It also can include everyday activities such as active gardening, climbing stairs, or brisk housework. People with heart disease or risk factors should consult a doctor before beginning an exercise program.

Maintaining a desirable body weight

People who are 20 percent or more above their ideal body weight have an increased risk of developing heart disease. Losing weight can help decrease total and LDL cholesterol, reduce triglycerides, and boost HDL cholesterol. It may also reduce blood pressure. Eating right and exercising are two essential components of losing weight.

Quitting smoking

Smoking has many adverse effects on the heart. It increases the heart rate, constricts major arteries, and can create irregular heartbeats. It also raises blood pressure, contributes to the development of plaque, increases the formation of blood clots, and causes blood platelets to cluster and impede blood flow. When smokers quit the habit, heart damage can be repaired. Several studies have shown that ex-smokers face the same risk of heart disease as non-smokers within 5 to 10 years after they quit.

Drinking in moderation

Modest consumption of alcohol may actually protect against heart disease because alcohol appears to raise levels of HDL cholesterol. The American Heart Association defines moderate consumption as one to two daily drinks for men, and one daily drink for women. The association defines one drink as 4 ounces of wine, 12 ounces of beer, 1.5 ounces of 80-proof spirits, or 1 ounce of 100-proof spirits.

Seeking diagnosis and treatment for hypertension

High blood pressure, one of the most common and serious risk factors for heart disease, can be completely controlled through lifestyle changes and medication. Seeking diagnosis and treatment is critical because hypertension often exhibits no symptoms, so many people do not know they have it. Moderate hypertension can be controlled by reducing dietary intake of sodium and fat, exercising regularly, managing stress, abstaining from smoking, and drinking alcohol in moderation.

Managing stress

Everyone experiences stress. Stress can sometimes be avoided and, when it is inevitable, it can be managed through relaxation techniques, exercise, and other methods.

Prevention

The only way to prevent rheumatic heart disease is to prevent rheumatic fever or successfully treat rheumatic fever before it can damage heart valves. There is no way

KEY TERMS

Angina—Chest pain.

Angiogram—An x-ray image of one or more blood vessels.

Angioplasty—A surgical operation to clear a narrowed or blocked artery.

Arrhythmia—An irregular heartbeat.

Atherosclerosis—A buildup of plaque in the arteries, also called hardening of the arteries.

Beta-blocker—A drug that blocks some of the effects of fight-or-flight hormone adrenaline (epinephrine and norepinephrine), slowing the heart rate and lowering the blood pressure.

Calcium channel blocker—A drug that blocks the entry of calcium into the muscle cells of small blood vessels (arterioles) and keeps them from narrowing.

Coronary arteries—The main arteries that provide blood to the heart. The coronary arteries surround the heart like a crown, coming out of the aorta, arching down over the top of the heart, and dividing into two branches. These are the arteries in which heart disease occurs.

Echocardiogram—An image of the heart created by ultrasound waves.

Electrocardiogram—A test that measures the electrical activity of the heart. Also called an ECG or EKG.

HDL cholesterol—High-density lipoprotein cholesterol is a component of cholesterol that helps protect against heart disease. HDL is nicknamed "good cholesterol."

LDL cholesterol—Low-density lipoprotein cholesterol is the primary cholesterol molecule. High levels of LDL increase the risk of coronary heart disease. LDL is nicknamed "bad cholesterol."

Plaque—A mass of material made up of fat, cholesterol, calcium, and other substances found in the blood. It can stick to the walls of arteries, partially or totally blocking blood flow.

Triglyceride—A fat that comes from food or is made from other energy sources in the body. Elevated triglyceride levels contribute to the development of atherosclerosis.

Ultrasound—A technique that uses high-frequency sound waves for medical diagnosis and treatment by creating images of internal organs.

Vasodilator—A class of drugs that widen the blood vessels, in turn decreasing resistance to blood flow and lowering blood pressure.

to prevent congenital heart disease, since it is an inherited (genetic) disorder that develops in the womb.

People can lower their risk of coronary artery disease and heart attack by knowing and controlling their blood pressure, diabetes, and cholesterol. It is also important to lead a healthy lifestyle by not smoking and being physically active (exercising regularly), eating a healthy diet that is lower in fat, especially saturated and trans fat, achieving and maintaining a healthy weight, limiting alcohol use, and reducing stress. Seniors can reduce stress by regularly socializing with friends and family and with such activities as yoga and meditation. Many doctors also recommend taking a low-dose (81mg) of aspirin daily.

A healthy lifestyle can help prevent heart disease and slow its progress. A heart-healthy lifestyle includes maintaining a healthy diet and weight, performing regular exercise, refraining from smoking, engaging in moderate drinking, controlling hypertension, and managing stress. Cardiac rehabilitation programs are excellent ways to help prevent recurring coronary problems for people who are at risk and who have had coronary events and procedures.

Caregiver concerns

Patients with heart disease may have as many as five (or more) medications that need to be taken daily. Caregivers should have a system to make sure that the patient takes the medications when and how they are prescribed. Alarms or timers can be used to remind the patient when to take each pill. Also, weekly pill dispensers can help to ensure that patients only take the dose that is prescribed. Caregivers may want to keep a medicine calendar and note every time the patient takes a dose, or have the patient do it themselves. It is vital that the caregiver makes sure that prescriptions are refilled before they run out. Make sure that the patient is not taking anything that is contraindicated by their condition or that may interact with their medication. Examples include such things as herbal supplements, antihistamines, and analgesics. Check with the patient's doctor or pharmacist for possible drug interactions. Also, people who take nitrates (such as nitroglycerine) should not take medications for erectile dysfunction (ED), including sildenafil (Viagra), vardenafil (Levitra), and tadalafil (Cialis).

Helping a patient stick to their diet and exercise routine is critical to their overall health. One way to ensure adherence to a restricted diet is to prepare meals for the patient. If this is not feasible, the caregiver can try to limit the amount of forbidden foods that are present in the patient's home. The level of exercise required of a patient will depend on their overall health, but for most patients, frequent walks are beneficial. If the caregiver can accompany them on their walks, it will make the experience more enjoyable and increase adherence. Perhaps the most important role of a caregiver is providing emotional support. Simply being there to listen to the patient's concerns and to provide encouragement can keep them on the path toward better health. In some cases, the patient may require at-home oxygen therapy. The caregiver should learn how the oxygen equipment is used and to make sure more oxygen is ordered well before the patient's current supply runs out.

Prognosis

Advances in medicine and the adoption of healthier lifestyles have caused a substantial decline in death rates from heart disease since the mid-1980s. New diagnostic techniques enable doctors to identify and treat heart disease in its earliest stages. New technologies and surgical procedures have extended the lives of many patients who otherwise would have died. Research continues, and valuable organizations continue to educate clinicians, patients, and healthy individuals alike, in the fight against heart disease

Resources

BOOKS

DeBakey, Michael E. *The Living Heart in the 21st Century*. Amherst, NY: Prometheus Books, 2012.

DeSilva, Regis. *Heart Disease*. Santa Barbara, CA: Greenwood, 2012.

Pollock, Anne. *Medicating Race: Heart Disease and Durable Preoccupations with Difference*. Durham, NC: Duke University Press, 2012.

Sato, Atsuko, and Seiji Hayashi. *Coronary Artery Disease, Cardiac Arrest and Bypass Surgery: Risk Factors, Health Effects and Outcomes*. New York: Nova Science Publishers, 2012.

PERIODICALS

Adams, Scott, Chad Cotti, and Daniel Fuhrmann. "The Short-term Impact of Smoke-free Workplace Laws on Fatal Heart Attacks." *Applied Economics* 45, 11. (2013): 1381–93.

Cohen, M. S. "Clinical Practice: The Effect of Obesity in Children with Congenital Heart Disease." *European Journal of Pediatrics* 171, 8. (2012): 1145–50.

Fuster, Valentin, and Jagat Narula, eds. "Coronary Risk Factors, Update." *Medical Clinics of North America* 96, 1. (2012): all.

Oldridge, Neil. "Exercise-based Cardiac Rehabilitation in Patients with Coronary Heart Disease: Meta-analysis Outcomes Revisited." *Future Cardiology* 8, 5. (2012): 729–51.

OTHER

"Coronary Heart Disease." PubMedHealth. http://www.ncbi.nlm.nih.gov/pubmedhealth/PMH0004449/. Accessed on October 22, 2012.

"Heart Disease." Mayo Clinic. http://www.mayoclinic.com/health/heart-disease/DS01120. Accessed on October 22, 2012.

"Heart Disease Health Center." WebMD. http://www.webmd.com/heart-disease/default.htm. Accessed on October 22, 2012.

"What Is Cardiovascular Disease (Heart Disease)?" American Heart Association. http://www.heart.org/HEARTORG/Caregiver/Resources/WhatisCardiovascularDisease/What-is-Cardiovascular-Disease_UCM_301852_Article.jsp. Accessed on October 22, 2012.

ORGANIZATIONS

Adult Congenital Heart Association, 6757 Greene St., Suite 335, Philadelphia, PA 19119-3508, (215) 849-1260, (888) 921-2242, Fax: (215) 849-1261, info@achaheart.org, http://www.achaheart.org

American Heart Association, 7272 Greenville Ave., Dallas, TX 75231, (301) 223-2307, (800) 242-8721, http://www.heart.org/HEARTORG/General/General-Questions-and-Latest-Research-Information_UCM_308883_Article.jsp, http://www.americanheart.org

Association of Black Cardiologists, 5355 Hunter Road, Atlanta, GA 30349, (404) 201-6600, (800) 753-9222, Fax: (404) 201-6601, abcardio@abcardio.org, http://www.abcardio.org

European Society of Cardiology, The European Heart House, 2035 Route des Colles, B.P. 179-Les Templiers, Sophia-Antipolis, France 06903, 33 4 9294 7600, Fax: 33 4 9294 7601, http://www.escardio.org/Pages/contactus.aspx, http://www.escardio.org

Heart Foundation, 80 William St., Level 3, SydneyNSW Australia 2011, 02 9219 2444, 300 36 27 87, http://www.heartfoundation.org.au/about-us/contact-us/Pages/contact-form.aspx, http://www.heartfoundation.org.au

National Heart, Lung, and Blood Institute, P.O. Box 30105, Bethesda, MD 20824-0105, (301) 592-8573, Fax: (204) 629-3246, nhlbiinfo@nhlbi.nih.gov, http://www.nhlbi.nih.gov.

Paula Ford-Martin
Ken R. Wells
Laura Jean Cataldo, RN, Ed.D.

Helminthiasis

Definition

Helminthiasis is a disease caused by infection of the body by some type of parasitic worm, such as pinworms, roundworms, tapeworms, or whipworms. Some of the more common types of helminthiasis are ancylostomiasis (a hookworm infection); ascariasis, **filariasis**, and trichuriasis (nematode infections); and **schistosomiasis** (a platyhelminth infection). The disease is sometimes called soil-transmitted helminthiasis (STH) because **parasites** that cause the disease spend at least some portion of their life cycle on or in the soil.

Description

Helminthiasis is transmitted when a person infected with the disease defecates into an area available to other humans. The feces of the infected person contain helminth eggs, which can then be ingested by a second individual who comes into contact with the feces or with foods grown in the soil where the feces were left. Larvae produced by maturation of the helminth eggs may also enter the body through openings in the skin. The symptoms associated with helminthiasis range from mild to severe, and can result in death of the infected individual.

Demographics

The **World Health Organization (WHO)** has called helminthiasis the most common infection in the world. **WHO** estimates that more than a billion people are infected with one form of the disease caused by the roundworm *Ascaris lumbricoides*, another 795 million by the whipworm *Trichuris trichiura*, and 740 million more by the two hookworms, *Ancylostoma duodenale* and *Necator americanus*). The first two diseases are caused by ingestion of worm eggs, while the latter is caused by penetration of the skin by means of the worm larvae. The region with the greatest number of cases of helminthiasis is the Western Pacific area, followed by Africa, South and Central America, and southeast Asia.

Causes and symptoms

Causes

In all forms of helminthiasis, parasitic worms are resident in the small intenstine of an individual infected with the disease. Those worms produce eggs, which are then excreted with a person's feces. If defecation occurs in some sanitary facility, such as a flush toilet, risk of transmitting the disease is greatly reduced. If defection occurs in an open area, such as a field, however, eggs remain on or in the soil, where they mature over a period of two to three weeks. After that point, they become infective and may be taken up by a person in a number of ways. For example, eggs may adhere to the surface of fruits and vegetables grown on soil containing the eggs, after which they may be ingested by other humans. Even if dried and stored, the eggs remain infective for a period of time. Infection may also occur if an individual touches the soil or plant material in the soil where eggs have been deposited. In such cases, infection may occur when larvae of worms enter the body through sores, wounds, or other breaks in the skin. After eggs or larvae have entered the body, they travel through the digestive system, where they become lodged in the small intestine and mature to adult worms. At that point, the cycle may repeat itself.

KEY TERMS

Helminth—A parasitic worm.

Pulmonary eosinophilia—Swelling of lung tissue as a result of increase production of white blood cells.

Symptoms

Symptoms of helminthiasis vary depending on the causative agent. A first or mild infection may be entirely asymptomatic, although the number or severity of symptoms tends to increase with further or more extensive infections. Some of the most common symptoms include nausea, lethargy, tiredness, abdominal **pain**, and loss of appetite. As the level of infection increases, these symptoms become more noticeable and more serious, including disorders of the gastrointestinal and circulatory systems. Blood loss and anemia are common later symptoms of an infection. As worms spread to other parts of the body, other symptoms may also develop. For example, the migration of worms into the lungs can result in pulmonary eosinophilia (Loeffler's syndrome), **pneumonia**, and other respiratory disorders. Migration of worms to other organs may cause other conditions also, such as liver disorders and pancreatic obstruction. In the most severe instances, death may result from severe nutritional stress, obstruction of organ function, tissue reactions, or rectal prolapse.

Diagnosis

Diagnosis of helminthiasis is generally based on microscopic examination of feces, which reveals the presence of eggs. In some cases, worms themselves may be observed visually in the feces. More advanced

QUESTIONS TO ASK YOUR DOCTOR

- What is the risk of developing helminthiasis in the region where we live?
- To what extent should I be concerned about contracting helminthiasis on our trip to Africa?
- What precautions can I take in advance of and during our trip against the disease?

diagnostic techniques, such as x-ray and endoscopy may be needed to detect the worms themselves or the anatomical changes caused by their presence in the body.

Prevention

Probably the most effective single approach to the **prevention** of helminthiasis is provision of sanitary facilities, such as flush toilets, to reduce the spread of eggs on common grounds. Educational programs that explain the **epidemiology** of the disease and ways to avoid its transmission are also essential. Widespread use of anthelmintics such as albendazole and mebendazole has been very effective in clearing a **population** of the causative agents of the disease, but without improved **sanitation** facilities, the disease is generally re-established in a relatively short period of time.

Treatment

Albendazole and mebendazole are also the drugs of choice for treatment of all forms of helminthiasis although, once more, such treatments are of only limited value if improvements in sanitation are not made in a community. Other forms of treatment are needed for secondary infections and other health problems that develop secondary to a helminth infection itself.

Prognosis

With early detection and treatment, prognosis for all forms of helminthiasis is good. As noted, the longer the condition goes untreated, or the greater the burden of the disease, the more serious the problem becomes and the more problematic the prognosis.

Resources

BOOKS

Cafrey, Conor R., ed. *Parasitic Helminths: Targets, Screens, Drugs, and Vaccines*. Berlin: Wiley-VCH Verlag, 2012.

Crompton, D. W. T., and Lorenzo Savioli. *Handbook of Helminthiasis for Public Health*. Boca Raton, FL: CRC/Taylor & Francis, 2007.

Helminth Control in School-age Children: A Guide for Managers of Control Programmes, 2nd ed. Geneva: World Health Organization, 2011.

PERIODICALS

Geary, T. G., et al. "A New Approach for Anthelmintic Discovery for Humans." *Trends in Parasitology* 28, 5. (2012): 176–81.

Minamoto, K., et al. "Short- and Long-term Impact of Health Education in Improving Water Supply, Sanitation and Knowledge about Intestinal Helminths in Rural Bangladesh." *Public Health* 126, 5. (2012): 437–40.

Piedrafita, P., and J. B. Matthews. "A Grand Scale Challenge: Vaccine Discovery for Helminth Control in Definitive Hosts." *Parasite Immunology* 34, 5. (2012): 241–2.

WEBSITES

"Common Helminthiasis" http://www.slideshare.net/kiran-chandranrox/helminthiasis#btnNext. Accessed on December 3, 2012.

"Helminthiasis." World Health Organization. http://www.who.int/topics/helminthiasis/en/. Accessed on December 3, 2012.

"Soil-Transmitted Helminthiasis." USAID Neglected Tropic Diseases. http://www.neglecteddiseases.gov/target_diseases/soil transmitted_helminthiasis/index.html. Accessed on December 3, 2012.

ORGANIZATIONS

World Health Organization (WHO), Avenue Appia 20, 1211 Geneva 27, Switzerland, +41 22 791 21 11, Fax: +41 22 791 31 11, http://www.who.int/about/contact_form/en/index.html, http://www.who.int/en/.

David E. Newton, Ed.D.

Hepatitis

Definition

Hepatitis is an inflammation of the liver caused by a virus, a toxic agent, or some other cause.

Description

Hepatitis is a medical condition characterized by loss of appetite, feelings of malaise, and a jaundiced appearance. It may occur as either an acute or a chronic condition. Acute hepatitis generally resolves spontaneously in less than six months, while chronic hepatitis extends for many years and may end in death. The disease is caused by a number of factors, most commonly a group of viruses known as the hepatitis viruses. The disease may also be caused by a variety of toxins, most commonly alcohol, by an autoimmune reaction in which the body's immune system attacks and destroys liver cells as if they were foreign bodies.

Causes and symptoms

Causes

The most common cause of hepatitis is one of five taxonomically unrelated viruses, known as the hepatitis A (HAV), hepatitis B (HBV), hepatitis C (HCV), hepatitis D (HDV), and hepatitis E (HEV) viruses. A number of other viruses have been suspected or hypothesized as causative agents, but confirmatory evidence for such hypotheses is as yet unavailable. One such virus, previously known as the hepatitis G virus, has recently been found not to be infective in humans and has been reclassified as GB virus C. Each of the five hepatitis viruses has its own genomic structure, method of transmission, incubation period, severity, duration, and other characteristics.

- Hepatitis A was previously known as infectious hepatitis because it is spread relatively easily from those infected to close household contacts. It has an acute, but not a chronic, stage. Even though people can take several weeks or months to recover completely from hepatitis A, they have lifelong immunity afterward. Complications from hepatitis A are rare and usually limited to people with chronic liver disease or those who have received a liver transplant.
- Hepatitis B was once known as serum hepatitis because the primary mode of transmission is blood. The disease has two forms: an acute form that lasts a few weeks, and a chronic form that can last for years, leading to cirrhosis, liver failure, liver cancer, and even death. Acute hepatitis B has a 5 percent chance of leading to the chronic form of the infection in adults. However, infants infected during the mother's pregnancy have a 90 percent chance of developing chronic hepatitis B, and children have a 25–50 percent chance.
- Hepatitis C is most commonly transmitted from person to person through contaminated blood. It is sometimes called non-A non-B hepatitis. Hepatitis C is an infection that often goes undetected until it has done significant damage to a patient's liver. The infection is divided into two phases, an acute phase (the first six months) and a chronic phase (after the first six months). A minority of patients clear the virus from their bodies during the acute phase, but 60–85 percent have a chronic HCV infection.
- Hepatitis D infections occur at the same time as hepatitis B develops or subsequent to infection by HBV's entering the chronic stage. The HDV virus is a small and incomplete viral particle. Perhaps this is the reason it cannot cause infection on its own. Its companion virus, HBV, actually forms a covering over the HDV particle. In chronically ill patients, the combined viruses cause inflammation throughout the liver and eventually destroy the liver cells, which are then replaced by scar tissue. This scarring is called cirrhosis. When HBV and HDV infections develop at the same time, a condition called coinfection, recovery is the rule. Only 2–5 percent of patients become chronic carriers. It may be that HDV actually keeps HBV from reproducing as rapidly as it would if it were alone, so chronic infection is less likely.
- Hepatitis E is transmitted via the intestinal tract, most often by contaminated drinking water. It is also known as epidemic non-A, non-B hepatitis. There are at least two strains of HEV, one found in Asia and another in Mexico. The virus may start dividing in the gastrointestinal tract, but it grows mostly in the liver. After an incubation period of two to eight weeks, infected persons develop a fever, may feel nauseous, lose their appetite, and often have discomfort or actual pain in the right upper part of the abdomen where the liver is located. Some develop jaundice. Most often the illness is mild and disappears within a few weeks with no lasting effects. Children younger than 14 years and persons over age 50 seldom have jaundice or show other clinical signs of hepatitis. On rare occasions the acute illness damages and destroys so many liver cells that the liver can no longer function. This condition is called fulminant liver failure and may cause death. Pregnant women are at much higher risk of dying from fulminant liver failure; this increased risk is not true of any other type of viral hepatitis. The great majority of patients who recover from acute infection do not continue to carry HEV and cannot pass on the infection to others.

Symptoms

Since all forms of hepatitis involve damage to the liver, symptoms are generally similar in all five types of infection. The first symptoms to appear are usually fatigue and general achiness. Those who like to drink coffee or smoke cigarettes may lose their taste for these products. The liver often enlarges, causing **pain** or tenderness in the right upper part of the abdomen. Other common symptoms of the disease include:

- low-grade fever (101°F)
- nausea, vomiting, and diarrhea
- loss of appetite and weight loss

- swelling of the liver and pain in the area of the abdomen over the liver
- tea- or coffee-colored urine
- jaundice
- an itchy rash or a generalized sensation of itching
- pale or clay-colored stools
- muscle pains

Many individuals with hepatitis may be asymptomatic. For example, as many as three out of four children have no symptoms of HAV infection, although about 85% of adults will have symptoms. Less than half of those infected with HBV show any symptoms at all and do not know they have the disease unless or until it is discovered during routine blood tests conducted for other purposes. The majority of individuals infected with HCV also have no symptoms. The absence of symptoms for a hepatitis infection do not, however, mean that a person cannot transmit the disease to others, either through blood products or through contact with urine, feces, and other bodily materials.

Demographics

The demographics for each form of hepatitis differ from each other. Hepatitis A is much more common in Africa, Asia, and South America than in the United States. The rates of hepatitis A in North America have been steadily dropping since the 1980s due to improvements in public health policies and sanitation; on the other hand, the rates of hepatitis A among frequent travelers have been rising during the same time period. In 1988 the Centers for Disease Control (now the Centers for Disease Control and Prevention; CDC) reported 32,000 cases in the United States; in 2003, 7,653 cases were reported. In 2010, the total number of cases of hepatitis A reported in the United States was 1,670. This number may not be an accurate representation of the actual number of hepatitis A cases, however, because many people do not show symptoms of the disease. In developing countries, children below the age of 2 account for most new cases of hepatitis A; in the United States, the age group most often affected is children between the ages of 5 and 14. Males and females are equally likely to get hepatitis A, as are people from all races and ethnic groups in the United States.

According to the most recent data available, there are about 2.2 million people in the United States living with chronic hepatitis B infection. The majority of these individuals (1.04–1.61 million) were born in foreign countries and did not, therefore, have access to childhood vaccinations against the disease that most native-born American receive. Hepatitis B causes about 5,000 deaths annually in the United States. In the rest of the world, as many as a third of the population (2 billion people) are chronic carriers of the disease. Chronic hepatitis B affects approximately 400 million people around the world as of 2012 and contributes to an estimated 1 million deaths worldwide each year. The age group most commonly affected by hepatitis B in the United States is adults between the ages of 20 and 50. The routine immunization of children against the disease since 1990 has led to a decline in the rate of acute hepatitis in North America for the past two decades. African Americans are more likely to be infected than either Hispanics or Caucasians; however, Alaskan Eskimos and Pacific Islanders have higher rates of carrier status than members of other racial groups. Asian Americans are at increased risk of severe liver damage from hepatitis B compared to members of other racial groups. More males than females are infected with hepatitis B in all races and age groups.

Hepatitis C is the major source of chronic liver infection in North America. It accounts for about 15 percent of cases of acute viral hepatitis, 60 to 70 percent of cases of chronic hepatitis, and up to 50 percent of cases of cirrhosis, end-stage liver disease, and liver cancer. There are approximately 20,000–30,000 new infections and 8,000–10,000 deaths from hepatitis C each year in the United States. It is estimated that 4 million persons in the United States have been infected by the virus and 3.2 million of these have the chronic form of the infection as of 2009. HCV infection presently accounts for 40 percent of referrals to liver clinics. The cost of treating hepatitis C in the United States is estimated to be more than $600 million a year. Hepatitis C is more common among Hispanics and African Americans than among Caucasians, Asian Americans, or Native Americans. In terms of age groups, 65 percent of persons with HCV infection are between the ages of 30 and 49 years. According to the CDC, the rates of hepatitis C infection are highest among people born between 1945 and 1965. Most of these persons were likely infected during the 1970s and 1980s, when rates of hepatitis C in North America were at their peak. The World Health Organization (WHO) estimates that 170 million individuals worldwide are infected with the hepatitis C virus. The rates vary considerably from country to country, however, from 0.02% of the population in the United Kingdom to 6.5% in Africa to 22% in Egypt.

As noted previously, hepatitis D affects only individuals who have also been infected with the hepatitis B virus. WHO estimates that about 5 percent of all HBV carriers in the world are also infected with HDV. The disease occurs most commonly in the Mediterranean Basin, the Middle East, Central Asia,

West Africa, the Amazon Basin of South America and certain South Pacific islands. The disease is most serious among indigenous people of Venezuela, Colombia, Brazil, and Peru, where both acute and chronic forms of the infection may be responsible for death. HDV infections in the United States are rare.

WHO estimates that there are about 20 million cases of hepatitis E infection worldwide at any one time, of which about 15 percent are acute cases. The disease is thought to be responsible for about 70,000 deaths a year, primarily in East and South Asia. The disease occurs most commonly in regions with poor sanitation, such as Egypt, where an estimated half of the adult population has been found to be positive for HEV antibodies. The disease is rare in the United States, with only about a dozen cases reported to the CDC each year. Most such cases occur among travelers who have visited foreign countries with poor sanitation systems.

Risk factors

Some people are at increased risk of contracting hepatitis, including:

- people who travel to parts of the world with high rates of the disease and poor sanitation, including the Middle East, South America, Eastern Europe, Mexico and Central America, Africa, Southeast Asia, and the Caribbean.
- male homosexuals.
- people who use illicit drugs, whether injected or taken by mouth.
- medical researchers and laboratory workers who may be exposed to HAV.
- child care workers and children in day care centers. Children at day care centers make up an estimated 14–40% of all cases of hepatitis infection in the United States. Changing diapers transmits infection through fecal-oral contact. Toys and other objects may remain contaminated for some time. Often a child without symptoms brings the infection home to siblings and parents.
- troops living under crowded conditions at military camps or in the field.
- homeless people.
- healthcare workers who routinely come into contact with blood products.

Costs to Society

The cost of all forms of hepatitis infection to societies can be substantial. In the United States, for example, the total costs for all aspects of hepatitis A infections in the United States (treatment, morbidity and mortality) in the late 1990s was estimated at $488 million annually. The availability of a vaccine against the disease since that time has dramatically reduced those costs as the number of new cases annually has decreased to fewer than 2,000 per year. However, in nations where the vaccine is not available or is too costly for widespread use, hepatitis A infections remain a substantial part of national health costs. Comparable estimates for the total financial burden for hepatitis B in the United States in 2008 was more than $1 billion, and a study of the financial costs of hepatitis C found that the disease more than doubled the cost of care of patients with the disease compared to those without the disease.

Diagnosis

The diagnosis of hepatitis can often be made only a short time after exposure to the disease, or it can be delayed for months or even years if a person is asymptomatic. The diagnostic procedure tends to be relatively similar for all forms of the disease and involves results of the patient's medical history, findings during an office examination, and a blood test for the disease.

Examination

The doctor may suspect that a patient has hepatitis during a physical examination in the office by feeling the area over the liver for signs of swelling and pain; taking the patient's temperature; and checking the skin and eyes for signs of jaundice.

Tests

A definite diagnosis is provided by a blood test for antibodies to one or another of the hepatitis viruses. For each virus, there is a specific antibody that develops when the virus is present in the body. This test always registers positive when a patient has symptoms and should continue to register positive for four to six months. In some cases the doctor may also have the sample of blood checked for abnormally high levels of liver enzymes.

Treatment

Treatments for the various forms of hepatitis vary somewhat.

There is no specific drug treatment for hepatitis A, as antibiotics cannot be used to treat virus infections. Most people can care for themselves at home by making sure they get plenty of fluids and adequate nutrition. People whose appetite has been affected may benefit from eating small snacks throughout the day rather than three main meals and by eating soft and easily digested foods. Patients with hepatitis A should avoid drinking alcohol, which makes it harder for the liver to recover from inflammation. Patients should also tell their doctor about any over-the-counter or prescription drugs they are taking because the drugs may need to be stopped temporarily or have the dosages changed. Patients may also take acetaminophen to reduce fever and relieve pain. Patients with mild nausea and vomiting may be prescribed antiemetics (drugs to control nausea); the drug most commonly prescribed for hepatitis patients is metoclopramide (Reglan). Those with severe vomiting may need to be hospitalized in order to receive intravenous fluids.

There are few treatment options for chronic hepatitis B. If the patient has no symptoms and little sign of liver damage, the doctor may suggest monitoring the levels of HBV in the patient's blood periodically rather than starting drug treatment right away. If the patient develops fulminant hepatitis B or the liver is otherwise severely damaged by HBV, the only option is a liver transplant. This is a serious operation with a lengthy recovery period; its success also depends on finding a suitable donor liver. Patients who know that they have been exposed to the hepatitis B virus can be treated by administering three shots of the HBV vaccine to prevent them from developing an active infection. Those who have already developed symptoms of the acute form of the disease may be given intravenous fluids to prevent dehydration or antinausea medications to stop vomiting. There is no medication as of late 2012 that can prevent acute hepatitis B from becoming chronic once the symptoms begin. There are seven different drugs approved in the United States to treat chronic hepatitis B in adults as of 2012, but they do not work in all patients and may produce severe side effects. These drugs include adefovir dipivoxil (Hepsera), alpha interferon (Intron A), pegylated interferon (Pegasys), entecavir (Baraclude), telbivudine (Telzeka), tenofovir (Viread), and lamivudine (Zeffix or Epivir-HBV). The two interferons are given by injection; the other five drugs are taken by mouth in pill form once a day. Most doctors will wait until the patient's liver function begins to worsen before administering these drugs. The drugs do not cure the infection; they lower the patient's risk of severe liver damage by slowing or preventing the hepatitis B virus from reproducing further.

The only drugs approved as of 2012 for treating chronic hepatitis B in children are alpha interferon (Intron A) and lamivudine (Zeffix or Epivir-HBV).

The first line of treatment in hepatitis C is two medications known as Intron A, a drug that resembles the antibodies that the body makes naturally to fight viruses; and Virazole, which is an antiviral drug. The combination of these drugs works better than Intron A alone. Combination therapy with these drugs is not recommended for patients who have already developed cirrhosis due to hepatitis C, or for patients who have received kidney, liver, or heart transplants. Other patients who should not be given these drugs include those with lupus or other autoimmune diseases, severe psychiatric disorders, coronary artery disease, inability to practice birth control, and active alcohol or substance abuse. There are few treatment options for patients who do not respond to drug therapy or have a relapse. The only treatment for cirrhosis or severe liver disease as of 2012 is liver transplantation. Chronic HCV infection, in fact, is the leading indication for liver transplants in the United States. The problem, however, is that there are many more patients waiting for donated livers than there are suitable organs available. In addition, liver transplantation does not cure HCV infection; most people who receive transplanted livers will develop a recurrence of the virus. About 30% of recipients die, develop cirrhosis, or have the transplanted liver fail within five years of surgery, with the rate of failure increasing with each year of follow-up.

As in any form of hepatitis, patients in the acute stage of HDV and HEV infection should rest in bed as needed, eat a balanced diet, and avoid alcohol. Alpha-interferon, the natural body substance which helps control hepatitis C, has generally not been found helpful in treating hepatitis D or hepatitis E. If the liver is largely destroyed and has stopped functioning, liver transplantation is an option. Even when the procedure is successful, the disease often recurs and cirrhosis may actually develop more rapidly than before.

Prevention

A single vaccine is now available for both hepatitis A and hepatitis B. It is called Twinrix because it is a combination of the two vaccines previously used independently for the two diseases, Havrix and Energix-B. The vaccine is administered shortly after birth and at ages one and six months, although alternative schedules are also available for special circumstances. The vaccine provides immunity approaching 99.9 percent against both forms of hepatitis shortly after administration and lasting as long as 20 years or more. No vaccine is currently available for hepatitis C, D, or E. Everyone can reduce their risk of all forms of hepatitis by observing the following precautions:

- Practice good personal hygiene; wash hands frequently, especially after using the toilet or changing a child's diaper.

- When traveling, drink only bottled water; avoid raw or undercooked meat or shellfish; and avoid eating fresh fruits or vegetables unless you have washed and peeled them yourself.
- Avoid sharing drinking glasses and eating utensils. If someone in the family has hepatitis A, wash their glasses and utensils separately in hot, soapy water.
- Avoid sexual contact with anyone who has hepatitis A.
- Practice safer sex.
- Do not share needles, razors, toothbrushes, or any other personal item that might have blood on it.
- Avoid getting a tattoo or body piercing, as some people who perform these procedures do not sterilize their needles and other equipment properly.
- Get tested for hepatitis infection if pregnant, as the virus can be transmitted from a mother to her unborn baby.
- Consult a doctor before taking an extended trip to any country with high rates of hepatitis.
- Carefully disinfect any bloodstained surface or material with a mixture of chlorine bleach and water

Prognosis

Prognosis differs for various forms of hepatitis. Most people recover fully from hepatitis A within a few weeks or months. Between 3 and 20% have relapses for as long as six to nine months after infection. In the United States, serious complications are infrequent and deaths are very rare. As many as 75% of adults over 50 years of age in North America will have blood test evidence of previous hepatitis A infection. About one percent of patients develop liver failure following HAV infection, mostly those over 60 or those with chronic liver disease. In these cases liver transplantation may be necessary for the patient's survival. There are about 100 deaths from hepatitis A reported each year in the United States.

Each year an estimated 150,000 persons in the United States get hepatitis B. More than 10,000 will require hospital care, and as many as 5,000 will eventually die from complications of the infection. About 90% of all those infected will have acute disease only. It is the remaining 10% with chronic infection who account for most serious complications and deaths from HBV infection. Even when no symptoms of liver disease develop, chronic carriers remain a threat to others by serving as a source of infection. Patients with acute hepatitis B usually recover; the symptoms go away in 2–3 weeks, and the liver itself returns to normal in about 4 months. Other patients have a longer period of illness with very slow improvement. The course of chronic HBV infection in any particular patient is unpredictable. Some patients who do well at first may later develop serious complications. Chronic hepatitis leads to an increased risk of cirrhosis and liver cancer, and eventual death in about 1 percent of cases.

The prognosis for hepatitis C is guarded for most patients. The antiviral drugs presently used to treat the infection cure only about 60% of patients. According to the CDC, between 75 and 85 percent of people infected with HCV will develop chronic HCV infection, and 60–70 percent will develop some form of chronic liver disease. Twenty percent of these chronically infected persons will develop cirrhosis of the liver within 20 years of infection; 1–5 percent of chronically infected people will eventually die of liver disease. Women with chronic hepatitis C have better outcomes than men, and patients infected at younger ages have better outcomes than those infected in middle age. The reason for these differences is not clear as of 2012. A small percentage of patients with hepatitis C develop medical conditions that are not related to the liver. It is thought that these conditions result from the body's immune response to the HCV virus. These conditions include diabetes mellitus; skin rashes; inflammation of the kidney glomerulonephritis; non-Hodgkin lymphoma; and essential mixed cryoglobulinemia, a condition marked by the presence of abnormal proteins in the blood.

A large majority of patients with coinfection of HBV and HDV recover from an episode of acute hepatitis. However, about two-thirds of patients chronically infected by HDV go on to develop cirrhosis of the liver. In one long-term study, just over half of patients who became carriers of HDV had moderate or severe liver disease, and one-fourth of them died. If severe liver failure develops, the patient has a 50% chance of surviving. A liver transplant may improve this figure to 70%. When transplantation is done for cirrhosis, rather than for liver failure, nearly 90% of patients live five years or longer. The major concern with transplantation is infection of the transplanted liver; this may occur in as many as 40% of transplant patients.

In the United States hepatitis E is not a fatal illness, but elsewhere about 1–2% of those infected die of advanced liver failure. In pregnant women the death rate is as high as 20%. It is not clear whether having hepatitis E once guarantees against future HEV infection.

Alcoholic hepatitis

Alcoholic hepatitis is an inflammation of the liver caused by alcohol. Whether it comes from toxins or infections, inflammation causes a similar response in body organs. The response consists of:

- an increase in the blood to the affected organ
- redness and swelling of the organ

- influx of immune agents like white blood cells and their arsenal of chemical weapons
- pain

As the acute process subsides, there is either healing or lingering activity. Lingering activity—chronic disease—has a milder presentation with similar ingredients. Healing often takes the form of scarring, wherein normal functioning tissue is replaced by tough, fibrous, and non-productive scar. Both chronic disease and healing can happen simultaneously, so that scar tissue progressively replaces normal tissue. This leads to cirrhosis, a liver so scarred it is unable to do its job adequately. Alcohol can cause either an acute or a chronic disease in the liver. The acute disease can be severe, even fatal, and can bring with it hemolysis–blood cell destruction. Alcohol can also cause a third type of liver disease, fatty liver, in which the continuous action of alcohol turns the liver to useless fat. This condition eventually progresses to cirrhosis if the **poisoning** continues.

Inflammation of the liver can be caused by a great variety of agents—poisons, drugs, viruses, bacteria, protozoa, and even larger organisms like worms. Alcohol is a poison if taken in more than modest amounts. It favors destroying stomach lining, liver, heart muscle, and brain tissue. The liver is a primary target because alcohol travels to the liver after leaving the intestines. Those who drink enough to get alcohol poisoning have a tendency to be undernourished, since alcohol provides ample calories but little **nutrition**. It is suspected that both the alcohol and the poor nutrition produce alcoholic hepatitis.

Hepatitis of all kinds causes notable discomfort, loss of appetite, nausea, pain in the liver, and usually jaundice. Blood test abnormalities are unmistakably those of hepatitis, but selecting from so many the precise cause may take additional diagnostic work.

As with all poisonings, removal of the offending agent is primary. There is no specific treatment for alcohol poisoning. General supportive measures must see the patient through until the liver has healed by itself. In the case of fulminant (sudden and severe) disease, the liver may be completely destroyed and have to be replaced by a transplant.

Autoimmune hepatitis

Autoimmune hepatitis is a form of liver inflammation in which the body's immune system attacks liver cells. It is similiar in many ways to viral hepatitis. It can be an acute disease that kills over a third of its victims within six months, can persist for years, or can return periodically. Some patients develop cirrhosis of the liver which, over time, causes the liver to cease functioning.

QUESTIONS TO ASK YOUR DOCTOR

- How did I contract hepatitis?
- What steps can I take to avoid spreading the infection to others?
- Should I continue working and maintaining my daily routines around the house?
- Should my spouse and children be vaccinated against hepatitis?
- What community resources are available for learning more about hepatitis infection?

Symptoms of autoimmune hepatitis resemble those of other types of hepatitis. Patients who develop autoimmune hepatitis experience pain under the right ribs, fatigue and general discomfort, loss of appetite, nausea, and sometimes vomiting and jaundice. In addition, other parts of the body may be involved and contribute their own symptoms.

Extensive laboratory testing may be required to differentiate this disease from viral hepatitis. The distinction may not even be made during the initial episode. There are certain markers of autoimmune disease in the blood that can lead to the correct diagnosis if they are sought. In advanced or chronic cases a liver biopsy may be necessary.

Autoimmune hepatitis is among the few types of hepatitis that can be treated effectively. Since treatment itself introduces problems in at least 20% of patients, it is reserved for the more severe cases. Up to 80% of patients improve with cortisone treatment, although a cure is unlikely. Another drug—azathioprine—is sometimes used concurrently. Treatment continues for over a year and may be restarted during a relapse. At least half the patients relapse at some point, and most will still continue to have progressive liver scarring. If the liver fails, transplant is the only recourse.

In spite of treatment, autoimmune hepatitis can re-erupt at any time and may continue to damage and scar the liver. The rate of progression varies considerably from patient to patient.

Resources

BOOKS

Dworkin, Mark S. *Outbreak Investigations around the World: Case Studies in Infectious Disease Field Epidemiology.* Sudbury, MA: Jones and Bartlett, Publishers, 2010.

KEY TERMS

Antibody—A substance made by the body in response to a foreign body, such as a virus, which is able to attack and destroy the invading virus.

Antiemetic—A type of drug given to control nausea and vomiting.

Bile—A yellow-green fluid secreted by the liver that aids in the digestion of fats.

Carrier—A person who is infected with a virus or other disease organism but does not develop the symptoms of the disease.

Chronic—Long-term or recurrent.

Cirrhosis—Disruption of normal liver function by the formation of scar tissue and nodules in the liver.

Coinfection—Invasion of the body by two viruses at about the same time.

Contamination—The process by which an object or body part becomes exposed to an infectious agent such as a virus.

Epidemic—A situation where a large number of infections by a particular agent, such as a virus, develops in a short time. The agent is rapidly transmitted to many individuals.

Fulminant—Referring to a disease that comes on suddenly with great severity.

Hepatitis—The medical term for inflammation of the liver. It can be caused by toxic substances or alcohol as well as infections.

Immune globulin—A preparation of antibodies that can be given before exposure for short-term protection against hepatitis A and for persons who have already been exposed to hepatitis A virus. Immune globulin must be given within two weeks after exposure to hepatitis A virus for maximum protection.

Incubation period—The interval from initial exposure to an infectious agent, such as a virus, and the first symptoms of illness.

Jaundice—A yellowish discoloration of the skin and whites of the eyes caused by increased levels of bile pigments from the liver in the patient's blood.

Pathogen—Any biological agent that causes illness or disease in its host. A pathogen may be a virus, bacterium, fungus, or prion.

Relapse—A temporary recurrence of the symptoms of a disease.

Vaccine—A substance prepared from a weakened or killed microorganism which, when injected, helps the body to form antibodies that will prevent infection by the natural microorganism.

Feigin, Ralph D., et al, eds. *Feigin and Cherry's Textbook of Pediatric Infectious Diseases*, 6th ed. Philadelphia, PA: Saunders/Elsevier, 2009.

Koff, Raymond S. *Hepatitis Essentials*. Sudbury, MA: Jones and Bartlett Leaning, 2011.

Richman, Douglas D., Richard J. Whitley, and Frederick G. Hayden, eds. *Clinical Virology*, 3rd ed. Washington, DC: ASM Press, 2009.

Younossi, Zobair M., ed. *Practical Management of Liver Diseases*. New York: Cambridge University Press, 2008.

PERIODICALS

Borgia, G., et al. "Hepatitis B in Pregnancy." *World Journal of Gastroenterology* 18, 34. (2012): 4677–83.

Choi, G., and B. A. Runyon. "Alcoholic Hepatitis: A Clinician's Guide." *Clinics in Liver Disease* 16, 2. (2012): 371–85.

Czaja, A. J. "Autoimmune Hepatitis: Focusing on Treatments other than Steroids." *Canadian Journal of Gastroenterology* 26, 9. (2012): 615–20.

Kamar, N., et al. "Hepatitis E." *Lancet* 379, 9835. (201): 2477–88.

Mackinney-Novelo, I., et al. "Clinical Course and Management of Acute Hepatitis A Infection in Adults." *Annals of Hepatology* 11, 5. (2012): 652–57.

Miller, L., et al. "Improving Access to Hepatitis C Care for Urban, Underserved Patients using a Primary Care-based Hepatitis C Clinic." *Journal of the National Medical Association* 104, 5-6. (2012): 244–50.

"WHO Position Paper on Hepatitis A Vaccines." *Weekly Epidemiological Record* 87, 28/29 (2012): 261–76.

WEBSITES

"Hepatitis." National Digestive Diseases Information Clearinghouse. http://digestive.niddk.nih.gov/ddiseases/pubs/hepatitis/index.aspx. Accessed on September 28, 2012.

"Hepatitis." PubMed Health. http://www.ncbi.nlm.nih.gov/pubmedhealth/PMH0002139/. Accessed on September 28, 2012.

"Hepatitis. World Health Organization."http://www.who.int/topics/hepatitis/en/. Accessed on September 28, 2012.

"Viral Hepatitis. Centers for Disease Control and Prevention." http://www.cdc.gov/hepatitis/. Accessed on September 28, 2012.

ORGANIZATIONS

American College of Gastroenterology (ACG), 6400 Goldsboro Rd., Suite 200, Bethesda, MD 20817, (301) 263-9000, info@acg.gi.org, http://www.acg.gi.org/

American Liver Foundation (ALF), 39 Broadway, Suite 2700, New York, NY 10006, (212) 668-1000, Fax: (212) 483-8179, http://www.liverfoundation.org/contact/, http://www.liverfoundation.org/

Centers for Disease Control and Prevention (CDC), 1600 Clifton Rd., Atlanta, GA 30333, (800) 232-4636 cdcinfo@cdc.gov, http://www.cdc.gov

National Institute of Allergy and Infectious Diseases (NIAID), 6610 Rockledge Dr., MSC 6612, Bethesda, MD 20892-6612, (301) 496-5717, (866) 284-4107, Fax: (301) 402-3573, ocpostoffice@niaid.nih.gov, http://www3.niaid.nih.gov

World Health Organization (WHO), Avenue Appia 20, 1211 Geneva 27, Switzerland, +41 22 791 21 11, Fax: +41 22 791 31 11, info@who.int, http://www.who.int/en/.

David E. Newton, Ed.D.

Herpes

Definition

Herpes viruses fall within the family Herpesviridae. This family includes the herpes simplex viruses: herpes simplex virus type 1 (HSV-1) and herpes simplex virus type 2 (HSV-2). These two viruses cause blister-like open sores, usually on the mouth (HSV-1) or genitals (HSV-2) of the infected person.

Description

HSV-2, or genital herpes, is a sexually transmitted disease (STD) and usually is associated with genital ulcers or sores. HSV-1, which is transmitted from person to person by close contact such as kissing or sharing eating utensils; usually is associated with infections of the lips, mouth, and face; and its sores are referred to as "oral herpes," "cold sores," or "fever blisters." HSV-1 can also cause genital herpes, but HSV-2 is the main cause of genital herpes. Other herpes viruses that infect humans include:

- Human herpes virus 3 (HHV-3), also known as herpes zoster virus or varicella zoster virus, is the cause of chickenpox. This virus lies dormant in the body, and in some cases may reactivate later in life, causing shingles (herpes-zoster), which results in a painful rash, and in some cases, continuing nerve pain (postherpatic neuralgia), temporary partial facial paralysis, or other problems.
- Human herpes virus 4 (HHV-4), also known as "Epstein Barr virus," causes infectious monoucleosis, or "mono" (sometimes known as "the kissing disease"). It is also associated with Hodgkin's lymphoma and specific other cancers.
- Human herpes virus 5 (HHV-5) is also known as "cytomegalovirus." Most people have no symptoms from infection with this virus, but birth defects can occur in infants born to women who have primary (first) infections with cytomegalovirus during pregnancy. In addition, individuals who are immunocompromised can develop infection-related illness.
- Human herpes virus 6 (HHV-6) is actually a set of two viruses, HHV-6A and HHV-6B. Infection with HHV-6B can cause roseola (exanthem subitum rash) as well as fever and diarrhea in infants. Although rare, some infants experience seizures and/or encephalitis. If reactivated later in life, the virus can cause symptoms, which occasionally include infection of the brain, leading to cognitive dysfunction and even death.
- Human herpes virus 7 (HHV-7) is similar to HHV-6, although it causes roseola less frequently.
- Human herpes virus 8 (HHV-8), also known as "Kaposi's sarcoma-associated herpes virus (KSHV)," because it causes Kaposi's sarcoma, a type of cancer that commonly occurs in patients who have acquired immunodeficiency syndrome (AIDS).

Demographics

Herpes viruses are prevalent worldwide. As of 2010 in the United States, 16.2% of people aged 14–49 years had genital HSV-2 infection, according to the **Centers for Disease Control and Prevention**. The virus moves from an infected male to a female partner more easily than from an infected female to a male partner. It is therefore more common among women (about 20% of the population aged 14–49) than among men (about 11% of the population aged 14–49). Among African Americans, as of 2010, the prevalence was higher with 39.2% of the population experiencing HSV-2. Among African-American women, the prevalence of HSV-2 is 48%.

Exposure to other herpes viruses is even more common. Estimates of the infection rate for HSV-1 are as high as 90%. HHV-6 is similarly a nearly universal infection. It is responsible for up to 20% of all fever-associated, infant visits to U.S. emergency rooms. Between 50% and 80% of adults in the United States have had a CMV infection by age 40. About 90% of all Americans have been exposed to the chickenpox virus by the time they are 15 years old. Those who have had the chickenpox vaccine may have no or only mild symptoms.

Causes and symptoms

Causes

The herpes viruses are spread in many ways. HSV-1 is transmitted by close contact, including kissing. HSV-2 is sexually transmitted, and risk factors for HSV-2 infection include having many sexual partners and unprotected sex. HSV-2 can also be transmitted by oral sex and cause sores on the lips. People acquire HHV-3, the chickenpox virus, infections through direct contact with broken chickenpox blisters on an infected individual, through contact with a recently contaminated item (such as a ball that an infected person was handling), and through airborne droplets expelled via coughing or sneezing. Some herpes viruses may also be transmitted from a mother to her unborn child.

Symptoms

Symptoms vary among the different types of herpes. HSV-1 and HSV-2 cause sores on mucous membranes, most often in the mouth and in the genital region. Once HSV-1 and HSV-2 enter the body, they spread to nearby mucosal areas through nerve cells. Typically, 50–80% of people with oral herpes experience a prodrome (symptoms of oncoming disease) of **pain**, burning, itching, or tingling at the site where blisters will form. This prodrome stage may last anywhere from a few hours to one or two days. The herpes infection prodrome occurs in both the primary infection and recurrent infections.

Symptoms of the primary infection of HSV-1 and HAV-2 usually are more severe than those of recurrent infections. The primary infection can cause symptoms similar to those experienced in other viral infections, including lack of energy, headache, fever, and swollen lymph nodes in the neck. The first sign of infection is formation of fluid-filled blisters that may last up to two weeks. However, the pain in the area may last much longer.

Once an individual becomes infected with HSV-1 or HSV-2, the virus remains in the body for the life of that individual. (This is true of other herpes viruses, too.) During periods of latency, the patient has no symptoms. At times, the infected person may shed the virus into their saliva and genital secretions and infect others. Shedding can occur even in the absence of visible symptoms. Individuals infected with the virus can have recurrent infections or flare-ups; however, recurrent infections usually have milder and shorter symptoms. Nevertheless, **cancer** patients and others with compromised immune systems can have severe recurrences and serious complications.

Women who develop a primary HSV-2 infection during pregnancy are at greater risk of delivering babies with **birth defects**. An active genital herpes sore at the time of birth can cause extremely serious results for the baby. These include blindness, birth defects, and even death in the baby. Cesarean section may be advisable for mothers with active herpes sores at the time of delivery.

KEY TERMS

Reye's syndrome—A rare, but often fatal, disease that involves the brain, liver, and kidneys. It may brought on by giving salicylates to children (but not adults) who have a viral infection.

Roseola—A viral infection that typically affects infants and young children. Its common symptoms include a skin rash and fever.

Shingles—Also known as "herpes zoster,"it is a viral infection that causes a painful rash. The virus that causes shingles also causes chickenpox.

Diagnosis

Often, infection with HSV-1 or HSV-2 is diagnosed from the patient's description of symptoms and by visual examination of the sores. If uncertainty remains about the cause of a sore, a tissue sample or culture can be taken to determine what type of virus or other microorganism is responsible. For herpes, it is preferable to have this test done within the first 48 hours after symptoms first appear, for a more accurate result.

Testing for neonatal HSV infections may include special smears and/or viral cultures, blood antibody levels, and polymerase chain reaction (PCR) testing of spinal fluid. Cultures are usually obtained from skin vesicles, eyes, mouth, rectum, urine, stool, and blood.

Treatment

There is no cure for HSV infection. Usually, the sores clear without treatment. Until they do, it is important to keep the blisters or sores clean and dry with an agent such as cornstarch. One should avoid touching the sores, and wash hands frequently. Local application of ice may relieve the pain. Over-the-counter medication for fever, pain, and inflammation, such as aspirin, acetaminophen, or ibuprofen, may help. Children should never be given aspirin, because of the possible development of Reye's syndrome.

During an outbreak of HSV cold sores, that patient should avoid salty foods, citrus foods (e.g., oranges), and other foods that irritate the sores. Over-the-counter lip products that contain the chemical "phenol" (such as many medicated lip ointments) and numbing agents (such as the ointment Anbesol) help to relieve the pain of cold sores. A bandage may be placed over the sores to protect them and to prevent spreading the virus to other sites on the lips or face.

Sexual intercourse should be avoided during both the HSV active and prodrome stages.

Drugs

Antiviral drugs have some effect in lessening the symptoms of HSV infection, decreasing the length of herpes outbreaks, and preventing complications in immunocompromised individuals. For the best results, drug treatment should begin during the prodrome stage before blisters are visible. Depending upon the length of the outbreak, drug treatment could continue up to 10 days. Antiviral medications include acyclovir (Zovirax), famciclovir (Famvir), and valacyclovir (Valtrex). All are administered in pill form. For severe cases, acyclovir may also be administered intravenously. Acyclovir, a commonly prescribed medication, is effective in treating both the primary infection and recurrent outbreaks and can reduce the frequency of herpes outbreaks.

Prognosis

Infection with HSV is permanent. Although symptom-free periods are common, during these times individuals may still shed the virus and infect others. Life-threatening neurological complications may occur in individuals who are immunocompromised, and HSV-2 infection during pregnancy and delivery can cause birth defects or serious harm to the infant.

Prevention

It is almost impossible to prevent HSV-1 infection. Limiting the number of sexual partners reduces the likelihood of becoming with HSV-2. Using a condom may help discourage infection but does not fully protect against spread of the virus.

Effects on public health

Genital herpes, in particular, is a public health concern because it is one of the most prevalent **sexually transmitted diseases** in the United States. In addition, many people who have the disease fail to recognize that their symptoms are related to genital herpes, and therefore continue their normal sexual behavior, which can transmit it to their partners. Even those who have the disease and are vigilant about avoiding sexual relations while they have outbreaks, however, may spread the virus to their partners. Genital herpes is especially common in some populations (almost 40% of African Americans overall, and almost 50% of African-American women are infected with HSV-2). Such a high incidence of this disease hampers its containment.

Costs to society

The United States' annual direct medical costs for genital herpes has been estimated as high as $984 million, with nearly half going to drug expenditures, and another 48% to outpatient medical care. Lost productivity due mainly to days off for sickness or time spent for treatment accounted for a further $214 million. A single case of neonatal herpes was estimated to result in $60,000 in medical costs.

QUESTIONS TO ASK YOUR DOCTOR

- How do I know whether I have HSV-1 or HSV-2?
- How will HSV infection affect my sex life?
- What can I do to help prevent spreading HSV-1 to family members?
- What are the possible serious complications of this infection, and when should I call the doctor?

Efforts and solutions

A vaccine for HSV-1, and especially for HSV-2, would help to stem the incidence of genital herpes. Work on that front is continuing. Hopes were high for an investigational HSV-2 vaccine, but a research article in a 2012 issue of the *New England Journal of Medicine* found that while the vaccine was effective in preventing HSV-1 genital disease and infection, it was ineffective against HSV-2, which causes most genital herpes.

A study that appeared in a 2012 issue of *The Lancet* demonstrated that the frequency of HSV-2 shedding was reduced in individuals who used acyclovir, compared to those who used no medication. It also showed an advantage for high doses of antiviral drugs: High-dose acyclovir and high-dose valaciclovir each resulted in less-frequent shedding than standard doses of the medications. Nonetheless, shedding occurred even with high doses of the drugs, and transmission of the virus between sexual partners still occurred, although at a lower rate. The authors concluded, "Short bursts of subclinical genital HSV reactivation are frequent, even during high-dose antiherpes therapy, and probably account for continued transmission of HSV during suppressive antiviral therapy. More potent antiviral therapy is needed to eliminate HSV transmission."

Another intriguing avenue of research involves Alzheimer's disease, which affects about 20 million people worldwide. Researchers have uncovered a potential link between HSV-1 infection and an increased risk for Alzheimer's disease, especially in individuals who have a specific genetic factor. Additional studies on the possible connection are under way. One study, published in 2011 by researchers in the United Kingdom, considered the possibility that antiviral agents against HSV1 might slow the progression of Alzheimer's disease, and found evidence that it might do just that. Their findings suggested that the antiviral agents significantly reduced the levels of proteins associated with Alzheimer's disease, and could therefore be a potential treatment vector.

Resources

PERIODICALS

Belshe, Robert B., et al. "Efficacy Results of a Trial of a Herpes Simplex Vaccine." *New England Journal of Medicine* 366 no. 1 (2012): 34–43.

Johnston, Christine, et al. "Standard-dose and high-dose daily antiviral therapy for short episodes of genital HSV-2 reactivation: three randomised, open-label, cross-over trials." *The Lancet* 379 no. 9816 (2012): 641–647.

Wozniak, Matthew A., et al. "Antivirals Reduce the Formation of Key Alzheimer's Disease Molecules in Cell Cultures Acutely Infected with Herpes Simplex Virus Type 1." *PLoS ONE* 6 no. 10 (2011): e25152. http://www.plosone.org/article/info%3Adoi%2F10.1371%2Fjournal.pone.0025152 (accessed September 18, 2012).

WEBSITES

"Genital Herpes." U.S. Center for Disease Control and Prevention. http://www.cdc.gov/std/Herpes (accessed September 18, 2012).

"Herpes simplex." MedlinePlus. August 14, 2009 [August 29, 2009]. http://www.nlm.nih.gov/medlineplus/herpessimplex.html (accessed September 18, 2012).

"Herpes simplex." American Academy of Dermatology. http://www.aad.org/skin-conditions/dermatology-a-to-z/herpessimplex (accessed September 18, 2012).

"CDC Analysis of National Herpes Prevalence." Centers for Disease Control and Prevention. http://www.cdc.gov/std/herpes/herpes-NHANES-2010.htm (accessed September 18, 2012).

ORGANIZATIONS

Centers for Disease Control and Prevention (CDC), 1600 Clifton Road, Atlanta, GA 30333, (800) 232-4636, cdcinfo@cdc.gov, http://www.cdc.gov

American Social Health Association, P.O. Box 13827, Research Triangle Park, NC 27709, (919) 361-8400, (800) 227-8922, Fax: (919) 361-8425, http://www.ashastd.org

National Institute of Allergy and Infectious Diseases (NIAID), 6610 Rockledge Drive, MSC 6612, Bethesda, MD 20892, (866) 284-4107, http://www.niaid.nih.gov/Pages/default.aspx.

Belinda M. Rowland, Ph.D.
Tish Davidson, A.M.
Leslie Mertz, Ph.D.

High blood pressure *see* **Hypertension**

Hill-Burton Act

Definition

The Hill-Burton Act is the name given to legislation adopted by the U.S. Congress in 1946 in an attempt to meet the growing demand for health and medical care in the United States following World War II.

Purpose

The purpose of the Hill-Burton Act was to encourage the construction of health and medical facilities needed for a growing U.S. **population** in the second half of the twentieth century.

Description

The end of World War II saw a return in the United States to issues regarding peacetime needs for infrastructure growth and development. One area of particular concern was the demand for health and medical facilities, such as clinics, nursing homes, and hospitals. In an effort to address this problem, Senator Harold Burton (R-OH) and Senator Lister Hill (D-AL) introduced Senate bill S. 191, providing federal grants for construction and improvement of health and medical facilities in the United States. Congress passed the bill, which was then signed by President Harry S Truman. The bill became part of the U.S. Code as 42 CFR 124. In general, the law authorized grants and loans to local communities for improvement of health care facilities. Funds were allocated to individual communities with the goal of producing 4.5 new beds for each 1,000 individuals in a community. In order to receive these funds, communities had to abide by certain regulations and restrictions, namely:

- A facility could not discriminate against an individual on the basis of race, creed, color, or national origin. The construction of so-called "separate-but-equal" facilities was permitted, so that all-white or all-black hospitals were permitted at the time. The "separate-but-equal" provision was later invalidated with the U.S. Supreme Court ruling against the practice in 1963.
- A facility was required to offer some "reasonable volume" of free care to individuals who could not afford to pay for their own health and medical care. This provision was to remain intact for a period of 20 years after issuance of the grant. (S. 191 provided no specific standard for "reasonable volume," an issue that was eventually to require wholesale revision of the bill.)
- Communities were required to provide matching funds for each Hill-Burton grant, so that, for most projects,

federal funds accounted for no more than about a third of the total cost of construction.

- Local communities were required to confirm the economic viability of the area in which construction was to occur. Since this provision could be satisfied only in areas with sound economies, construction tended to take place in middle- and upper-class neighborhoods, with lower-class areas left out of the program.

The original Hill-Burton bill obviously had a number of problems, such as the lack of a standard for a "reasonable volume," of health care and the failure to provide new facilities in economic regions that needed such construction the most. As a result, the law was revised and amended in 1975 when it became Title XVI of the Public Health Service Act. (That act constitutes Title 42 of the U.S. Code.) Two major changes made in the original act were a clear statement as to the standard for a person's inability to pay for health and medical care and an extension for some facilities of their obligation to offer free care into perpetuity, rather than for the original 20-year period. The federal government discontinued providing funds under Hill-Burton in 1977, but institutions that took advantage of the program in the first three decades are still obligated to abide by provisions for offering free health and medical care that was part of the original agreement.

Overall, the Hill-Burton Act has had a powerful influence on health and medical care in the United States. In its earliest history, between 1946 and 1973, the act provided more than $12 billion toward construction projects for new and improved facilities. In total, the program has paid more than $6 billion since 1980 for otherwise uncompensated medical care at Hill-Burton facilities. Today, 175 clinics, nursing homes, and hospitals are still classified as designated Hill-Burton facilities, with the obligation to continue offering free medical care as long as they remain in operation. Those facilities are found in every state except Alaska, Indiana, Minnesota, Nebraska, Nevada, North Dakota, Rhode Island, South Dakota, Utah, and Wyoming. An interactive directory of designated facilities is available at the U.S. **Department of Health and Human Services** (HHS) website at http://www.hrsa.gov/gethealthcare/affordable/hillburton/facilities.html#alternative. Each Hill-Burton facility must agree to certain basic provisions as a participant in the program. They are:

- The facility will not discriminate on the basis of race, color, creed, or national origin.
- The facility must participate in the federal Medicare and Medicaid programs unless they are ineligible to do so for some other reason.

KEY TERMS

Poverty level—A minimum amount of income for an individual or family that allows adequate lifestyle in any particular country, state, or region.

Reasonable volume—The number of indigent clients a clinic, nursing home, hospital, or other healthcare facility is required to treat in order to qualify for Hill-Burton grants and loans. The term has been interpreted by courts in specific cases, but never defined specifically by the U.S. Congress.

Separate-but-equal—A now illegal doctrine that posits that individuals of different race, class, ethnicity, or other traits may be treated equally even if services are provided in physically separate facilities, such as schools or hospitals.

- The facility must post a notice of its participation in the Hill-Burton program in English and Spanish, and in any other language spoken by at least 10 percent of the residents of the community.
- The facility may not withhold emergency services for any member of the community, whether or not he or she can pay for those services.
- The facility may not impose any restrictions on admission to the facility based on any of the factors listed above, including one's ability to pay for those services.
- Eligibility for free service at a Hill-Burton facility is determined by individual or family income. Each facility develops its own specific policies, but generally speaking, free service is available to anyone whose income falls within the U.S. Department of Health and Human Services poverty guidelines, which are revised annually. Individuals and families with incomes twice or three times that of the poverty level may be eligible for some, but not necessarily all, health and medical services. Each facility is permitted to decide which services will be included in its free or reduced-rate program. The Hill-Burton program covers only facility expenses, and does not cover private physician bills. The process by which an individual can determine the services for which she or he may be eligible and the procedure for applying for those services is described on the HHS website at http://www.hrsa.gov/gethealthcare/affordable/hillburton/FAQ/getcarefaq.html.

Resources

BOOKS

Almond, Douglas, Janet Currie, and Emilia Simeonova. *Public vs. Private Provision of Charity Care? Evidence from the*

Expiration of Hill-Burton Requirements in Florida. Cambridge, MA: National Bureau of Economic Research, 2010.

Rovner, Julie. *Health Care Policy and Politics A to Z.* Washington, DC: CQ Press, 2003.

PERIODICALS

Almond, Douglas, Janet Currie, and Emilia Simeonova. "Public vs. Private Provision of Charity Care? Evidence from the Expiration of Hill-Burton Requirements in Florida." *Journal of Health Economics* 30, 1. (2011): 189–99.

"The Hill-Burton Act: The 1946 Hospital Survey and Construction Act, Still on the Books, Says Simply and Clearly What Needs to Be Done." *Executive Intelligence Review* 36, 21. (2009): 14–15.

"A Hill-Burton Act for the 21st Century Could Be Just the Ticket." *Modern Healthcare* 38, 48. (2008): 28–29.

WEBSITES

"Hill-Burton Act Stimulates Licensing of Healthcare." ElderWeb. http://www.elderweb.com/book/1940-1949/hill-burton-act-stimulates-licensing-healthcare. Accessed on October 22, 2012.

"Hill-Burton Free and Reduced-Cost Health Care." Health Resources and Services Administration. http://www.hrsa.gov/gethealthcare/affordable/hillburton/. Accessed on October 22, 2012.

Wing, Kenneth R. "The Community Service Obligation of Hill-Burton Health Facilities."http://lawdigitalcommons.bc.edu/cgi/viewcontent.cgi?article=1702&context=bclr. Accessed on October 22, 2012.

ORGANIZATIONS

Health Resources and Services Administration, U.S. Department of Health and Human Services, 5600 Fishers Lane, Rockville, MD USA 20857, (888) 275–4772, ask@hrsa.gov, http://www.hrsa.gov/.

David E. Newton, Ed.D.

Holistic medicine *see* **Alternative medicine**

Homeopathic medicine *see* **Alternative medicine**

Human papilloma virus (HPV)

Definition

HPV infection is a sexually transmitted disease (STD) caused by 30–40 of the 130 or so known strains of human papillomavirus, the name of a group of viruses that infect the skin and mucous membranes of humans and some animals. In humans these sexually transmitted strains can cause genital warts, precancerous changes in the tissues of the female vagina, or cervical **cancer**. Other strains of HPV are responsible for warts on the soles of the feet (plantar warts), common warts on the hands, and flat warts on the face or legs.

Demographics

In recent years HPV infection has become the most common STD in the United States. The most recent statistics show approximately 20 million Americans are infected with HPV, and another 6.2 million people become newly infected each year. According to one study, 27 percent of women between the ages of 14 and 59, and 35% of homosexual men, are infected with one or more types of HPV. The **Centers for Disease Control and Prevention (CDC)** estimates that more than 80 percent of American women will contract at least one strain of genital HPV by age 50. About 75–80 percent of sexually active Americans of either sex will be infected with HPV at some point in their lifetime.

As far as is known, men and women are at equal risk of being infected with HPV, as are members of all races and ethnic groups.

In terms of specific illnesses associated with HPV, 11,000 women are diagnosed with cervical cancer each year in the United States and 4,000 women die of the disease. Another 5,800 women are diagnosed with cancers of the vagina and the external female genitals, while 3,300 men are diagnosed with cancer of the penis or the anal area. The risk of anal cancer is 17 to 31 times higher among gay and bisexual men than among heterosexual men.

Description

The family of human papilloma viruses includes a large number of genetically-related viruses. Many of these cause warts, including the warts commonly found on the skin. Another group of HPV preferentially infect the mucosal surfaces of the genitals, including the penis, vagina, vulva, and cervix. These are spread among adults by sexual contact. One group of HPV that infect the genitals causes soft warts, often designated condylomata acuminata. These genital warts are quite common and rarely, if ever, become cancerous. The most common of these low-risk HPV types are designated HPV 6 and 11.

The second group of viruses, termed high-risk HPV types, is associated with the development of cervical cancer. Individuals infected with these viruses are at higher risk for the development of precancerous lesions. Typically, infection with these viruses is common in adolescents and women in their twenties and usually does not result in cancerous growth. The most common high-risk HPV is type 16. The appearance of abnormal cells containing high-risk HPV types is seen most frequently in women over the age of 30 who have abnormal Pap smears.

It is possible that other viruses work together with human papilloma viruses to produce precancerous changes in tissue. Cases of tongue cancer have been reported in which HPV was found together with **Epstein-Barr virus**, or EBV. **Smoking**, the use of oral contraceptives for birth control for longer than five years, and suppression of the immune system are also thought to be factors that combine with HPV infection to lead to precancerous lesions in tissue.

Risk factors

Some people are at greater risk of sexually transmitted HPV than others:

- Gay and bisexual men.
- People with HIV or other diseases that weaken the immune system.
- Males or females below age 25. Younger people appear to be more biologically vulnerable to the HPV virus.
- People who have large numbers of sexual partners.
- People in relationships with partners who have sex with many other people.
- People who must take drugs that suppress the immune system.

Causes and symptoms

Causes

The cause of sexually transmitted HPV infection is one or more strains of the human papillomavirus. The virus enters the body through small breaks in the skin surface or in the mucous membranes lining the genitals. In most cases the body fights off the virus within a few weeks. In some people, however, HPV remains dormant for a period ranging from a few weeks to three years, in one of the lower layers of skin cells. The virus then begins to replicate (copy itself) when these cells mature and move upward to the surface of the skin. The virus affects the shape of the cells, leading to the formation of noticeable warts, precancerous changes in skin cells, or cervical cancer. About 1% of sexually active adults in the United States have genital warts at any one time; about 10% of women with high-risk HPV in the tissues of their cervix will develop long-lasting HPV infections that put them at risk for cervical cancer.

The percentages of cancers caused by high-risk types of HPV are as follows:

- Cervical cancer: nearly 100%
- Anal cancer: 90%
- Cancer of the vulva: 40%
- Vaginal cancer: 40%
- Oropharyngeal cancer: 12%
- Oral cancer: 3%

Symptoms in adults

Symptoms of sexually transmitted HPV infection may include:

- Genital warts. These appear as bumps or clusters of fleshy outgrowths around the anus or on the genitals. Some may grow into large cauliflower-shaped masses. Genital warts usually appear within weeks or months after sexual contact with an infected person. If left untreated, genital warts may go away, remain unchanged, or increase in size or number but will not turn into cancers. It is possible, however, for a person to be infected with a high-risk strain of HPV as well as one of the strains that cause genital warts; therefore the appearance of genital warts does not necessarily mean that the person is not at risk of cancer.
- Precancerous changes in the tissues of the female cervix. These are flat growths on the cervix that cannot be seen or felt by the infected woman.
- Cancer. High-risk strains of HPV can cause cancers of the mouth and throat as well as cancers of the anal area and the male and female genitals. These typically take years to develop after infection. In men, symptoms of anal cancer may include bleeding, pain, or a discharge from the anus, or changes in bowel habits. Early signs of cancer of the penis may include thickening of the skin, tissue growths, or sores.

It was not fully understood as of 2012 why most infections with high-risk HPV are of short duration, while a small percentage persist and eventually transform cervical cells to a state of cancerous growth.

Symptoms in children

In addition to producing precancerous lesions in some patients, HPV infections in women are a health concern because they can be transmitted to the respiratory tract of a baby during childbirth. This type of HPV infection may lead to a rare disorder known as juvenile-onset recurrent respiratory papillomatosis (JO-RRP) or laryngeal papillomatosis, in which papillomas or warts form in the child's airway, producing hoarseness or partial blockage of the windpipe. Although laryngeal papillomatosis can occur in HPV-infected adults, 60–80% of cases occur in children, most of them younger than three years.

Laryngeal papillomatosis is usually diagnosed by laryngoscopy. Surgery, whether traditional or laser surgery, is the usual treatment for JO-RRP, but the warts often recur and require additional surgery to remove them. In extreme cases, the patient may be given a tracheotomy, a procedure in which a hole is cut through the throat into the windpipe and a tube is inserted to keep the breathing hole open. A new treatment for the disorder is photodynamic therapy or PDT. In PDT, a special light-sensitive dye is injected into the patient's blood. The dye collects in the tumors rather than in healthy tissue. When bright light of a specific wavelength is shined on the throat, it destroys the tumors containing the dye.

Cidofovir and interferon are often given as adjuvant treatments for this disease as of the early 2000s. JO-RRP is a serious illness, leading to death in a significant number of affected children. In a very few cases, respiratory papillomatosis can lead to cancer as well as breathing difficulties.

Diagnosis

There is no general blood, urine, or imaging test for HPV infection. The diagnosis of genital warts is obvious based on their location and appearance. The doctor may, however, use a vinegar solution to identify HPV-infected areas on the skin of the genitals. The vinegar solution will turn white if HPV is present. Since genital warts are caused by low-risk strains of HPV, the doctor does not need to identify the specific strain of the virus that is present.

Sexually active women should be screened periodically for the presence of changes in the tissues of the cervix. The most common test is the Papanikolaou test or Pap smear, invented by a Greek physician in the 1940s. To perform a Pap smear, the doctor takes a small spatula to obtain cells from the outer surface of the cervix and smears the collected cells on a slide that is then examined in a laboratory for signs of any abnormal cells. If abnormal or questionable cells are found, the doctor may order an HPV DNA test, which can identify the DNA of 13 high-risk types of HPV in cells taken from the cervix.

There were no HPV screening tests for men as of 2012; however, some doctors suggested that anal Pap smears for men who have sex with men would be useful in early detection of anal cancer.

KEY TERMS

Ablative—Also known as "ablation" and referring to the surgical removal of lesions associated with HPV.

Biopsy—The removal of a small bit of tissue for diagnostic examination.

Cervical intra-epithelial neoplasia (CIN)—A precancerous condition in which a group of cells grow abnormally on the cervix but do not extend into the deeper layers of this tissue.

Cervix—The narrow neck or outlet of a woman's uterus.

Colposcopy—Procedure in which the cervix is examined using a special microscope.

Condylomata acuminata (singular, condyloma acuminatum)—The medical term for infectious warts on the genitals caused by HPV.

Cryotherapy—The use of liquid nitrogen or other forms of extreme cold to destroy tissue.

Epithelial—Referring to the epithelium, the layer of cells forming the epidermis of the skin and the surface layer of mucous membranes.

High-risk HPV type—A member of the HPV family of viruses that is associated with the development of cervical cancer and precancerous growths.

Pap test—A screening test for cervical cancer devised by Giorgios Papanikolaou (1883–1962) in the 1940s.

Photodynamic therapy (PDT)—A treatment for tumors in which a light-sensitive dye is injected into the blood (or skin) to be taken up selectively by the tumors. Light of a specific wavelength is then applied to the affected area to kill the tumors.

Topical—Referring to a type of medication applied directly to the skin or outside of the body.

Tracheotomy—A surgical procedure in which a hole is cut through the neck to open a direct airway through an incision in the trachea (windpipe).

Tests

The relationship among HPV, precancerous cellular changes, and cervical cancer have led to the suggestion that testing for the presence of HPV can be a useful addition to Pap smears. Pap smears involve microscopic analysis of cells removed from the cervix. The results of these tests are generally reported as either normal or consistent with the presence of cancer or a precancerous condition. Patients receiving the latter diagnosis usually are treated either by excisional or ablative therapy surgery or some other means in order to remove the tumor or precancerous lesion.

In some cases the cytologist or pathologist examining a Pap smear reports a "borderline" result when abnormal cells are observed, but it is not possible to distinguish whether the changes seen are due to early precancerous changes or to inflammation caused by some infectious agent or irritant. In these cases, some physicians and scientists believe that testing for the presence of HPV can help to identify those women who should be closely followed for the development of early cancerous lesions, or who should undergo colposcopy, a procedure to examine the cervix for precancerous lesions. These cancer precursors, termed cervical intraepithelial neoplasia (CIN) when identified early, before they have become invasive, can almost always be completely removed by minor surgery, essentially curing the patient before the cancer has had a chance to develop. The cervical tissue removed, which includes the precancerous tissue, is examined as part of a biopsy to confirm the diagnosis, and if requested by a doctor, can be tested for the presence of high-risk HPV types.

Treatment

Traditional

Patients with genital warts should *never* use over-the counter-preparations designed to remove common or flat warts from the hands or face. Doctors can treat genital warts with various medical or surgical techniques, including:

- Cryotherapy. Cryotherapy uses liquid nitrogen to freeze the warts. The dead tissue in the wart falls away from the skin beneath in about a week.
- Imiquimod. Imiquimod (Aldara) is a topical cream that gets rid of genital warts by stimulating the body's immune system to fight the virus that causes the warts.
- Podofilox. Podofilox (Condylox) is a topical medication available in liquid or gel form that destroys the wart tissue.
- Surgery. The doctor can remove the wart by drying it out with an electric needle and then scraping the tissue with a sharp instrument called a curette. Lasers can also be used to remove genital warts.

Low-grade precancerous changes in the tissue of the female cervix are not usually treated directly because most of them will eventually go away on their own without developing into cancer. The patient should, however, see the doctor for follow-up Pap smears to make sure that the tissues are returning to normal. High-risk precancerous lesions are removed, usually by surgery, cryotherapy, electrocauterization, or laser surgery.

Since the incidence of latent and recurrent infections is high, the eradication of HPV is not always 100% effective. It is essential to be aware that HPV is a sexually transmitted disease and women must engage in **safe sex** practices to decrease the risk of spreading the virus or becoming reinfected. A vaccine effective against four of the HPV types most likely to cause genital warts or cervical cancer was approved for use in 2006; it is described more fully in the **Prevention** section of this article. As of 2012, there are two similar HPV vaccines—Gardasil and Cervarix, and researchers were working on developing vaccines to protect against additional types of the HPV virus.

Prognosis

The prognosis of sexually transmitted HPV infections depends on the patient's age, number of sexual partners, gender, and the condition of his or her immune system. Women are significantly more likely than men to develop cancers following HPV infection. However, most people of either sex with normally functioning immune systems who are infected with HPV will clear the infection from their bodies within two years.

Prevention

Preventive measures that people can take to lower their risk of HPV infection include:

- Abstaining from sex or having sex only with an uninfected partner who is faithful.
- Reducing the number of sexual partners.
- Using condoms regularly during sexual intercourse.
- For women, using a vaccine called Gardasil. Approved by the Food and Drug Administration (FDA) in 2006, Gardasil protects against four of the types of HPV that cause most cervical cancers and genital warts. The vaccine is recommended for 11- and 12-year-old girls. It is also recommended for girls and women age 13 through 26 who have not yet been vaccinated or completed the vaccine series. Gardasil works best in girls who have not yet been sexually active. It is given as a series of three shots over a six-month period.

A second human papillomavirus vaccine, Cervarix, was approved in Europe, Australia, and the Philippines in 2007. It received FDA approval for use in the United States in October 2009.

In addition to giving the available preventive vaccines to women, some doctors think it might be a useful preventive measure to vaccinate men as well to protect their female partners against infection. As of 2012, the **CDC** recommends Gardasil **vaccination** for boys from 11 to 21 years of age, and can be received through age 26.

Efforts and solutions

As of 2012, researchers are still working to develop more advanced testing for HPV, such as a general HPV test for men and women, and a test to locate HPV on the genitals, mouth, or throat. Researchers are still learning about how pregnant women respond to the HPV vaccine. The CDC suggests that if a woman believes she was pregnant while receiving any of her HPV vaccine shots, she should wait until after the pregnancy to complete the remaining dosages, and work with her physician to report the case to the correct registry—Gardasil or Cervarix.

Resources

BOOKS

Gonzales, Lissette. *Frequently Asked Questions about Human Papillomavirus*. New York: Rosen, 2009.

Krueger, Hans, et al. *HPV and Other Infectious Agents in Cancer: Opportunities for Prevention and Public Health*. New York: Oxford University Press, 2010.

Marr, Lisa. *Sexually Transmitted Diseases: A Physician Tells You What You Need to Know*, 2nd ed. Baltimore, MD: Johns Hopkins University Press, 2007.

Nardo, Don. *Human Papillomavirus (HPV)*. Detroit, MI: Lucent Books, 2007.

Rosenblatt, Alberto. *Human Papillomavirus*. New York: Springer, 2009.

PERIODICALS

Burki, T. "Should Males Be Vaccinated against HPV?" *Lancet Oncology* 10 (September 2009): 845.

Haug, C. "The Risks and Benefits of HPV Vaccination." *Journal of the American Medical Association* 302 (August 19, 2009): 795–95.

Hershey, J.H., and L.F. Velez. "Public Health Issues Related to HPV Vaccination." *Journal of Public Health Management and Practice* 15 (September-October 2009): 384–92.

Lindsey, K., et al. "Anal Pap Smears: Should We Be Doing Them?" *Journal of the American Academy of Nurse Practitioners* 21 (August 2009): 437–43.

O'Connor, M. B., and C. O'Connor. "The HPV Vaccine for Men." *International Journal of STD and AIDS* 20 (April 2009): 290–91.

Printz, C. "HPV Status Predicts Survival of Oropharyngeal Cancer Patients." *Cancer* 115 (September 15, 2009): 4045.

Samara, R. N., and S. N. Khleif. "HPV as a Model for the Development of Prophylactic and Therapeutic Cancer Vaccines." *Current Molecular Medicine* 9 (August 2009): 766–73.

Wang, Z., et al. "Detection of Human Papilloma Virus Subtypes 16 and P16(ink4a) in Invasive Squamous Cell Carcinoma of the Fallopian Tube and Concomitant Squamous Cell Carcinoma in Situ of the Cervix." *Journal of Obstetrics and Gynaecology Research* 35 (April 2009): 385–89.

WEBSITES

Centers for Disease Control and Prevention (CDC). *HPV Vaccine Questions & Answers*. http://www.cdc.gov/vaccines/vpd-vac/hpv/vac-faqs.htm. Accessed August 19, 2012.

Centers for Disease Control and Prevention (CDC). *Human Papillomavirus (HPV) Infection*. http://www.cdc.gov/std/hpv/default.htm. Accessed August 19, 2012.

Centers for Disease Control and Prevention (CDC) Fact Sheet. *HPV and Men*. http://www.cdc.gov/std/hpv/STDFact-HPV-and-men.htm. Accessed August 19, 2012.

Gearhart, Peter A., and Thomas C. Randall. "Human Papillomavirus." *eMedicine*, August 4, 2009. http://emedicine.medscape.com/article/219110-overview.

Mayo Clinic. *HPV Infection*. http://www.mayoclinic.com/health/hpv-infection/DS00906.

National Cancer Institute (NCI). http://www.cancer.gov/cancertopics/factsheet/Risk/HPV.

National Institute of Allergy and Infectious Diseases (NIAID). *Human Papillomavirus and Genital Warts*. http://www3.niaid.nih.gov/topics/genitalWarts.

National Institute on Deafness and Other Communication Disorders (NIDCD). *Laryngeal Papillomatosis*. http://www.nidcd.nih.gov/health/voice/laryngeal.htm.

ORGANIZATIONS

American College of Obstetricians and Gynecologists (ACOG), 409 12th St., S.W., P.O. Box 96920, Washington, DC 20090-6920, 202-638-5577, resources@acog.org, http://www.acog.org/

American Social Health Association (ASHA), P.O. Box 13827, Research Triangle Park, NC 27709, 919-361-8400, 800-227-8922, Fax: 919-361-8425, http://www.ashastd.org/index.cfm

Centers for Disease Control and Prevention (CDC), 1600 Clifton Road, Atlanta, GA 30333, 800-232-4636, cdcinfo@cdc.gov, http://www.cdc.gov

National Cancer Institute, 6116 Executive Blvd., Room 3036A, Bethesda, MD 20892-8322, 800-422-6237, cancergov-staff@mail.nih.gov, http://www.cancer.gov

National Institute of Allergy and Infectious Diseases (NIAID), 6610 Rockledge Drive, MSC 6612, Bethesda, MD 20892-6612, 301-496-5717, 866-284-4107, Fax: 301-402-3573, http://www3.niaid.nih.gov

National Institute on Deafness and Other Communication Disorders (NIDCD), 31 Center Drive, MSC 2320, Bethesda, MD 20892-2320, 800 241-1044, Fax: 301 770-8977, nidcdinfo@nidcd.nih.gov, http://www.nidcd.nih.gov/index.asp.

Warren Maltzman, Ph.D
Rebecca J. Frey, Ph.D
Andrea Nienstedt, MA

Human rights

Definition

Human rights are the fundamental freedoms to which everyone is entitled merely because they are human. These rights are universal and the same for everyone, regardless of race, religion, ethnicity, or sexual orientation.

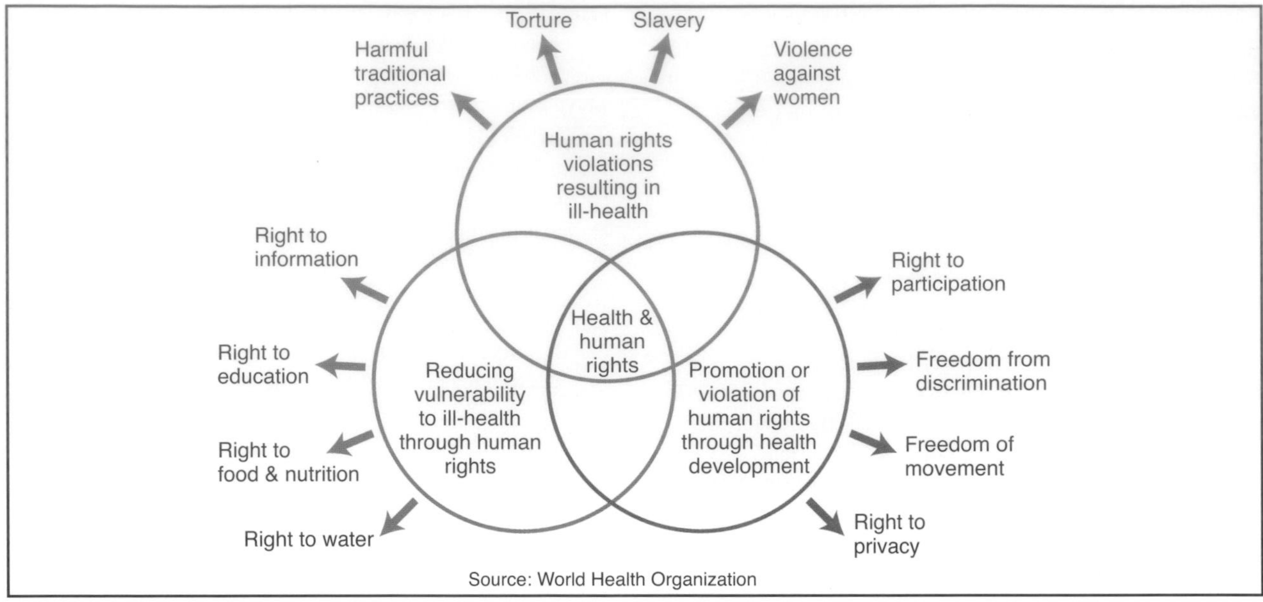

(Illustration by Electronic Illustrators Group. © 2013 Cengage Learning)

Description

Human rights are the inalienable rights entitled to every human. These rights are the same for all people, all around the world, regardless of individual differences such as language, religion, ethnicity, sexual preferences, or race. The United Nations Declaration of Human Rights lists 30 basic rights that are inalienable and universal. These rights include the right to life, the right to not be tortured, the right to be equal before the law, and the right to privacy. Although this declaration has been signed by all 192 member states of the United Nations, it is not binding and therefore not law. The International Covenant on Civil and Political Rights (ICCPR) and the International Covenant on Economic, Social, and Cultural Rights (ICESCR), were written later in order to have a way to enforce the rights listed. These laws are binding on the countries that ratify them.

Not all nations agree on what should be considered to be human rights and who should have the power to determine what rights should be recognized. Although the United Nations Declaration of Human Rights forbids acts such as torture and genocide, these acts still take place around the world. Additionally, many smaller violations of human rights take place on a daily basis, such as people living without access to shelter, clean **water**, or affordable health care. Many international bodies such as the United Nations Human Rights Council, individual governments, non-governmental organizations such as Amnesty International and Human Rights Watch, and corporations, work together to monitor the rights of humans worldwide and to stop and punish those who violate people's human rights.

Origins

The belief that there are inalienable fundamental rights to which every person is entitled is not a new concept. The first charter of human rights was written in 539 BC, on a baked clay cylinder. These rights were determined by Cyrus the Great, a king who, after conquering Babylon, freed the slaves and declared racial equality, and the right of citizens to choose their own religion. The ideas written on the Cyrus cylinder spread to other nations including India, Rome, and Greece. Rome called these basic inalienable rights natural law.

As the idea of basic human rights spread, it began to be included in important documents. In 1215, King John of England was forced to sign the Magna Carta when he broke many of the basic laws and customs by which the people of England lived. Basic rights mentioned in the Magna Carta included the right for free citizens to inherit and own property, the right for the church to be free from government interference, and the right for citizens to be protected from excessive taxation. The Magna Carta became a model for many other important documents including the Petition of Rights in 1628, and the United States Constitution in 1787.

The idea of human rights was expanded on at the first Geneva Convention in 1864. Sixteen European countries and a several American states came together in Geneva, Switzerland, to discuss certain rights of man.

The focus of the first Geneva conference was the treatment of wounded soldiers during war. The Geneva Convention was important in the foundation of international standards of how victims of war should be treated.

In April 1945, 50 countries sent delegates to the United Nations Conference on International Organization in San Francisco, California. This conference took place toward the end of World War II, when the mass destruction and terror caused by war was fresh in the minds of governments and the public. The goal was to develop an international body to promote peace and prevent future wars. The charter to create the United Nations went into effect on October 24, 1945.

Although the United Nations is involved in many different aspects of international peace, human rights was, and still is, one of its main focuses. Beginning in 1945, Eleanor Roosevelt, the widow of President Franklin Roosevelt, was a delegate to the United Nations General Assembly and chaired the United Nations Human Rights Commission. With the help of the other members of the Human Rights Commission, the Universal Declaration of Human Rights was developed. This document stated there are certain inherent rights for all humans and listed 30 of these rights. Examples of the rights described in the document included the freedom of thought, the right to food and shelter, and the right to an education. This declaration was adopted on December 10, 1948, with 48 countries voting for the declaration, zero against it, and eight countries abstaining from voting. As of 2012, all 192 member states of the United Nations have signed the United Nations Declaration of Human Rights.

Although the Universal Declaration of Human Rights is a non-binding agreement, meaning that it is not enforceable because it is not a law, the rights put forth by the document are considered by many to have become a part of customary law, meaning those who are involved consider them to be law. Additionally, two law-binding treaties were written after the declaration was adopted. These include the International Covenant on Civil and Political Rights (ICCPR) and the International Covenant on Economic, Social, and Cultural Rights (ICESCR). The goal of these two covenants was to establish a way to enforce the Universal Declaration of Human Rights. Together, these three documents form the International Bill of Human Rights. As of 2012, 167 countries have ratified the ICCPR and 160 countries have ratified the ICESCR.

Effects on public health

Many of the rights put forth in the United Nations Declaration of Human Rights focus on aspects involving public health. Examples include the right to food, affordable housing, medicine, and medical help. Almost always when a group of people's human rights are violated there is a major negative public health effect. For example, genocide, such as what took place during the Holocaust and in Darfur, left thousands of people sick, injured, and dead. In cases like the Holocaust, people's basic rights of freedom, food, and shelter were violated. Victims were forced to do manual labor, became ill from living in crowded and unsanitary conditions, and were not offered proper medical treatment when sick. Even though not all concentration camps were extermination camps, millions of victims died as a consequence of their human rights being violated. During genocide in places such as Darfur, ethnic groups were not only systematically killed, but many citizens went hungry and got sick because of a shortage of food and resources. People within the victim groups may be stopped from giving birth and bodily and mental harm is inflected. Many organizations that focus on human rights are also focused on public health because the two go hand in hand. These organizations work to protect the rights of all people and to promote good public health standards around the world.

Costs to society

When human rights are violated there is a huge cost to society. Entire communities and ethnic groups can be destroyed because of the violation of their human rights. Millions of people have been killed over the centuries due to human rights violations. During World War II alone, more than 12 million people were deliberately killed. Even when human rights are restored to an area, the physical and mental health problems can last for years. Communities must be put back together, many times from scratch, and community members often live in fear that their rights will be violated again. Entire generations may be lost due to the violation of human rights, such as in genocide when a particular ethnic, religious, or racial group is specifically targeted. These communities are also hurt financially, which adds to the time it takes to recover and rebuild.

The protection of human rights also has an economic cost. Many of the rights laid out in the United Nations Declaration of Human Rights take governmental money to make sure that every person's rights are met. This is not possible for all countries due to the economic hardship many nations face. Rights such as access to affordable healthcare, clean water, food, and even shelter, may be unaffordable for all countries to provide. For this reason, not everyone agrees that rights that cost governments money should be considered part of human rights.

The promotion and protection of human rights is also costly. Governments and organizations that try to enforce human rights around the world and to stop and punish human rights violators spend billions of dollars each year. Government resources to fight violations such as **human trafficking**, war, and genocide are costly and add up, often being paid for with taxpayers' money. According to a 2010 study, Britain's membership to the European Court of Human Rights has cost United Kingdom taxpayers over £42 billion since 1950. Non-governmental organizations receive money through grants and personal and corporate donations. This money is often used to keep track of human rights violations, legislation, and program success both locally and around the world. Many people question how much money should go toward human rights campaigns in other countries when the money could be spent toward improving life for citizens at home. Others believe that there is no cost too high to promote and protect the rights of all humans.

Efforts and solutions

The fight to maintain human rights around the world is ongoing. Hundreds of organizations, both big and small, are involved in human rights campaigns. Eleanor Roosevelt once said that human rights begin, "In small places, close to home—so close and so small that they cannot be seen on any maps of the world. Yet they are the world of the individual people; the neighborhoods they live in; the school or college they attend; the factory, farm or office where they work." This idea has continued, and while many governments and organizations focus on the promotion and protection of human rights internationally, many have followed Eleanor Roosevelt's advice and work to support human rights in their own communities.

Since the Universal Declaration of Human Rights, many additional documents, treaties, and laws have gone into effect to protect the rights of everyone. Sometimes these laws are local, only affecting a few thousand people. Other times these laws are international, affecting an entire country or continent. Thousands of human rights projects are currently underway working to improve the quality of life for those whose rights are not being met and making sure that no one loses the rights they currently have.

KEY TERMS

Customary law—A law that has been established due to the belief among those involved that a practice is legally binding and the evidence of widespread and consistent practice in a particular social setting.

Inalienable rights—privileges to which all humans are entitled, just because they are human. These are unlike legal rights, which can be taken away and may not be equal for everyone.

Genocide—The deliberate killing of a racial or ethnic group.

Resources

BOOKS

Neier, Aryeh. *The International Human Rights Movement: A History.* Princeton, NJ: Princeton University Press, 2012.

WEBSITES

United for Human Rights. "A Brief History of Human Rights." http://www.humanrights.com/what-are-human-rights/brief-history/cyrus-cylinder.html (accessed September 22, 2012).

United Nations Office of the High Commissioner for Human Rights. "What are Human Rights?" http://www.ohchr.org/en/issues/Pages/WhatareHumanRights.aspx (accessed September 22, 2012).

United Nations Treaty Collection. "International Covenant on Economic, Social and Cultural Rights." http://treaties.un.org/Pages/ViewDetails.aspx?src=TREATY&mtdsg_no=IV-3&chapter=4&lang=en#10 (accessed September 22, 2012).

Youth for Human Rights International. "Universal Declaration of Human Rights." http://www.youthforhumanrights.org/what-are-human-rights/universal-declaration-of-human-rights/articles-1-15.html (accessed September 22, 2012).

ORGANIZATIONS

Amnesty International, 1 Easton Street, London, United Kingdom WC1X 0DW, 44 20 74135500, Fax: 44 20 79561157, http://www.amnesty.org

Human Rights Watch, 350 Fifth Avenue, 34th Floor, New York, NY 10118, (212) 290 4700, Fax: (212) 736 1300, http://www.hrw.org

Office of the United Nations High Commissioner for Human Rights, Palais des Nations, Geneva, Switzerland CH-1211, 41 22 917 9220, InfoDesk@ohchr.org, http://www.ohchr.org.

Tish Davidson, AM

Human trafficking

Definition

Human trafficking is the illegal recruitment, transportation, and trading of humans for sexual exploitation, forced labor, or the removal of organs. Human trafficking is also commonly known as modern-day slavery.

Description

Human trafficking is considered one of the fastest growing crime industries. It is the second largest crime industry in the world, directly behind the drug trade. Although similar in name, human smuggling is different from human trafficking. In human trafficking, victims are forced or coerced with deception to be taken to a new city or country. They are then held against their will and exploited. In human smuggling, a person voluntarily hires people, without deception, to get them into a new country. They are then free to go their own way once they reach the destination. Although victims of human trafficking are often taken to a new country, many victims remain in their country of origin. Human smuggling, on the other hand, always takes place across borders.

Each year, an estimated 700,000 to 4 million women and children are trafficked. Most trafficked women and children are sexually exploited, forced to work as prostitutes, strippers, or participate in pornography. Women and children may also be exploited for labor, forced to work for no or very little pay, used for their organs, or forced to be soldiers in armed conflicts. Men can also be victims of human trafficking, and are most often forced into labor, used for their organs, or forced to become soldiers.

Human trafficking is a large industry generating an estimated $32 billion each year. On average, each forced labor victim generates $13,000 each year, some generating up to $67,200 a year.

Demographics

Human trafficking takes place around the world. Victims of human trafficking come from over 127 countries and are sent to more than 137 countries. In total, as many as 161 countries are believed to be affected by human trafficking through being a source, transit, or destination country. Although the majority of victims are between the ages of 18 and 24, over 1.2 million children are also trafficked each year. Estimates for the number of victims trafficked vary. The United Nations (UN) estimates that between 700,000 to 4 million women and children alone are trafficked each year. Another UN statement estimated that 2.4 million people are suffering from human trafficking at any one time, with two out of every three victims being a woman or child.

Victims of human trafficking come from all racial and ethnic groups. The largest number of victims come from Asia and the Pacific. A majority of victims have vulnerable backgrounds and come from war-torn or economically poor areas. Often, human traffickers deceive people looking for work, promising a good job and better life in another country. These people are then held against their will once they arrive in the new country. Other victims may be runaway teens, kidnap victims, drug addicts, tourists, refugees, or the homeless. As unemployment around the world rises, more people are in danger of becoming victims of human trafficking.

Origins

There is no one time or event agreed upon as to when human trafficking began. Although slavery has been around for thousands of years, many feel that human trafficking did not get its start until the time of white slavery. White slavery is the name given for the use of deceit, force, or drugs to entrap women or children into prostitution. White slavery first got attention during the same time black slavery was beginning to be abolished in countries such as the United Kingdom. Although now it is believed that the actual number of white slavery cases was small, during this same period, there was an increase in women migrants from Europe travelling abroad to search for work making them more vulnerable.

What to do about white slavery was first discussed at a conference in Paris in 1895, and was again a topic at conferences in London and Budapest in 1899. In 1899, and again in 1902, an international conference against white slavery was held in Paris. An agreement was signed in Paris in 1904, known as the International Agreement for the Suppression of the White Slave Traffic. This agreement focused not only on the safety of women and children, but also the repatriation of migration workers.

Policy against white slavery continued to develop. In 1910, 13 countries signed the International Convention for the Suppression of the White Slave Trade. However, no real changes were made because the start of World War I put an end to the work this convention set out to do. Over time, the name white slavery began to be replaced by traffic in women. This name change officially took place at a 1921 conference of the League of Nations. This also began a change in focus from just women and girls to children of both sexes. Thirty-three countries signed the International Convention for the Suppression of the Traffic in Women and Children at this conference.

A study done by the League of Nations in 1927 focused on trafficking in the West and found that the most common source countries included Austria, France, Germany, Greece, Hungary, Italy, Poland, Romania, Spain, and Turkey. The most common destination countries included Algeria, Argentina, Brazil, Egypt, Mexico, Panama, Tunis, and Uruguay. This is the reverse of the pattern seen in the twenty-first century. A second study that focused on trafficking in the East was released in 1932. This study found similar countries of origin and that the most popular destinations included Beirut, Bombay, Calcutta, Hong Kong, Saigon, and Shanghai. This study also discovered that many Asian women were trafficked within Asia.

Adopted in 1949 and effective starting in 1951, the United Nations Convention for the Suppression of the Traffic in Persons and of the Exploitation of the Prostitution of Others, was the first legally binding agreement dealing with the trafficking of women and children internationally. As of 2010, only 66 countries had ratified this agreement. Other non-binding instruments have been passed since 1949. In 1995, the Beijing Platform for Action was adopted with the goal of effectively suppressing human trafficking of women and children. The Optional Protocol on the Sale of Children, Child Prostitution and Child Pornography was at first a non-binding agreement, but was later ratified in 2002 to become binding. As of 2012, more than 100 countries had signed and ratified this law-binding agreement.

The largest law-binding step took place in 2000, when the UN adopted the Convention against Transnational Organized Crime. This included multiple protocols, two with a specific focus on human trafficking. The first dealt with the prevention of trafficking of persons, especially women and children. The second was against the smuggling of migrants by land, sea, and air. These protocols went into effect in 2003 and 2004, respectively. As of 2012, this convention has been signed by 147 countries and 171 parties.

Effects on public health

Human trafficking can have devastating consequences on the physical and mental health of its victims and the public. Victims of human trafficking often live in crowded and unsanitary conditions, leading to the possible spread of communicable diseases, such as **tuberculosis** and scabies. Victims forced to do labor may suffer from back problems or **stress** injuries due to repetitive motion. Hearing, vision, cardiovascular, and respiratory problems can also be linked to working in harsh conditions such as in sweatshops or agricultural labor.

Malnourishment can be a problem faced by victims, especially children, who do not have their basic needs taken care of such as health and dental care. Depression, anxiety, panic attacks, and other mental disorders are common among trafficking victims who are forced to live and work in fear. Sexually exploited victims risk being infected by sexually transmitted and other communicable diseases such as human immunodeficiency virus (HIV), tuberculosis, and **hepatitis** B. These diseases can become a larger public health threat when they are transmitted across borders through the transportation of human trafficking victims. Victims may also be forced or willingly participate in drug use, adding to the spread of disease.

Costs to society

Human trafficking has a large cost to individual victims and society as a whole. Human trafficking is negative for public health, leading to the spread of disease throughout communities and between countries. Human trafficking also disrupts families and communities who lose their own to the trafficking trade and may discriminate against, or completely reject, those victims who are able to return home. Additionally, human trafficking deprives people of basic **human rights**, fuels organized crime, encourages corruption, and can damage a government's authority. Both local and national labor markets can also be negatively impacted by human trafficking. Communities can find themselves with depressed wages, an undereducated generation, and a shortage of people to care for the elderly. Around the world, billions of dollars are spent trying to stop human trafficking and to rehabilitate victims who have been able to escape, costing governments, private organizations, and public healthcare systems.

Efforts and solutions

Hundreds of organizations throughout the world are working to combat human trafficking. These groups include both governmental and non-governmental organizations. While some groups are quite small, others have branches throughout the world such as Amnesty International and Human Rights Watch. Governmental organizations at all levels have worked to pass legislation and develop action plans to fight human trafficking. The United Nations Office on Drugs and Crime participates in research and holds conferences and seminars to discuss human trafficking and the successes and failures of their action plans.

Individual countries and states also participate in the fight against human trafficking by passing legislation to increase the sentences given to people convicted of human trafficking and the funds available to help victims. Education also plays a large role in the fight against human trafficking. Potential victims are educated about the warning signs of job offers that may be a cover-up for a human trafficking operation and medical professionals, law enforcement agencies, and the public are educated about the signs of human trafficking operations or human trafficking victims. Unfortunately, due to the large and

KEY TERMS

Anxiety—Worry or tension in response to real or imagined stress, danger, or dreaded situations. Physical reactions, such as fast pulse, sweating, trembling, fatigue, and weakness may accompany anxiety.

Human immunodeficiency virus (HIV)—A transmissible retrovirus that causes AIDS in humans. Two forms of HIV are now recognized: HIV-1, which causes most cases of AIDS in Europe, North and South America, and most parts of Africa; and HIV-2, which is chiefly found in West African patients. HIV-2, discovered in 1986, appears to be less virulent than HIV-1 and may also have a longer latency period.

Panic attack—A time-limited period of intense fear accompanied by physical and cognitive symptoms. Panic attacks may be unexpected or triggered by specific internal or external cues.

Tuberculosis—An infectious disease that primarily infects the lungs. Tuberculosis can cause weight lost, chest pain, fever, and death. Tuberculosis is caused by various strains of bacteria and is passed from one person to another through the air.

White slavery—A term first used in 19th century Britain to describe forced prostitution. White slavery is sometimes still used to describe sexual slavery today.

corrupt nature of human trafficking, organizations struggle to capture and convict all criminals involved. In 2006, only 3,160 people were convicted of human trafficking, averaging one person for every 800 trafficked. In 2012, it was estimated that only one out of every 100 victims is ever rescued.

Resources

BOOKS

United Nations. *Human Trafficking: An Overview*. New York: UN, 2008.

United Nations Independent Evaluation Unit. *In-Depth Evaluation of the United Nations Global Initiative to Fight Human Trafficking*. New York: UN, 2011.

WEBSITES

Kangaspunta, Kristina. "A Short History of Trafficking in Persons." http://www.freedomfromfearmagazine.org/index.php?option=com_content&view=article&id=99:a-short-history-of-trafficking-in-persons&catid=37:issue-1&Itemid=159 (accessed September 21, 2012).

Polaris Project. "Increasing Awareness and Engagement: Strengthening the National Response to Human Trafficking in the U.S." https://na4.salesforce.com/sfc/p/300000006E4S11Sv6mFa.D_CBl0UueofejFjNL0= (accessed September 21, 2012).

Polaris Project. "Human Trafficking Statistics." http://www.cicatelli.org/titlex/downloadable/Human%20Trafficking%20Statistics.pdf (accessed September 21, 2012).

United Nations Office on Drugs and Crime. "Human Trafficking." http://www.unodc.org/unodc/en/human-trafficking/what-is-human-trafficking.html (accessed September 21, 2012).

ORGANIZATIONS

Amnesty International, 1 Easton Street, London, United Kingdom WC1X 0DW, 44 20 74135500, Fax: 44 20 79561157, http://www.amnesty.org

Human Rights Watch, 350 Fifth Avenue, 34th Floor, New York, NY 10118, (212) 290 4700, Fax: (212) 736 1300, http://www.hrw.org

United Nations Office on Drugs and Crime, PO Box 500, Vienna, Austria A 1400, 43 (1) 26060, Fax: 43 (1) 263 3389, info@unodc.org, https://www.unodc.org.

Tish Davidson

Hunger and undernutrition

Definition

Hunger is the lack of availability of food in a country. Over time, hunger leads to undernutrition, which is the result of extremely inadequate intake of calories, protein, or micronutrients. Although "undernutrition" and malnutrition often are used interchangeably, "malnutrition" is a more inclusive term that includes overnutrition.

Demographics

Undernutrition affects 925 million people in the world. This number is broken down geographically as follows:

- Asia and the Pacific—578 million
- Sub-Saharan Africa—239 million
- Latin America and the Caribbean—53 million
- Near East and North Africa—37 million
- Developed nations—19 million

The United Nations Children's Fund (UNICEF) estimates that about 195 million children have stunted growth as a direct result of undernutrition. Of these, about 90% are in Africa and Asia. India has the largest absolute number of stunted children, while Afghanistan

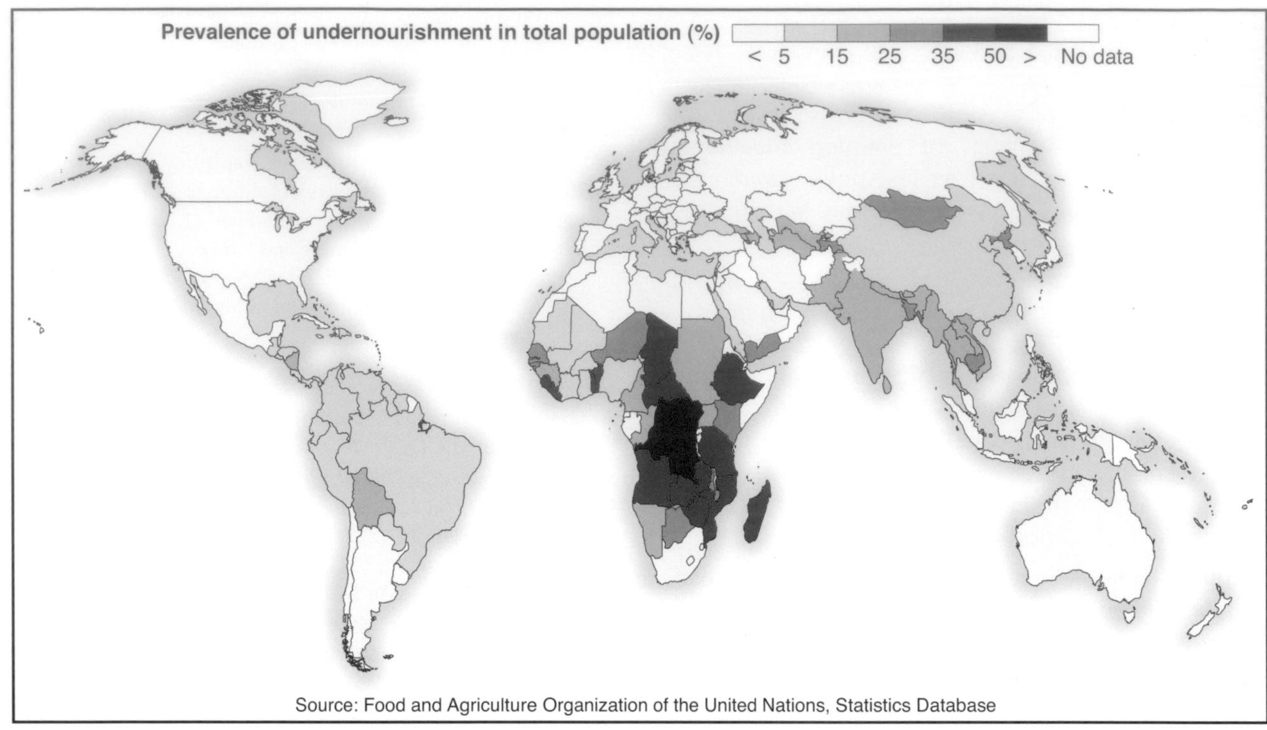

(Illustration by Electronic Illustrators Group. © 2013 Cengage Learning)

has the highest percentage of stunted children. Undernutrition is uncommon in the developed world, but the British **Nutrition** Foundation estimates that about two million people in the United Kingdom are undernourished. Undernutrition has the most severe impact on children under age five.

Undernutrition in children is much less common in the United States than in developing countries. Estimates suggest that only about 1% of all children in the United States experience undernutrition. The highest-risk children in the United States are those living in homeless shelters, where an estimated 10% of children are undernourished. Estimates also suggest that one in every seven elderly individuals in the United States consumes fewer than 1,000 calories per day and is undernourished.

Approximately half of the hungry people in the world live in rural communities with land that tends to be subject to **natural disasters**. One-fifth of hungry people live in shanty towns on the edges of larger cities in developing nations.

Description

There is enough food produced to feed everyone in the world 2,720 kilocalories each day. However, some people do not have access to enough food in their region, while others cannot afford to purchase food. **Poverty** is the primary cause of hunger in the world.

Undernutrition is a serious problem in developing countries, especially in children under age five years. It is estimated that 146 million children in developing nations weigh less than their ideal weight because they suffer from hunger, on either a short- or long-term basis. Undernutrition can begin before a baby is born. Deficiencies in calories, protein, minerals, and/or **vitamins** often affect the fetus during pregnancy because the mother does not consume enough calories and micronutrients. This often results in the delivery of a low-birthweight baby. According to the **World Health Organization (WHO)**, low-birthweight accounts for about 60% of deaths in newborns in developing countries or 3.3% of all child deaths.

Undernutrition frequently continues into early childhood. It is estimated that children who are not properly nourished are sick 160 days out of the year. There is a strong relationship between undernutrition and failure to survive. Undernutrition intensifies the diseases a child may develop, such as **measles**. Children might not directly starve to death from undernutrition, although some do die of disorders such as marasmus, which is a severe deficiency in calories and protein. Instead, undernourished children tend to have weak immune systems that leave them highly susceptible to common diseases such as diarrhea, **pneumonia**, **malaria**, and measles, all of which are common in the developing world. Often, undernourished children go through a downward cycle of repeated disease and recovery before they die; if they do survive, this cycle exacts a heavy toll on their development. Exact figures are difficult to obtain from developing countries, but estimates suggest that maternal and child undernutrition is the cause of 3–5 million deaths annually. Zinc and vitamin A deficiency are the most common micronutrient deficiencies, while iron and iodine deficiencies also contribute to undernutrition.

A critical window for development exists between birth and age two years. Even when children survive these critical years, the effects of undernutrition remain. Often, these children are stunted (short stature) or wasted (seriously underweight). In addition to physical effects, undernutrition can restrict a child's mental development.

Undernutrition in the elderly is a greater problem in the United States than undernutrition in children. Declining appetite, limited funds, difficulty in preparing and eating food, and disease all contribute to undernutrition in the elderly. Elderly people living in nursing homes or hospitalized for prolonged periods are at high risk for undernutrition. Individuals of any age who have had gastric bypass surgery may experience undernutrition unless they take prescribed vitamin and mineral supplements.

Risk factors

Risk factors for undernutrition include inadequate food supply (e.g., **famine**), inadequate variety of food (i.e., food does not contain all the required micronutrients), living in a war zone, poverty, HIV/AIDS, low maternal status, poor breastfeeding habits, and cultural attitudes (e.g., boy infants may be fed more than girl infants).

Homelessness is a major cause of undernutrition in the United States, as is **alcoholism**. Diseases such as depression or other mental illness can cause individuals to stop eating or to refuse to eat a variety of foods. Certain medications can also inhibit the uptake of nutrients from the digestive system, resulting in undernutrition. Certain diseases, such as some cancers and **AIDS**, can cause the body to increase the amount of calories used, resulting in severe wasting, called "cachexia." Protein-energy malnutrition (PEM) is the most dangerous level of undernutrition caused by a shortage of calories and protein.

Causes and symptoms

The root cause of undernutrition is inadequate intake of calories, protein, and micronutrients. Secondary causes are the same as the risk factors previously described. Food shortages, particularly in developing countries, contribute to hunger. Drought is the most common cause of food shortage. Human causes of food shortages accounted for 15% of the problem prior to 1992. Since that year, human causes, such as war, have risen to the point where they account for 35% of food shortages.

Symptoms of undernutrition in children include low birth weight, stunting, wasting, low energy level, slowed physical development, impaired mental development, and frequent serious illnesses. In the elderly, undernutrition can cause weight loss, thinning and drying of the skin, hair loss, constantly feeling cold, confused thinking, frequent falls, and frequent infections. These symptoms often go unrecognized and are attributed to a general decline due to **aging**.

KEY TERMS

Micronutrients—Minerals and vitamins needed in small quantities to maintain health (e.g., iodine).

Stunting—A height more than two standard deviations from the median height for the age in the reference population.

Wasting—Weight more than two standard deviations below that of the median weight for the reference population.

Diagnosis

Examination

Diagnosis is most often made by examination and by comparing the height and weight of the individual to the median height and weight of the reference population. The physician will review drugs the individual is taking and will ask questions about alcohol and food consumption.

Tests

A complete blood count (CBC) generally is done to assess the individual's general health and to look for signs of infections. Blood tests may be done to measure the amount of albumin in the blood. Albumin is a blood protein that decreases when there is an inadequate amount of protein in the diet. Additional tests may be done when a specific vitamin or mineral deficiency is suspected.

Treatment

The only treatment for undernutrition is to increase calories and protein and to replace the micronutrients missing from the diet. In healthcare settings, such as a nursing home or hospital, this can be done in consultation with a registered dietitian. Long-term success in reducing undernutrition generally requires overcoming the barriers that prevent the individual from getting enough calories and enough food variety. This may involve:

- treating any underlying disease or mental condition contributing to the undernutrition
- overcoming barriers to food preparation, for example, by enrolling the individual in Meals on Wheels
- providing a wide range of nutritious food through meals for the homeless, the establishment of inner-city farmers's markets, or providing transportation to local food banks
- using drugs to stimulate the appetite
- enrolling individuals in food-support programs, such as Women Infants and Children (WIC), the Supplementary Nutrition Program (SNAP, formerly food stamps), and the Federal School Lunch program in the United States

In 2010, the **World Health Organization** studied the use of Ready to Use Therapeutic Foods (RUTF) in children who suffered undernutrition during treatment for HIV/AIDS. The researchers concluded that the use of RUTF was associated with a reduction in undernutrition.

Individuals who cannot eat, for example, those who cannot swallow because they have had a **stroke**, may be fed through a tube inserted into the nose and down the esophagus to the stomach. Individuals who do not absorb enough nutrients from the digestive tract may be fed intravenously (total parenteral nutrition). Both of these feeding methods have drawbacks and potentially serious side effects.

Prognosis

Some early effects of undernutrition cannot be reversed. Consistent undernutrition before birth and during the first five years of life often leads to childhood death. In survivors, it has permanent physical and developmental effects. Even if the child later receives adequate nutrition, he or she may remain short of stature and have permanent cognitive deficits. Undernutrition during pregnancy can lead to miscarriage, premature delivery, a low-birthweight baby, maternal susceptibility to disease, and maternal death. Undernutrition in the elderly results in more frequent and more severe illness and infection.

Prevention

The problem of preventing undernutrition is complex. Many international aid agencies work to prevent undernutrition, especially in children. Their goal is to eventually help developing countries develop adequate food resources for the entire population. To do this, they must overcome food delivery, storage, and distribution problems; regional warfare; poverty; illiteracy; and cultural attitudes. UNICEF and **WHO** have made reducing child undernutrition one of their priorities for the twenty-first century.

Exclusive breastfeeding for at least six months with supplemental breastfeeding until age two is recommended for all babies. This is especially important in developing countries where supplies of clean **water** and adequate infant food are limited. According to WHO, appropriately breastfed children in developing countries are six times more likely to survive to age five than those who are not breastfed.

In the United States, treating homelessness, alcoholism, and drug abuse, as well as educating individuals about food security programs that are available to them, are the most effective ways of preventing undernutrition.

Resources

BOOKS

Boyle, Marie A., and Sara Long. *Personal Nutrition.* Belmont, CA: Wadsworth, 2013.

Leathers, Howard D. *The World Food Problem: Toward Ending Undernutrition in the Third World.* Boulder, CO: Lynne Rienner Publishers, 2009.

PERIODICALS

Black, Robert E., et al. "Maternal and Child Undernutrition: Global and Regional Exposures and Health Consequences." *The Lancet.* 371, no. 9608 (January 19, 2008): 243–260. http://www.thelancet.com/journals/lancet/article/PIIS0140-6736%2807%2961690-0/fulltext (accessed October 10, 2010).

Caufield, Laura E., et al. "Undernutrition as an Underlying Cause of Child Death in Diarrhea, Pneumonia, Malaria, and Measles." *American Journal of Clinical Nutrition.* 80 (2004): 193–198. http://www.who.int/nutgrowthdb/publications/risk/en/index.html (accessed October 10, 2010).

Sunguya, Bruno F., et al. "Ready to Use Therapeutic Foods (RUTF) Improves Undernutrition among ART-treated, HIV-positive Children in Dar es Salaam, Tanzania." *Nutrition Journal.* 11:60 (2012).

WEBSITES

World Food Programme. http://www.wfp.org/hunger/who-are (accessed September 25, 2012).

Thomas, David R. "Undernutrition." *Merck Manuals Online.* http://www.merck.com/mmhe/sec12/ch153/ch153a.html (accessed October 10, 2010).

"Tracking Progress on Child and Maternal Nutrition: A Survival and Development Priority." UNICEF. http://www.unicef.org/publications/index_51656.html (accessed October 10, 2010).

"2012 World Hunger and Poverty Facts and Statistics" World Hunger Education Service. http://www.worldhunger.org/articles/Learn/world%20hunger%20facts%202002.htm (accessed September 25, 2012).

ORGANIZATIONS

American Dietetic Association, 120 South Riverside Plaza, Suite 2000, Chicago, IL 60606-6995, (800) 877-1600, http://www.eatright.org

British Nutrition Foundation, High Holborn House, 52-54 High Holborn, London, United Kingdom WC1V 6RQ, 020 7404 6504, Fax: 020 7404 6747, postbox@britishnutrition.org.uk, http://www.britishnutrition.org.uk

World Health Organization, Avenue Appia 20, 1211 Geneva 27, Switzerland, +22 41 791 21 11, Fax: +22 41 791 31 11, info@who.int, http://www.who.int.

Tish Davidson, AM
Rhonda Cloos, RN

Hygiene

Definition

Hygiene is a very general term that refers to any practice that helps to maintain health and prevent the spread of disease. The term is also used in more specific connotations, such as personal hygiene, the maintenance of personal cleanliness; medical hygiene, practices that reduce the risk of spreading disease during the use of medical procedures; dental hygiene, the use of practices that maintain good **dental health**; industrial hygiene, practices that reduce the risk of disease and injury in the workplace; and culinary hygiene, which involves a number of practices involved in food storage, preparation, and service designed to reduce the risk of spreading disease to consumers and food workers.

Purpose

The purpose of all forms of hygiene is to help an individual or community of individuals maintain the highest possible level of health, while specifically avoiding to the greatest extent possible the spread of disease between individuals.

Demographics

Hygienic practices are essential for good health among all people of all races, sexes, ethnicities, and other characteristics, although the challenges in achieving this goal can vary considerably depending on individual circumstances. For example, people with physical handicaps and the elderly may find it significantly more difficult to maintain good personal hygiene because of their own physical and mental limitations.

Origins

Many researchers believe that hygienic practices, in one form or another, are as old as the human species, and perhaps very much older. Many animal species are known to practice cleaning or grooming procedures that could be classified as hygienic. For example, ants clean themselves of fungal **parasites**, bats groom to remove parasites, birds clean their nests of fecal matter, and chimpanzees have been observed cleaning their genitals after mating. Evidence also exists for the presence of hygienic practices among pre-humans. For example, tools and structures found during archeological excavations suggest that Neanerthals shaved, plucked their hair, and used primitive toilets. Within the earliest written records is abundant evidence of the importance placed on personal hygiene in many early civilizations, where ritual bathing and other hygienic practices were not only described, but were praised and even required by some early cultures. Of course, hygienic practices have not always been held in high regard, as some stories from the Middle Ages can attest. However, in most civilized cultures, at least some hygienic practices seem to have been expected among well-educated individuals.

The rise of the modern science of hygienics can be traced to the elucidation of the **germ theory** in the middle of the eighteenth century. One of the most significant events during this period was the effort by Hungarian physician Ignaz Philipp Semmelweis to reduce the death rate among women from puerperal fever by having physicians simply wash their hands between procedures. Semmelweiss had accumulated extensive evidence to show that this sanitary practice dramatically reduced the number of women who developed the disease after being infected by their physician during childbirth. Semmelweiss' suggestion was ignored and disparaged by the medical community, who felt their professionalism was being degraded by such a simplistic practice. Semmelweiss died a broken and despised man, although the value of his suggestion was recognized only shortly after his death. **Handwashing** is now regarded as perhaps the most important single hygienic procedure available both to the medical community and to the general public.

Description

The specific procedures that constitute good hygienic practice differ to some extent depending on the setting in which they are carried out.

EDWIN CHADWICK (1800–1890)

Chadwick's contemporaries called him boring, unreasonable, and overbearing, but he was, in fact, an effective crusader for social change. He devoted his considerable talents to solving public health problems engendered by the Industrial Revolution, and he had the satisfaction of seeing steps taken to address most of the wrongs he sought to correct.

Chadwick was born on January 24, 1800, at Longsight, near the city of Manchester. When he was ten, he and his family moved to London, where he was initially trained in the legal profession. He became acquainted with the great utilitarian philosophers of his time, Jeremy Bentham (1748–1832) and John Stuart Mill (1806–1873), and for a time served as Bentham's personal secretary. Medical reformer Neil Arnott, Chadwick's personal physician, introduced him to the social implications of public hygiene. In 1834, Chadwick was appointed to the Poor Law Commission, which the government established to reform the distribution of relief to the poor. In particular, the commission was appointed to discourage the poor from taking advantage of charity. Maintaining that people without work were just lazy, Parliament had decreed that government relief would be distributed only to people so destitute that their sole option was living in unpleasant workhouses, where they were given onerous and distasteful tasks designed to motivate them to seek other employment. After epidemics of cholera and typhoid broke out in 1837 and 1838, the government turned its attention to the health and hygiene of the working classes, assigning the Poor Law Commission to investigate hygienic conditions in the manufacturing towns of the country.

Because he was unable to get along with the three other members of the Poor Law Commission, Chadwick, who was its secretary, researched and wrote *The Report on the Sanitary Condition of the Labouring Population of Great Britain* (1842) by himself, taking several years to complete it. He sent detailed questionnaires to poor-law guardians throughout the country, and he buttressed the data he collected from them with many eyewitness accounts from doctors who treated the poor. Chadwick also participated personally in inspecting workers' housing in parts of London, Edinburgh, Glasgow, Manchester, Leeds, and Macclesfield. His conclusions represented significant disagreement with the government policy, as well as a departure from his own earlier thinking about the dimensions of poverty, the necessity of poor relief, and how it should be distributed. In fact, his fellow commissioners considered his conclusions too radical and refused to be associated with the report. In particular, Chadwick's approach to sanitary reform called for the greatly increased involvement of local and national governments.

The main purpose of Chadwick's report was to influence public attitudes toward the poor. Because of his controversial conclusions, however, the government would not sponsor its publication, and to take his case to the public Chadwick had to arrange for private publication. As many as 20,000 copies were subsequently sold or given away. *The Times* and *The Morning Chronicle* also published features on Chadwick's report. His first aim was to establish irrefutable evidence of how poor drainage, inadequate water supplies, and overcrowded housing were linked to disease, high mortality rates, and low life expectancy. Chadwick then turned to the economic costs of ill health among the poor before addressing what he felt to be the most damaging effect of poor hygienic conditions: the connection of inadequate housing to gambling, drunkenness, and immorality. Such thinking was profoundly different from his attitudes in the mid 1830s. Like the other Poor Law Commissioners, he had then considered poverty and the resort to charity a result of moral failings, rather than their cause. By the 1840s he had concluded that moral reform could not be accomplished by making work-houses inhospitable, but rather by government programs to improve the housing of the working class.

Chadwick's report instigated a struggle in Parliament that lasted nearly 10 years, and it was a model for later investigations of housing in France and the United States. The most important legislation resulting from Chadwick's report was the Public Health Act of 1848. Although this law only partially addressed the concerns raised by Chadwick's report, it was a step toward reforming the living conditions of the laboring poor. For historians Chadwick's enormous report has provided valuable information about working-class living conditions during the early period of industrialization.

Personal hygiene

The most basic principle in good hygienic practice is to interrupt the pathway by which infectious organisms are transferred from one person or animal to a second person or animal. In the home, this principle leads to the following practices:

- Handwashing, which should be practiced each time a person comes into contact with a possible source of pathogens, such as using the toilet, working in the yard, brushing a pet dog or cat, handling raw food, shaking hands with a stranger, touching a door knob or other object that others may have touched, and similar everyday events. Handwashing generally means washing hands thoroughly with warm, soapy water, but it can also mean using other antimicrobial agents, such as alcoholic solutions.
- Respiratory hygiene, which involves the use of tissues to cover the nose and mouth during sneezing, coughing,

and other actions that result in the release of pathogens from one's respiratory system into the surrounding air. Proper disposal of tissues and handwashing following their use are components of respiratory hygiene.

- Food hygiene, which involves an understanding of the conditions under which pathogens can survive on the food one eats and ways in which to destroy those pathogens. For example, frozen meats should not be allowed to thaw on the kitchen counter as they will go through a temperature range during the process that encourages the growth of any pathogens present in or on the food. Equipment used to prepare one kind of food (such as raw chicken) should not be used to prepare other types of foods (such as salads) because the equipment provides a mechanism for transferring pathogens from one food to the other. In general, the consumption of raw foods should be avoided since no procedure has been used on such foods to kill pathogens that may be present. It should be noted that these "at home" hygienic practices also form the food quality standards required of commercial establishments throughout the United States where food is served (such as restaurants). The difference is that commercial food safety requirements are established by law, are much more stringent, and are much more comprehensive than those that apply to a home kitchen.
- Environmental hygiene refers to any and all practices designed to maintain pathogen-free surfaces within the home. Cleaning around a toilet, for example, is done not just to make a room smell and look better, but, far more important, to destroy pathogens that may be present and might be transferred to human occupants. The full arsenal of cleaning products maintained by a conscientious housekeeper all serve this function in one way or another.
- Animal control hygiene addresses the fact that more than half of the homes in the United States have one or more animal pets, ranging from dogs and cats to guinea pigs and parrots. As beloved as they may be, pets are a reliable repository of a variety of pathogens that can transmit diseases to their human hosts. For this reason, pet-loving should always be paired with handwashing and, from time to time, with animal cleanliness.
- Laundry hygiene involves the routine of washing clothing, bedding, curtains, and other household objects that may provide a habitat for pathogens.
- Water sources include any locations in which water has a tendency to pool because these provide breeding sites for mosquitoes and other disease-carrying vectors. Virtually all households in the United States now have access to potable water. The availability of potable water has somewhat reduced the importance of this factor. Access to potable water is not quite universal for all homes in the United States, In other parts of the world, the majority of inhabitants do not have access to potable water. Experts estimate that only four persons in ten around the world have access to potable water on demand. The majority (six of every ten) must treat their water to render it potable or safe to drink.
- Dental hygiene refers to all activities such as regular flossing and brushing involved in keeping one's teeth and mouth clean. Dental problems are less likely to be of the severity of health issues caused by pathogens found in water, food, and air, but are serious enough considerations in dental health to make dental hygiene a high priority.

KEY TERMS

Hygiene—Any practice or set or practices that maintains good health and prevents the spread of disease.

Pathogen—A microorganisms that causes disease.

Puerperal fever—An infection in women who have just undergone childbirth.

Standard precautions—A minimum set of hygienic practices designed to prevent the spread of infection; also known as universal precautions.

Medical hygiene

Hygienic procedures for medical personnel are more extensive and more stringent than those used in private homes because the very nature of health and medical professions involves contact with individuals who are actual or potential carriers of pathogens. In 1985, largely in response to the HIV/AIDS epidemic, the medical community developed the concept of *standard precautions*, also known as *universal precautions*. These terms refer to a minimum set of hygienic practices designed to prevent the spread of infection. Those minimum practices include:

- hand hygiene, which includes but is not limited to vigorous handwashing
- use of personal protective equipment, such as masks, gloves, and gowns
- safe injection procedures
- safe handling and processing of potentially contaminated surfaces and equipment
- respiratory hygiene of the types previously described

A more detailed description of standard procedures is available from the **World Health Organization** at http://www.who.int/csr/resources/publications/EPR_AM2_E7.pdf.

QUESTIONS TO ASK YOUR DOCTOR

- Are there circumstances in which a person should exceed reasonable boundaries associated with hygienic practices? If so, what are they?
- Do I have reporting obligations or options if I observe members of a health or medical team's NOT adhering or practicing standard precautions?
- How can I know that the restaurants at which I eat maintain proper culinary hygienic standards?
- Are there federal or state standards for hygienic conditions in various types of workplaces? If so, how can I get access to those standards?

Occupational hygiene

Also known as *industrial hygiene*, this field of hygiene encompasses a variety of substances and circumstances encountered within certain industries, but generally not in one's everyday life. Some of the special health concerns with which the occupational hygienist must be concerned and remediate if encountered are dust from wood, metals, earths (soils and clays), and other substances; **radiation** in various forms and emitted from various sources; electrical devices; lights of high intensity; noise; a broad range of solid, liquid, and gaseous chemicals; unusually high or low temperatures; physically restrictive environments; repetitive motion situations; and exposure to a host of potential biological agents.

Resources

BOOKS

Dingwall, Lindsay. *Personal Hygiene Care*. Chichester, UK; Ames, IA: Wiley-Blackwell, 2010.

Roller, Sibel. *Essential Microbiology and Hygiene for Food Professionals*. London: Hodder Arnold, 2012.

Rose, Vernon E., et al. *Patty's Industrial Hygiene*. Hoboken, NJ: Wiley, 2011.

Selendy, Janine M. H. *Water and Sanitation-related Diseases and the Environment: Challenges, Interventions, and Preventive Measures*. Hoboken, NJ: Wiley-Blackwell, 2011.

PERIODICALS

Brown, J., et al. "Water, Sanitation, and Hygiene in Emergencies: Summary Review and Recommendations for Further Research." *Waterlines* 31. 1-2. (2012): 11–29.

Curtis, Valerie A. "A Natural History of Hygiene." *Canadian Journal of Infectious Diseases and Medical Microbiology*. 18. 1. (2007): 11–14.

Gueits, L. "It Takes a Hygiene Village: Together, We Can Turn Hygiene Around." *RDH* 32. 6. (2012): 20–25.

Kelcikova, S., Z. Skodova, and S. Straka. "Effectiveness of Hand Hygiene Education in a Basic Nursing School Curricula." *Public Health Nursing* 29. 2. (2012): 152–9.

WEBSITES

Hand Hygiene in Healtcare Settings. Centers for Disease Control and Prevention. http://www.cdc.gov/handhygiene/ . Accessed on September 14, 2012.

Hygiene. World Health Organization. http://www.who.int/topics/hygiene. Accessed on September 14, 2012.

Personal Hygiene. WebHealthCentre. http://www.webhealthcentre.com/HealthyLiving/personal_hygiene_index.aspx. Accessed on September 14, 2012.

ORGANIZATIONS

Association for Professionals in Infection Control and Epidemiology (APIC), 1275 K St., N.W., Suite 1000, Washington, DC USA 20005–4006, 1 (202) 789–1890, Fax: 1 (202) 789–1899, http://www.apic.org/About-APIC/Contact-Us/Form, http://www.apic.org/.

David E. Newton, Ed.D.

Hypertension

Definition

Hypertension is high blood pressure. Blood pressure is the force of blood pushing against the walls of arteries as it flows through them. Arteries are the blood vessels that carry oxygenated blood from the heart to the body's tissues.

Demographics

Hypertension is a major health problem, especially because it has no symptoms. Many people have hypertension without knowing it. In the United States, about 50 million people age six and older have high blood pressure. Hypertension is more common in men than women and in people over the age of 65 than in younger persons. More than half of all Americans over the age of 65 have hypertension. It also is more common in African Americans than in white Americans.

Description

As blood flows through arteries it pushes against the inside of the artery walls. The more pressure the blood exerts on the artery walls, the higher the blood pressure will be. The size of small arteries also affects the blood pressure. When the muscular walls of arteries are relaxed, or dilated, the pressure of the blood flowing through them is lower than when the artery walls narrow, or constrict.

Blood pressure is highest when the heart beats to push blood out into the arteries. When the heart relaxes to fill with blood again, the pressure is at its lowest point. Blood pressure when the heart beats is called systolic pressure. Blood pressure when the heart is at rest is called diastolic pressure. When blood pressure is measured, the systolic pressure is stated first and the diastolic pressure second. Blood pressure is measured in millimeters of mercury (mm Hg). For example, if a person's systolic pressure is 120 and diastolic pressure is 80, it is written as 120/80 mm Hg. The American Heart Association has long considered blood pressure less than 140 over 90 normal for adults. However, the National Heart, Lung, and Blood Institute in Bethesda, Maryland, released new clinical guidelines for blood pressure in 2003, lowering the standard normal readings. A normal reading was lowered to less than 120 over less than 80.

Hypertension is serious because people with the condition have a higher risk for heart disease and other medical problems than people with normal blood pressure. Serious complications can be avoided by getting regular blood pressure checks and treating hypertension as soon as it is diagnosed.

If left untreated, hypertension can lead to the following medical conditions:

- arteriosclerosis, also called atherosclerosis
- heart attack
- stroke
- enlarged heart
- kidney damage

Arteriosclerosis is hardening of the arteries. The walls of arteries have a layer of muscle and elastic tissue that makes them flexible and able to dilate and constrict as blood flows through them. High blood pressure can make the artery walls thicken and harden. When artery walls thicken, the inside of the blood vessel narrows. Cholesterol and fats are more likely to build up on the walls of damaged arteries, making them even narrower. Blood clots also can get trapped in narrowed arteries, blocking the flow of blood.

Arteries narrowed by arteriosclerosis may not deliver enough blood to organs and other tissues. Reduced or blocked blood flow to the heart can cause a heart attack. If an artery to the brain is blocked, a **stroke** can result.

Hypertension makes the heart work harder to pump blood through the body. The extra workload can make the heart muscle thicken and stretch. When the heart becomes too enlarged it cannot pump enough blood. If the hypertension is not treated, the heart may fail.

The kidneys remove the body's wastes from the blood. If hypertension thickens the arteries to the kidneys, less waste can be filtered from the blood. As the condition worsens, the kidneys fail and wastes build up in the blood. Dialysis or a kidney transplant are needed when the kidneys fail. About 25% of people who receive kidney dialysis have kidney failure caused by hypertension.

Risk factors

Even though the cause of most hypertension is not known, some people have risk factors that increase their chance of developing hypertension. Many of these risk factors can be avoided to lower the chance of developing hypertension or as part of a treatment program to lower blood pressure.

Risk factors for hypertension include:

- age over 60
- male sex
- race
- heredity
- salt sensitivity
- obesity
- inactive lifestyle
- heavy alcohol consumption
- use of oral contraceptives

Some people inherit a tendency for hypertension. People with family members who have hypertension are more likely to develop it than those whose relatives are not hypertensive. People with these risk factors can avoid or eliminate other risk factors to lower their chance of developing hypertension. A 2003 report found that the rise in incidence of high blood pressure among children is most likely due to an increase in the number of overweight and obese children and adolescents.

Causes and symptoms

Many different actions or situations can normally raise blood pressure. Physical activity can temporarily raise blood pressure. Stressful situations can make blood pressure go up; when the **stress** goes away, blood pressure usually returns to normal. These temporary increases in blood pressure are not considered hypertension. A diagnosis of hypertension is made only when a person has multiple high blood pressure readings over a period of time.

The cause of hypertension is not known in 90–95% of the people who have it. Hypertension without a known cause is called primary or essential hypertension.

When a person has hypertension caused by another medical condition, it is called secondary hypertension. Secondary hypertension can be caused by a number of different illnesses. Many people with kidney disorders have secondary hypertension. The kidneys regulate the balance of salt and water in the body. If the kidneys cannot rid the body of excess salt and water, blood pressure goes up. Kidney infections, a narrowing of the arteries that carry blood to the kidneys, called renal artery stenosis, and other kidney disorders can disturb the salt and water balance.

Cushing's syndrome and tumors of the pituitary and adrenal glands often increase levels of the adrenal gland hormones cortisol, adrenalin, and aldosterone, which can cause hypertension. Other conditions that can cause hypertension are blood vessel diseases, thyroid gland disorders, some prescribed drugs, **alcoholism**, and pregnancy.

One of the most dangerous features of hypertension is the fact that it does not usually cause any symptoms. Individuals may not be aware that they have the condition, or they may mistakenly downplay its importance, simply because it is not causing any discernible problems. Without treatment, the deleterious effects of hypertension progress unchecked.

When blood pressure becomes extremely high, for example over 180/110 mmHg (termed malignant hypertension), symptoms such as headache, visual disturbances, anxiety, and shortness of breath may occur. If left untreated, stroke may supervene, or a hypertensive crisis, in which organs cannot receive an adequate blood supply and begin to fail, may occur.

Diagnosis

Examination

Because hypertension does not cause symptoms, it is important to have blood pressure checked regularly. Blood pressure is measured with an instrument called a sphygmomanometer. A cloth-covered rubber cuff is wrapped around the upper arm and inflated. When the cuff is inflated, an artery in the arm is squeezed to momentarily stop the flow of blood. Then, the air is let out of the cuff while a stethoscope placed over the artery is used to detect the sound of the blood spurting back through the artery. This first sound is the systolic pressure, the pressure when the heart beats. The last sound heard as the rest of the air is released is the diastolic pressure, the pressure between heart beats. Both sounds are recorded on the mercury gauge on the sphygmomanometer.

Normal blood pressure is defined by a range of values. Blood pressure lower than 120/80 mm Hg is considered normal. A number of factors such as pain, stress, or anxiety can cause a temporary increase in blood pressure. For this reason, hypertension is not diagnosed on one high blood pressure reading. If a blood pressure reading is 120/80 or higher for the first time, the physician will have the person return for another blood pressure check. Diagnosis of hypertension usually is made based on two or more readings after the first visit.

Systolic hypertension of the elderly is common and is diagnosed when the diastolic pressure is normal or low, but the systolic is elevated, e.g., 170/70 mm Hg. This condition usually co-exists with hardening of the arteries (atherosclerosis).

Blood pressure measurements are classified in stages, according to severity:

- normal blood pressure: less than 120/80 mm Hg
- pre-hypertension: 120–129/80–89 mm Hg
- Stage 1 hypertension: 140–159/90–99 mm Hg
- Stage 2 hypertension: at or greater than 160–179/100–109 mm Hg

A typical physical examination to evaluate hypertension includes:

- medical and family history
- physical examination
- ophthalmoscopy: Examination of the blood vessels in the eye
- chest x-ray
- electrocardiograph (ECG)
- blood and urine tests

The medical and family history help the physician determine if the patient has any conditions or disorders that might contribute to or cause the hypertension. A family history of hypertension might suggest a genetic predisposition for hypertension.

The physical exam may include several blood pressure readings at different times and in different positions. The physician uses a stethoscope to listen to sounds made by the heart and blood flowing through the arteries. The pulse, reflexes, and height and weight are checked and recorded. Internal organs are palpated, or felt, to determine if they are enlarged.

Because hypertension can cause damage to the blood vessels in the eyes, the eyes may be checked with a instrument called an ophthalmoscope. The physician will look for thickening, narrowing, or hemorrhages in the blood vessels.

Tests

A chest x-ray can detect an enlarged heart, other vascular (heart) abnormalities, or lung disease.

An electrocardiogram (ECG) measures the electrical activity of the heart. It can detect if the heart muscle is enlarged and if there is damage to the heart muscle from blocked arteries.

Urine and blood tests may be done to evaluate health and to detect the presence of disorders that might cause hypertension.

Treatment

Traditional

There is no cure for primary hypertension, but blood pressure can almost always be lowered with the correct treatment. The goal of treatment is to lower blood pressure to levels that will prevent heart disease and other complications of hypertension. In secondary hypertension, the disease that is responsible for the hypertension is treated in addition to the hypertension itself. Successful treatment of the underlying disorder may cure the secondary hypertension.

Guidelines advise that clinicians work with patients to agree on blood pressure goals and develop a treatment plan for the individual patient. Actual combinations of medications and lifestyle changes will vary from one person to the next. Treatment to lower blood pressure may include changes in diet, getting regular exercise, and taking antihypertensive medications. Patients falling into the pre-hypertension range who do not have damage to the heart or kidneys often are advised to make lifestyle changes only. A 2003 report of a clinical trial showed that adults with elevated blood pressures lowered them as much as 38% by making lifestyle changes and participating in the DASH diet, which encourages eating more fruit and vegetables.

Drugs

Patients with stage 1 hypertension may be advised to take antihypertensive medication. Numerous drugs have been developed to treat hypertension. The choice of medication depends on the stage of hypertension, side effects, other medical conditions the patient may have, and other medicines the patient is taking.

If treatment with a single medicine fails to lower blood pressure enough, a different medicine may be tried or another medicine may be added to the first. Patients with more severe hypertension may initially be given a combination of medicines to control their hypertension. Combining antihypertensive medicines with different types of action often controls blood pressure with smaller doses of each drug than would be needed for just one.

Antihypertensive medicines fall into several classes of drugs:

- diuretics
- beta-blockers
- calcium channel blockers
- angiotensin converting enzyme inhibitors (ACE inhibitors)
- alpha-blockers
- alpha-beta blockers
- vasodilators
- peripheral acting adrenergic antagonists
- centrally acting agonists

Diuretics help the kidneys eliminate excess salt and water from the body's tissues and the blood. This reduces the swelling caused by fluid buildup in the tissues. The reduction of fluid dilates the walls of arteries and lowers blood pressure. Diuretics are recommended as the first drug of choice for most patients with high blood pressure and as part of any multi-drug combination.

Beta-blockers lower blood pressure by acting on the nervous system to slow the heart rate and reduce the force of the heart's contraction. They are used with caution in patients with heart failure, **asthma**, diabetes, or circulation problems in the hands and feet.

Calcium channel blockers block the entry of calcium into muscle cells in artery walls. Muscle cells need calcium to constrict, so reducing their calcium keeps them more relaxed and lowers blood pressure.

ACE inhibitors block the production of substances that constrict blood vessels. They also help reduce the build-up of water and salt in the tissues. They often are given to patients with heart failure, kidney disease, or diabetes. ACE inhibitors may be used together with diuretics.

Alpha-blockers act on the nervous system to dilate arteries and reduce the force of the heart's contractions.

Alpha-beta blockers combine the actions of alpha and beta blockers.

Vasodilators act directly on arteries to relax their walls so blood can move more easily through them. They lower blood pressure rapidly and are injected in hypertensive emergencies when patients have dangerously high blood pressure.

Peripheral acting adrenergic antagonists act on the nervous system to relax arteries and reduce the force of the heart's contractions. They usually are prescribed together with a diuretic. Peripheral acting adrenergic antagonists can cause slowed mental function and lethargy.

Centrally acting agonists also act on the nervous system to relax arteries and slow the heart rate. They are usually used with other antihypertensive medicines.

Home remedies

Lifestyle changes that may reduce blood pressure by 5 to 10 mm Hg include:

- reducing salt intake
- reducing fat intake
- losing weight
- getting regular exercise
- quitting smoking
- reducing alcohol consumption
- managing stress

Prognosis

There is no cure for hypertension. However, it can be well controlled with proper treatment. Therapy with a combination of lifestyle changes and antihypertensive medicines can keep blood pressure at levels that will not cause damage to the heart or other organs. The key to avoiding serious complications of hypertension is to detect and treat it before damage occurs. Because antihypertensive medicines control blood pressure, but do not cure it, patients must continue taking the medications to maintain reduced blood pressure levels and avoid complications.

Prevention

Prevention of hypertension centers on avoiding or eliminating known risk factors. Even persons at risk because of age, race, or sex or those who have an inherited risk can lower their chance of developing hypertension.

Resources

BOOKS

Goldman, L., and D. Ausiello, eds. *Cecil Textbook of Internal Medicine*, 23rd ed. Philadelphia: Saunders, 2008.

Libby, P., et al. *Braunwald's Heart Disease*, 8th ed. Philadelphia: Saunders, 2007.

PERIODICALS

McNamara, Damian. "Obesity Behind Rise in Incidence of Primary Hypertension." *Family Practice News*, April 1, 2003: 45–51.

McNamara, Damian. "Trial Shows Efficacy of Lifestyle Changes for BP: More Intensive Than Typical Office Visit." *Family Practice News*, July 1, 2003: 1–2.

"New BP Guidelines Establish Diagnosis of Pre-hypertension: Level Seeks to Identify At-risk Individuals Early." *Case Management Advisor*, July 2003: S1.

"New Hypertension Guidelines: JNC-7." *Clinical Cardiology Alert*, July 2003: 54–63.

ORGANIZATIONS

American Heart Association, 7272 Greenville Avenue, Dallas, TX 75231, (800) 242-8721, http://www.americanheart.org

National Heart, Lung and Blood Institute, P.O. Box 30105, Bethesda, MD 20824-0105, (301) 592-8573, Fax: (240) 629-3246, nhlbiinfo@nhlbi.nih.gov, http://www.nhlbi.nih.gov

Texas Heart Institute, P.O. Box 20345, Houston, TX 77225-0345, (800) 292-2221, hic@heart.thi.tmc.edu, http://www.texasheart.org.

Toni Rizzo
Teresa G. Odle

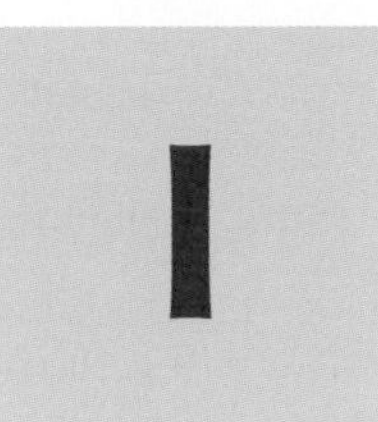

Immunization

Definition

Immunization is the process that makes an individual immune to infection. A **vaccination** is a type of immunization.

Demographics

Certain types of immunizations are administered in infancy and childhood and offer lifelong protection, while other types of immunization, such as the vaccine for **tetanus**, must be given according to a certain schedule throughout life.

Description

When an immunization enters a person's body, the body reacts as if it received a major attack by the infectious agent, even though, in reality, it received a small, and likely, an inactive amount of that agent. This process creates a response that builds immunity to the infectious agent.

Origins

The first vaccination, which was for **smallpox**, was invented by Edward Jenner, an army surgeon, in 1796. Jenner came up with the term "vaccination" based on the latin *vacca*, which means "cow" because the inoculation he used was cow-pox.

Precautions

Immunization carries some risk of side effects, mostly minor, but which may be more serious. A person who has an allergy to any component in a vaccination should not have that vaccine. Pregnant women or any person with a chronic disease should check with a physician or health care provider before receiving a vaccine. There may be side effects and risks with a vaccination. Before having a vaccination, a person should discuss these risks with his or her physician or health care provider.

The National Injury Compensation Program has been established to help families cover costs associated with caring for persons who have experienced harmful reactions to vaccines. The website for this program is www.hrsa.gov/vaccinecompensation.

Effect on public health

In the **Center for Disease Control and Prevention's** list of the 10 great public health achievements in the 20th century in the United States, vaccination was ranked number one. Cited were the elimination of smallpox and **polio**, as well as the control of numerous other infectious diseases in the United States and other portions of the world.

Vaccinations

Vaccination is a common way to immunize.

Bucillus Calmette-Gužrin (BCG)

BCG is a vaccine that provides immunity against **tuberculosis** (TB). It may be given to a person who has a high likelihood of contracting TB. BCG is also used as a treatment for **cancer** of the bladder. In the United States, BCG, which is a live vaccine, is only given to persons who are at high risk of tuberculosis. It was first given to humans in 1921.

Used as a vaccine against TB, BCG is injected by needle into the skin. The area where the vaccine was injected must be kept dry for 24 hours. BCG is usually given in one dose, and immunity is later detected via a tuberculin skin test. Two to three months after the vaccine is administered, it may be repeated if the skin test does not indicate immunity.

Side effects that may result from BCG include swelling of the lymph nodes, small red areas at the injection site, fever, blood in urine, painful or frequent urination, stomach upset, and vomiting. Serious side effects, which must be reported to a health care professional immediately, include a severe skin rash, difficulty swallowing or breathing, or wheezing.

TUBERCULOSIS. Tuberculosis (TB) is a disease caused by *Mycobacterium tuberculosis*. TB bacteria may attack any part of the body (kidney, spine, and brain), but they usually attack the lungs. If a person with TB does not receive adequate treatment, he or she may die as a result of the disease.

TB spreads via the air when infected persons sneeze, cough, talk, or sing. A person may be infected with TB without becoming ill; therefore, there are two forms of the disease: latent TB infection and TB disease.

Symptoms include a serious cough that persists for three weeks or longer, chest **pain**, blood or sputum in the cough, weakness, fatigue, loss of weight, lack of appetite, chills, fever, and night sweats.

A person is at higher risk for TB if he or she has HIV, has been infected with TB bacteria within two years, experiences other health problems such as diabetes, is a substance abuser, or has a past history of improperly treated TB. TB is diagnosed via skin testing and blood tests. Treatment is achieved through medications that must be taken for six to nine months.

BCG EFFECTIVENESS. In a United Kingdom study that spanned eight years (1999 to 2007) and involved children ages seven to 14 years, BCG vaccine's effectiveness was 25%.

Chickenpox vaccine

Chickenpox vaccine prevents chickenpox, which is a viral disease that is also called varicella. The vaccine is given in two doses: once at 12 to 15 months and the second dose at four to six years of age. Persons who are at least 13 years of age and who have never had chickenpox or the vaccine should be vaccinated in two doses. The dosing should be at least 28 days apart.

Those who have had a life-threatening allergic reaction to a previous dose of the vaccine or to gelatin or to neomycin (antibiotic) should not have the vaccine. The vaccine should not be given to pregnant women until after childbirth. Women should not become pregnant for one month after the vaccine. Persons with certain risks such as lowered immunity should check with their health care provider before receiving the vaccine.

The vaccine may lead to soreness or swelling at the injection site, fever, or a mild rash. More serious side effects include seizure related to the fever and **pneumonia**, which is very rare. There have been reports of serious brain reactions and low blood count following vaccine administration. The incidence is very rare and experts in the field are unable to determine whether or not they were related to the vaccine.

In 2005, the MMRV (measles/mumps/rubella/varicella) vaccine was licensed.

CHICKENPOX. Chickenpox is a viral illness, which is common during childhood. Symptoms include a rash that itches as well as fever and fatigue. It is spread through the air or via contact with fluid from the chickenpox blisters. Later in life, a person who previously had chickenpox can get **shingles**, which is a painful rash.

CHICKENPOX VACCINE EFFECTIVENESS. Prior to the chickenpox vaccine, approximately 11,000 people were hospitalized for the illness in the United States each year, and 100 died per year. According to the **Centers for Disease Control and Prevention (CDC)**, most people who receive the chickenpox vaccine will not get the disease. If a vaccinated person does get the illness, he or she usually has a very mild case with fewer blisters, less likelihood of fever, and a more rapid recovery.

Influenza vaccine (seasonal flu vaccine)

According to the CDC, the seasonal flu vaccine is recommended yearly for persons ages six months and up. It is particularly important for persons who are at increased risk of **influenza** and their close contacts, including persons who work in the healthcare industry as well as those who are in close contact with infants younger than six months of age. People should not get the vaccine if they are ill, and should wait until they recover. A brand of inactivated flu vaccine, which is called Afluria, should not be given to children under eight years of age unless special circumstances exist. This type of vaccine was related to fevers and fever-related seizures in Australia. A parent should discuss this issue with the child's physician.

The vaccine is given in one dose. It is available as an inactivated vaccine in injection form or as a live, attenuated (weakened) form via nasal spray. The nasal spray version is not recommended for certain age groups or individuals who have certain chronic diseases, including persons under age two or age 50 and older. Persons age 65 and up should ask their physician for information regarding a high dose influenza vaccine. Depending on the strain of flu that is prevalent during a flu season, the vaccination changes, explaining why it is necessary to have a vaccination yearly.

The flu vaccine takes approximately two weeks to become effective, and is administered yearly because protection lasts about 12 months.

Persons should discuss risks with their doctor. A person who has an allergy to eggs or to any ingredient (including thimerosal) may be advised not to have the vaccine. A thimerosal-free version is available. One who has had Gullain-Barrž syndrome must discuss with a physician whether or not to have the vaccine.

Seasonal influenza

Mild side effects include soreness, redness or swelling at the site of injection; hoarseness; itchy, sore, red eyes; cough; fever; aches; headache; fatigue; or itching. These issues usually appear shortly after the injection is given, and last a few days.

If a child has an inactivated flu vaccine at the same time he or she has a pneumococcal vaccine, there is a higher risk for seizure caused by fever. A parent should ask the child's physician for information on this topic.

Severe side effects include allergic reactions that are life-threatening. This is very rare and usually occurs within a few minutes to a few hours following the injection. In 1976, Guillain-Barrž Syndrome was associated with a type of flu vaccine. Risk in current vaccines, if it exists, is one or two cases per million people who get the vaccine. Consumers should discuss this with their physician prior to having the vaccine.

Influenza can strike anyone; children are most vulnerable. Those at highers risk of complications from influenza are young children, people with certain chronic health conditions, those 65 and up, and pregnant women.

Symptoms generally come on suddenly and include sore throat, fever and chills, achy muscles, cough, fatigue, headache, and runny nose or congestion. Pneumonia is a complication that can be very serious. Thousands of people die each year from the flu.

Influenza vaccine effectiveness

The effectiveness of the flu vaccine varies by year, depending on how closely the vaccine matches the virus circulating in a given year. More data exists for the live attenuated version (nasal spray) than the inactivated flu vaccine. According to one large study reported by the CDC, the nasal spray effectiveness was 92% when compared with a placebo.

Tdap

Tdap is a vaccine that protects against tetanus (lockjaw), **diphtheria**, and pertussis (**whooping cough**). A form of the vaccine has been used for decades, although the Tdap vaccine was licensed in 2005. Another form of the vaccine, Td, protects against tetanus and diphtheria (not pertussis).

Vaccination begins in infancy. DTaP is a vaccine that helps children younger than age 7 develop immunity to three deadly diseases caused by bacteria: diphtheria, tetanus, and whooping cough (pertussis). Tdap is a booster immunization given at age 11 that offers continued protection from those diseases for adolescents and adults. Adults receive a Td booster (tetanus-diptheria) every 10 years; however, they may have a Tdap or Td booster following a serious laceration or burn. Tdap is used for any person who did not previously have the vaccine. Td is used if Tdap is unavailable or if a person already had a Tdap vaccine, for children ages seven to nine years who already finished the DTaP series, or adults age 65 and up. Pregnant women who never received Tdap should have the vaccine after week 20 of gestation or, preferably, in the third trimester. If a pregnant woman already received Tdap and the need for a tetanus or diphtheria vaccine arises during pregnancy, she should receive the Td vaccine.

Tdap or Td should not be given to those who had a life-threatening allergic reaction to a previous vaccine containing tetanus, diphtheria, or pertussis; or any person who experienced a coma or long or multiple seizures within a seven day period after DTP or DTaP (these individuals may receive Td).

After Td, a person may rarely experience a fever higher than 102F. In Tdap or Td, the person may have significant swelling of the arm where the injection was given.

TETANUS, DIPHTHERIA, AND PERTUSSIS. Tetanus, also called lockjaw, consists of painful spasms of the muscles, as well as stiffness, in all parts of the body. The muscles in the head and neck may tighten to the extent that the person infected cannot open his or her mouth to swallow or breathe. One out of five people with tetanus die as a result of the infection. A person becomes infected with tetanus, which is caused by bacteria, after the pathogen gains entry to the body via a cut, scratch, or wound.

Diphtheria, which is also caused by bacteria, causes the formation of a thick membrane, which covers the back of the throat. The disease leads to problems breathing, paralysis, heart failure, and death.

Pertussis is an infection in which severe coughing can make breathing difficult and lead to vomiting and difficulty sleeping. Up to two out of 100 adolescents with pertussis and up to five out of 100 adults with the disease are hospitalized or experience complications such as pneumonia and death. The coughing is so violent that it may result in fractured ribs, incontinence, and loss of weight.

DTAP EFFECTIVENESS. In the United States, there were up to 200,000 cases of diphtheria and pertussis before the vaccines were readily available, as well as hundreds of tetanus cases. Now that the vaccines are routinely administered, cases of diphtheria and tetanus have been reduced by approximately 99% and pertussis cases have gone down by approximately 92%.

Haemophilus influenza type b (Hib) vaccine

Haemophilus influenza (Hib) vaccines are recommended for children in three to four doses (depending on the brand of Hib vaccine used) beginning at two months of age and ending at 12 to 15 months of age. In some cases, older children or adults who have certain health conditions should get the vaccine.

The most common side effects of Hib vaccination are redness, warmth, or swelling at the injection site, and fever. These issues may last two to three days. A severe reaction would be a serious allergic reaction, high fever, or changes in behavior.

***HAEMOPHILUS INFLUENZA* TYPE B ILLNESS.** *Haemophilus influenza* (Hib) disease is a serious bacterial infection that usually occurs in children under five years of age. It is a serious form of **meningitis** that can result in brain damage and deafness. Hib may also cause pneumonia; severe swelling of the throat so that it is difficult to breathe; infections of the blood, joints, bones, and covering of the heart; and death.

***HAEMOPHILUS INFLUENZA* TYPE B VACCINE EFFECTIVENESS.** Prior to the Hib vaccine, the disease was the leading cause of bacterial meningitis in children under five years of age in the United States. Each year, approximately 20,000 children in the United States developed severe cases of Hib and nearly 1,000 died. The vaccine has significantly reduced the number of cases.

Hepatitis A and B vaccines

The vaccine for **hepatitis** A prevents hepatitis A. The vaccine is given to children at 12 months of age through 23 months, as well as others who are at high risk of infection. Travelers should start the series of hepatitis A vaccines at least one month prior to travel. Some travelers who cannot obtain the vaccine prior to leaving may get an injection of immune globulin (IG), for temporary, but immediate, protection.

Hepatitis A vaccine should not be given to those with an allergic reaction to a previous dose, or to others who have a serious (life threatening) allergy to a component, or to latex. Hepatitis A vaccines contain alum, and some contain 2-phenoxyethanol. Persons who are ill should not receive the vaccine until they are well. A pregnant woman should discuss hepatitis A vaccination with her doctor.

Two doses of the hepatitis A vaccine are needed for long-term protection. The doses should be administered six months apart.

The vaccine for hepatitis B disease prevents hepatitis B. Starting in 1982, the vaccine was recommended for some adults and children in the United States. As of 1991, it has been recommended for all children in the United States.

HEPATITIS A AND B ILLNESSES. Hepatitis A is a severe liver disease, which is caused by the hepatitis A virus (HAV). HAV may be present in the feces of infected people. It is spread via close personal contact or ingesting food or **water** containing HAV. It appears as a flu type of illness. Yellowing skin and eyes (jaundice) and dark colored urine are present. Children may have severe stomach pain and diarrhea. The disease is so serious that it leads to hospitalization in 10% of its victims. Approximately three to six out of 1,000 people who have hepatitis die as a result of the disease.

Hepatitis B is a viral infection of the liver. The infection is quite serious and can lead to cirrhosis or cancer of the liver, which kills approximately 2,000 to 4,000 people each year. In 2009, hepatitis B infected approximately 39,000 people.

Hepatitis B can be an acute (short-term) illness or a chronic (long-term) infection. Symptoms of the acute form are lack of appetite; fatigue; muscle, joint, and stomach pains; vomiting and diarrhea; and yellowing of the skin or eyes (jaundice). The chronic form of hepatitis B is more commonly seen in infants and children rather than adults. In the United States, up to 1.4 million people have chronic hepatitis B. It is spread through contact with an infected person's blood or body fluids. A person may also be infected after contact with an object that has been contaminated, such as a needle.

Persons up to age 18 years who have not received the vaccine should get it. Adults at risk for hepatitis B should have the vaccination. This group includes sexual partners of persons with hepatitis B as well as those who use injectable street drugs; people who have had more than one sexual partner; those with chronic diseases of the liver or kidney; people under age 60 who have diabetes; and people whose employment exposes them to human blood or body fluids.

HEPATITIS A AND B VACCINE EFFECTIVENESS. The vaccine for hepatitis A is effective in preventing the disease.

Since 1990, new cases of hepatitis B in children and adolescents have dropped by more than 95%. New cases have dropped by 75% in other age categories.

The hepatitis B vaccine provides long-term protection from hepatitis B; in fact, protection may be lifelong.

HPV

Bivalent vaccine (Cervarix) and quadrivalent vaccine (Gardisil) are the two vaccines that prevent human papillomavirus (**HPV**). This virus is the cause behind most cancers of the cervix. Gardisil also prevents the type of HPV that causes most genital warts.

HPV vaccination is recommended for females ages 13 through 26 years who have not been vaccinated. The vaccine can be given as young as nine years of age. It is ideal to administer it before a girl becomes sexually active, although girls who are sexually active may find some benefit from the vaccine. The vaccine is not recommended for pregnant women.

As of June 2012, more than 46 million doses of HPV vaccine have been administered.

Side effects include pain at the injection site, fever, dizziness, nausea, and fainting. Because fainting can cause an injury, the patient sits or lies down for 15 minutes after the vaccine is administered.

Gardisil is safe and effective for males ages nine to 26 years. It is recommended for males ages 13 to 21 years who have not been previously vaccinated.

As of July 2012, the vaccine has a retail cost of $130 per dose in the United States, or $390 for the full series of three doses. Most health insurances cover the cost, but consumers should contact their health insurance company to determine coverage.

HPV DISEASE. HPV is the most common sexually transmitted disease. More than 40 types of HPV can infect males and females in their genitals, mouth, and throat. HPV is not the same as **herpes** or HIV, but it can be transmitted via sexual activity.

In 90% of cases, the infection resolves within two years. In some cases, the infection persists and appears as genital warts or warts in the throat (rare), which is called recurrent respiratory papillomatosis, or RRP. HPV can also lead to cancer of the cervix, as well as less common cancers such as cancer of the vulva, vagina, penis, anus, and back of the throat.

HPV EFFECTIVENESS. Both of the HPV vaccines are highly effective in preventing the HPV types for which they were designed, along with the common health issues that arise with these forms of HPV. The effectiveness is less if the female has already been exposed to at least one type of HPV. The vaccine does not treat existing HPV infection. The vaccine is believed to offer long-term protection.

MMR

The MMR vaccine protects individuals against **measles**, **mumps**, and **rubella**, which are all viruses. In 2005, the MMRV (measles/mumps/rubella/varicella) vaccine was licensed, which also protects against varicella (chickenpox). MMRV may be given in two doses to children between 12 to 15 months of age (first dose) and four to six years of age (second dose).

Most common side effects of the vaccine are fever, mild rash, and swollen glands in the cheeks or the neck. There is a small increased risk of seizure associated with the fever in children who are younger than seven years of age. The three vaccines are given in one injection.

MEASLES, MUMPS AND RUBELLA DISEASES. Measles, mumps, and rubella are viral illnesses, which were common in childhood prior to the availability of vaccines. Outbreaks still occur in Western Europe, Asia, the South Pacific, and Africa.

Measles is highly contagious and affects the respiratory system. It is also called rubeola. Symptoms include fever, runny nose, cough, and rash that covers the body. About 10% of children with measles also get an ear infection and about 5% get pneumonia.

Rubella, which is also known as German measles, is a mild, three-day form of measles. The child may have a sore throat, while an adult may a headache, conjunctivitis, and discomfort for about one to five days before a rash appears. Adults may also have complications such as swollen joints. A very rare complication, called **encephalitis**, may occur in adults who have rubella. The most serious consequence of rubella in adults is its affect on the fetus of a pregnant woman. It can cause serious **birth defects**, such as heart problems, loss of hearing and vision, intellectual disability, and damage to the liver or spleen. If the woman gets rubella earlier in pregnancy, the birth defects are likely to be more serious. Rubella during pregnancy can also cause a woman to have a miscarriage or premature birth.

Mumps is a contagious childhood disease, which is caused by the mumps virus. It begins with fever, headache, muscle aches, fatigue, and lack of appetite. The next stage involves swelling of the salivary glands.

MMR EFFECTIVENESS. The vaccines stopped cases of measles from developing in the United States. Between 2001 and 2010, there were about 70 cases per year. In 2011, there were more than double the cases because of an increase in measles in Europe, Asia, and Africa. Most of these cases were seen in persons in the United States who were not vaccinated.

According to the CDC, people in the United States are protected from measles if they tested positive in a measles antibody test or were born in the United States prior to 1957 or had two doses of MMR vaccine.

In 2004, it was declared that rubella was eliminated from the United States; however, it is still common in other countries and can be carried to the United States by visitors.

Mumps was quite common in the United States prior to vaccination. At this point, it is very rare in the United States.

Polio vaccination

There are two main types of polio vaccination: inactivated (IPV) and oral polio vaccine (OPV). IPV has been used in the United States since 2000, and is given by injection into the leg or arm, depending on the age of the patient. OPV, which was given by mouth, has not been used in the United States since 2000, but this form of the vaccination is still used in other areas of the world.

Polio vaccination is given to children, who get four doses of IPV, and then a booster dose between the ages of four and six years.

POLIO DISEASE. Polio is an **infectious disease** caused by a virus, which survives in the throat and intestines of its victims. It is spread through contact with the stool of an infected person as well as through oral or nasal secretions.

In the United States, most people who had polio had no symptoms. Less than 1% developed paralysis from the disease, resulting in permanent disability.

POLIO VACCINE EFFECTIVENESS. Polio was very common in the United States before the introduction of the vaccine in 1955, infecting thousands of people. At the peak of the disease in 1952, there were 21,000 reported cases and many deaths from the disease. The number of cases dropped dramatically after the Salk vaccine was issued in 1955, and was further reduced when the oral Sabin vaccine came about in 1961. The last cases of paralytic polio in the United States were in 1979. The most recent case, from outside the country, was in 1993. The disease has been eliminated from the United States and the Western Hemisphere.

Pneumococcal vaccine

Pneumococcal conjugate vaccine is recommended for children less than five years of age as well as children at high risk who are more than two years of age. It is also given to adults age 65 years and up, and younger adults with certain risk factors such as certain chronic illnesses or immune disorders.

PNEUMOCOCCAL DISEASE. Pneumococcal disease is an infection that is caused by *Streptococcus pneumonia*. Symptoms of pneumococcal pneumonia include fever, cough, shortness of breath, and chest pain. Symptoms of pneumococcal meningitis include stiff neck, fever, mental confusion and disorientation, and photophobia (sensitivity to light). Symptoms of pneumococcal bloodstream infection are similar to the symptoms found in pneumonia and meningitis, and also include joint pain and chills. Symptoms of otitis media (ear infection) are pain in the ear, red or swollen eardrum, and fever, irritability, and inability to sleep.

Pneumococcal disease can result in long-term health problems such as brain damage, loss of hearing, and loss of limb. It can also be fatal. The disease, which is caused by a type of bacteria, is spread by coughing, sneezing, or contact with respiratory secretions.

PNEUMOCOCCAL VACCINE EFFECTIVENESS. The pneumococcal vaccine is effective at preventing severe forms of the disease, hospitalization, and death, but it does not prevent the infection and symptoms in all people who have the vaccine.

In a severe **pandemic**, vaccination may prevent more than one million deaths from pneumococcal disease.

Resources

BOOKS

Brunette, Gary W., Ed. *CDC Health Information for International Travel 2012: The Yellow Book*. New York, NY: Oxford University Press, 2012.

PERIODICALS

Pereira, Susan M., et.al. "Effectiveness and Cost-Effectiveness of First BCG Vaccination Against Tuberculosis in School-Age Children Without Previous Turberculin Test (BCG-REVAC trial): A Cluster-Randomized Trial." *The Lancet Infectious Diseases* 12, no. 4 (2012).

Rubin, Jaime L., et.al. "Public Health and Economic Impact of Vaccination with 7-valent pneumococcal vaccine (PCV7) in the Context of the Annual Influenza Epidemic and a Severe Influenza Pandemic." *BMC Infectious Diseases* 10, no. 14 (2010): 300-306.

WEBSITES

Chickenpox Vaccine: What You Need to Know. Centers for Disease Control and Prevention. http://www.cdc.gov/vaccines/pubs/vis/downloads/vis-varicella.pdf (accessed September 30, 2012).

Edward Jenner and the Discovery of Vaccination. University Libraries Rare Books & Special Collections, University of South Carolina. library.sc.edu/spcoll/nathist/jenner.html (accessed September 30, 2012).

Flu Vaccine Effectiveness: Questions and Answers for Health Professionals. http://www.cdc.gov/flu/professionals/vaccination/effectivenessqa.htm (accessed September 30, 2012).

Hepatitis A Vaccine: What You Need to Know. Centers for Disease Control and Prevention. http://www.cdc.gov/vaccines/pubs/vis/downloads/vis-hep-a.pdf (accessed September 30, 2012).

Hepatitis B Vaccine: What You Need to Know. Centers for Disease Control and Prevention. http://www.cdc.gov/

vaccines/pubs/vis/downloads/vis-hep-b.pdf (accessed September 30, 2012).

HPV Vaccine Information for Young People. Centers for Disease Control and Prevention. http://www.cdc.gov/std/hpv/stdfact-hpv-vaccine-young-women.htm (accessed September 30, 2012).

Influenza Vaccine Inactivated: What You Need to Know. Centers for Disease Control and Prevention.http://www.cdc.gov/vaccines/pubs/vis/downloads/vis-flu.pdf (accessed September 30, 2012).

MMR: What You Need to Know. Centers for Disease Control and Prevention.http://www.cdc.gov/vaccines/pubs/vis/downloads/vis-mmr.pdf (accessed September 30, 2012).

MMRV: What You Need to Know. Centers for Disease Control and Prevention.http://www.cdc.gov/vaccines/pubs/vis/downloads/vis-mmrv.pdf (accessed September 30, 2012).

Pneumococcal Disease in Short. Centers for Disease Control and Prevention.http://www.cdc.gov/vaccines/vpd-vac/pneumo/in-short-both.htm (accessed September 30, 2012).

Polio. National Network for Immunization Information. http://www.immunizationinfo.org/vaccines/polio (accessed September 30, 2012).

Polio Vaccination. Centers for Disease Control and Prevention. http://www.cdc.gov/vaccines/vpd-vac/polio/default.htm (accessed September 30, 2012).

Seasonal Influenza (Flu). Centers for Disease Control and Prevention.http://www.cdc.gov/flu/about/qa/nasalspray.htm (accessed October 1, 2012).

Td or Tdap: What You Need to Know. Centers for Disease Control and Prevention. http://www.cdc.gov/vaccines/pubs/vis/downloads/vis-td-tdap.pdf (accessed September 30, 2012).

ORGANIZATIONS

Centers for Disease Control and Prevention, 1600 Clifton Road, Atlanta, GA 30333, (800) CDC-INFO (232-4636), cdcinfo@cdc.gov, http://www.cdc.gov

National Vaccine Injury Compensation Program, Parklawn Building, Room 11C-26, 5600 Fishers Lane, Rockville, MD 20857, (800) 338-2382, http://www.hrsa.gov/vaccinecompensation/index.html.

Rhonda LAST, RN

Required nutrients for infant formula

Nutrient	Minimum per 100 calories	Maximum per 100 calories
Protein (g)[1]	1.8 g	4.5 g
Fat	3.3 g 30% calories	6 g 54% calories
Essential fatty acids (linoleate)	300 mg 2.7% calories	
Vitamins		
A	250 IU (75 mcg)	750 IU (225 mcg)
D	40 IU	100 IU
K[2]	4 mcg	
E[3]	0.7 IU	
C (ascorbic acid)	8 mg	
B1 (thiamine)	40 mcg	
B2 (riboflavin)	60 mcg	
B6 (pyridoxine)[4]	35 mcg	
B12	0.15 mcg	
Niacin[5]	250 mcg	
Folic acid	4 mcg	
Pantothenic acid	300 mcg	
Biotin[6]	1.5 mcg	
Choline[6]	7 mg	
Inositol[6]	4 mg	
Minerals		
Calcium[7]	60 mg	
Phosphorus[7]	30 mg	
Magnesium	6 mg	
Iron	0.15 mg	3 mg
Iodine	5 mcg	75 mcg
Zinc	0.5 mg	
Copper	60 mcg	
Manganese	5 mcg	
Sodium	20 mcg	60 mcg
Potassium	80 mg	200 mg
Chloride	55 mg	150 mg

[1]Amounts apply to proteins with a biological quality equivalent to or better than that of casein. If the quality is less than that of casein, the minimum amount must be increased—e.g., formula containing protein with a biological quality of 75% of casein will need at least 2.4 grams of protein (1.8/0.75). All formulas must use a protein with a biological quality of at least 70% of casein's.
[2]Added vitamin K must be in the form of phylloquinone.
[3]Must be 0.7 IU per gram of linoleic acid.
[4]At least 15 mcg for each gram of protein (past the required 1.8 g).
[5]Includes niacin (nicotinic acid) and niacinamide (nicotinamide).
[6]Required only for non-milk-based infant formulas.
[7]The ratio of calcium to phosphorus in infant formula must be no less than 1.1 but not more than 2.0.

SOURCE: U.S. Food and Drug Administration.

(Table by PreMediaGlobal. © 2013 Cengage Learning.)

Infant nutrition

Definition

Children between the ages of birth and one year are considered infants. Infants grow rapidly and have special nutritional requirements that are different from other age groups.

Purpose

Infant **nutrition** is designed to meet the special needs of very young children and to give them a healthy start in life. Children under one year old do not have fully mature organ systems. They need nutrition that is easy to digest and contains enough calories, **vitamins**, minerals, and other nutrients to allow them to grow and develop

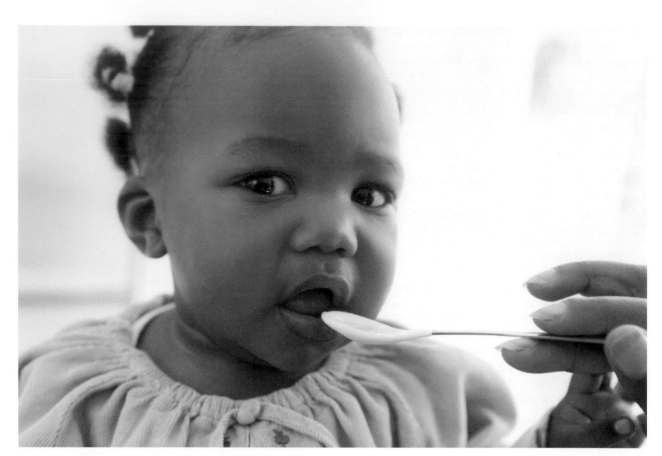

An infant being fed. *(Monkey Business Images/Shutterstock.com)*

normally. Infants also need to receive the proper amount of fluids for their immature kidneys to process wastes. In addition, infant nutrition involves avoiding exposing infants to substances that are harmful to their growth and development.

Description

Infancy is a time of incredibly rapid growth and development. Ensuring that infants get the right kinds of nutrients in the right quantities and avoid the wrong kinds of substances gives them their best chance at a healthy start to life. Parents and caregivers are responsible for seeing that their infant's nutritional needs are met. Infant nutrition is so important that the U.S. Department of Agriculture (USDA) has developed the Women, Infants, and Children (WIC) program. This program provides free health and social service referrals, nutrition counseling, and vouchers for healthy foods to supplement the diet of pregnant and breastfeeding women, infants, and children up to age five who are low-income and nutritionally at risk. In 2010, WIC served about 9.17 million people, including 2.17 million infants, 4.86 million children, and 2.14 million pregnant and nursing women.

Breast-feeding

Human milk is uniquely suited to meet the nutrition needs of newborns. Many health organizations, including the American Academy of Pediatrics (AAP), the American Medical Association (AMA), the Academy of Nutrition and Dietetics (formerly the American Dietetic Association), and the **World Health Organization (WHO)** support the position that breast milk is the best and most complete form of nutrition for infants. The AAP recommends that infants be exclusively breastfed for the first 6 months of life and that breast-feeding should continue for at least 12 months.

Breast-feeding in the United States slowly increased in acceptance in the last decade of the twentieth century. In 1998, 64% of American mothers breastfed their babies for a short time after birth, but only 29% were still breast-feeding by the time their baby was 6 months old. One of the goals of Healthy People 2000, a set of health goals for the nation developed by the U.S. **Department of Health and Human Services**, was for 75% of American women to breast-feed their babies for a period immediately after birth and for 50% to breast-feed for the first 6 months of their infant's life. Women were divided into groups based on ethnicity, but none of the groups met the target. The next initiative, Healthy People 2010, eliminated the ethnic categories, but the goals stayed the same, with the addition of a third target: 75% to breast-feed for a period after birth, 50% to breast-feed for 6 months, and 25% to breast-feed for a full year.

ADVANTAGES OF BREAST-FEEDING. Research comparing formula-fed and breast-fed babies convincingly shows that both full-term and premature breast-fed infants have certain advantages over formula-fed infants. One of the most important advantages conferred by breast milk is an increased resistance to infection.

Infants are born with immature immune systems that do not become fully functional for about two years. Since immune system cells make antibodies to fight infection, having incompletely developed immune systems leaves infants vulnerable to many bacterial and viral infections. However, nursing mothers have fully developed immune systems, and many of the antibodies and other components of the immune system are passed into breast milk. Nursing infants take in their mother's antibodies along with the other nutrients when they nurse. These antibodies survive passage through the infant's digestive system and are absorbed into the infant's blood, where they help protect against infection. Well-designed studies have repeatedly documented the fact that breast-fed babies have fewer ear infections, bouts of diarrhea, respiratory infections, and cases of **meningitis** than formula-fed babies. Overall, the death rate of breast-fed babies during the first year of life is lower than the death rate of formula-fed babies.

Another way that breast-feeding protects against infection is by helping prevent exposure to waterborne contaminants. In developing countries, **water** supplies are often contaminated with bacteria and chemicals. Using this water to mix formula increases the risk of the baby ingesting these pathogens and toxins. Breast-fed babies are not exposed to this type of contamination.

Another advantage of breast-feeding is that infants are unlikely to gain excess weight. **Childhood obesity** is a major concern in the United States. Since mothers are unable to measure how much breast milk their baby consumes, they are less likely to encourage overfeeding. Research suggests that breast-fed babies have a lower risk of developing type 2 diabetes. Other research suggests that the rate of other chronic diseases such as **asthma**, celiac disease, inflammatory bowel disease, and various **allergies** appears to be lower in breast-fed babies than in babies fed with formula. Premature babies especially appear to benefit from reduced chronic disease as a result of breast-feeding.

Breast-feeding also provides benefits to the nursing mother. Breast-feeding is more economical than buying formula, even taking into account the extra food—about 500 calories daily—that the mother needs to eat when she is nursing. Since breast-fed babies on average get sick less than formula-fed babies, the family is also likely to save money on doctor visits, medicine, and time off from work to care for a sick child.

The mother's health also benefits from breast-feeding. Nursing mothers tend to lose the weight they put on during pregnancy faster than mothers who do not nurse. The hormones that are released in the mother's body when her infant nurses also help her uterus contract and become closer to the size it was before pregnancy. Mothers who nurse their babies also seem to be less likely to develop breast, ovarian, or uterine **cancer** early in life. Finally, breast-feeding offers psychological benefits to the mother as she bonds with her baby and may reduce the chance of postpartum depression.

DISADVANTAGES OF BREAST-FEEDING. Although breast milk is the best food for an infant, breast-feeding does have some disadvantages for the mother. Initially, babies breast-feed about every two to three hours. Some women find it exhausting to be available to the baby so frequently. When the infant is older, the mother may need to pump breast milk for her child to eat while she is away or at work. Fathers sometimes feel shut out during the early weeks of breast-feeding because of the close bond between mother and child. In addition, women who are breast-feeding must watch their diet carefully. Some foods or substances such as caffeine can pass into breast milk and cause the baby to be restless and irritable. Finally, some women simply find the idea of breast-feeding messy and distasteful, and resent the fact that they need to be available much of the time for feeding. For women who cannot or do not want to breast-feed, infant formula provides an adequate alternative.

Formula feeding

Although infant formula is not as perfect a food as breast milk for infants (it is harder for them to digest and is not a chemical replica of human milk), formula does provide all of the nutrients that babies need to grow up healthy. The U.S. Food and Drug Administration (FDA) regulates infant formula under the Federal Food, Drug, and Cosmetic Act (FFDCA). The FDA sets the minimum amounts of nutrients (29) that must be present in infant formula and sets maximum amounts for 9 other nutrients. Some of these nutrients include vitamins A, D, E, and K, and calcium. Some formulas contain iron, while others do not.

Substances used in infant formulas must be foods on the FDA-approved "Generally Recognized as Safe"

(GRAS) list. Facilities that manufacture infant formula are regularly inspected by the FDA and are required to keep process and distribution records for each batch of formula. Every container of formula must show an expiration or use-by date. The FDA must be informed of any changes made to the formula.

Infant formulas are either cow's milk based or soy based. Infants who show signs of lactose intolerance (colicky, restless, gassy, spitting up) usually do well on soy-based formula. Formula comes in three styles: ready-to-feed, concentrated liquid, and powder. Ready-to-feed formulas are the easiest to use and can be poured straight from the can into a bottle; however, they are also the most expensive. Concentrated liquids need to be mixed with an equal portion of water. Powder formulas, which also need to be mixed with water, are the least expensive and keep longer than the liquid varieties.

REASONS TO FORMULA FEED. Not every woman wants or is able to breast-feed. Aside from personal preference, women should formula feed if they:

- are adoptive parents
- have HIV, active tuberculosis, or hepatitis C, which all can be passed on to their infants through breast milk
- use street drugs or abuse prescription medicines, which can pass to the infant and permanently damage a baby's health
- are taking chemotherapy drugs, certain mood stabilizers, migraine headache medications, or any other drugs that may pass into breast milk
- have alcoholism or are binge drinkers, as the alcohol will be present in their breast milk
- have difficult-to-control diabetes, as blood sugar levels may be even harder to control if breast-feeding
- are going to be separated from their baby for significant periods of time
- have had breast surgery that interferes with milk production
- are emotionally repelled by the idea of breast-feeding

A few babies are born with a genetic inborn error in metabolism that prevents them from digesting any mammalian milk. These babies must be fed soy-based formula in order to survive.

PROS AND CONS OF FORMULA FEEDING. Formula feeding has some definite advantages. Anyone, not just the mother, can feed the infant. This gives the mother more flexibility in her schedule and allows the father or other relatives to enjoy a special closeness with the baby that comes with feeding. Also, the mother does not need to be concerned about how her diet affects her baby, and she does not need to worry about breast milk leakage. Since formula is digested more slowly than breast milk, feedings are less frequent. Some women feel uncomfortable nursing in front of other people or find it difficult to locate places to nurse in private. Formula feeding eliminates this problem.

There are also disadvantages to formula feeding. Aside from the fact that formula is not an exact duplicate of breast milk and is harder to digest, it also costs more and requires more advance preparation. Bottles need to be washed, and the water used to mix formula, at least in the early months, needs to be boiled or be special bottled water suitable for infants. The Academy of General Dentistry warns that some public water supplies are fluoridated at levels too high for infants, and that fluorodosis of the primary (baby) teeth may result. Finally, formula must be refrigerated once it is mixed or a can is opened. It can only be kept about two days in the refrigerator, so waste is more likely to occur. Likewise, when traveling, bottles need to be refrigerated. Although most babies do not mind cold formula, many parents like to heat their child's bottles to body temperature, another inconvenience when traveling.

TRANSITIONING TO SOLID FOODS. When an infant is between four and six months old, most pediatricians recommend introducing the infant to some baby foods. By this age, infants begin to have the muscle coordination to swallow stage one, or pureed, baby foods. Stage one baby foods are essentially thick liquids, with stage two foods progressing in consistency and stage three foods introducing small pieces. If there is a family history of food allergies, some pediatricians recommend waiting until six months or older to add in additional foods.

The introduction of foods normally begins with a small amount of iron-fortified rice cereal or other single-grain cereal mixed into a slurry the consistency of thin gravy with formula or breast milk. The infant is then offered a small amount of cereal on a small spoon; it should never be offered in a bottle. It may take many attempts before the infant will eat the new food. After runny cereal is accepted, a thicker cereal can be offered. When the child eats this with ease, parents can begin feeding one new pureed food every week. Commercial baby food is available in jars or frozen. Baby food can also be made at home using a blender or food processor. Portions can be frozen in an ice cube tray and thawed as needed.

About the same time babies begin eating solid food, they are ready to take small sips of apple, grape, or pear juice (but not citrus juices) from a cup. Juice should not be served in a bottle. By the end of the first year, infants can eat a variety of ground or chopped soft foods that the rest of the family eats.

Foods that should not be fed to infants

Some foods are not appropriate for children during their first year. These include:

- Homemade formula. The nutrient requirements for infants are very specific, and even small excesses or deficits of a particular nutrient can permanently harm the child's development.
- Cow's milk. Plain cow's milk should not be offered before six months. After this, it can be introduced in small amounts as part of weaning foods, but it should not be offered as the main drink before age one. The cow's milk used in some formulas has been altered to make it acceptable for infants.
- Honey. Honey can contains spores of the bacterium *Clostritium botulinum*. This bacterium causes a serious, potentially fatal disease called infant botulism. Older children and adults are not affected. *C. botulinum.* can also be found in maple syrup, corn syrup, and undercooked foods.
- Well-cooked eggs, fish, shellfish, and peanut butter. Opinions differ on how early to introduce these foods into the diet, as young children may be more prone to allergic reactions, especially during the first year.
- Orange, grapefruit, or other citrus juices. These often cause a painful diaper rash during the first year.
- Home-prepared spinach, collard greens, turnips, or beets. These may contain high levels of harmful nitrates from the soil. Jarred versions of these foods are okay.
- Raisins, whole grapes, hot dog rounds, hard candy, popcorn, raw carrots, nuts, and stringy meat. These and similar foods can cause choking, a major cause of accidental death in infants and toddlers.

Precautions

Mothers with certain health conditions or using certain drugs should not breast-feed. Women with chronic diseases should consult with their healthcare providers before breast-feeding.

Parents using concentrated liquid and powdered formulas must measure and mix formula accurately. Inaccurate measuring can harm the infant's growth and development. Water used in mixing formula must be free of pathogens, contaminants, and excessive levels of fluoride.

Interactions

Street drugs, many prescription and over-the-counter drugs, and alcohol can all pass into breast milk and have the potential to permanently harm an infant's growth and development. Pregnant or breast-feeding women should consult their healthcare providers before taking any drug or supplement. Caffeine also passes into breast milk. Some women find that even moderate amounts of coffee or caffeinated sodas cause their infants to become restless and irritable, while others find little effect. Breast-feeding women should monitor their caffeine intake and try to keep it to a minimum.

KEY TERMS

Atopy—An inherited tendency toward strong and immediate hypersensitivity reactions to substances in the environment. Examples include severe food allergies, allergic skin reactions, and bronchial asthma.

Colic—Excessive crying in an otherwise healthy infant.

Fluorodosis—A cosmetic dental problem that can be caused by the presence of too much fluoride in drinking water. Fluorodosis causes brown spots on the teeth but does not weaken them in any way.

Complications

Many women have trouble getting newborn infants to latch on and begin breast-feeding. This can usually be overcome with the help of a lactation consultant or pediatric nurse. Breast-feeding can cause the mother to develop sore, infected nipples. This is usually a temporary condition and should not be a reason to stop breast-feeding.

Complications from bottle feeding tend to be related to the infant's difficulty with digesting formula. Some infants become gassy and colicky and may fuss, cry for long periods, and spit up cow's milk-based formula. A switch to soy-based formula, if approved by a healthcare professional, usually relieves this problem. Other complications of formula feeding are generally related to improper mixing of formula.

Parental concerns

Breast-feeding parents often are concerned about whether their baby is getting enough milk, since there is no way to directly measure how much milk a baby consumes when nursing. Newborns should have a minimum of six to eight wet diapers and four bowel movements per day during the first two weeks of life. As the child grows, these numbers will gradually decrease. In addition, a woman's breasts should feel hard and full (sometimes even painful) before nursing, and softer after

QUESTIONS TO ASK YOUR DOCTOR

- Are there any medical reasons why I should not breast-feed?
- Is there a particular type of formula you recommend?
- If my baby is bottle fed, how many ounces of formula should he/she be drinking at every feeding?
- What are some signs that my formula-fed baby is full?
- What food should I introduce first after cereal?
- When is my infant ready for table food, or the same food that I am eating?

nursing. Newborns nurse every two to three hours, and they should seem satisfied after nursing. The most definite sign that the baby is getting enough food is that he or she is gaining weight.

Infants grow in irregular spurts. They may eat hungrily for a few days and then eat little few days later. Parents often worry about this, but it is a normal pattern.

The transition to solid food is often a slow process. Infants eat very small amounts and often must be exposed to a new food multiple times before they will eat it willingly. Parents should avoid strictly feeding an infant only foods that they like, as the infant should be allowed to form his or her own taste preferences. Since childhood **obesity** is a major problem in the United States, parents and caregivers should avoid encouraging the infant to overeat.

Resources

BOOKS

Behan, Eileen. *The Baby Food Bible: A Complete Guide to Feeding Your Child, from Infancy On*. New York: Ballantine Books, 2008.

Dietz, William H., and Loraine Stern, eds. "What's Best for my Newborn?" In *Nutrition: What Every Parent Needs to Know*. 2nd ed. Elk Grove Village, IL: American Academy of Pediatrics, 2012.

Meek, Joan Younger, ed. *The American Academy of Pediatrics New Mother's Guide to Breast-feeding*. 2nd ed. New York: Bantam Books, 2011.

Samour, Patricia Q. and Kathy King, eds. *Pediatric Nutrition*. 4th ed. Sudbury, MA: Jones and Bartlett Learning, 2010.

PERIODICALS

American Academy of Pediatrics. "Breastfeeding and the Use of Human Milk (Policy Statement)." *Pediatrics* 129, no. 3 (2012): e827–41. http://dx.doi.org/10.1542/peds.2011-3552 (accessed April 27, 2012).

WEBSITES

American Academy of Pediatricians. "Breastfeeding Initiatives." http://www2.aap.org/breastfeeding (accessed April 27, 2012).

International Food Information Council. "Questions and Answers About the Nutritional Content of Processed Baby Food." FoodInsight.org. http://www.foodinsight.org/Resources/Detail.aspx?topic=Questions_and_Answers_About_the_Nutritional_Content_of_Processed_Baby_Food_ (accessed April 26, 2012).

MedlinePlus. "Infant and Toddler Nutrition." U.S. National Library of Medicine, National Institutes of Health. http://www.nlm.nih.gov/medlineplus/infantandnewbornnutrition.html (accessed April 26, 2012).

ORGANIZATIONS

American Academy of Pediatrics, 141 Northwest Point Boulevard, Elk Grove Village, IL 60007-1098, (847) 434-4000, Fax: (847) 434-8000, http://www.aap.org

La Leche League International, 957 N Plum Grove Rd, Schaumburg, IL 60173, (847) 519-7730, (800) LA-LECHE (525-3243), Fax: (847) 969-0460, http://www.llli.org

Women, Infants, and Children, Supplemental Food Programs Division, Food and Nutrition Service, USDA, 3101 Park Center Dr., Rm. 520, Alexandria, VA 22302, (202) 305-2746, Fax: (703) 305-2196, http://www.fns.usda.gov.

Tish Davidson, AM

Infection control

Definition

Infection control refers to policies and procedures used to minimize the risk of spreading infections, especially in hospitals and human or animal health care facilities.

Purpose

The purpose of infection control is to reduce the occurrence of infectious diseases. Usually caused by bacteria or viruses, these diseases can be spread by human-to-human contact, animal-to-human contact, human contact with an infected surface, airborne transmission through tiny droplets of infectious agents suspended in the air, and, finally, by such common vehicles as food or **water**. Diseases that are spread from animals to humans are known as "zoonoses." Animals

ELIZABETH LEE HAZEN (1885–1975)

Elizabeth Lee Hazen was born on August 24, 1885, in Rich, Mississippi. Orphaned before she turned 4, she and her older sister went to live with their aunt and uncle shortly after her younger brother died. Hazen eventually went to college, where she became interested in science, ultimately earning her M.S. in biology from Columbia University in 1917, and after working in the U.S. Army laboratories during World War I, receiving her Ph.D. in microbiology from Columbia in 1927. After serving as an instructor at Columbia, Hazen accepted a position with the New York Department of Health, where she researched bacterial diseases.

In 1948, Hazen and colleague Rachel Brown began studying fungal infections and antibiotics. Some of the antibiotics they discovered did indeed kill the fungus; however, they also killed the test mice. Finally, Hazen located a micro-organism on a farm in Virginia, and Brown's tests indicated that the micro-organism produced two antibiotics, one of which proved effective for treating fungus and candidiasis in humans. Brown purified the antibiotic, which was patented under the name *nystatin*. In 1954, the antibiotic became available in pill form. Hazen and Brown continued their research and discovered two other antibiotics. Hazen received numerous awards individually and together with Brown. Elizabeth Hazen died on June 24, 1975.

that carry disease agents from one host to another are known as "vectors."

Description

The goals of infection control programs are: immunizing against preventable diseases, defining precautions that can prevent exposure to infectious agents, and restricting the exposure of healthcare workers to an infectious agent. An infection-control practitioner is a specially trained professional, often a nurse, who oversees infection control programs.

Infection control in hospitals and other health care settings

Infections contracted in hospitals are also called "nosocomial infections." They occur in approximately 5–10% of all hospital patients. These infections result in increased time spent in the hospital and, in some cases, death. There are many reasons why nosocomial infections are common, one of which is that many hospital patients have a weakened immune system, which makes them more susceptible to infections. This weakened immune system can be caused either by the patient's diseases or by treatments given to the patient. Second, many medical procedures can increase the risk of infection by introducing infectious agents into the patient. Thirdly, many patients are admitted to hospitals because of **infectious disease**. These infectious agents can then be transferred from patient to patient by hospital workers or visitors.

Infection control has become a formal discipline in the United States since the 1950s, due to the spread of **staphylococcal infections** in hospitals. Because health care providers both risk acquiring infections themselves, and then passing infections on to patients, the **Centers for Disease Control and Prevention (CDC)** established guidelines for infection-control procedures. In addition to hospitals, infection control is important in nursing homes, clinics, child care centers, and restaurants, as well as in the home.

To lower the risk of nosocomial infections, the CDC's National Healthcare Safety Network includes a patient-safety component that tracks the occurrence of infectious disease in hospitals. Data collected through this program and its previous National Nosocomial Infections Surveillance program, which began in 1970, show that infection-control programs can significantly improve patient safety, lower infection rates, and lower patient mortality.

Dental healthcare settings are similar to hospitals in that both personnel and equipment can transmit infection if proper safeguards are not observed. The **CDC** issued new guidelines in 2003 for the proper maintenance and sterilization of dental equipment; hand **hygiene** for dentists and dental hygienists; dental radiology; medications; oral surgery; as well as environmental infection control and standards for dental laboratories.

Problems of antibiotic resistance

Because of the overuse of **antibiotics**, many bacteria have developed a resistance to common antibiotics, making ever-newer antibiotics necessary to counter what were previously simple-to-treat infections. The use of antibiotics outside of medicine also contributes to increased antibiotic resistance. Repeated use of antibiotic cleaners on a surface, for instance, kills off those bacteria that are susceptible to it, leaving behind the few bacteria that are resistant. Without competition from the susceptible bacteria, those resistant bacteria can multiply more quickly, leaving behind a greater percentage of resistant bacteria on that surface. More rational use of antibiotics through treatment guidelines will help stem this trend.

Bioterrorism

The events of September 11, 2001, and the **anthrax** scare that followed in October 2001 alerted public health officials as well as the general public to the possible use of infectious disease agents as weapons of terrorism. The **Centers for Disease Control and Prevention** (CDC) now maintains a list of topics and resources related to bioterrorism on its web site.

Prevention

Commonly recommended precautions to avoid and control the spread of infections include:

- Vaccinate people and pets against diseases for which a vaccine is available. The vaccines used against infectious diseases are very safe compared to most drugs.
- Wash hands often.
- Cook food thoroughly.
- Use antibiotics only as directed.
- See a doctor for infections that do not heal.
- Avoid areas with a lot of insects.
- Be cautious around wild or unfamiliar animals, or any animals that are unusually aggressive. Do not purchase exotic animals as pets.
- Do not engage in unprotected sex or in intravenous drug use.
- Find out about infectious diseases when you make travel plans. Travelers' advisories and adult vaccination recommendations are available on the CDC web site or by calling the CDC's telephone service at 404-332-4559.

Because of the higher risk of spreading infectious disease in a hospital setting, higher levels of precautions are taken there. Typically, health care workers wear gloves with all patients, since it is difficult to know whether a transmittable disease is present or not. Patients who have a known infectious disease are isolated to decrease the risk of transmitting the infectious agent to another person. Hospital workers who come in contact with infected patients must wear gloves and gowns to decrease the risk of carrying the infectious agent to other patients. All articles of equipment that are used in an isolation room are decontaminated before reuse. Patients who are immunocompromised may be put in protective isolation to decrease the risk of infectious agents being brought into their room. Any hospital workers with infections, including colds, are restricted from that room.

Hospital infections can also be transmitted through the air, so it is important for healthcare workers to handle infected materials with care to reduce opportunities for infectious agents to become airborne. Hospitals must also take special care with hospital ventilation systems to prevent recirculation of contaminated air.

Effects on public health

Emerging and re-emerging infectious diseases are a global health threat. Scientists and medical professionals have identified many new contagious diseases in the past 30 years. These include **AIDS**, Ebola, and hantavirus. Increased travel between continents makes the worldwide spread of disease a bigger concern than it once was, because individuals can easily and unknowingly carry infectious agents from one location to another. Additionally, many common infectious diseases have become resistant to known treatments.

The emergence of the **severe acute respiratory syndrome (SARS)** epidemic in Asia in February 2003 was a classic instance of an emerging disease that spread rapidly because of the increased frequency of international and intercontinental travel. In addition, the **SARS** outbreak demonstrated the vulnerability of hospitals and healthcare workers to **emerging diseases**. Clusters of cases within hospitals occurred in the early weeks of the epidemic when the disease had not yet been recognized, and the first SARS patients were admitted without isolation precautions.

Costs to society

Infectious diseases can have devastating consequences. This is especially evident in developing countries, where infectious disease affects a higher proportion of the **population**. Sickness results not only in increased inpatient and outpatient health care costs, but also in indirect economic costs associated with lost productivity when individuals cannot work, are prevented from ever working, or die. Costs also mount when people must cut back on their own employment to care for an ailing family member.

Vaccines are typically a cost-effective way to control infectious disease. Vaccines have, for instance, eradicated **smallpox** and eliminated **polio** from the United States and many other parts of the world. Infection-control measures in healthcare facilities can also reduce the spread of infectious disease, which, in turn, lowers the cost of healthcare.

Efforts and solutions

Many efforts are under way to control infectious diseases. Individual labs at universities are working alongside and often in concert with government initiatives to develop novel treatments. Many agencies, some of them global, are improving their disease-surveillance methods so they can spot potential infectious-disease

KEY TERMS

Acquired immune deficiency syndrome (AIDS)—A disease that weakens the body's immune system. It is also known as "HIV infection."

Antibiotic—A substance, such as a drug, that can stop bacteria from growing, or destroy the bacteria.

Antibiotic resistance—The ability of infectious agents to change their biochemistry in such a way as to make an antibiotic no longer effective.

Bioterrorism—The intentional use of disease-causing microbes or other biologic agents to intimidate or terrorize a civilian population for political or military reasons.

Ebola—The disease caused by the newly described and very deadly Ebola virus found in Africa.

Epidemiology—The branch of medicine that deals with the transmission of infectious diseases in large populations and with detection of the sources and causes of epidemics.

Hantavirus—A group of arboviruses that cause hemorrhagic fever (characterized by sudden onset, fever, aching, and bleeding in the internal organs).

Immunization—Immunity refers to the body's ability to protect itself from a certain disease after it has been exposed to that disease. Through immunization, also known as "vaccination," a small amount of an infectious agent is injected into the body to stimulate development of immunity.

Immunocompromized—Refers to the condition of having a weakened immune system. This can happen due to genetic factors, drugs, or disease.

Nosocomial infection—An infection acquired in a hospital setting.

Staphylococcal infection—An infection caused by the organism *Staphylococcus*. Infection by this agent is common and is often resistant to antibiotics.

Vector—An animal carrier that transfers an infectious organism from one host to another.

Zoonosis (plural: zoonoses)—Any disease of animals that can be transmitted to humans under natural conditions. Lyme disease, rabies, psittacosis (parrot fever), cat-scratch fever, and monkeypox are examples of zoonoses.

outbreaks as early as possible. They are also developing strategies to react to those outbreaks, including the dissemination of vaccines. Beyond these activities, medical centers are implementing procedures to keep patient and healthcare-worker exposure to infectious organisms to a minimum. Increased publicity has also made members of the general public more aware of infectious diseases and what they can do to protect themselves and their families.

Resources

BOOKS

Bartlett, John G., Paul G. Auwaerter, Paul A. Pham. *Johns Hopkins ABX Guide 2012,* 3rd ed. Burlington, MA: Jones & Bartlett Learning, 2011.

Shannon, Joyce Brennfleck. *Contagious Diseases Sourcebook: Basic Consumer Information About Disease Spread from Person to Person,* 2nd ed. Detroit: Omnigraphics, 2010.

PERIODICALS

Endy, Timothy P. et al. "Emerging Infectious Diseases as Global Health Threat." *Experimental Biology and Medicine* 236, no. 8 (2011): 897–898.

Grady, Denise. "Gut Infections Are Growing More Lethal." *New York Times* (March 19, 2012). http://www.nytimes.com/2012/03/20/health/gut-infections-are-growing-much-more-lethal.html (accessed December 4, 2012).

WEBSITES

"An Ounce of Prevention Keeps the Germs Away: Seven Keys to a Safer Healthier Home." Centers for Disease Control and Prevention. http://www.cdc.gov/ounceofprevention/docs/oop_brochure_eng.pdf (accessed September 17, 2012).

"Infectious Disease Cost Calculator." Center for Biosecurity of UPMC (University of Pittsburgh Medical Center). http://www.idcostcalc.org/Hold_May2012/index.html (accessed September 18, 2012).

"Infectious Diseases." World Health Organization. http://www.who.int/topics/infectious_diseases/en/ (accessed September 17, 2012).

MedlinePlus "Infectious Diseases." U.S. National Library of Medicine. http://www.nlm.nih.gov/medlineplus/infectiousdiseases.html (accessed September 17, 2012).

"Methicillin-resistant Staphylococcus Aureus (MRSA) Infections." Centers for Disease Control and Prevention. http://www.cdc.gov/mrsa/ (accessed September 17, 2012).

"National Healthcare Safety Network (NHSN) Data and Statistics." Centers for Disease Control and Prevention. http://www.cdc.gov/nhsn/datastat.html (accessed September 17, 2012).

"Recommended Infection-Control Practices for Dentistry." Centers for Disease Control and Prevention. http://www.cdc.gov/oralhealth/infectioncontrol/guidelines/index.htm (accessed September 17, 2012).

"Understanding Microbes in Sickness and in Health." National Institute of Allergy and Infectious Diseases. http://www.niaid.nih.gov/topics/microbes/documents/microbesbook.pdf (September 17, 2012).

ORGANIZATIONS

American College of Epidemiology, 1500 Sunday Drive, Suite 102, Raleigh, NC 27607, (919) 861-5573, info@acepidemiology.org, http://www.acepidemiology.org/

American Public Health Association (APHA), 800 I Street NW, Washington, DC 20001-3710, (202) 777-APHA, http://www.apha.org

American Veterinary Medical Association (AVMA), 1931 North Meacham Road, Suite 100, Schaumburg, IL 60173-4360, Fax: (847) 925-1329, (800) 248-2862, http://www.avma.org/

Centers for Disease Control and Prevention (CDC), 1600 Clifton Road, Atlanta, GA 30333, (800) 232-4636, cdcinfo@cdc.gov, http://www.cdc.gov

National Institute of Allergies and Infectious Diseases, 6610 Rockledge Drive, MSC 6612, Bethesda, MD 20892-6612, (301) 496-5717, Fax: (301) 402-3573, (866) 284-4107, ocpostoffice@niaid.nih.gov, http://www.niaid.nih.gov.

Cindy L. A. Jones, Ph.D.
Rebecca J. Frey, Ph.D.
Leslie Mertz, Ph.D.

Infectious disease

Definition

Infectious disease—also called communicable disease—is any illness caused by an infective agent—a germ, microbe, or parasite. Infective agents include bacteria, viruses, fungi, parasitic protozoa, and worms.

Demographics

Virtually all children contract infectious disease, especially during infancy and early childhood. Respiratory and gastrointestinal infections are the most common causes of illness in children. For instance, children develop three to eight colds or respiratory infections per year.

Worldwide, more children and adults die from infectious disease than any other single cause. The vast majority of these deaths occur in poorer counties with limited access to **prevention**, medical care, and drugs.

Among American children, the frequency and severity of infectious disease have declined dramatically in recent decades, primarily due to the development of vaccines for common childhood infections. The United States is one of the few places in the world where **polio** has been completely eradicated. Childhood pneumococcal infections caused by vaccine–targeted bacterial strains have been almost completely eliminated.

Description

When an infective agent enters the body and begins to multiply, the immune system responds with various defensive mechanisms that protect against most infectious disease. However when an infective agent temporarily evades or overwhelms the immune system and begins to damage tissues, signs and symptoms of disease develop.

The most common infectious diseases are contagious—they spread via direct transfer of an infective agent from one person to another. Shaking hands, kissing, or coughing or sneezing on someone can directly transmit contagious diseases such as colds, flu, or **tuberculosis** (TB). Some infective agents, including cold viruses, can be contracted by indirect contact with a contaminated surface such as a faucet, doorknob, or computer keyboard. International airplane travel is responsible for the spread of contagious diseases around the world. Infant diarrhea caused by **rotavirus** or the protozoan *Giardia lamblia* often spreads among babies and young children through the accidental transferring of feces from hand to mouth after diaper changes. Some infectious diseases can be passed from a mother to her unborn child across the placenta or during birth.

Other infectious diseases can be transmitted from animals or animal waste to humans. Dog and cat saliva may contain more than 100 different types of infective agents. *Pasteurella* bacteria are the most common microbes transmitted via pet bites. These bacteria can cause serious—sometimes fatal—infectious diseases such as **meningitis**, an inflammation of the lining of the brain and spinal cord. Toxoplasmosis is a bacterial infection that is transmitted via cat feces. Pet reptiles, such as turtles, snakes, and iguanas, can transmit *Salmonella* bacteria. Wild animals can directly or indirectly transmit a wide variety of infectious disease.

Some infectious diseases are transferred between human hosts by insect and other invertebrate vectors:

- Mosquitoes transfer the protozoan that causes malaria, as well as West Nile virus, dengue fever, and viral encephalitis.
- Body lice can transmit typhus.

Selected infectious diseases and corresponding treatment

Disease	Symptoms	Transmittal	Treatment
Chicken pox	Rash, low-grade fever	Person to person	None; acetaminophen may treat fever or discomfort
Common cold/influenza	Runny nose, sore throat, cough, fever, headache, muscle aches	Person to person	None, although various remedies may help relieve symptoms
Hepatitis A	Jaundice, flu-like symptoms	Sexual contact with an infected person or contact with contaminated blood, food, or water	None; acetaminophen may treat fever or pain
H1N1 influenza	Fever, cough, sore throat, body aches, loss of appetite, fatigue	Person to person	Antiviral drugs
Measles	Skin rash, runny nose and eyes, fever, cough	Person to person	None; acetaminophen may treat fever or discomfort
Meningitis	Neck pain, headache, pain caused by exposure to light, fever, nausea, drowsiness	Person to person	Antibiotics for bacterial meningitis, hospital care for viral meningitis
Methicillin-resistant Staphylococcus aureus (MRSA)	Rash, shortness of breath, fever, chest pain, headache	Person to person or contact with contaminated surfaces	Antibiotics
Mumps	Swelling of salivary glands	Person to person	Anti-inflammatory drugs
Ringworm	Skin rash	Contact with infected animal or person	Antifungal drugs applied topically or taken orally
Tetanus	Lockjaw, other spasms	Soil infection of wounds	Antibiotics, antitoxins, muscle relaxants

(Table by PreMediaGlobal. Reproduced by permission of Gale, a part of Cengage Learning.)

- Fleas can transmit typhus and transfer plague bacteria from rodents to humans.
- Deer ticks—which are actually more closely related to crabs than to insects—can transfer the bacterium that causes Lyme disease from mice to humans.
- Ticks can also transmit the bacterium that cause Rocky Mountain spotted fever and tularemia, and the protozoan that causes babesiosis.

Some infectious diseases are spread from a single source to many people through contaminated food or **water**. For example, the bacterium *Escherichia coli* (*E. coli*) can be transmitted via unwashed fruit or vegetables or undercooked meat.

Some infectious diseases have recently emerged, re–emerged, or become much more widespread and dangerous by acquiring **drug resistance**. Examples include:

- methicillin–resistant *Staphylococcus aureus* (MRSA) bacteria
- multi–and extensively drug–resistant TB bacteria
- 2009 H1N1 influenza virus
- H5N1 avian influenza virus
- West Nile virus
- Ebola virus
- Marburg virus
- Nipah virus
- SARS (severe acute respiratory syndrome) virus
- dengue virus
- polio virus
- malaria parasite

Risk factors

Risk factors for respiratory or gastrointestinal infectious diseases in babies include:

- premature birth
- low birth weight
- low socioeconomic status
- multiple siblings
- daycare
- parental smoking

Children with weakened immune systems are at increased risk for infectious disease. Infection can occur if a child:

- has HIV/AIDS
- has an autoimmune disease
- is taking steroids or anti–rejection drugs for a transplanted organ
- is being treated for cancer

ELIZABETH LEE HAZEN (1885–1975)

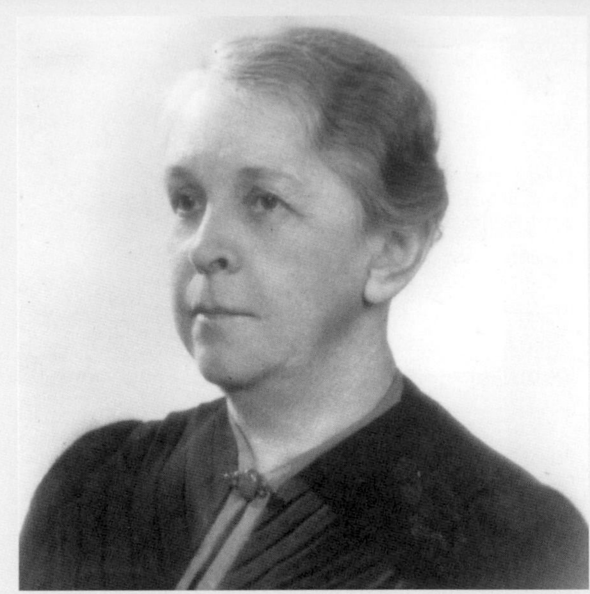

(© Bettmann/CORBIS)

Elizabeth Lee Hazen was born on August 24, 1885, in Rich, Mississippi. Hazen, born the middle of three children to Maggie (Harper) and William Edgar Hazen, was orphaned before she turned four. She and her sister went to live with their aunt and uncle shorly after her younger brother died. Hazen attended the Mississippi Industrial Institute and College at Columbus, receiving her B.S. degree in 1910. During college, Hazen became interested in science and she studied biology at Columbia University, earning her M.S. in 1917. After working in the U.S. Army laboratories during World War I, she returned to Columbia where she received her Ph.D. in microbiology in 1927. Following her work as an instructor at Columbia, Hazen accepted a position with the New York Department of Health where she researched bacterial diseases.

In 1948, Hazen and Rachel Brown began researching fungal infections found in humans due to antibiotic treatments and diseases. Some of the antibiotics they discovered did indeed kill the fungus; however, they also killed the test mice. Finally, Hazen located a microorganism on a farm in Virginia, and Brown's tests indicated that the microorganism produced two antibiotics, one of which proved effective for treating fungus and candidiasis in humans. Brown purified the antibiotic which was patented under the name *nystatin*. In 1954, the antibiotic became available in pill form. Hazen and Brown continued their research and discovered two other antibiotics. Hazen received numerous awards individually and with her research partner, Rachel Brown. Elizabeth Hazen died on June 24, 1975.

In 2010, scientists reported the discovery of mutations that increase susceptibility to infectious disease. The mutations are in a gene called CISH that encodes a protein that regulates the immune system's response to infectious disease. A child who inherits one of these mutations from a parent has an 18% increased risk for infectious disease. Inheriting four or more of the mutations increases the risk to 81%.

Causes and symptoms

Causes

Although most bacteria are not harmful—and some types are essential for proper functioning of the human body—some bacteria produce toxins that cause infectious disease. *Streptococcus* can cause infections ranging from relatively mild ear infections to strep throat to potentially fatal pneumococcal **pneumonia**, meningitis, and sepsis or blood **poisoning**. Children can be especially vulnerable to bacteria that cause:

- diphtheria
- pertussis or whooping cough
- tetanus
- urinary tract infections

Viruses cause many childhood diseases, including:

- common colds
- influenzas
- diarrhea from rotaviruses
- measles
- mumps
- rubella (German measles)
- chicken pox
- polio
- hepatitis
- human papillomavirus (HPV)
- herpes
- HIV/AIDS

Fungi cause various infectious diseases, including:

- thrush, a mouth and throat infection in infants caused by *Candida albicans*

- skin conditions, such as ringworm and athlete's foot
- pneumonia caused by *Pneumocystis carinii*

Protozoan **parasites** cause infectious diseases such as **malaria**, giardiasis, and toxoplasmosis. Helminths are larger parasites—such as tapeworms and roundworms—that can infect the intestinal tract, lungs, liver, skin, or brain.

SYMPTOMS. Symptoms of infectious disease vary with the type of infection. However many infectious diseases have symptoms that include:

- fever and chills
- loss of appetite
- muscle aches
- fatigue

Diagnosis

Examination

A medical history and physical exam—including the patient's breathing pattern and respiratory rate, body temperature, and other symptoms—may be sufficient for diagnosing an infectious disease. Sometimes an infectious organism in a blood or urine sample can be seen under a microscope.

Tests

Blood, urine, throat swabs, or other bodily secretions may be cultured in a laboratory to identify the infective agent. Diagnosis of some infectious diseases requires a lumbar puncture or spinal tap to obtain a sample of cerebrospinal fluid.

Procedures

Diagnostic procedures may include:

- a chest x ray to diagnose pneumonia
- computerized tomography (CT) scans or magnetic resonance imaging (MRI)
- a biopsy—the removal of a tiny amount of tissue from an infected area, such as the lung, for diagnosing fungal pneumonia

Treatment

Treatment depends on the type of infectious disease. Some diseases resolve on their own without any treatment other than possibly relieving symptoms.

Drugs vary based on the infecting organism and specific disease:

- Bacterial infections are treated with antibiotics.
- A very few antiviral drugs, such as acyclovir, are available for treating viral infections such as flu and herpes.
- Various drugs may be used to treat hepatitis B and C.
- HIV/AIDS is treated with a combination of drugs, commonly known as highly active antiretroviral therapy (HAART).
- Fungal infections of the skin and nails may be treated with over-the-counter or prescription medications applied directly to the affected area.
- Oral antifungal medications are used to treat systemic fungal infections, such as histoplasmosis, or severe infections of the mouth and throat in children with weakened immune systems.
- Only a very few anti–parasitic drugs are available, and some of these are either very toxic or are becoming less effective with the spread of drug–resistant parasites.

A wide variety of home or alternative therapies are also used to treat infectious disease, although bacterial infections usually require **antibiotics**. Yogurt containing healthy gut bacteria can ease gastrointestinal symptoms and has been shown to reduce the incidence of some common infections in children. Many mild infectious

KEY TERMS

Bacteria—Single–celled microorganisms that live in soil, water, organic matter, plants, and animals, and are associated with a number of infectious diseases.

Fungi—A kingdom of saprophytic and parasitic spore–producing organisms that include mushrooms and yeast.

Helminths—Parasitic worms, such as tapeworms or liver flukes, that can live in the human body.

Immunization—Treatment, usually by vaccination, to produce immunity to a specific infective agent.

Meningitis—An infection or inflammation of membranes surrounding the brain and spinal cord.

Pneumococcal—Infection by the bacterium *Streptococcus pneumoniae* that causes acute pneumonia.

Pneumonia—Inflammation of the lungs, usually caused by infection with a bacterium, virus, or fungus.

Protozoa—Single–celled microorganisms of the Kingdom Protista, some of which can cause infectious disease in humans.

Vaccine—A preparation of live, weakened, or killed microorganisms that is administered to produce or increase immunity to specific diseases.

diseases respond well to home remedies. Bed rest and drinking plenty of fluids are the most common remedies.

Prognosis

Prognosis varies greatly, depending on the type of infectious disease. Some, such as the **common cold**, usually resolve quickly without medical treatment, and most infectious diseases have only minor complications. However some—such as pneumonia or meningitis—can be life-threatening. Even some common and usually mild infectious diseases—such as **measles**, **mumps**, chicken pox, or seasonal flu—can be dangerous or life–threatening in very young children.

Prevention

Many common infectious diseases are preventable with good **hygiene** and vaccines. The best protection is frequent and thorough hand washing:

- before, during, and after handling food
- before eating
- after using the toilet
- after changing diapers
- after touching animals or their toys, leashes, or waste
- after touching trash, cleaning rags, drains, or soil
- after contact with body fluids, including blood, vomit, saliva, or nasal secretions
- before cleaning a wound, administering medicine, or inserting contact lenses
- more often, if someone in the home is ill

Hands should be washed thoroughly and vigorously with soap and water for 20 seconds. If soap and water are not available, alcohol–based disposable hand wipes or sanitizers are an alternative.

Other practices for preventing infectious disease include:

- breastfeeding infants, which helps protect babies from respiratory and gastrointestinal infections
- avoiding touching one's eyes, nose, and mouth
- covering one's mouth and nose when coughing or sneezing
- rinsing fresh fruit and vegetables under running water and scrubbing firm-skinned produce with a vegetable brush
- keeping meat, poultry, seafood, and eggs separated from other foods at all times
- refrigerating foods promptly at a constant temperature of 40°F (4°C) or below, with enough room for cold air to circulate freely
- freezing foods at 0°F (-18°C) or below
- using separate cutting boards for produce and meat, poultry, seafood, or eggs
- washing cutting boards, dishes, utensils, and counter tops with hot, soapy water between preparation of each food item
- never reusing marinades from raw foods without boiling first
- thoroughly cooking all foods, especially meat, at the correct temperature
- cleaning with disposable paper towels or wipes, cloth towels that are washed in hot water, or sponges that are washed in the dishwasher or microwaved daily for 30 seconds
- cleaning and disinfecting all bathroom surfaces, especially when someone in the home has an infectious disease
- avoiding sharing personal items, including toothbrushes, combs, drinking glasses, and eating utensils
- keeping children home when they are sick
- not flying when ill
- practicing safe sex or abstaining from sex entirely to avoid sexually transmitted infections that can be passed to unborn children

Precautions against contracting infectious disease from animals include:

- adopting pets from an animal shelter or purchasing from a reputable store or breeder
- obtaining routine care and immunizations for your pet from a veterinarian
- obeying leash laws
- cleaning litter boxes daily, except when a person is pregnant
- keeping children away from pet waste
- keeping sandboxes covered
- washing one's hands thoroughly after contact with animals
- keeping wild animals away from the house
- using insect repellent and routinely checking for ticks and removing them immediately by applying gentle, steady pressure with tweezers

Children should receive all recommended vaccinations on schedule. Adults should receive vaccinations and booster shots (such as **tetanus** booster shots) as necessary. Travelers should also consult a healthcare professional about recommended immunizations for travel.

Effects on public health

More than a quarter of the annual global death rate can be traced to infectious diseases. In developing countries, the impact is even greater. As the world **population** grows, people move freely between geographic areas, and infectious agents evolve into virulent strains (some of which are difficult to treat), new and resurging infectious diseases will continue to emerge, and some will pose serious threats to public health. With international air travel, these diseases have the potential to become reach epidemic levels in a matter of days.

Costs to society

Infectious diseases can have devastating consequences. This is especially evident in developing countries, where infectious disease affects a higher proportion of the population. Sickness not only results in increased inpatient and outpatient health care costs, but also in indirect economic costs associated with lost productivity when individuals cannot work, are prevented from ever working, or die. Costs also mount when people must cut back on their own employment to care for an ailing family member.

Infectious disease can be particularly detrimental to the youngest members of society. According to a 2010 research article in *Lancet*, infectious disease in 2008 killed 5,970,000 children under the age of five, accounting for 68% of all deaths in that age group: an estimated 18% died of pneumonia, 15% of diarrhea, and 8% of malaria.

Efforts and solutions

Many efforts are under way to curb the health threats posed by infectious diseases. The task is great, but the global health community has made headway. For instance, thanks in great part to the Maternal and Neonatal Tetanus (MNT) Elimination Initiative of the **World Health Organization (WHO)**, United Nations Children's Fund (UNICEF), and the United Nations Population Fund (UNFPA), the number of deaths due to neonatal tetanus has dropped from 787,000 in the late 1980s to 59,000 in 2008 (the latest data available). In 1979, **smallpox** was officially and completely eradicated. A vaccine for polio has eliminated the disease from most of the world.

Efforts continue. Labs are developing new antimicrobials and other novel treatments; governments and agencies are reviewing and improving disease surveillance measures; researchers are studying how diseases spread and developing computer models to predict epidemics; molecular biologists are uncovering the genomes of disease organisms and identifying vulnerabilities; and health organizations are working on means to disseminate vaccines, both widely and rapidly.

Resources

BOOKS

Bartlett, John G., Paul G. Auwaerter, Paul A. Pham. *Johns Hopkins ABX Guide 2012,* 3rd ed. Burlington, MA: Jones & Bartlett Learning, 2011.

Shannon, Joyce Brennfleck. *Contagious Diseases Sourcebook: Basic Consumer Information About Disease Spread from Person to Person,* 2nd ed. Detroit: Omnigraphics, 2010.

PERIODICALS

Black, Robert E. et al. “Global, Regional, and National Causes of Child Mortality in 2008: A Systematic Analysis.” *Lancet* 375, no. 9730 (June 5–11, 2010): 1969–87.

Endy, Timothy P. et al. “Emerging Infectious Diseases as Global Health Threat.” *Experimental Biology and Medicine* 236, no. 8 (2011): 897–898.

Grady, Denise. “Gut Infections Are Growing More Lethal.” *New York Times*. (March 19, 2012). http://www.nytimes.com/2012/03/20/health/gut-infections-are-growing-much-more-lethal.html

Khor, Chiea C., et al. “CISH and Susceptibility to Infectious Diseases.” *New England Journal of Medicine* 362, no. 22 (June 3, 2010): 2092.

Rockoff, Jonathan D. “More Parents Seek Vaccine Exemption.” *Wall Street Journal* (July 6, 2010): A19.

WEBSITES

“An Ounce of Prevention Keeps the Germs Away: Seven Keys to a Safer Healthier Home.” Centers for Disease Control and Prevention. http://www.cdc.gov/ounceofprevention/docs/oop_brochure_eng.pdf (accessed September 17, 2012).

“Infectious Disease Cost Calculator.” Center for Biosecurity of UPMC (University of Pittsburgh Medical Center). http://www.idcostcalc.org/Hold_May2012/index.html (accessed September 18, 2012).

“Infectious Diseases.” World Health Organization. http://www.who.int/topics/infectious_diseases/en/ (accessed September 17, 2012).

MedlinePlus“Infectious Diseases.” U.S. National Library of Medicine. http://www.nlm.nih.gov/medlineplus/infectiousdiseases.html (accessed September 17, 2012).

“Understanding Microbes in Sickness and in Health.” National Institute of Allergy and Infectious Diseases. http://www.niaid.nih.gov/topics/microbes/documents/microbesbook.pdf (September 17, 2012).

ORGANIZATIONS

Centers for Disease Control and Prevention (CDC), 1600 Clifton Road, Atlanta, GA 30333, (800) 232-4636, cdcinfo@cdc.gov, http://www.cdc.gov

National Foundation for Infectious Diseases (NFID), 4733 Bethesda Avenue, Suite 750, Bethesda, MD 20814, (301) 656-0003, http://www.nfid.org

National Institute of Allergy and Infectious Diseases (NIAID), 6610 Rockledge Drive, MSC 6612, Bethesda, MD 20892, (866) 284-4107, http://www.niaid.nih.gov/Pages/default.aspx

World Health Organization, Avenue Appia 20, 1211 Geneva 27, Switzerlandhttp://www.who.int/.

Margaret Alic, Ph.D.
Leslie Mertz, Ph.D.

Infertility

Definition

Infertility is the biological failure of a couple to conceive a pregnancy after trying to do so frequently and without the use of contraceptives for at least one full year.

Description

Most couples in the United States, when they are not using contraceptive devices and techniques, conceive within the first six months of trying. However, infertility is a problem for about 10% of couples at any given time. In primary infertility, pregnancy has never occurred. In secondary infertility, one or both members of the couple have previously conceived, but are unable to conceive again after a full year of trying. The inability to conceive may be due to a single cause or multiple causes in either the female or the male, or both. Medical treatments are available that are safe and effective, and allow many couples to eventually become pregnant.

Demographics

About 10 percent of American women (6.1 million) between the ages of 15 and 44 have difficulty getting pregnant or staying pregnant, according to the **Centers for Disease Control and Prevention (CDC)**. The main factors involved in causing infertility include:

- Male problems: 20%
- Male and female problems: 30–40%
- Female problems: 40–50%

Fertility also decreases with increasing age. Numerous studies have documented this drop. A major study by the National Institute of **Environmental Health** Sciences in 2002, for instance, found that couples aged 19–26 had about a 50% chance of becoming pregnant if they had intercourse two days before ovulation, whereas couples aged 27–34 had a 40 percent chance, and couples aged more than 35 had a 30 percent chance.

Causes and symptoms

Causes

Unlike most medical problems, infertility is an issue requiring the careful evaluation of two separate partners, as well as an evaluation of their interactions with each other. In about 3%–4% of couples, no cause for infertility is discovered.

Male factors

Male infertility can be caused by a number of different characteristics of the sperm. These include low sperm count, abnormal sperm function or structure, and low volume of semen. Any number of conditions result in abnormalities. Genetic problems at birth can lead to improper growth of the testicles and, thus, infertility. Men can be born with one or both testicles that have not descended properly from the abdominal cavity (where testicles develop originally) into the scrotal sac, or may be born with only one instead of the normal two testicles. When testicles have not descended from the abdominal cavity, they are exposed to a higher body temperature than when they are descended. The higher temperature reduces the production of sperm.

In addition, testicle size can be smaller than normal. Past infections (including **mumps**) can affect testicular function, as can a past injury. For instance, exposure to sexually transmitted infections (STIs), such as gonorrhea and chlamydia, can result in infertility. The presence of abnormally large veins (varicocele) in the testicles can increase testicular temperature, which decreases sperm count.

History of exposure to various toxins, drug use, excess alcohol use, use of anabolic steroids, certain medications, diabetes, thyroid problems or other endocrine disturbances, and prostate problems can have direct effects on the formation of sperm (spermatogenesis). Problems with the male anatomy can cause sperm to be ejaculated not out of the penis, but into the bladder (a process known as retrograde ejaculation). Prostate, urethral, and bladder surgeries are three procedures that can lead to retrograde ejaculation. In addition, scarring from past infections can interfere with ejaculation. A condition called hypospadias can also cause infertility. Hypospadias occurs when the urinary opening on a man's penis is incorrectly located on its underside so that sperm cannot reach the cervix of a woman.

Sexual issues, such as erectile dysfunction, premature ejaculation, and dyspareunia (painful intercourse) can contribute to a male's infertility. Various psychological problems can also lead to a diminished level of fertility. **Stress** and depression can interfere with hormones that

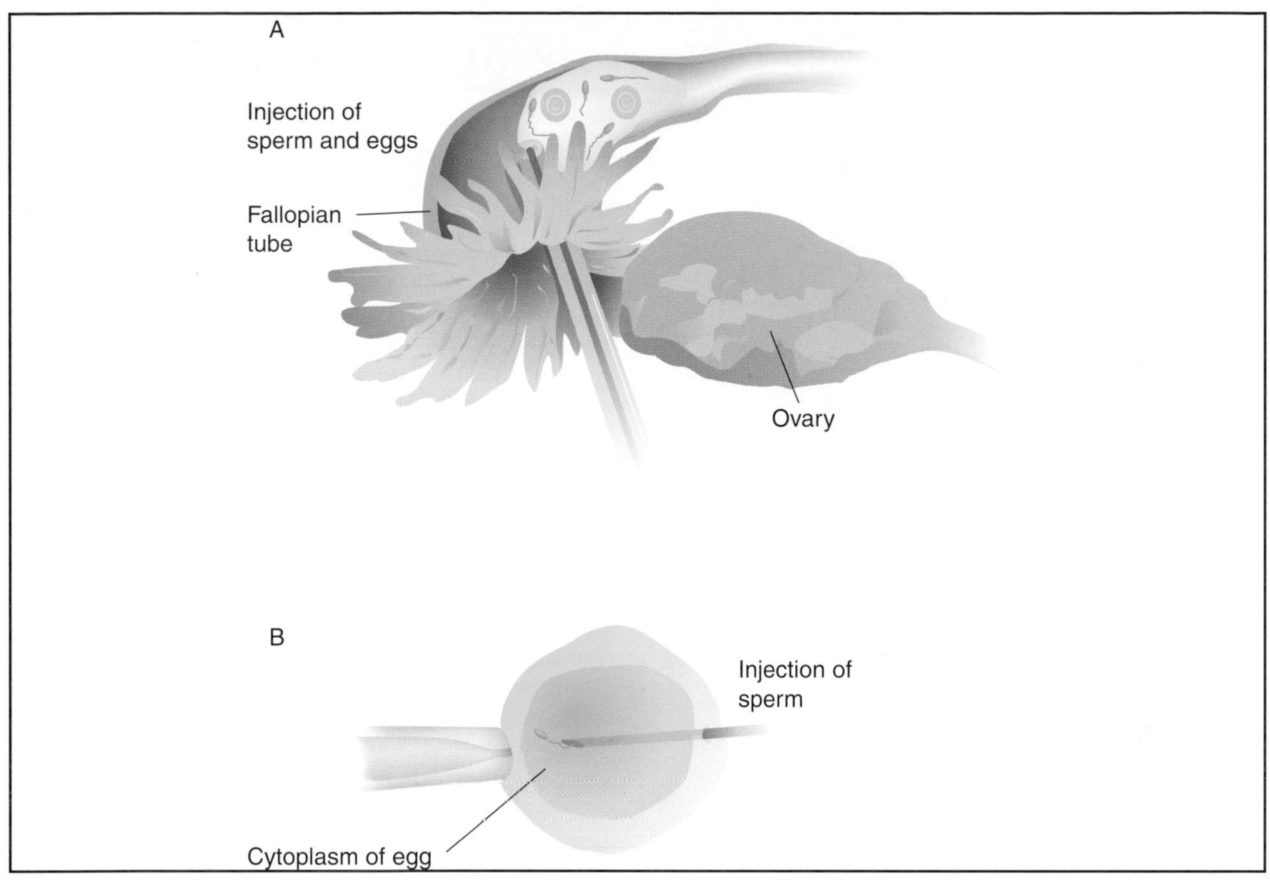

Gamete intrafallopian transfer (GIFT) *(Illustration by Argosy, Inc. Reproduced by permission of Gale, a part of Cengage Learning.)*

help to produce sperm. Men with long-term depression may have a reduced sperm count. Dietary deficiencies, such as insufficient vitamin C, zinc, and folate, may lead to infertility. **Obesity** (being extremely overweight) in males can also be a contributing factor in infertility. In addition, **radiation** treatment and chemotherapy for **cancer**, as well as **environmental toxins** (e.g., pesticides and lead) can reduce fertility.

Female factors

Pelvic adhesions and endometriosis are two causes of infertility in women, and can result in infertility by preventing the sperm from reaching the egg or interfering with fertilization. Pelvic adhesions are fibrous scars. These scars may result from past infections, such as pelvic inflammatory disease, or infections following abortions or prior births, or from previous surgeries.

Endometriosis may lead to pelvic adhesions. Endometriosis is the abnormal location of uterine tissue outside of the uterus. When uterine tissue is planted elsewhere in the pelvis, it still bleeds on a monthly basis with the start of the normal menstrual period. This leads to irritation within the pelvis around the site of this abnormal tissue, and may cause scarring, along with pelvic **pain**.

Pelvic adhesions cause infertility by blocking the Fallopian tubes. The ovum may be prevented from traveling down the Fallopian tube from the ovary, or the sperm may be prevented from traveling up the Fallopian tube from the uterus.

Cervical factors may affect a woman's ability to conceive. The cervix is the opening from the vagina into the uterus through which the sperm must pass. Mucus produced by the cervix helps to transport the sperm into the uterus. Injury to the cervix, or scarring of the cervix after surgery or infection can result in a smaller-than-normal cervical opening, making it difficult for the sperm to enter. Injury or infection can also decrease the number of glands in the cervix, leading to a smaller amount of cervical mucus. In other situations, the mucus produced is the wrong consistency (perhaps too thick) to allow sperm to travel through the cervix. In addition, some women produce antibodies (immune cells) that identify sperm as foreign invaders and kill them.

Other causes of female infertility include: Fallopian-tube damage or blockage (usually caused by

PATRICK CHRISTOPHER STEPTOE (1913–1988)

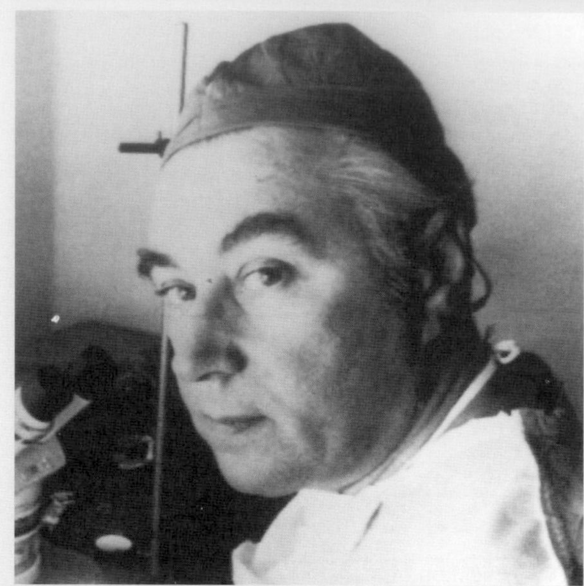

(Steptoe, Patrick, photograph. AP/Wide World Photos. Reproduced by permission.)

Patrick Christopher Steptoe was born in Oxfordshire, England, on June 9, 1913. His mother was a social worker and his father was a church organist. Steptoe entered the University of London's St. George Hospital Medical School, earning his physician's license in 1939 and becoming a member of the Royal College of Surgeons. When Steptoe volunteered as a naval surgeon during World War II, he was captured and held as a prisoner until his release in 1943. Following his release, Steptoe studied obstetrics and gynecology and moved to Manchester to start a private practice in 1948. In 1951, Steptoe accepted a position at Oldham General and District Hospital in England.

During his time at Oldham, Steptoe continued his study of fertility problems. Using a laparoscope, he developed a method to remove eggs from a woman's ovaries. In 1966, Steptoe teamed with physiologist Robert G. Edwards who had successfully fertilized eggs outside of the body. In 1968, the pair had a breakthrough when Edwards successfully fertilized an egg that Steptoe had removed, but their attempts to implant the embryo failed repeatedly. However, Steptoe and Edwards experienced success when a fertilized egg was implanted into the uterus of Leslie Brown. Brown gave birth to a healthy baby girl, Louise, on July 25, 1978.

Steptoe retired and built a clinic in Cambridge. He and Edwards were named Commanders of the British Empire, and Steptoe was honored with fellowship in the Royal Society. He and his wife had two children. Steptoe died on March 21, 1988.

inflammation), elevated prolactin (hyperprolactinemia), polycystic ovary syndrome (which results in the production of too much androgen hormone), early menopause (premature ovarian failure), uterine fibroids (benign tumors on the wall of the uterus), and various other medical problems (such as sickle cell disease, kidney disease, and diabetes).

A phenomenon of the past several decades, individuals often have multiple sexual partners before they try to have children. This increase in numbers of sexual partners has led to a rise in sexually transmitted infections. Scarring from these infections, especially from pelvic inflammatory disease (a serious infection of the female reproductive organs, most commonly caused by gonorrhea) seems to be in part responsible for the increase in infertility. Furthermore, use of a form of contraceptive called the intrauterine device (IUD) at one time contributed to an increased rate of pelvic inflammatory disease, with subsequent scarring. Newer IUDs do not lead to this increased rate of infection.

Symptoms

Infertility occurs upon the biological failure of a couple to conceive a pregnancy after trying to do so frequently and without the use of contraceptives for at least one full year.

Diagnosis

For men

To check for male infertility, a sample of semen is obtained and examined under the microscope, a procedure known as semen analysis. Four basic characteristics are usually evaluated:

- Sperm count, which refers to the number of sperm present in a semen sample. The normal number of sperm present in one milliliter (mL) of semen is more than 20 million. An individual with five to 20 million sperm per milliliter of semen is considered subfertile, and an individual with fewer than five million sperm per milliliter of semen is considered infertile.
- Sperm motility. Sperm are examined to see how well they swim.
- Abnormal sperm. Not all sperm within a specimen of semen will be perfectly normal. Some may be immature, and some may have abnormalities of the head or tail. A normal semen sample will contain no more than 25% abnormal forms of sperm.

• Volume of the semen sample. An abnormal amount of semen could affect the ability of the sperm to successfully fertilize an ovum.

Another test can be performed to evaluate the ability of the sperm to penetrate the outer coat of the ovum. This test is conducted by observing whether sperm in a semen sample can penetrate the outer coat of a guinea pig ovum. Fertilization cannot occur, of course, but this test is useful in predicting the ability of the individual's sperm to penetrate a human ovum.

For women

For pelvic adhesions, a hysterosalpingogram (HSG) can show if the Fallopian tubes are blocked. This is an x-ray examination that follows the movement of dye material through the patient's Fallopian tubes. A few women become pregnant following this x-ray exam. It is thought that the dye material in some way helps flush out the tubes, decreasing any existing obstruction. Scarring may be diagnosed by examining the pelvic area with a scope that can be inserted into the abdomen through a tiny incision made near the naval. This scoping technique is called laparoscopy.

Cervical mucus can be examined under a microscope to diagnose whether cervical factors are contributing to infertility. The interaction of a live sperm sample from the male partner and a sample of cervical mucus from the female partner can also be examined. This procedure is called a post-coital test.

The first step in diagnosing ovulatory problems is to make sure that an ovum is being produced each month. A woman's morning body temperature is slightly higher around the time of ovulation. A woman can measure and record her temperatures daily and a chart can be drawn to show whether or not ovulation has occurred. Luteinizing hormone (LH) is released just before ovulation. A simple urine test can be done to check if LH has been released around the time that ovulation is expected.

Treatment

Male infertility

Treatment of male infertility includes addressing known reversible factors first. These may include discontinuing any medication known to have an effect on spermatogenesis or ejaculation, as well as decreasing alcohol intake, quitting **smoking**, and treating thyroid or other endocrine disease. Varicoceles can be treated surgically. Testosterone in low doses can improve sperm motility.

Other treatments of male infertility include collecting semen samples from multiple ejaculations, after which the semen is put through a process that allows the most motile sperm to be sorted out. These motile sperm are pooled together to create a concentrate that can be deposited into the female partner's uterus at a time that coincides with ovulation. In cases where the male partner's sperm is proven to be absolutely incapable of causing pregnancy in the female partner, and with the consent of both partners, donor sperm may be used for this process. Depositing the male partner's sperm or donor sperm by mechanical means into the female partner are both forms of artificial insemination.

Female infertility

Pelvic adhesions can be treated during laparoscopy. The adhesions are cut using special instruments. Endometriosis can be treated with certain medications, but may also require surgery to repair any obstruction caused by adhesions.

Treatment of cervical factors includes **antibiotics** in the case of an infection, steroids to decrease production of anti-sperm antibodies, and artificial insemination techniques to completely bypass the cervical mucus.

Treatment of ovulatory problems depends on the cause. If a thyroid or pituitary problem is responsible, simply treating that problem can restore fertility. (The thyroid and pituitary glands release hormones that also are involved in regulating a woman's menstrual cycle.)

Prescribed medication can also be used to stimulate fertility:

• Clomiphene citrate (Clomid, Milophene, and Serophene), which is used to increase the natural production of the hormones that stimulate ovulation in otherwise healthy women. When clomiphene is administered, the body produces higher levels of luteinizing hormone (LH), follicle stimulating hormone (FSH), and gonadotropins. These hormones induce ovulation. In some cases, FSH may be administered by injection to stimulate the follicle growth directly.

• Human chorionic gonadotropin (hCG), which is sold under many brand names including Gonic, Pregnyl, Ovidrel, Chorex, Chorigon, and Profasi. This hormone stimulates the gonads in both men and women. In men, hCG increases androgen production. In women, it increases the levels of progesterone. Human chorionic gonadotropin can help stimulate ovulation in women.

• Other natural and synthetic hormones, which are used to induce ovulation. Urofollitropin (Bravelle, Fertinex) is a concentrated preparation of human hormones, while follitropin alfa (Gonal-F) and follitropin beta (Follistim) are human FSH preparations of recombinant DNA (deoxyribonucleic acid) origin.

• Menotropins (Pergonal, Humegon, Repronex) are often given with human chorionic gonadotropin to stimulate ovulation in women and sperm production in men. Human menopausal gonadotropins (hMG) may be used be administered by injection to stimulate the ovaries to produce more than one egg during a cycle.

- Bromocriptine and cabergoline are medications given orally to reduce prolactin levels. Prolactin is a hormone that inhibits FSH and gonadotropin-releasing hormone.

Assisted reproductive techniques

Assisted reproductive techniques include *in vitro* fertilization (IVF), gamete intrafallopian transfer (GIFT), and zygote intrafallopian tube transfer (ZIFT). These are usually used after other techniques to treat infertility have failed. According to the CDC's 2010 statistics (the latest available), IVF is successful in leading to a live birth in 41.5% of women 34 years old and younger; 31.9% of those 35–37 years old; 22.1% of those 37–40 years old; and 12.4% of those 41–42 years old. (In comparison, the 1997 rates were 30.7%, 25.5% 17.1% and 7.6%, respectively.) As of 2010, the **CDC** reports that more than 1% of infants born in the United States are conceived using assisted reproductive techniques.

In vitro fertilization involves the use of a drug to induce the simultaneous release of many eggs from the female's ovaries, which are retrieved surgically. Meanwhile, several semen samples are obtained from the male partner, and a sperm concentrate is prepared. The ova and sperm are then combined in a laboratory, where several of the ova may be fertilized. Cell division is allowed to take place up to the embryo stage. While this takes place, the female may be given drugs to ensure that her uterus is ready to receive an embryo. Three or four of the embryos are transferred to the female's uterus, and the wait begins to see if any or all of them implant and result in an actual pregnancy.

IVF procedures typically put more than one embryo into the uterus, so the chance for a multiple birth (twins or more) is greatly increased in couples undergoing IVF. Couples should discuss this possibility with their healthcare professionals.

According to the American Pregnancy Association, The success rate (a live birth) for each cycle of IVF varies with the age of the mother: 30–35% for women age 34 or younger; 25% for women ages 35–37; 15–20% for women ages 38–40; and 6–10% for women more than 40 years old. As of 2012, an estimated five million babies around the world had been born with the help of in vitro fertilization.

GIFT involves retrieval of both multiple ova and semen, and the mechanical placement of both within the female partner's Fallopian tubes. ZIFT involves the same retrieval of ova and semen, and fertilization and growth in the laboratory up to the zygote stage, at which point the zygotes are placed in the Fallopian tubes.

For serious problems with the sperm, or for older couples who have not had success with IVF, doctors may recommend intracytoplasmic sperm injection (ICSI). In this method, a single sperm is injected into a mature egg, which is then transferred to the uterus or Fallopian tube.

KEY TERMS

Blastocyst—A cluster of cells representing multiple cell divisions that have occurred in the Fallopian tube after successful fertilization of an ovum by a sperm. This is the developmental form which must leave the Fallopian tube, enter the uterus, and implant itself in the uterus to achieve actual pregnancy.

Cervix—The opening from the vagina, which leads into the uterus.

Embryo—The stage of development of a baby between the second and eighth weeks after conception.

Endometrium—The lining of the uterus.

Fallopian tube—The tube leading from the ovary into the uterus. Just as there are two ovaries, there are two Fallopian tubes.

Fetus—A baby developing in the uterus from the third month to birth.

Ovary—The female organ in which eggs (ova) are stored and mature.

Ovum (plural: ova)—The reproductive cell of the female, which contains genetic information and participates in the act of fertilization. Also popularly called the egg.

Semen—The fluid that contains sperm, which is ejaculated by the male.

Sperm—The reproductive cell of the male, which contains genetic information and participates in the act of fertilization of an ovum.

Spermatogenesis—The process by which sperm develop to become mature sperm, capable of fertilizing an ovum.

Zygote—The result of the sperm successfully fertilizing the ovum. The zygote is a single cell that contains the genetic material of both the mother and the father.

Other options for infertile couples include the use of a surrogate or a gestational carrier. In surrogacy, the woman's cannot produce a healthy egg, so the man's sperm is used to fertilize the egg of another woman, called the surrogate, and implanted in her womb. Once the surrogate delivers the baby, the couple adopts the baby. A gestational carrier is similar to a surrogate, except that the implanted embryo is biologically the couple's (the sperm and egg are both from the couple).

Individuals who undergo assisted reproductive techniques may wish to consider preimplantation genetic diagnosis, which are procedures that screen the egg or embryo for specific genetic diseases.

RECOMMENDED DOSAGE. Dosage varies for different patients. The physician who prescribes the drug or the pharmacist who fills the prescription will recommend the correct dosage. For instance, clomiphene must be taken at certain times during the menstrual cycle.

PRECAUTIONS. Seeing a physician regularly while taking infertility drugs is important because side effects and complications can occur. A patient should inform her doctor at once if she becomes pregnant while taking the drugs. In addition, patients should inform their doctors about any other drugs they are taking, any **allergies** and additional medical conditions they may have.

Infertility treatments may increase the chance of multiple births, which can cause problems during pregnancy and delivery, and can even threaten the babies' survival.

SIDE EFFECTS. When used in low doses for a short time, clomiphene and HCG rarely cause side effects. However, anyone who has stomach or pelvic pain or bloating while taking either medicine should check with a physician immediately. Each of the infertility drugs carries some side effects, so patients should get complete information from their physicians before beginning these medications. These side effects usually go away as the body adjusts to the drug and do not require medical treatment unless they continue or they interfere with normal activities. However, anyone who has unusual symptoms after taking infertility drugs should contact a physician.

Some studies suggest that the risk for certain cancers may increase or decrease following the use of certain fertility drugs. A 2012 study, for instance, suggested that women who used the fertility drugs clomiphene and FSH, but who did not conceive a 10-plus week pregnancy, experienced a reduced risk of young-onset breast cancer (diagnosed at 49 years old or younger) compared to nonusers. Those women who used the drugs and did conceive a 10-plus week pregnancy, however, showed no similar benefit.

Prevention

Couples can naturally increase the chances of becoming pregnant by having regular sexual intercourse, particularly between the 10th day and 18th days after the beginning of a woman's menstrual period. Among women who have regularly spaced menstruation periods, ovulation normally occurs about 14 days before menstruation begins. Therefore, sexual activity should be especially frequent from three days before to three days after ovulation. For additional help, a physician may recommend using an ovulation prediction test kit to help determine the best times for intercourse.

Prognosis

Prognosis varies greatly and is based on the different problems that exist within an individual or couple trying to conceive. In general, about half of all couples that undergo a complete evaluation of infertility followed by treatment and therapies will ultimately have a successful pregnancy. Of those couples who do not choose to undergo evaluation or treatment, about 5% go on to conceive after a year or more of infertility.

Prevention

Individuals can take a number of steps to reduce their future chances of infertility. These include:

- Having fewer sexual partners and using contraceptive devices (such as condoms) that reduce the chances of contracting sexually transmitted infections, such as chlamydia and gonorrhea
- Getting a mumps vaccination
- Quitting smoking
- Maintaining a healthy lifestyle with respect to diet and exercise.

Effects on public health

Challenges to fertility may arise for any number of reasons, but regardless of the reason, infertility can be devastating to individuals who want to have children, and may lead to psychological stress, anxiety, and depression. As described in a 2010 article in *Fertility and Sterility*, "The journey for those people who are infertile may begin with unrecognized health problems; continue with difficulties in obtaining services that often are not covered by health insurance; and even after success with physically demanding and expensive medical procedures, it may lead to unexpected adverse effects on the health and quality of life of the patients and their children."

QUESTIONS TO ASK THE DOCTOR

- What can I and my partner do to increase our chances of becoming pregnant?
- What are the potential side effects of fertility drugs?
- What is the likelihood that in vitro fertilization will lead to multiple fertilizations? What are my options if that occurs?
- Does in vitro fertilization carry any additional health risks for babies born with this method?

Costs to society

The financial costs for treatment options vary. According to estimates from RESOLVE, the National Infertility Association, the average cost for various assisted reproductive techniques are: one cycle of IVF using fresh embryos (not including medications): $8,158, plus an additional $1,544 for intracytoplasmic sperm injection and/or $3,550 for preimplantation genetic diagnosis, if necessary and available.

In addition, infertility may take a psychological toll on individuals, and affect overall quality of life.

Efforts and solutions

The **Centers for Disease Control and Prevention (CDC)** monitors the prevalence of infertility and the use of infertility services and treatments; conducts and promotes research on causes of infertility and the efficacy and safety of infertility treatments; and develops public-health programs that address the causes of infertility, especially **sexually transmitted diseases** and reproductive-tract infections. In addition to those efforts, the Centers for Disease Control is drafting "A National Public Health Action Plan for the Detection, **Prevention**, and Management of Infertility." Developed with many governmental and nongovernmental partners, the draft plan addresses male and female infertility, and outlines actions needed promote, preserve, and restore the ability of women to have healthy babies. The full draft plan is available at http://www.cdc.gov/reproductivehealth/Infertility/PDF/CDC-2012-0004-0002.pdf.

Fertility treatments can be very expensive, and they are usually not covered by medical insurance. In answer to the demand for infertility treatments, and in recognition of the large financial outlay that is typically required, a network of fertility clinics, called Advanced Reproductive Care, offers a program called "The ARC Affordable Payment Plan." It offers a financing plan for fertility treatments, and also a money-back guarantee for patients who do not have a baby at the end of their fertility care.

In addition, research is underway at universities, in drug-company laboratories, and other venues around the country and around the world to test the efficacy and safety of current infertility drugs, and to develop new options for infertile couples.

Resources

PERIODICALS

Centers for Disease Control and Prevention. "A National Public Health Action Plan for the Detection, Prevention, and Management of Infertility." (2012). http://www.cdc.gov/reproductivehealth/Infertility/PDF/CDC-2012-0004-0002.pdf.

Cui, Weiyuan W. "Mother or Nothing." *Bulletin of the World Health Organization.* 88, no. 12 (2010): 877–953.

Falco, Miriam. "5 Million Babies Born So Far, Thanks to IVF," CNN Health, CNN. http://thechart.blogs.cnn.com/2012/07/02/5-million-babies-born-so-far-thanks-to-ivf/ (accessed September 18, 2012).

Fei, C., et al., "Fertility Drugs and Young-Onset Breast Cancer: Results from the Two-Sister Study." *Journal of The National Cancer Institute* 104, no. 13 (2012): 1021–1027.

Macaluso, Maurizio, et al. "A Public Health Focus on Infertility Prevention, Detection, and Management." *Fertility and Sterility.* 93, no. 1 (2010): 16.e1–16.e10.

WEBSITES

"Fertility Drugs Impact on U.S. Births." Centers for Disease Control. http://www.cdc.gov/reproductivehealth/infertility/index.htm (accessed September 18, 2012)

"Infertility" Medline Plus, U.S. National Library of Medicine and National Institutes of Health. http://www.nlm.nih.gov/medlineplus/infertility.html (accessed September 18, 2012)

"Infertility FAQs" Centers for Disease Control. http://www.cdc.gov/reproductivehealth/infertility/index.htm (accessed September 18, 2012)

"Infertility Medications" American Pregnancy Association. http://www.americanpregnancy.org/infertility/infertility-medications.html (accessed September 18, 2012).

"In vitro Fertilization: IVF" American Pregnancy Association. http://www.americanpregnancy.org/infertility/ivf.html (accessed September 18, 2012)

"Male Infertility FAQs" American Fertility Association. http://www.theafa.org/family-building/male-infertility/ (accessed September 18, 2012)

"Optimizing My Fertility" RESOLVE: The National Infertility Association. http://www.resolve.org/infertility-overview/optimizing-fertility/ (accessed September 18, 2012)

PubMed Health. "Infertility" U.S. National Library of Medicine. http://www.ncbi.nlm.nih.gov/pubmedhealth/PMH0002173/ (accessed September 18, 2012)

"What Is Assistive Reproductive Technology" Centers for Disease Control. http://www.cdc.gov/art/ (accessed September 18, 2012)

Women'sHealth.gov. "Infertility Fact Sheet" U.S. Department of Health and Human Services. http://www.womenshealth.gov/publications/our-publications/fact-sheet/infertility.cfm#b (accessed September 18, 2012)

ORGANIZATIONS

American Fertility Organization, 315 Madison Avenue, Suite 901, New York, NY 10017, (888) 917-3777, http://www.theafa.org/

American Pregnancy Association, 1425 Greenway Drive, Suite 440., Irving, TX 75038, (972) 550-0800, Questions@AmericanPregnancy.org, http://www.americanpregnancy.org/

American Society for Reproductive Medicine, 1209 Montgomery Hwy., Birmingham, AL 35216-2809, (205) 978-5000, asrm@asrm.org, http://www.asrm.org

Centers for Disease Control and Prevention (CDC), 1600 Clifton Road, Atlanta, GA 30333, (800) 232-4636, cdcinfo@cdc.gov, http://www.cdc.gov

Planned Parenthood Federation of America, 434 West 33rd Street, New York, NY 10001, (212) 541-7800, http://www.plannedparenthood.org/

RESOLVE, The National Infertility Association, 1760 Old Meadow Rd., Suite 500, McLean, VA 22102, (703) 556-7172, info@resolve.org, http://www.resolve.org.

Rosalyn Carson-DeWitt, M.D.
Teresa G. Odle
Leslie Mertz, Ph.D.

Infestations

Definition

Infestation can describe any presence of living organisms—including animals, plants, or **parasites**—in such large quantities that the organisms become overwhelming, dangerous, or cause damage. Organisms likely to cause infestation often have a tendency to reproduce rapidly.

Description

Infestations occur when a given area is overrun by abnormally large quantities of a pest. Large populations often become infestations when the pests begin to cause damage to property or health. The excessively invasive nature of such pests differentiates them from other organisms that may be a nuisance. Some common infestations include: bed bugs, bats, rodents, lice, tapeworms, termites, zebra mussels, kudzu, and scabies.

The scope of an infestation varies—often depending upon the type of pest involved. Some infestations damage only the person or location that they are inhabiting (like tapeworms, or bats), some infestations require specific types of contact to spread (like pubic lice, also known as "crabs"), other infestations grow and expand rapidly to surrounding areas with little assistance (like zebra mussels, kudzu, or rodents). Despite the many different types of infestations, they can be generically categorized based on the types of organisms that cause them: infestations of the human body, botanical (plant) infestations, and animal infestations.

Infestations of the human body

Some infestations are localized on or within the human body. Infestations should be differentiated from infections. Infestations harm or molest the areas they occupy, whereas infections contaminate and feed off of their host. Some infections can kill their host. Most organisms that infest the human body do so externally, without invading the blood or respiratory system. Tapeworms (cestoid worms) are examples of an infestation that can occur internally—tapeworms are an infestation that affects the digestive tract of humans and animals. Some examples of external infestations are scabies, ringworm, and lice (including head lice, body lice, and pubic lice).

Treatments for infestations of the human body vary depending on the type of infestation. There are pharmaceutical treatments available for these infestations, and many infestations have corresponding alternative treatments. When dealing with all forms of lice, neither pharmaceutical nor alternative treatments have proven 100% effective on first use—lice nits (eggs) and live lice must be removed manually, in addition to the application of a pharmaceutical or alternative treatment. Most infestations on or affecting the human body (including lice, scabies, and bed bugs) require sterilization or disposal of personal items and clothing.

DELUSIONAL INFESTATION. In addition to the physical presence of an infestation on the human body, there is a psychological or dermatological condition in which a patient has the sensation of a skin infestation (usually involving sensations of itching, crawling on the skin, and **pain**) yet doctors can locate no organism causing infestation. There have been attempts to create an official diagnosis—Morgellens disease—for this condition, though this diagnosis has not been officially approved by a medical body. Dermatologists and emergency room physicians are often the first to treat patients with these symptoms. These doctors then conduct various tests and screenings to attempt to locate bacteria, fungus, parasites, or other potential causes of infestation. Even if no cause is found, sometimes precautionary medication will be prescribed or medication to treat presenting inflammatory symptoms. If the patient continues to declare symptoms in the absence of a detectable cause, these doctors will usually attempt to get the patient psychiatric help.

Botanical infestation

Plants that pose a risk to property, ecosystems, and other plants are often dubbed "invasive." Some plants are invasive enough that they are categorized as infesting the areas that they take over. These plants are introduced to a non-native region from a foreign source, sometimes intentionally (kudzu was important to help with soil erosion), sometimes accidentally (seeds are sometimes mistakenly transported or planted). The effects of botanical infestations can vary, but they tend to be far-reaching and hard to contain. Plant infestations usually displace native vegetation, thereby disrupting the area's ecosystem. One example of a botanical infestation is the Japanese kudzu (*Pueraria Montana*), which is a vine in the pea family that can grow up to 60 feet per season, with tap roots that can grow to more than six feet in length and can weigh as much as 400 pounds. Kudzu grows over anything in its path, choking out any vegetation it overtakes. Another botanical infestation is leafy spurge (*Euphorbia esula L.*), which appears to be a yellow wildflower, but displaces nutrients and **water** from the surrounding soil and releases a toxin, the combined effect of which is destruction of native vegetation in the area. Many plant infestations are treated through pesticides, mechanical removal, and/or burning. Some plants, such as cogon grass (*Imperata cylindrical*) actually thrive after burning—it prohibits other vegetation from emerging after the fire and comes back more heartily.

Animal infestations

Like other infestations, animal infestations can vary in severity. Bat infestations, for instance, are often more localized; even as contained as within a single house. Other infestations—like the boll weevil infestation of the early twentieth century—can span thousands of miles and wreak havoc on property and economies. Rodent infestations, though dangerous to property and health, are more common and often systemic. Many urban areas in the United States and abroad, particularly developing countries, have problems with rodent infestations and subsequent damage and disease. Some animal infestations are natural results of cycles in the dominance of various predators, prey, and even weather.

As a result of the many types of animal infestations and their many causes, there are many ways to deal with animal infestations. Bat infestations tend to be more of a nuisance to property than to health—though depending on the size of the infestation, bat feces and **rabies** may become issues—and there are a variety of removal experts that can trap and remove bats. Smaller rat infestations in an individual residence or business can usually be dealt with by the same pest removal companies that handle bat removal. Municipal infestations are harder to control and are often ongoing, though they may take on an ebb and flow pattern.

KEY TERM

Morgellons Disease—a mysterious medical condition first described in the seventeenth century featuring the sensation of itching and/or crawling on the skin, where no cause can be found medically. Some Morgellons patients have additional health side effects or conditions and many show an inflammatory response though no cause can be located. Despite being described for hundreds of years, Morgellons Disease has not yet been recognized by any official medical body in the United States.

Effects on public health

Infestations of the human body are particularly damaging to public health. Many infestations that can occur on or affect the human body spread easily with contact. Head and body lice are prone to spread, particularly among schoolchildren who spend prolonged periods of time together and frequently exchange clothing and other personal belongings. Luckily lice infestations do not pose a serious health threat and both pharmaceutical and alternative treatments for lice are relatively inexpensive. Scabies infestations are frequently transmitted in nursing homes, prisons, and child care facilities. Crusted (Norwegian) scabies are particularly dangerous as they indicate an excessive number of the mites which cause scabies. Persons with crusted scabies are much more contagious and pose a greater risk to the public until medication has neutralized the infestation.

Animal infestations—particularly when they cover larger areas—can become public health concerns. With many animal infestations—like those of bats and rodents—there are peripheral concerns for public health. Animal feces and bites can cause disease and infection to spread rapidly. Historically, many plagues and large disease outbreaks were spread through animal infestations.

Costs to society

Any widespread infestation has the potential to be costly to society. Botanical infestations often move quickly, cover large areas, and are difficult or impossible to completely eradicate. Botanical infestations often have long-lasting effects by affecting the components and viability of entire ecosystems. Botanical infestations also interfere with the growth of crops that are depended upon for food and income—for instance, jointed goatgrass has been detrimental to American wheat crops, and the boll weevil infestation of the early 1900s devastated cotton crops across the south. Additionally, removal methods for botanical infestations tend to be costly and require multiple applications without guarantee of success. When infestations of the human body or the peripheral effects of animal infestations become widespread, society bears the health costs involved.

Resources

BOOKS

"Boll Weevil Infestation." *Gale Encyclopedia of U.S. Economic History*. Ed. Thomas Carson and Mary Bonk. Vol. 1. Detroit: Gale, 1999.

Cancedda, Corrado. "Tapeworm Infestation." *Encylopedia of Diseases and Disorders*. New York: Marshall Cavendish Reference, 2011.

Davidson, Tish. "Bedbug Infestation." *The Gale Encyclopedia of Medicine*. Ed. Laurie J. Fundukian. 4th ed. Vol. 1. Detroit: Gale, 2011.

Frey, Rebecca J., and Margaret Alic. "Lice Infestation." *The Gale Encyclopedia of Medicine*. Ed. Laurie J. Fundukian. 4th ed. Vol. 4. Detroit: Gale, 2011.

"Morgellons Disease." *Magill's Medical Guide*. Ed. Brandon P. Brown, et al. 6th ed. Vol. 4: Kinesiology–Parasitic diseases. Pasadena, CA: Salem Press, 2011.

"Skin Infections and Infestations." *Skin and Connective Tissue*. Ed. Kara Rogers. New York: Britannica Educational Publishing with Rosen Educational Services, 2012.

Weinstein, Philip, and David Slaney. "Psychiatry and Insects: Phobias and Delusions of Insect Infestations in Humans." *Encyclopedia of Entomology*. Ed. John L. Capinera. 2nd ed. Dordrecht, The Netherlands: Springer, 2008.

PERIODICALS

Bostwick, J. Michael, et al. "Delusional infestation: Clinical presentation in 147 patients seen at Mayo Clinic." *Journal of the American Academy of Dermatology*. Oct. 2012: 673.e1-673.e10.

Kavita, Tarun Narang, and Shubh Singh. "Delusional infestation with fungus." *Indian Journal of Dermatology, Venereology and Leprology* 78.5 (2012): 645.

WEBSITES

Center for Disease Control and Prevention "Scabies."http://www.cdc.gov/parasites/scabies/gen_info/index.html Accessed September 25, 2012.

Center for Invasive Species and Ecosystem Health"Invasive and Exotic Plants."http://www.invasive.org/species/weeds.cfm Accessed September 25, 2012.

National Park Service"Alien Plant Invaders of Natural Areas." http://www.nps.gov/plants/alien/fact.htm Accessed September 25, 2012.

ORGANIZATIONS

Centers for Disease Control and Prevention, 1600 Clifton Road, Atlanta, GA USA 30333, (800) 232-4636, cdcinfo@cdc.gov, www.cdc.gov.

Andrea Nienstedt, MA

Influenza

Definition

Usually referred to as "the flu" or "grippe," influenza is a highly infectious respiratory disease. The disease is caused by certain strains of the influenza virus. When the virus is inhaled, it attacks cells in the upper respiratory tract, causing typical flu symptoms such as fatigue, fever and chills, a hacking cough, and body aches. Influenza victims are also susceptible to potentially life-threatening secondary infections. Although the stomach or intestinal "flu" is commonly blamed for stomach upsets and diarrhea, the influenza virus rarely causes gastrointestinal symptoms. Such symptoms are most likely due to other organisms, such as **rotavirus**, *Salmonella*, *Shigella*, or *Escherichia coli*.

Description

The flu is considerably more debilitating than the **common cold**. Influenza outbreaks occur suddenly, and infection spreads rapidly. The annual death toll attributable to influenza and its complications ranges from 3,000 to about 49,000 in the United States alone, according to the **Centers for Disease Control and Prevention (CDC)**.

Demographics

Each year, between 5 and 20% of U.S. residents get the flu, and on average, more than 200,000 are hospitalized for flu-related complications. Between 1976 and 2006, estimates of flu-associated deaths in the United States ranged from a low of about 3,000 to a high of about 49,000 people. In the United States, an estimated 90% of all deaths from influenza occur among persons older than 65. In addition, 60% of seasonal flu-related hospitalizations occur in this older population. Flu-related deaths have increased substantially in the United States since the 1970s, largely because of the **aging** of the American population. In addition, elderly persons are vulnerable because they are often reluctant to be vaccinated against flu.

Causes and symptoms

Causes

There are three types of influenza viruses, identified as A, B, and C. Influenza A can infect a range of animal species, including humans, pigs, horses, and birds, but only humans are infected by types B and C. Influenza A is responsible for most flu cases, while infections with types B and C are less common and cause a milder illness.

Symptoms

Approximately one to four days after infection with the influenza virus, the victim is hit with an array of symptoms. "Hit" is an appropriate term, because symptoms are sudden, harsh, and unmistakable. Typical influenza symptoms include the abrupt onset of a headache, dry cough, and chills, rapidly followed by overall achiness and a fever that may run as high as 104°F (40°C). As the fever subsides, nasal congestion and a sore throat become noticeable. Flu victims feel extremely tired and weak and might not return to their normal energy levels for several days or even a couple of weeks.

Influenza complications usually arise from bacterial infections of the lower respiratory tract. Signs of a secondary respiratory infection often appear just as the victim seems to be recovering. These signs include high fever, intense chills, chest pains associated with breathing, and a productive cough with thick, yellowish-green sputum. If these symptoms appear, medical treatment is necessary. Other secondary infections, such as sinus or ear infections, may also require medical intervention. Heart and lung problems, and other chronic diseases, can be aggravated by influenza, which is a particular concern with elderly patients.

With children and teenagers, it is advisable to be alert for symptoms of Reye's syndrome, a rare but serious complication. Symptoms of Reye's syndrome are nausea and vomiting, and more seriously, neurological problems such as confusion or delirium. The syndrome has been associated with the use of aspirin to relieve flu symptoms.

Origins

The earliest existing descriptions of influenza were written nearly 2,500 years ago by the ancient Greek physician Hippocrates. Historically, influenza was ascribed to a number of different agents, including "bad air" and several different bacteria. In fact, its name comes from the Italian word for "influence," because people in 18th-century Europe thought that the disease was caused by the influence of bad weather. It was not until 1933 that the causative agent was identified as a virus.

Influenza is frequently associated with pandemics, which affect millions of people worldwide and last for several months. In the 1918–1919 Spanish flu **pandemic**, for instance, the death toll reached a staggering 20 million—40 million worldwide. Approximately 500,000 of these fatalities occurred in the United States. Influenza outbreaks occur on a regular basis. The 1918–1919 influenza outbreak serves as the primary example of an influenza pandemic. Pandemics also occurred in 1957 and 1968 with the Asian flu and Hong Kong flu, respectively. The Asian flu was responsible for 70,000 deaths in the United States, while the Hong Kong flu killed 34,000.

Epidemics are widespread regional outbreaks that affect 5–10% of the population. The Russian flu in the winter of 1977 was an example of an epidemic. A regional epidemic is shorter-lived than a pandemic, lasting only several weeks. Smaller outbreaks that are confined to specific locales also occur each winter.

Diagnosis

Although specific tests are available to identify the flu virus strain from respiratory samples, doctors typically rely on the set of symptoms and the presence of influenza in the community for diagnosis. Specific tests are useful to determine the type of flu in the community, but they do little for individual treatment. Doctors may administer tests, such as throat cultures, to identify secondary infections.

Rapid diagnostic tests for flu have become commercially available. As of 2012, The U.S. Food and Drug Administration had approved more than 10 of them. The tests provide results within 15 minutes. According to the **CDC**, they are useful for determining whether influenza is the cause of an outbreak of acute respiratory disease and for confirming that the flu is the cause of respiratory illness in specific patients and helping healthcare personnel decide the best course of action. Rapid diagnostic tests are not necessary for most flu patients.

Treatment

Essentially, a bout of influenza must be allowed to run its course. Symptoms can be relieved with bed rest and by keeping well hydrated. A steam vaporizer may make breathing easier, and **pain** relievers will take care of the aches and pain. Food might not seem very appetizing, but an effort should be made to consume nourishing food. Recovery should not be pushed too rapidly. Returning to normal activities too quickly invites a possible relapse or complications.

Drugs

Since influenza is a viral infection, **antibiotics** are useless in treating it. However, antibiotics are frequently used to treat secondary infections.

Over-the-counter medications are used to treat flu symptoms, but it is not necessary to purchase a medication marketed specifically for flu symptoms. Any medication that is designed to relieve symptoms, such as pain and coughing, will provide some relief. Medications containing alcohol, however, should be avoided because of the dehydrating effects. The best medicine for symptoms is simply an analgesic, such as aspirin, acetaminophen, or naproxen. Without a doctor's approval, aspirin is generally not recommended for people under 18, owing to its association with Reye's syndrome, a rare aspirin-associated complication seen in children recovering from the flu. To be on the safe side, children should instead receive acetaminophen or ibuprofen to treat their symptoms.

Antiviral drugs are available for treating influenza and are typically prescribed for patients who have weakened immune systems or who are at risk for developing serious complications. The drugs include amantadine (Symmetrel, Symadine) and rimantadine (Flumandine), which work against Type A influenza, and zanamavir (Relenza) and oseltamavir phosphate (Tamiflu), which work against both Types A and B influenza. Amantadine and rimantadine can cause side effects such as nervousness, anxiety, lightheadedness, and nausea. Severe side effects include seizures, delirium, and hallucination but are rare and are nearly always limited to people who have kidney problems, seizure disorders, or psychiatric disorders. The new drugs zanamavir and oseltamavir phosphate have few side effects but can cause dizziness, jitters, and insomnia.

Alternative treatments

Several alternative treatments may help in fighting off the virus and recovering from the flu, in addition to easing flu symptoms. These include:

- Acupuncture and acupressure. Both are said to stimulate natural resistance, relieve nasal congestion and headaches, fight fever, and calm coughs, depending on the acupuncture and acupressure points used.
- Aromatherapy. Aromatherapists recommend gargling daily with one drop each of the essential oils of tea tree (*Melaleuca* spp.) and lemon mixed in a glass of warm water. If already suffering from the flu, two drops of tea tree oil in a hot bath may help ease the symptoms. Essential oils of eucalyptus (*Eucalyptus globulus*) or peppermint (*Mentha piperita*) added to a steam vaporizer may help clear chest and nasal congestion.
- Herbal remedies. Herbalists may suggest remedies to stimulate the immune system (echinacea), or to fight the virus (*Hydrastis canadensis*), goldenseal and garlic (*Allium sativum*). They may recommend additional herbs to fight other symptoms that arise as a result of the flu: an infusion of boneset (*Eupatroium perfoliatum*) for counteracting aches and fever, and yarrow (*Achillea millefolium*) or elderflower tinctures for combating chills.
- A wide variety of additional alternative treatments are also used. These include homeopathic remedies, hydrotherapy (hot-water baths), and traditional Chinese medicine.
- Vitamins. Some people take vitamin C every day to help prevent the flu and to hasten recovery when they get the flu.

Prognosis

Following proper treatment guidelines, healthy people under the age of 65 usually suffer no long-term consequences associated with flu infection. The elderly and the chronically ill are at greater risk for secondary infection and other complications, but they can also enjoy a complete recovery.

Most people recover fully from an influenza infection, but it should not be viewed complacently. Influenza is a serious disease and sometimes proves fatal.

Prevention

In February 2010, the CDC's Advisory Committee on **Immunization** Practices (ACIP) voted for "universal" flu **vaccination**, which means that everyone aged 6 months or older should get a flu vaccine each year. Through this action, the committee hoped to expand protection against the flu to more people. In the United States, flu season typically runs from late December to early March, but it may begin as early as October. As of 2012, three flu shots are available in the United States:

- The regular seasonal flu shot, which is injected into muscle (usually in the upper arm), is for use in people who are 6 months of age or older, including healthy people, people with chronic medical conditions and pregnant women. This regular seasonal flu shot is the main vaccine supply produced for the United States.
- A high-dose vaccine for people 65 and older. This vaccine, which is injected into muscle (intramuscular) first became available during the 2010–2011 season.
- An intradermal vaccine (a vaccine that is injected into the skin) for people aged 18–64 years old. This vaccine first became available during the 2011–2012 season.

In addition, patients may opt to receive the vaccine as a mist, which is sprayed into the nostrils. Because it is made with live, weakened flu viruses, it is known as "live attenuated influenza vaccine" (LAIV). These weakened viruses do not cause the flu. LAIV is an option for healthy, non-pregnant individuals who between two and 49 years old.

Each season's flu vaccine typically contains three virus strains that are the most likely to be encountered in the coming flu season: two of type A virus and one of type B virus. The strains of viruses included in the vaccine change yearly based on international surveillance data of influenza cases and estimations by scientists on what types and strains of viruses will be prevalent in the coming influenza season. When the strains included in the vaccine are well matched to the strains present in the community, the vaccine is 70–90% effective in people who are less than 65 years old. Because immune response diminishes somewhat with age, people 65 and older may not receive the same level of protection from the vaccine. Even if they do contract the flu, however, the vaccine diminishes the flu's severity and helps prevent complications.

The virus strains used to make the vaccine are inactivated and will not cause the flu. In the past, flu symptoms were associated with vaccine preparations that were not as highly purified as modern vaccines. (They were not associated with the virus itself.) In 1976, the swine flu vaccine carried a slightly increased risk of developing Guillain-Barré syndrome, a very rare disorder. This association between the syndrome and the vaccine occurred only with the 1976 swine flu vaccine preparation and has never recurred.

Serious side effects with modern vaccines are extremely unusual. Some people experience a slight soreness at the point of injection, which resolves within a day or two. People who have never been exposed to influenza, particularly children, may experience one to two days of a slight fever, tiredness, and muscle aches. These symptoms start within 6–12 hours after the vaccination.

It should be noted that certain people should not receive an influenza vaccine. Infants six months and younger have immature immune systems and will not benefit from the vaccine. Since the vaccines are prepared using hen eggs, people who have severe **allergies** to eggs or to other vaccine components should not receive the influenza vaccine. As an alternative, they may receive a course of amantadine or rimantadine, which are also used as a protective measure against influenza. Other people who might receive these drugs are those who have been immunized after the flu season has started or those who are immunocompromised, such as people with advanced HIV disease. Amantadine and rimantadine are 70–90% effective in preventing influenza.

H1N1 Influenza

In April 2009, the United States **Department of Health and Human Services** declared a public health emergency regarding human cases of **H1N1 influenza A**, more commonly called "swine flu."

Swine flu was of special concern for several reasons. Experts believed that the virus was a new strain of influenza with a genetic composition unlike the familiar viruses that cause seasonal influenza. Individuals were especially susceptible to developing serious illness. In addition, the virus was different from the familiar viruses in that it often caused more intense symptoms in young, healthy people than in the elderly or the very young who are the greatest target of seasonal flu.

Because the decision had already been made about which strains of seasonal flu were to be included in the vaccine for the next flu season, and manufacture had already begun, a special push was made to make a separate vaccine against the swine flu. Thus, in the winter of 2009 and through the 2010 flu season, people were advised to get two separate flu shots: one against seasonal flu and one against the new H1N1 influenza A.

The CDC's Advisory Committee on Immunization Practices (ACIP) recommends that everyone aged 6 months or older get a flu vaccine each year. Those at increased risk for influenza-related complications include:

- all people 65 years and older
- residents of nursing homes and chronic-care facilities, regardless of age

KEY TERMS

Bioterrorism—The intentional use of disease-causing microbes or other biologic agents to intimidate or terrorize a civilian population for political or military reasons. Type A influenza virus could be used as an agent of bioterrorism.

Common cold—A mild illness caused by a upper respiratory viruses. Usual symptoms include nasal congestion, coughing, sneezing, throat irritation, and a low-grade fever.

Epidemic—A widespread regional disease outbreak.

Guillain-Barré syndrome—Also called "acute idiopathic polyneuritis," this condition is a neurologic syndrome that can cause numbness in the limbs and muscle weakness following certain viral infections.

Pandemic—Worldwide outbreak of an infection, afflicting millions of victims.

Vaccination—Injection of a killed or weakened microbe in order to stimulate the immune system against the microbe, thereby preventing disease. Vaccinations, or "immunizations," work by stimulating the immune system so that it will recognize invading bacteria and viruses, and produce substances (antibodies) to destroy or disable them. Vaccinations therefore prepare the immune system to ward off a disease.

- adults and children who have chronic heart or lung problems, such as asthma
- adults and children who have chronic metabolic diseases, such as diabetes and renal dysfunction, as well as severe anemia or inherited hemoglobin disorders
- children and teenagers who are on long-term aspirin therapy
- pregnant women who will be in their second or third trimester during flu season or women who are nursing
- anyone who is immunocompromised, including HIV-infected persons, cancer patients, organ transplant recipients, and patients receiving steroids, chemotherapy, or radiation therapy
- anyone in contact with the above groups, such as teachers, care givers, health-care personnel, and family members
- travelers to foreign countries

A person need not be in one of the at-risk categories listed above, however, to receive a flu vaccination. Anyone who wants to forego the discomfort and inconvenience of an influenza attack may receive the vaccine.

Effects on public health

The flu is a public health concern because it is a recurring illness that affects a large number of people every year. It can be a serious illness, especially for older individuals, when potentially life-threatening secondary infections occur. Flu pandemics have occurred in the past, and although surveillance measures are in place, the potential for another pandemic exists.

In addition, one new concern regarding influenza is the possibility that hostile groups or governments could use the virus as an agent of bioterrorism and trigger a flu pandemic.

Costs to society

The average seasonal influenza epidemic results in direct medical costs of about $10.4 billion, and lost earnings due to illness and loss of life of $16.3 billion, according to a 2007 study in the journal *Vaccine*. Vaccine development typically runs about $700 million per vaccine.

Efforts and solutions

Each year, global surveillance keeps tabs on the new strains of influenza virus that will strike in the upcoming flu season. The findings help researchers to develop flu vaccines that will help protect people from those strains. This effort not only keeps people from getting sick, it also saves lives.

As of 2012, a major debate was still under way over research that, on the one hand, would be helpful in developing new flu vaccines, but on the other hand, could provide a roadmap for turning the flu into a weapon. The controversy arose when researchers announced that they had been able to genetically modify the bird flu H5N1 virus into a highly contagious form that could jump from mammal to mammal. They used ferrets, because ferrets and humans react to the flu similarly. The point of the research was to learn how the flu spreads, so they could use that knowledge to develop a vaccine or other treatments, and possibly other preventative measures. Many members of the scientific and medical community, including the **World Health Organization**, recommended that the research not be published over fears that terrorists would use the information for nefarious purposes. Others, including the Center for Biosecurity of UPMC (University of

QUESTIONS TO ASK YOUR DOCTOR

- How long will my flu last?
- How should I monitor my child's flu symptoms so that it doesn't progress to something more dangerous?
- If antibiotics are not useful for treating the flu, why are you prescribing them for my child?
- Which over-the-counter flu medications, if any, do you recommend?

Pittsburgh Medical Center), worry that the newly created and highly contagious mutated strains could escape the lab. On the other side, some believe that the research is very important in flu-prevention work and that it is impossible to put a cap on research.

Resources

BOOKS

Brouwer, Emma S.*Influenza Pandemic: Preparedness and Response to a Health Disaster*. Hauppauge, NY: Nova Science, 2010.

PERIODICALS

WEBSITES

"Key Facts about Influenza (Flu) & Flu Vaccine." Centers for Disease Control and Prevention. http://www.cdc.gov/flu/keyfacts.htm (accessed September 18, 2012).

"Key Facts about Influenza (Flu) & Flu Vaccine." National Institute of Allergy and Infectious Diseases (NIAID). http://www.niaid.nih.gov/topics/Flu/understandingFlu/Pages/keyFacts.aspx (accessed September 20, 2012).

"Flu and You." Centers for Disease Control and Prevention. www.cdc.gov/flu/pdf/freeresources/family/fluandyou_press.pdf (accessed September 18, 2012).

MedlinePlus "Infectious Diseases." U.S. National Library of Medicine. http://www.nlm.nih.gov/medlineplus/infectiousdiseases.html (accessed September 17, 2012).

Inglesby, Thomas V., Anita Cicero, and D.A. Henderson. "The Risk of Engineering a Highly Transmissible H5N1 Virus" Center of Biosecurity of UPMC (University of Pittsburgh Medical Center). http://www.upmc-biosecurity.org/website/resources/publications/2011/2011-12-15-editorial-engineering-H5N1 (September 18, 2012).

"Rapid Diagnostic Testing for Influenza." Centers for Disease Control and Prevention. http://www.cdc.gov/flu/professionals/diagnosis/rapidlab.htm#table (accessed September 18, 2012).

"Seasonal Influenza." Centers for Disease Control and Prevention. http://www.cdc.gov/flu/about/qa/disease.htm (accessed September 18, 2012).

"Understanding Microbes in Sickness and in Health." National Institute of Allergy and Infectious Diseases. http://www.niaid.nih.gov/topics/microbes/documents/microbesbook.pdf (September 17, 2012).

"What You Should Know and Do this Flu Season If You Are 65 Years and Older." Centers for Disease Control and Prevention. http://www.cdc.gov/flu/about/disease/65over.htm (accessed September 18, 2012).

ORGANIZATIONS

American Public Health Association (APHA), 800 I Street NW, Washington, DC 20001-3710, (202) 777-APHA, http://www.apha.org

Centers for Disease Control and Prevention (CDC), 1600 Clifton Road, Atlanta, GA 30333, (800) 232-4636, cdcinfo@cdc.gov, http://www.cdc.gov

National Institute of Allergy and Infectious Diseases, 6610 Rockledge Drive, MSC 6612, Bethesda, MD 20892-6612, (301) 496-5717, (866) 284-4107, ocpostoffice@niaid.nih.gov, http://www.niaid.nih.gov.

Julia Barrett
Rebecca J. Frey, Ph.D.
Judith L. Sims
Tish Davidson, AM
Leslie Mertz, Ph.D.

Insecticide poisoning

Definition

Insecticide **poisoning** is exposure to a group of chemicals designed to eradicate insects that cause affected persons to develop clinical signs that can progress to death.

Description

Insecticides belong to a group of chemicals called organophosphates used to protect against insects. Their use is popular since they are effective and do not remain in the environment, disintegrating within a few days. Organophosphates act to inhibit an enzyme in humans called acetyl cholinesterase. This enzyme functions to degrade a chemical called acetylcholine, which excites nerve cells. The resultant effect of organophosphates would be an increase in acetylcholine, thus causing initial excitation of nerve cells. Insecticide poisoning is often called carbamate poisoning and pesticide poisoning as well.

Poisoning can occur with a broad range of symptoms affecting the functioning of nerves and initial symptoms similar to the flu such as vomiting, abdominal **pain**, dizziness, and headache. Common names for insecticides are dichlorvos, chlorpyrifos, diazinon, fenthion, malathion, parathion, and carbamate. A special type of insecticide called paraquat is lethal and responsible for approximately 1,000 deaths per year in Japan alone. Paraquat poisoning releases oxygen free radicals that destroy lung and kidney tissues. When poisoning is suspected, a comprehensive management and assessment plan should be performed. This initial assessment should include:

- description of toxins: names of chemical(s)
- magnitude of exposure: determination of amount of exposure
- progression of symptoms: determination of the progression of symptoms to provide information concerning life support and overall outcome
- time of exposure: determination of the time of exposure given that symptoms may be delayed and time information helps determine a management plan.
- medical history: given that underlying diseases and therapeutic mediations may worsen toxic manifestations

Demographics

As of 2012, the **Environmental Protection Agency** estimated that 10,000-20,000 physician-diagnosed pesticide poisonings occurred each year among the approximately two million U.S. agricultural workers. Agricultural workers, groundskeepers, pet groomers, fumigators, and a variety of other occupations are at risk for exposure to pesticides, including fungicides, herbicides, insecticides, rodenticides, and sanitizers.

Causes and symptoms

Exposure to insecticides can occur by ingestion, inhalation, or exposure to skin or eyes. The chemicals are absorbed through the skin, lungs, and gastrointestinal tract and then widely distributed in tissues. Symptoms cover a broad spectrum and affect several organ systems:

- gastrointestinal: nausea, vomiting, cramps, excess salivation, and loss of bowel movement control
- lungs: increases in bronchial mucous secretions, coughing, wheezing, difficulty breathing, and water collection in the lungs (this can progress to breathing cessation)
- skin: sweating
- eyes: blurred vision, smaller sized pupil, and increased tearing
- heart: slowed heart rate, block of the electrical conduction responsible of heartbeat, and lowered blood pressure
- urinary system: urinary frequency and lack of control
- central nervous system: convulsions, confusion, paralysis, and coma

KEY TERMS

Acetylcholine—A chemical called a neurotransmitter that functions to excite nerve cells.

Acetylcholinesterase—An enzyme that breaks down acetylcholine.

Central nervous system—Consists of the brain and spinal cord and integrates and processes information.

Enzyme—A protein that speeds up a chemical reaction but is not consumed during the process.

Oxygen free radicals—Reactive molecules containing oxygen and can cause cell damage.

Diagnosis

A confirmed diagnosis for insecticide poisoning is the measurement of blood acetyl cholinesterase less than 50% of normal. The chemicals can also be detected by specific urine testing. Signs and symptoms in addition to a comprehensive poisoning assessment are essential for diagnosis. Carbamate insecticide poisoning exhibits symptoms similar to organophosphate poisoning but without central nervous system signs.

Treatment

Individuals should decontaminate exposed clothing and wash with soap and water immediately. Emergency measures may focus on ventilator support and heart monitoring. If inhalation is suspected, the patient should be removed from the site of exposure. If the eyes were the entry site, they should be flushed with large amounts of water. If the chemicals were ingested, the stomach may be washed out and activated charcoal may be administered. Atropine or glycopyrrolate (Robinul) is the drug of choice for carbamate insecticide poisoning. It reverses many symptoms but is only partially effective for central nervous symptom effects such as coma and convulsions. Pralidoxime is also commonly indicated to reactivate acetylcholinesterase and to reverse typical symptoms due to organophosphate poisoning. Additionally, the patient is monitored for heart, lung, liver functioning, specific blood tests, and oxygen levels in blood.

QUESTIONS TO ASK YOUR DOCTOR

- How much DEET is harmful to my children?
- Does insecticide poisoning pose any other health risks?
- Can I infect others?
- What is the best treatment option for me?
- How helpful are poison control centers?

Prognosis

Prognosis depends on the specific chemical of exposure, magnitude and time of exposure, progression of symptoms (severity), and onset for medical attention.

Prevention

Adherence to accepted guidelines for handling and management is the key to preventing insecticide poisoning. These may include using masks, gowns, gloves, goggles, respiratory breathing machines, or hazardous material suits.

Public health role and response

The National Institute for Occupational Safety and Health (NIOSH) established the Sentinel Event Notification System for Occupational Risks-Pesticides Program (SENSOR-Pesticides) in 1987 to reduce the number of injuries and illnesses associated with occupational pesticide exposure.

The program is a U.S. state-based surveillance effort that monitors pesticide-related illness and injury in 11 states. Under this program, NIOSH provides technical support and funding to state **health departments** to build and maintain surveillance capacity and to bolster pesticide-related illness and injury surveillance. The U.S. **Environmental Protection Agency (EPA)** also provides funding for the program.

The SENSOR-supported surveillance systems tabulate the number of acute occupational pesticide poisonings, allowing for the timely identification of outbreaks. The program also helps develop preventive interventions and maintains a national database that compiles information from participating states. Researchers and government officials from the SENSOR-Pesticides Program publish articles highlighting findings from the data and build state and national capacity by facilitating communication across participating states. Publications discuss issues as diverse as pesticide poisoning among agricultural workers, pesticide poisoning in schools, **birth defects**, and residential use of total release foggers (bug bombs, devices that release an insecticide mist).

Resources

BOOKS

Borron, S. W. "Pyrethins, Repellants, and Other Pesticides." In *Haddad and Winchester's Clinical Management of Poisoning and Drug Overdose.* 4th ed. Edited by M. W. Shannon, S. W. Borron, M. J. Burns, chap. 77. Philadelphia: Saunders Elsevier, 2007.

Goldman, Lee, and Andrew I. Schafer, eds. Cecil Medicine. 24th ed. Philadelphia: Saunders, 2011.

ORGANIZATIONS

American Associations of Poison Control Centers, 515 King St., Ste. 510, Alexandria, VA 22314, (703) 894-1858, Fax: (703) 683-2812, http:// info@aapcc.org

Occupational Safety & Health Administration, 200 Constitution Ave. NW, Washington, DC 20210, http://www.osha.gov.

Laith Farid Gulli, M.D.
Karl Finley

Intestinal disorders

Definition

Intestinal disorders are maladies that interfere with the ingestion, digestion, or absorption of nutrients. They include a number of specific conditions, such as gastroesophageal reflux disorder (GERD), peptic ulcer, short bowel syndrome, inflammatory bowel disease (ulcerative colitis and Crohn's disease), biliary tract diseases, pancreatitis, and cancers of the esophagus, pancreas, liver, colon, and other intestinal organs.

Description

Intestinal disorders are also known by a variety of other names, including intestinal diseases, digestive diseases or disorders, and gastrointestinal diseases or disorders, terms which are not necessarily identical, but which refer to a cluster of conditions affecting all or part of the gastrointestinal tract. The gastrointestinal (GI) tract is a body system whose function it is to break food down into its nutritional components (such as sugars and amino acids), provide a mechanism for the absorption of those nutrients into the bloodstream, and transport waste products of digestion out of the body. Authorities differ somewhat as to the components of the GI tract. By its most comprehensive definition, it includes the mouth (salivary glands, tongue, and pharynx), esophagus,

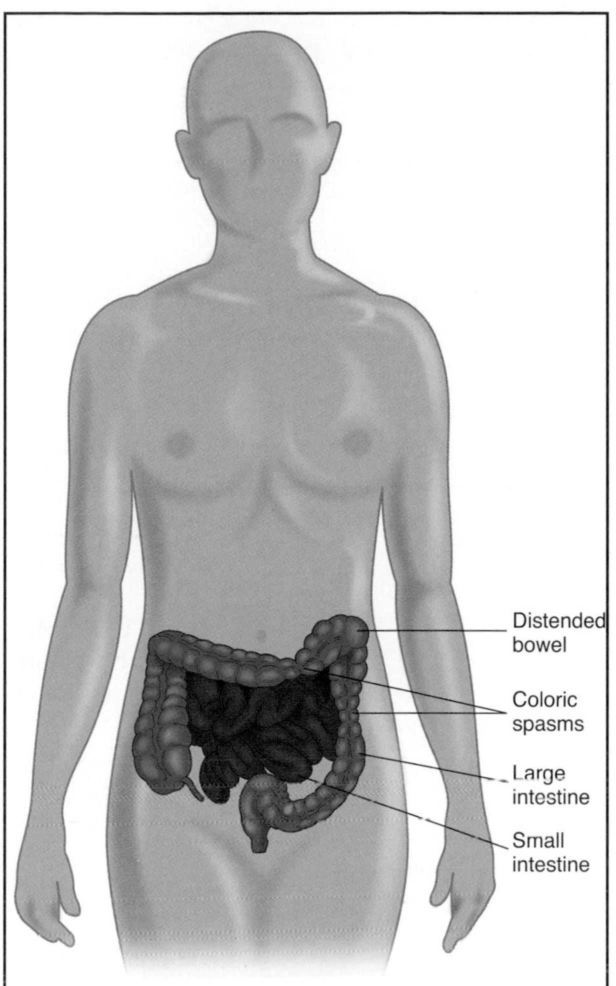

Locations affected by Irritable Bowel Syndrome. *(Illustration by Electronic Illustrators Group. © 2013 Cengage Learning)*

stomach, duodenum, small and large intestine, and anus. The term *upper gastrointestinal tract*, or *upper GI tract* is sometimes used to describe the esophagus, stomach, and duodenum, and the *lower gastrointestinal tract*, or *lower GI tract* is reserved for the small and large intestines, which together are called the *bowel*.

A very large range of disorders fall under the category of intestinal diseases, including conditions as relatively common and benign as nausea and vomiting to potentially fatal conditions such as a variety of cancers. Some specific intestinal disorders are:

- esophagitis
- gastroesophageal reflux disorder (GERD) and laryngopharyngeal reflux disorder
- gastritis
- gastric (peptic) ulcer
- dyspepsia
- emesis (nausea and vomiting)
- pyloric stenosis
- gastric dumping syndrome
- enteritis (duodenitis, jejunitis, ileitis)
- malabsorption
- celiac disease (sprue)
- appendicitis
- colitis
- irritable bowel syndrome
- Crohn's disease
- diverticulitis and diverticulosis
- obstructive bowel disorder
- diarrhea and constipation
- anal fissures and anal fistulas
- proctitis
- rectal prolapse
- hepatitis and cirrhosis and many other liver diseases
- pancreatitis and other pancreatic disorders
- cholecystitis, cholesterolosis, gallstones, and other gallbladder disorders
- hiatal and abdominal hernias
- peritonitis
- idiopathic intestinal bleeding
- cancers of the liver, pancreas, stomach, and other organs

Demographics

According to the most recent data available, approximately 60 to 70 million Americans experience some form of digestive disease at any one time. Digestive diseases were responsible for 104.7 million ambulatory visits to doctors, nurses, and other healthcare personnel in 2004, requiring 5.5 million inpatient diagnostic and therapeutic procedures, 12 percent of all such procedures conducted in 2006. In addition, ambulatory visits also involved about 20 million inpatient surgical procedures, 31 percent of all such procedures conducted in 2006. The total estimated cost of all procedures related to digestive disease complaints amounted to $141.8 billion in 2004, of which almost 70 percent were direct medical costs for treatment of a condition and the rest were indirect costs related to mortality and long-term disability from a disease. Digestive diseases also resulted in 13.5 million hospitalizations and an estimated 236,000 deaths in 2004.

Causes and symptoms

The causes and symptoms of intestinal disorders vary depending on the specific type of disease involved.

Causes

The causes of most intestinal disorders can be classified into one of two categories: structural causes and functional causes. Structural causes are those conditions in which an organ or some other part of the GI tract both looks abnormal and does not function normally. By contrast, functional causes are those conditions in which the GI tract looks normal, but it does not function as it supposed to. Some examples of intestinal disorders caused by structural changes are the following:

- Diverticulosis is a condition in which small pockets (diverticula) appear the wall of the large intestine. If these pockets become infected or inflammed, the intestine may become blocked producing more serious complications in a condition known as diverticulitis.
- Cancers are rapid, uncontrolled growths that occur in an organ or tissue, resulting in one or another of the more serious types of intestinal disease. One of the most common types of intestinal cancers is colon cancer, which is often preceded by the development of small protrusions in the colon wall called polyps.
- Anal fissures are cracks that form in the lining of the anal opening, producing pain and bleeding, especially during bowel movements.
- Anal fistulas are tiny tube-like structures that open in the skin near the anal opening, causing itching, bleeding, and general discomfort.
- Colitis is a general term that refers to inflammation of the bowel. For two of the most common forms of colitis, ulcerative colitis and Crohn's disease, there is no known cause.

The two most common intestinal disorders caused by functional factors are chronic constipation and irritable bowel syndrome (IBS), also known as nervous stomach, irritable colon, or spastic colon. All of these conditions are caused by lifestyle choices, such as:

- eating a diet low in fiber
- not getting enough physical exercise
- not drinking enough fluids
- including too much dairy products in the diet
- delaying bowel movements
- taking certain over-the-counter or prescription medications
- overusing laxatives
- experiencing mental or emotional stress
- being pregnant

Symptoms

As with causes, the specific symptoms for various intestinal disorders may vary from disease to disease. However, a few general symptoms tend to be associated with all or most types of GI tract disorders. They include fever, nausea and/or vomiting with or without loss of blood, loss of appetite, weight loss, jaundice (yellowing of the skin and whites of the eyes), bronzing of the skin, changes in color of the urine, itchiness, and certain characteristic symptoms associated with vitamin deficiencies related to malabsorption, such as bruising, numbness and tingling of the skin, muscles spasms, bone **pain**, and scaling skin.

KEY TERMS

Dyspepsia—Indigestion.

Emesis—Nausea and vomiting.

Enteritis—Inflammation of the intestines.

Gastritis—Inflammation of the lining of the stomach.

Gastrointestinal tract—That portion of the body through which food passes, is broken down, and is absorbed into the bloodstream.

Hernia—Protrusion of an organ through the structure or muscle in which it is usually contained.

Malabsorption—Impaired absorption of nutrients within the intestines.

Peritonitis—Inflammation of the peritonium, the membrane which lines the inside of the abdomen and other internal organs.

Proctitis—Inflammation of the lining of the anus and/or the rectum.

Pyloric stenosis—Narrowing of the pyloric sphincter that blocks the passage of food from the stomach into the duodenum.

Rectal prolapse—Protrusion of rectal tissue through the anus to the exterior of the body.

Diagnosis

A host of diagnostic techniques are available for identifying the presence of an intestinal disorder. The presence of one or more of the symptoms listed previously provides the first suggestion of a GI tract disorder. Obtaining a patient history is also an essential part of the diagnosis since information about diet, exercise, **stress**, and other factors may help confirm a tentative diagnosis. Procedures are also available for confirming an initial diagnosis of a functional disorder, such as the use of manometry. Manometry involves inserting a sensitive pressure-measuring device into the patient's GI tract to look for blockages that may reduce motility in the tract. Structural disorders generally require more extensive testing in order to obtain a differential diagnosis. X rays and other types of imaging procedures can be used to obtain a full GI image or to focus on some specific region of the intestinal tract. Imaging often makes use of some material to provide greater contrast in the final picture, giving greater detail to the image. The so-called "barium enema," for example, makes use of a barium compound that is largely opaque to x rays. A number of variations to the procedure are available for obtaining higher definition images of specific portions of the GI tract. Among these is the CT colonography, which involves the use of computed tomography technology to obtain 2D and 3D images of the colon. A number of endoscopic variations are also available for diagnosis. Endoscopes are devices that contain small cameras at the end of long tubes that can be inserted into the throat or the rectum for viewing various parts of the GI tract. An anoscope, for example, is used to examine the anus and the distal rectal region, while a sigmoidoscope allows deeper penetration into the sigmoid for examination. Full-size endoscopes can be used for the study of the upper GI tract with insertion through the throat, and for the lower GI tract with insertion through the rectum. Endoscopes can also be outfitted with devices for removing small samples of tissue for biopsies to determine the presence of malignant tumors. Endoscopes can also be adapted to carry small ultrasound devices to measure blood flow and to obtain images of GI lesions for further study.

QUESTIONS TO ASK YOUR DOCTOR

- How can we determine the cause of my chronic constipation?
- What treatments are available for my gastroesophageal reflux disorder, and what are the possible risks and benefits of each treatment?
- Based on your tests, what is your prognosis for the progress of my ulcerative colitis over the next 10 years?
- What is your recommendation for colonoscopy screening for me?
- What other screening tests or other routine procedures do you recommend for potential intestinal diseases?
- What is your opinion of the use of complementary or alternative treatments for my GI tract disorder?
- What services does a gastroenterologist offer that a primary physician does not offer?
- What diagnostic or therapeutic intestinal procedures can you perform in your office rather than having to refer me to a gastroenterologist?

Prevention

No recommendations for **prevention** can be made for some types of intestinal disorders because there are no known causes for the disorders. Ulcerative colitis and Crohn's disease are two such conditions. Other types of intestinal disorders can often be detected by early screening programs even if no proximate cause for the condition is known. For example, the **Centers for Disease Control and Prevention (CDC)** recommends regular colorectal screening tests for men and women between the ages of 50 and 75, using sigmoidoscopy, colonoscopy, or a fecal occult blood test. Detection and removal of polyps has proved to be one of the most effective methods for reducing a person's risk for colon **cancer**. Attention to lifestyle choices is also commonly recommended as a critical way of preventing most functional disorders. This recommendation means more attention to the role of fiber in one's diet, increased levels of exercise, efforts to reduce stress in one's life, and attention to the medications and other drugs one uses. The American College of Gastroenterology has a number of specific suggestions for avoiding GI tract disorders on its website at http://patients.gi.org/topics/digestive-health-tips/.

Treatment

Most types of functional intestinal disorders can be treated quite successfully with lifestyle choices, such as improving one's diet, increasing **physical activity**, and reducing stress in one's daily life. Structural disorders generally require some form of medical intervention, the use of a variety of medications and/or surgery to remove or repair a damaged section of the GI tract. For example, both internal and external hemorrhoids often respond to simple treatments, such as the use of warm sitz baths, dietary changes, the use of stool softeners, and over-the-counter medications, such as Preparation H. Cases that do not respond to these treatments may require more aggressive attention, which can include treatment with lasers, chemicals that will reduce the size of the hemorrhoids, or surgical removal of the hemorrhoids. Similarly, treatment of diverticulitis begins with conservative approaches, such as bowel resting for a few days and the use of **antibiotics**. If these procedures are unsuccessful, surgery may be necessary in which a portion of the GI tract where the diverticula are located is removed or bypassed.

Complementary and alternative treatments

A number of complementary and alternative procedures have been recommended for treating the whole range of gastrointestinal disorders, including acupuncture, aromatherapy, traditional Chinese medicine, homeotherapy, naturopathy, and herbal formulations. Among the herbal treatments suggested for GI tract disorders are aloe vera, boswellia, calendula, flaxseed, marshmallow, and slippery elm. Scientific studies on the safety and efficacy of most complementary and alternative treatments are generally not available, so they should be used only with the advice and supervision of a medical professional.

Prognosis

Many GI tract disorders resolve spontaneously, especially when the causative agents are removed. For example, a person who experiences gastric discomfort because of stress at the workplace may feel much better when that stress disappears. Similarly, switching to a healthier diet, reducing one's consumption of alcohol, stopping **smoking**, increasing physical activity, and adopting other lifestyle changes may be all that is needed to achieve a complete recovery or to reduce symptoms to a manageable level. With the exception of cancers, most forms of GI tract disease are not life-threatening. Some types of disease are persistent, however, and require efforts by patients to learn how to adjust to and live with their conditions. Still other disorders tend to be recurrent, characterized by periods of remission and reoccurence.

Resources

BOOKS

Everhart, James E., ed. *The Burden of Digestive Diseases in the United States*. Washington, DC: US Government Printing Office, 2008.

Hay, David W. *The Little Black Book of Gastroenterology*. Sudbury, MA: Jones & Bartlett Learning, 2011.

Tulassay, Z., et al., eds. *Intestinal Disorders*. Dordrecht, Netherlands: Springer, 2009.

PERIODICALS

Beamish, Leigh A., Alvaro R. Osornio-Vargas, and Eytan Wine. "Air Pollution: An Environmental Factor Contributing to Intestinal Disease." *Journal of Crohn's and Colitis* 5. 4. (2011): 279–86.

Nolan, Jonathan D., Ian M. Johnston, and Julian R. F. Walters. "Physiology of Malabsorption." *Surgery* 30. 6. (2012): 268–74.

Sanger, Gareth, et al. "Challenges and Prospects for Pharmacotherapy in Functional Gastrointestinal Disorders." *Therapeutic Advances in Gastroenterology* 3. 5. (2010): 291–305.

Yan, F., and D. B. Polk. "Probiotics: Progress toward Novel Therapies for Intestinal Diseases." *Current Opinion in Gastroenterology* 36. 2. (2010): 95–101.

WEBSITES

Digestive Disorders Health Center. WebMD. http://www.webmd.com/digestive-disorders/gastrointestinal-disorders. Accessed on September 15, 2012.

Gastrointestinal Disorders. The Cleveland Clinic. http://my.clevelandclinic.org/disorders/gastrointestinal_tract_disorders/hic_gastrointestinal_disorders.aspx. Accessed on September 15, 2012.

Intestinal Diseases. Health Insite. http://www.healthinsite.gov.au/topics/Intestinal_diseases. Accessed on September 15, 2012.

Intestinal Diseases, Parasitic. World Health Organization. http://www.who.int/topics/intestinal_diseases_parasitic/en/. Accessed on September 15, 2012.

ORGANIZATIONS

Office of Communications and Public Liaison, National Institute of Diabetes and Digestive and Kidney Diseases (NIDDKD), 31 Center Dr., MSC 2560, Bldg. 31, Rm. 9A06, Bethesda, MD USA 20892–2560, 1 (301) 496–3583, http://www2.niddk.nih.gov/Footer/ContactNIDDK, http://www2.niddk.nih.gov/.

David E. Newton, Ed.D.

Ionizing radiation

Definition

Ionizing **radiation** is the high-energy form of electromagnetic radiation found in X-rays and Gamma rays. Ionizing radiation causes changes in living material. Ionizing radiation is both naturally-occurring and can be constructed through man-made means.

Description

Molecules are bound to each other, usually with an even number of electrons. The penetration of ionizing radiation causes the division of molecules. The result is atoms with unpaired electrons, which are commonly known as "free radicals." The free radicals are then said to be "ionized"—they are very reactive and when in contact with macromolecules (like the DNA) of living cells, these free radicals can cause cell damage and cell death. Ionizing radiation is recognized as a carcinogen and is able to act on its own or in accordance with other carcinogens to cause cell mutations, cell damage, or cell death.

There are multiple units for measuring ionizing radiation. The roentgen (R), is the oldest unit used to measure charge under standard conditions. The grey (Gy) and the rad are the units used to measure the amount of radiation absorbed by living tissue. Finally, the sievert (Sv) and the rem are the units used to normalize doses of radiation based on relative biologic effectiveness (RBE).

There are many types of electromagnetic waves producing radiation on the electromagnetic spectrum. These waves include: radio, microwave, infrared, visible, ultraviolet, X-ray, and Gamma ray. Each of these types of waves has a different intensity and wavelength. Electromagnetic waves with high frequencies have short but intense wavelengths, whereas low-frequency electromagnetic waves have long but less intense wavelengths. The high-frequency electromagnetic waves with short wavelengths have more potential for biological harm. Lower frequency electromagnetic waves that do not cause ionization include the spectrum of UV, visible light, infrared (IR), microwave (MW), and radio frequency (RF).

All humans are exposed to certain levels of radiation, called background radiation. These types of radiation are naturally-occurring and include cosmic radiation, radiation from elements in the Earth's surface, and radiation from atoms normally present in food or the air.

Survivors of nuclear disaster—including nuclear bombs—are especially susceptible to cell mutation, cell death, and the carcinogenic properties of ionizing radiation. The greater the dose of radiation an individual is exposed to, the greater the likelihood of **cancer** and death. Scientists have conducted research and concluded that this type of radiation exposure produces tendencies to certain types of cancers—like stomach, lung, and liver—more than others—like pancreas, prostate, and rectum.

Those suffering from certain medical conditions (especially conditions that are genetically inherited), are more susceptible to the damaging risks of ionizing radiation than the general population. A medical condition called ataxia telangiectasia (AT) is the most well known medical condition contributing to such a susceptibility to ionizing radiation. AT patients are especially susceptible to ionizing radiation and between 10–20% of AT patients contract cancer in their teens or early 20s.

The radiation used to treat cancerous tumors can cause additional damage to the body through its ionizing effects. Both bone and cartilage tissues can be damaged by cancer-treating radiation, resulting in fractures of the bone, which cannot always be prevented. These types of fractures are most common during radiation treatments to address cancerous tumors on the uterus or bladder. Patients suffering from these radiation-induced fractures will often feel the **pain** of the fracture before it can be detected by X-ray.

Demographics

According to the United Nations Scientific Committee on the Effects of Atomic Radiation, roughly 82% of the radiation all humans are exposed to is naturally-occurring background radiation. The remaining 18% of radiation exposure comes from man-made sources including medical X-rays, nuclear medicine, consumer products, occupational hazards, fallout, and the nuclear fuel cycle.

Precautions

Exposure to background radiation is universal and cannot be avoided. There are steps that can be taken, however, to reduce other exposure to ionizing radiation, thereby reducing the potential for the generation of free radicals and the subsequent health risks like cell damage, cell death, cancer, and death.

Medical exposures to ionizing radiation are the greatest man-made sources of ionizing radiation. The exposure of ionizing radiation from a 10 second chest X-ray is 20,000 microsieverts, the exposure of ionizing radiation from a 20 second CT scan is 800,000 microsieverts. This is compared with the total dose rate from background radiation which is between 0.3 and 1.5 microsievert or the exposure from an airplane flight which is around 3 microsieverts. Therefore, minimizing unnecessary exposure to ionizing radiation associated with diagnostic tests like X-rays and CT scans is desirable. These tests are often used more frequently than is necessary given the risk of ionizing radiation exposure. Before receiving such a diagnostic test, individuals should compare the risk of identifying a potential illness or injury being detected with the risks associated with the level of ionizing radiation to which they will be exposed during such a test. Until the causes of various forms of cancer are fully understood, preventing unnecessary exposure to all carcinogens—including ionizing radiation—may help reduce the likelihood of developing cancer.

The Occupational Safety & Health Administration (OSHA)—a division of the U.S. Department of Labor—has regulations in place to help protect individuals whose jobs put them in contact with sources of ionizing radiation. Additionally, 25 states, Puerto Rico, and the Virgin Islands have their own standards and policies of enforcements to help protect workers within their borders. These regulations also dictate how potentially dangerous materials and machinery should be handled, which helps reduce exposure to ionizing radiation for employees and the general public by standardizing necessary safety standards.

Effects on public health

Medical X-rays and CT scans are necessary and life-saving diagnostic tools used around the world and

KEY TERMS

Electromagnetic Radiation (EMR)—A type of energy that is both absorbed and emitted by particles. Forms of EMR demonstrate wave-like movement as they travel through space and can be measured along the electromagnetic spectrum based on the frequency of wavelengths of emitted light or energy. Forms of EMR include radio radiation, infrared radiation, light on the visible spectrum, ultraviolet light, X-rays and Gamma rays.

Ionize—To transform a molecule or atom—a neutral particle—into an ion—a particle with a positive or negative charge.

particularly in the United States. The diagnostic capabilities of these tests save lives, detect injuries, and help doctors locate causes of illness and discomfort. The availability of this technology has caused these diagnostic tools to be relied upon heavily, often used before or in place of other diagnostic tools.

It is important that these tests remain readily available to assist in detecting disease and injury; however, it is also important to recognize the potential for adverse health risks posed by these tests. Better education and awareness is needed to help doctors and patients when making informed decisions regarding the necessity and frequency of using diagnostic tools that emit ionizing radiation.

Efforts and solutions

Research out of France suggests that it may be possible to determine the relative efficacy of radiation cancer treatments on a patient based on genetic biomarkers. This could help doctors plan more effective cancer treatments and limit unnecessary exposure to ionizing radiation through radiation treatments for cancer patients that may not be likely to respond well to these treatments.

Resources

BOOKS

"The Difference Between Ionizing and Non-Ionizing Radiation." *Cancer Sourcebook.* Ed. Karen Bellenir. 6th ed. Detroit: Omnigraphics, 2011.

"Ionizing Radiation." *Environmental Encyclopedia.* 4th. ed. Vol. 1. Detroit: Gale, 2011.

Jones, J A, R C Casey, and F Karouia. "Ionizing Radiation as a Carcinogen." *Comprehensive Toxicology.* Ed. Charlene A. McQueen. 2nd ed. Vol. 14: Carcinogenesis. Oxford, United Kingdom: Elsevier, 2010.

"Ionizing Radiation Injury to Bone." *Bone and Muscle: Structure, Force, and Motion.* Ed. Kara Rogers. New York: Britannica Educational Publishing with Rosen Educational Services, 2011.

"Units for Measuring Ionizing Radiation." *The Britannica Guide to The Atom.* Ed. Erik Gregersen. New York: Britannica Educational Publishing with Rosen Educational Services, 2011.

PERIODICALS

Borchiellini, Delphine, et al. "The impact of pharmacogenetics on radiation therapy outcome in cancer patients. A focus on DNA damage response genes." *Cancer Treatment Reviews* 28.6 (2012).

"Ionizing radiation biomarkers for potential usein epidemiological studies." *Mutation Research — Reviews in Mutation Research* 751.2 (2012).

WEBSITES

Occupational Safety & Health Administration. "Ionizing Radiation."http://www.osha.gov/SLTC/radiationionizing/index.htmlAccessed September 25, 2012.

United Nations Scientific Committee on the Effects of Atomic Radiation. "Answers to Frequently Asked Questions (FAQs)."http://www.unscear.org/unscear/en/faq.html#Effects%20of%20radiation%20exposure Accessed September 25, 2012.

ORGANIZATIONS

American Cancer Society, 250 Williams Street NW, Atlanta, GA USA 30303, (800) 227-2345, www.cancer.org.

Andrea Nienstedt, MA

Irradiated food

Definition

Irradiated foods are foods that have been exposed to a radiant energy source to kill harmful bacteria, insects, or **parasites**, or to delay spoilage, sprouting, or ripening.

Purpose

There are many reasons that foods are irradiated. The most common reason is for increased **food safety**. The United States Centers for Disease Control (**CDC**) estimates that there are about 76 million cases of foodborne illness each year in the United States, resulting in about 5,000 deaths annually. Irradiating foods can reduce the risk of many foodborne illnesses by killing the bacteria or pathogens responsible, or harming them to such an extent that they are not able to reproduce or cause disease. The National Aeronautics and Space Administration (NASA) exposes the food that astronauts eat while in space to a level of irradiation far higher than that approved for commercial use in order to reduce the risk that astronauts will develop illness while in space. Patients who have diseases that severely impair the functioning of the immune system are often fed irradiated foods to decrease the risk that they will develop a serious disease.

Irradiation can also be used to destroy insects and other pests that may be present on produce. When produce is shipped from Hawaii to the mainland United States, it must be fumigated to kill any insects or insect eggs that might be present so that they do not spread to the mainland. Irradiating this produce is sometimes used as an alternative to fumigation, and does not leave a residue of chemicals on the produce in the way that fumigation can.

Some fruits and vegetables can be kept fresh longer by the use of low to moderate levels of irradiation. When exposed to low levels of **radiation**, potatoes, onions, and other vegetables do not sprout as quickly. Strawberries and other berries can benefit from irradiation as well, as irradiation can significantly delay the growth of **mold**. Strawberries stay fresh from 3–5 days when they are not irradiated or treated in any way, but can stay fresh and unspoiled for up to three weeks after being irradiated.

Description

Irradiated foods are foods that have been exposed to **ionizing radiation**. Ions are electrically charged particles, and ionizing radiation is radiation that produces these charged particles. Nonionizing radiation is produced by microwaves, television and radio waves, and visible light. Ionizing radiation is higher in power than these types of radiation, although it is in the same spectrum. The kinds of ionizing radiation used for food irradiation include gamma rays, beams of high-energy electrons, and x-rays.

When foods are irradiated, they are exposed to the source of the ionizing radiation for a short time. This radiation produces short-lived compounds that damage the deoxyribonucleic acid (DNA) of living organisms, such as bacteria that are in the food. Because DNA makes up the genes that contain the instructions that tell an organism how to grow and reproduce, once the DNA is damaged the organism cannot do this correctly and will die.

The amount of radiation required to irradiate foods depends on the type and thickness of the food product and the types of organisms that are present. The larger the DNA of the organism, generally the less radiation is

KEY TERMS

Ion—An electrically charged particle.

Ionizing radiation—Radiation that produces ions.

Pathogen—An organism that causes a disease.

Vitamin—A nutrient that the body needs in small amounts to remain healthy but that the body cannot manufacture for itself and must acquire through diet.

Foods permitted to be irradiated under FDA regulations (21 CFR 179.26)

Food	Purpose	Dose
Fresh, non-heated processed pork	Control of *Trichinella spiralis*	0.3 kGy min. to 1 kGy max.
Fresh foods	Growth and maturation inhibition	1 kGy max.
Foods	Arthropod disinfection	1 kGy max.
Dry or dehydrated enzyme preparations	Microbial disinfection	10 kGy max.
Dry or dehydrated spices/seasonings	Microbial disinfection	30 kGy max.
Fresh or frozen, uncooked poultry products	Pathogen control	3 kGy max.
Frozen packaged meats (solely NASA)	Sterilization	44 kGy min.
Refrigerated uncooked meat products	Pathogen control	4.5 kGy max.
Frozen uncooked meat products	Pathogen control	7 kGy max.
Fresh shell eggs	Control of *Salmonella*	3.0 kGy max.
Seeds for sprouting	Control of microbial pathogens	8.0 kGy max.
Fresh or frozen molluscan shellfish	Control of *Vibrio* species and other foodborne pathogens	5.5 kGy max.
Fresh iceberg lettuce and fresh spinach	Control of food-borne pathogens, and extension of shelf-life	4.0 kGy max.

kGy = kiloGray

SOURCE: U.S. Food and Drug Administration.

(Table by PreMediaGlobal. © 2013 Cengage Learning)

required to irradiate it. Insects and parasites have the larger DNA and require the lowest levels of radiation, while bacteria generally require slightly more, and viruses have very small amounts of DNA and require very high levels of radiation. Most parasites, insects, and bacteria can be eliminated at levels of radiation approved for commercial use, but many viruses cannot.

Irradiating foods does not make the foods radioactive in any way. Irradiation done using beams of high-energy electrons or x-rays does not even use any radioactive material. Irradiation done using gamma rays involves exposure of the food to a radioactive substance, usually cobalt 60 or cesium 137, for a short period. The radioactivity of this substance is not in any way transferred to the food that is exposed to it.

QUESTIONS TO ASK YOUR DOCTOR

- What are the risks of handling irradiated food?
- Is eating irradiated food safe for me?
- How can I tell if I am getting the right nutrients?
- What tests or evaluation techniques can you perform to see if my diet and nutritional choices promote a healthy condition?
- What symptoms or adverse effects are important enough that I should seek immediate treatment?

Precautions

Irradiation is not a substitute for safe food handling practices. Although irradiation kills or disables many pathogenic organisms, these organisms can be reintroduced to the foods if cross contamination occurs. In addition, not every pathogen is completely destroyed by irradiation, and leaving foods such as raw meat out at room temperature can allow these pathogens to reproduce to significant levels. Irradiation should be viewed as an extra step to help ensure that the food supply is safe, not as a replacement for food safety practices that are already in place.

Interactions

Irradiated foods are not expected to interact with any other foods, medicines, or products.

Complications

There are no complications expected from consuming irradiated foods. Some concerned groups have expressed fears that the long-term effects of eating irradiated food are unknown. However, many different scientific studies have examined the effects on both animals and humans of consuming irradiated foods. There has not been any evidence that irradiated foods are harmful in either the short or the long term. One study even examined many generations of animals fed irradiated foods and found no harmful effects. Irradiating food is accepted as a safe practice and is endorsed by many organizations including the **World Health Organization**, the Centers for Disease Control, the United States Food and Drug Administration, and the American Medical Association.

Parental concerns

Some parents may have concerns that the vitamin and nutrient content of irradiated foods may be reduced compared to the content of the same foods that have not been irradiated. For most **vitamins**, minerals, and nutrients this is not the case. Studies have shown that the levels of most vitamins in irradiated foods are not significantly different from the levels in foods that have not been irradiated. Some vitamins however, such as thiamin (vitamin B_1), have been found to be sensitive to irradiation. The extent to which such vitamins are destroyed however, depends greatly on the type of food being irradiated. Thiamin was found to be decreased by 50% in a **water** solution that was exposed to radiation, but only decreased by 5% in a dried egg exposed to the same level of radiation. Many vitamins, like thiamin, that are sensitive to irradiation are as sensitive, or even more sensitive, to heat, and are broken down at least as much by the process of canning or heat treatments. Therefore, although levels of some vitamins may be decreased in irradiated foods compared to fresh foods, the levels of these vitamins may be higher in irradiated foods than in comparable canned or otherwise sterilized foods.

Resources

BOOKS

Bender, David A. *A Dictionary of Food and Nutrition*. New York: Oxford University Press, 2009.

Larsen, Laura, ed. *Diet and Nutrition Sourcebook*. 4th ed. Detroit, MI: Omnigraphics Inc, 2011.

Rodrigues, Sueli, and Fabiano Andre Narciso Fernandes, eds. *Advances in Fruit Processing Technologies*. Boca Raton, FL: CRC Press, 2012.

Sommers, Christopher H, and Xuetong Fan, eds. *Food Irradiation Research and Technology*. 2nd ed. New York: Wiley-Blackwell, 2012.

WEBSITES

Organic Consumers Association. "Information on Food Irradiation." 2012. http://www.organicconsumers.org/irradlink.cfm (accessed August 30, 2012).

ORGANIZATIONS

Centers for Disease Control, 1600 Clifton Rd., Atlanta, GA 30333, (800) 311-3435, http://www.cdc.gov

U.S. Department of Agriculture, 1400 Independence Avenue SW, Washington, DC 20250, http://www.usda.gov

U.S. Food and Drug Administration, 5600 Fishers Lane, Rockville, MD 20857-0001, (888) 463-6332, http://www.fda.gov

World Health Organization, Avenue Appia 20, Geneva, Switzerland, 41 22 791-2222, http://www.who.int/en

Tish Davidson, AM
Laura Jean Cataldo, RN, EdD

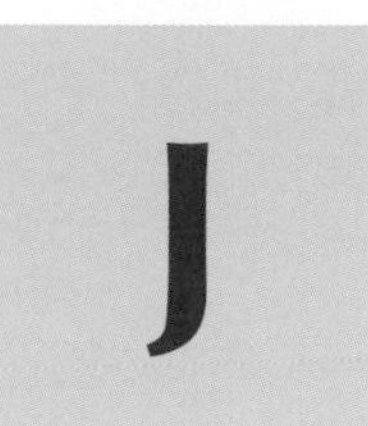

Joint replacement

Definition

Joint replacement is the surgical replacement of a joint with an artificial prosthesis.

Description

Great advances have been made in joint replacement since the first hip replacement was performed in the United States in 1969. Improvements have been made in the endurance and compatibility of materials used and the surgical techniques to install artificial joints. Custom joints can be made using a mold of the original joint that duplicates the original with a very high degree of accuracy.

The most common joints to be replaced are hips and knees. There is ongoing work on elbow and other joint replacement, but some joint problems are still treated with joint resection (the surgical removal of the joint in question) or interpositional reconstruction (the reassembly of the joint from constituent parts). In 2009, approximately 327,000 total hip replacements and 676,000 total knee replacements were performed in the United States. Since the lifetime of an artificial joint is limited, the best candidates for joint replacement are over age 60.

Joint replacements are performed under general or regional anesthesia in a hospital by an orthopedic surgeon. Some medical centers specialize in joint replacement, and these centers generally have a higher success rate than less specialized facilities. The specific techniques of joint replacement vary depending on the joint involved.

Hip Replacement

During a hip replacement, the surgeon makes an incision along the top of the thigh bone (femur) and pulls the thigh bone away from the socket of the hip bone (the acetabulum). An artificial socket made of metal coated with polyethylene (plastic) to reduce friction is inserted in the hip. The top of the thigh bone (femur) is cut, and a piece of artificial thigh made of metal is fitted into the lower thigh bone on one end and the new socket on the other.

The artificial hip can either be held in place by synthetic cement or by natural bone in-growth. The cement is an acrylic polymer. It assures good locking of the prosthesis to the remaining bone. However, bubbles left in the cement after it cures may act as weak spots, causing the development of cracks. This promotes loosening of the prosthesis later in life. If additional surgery is needed, all the cement must be removed before additional surgery can be performed.

An artificial hip fixed by natural bone in-growth requires more precise surgical techniques to assure maximum contact between the remaining natural bone and the prosthesis. The prosthesis is made so that it contains small pores that encourage the natural bone to grow into it. Growth begins 6–12 weeks after surgery. The short-term outcome with non–cemented hips is less satisfactory, with patients reporting more thigh **pain**, but the long-term outlook is better, with fewer cases of hip loosening in non–cemented hips. The current trend is to use the non–cemented technique. Hospital stays last from four to eight days.

Knee Replacement

The doctor puts a tourniquet above the knee, then makes a cut to expose the knee joint. The ligaments surrounding the knee are loosened, then the shin bone and thigh bone are cut and the knee removed. The artificial knee is then cemented into place on the remaining stubs of those bones. The excess cement is removed, and the knee is closed. Hospital stays range from three to six days.

As in all types of surgery, preventing infection is very important. **Antibiotics** are given intravenously and continued in pill form after the surgery. Fluid and blood loss can be great, and sometimes blood transfusions are needed.

Purpose

Seventy percent of joint replacements are performed because arthritis has caused the joint to stiffen and become painful to the point where normal daily activities are no longer possible. If the joint does not respond to conservative treatment such medication, weight loss, activity restriction, and use of walking aids such as a cane, joint replacement is considered appropriate.

Patients with rheumatoid arthritis or other connective tissue diseases may also be candidates for joint replacement, but the results are usually less satisfactory in those patients. Elderly people who fall and break their hips often undergo hip replacement when the probability of successful bone healing is low.

Preparation

Many patients choose to donate their own blood for transfusion during the surgery. This prevents any blood incompatibility problems or the transmission of blood-borne diseases.

Prior to surgery, all the standard preoperative blood and urine tests are performed, and the patient meets with the anesthesiologist to discuss any special conditions that affect the administration of anesthesia. Patients receiving general anesthesia should not eat or drink for ten hours prior to the operation.

KEY TERMS

Catheterization—Inserting a tube into the bladder so that a patient can urinate without leaving the bed.

Prosthesis—A synthetic replacement for a missing part of the body, such as a knee or a hip.

Rheumatoid arthritis—An autoimmune disease characterized by inflammation and degeneration of connective tissue in multiple joints at a young age. It also can affect additional organ systems.

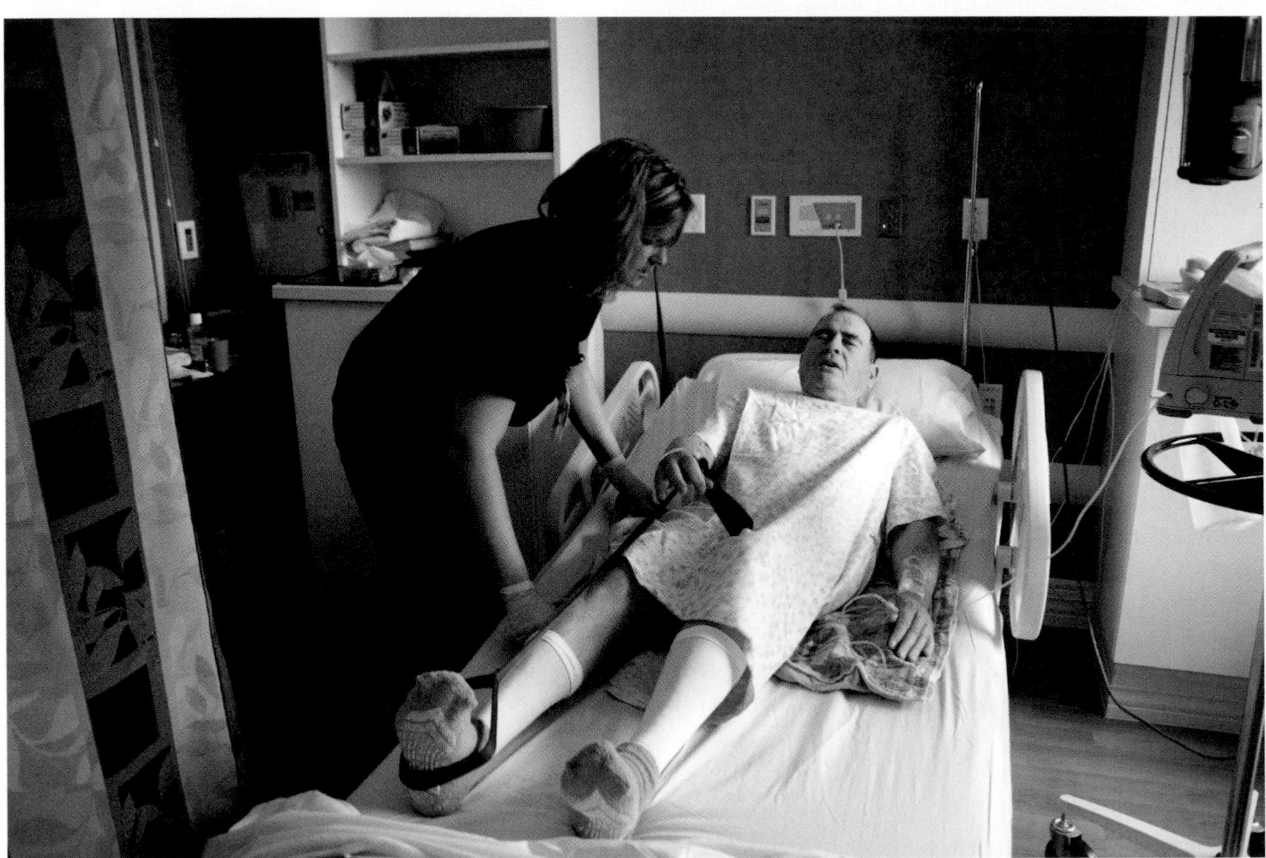

A therapist working with patient after total right hip arthroplasty or hip replacement. *(Inga Spence/Visuals Unlimited, Inc.)*

Aftercare

Immediately after the operation the patient will be catheterized so that he or she will not have to get out of bed to urinate. The patient will be monitored for infection. Antibiotics are continued and pain medication is prescribed. Physical therapy begins (first passive exercises, then active ones) as soon as possible using a walker, cane, or crutches for additional support. Long-term care of the artificial joint involves refraining from heavy activity and heavy lifting, and learning how to sit, walk, and get out of beds, chairs, and cars so as not to dislocate the joint.

Risks

The immediate risks during and after surgery include the development of blood clots that may come loose and block the arteries, excessive loss of blood, and infection. Blood-thinning medication is usually given to reduce the risk of clots forming. Some elderly people experience short-term confusion and disorientation from the anesthesia.

Although joint replacement surgery is highly successful, there is an increased risk of nerve injury. Dislocation or fracture of the hip joint is also a possibility. Infection caused by the operation can occur as long as one year later and can be difficult to treat. Some doctors add antibiotics directly to the cement used to fix the replacement joint in place. Loosening of the joint is the most common cause of failure in hip joints that are not infected. This may require another joint replacement surgery in about 12% of patients within a 15–year period following the first procedure.

Joint replacements are performed successfully on an older-than-average group of patients. People with diseases that interfere with blood clotting are not good candidates for joint replacement. Joint replacement surgery should not be done on patients with infection, or any heart, kidney, or lung problems that would make it risky to undergo general anesthesia.

Results

More than 90% of patients receiving hip replacements achieve complete relief from pain and significant improvement in joint function. The success rate is slightly lower in knee replacements, and drops still more for other joint replacement operations.

Effects on public health

Changing demographics will likely place new emphasis on joint replacement procedures in the healthcare system. For example, the demand for joint replacement surgery in younger people is rising dramatically as rising **obesity** rates stress younger joints.

QUESTIONS TO ASK YOUR DOCTOR

- What other options do I have besides total joint replacement?
- What activities will I be able to perform that I cannot now do if joint replacement is successful?
- Can you explain the rehabilitation process after joint replacement?
- How many of these operations have you performed?
- How many of your patients have serious complications from joint replacement surgery within three months after surgery? Within one year? Within five years?

According to the American Academy of Orthopedic Surgeons, more than half of patients needing hip or knee replacements will be under age 65 by 2016. Also, total joint replacement surgeries, now including shoulder and ankle replacements, are increasing at a time when fewer doctors are choosing orthopedic surgery as a career.

Costs to society

The **World Health Organization (WHO)** estimates that worldwide 10% of men and 18% of women have moderate to severe arthritis that interferes with daily functioning. Many of these people can have pain-free function restored with joint replacement surgery. In the developed world, hip replacement increased by 25% between 2000 and 2009, and knee replacement almost doubled during that time.

The cost to society for these joint replacements is substantial. In 2007, the average cost of a knee replacement was (all figures converted to U.S. dollars) $15,000 in the United States and Australia, $12,000 in France, and $10,000 in Germany, Sweden, and Canada. This creates a substantial healthcare expenditure whether the operations are paid for by private or government-provided health insurance. With an aging population that is living longer, it is likely that more healthcare dollars will be spent on joint replacement during the next decade.

Resources

BOOKS

Fischer, Stuart J. *100 Questions & Answers About Hip Replacement*. Sudbury, MA: Jones and Bartlett, 2011.

Hecht, M. E. *A Practical Guide to Hip Surgery: From Pre-op to Recovery*. North Branch, MN: Sunrise River Press, 2011.

WEBSITES

Foran, R. H., ed. "Joint Replacement." American Academy of Orthopaedic Surgeons. http://orthoinfo.aaos.org/menus/arthroplasty.cfm (accessed October 21, 2012).

National Institute of Arthritis and Musculoskeletal and Skin Diseases. "Joint Replacement Surgery: Information for Multicultural Communities." http://www.niams.nih.gov/Health_Info/Joint_Replacement/default.asp (accessed October 21, 2012).

ORGANIZATIONS

American Academy of Orthopaedic Surgeons (AAOS), 6300 North River Road, Rosemont, IL 60018-4262, (847) 823-7186, Fax: (847) 823-8125, http://orthoinfo.aaos.org

Arthritis Foundation, PO Box 7669, Atlanta, GA 30357-0669, (800) 283-7800, http://www.arthritis.org

National Institute of Arthritis and Musculoskeletal and Skin Diseases (NIAMS) Information Clearing house, 1 AMS Circle, Bethesda, MD 20892-3675, (301) 495-4484, (877) 22-NIAMS (226-4267), (301) 565-2966, Fax: (301) 718-6366, NIAMSinfo@mail.nih.gov, http://www.niams.nih.gov.

Tish Davidson, AM
Tish Davidson AM
Brenda W. Lerner

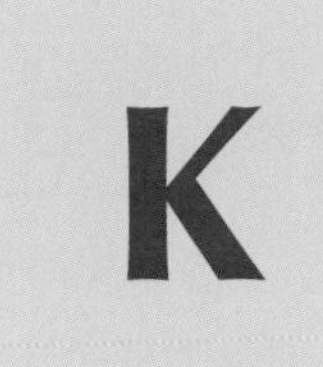

K

K-2 synthetic marajuana marijuana (spice)

Definition

Spice or K2 is a commercially-available blend of herbs and synthetic cannabinoid, or synthetic marijuana. Spice can be smoked, like marijuana, or mixed into an herbal drink to achieve psychoactive effects similar to marijuana, including relaxation, a blissful high, and hallucinations.

Description

Since the 2000s, synthetic cannabinoids have been mixed with a variety of potentially psychoactive herbs and sold under a variety of guises (including incense and plant food). Different brands of Spice are labeled to contain some variety of psychoactive herbs including (but not limited to): beach bean, white or blue water lily, dwarf skullcap, Indian warrior, lion's ear/tail, wild dagga, machonha brava, blue or sacred lotus, honeyweed, Siberian motherwart, marshmallow, dog rose, and rosehip.

Spice is known by many names and sold under many brands including (but not limited to): K2, fake weed, Yucatan Fire, Skunk, and Moon Rocks.

The human body has cannabinoid receptors, two of which were discovered in the 1980s and are associated with the central nervous and immune systems. When the tetrahydrocannabinol (THC) in marijuana (cannabis) connects with the receptors in the central nervous system, it creates psychoactive effects. When Spice or synthetic cannabinoids connect with the same receptors, the effects are the same and are often stronger than the effects of natural marijuana. Many users of Spice—especially those who use the drug for an extended period of time—report additional effects including aggression, anxiety, paranoia, and hallucinations, heart palpitations, vomiting, agitation, confusion, myocardial ischemia (reduced blood supply to the heart), and even heart attacks. Regular uses may also experience symptoms of withdrawal similar to those of other drug addicts.

Deaths have been attributed to Spice for a variety of reasons—including **suicide**, overdose, and homicide. Patients under the influence of Spice have been known to attack medical personnel. An individual's response to Spice seems to be unpredictable and, as of 2012, there have not been scientific studies to determine exactly how Spice works on the brain or the full range of its effects. The psychoactive effects of Spice have lead to a variety of bizarre incidents that have made national news. In a case in Detroit, a 19 year-old man—a long-time user of K2—and his 20 year-old friend beat the man's father to death with a baseball bat and nearly killed the man's mother and brother in the same manner. In another bizarre case in Texas, a 22 year-old man—who was under the influence of Spice—crawled on his hands and

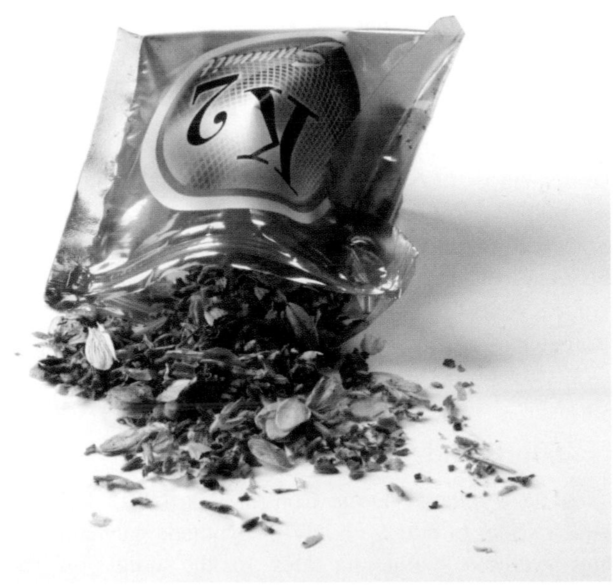

A pouch of dried herbal potpourri being used as "synthetic marijuana." *(Washington Post/Getty Images)*

knees, chasing a neighbor and barking like a dog. Shortly afterward, the same man captured a neighbor's dog, choked it, and then began to eat it.

Origins

Synthetic cannabinoids were originally developed from the 1960s–1990s in laboratories for a variety of pharmaceutical purposes. Since Spice is sold under so many names and for so many purposes, drug enforcement task forces in the United States and Europe have had difficulty tracking the origins of Spice and regulating its sale. The European Monitoring Centre for Drugs and Drug **Addiction** estimates that Spice or similar products first appeared on the market around 2004.

Demographics

According to the *Clinical Psychiatry News*'s interview with the American Association of Poison Control Centers (AAPCC), in 2011, calls related to synthetic marijuana were up to 6,959 from 2,906 in 2010.

According to a 2011 study by the University in Michigan and the National Institute on Drug Abuse (NIDA)—the first to question minors about their use of synthetic drugs)—roughly one in nine high school seniors reported having used Spice in 2011, which makes Spice the second most popular illicit drug (after marijuana) for this age group.

Effects on Public Health

Since Spice is a relatively new public health concern—the full range of its effects have yet to be realized. As of 2012, there are no existing scientific data to help the medical, law enforcement, and policy-making communities properly combat the threat. Until scientific tests are available, the human health and toxicity consequences of Spice remain unknown, though NIDA suspects harmful heavy metal residues may be present in Spice compounds. U.S. Customs and Border Protection believes that many of the Spice products available in the United States originate from overseas locales—increasing the potential for variation and inclusion of toxic substances or traces.

Efforts and Solutions

The Synthetic Drug Control Act (H.R. 1254)—which seeks to add a variety of synthetic cannabinoids and synthetic hallucinogenics to the drugs on the Controlled Substance Act—was passed by the U.S. House of Representatives in 2011, though it awaits Senate and Presidential approval as of September, 2012.

KEY TERMS

Psychoactive drug—A drug that affects the central nervous system by crossing the blood-brain barrier. These drugs cause alterations in the brain's ability to function normally.

Cannabinoid—Any one of a class of compounds that stimulate the cannabinoid receptor sites in the human body. In humans, cannabinoid receptors primarily affect the nervous system—including the brain, spinal cord, and peripheral nerves—and the immune system—which helps the body fight disease and infection. Cannabinoids are separated into three classifications: endocannabinoids (which are produced naturally within the body); phytocannabinoids (which are found in plants) including tetrahydrocannabinol (THC), the psychoactive component of cannabis; and synthetic cannabinoids (which are manufactured in a laboratory).

Designer drugs—a class of substances that are specifically created to avoid traditional means of detection, including drug laws and testing. Designer drugs often consist of multiple variations of an original compound or they are created to mimic the effects of other popular illicit drugs.

As of May 2012, at least 18 states had enacted a ban on synthetic marijuana and at least 13 additional states were considering such bans. The efficacy of these bans, however, remains unclear. The many product names, ingredients, and advertised uses for Spice make it a difficult substance to regulate effectively.

Spice falls into the category of "designer drug," and as such, its molecular structure frequently changes, leading to increased difficulty in detection. In addition to the multiple forms of synthetic cannabinoids, there are numerous psychoactive herbs with which the cannabinoids can be mixed. As a result, there are numerous formulations for the drug. This complexity makes it even harder to develop comprehensive tests to screen for Spice.

The tests currently available to screen for drugs are "structure-based," meaning that they detect certain structural elements of a known substance. The many potential and varying components of Spice make these types of tests ineffective. NIDA is offering funding to researchers who may be able to develop "biofluid" tests, which can detect ranges of a substances in bodily fluids for a predetermined amount of time.

As of May, 2012, Redwood Toxicology Laboratory (RTL) has developed an oral fluid (saliva) test for synthetic cannabis that is able to detect seven other synthetic cannabinoids. As RTL refines its processes and increases the number of compounds the tet is able to detect, the number of positive results for a specific compound fluctuate. RTL reports that after adding a particular synthetic cannabinoid compound to their detectable list, rates of positivity for that compound decline. From such results, RTL is able to document changes in manufacturer's ingredients.

Drugfree.org offers an awareness kit that features a slide presentation, podcast, and video about synthetic drugs, including Spice. The kit also includes a printable guide to synthetic drugs and street names.

Resources

BOOKS

"Spice and Other Legal Forms of Synthetic Marijuana Should Be Banned." *Drug Abuse.* Ed. Lauri S. Friedman. Detroit: Greenhaven Press, 2012. 77–81. Introducing Issues with Opposing Viewpoints.

EMCDDA 2009 Thematic paper—Understanding the 'Spice' phenomenon. European Monitoring Centre for Drugs and Drug Addiction. Luxembourg: Office for Official Publications of the European Communities, 2009.

PERIODICALS

Anderson, Jane. "Designer drug ID methods sought." *Pediatric News.* April 2012: 23.

Braiser, L.L. and Tammy Stables Battaglia. "Blame K2 drug for deadly baseball bat attack, lawyer says." *Detroit Free Press.* June 9, 2012.

Miller, Naseem S. "'Spice' and 'K2' are new drugs of abuse." *Clinical Psychiatry News.*Mar. 2012: 2.

"Michael Daniel Accused of Killing, Eating Dog On K-2-Fueled Rampage." *The Huffington Post.* June 26, 2012.

"'Synthetic Marijuana' Oral Fluid Drug Test Now Includes Four Next-Generation Drugs to Address Changing Abuse Patterns." *Obesity, Fitness & Wellness Week.* May 12, 2012.

WEBSITES

National Institute on Drug Abuse. "Drug Facts: Spice (Synthetic Marijuana)." http://www.drugabuse.gov/publications/drugfacts/spice-synthetic-marijuana Accessed September 01, 2012.

ORGANIZATIONS

National Institute on Drug Abuse (NIDA), 6001 Executive Boulevard, Room 5213, Bethesda, Maryland USA 20892-9561, 1 (301) 443-1124, information@nida.nih.gov, www.drugabuse.gov.

National Organization of State Alcohol/Drug Abuse Directors, 1025 Connecticut Avenue NW, Suite 605, Washington, DC USA 20036, (202) 293-0090.

Andrea Nienstedt, MA

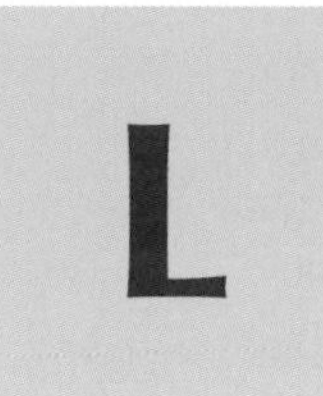

Legionnaires' disease

Definition

Legionnaires' disease is a type of **pneumonia** caused by *Legionella* bacteria. The bacterial species responsible for Legionnaires' disease is *L. pneumophila*. Major symptoms include fever, chills, muscle aches, and a cough that is initially nonproductive. Definitive diagnosis relies on specific laboratory tests for the bacteria, bacterial antigens, or antibodies produced by the body's immune system. As with other types of pneumonia, Legionnaires' disease poses the greatest threat to people who are elderly, ill, or immunocompromised.

Description

Legionella bacteria were first identified as a cause of pneumonia in 1976, following an outbreak of pneumonia among people who had attended an American Legion convention in Philadelphia, Pennsylvania. This eponymous outbreak prompted further investigation into *Legionella* and it was discovered that earlier unexplained pneumonia outbreaks were linked to the bacteria. The earliest cases of Legionnaires' disease were shown to have occurred in 1965, but samples of the bacteria exist from 1947.

Exposure to the *Legionella* bacteria doesn't necessarily lead to infection. According to some studies, an estimated 5–10% of the American population show serologic evidence of exposure, the majority of whom do not develop symptoms of an infection. *Legionella* bacteria account for 2–15% of the total number of pneumonia cases requiring hospitalization in the United States.

There are at least 40 types of *Legionella* bacteria, half of which are capable of producing disease in humans. A disease that arises from infection by *Legionella* bacteria is referred to as legionellosis. The *L. pneumophila bacterium*, the root cause of Legionnaires' disease, causes 90% of legionellosis cases. The second most common cause of legionellosis is the *L. micdadei* bacterium, which produces the Philadelphia pneumonia-causing agent.

Approximately 10,000–40,000 people in the United States develop Legionnaires' disease annually. The people who are the most likely to become ill are over age 50. The risk is greater for people who suffer from health conditions such as malignancy, diabetes, lung disease, or kidney disease. Other risk factors include immunosuppressive therapy and cigarette **smoking**. Legionnaires' disease does occur in children, but typically it has been confined to newborns receiving respiratory therapy, children who have had recent operations, and children who are immunosuppressed. People with HIV infection and **AIDS** do not seem to contract Legionnaires' disease with any greater frequency than the rest of the population, however, if contracted, the disease is likely to be more severe compared to other cases.

Cases of Legionnaires' disease that occur in conjunction with an outbreak, or epidemic, are more likely to be diagnosed quickly. Early diagnosis aids effective and successful treatment. During epidemic outbreaks, fatalities have ranged from 5% for previously healthy individuals to 24% for individuals with underlying illnesses. Sporadic cases (that is, cases unrelated to a wider outbreak) are harder to detect and treatment may be delayed pending an accurate diagnosis. The overall fatality rate for sporadic cases ranges from 10–19%. The outlook is bleaker in severe cases that require respiratory support or dialysis. In such cases, fatality may reach 67%.

Causes and symptoms

Legionnaires' disease is caused by inhaling *Legionella* bacteria from the environment. Typically, the bacteria are dispersed in aerosols of contaminated **water**. These aerosols are produced by devices in which warm water can stagnate, such as air-conditioning cooling towers, humidifiers, shower heads, and faucets. There have also been cases linked to whirlpool spa baths and water misters in grocery store produce departments. Aspiration of contaminated water is also a potential source of infection, particularly in hospital-acquired cases of Legionnaires' disease. There is no evidence of person-to-person transmission of Legionnaires' disease.

Once the bacteria are in the lungs, cellular representatives of the body's immune system (alveolar macrophages) congregate to destroy the invaders. The typical macrophage defense is to phagocytose the invader and demolish it in a process analogous to swallowing and digesting it. However, the *Legionella* bacteria survive being phagocytosed. Instead of being destroyed within the macrophage, they grow and replicate, eventually killing the macrophage. When the macrophage dies, many new *Legionella* bacteria are released into the lungs and worsen the infection.

Legionnaires' disease develops 2–10 days after exposure to the bacteria. Early symptoms include lethargy, headaches, fever, chills, muscle aches, and a lack of appetite. Respiratory symptoms such as coughing or congestion are usually absent. As the disease progresses, a dry, hacking cough develops and may become productive after a few days. In about a third of Legionnaires' disease cases, blood is present in the sputum. Half of the people who develop Legionnaires' disease suffer shortness of breath and a third complain of breathing-related chest **pain**. The fever can become quite high, reaching 104°F (40°C) in many cases, and may be accompanied by a decreased heart rate.

Although the pneumonia affects the lungs, Legionnaires' disease is accompanied by symptoms that affect other areas of the body. About half the victims experience diarrhea and a quarter have nausea and vomiting and abdominal pain. In about 10% of cases, acute renal failure and scanty urine production accompany the disease. Changes in mental status, such as disorientation, confusion, and hallucinations, also occur in about a quarter of cases.

In addition to Legionnaires' disease, *L. pneumophila* legionellosis also includes a milder disease, Pontiac fever. Unlike Legionnaires' disease, Pontiac fever does not involve the lower respiratory tract. The symptoms usually appear within 36 hours of exposure and include fever, headache, muscle aches, and lethargy. Symptoms last only a few days and medical intervention is not necessary.

Diagnosis

The symptoms of Legionnaires' disease are common to many types of pneumonia and diagnosis of sporadic cases can be difficult. The symptoms and chest x rays that confirm a case of pneumonia are not useful in differentiating between Legionnaires' disease and other pneumonias. If a pneumonia case involves multisystem symptoms, such as diarrhea and vomiting, and an initially dry cough, laboratory tests are done to definitively identify *L. pneumophila* as the cause of the infection.

If Legionnaires' disease is suspected, several tests are available to reveal or indicate the presence of *L. pneumophila* bacteria in the body. Since the immune system creates antibodies against infectious agents, examining the blood for these indicators is a key test. The level of immunoglobulins, or antibody molecules, in the blood reveals the presence of infection. In microscopic examination of the patient's sputum, a fluorescent stain linked to antibodies against *L. pneumophila* can uncover the presence of the bacteria. Other means of revealing the bacteria's presence from patient sputum

KEY TERMS

Antibody—A molecule created by the immune system in response to the presence of an antigen. It serves to recognize the invader and help defend the body from infection.

Antigen—A molecule, such as a protein, which is associated with a particular infectious agent. The immune system uses this molecule as the identifying characteristic of the infectious invader.

Culture—A laboratory system for growing bacteria for further study.

DNA probe—An agent that binds directly to a predefined sequence of nucleic acids.

Immunocompromised—Refers to conditions in which the immune system is not functioning properly and cannot adequately protect the body from infection.

Immunoglobulin—The protein molecule that serves as the primary building block of antibodies.

Immunosuppressive therapy—Medical treatment in which the immune system is purposefully thwarted. Such treatment is necessary, for example, to prevent organ rejection in transplant cases.

Legionellosis—A disease caused by infection with a Legionella bacterium.

Media—Substance which contains all the nutrients necessary for bacteria to grow in a culture.

Phagocytosis—The "ingestion" of a piece of matter by a cell.

samples include isolation of the organism on culture media or detection of the bacteria by DNA probe. Another test detects *L. pneumophila* antigens in the urine.

Public health response

In the United States and many other countries, legionellosis is a nationally notifiable disease. A health worker who learns of a case of the disease is required to notify officials of this fact, providing relevant information about the infection. Public health workers also interview individuals who have contracted the disease in order to obtain information about possible sources of the disease. When such sources are identified, arrangements can be made for cleaning that source, such as a dirty air conditioning unit. Public health workers can also reduce the risk to individuals of contracting the disease by informing healthcare workers and the general public about the conditions that lead to Legionnaires' disease and the steps that can be taken to reduce the risk of contracting the disease.

Treatment

Most cases of *Legionella* pneumonia show improvement within 12–48 hours of starting antibiotic therapy. The antibiotic of choice has been erythromycin, sometimes paired with a second antibiotic, rifampin. Tetracycline, alone or with rifampin, is also used to treat Legionnaires' disease, but has had more mixed success in comparison to erythromycin. Other **antibiotics** that have been used successfully to combat *Legionella* include doxycycline, clarithromycin, fluorinated quinolones, and trimethoprim/sulfamethoxazole.

The type of antibiotic prescribed by the doctor depends on several factors including the severity of infection, potential **allergies**, and interaction with previously prescribed drugs. For example, erythromycin interacts with warfarin, a blood thinner. Several drugs, such as penicillins and cephalosporins, are ineffective against the infection. Although they may be deadly to the bacteria in laboratory tests, their chemical structure prevents them from being absorbed into the areas of the lung where the bacteria are present.

In severe cases with complications, antibiotic therapy may be joined by respiratory support. If renal failure occurs, dialysis is required until renal function is recovered.

Prognosis

Appropriate medical treatment has a major impact on recovery from Legionnaires' disease. Outcome is also linked to the victim's general health and absence of complications. If the patient survives the infection, recovery from Legionnaires' disease is complete. Similar to other types of pneumonia, severe cases of Legionnaires' disease may cause scarring in the lung tissue as a result of the infection. Renal failure, if it occurs, is reversible and renal function returns as the patient's health improves. Occasionally, fatigue and weakness may linger for several months after the infection has been successfully treated.

QUESTIONS TO ASK YOUR DOCTOR

- How can you tell whether a case of pneumonia is caused by the *Legionella* bacterium, or by some other agent?
- How does this diagnosis affect the treatment you will recommend for the pneumonia?
- How is it possible to trace the source of the disease?
- How can you determine whether there is a sporadic case of the disease or an element of a wider ranging spread of the disease?
- To what extent is my child likely to be at risk for a *Legionella* infection from equipment not properly maintained at her school, and what can I do to reduce that risk?

Prevention

Since the bacteria thrive in warm stagnant water, regularly disinfecting ductwork, pipes, and other areas that may serve as breeding areas is the best method for preventing outbreaks of Legionnaires' disease. Most outbreaks of Legionnaires' disease can be traced to specific points of exposure, such as hospitals, hotels, and other places where people gather. Sporadic cases are harder to determine and there is insufficient evidence to point to exposure in individual homes.

Resources

BOOKS

Uzel, Atac, and E. Esin Hames-Kocabas. *Legionella Pneumophila: From Environment to Disease*. Hauppage, NY: Nova Science Publications, 2010.

PERIODICALS

Cristino, S., P. P. Legnani, and E. Leoni. "Plan for the Control of Legionella Infections in Long-term Care Facilities: Role of Environmental Monitoring." *International Journal of Hygiene and Environmental Health* 215, 3. (2012): 279–285.

PERIODICALS

Shuman, H. A., et al. "Intracellular Multiplication of Legionella pneumophila: Human Pathogen of Accidental Tourist?" Current Topics in Microbiology and Immunology 225 (1998): 99.

OTHER

Legionnaires' Disease. Medline Plus. http://www.nlm.nih.gov/medlineplus/legionnairesdisease.html (accessed August 18, 2012).

Patient Facts: Learn More about Legionnaires' Disease. http://www.cdc.gov/legionella/patient_facts.htm (accessed August 18, 2012).

Julia Barrett

Leishmaniasis

Definition

Leishmaniasis refers to several different illnesses caused by infection with a parasitic organism called a protozoan. Specifically, the organism belongs to the genus *Leishmania*. The disease is transmitted to humans from certain species of the infected female sand fly (order Dipteran) that are found in sandy areas. In the United States, the sand fly is often referred to by the terms of horse fly, greenhead, sand flea, sand gnats, and various other names. In the Balkans the disease is called the Balkan sore; in India, the Delhi boil; and in Iraq the Baghdad boil; while in Afghanistan it is called saldana.

Demographics

All ages of people are susceptible to the disease. However, children are at greater risk than are adults. In addition, it is more common in rural areas than in urban settings. The disease is also of greater risk to men than it is to women, probably because males tend to be outside more frequently than females and are more likely to be exposed to sand flies at a higher rate. The risk of getting the disease is higher during nighttime because sand flies are more active in darkness then in sunlight. People also at heightened risk for the disease are adventure travelers, ecotourists, and other tourists visiting areas where leishmaniasis is more common. Volunteers, missionaries, soldiers in such areas where the disease is common are also at higher risk, as are bird watchers, ornithologists (people who study birds), and people who frequently work and play outside.

Medical studies have shown that people with acquired immune deficiency syndrome (**AIDS**) have a much greater chance of developing visceral leishmaniasis, one of the four primary types of leishmaniasis.

The disease is found primarily in the tropics, subtropics, and southern Europe. In the Western Hemisphere, it is found in parts of Mexico, Central America, and South America (but not in Chile or Uruguay). In the Eastern Hemisphere, it is frequently located in parts of Asia, the Middle East, southern Europe, and Africa.

At any one time, about 12 to 20 million people throughout the world are infected with leishmaniasis. According to the U.S. **Centers for Disease Control and Prevention (CDC)**, about 1.5 million new cases of cutaenous leishmaniasis, the most common type of the disease, are reported yearly worldwide, while about a half million new cases of visceral leishmaniasis, the second most common type, are estimated annually. It is estimated that over 80,000 deaths occur annually from the disease.

While leishmaniasis exists as a disease in about 88 countries on five continents, some countries are hit harder than others. The vast majority of cases of cutaneous leishmaniasis take place in Afghanistan, Algeria, Brazil, Iran, Iraq, Peru, Saudi Arabia, and Syria. Almost all of the cases of visceral leishmaniasis happen in Bangladesh, Brazil, India, Nepal, and Sudan. Other areas that harbor the causative protozoa include China, many countries throughout Africa, Mexico, Central and South America, Turkey, and Greece. Cases of leishmaniasis occur in the United States but only from people who have traveled outside of the country. In addition, cases of cutaneous leishmaniasis have taken place in Texas and Oklahoma. Past cases of visceral leishmaniasis have not been reported in the United States, according to the **CDC**.

Description

Protozoa are considered to be the simplest organisms in the animal kingdom. They are all single-celled. The blood-sucking sand fly carries the types of protozoa that cause leishmaniasis. The sand fly is referred to as the disease vector, simply meaning that the infectious agent (the protozoan) is transported by the sand fly and passed on to other animals or humans in whom the protozoan will set up residence and cause disease. The animal or human in which the protozoan then resides is referred to as the host.

Once the protozoan is within the human host, the human's immune system is activated to try to combat the invader. Specialized immune cells called macrophages work to swallow up the protozoa. Usually, this technique kills a foreign invader, but these protozoa can survive and flourish within macrophages. The protozoa multiply within the macrophages, ultimately causing the macrophage to burst open. The protozoa are released, and take up residence within other neighboring cells.

At this point, the course of the disease caused by the protozoa is dependent on the specific type of protozoa, and on the type of reaction the protozoa elicits from the immune system. There are several types of protozoa that cause leishmaniasis, and they produce different patterns of disease progression.

There are four primary types of leishmaniasis. They are:

- Localized (simple) cutaneous leishmaniasis, which is the most common type, causes a skin sore at the site of the bite. This type can then proceed to become any of the other three types.
- Diffuse cutaneous leishmaniasis, which is difficult to treat, can produce large areas of skin lesions that resemble leprosy.
- Mucocutaneous leishmaniasis, which starts with skin ulcers, is especially troublesome for the nose and mouth.
- Visceral leishmaniasis, which is the second most common type and the most serious one because it usually affects some of the internal organs (such as liver and spleen), can be fatal if not treated promptly.

Causes and symptoms

There are a number of types of protozoa that can cause leishmaniasis. Each type exists in specific locations, and there are different patterns to the kind of disease each causes. All forms of the organism belong to the genus Leishmania. The specific disease-causing species include: *Leishmania donovani, L. infantum, L. chagasi, L. mexicana, L. amazonensis, L. tropica, L. major, L. aethiopica, L. brasiliensis, L. guyaensis, L. panamensis, and L. peruviana.* Some of the names are reflective of the locale in which the specific protozoan is most commonly found, or in which it was first discovered.

Localized cutaneous leishmaniasis

This type of disease, also called simple cutaneous leishmaniasis, occurs most commonly in China, India, Asia Minor, Africa, the Mediterranean Basin, and Central America. It has ranged in an area from northern Argentina all the way up to southern Texas. It is called different names in different locations, including chiclero ulcer, bush yaws, uta, oriental sore, Aleppo boil, and Baghdad sore.

This condition is perhaps the least drastic type of disease caused by any of the *Leishmania*. Several weeks or months after being bitten by an infected sand fly, the host may notice an itchy bump (lesion) on an arm, leg, or face. Lymph nodes in the area of this bump may be swollen. Within several months, the bump develops a crater (ulceration) in the center, with a raised, reddened ridge around it. There may be several of these lesions (sores) near each other, and they may spread into each other to form one large lesion. Often, individual lesions change in size and appearance as they develop. Eventually, they may have a raised edge and a central ulcerated area. People with sores also often have swollen glands near the infected areas. Although localized cutaneous leishmaniasis usually heals on its own, it may take as long as one year. A depressed, light-colored scar usually remains behind. Some lesions never heal, and may invade and destroy the tissue below. For example, lesions on the ears may slowly, but surely, invade and destroy the cartilage that supports the outer ear.

Diffuse cutaneous leishmaniasis

This type of disease occurs most often in Ethiopia, Brazil, Dominican Republic, and Venezuela. The lesions of diffuse cutaneous leishmaniasis are very similar to those of localized cutaneous leishmaniasis, except they are spread all over the body. The body's immune system apparently fails to battle the protozoa, which are free to spread throughout the body. The characteristic lesions resemble those of **leprosy**.

Mucocutaneous leishmaniasis

This type of leishmaniasis occurs primarily in the tropics of South America. With an incubation period of from one to three months, the disease begins with the same sores noted in localized cutaneous leishmaniasis. Sometimes these primary lesions heal, other times they spread and become larger. Some years after the first lesion is noted (and sometimes several years after that lesion has totally healed), new lesions appear in the mouth and nose, and occasionally in the area between the genitalia and the anus (the perineum). These new lesions, called mucosal lesions, are particularly destructive and painful. Sometimes their appearance is delayed twenty years from the first presence of the primary lesions.

The mucosal lesions erode underlying tissue and cartilage, frequently eating through the septum (the cartilage that separates the two nostrils). If the lesions spread to the roof of the mouth and the larynx (the part of the wind pipe which contains the vocal cords), they may prevent speech. Other symptoms include fever, weight loss, and anemia (low red blood cell count). There is always a large danger of bacteria infecting the already open sores.

Visceral leishmaniasis

This type of leishmaniasis occurs in India, China, the southern region of Russia, and throughout Africa, the Mediterranean, and South and Central America. It is frequently called kala-azar or Dumdum fever. In this disease, the protozoa use the bloodstream to travel to the liver, spleen, lymph nodes, and bone marrow. Fever may last for as long as eight weeks, disappear, and then reappear again. The lymph nodes, spleen, and liver are often quite enlarged. Weakness, fatigue, loss of appetite, diarrhea, and weight loss are common. Abnormal blood tests also result, including low red blood cell count, low white blood cell count, and low platelet count. Kala-azar translates (from the country of India) to mean "black fever." The name kala-azar comes from a characteristic of this type of leishmaniasis. Individuals with light-colored skin take on a darker, grayish skin tone, particularly of their face and hands. A variety of lesions appear on the skin.

Diagnosis

Diagnosis for each of these types of leishmaniasis involves taking a scraping from a lesion, preparing it in a laboratory, and examining it under a microscope to determine the causative protozoan. Other methods that have been used include:

- Culturing a sample piece of tissue in a laboratory to allow the protozoa to multiply for easier microscopic identification.
- Injecting a mouse or hamster with a solution made of scrapings from a patient's lesion to see if the animal develops a leishmaniasis-like disease.
- Demonstrating the presence in macrophages of the characteristic-appearing protozoan, called Leishman-Donovan bodies.

In some types of leishmaniasis, a skin test (similar to that given for **tuberculosis**, or TB) may be used. In this test, a solution containing a small bit of the protozoan antigen (cell marker that causes the human immune system to react) is injected or scratched into a patient's skin. In a positive reaction, cells from the immune system will race to this spot, causing a characteristic skin lesion. Not all types of leishmaniasis cause a positive skin test, however. The CDC states that diagnosis of leishmaniasis can be difficult. Results from laboratory tests frequently come back as negative even when the person has the disease.

KEY TERMS

Host—The organism (such as a monkey or human) in which another organism (such as a virus or bacteria) is living.

Larynx—The part of the airway lying between the pharynx and the trachea.

Leishman-Donovan body—A body of a (trypanosomatid) protozoa at a particular and characteristic stage in its life cycle; the infectious (trypanosomatid) protozoa can cause leishmaniasis, and is relatively easy to identify at that stage.

Lesion—A disruption of the normal structure and function of a tissue by some disease process.

Macrophage—A cell of the immune system that engulfs and digests foreign invaders such as bacteria and viruses in an attempt to stop them from causing disease within the body.

Protozoa—A group of organisms which are the smallest members of the animal kingdom, consisting of a single cell.

Ulceration—An area of pitting and irritation.

Vector—A carrier organism (such as a fly or mosquito) that delivers a virus (or other agent of infection) to a host.

Public health response

The control of leishmaniasis outbreaks depends critically on early detection and treatment. Public health response depends first of all on the host primarily involved in the outbreak. For cases in which humans are the primary host, early detection and treatment not only reduces **mortality and morbidity** in the short term, but also tends to eliminate the number of **parasites** remaining in the community, thus reducing the risk of further infections. When nonhuman animals are the primary or additional hosts, other treatments are also necessary. For example, dogs, who are a major vector for the disease in many areas, need to be tested for the parasite and treated or destroyed to reduce the risk to humans. Preventative measures such as the use of insect nets, spraying house and yards for insects, and initiating a program of rodent control are steps in reducing not only the immediate threat posed by these vectors, but also the long-term risks posed to human communities by the parasite. The effectiveness of these steps is somewhat limited in that some methods of **prevention** are too expensive to be employed in the poorest of communities. For example, providing all inhabitants with pesticide-impregnated mattresses is a powerful tool for reducing infection from insect bites, but the cost of such mattresses is often prohibitive.

Public health authorities are especially concerned about the co-infection of HIV and leishmania and have instituted a worldwide reporting system consisting of 28 institutions in 13 countries to receive, coordinate, and distribute data on such infections. No such reporting system yet exists for leishmaniasis itself, and the disease is a notifiable condition in only 33 of the 88 countries in which it occurs. Effective action against the disease probably depends to some extent on an expanded program of notification and surveillance.

Treatment

The treatment of choice for all types of leishmaniasis is a type of drug containing the element antimony. These include **sodium** sitogluconate, and meglumin antimonate. When these types of drugs do not work, other medications with anti-protozoal activity are utilized, including amphotericin B, pentamidine, flagyl, and allopurinol. In 2004, it was reported that the world's first non-profit drug company was seeking approval in India for a drug to cure visceral leishmaniasis. Historically, an estimated 200,000 people die annually from the disease in that country. The company, called One World Health, hoped to offer the drug called paromomycin for a three-week treatment course. In 2006, paromomycin was approved by the Drug Controller General of India for treatment of visceral leishmaniasis.

Prognosis

The prognosis for leishmaniasis is quite variable, and depends on the specific strain of infecting protozoan, as well as the individual patient's immune system response to infection. Localized cutaneous leishmaniasis may not require any treatment. Although it may take many months, these lesions usually heal themselves completely. Only rarely do these lesions fail to heal and become more destructive.

Diffuse cutaneous leishmaniasis may smolder on for years without treatment, eventually progressing to mucocutaneous leishmaniasis, and ultimately causing death when the large, open lesions become infected with bacteria.

Mucocutaneous leishmaniasis is often relatively resistant to treatment. Untreated visceral leishmaniasis has a 90% death rate, but only a 10% death rate with proper treatment.

Visceral leishmaniasis has been increasingly associated with human immunodeficiency virus (HIV). For example, the two have appeared together in southern Europe, primarily among intravenous drug users. If treated properly, the risk from death is minimal. However, the rates of mortality in untreated cases has been shown to range from 75% to 95%. Even when death does not occur from the disease, it can leave the person disfigured and with serious deformities. Advanced cases of visceral leishmaniasis can eventually cause death if left untreated.

QUESTIONS TO ASK YOUR DOCTOR

- To what extent are Americans who do not travel overseas at risk for leishmaniasis?
- When it is necessary to take precautions against leishmaniasis when traveling overseas?
- What is the best source of information about leishmaniasis for individuals who travel to off-the-main-road destinations overseas?
- Are there medications I should take ahead of time or carry with me for protection against leishmaniasis when traveling to India? To Africa? To South America?

Prevention

Prevention involves protecting against sand fly bites. Insect repellents used around homes, on clothing, on skin, and on bed nets (to protect people while sleeping) are effective measures.

Reducing the **population** of sand flies is also an important preventive measure. In areas where leishmaniasis is very common, recommendations include clearing the land of trees and brush for at least 1,000 feet (300 meters) around all villages, and regularly spraying the area with insecticides. Because rodents often carry the protozoan that causes leishmaniasis, careful rodent control should be practiced. Dogs, which also carry the protozoan, can be given a simple blood test.

Resources

BOOKS

Myler, Peter J., and Nicolas Fasel. *Leishmania: After the Genome.* Norfolk, UK: Caister Academic, 2008.

Tibayrenc, Michel, editor. *Encyclopedia of Infectious Diseases: Modern Methodologies.* Hoboken, NJ: Wiley-Liss, 2007.

Wertheim, Heiman, F. L., Peter Horby, and John P. Woodall. *Atlas of Human Infectious Diseases.* Oxford: Wiley-Blackwell, 2012.

OTHER

Leishmaniasis. New York Times Health Guide. http://health.nytimes.com/health/guides/disease/leishmaniasis/overview.html (accessed August 20, 2012).

Leishmaniasis. PubMed Health. http://www.ncbi.nlm.nih.gov/pubmedhealth/PMH0002362/ (accessed August 20, 2012).

Leishmaniasis. World Health Organization. http://www.who.int/leishmaniasis/en/ (accessed August 20, 2012).

ORGANIZATIONS

Centers for Disease Control and Prevention. 1600 Clifton Rd., NE, Atlanta, GA 30333. (800) CDC-INFO (800 232-4636) or (404) 639-3534. cdcinfo@cdc.gov. www.cdc.gov.

Rosalyn Carson-DeWitt, MD
Teresa G. Odle

Leprosy

Definition

Leprosy is a slowly progressing chronic bacterial infection that affects the skin, peripheral nerves in the hands and feet, upper respiratory tract, and mucous membranes of the nose, throat, and eyes. Destruction of the nerve endings causes the affected areas to lose sensation. Leprosy is a progressive disease; that is, one that takes anywhere from six months to 40 years to develop. If left untreated, it can cause skin lesions and inflammatory nodules (granulomas) on the skin and nerves and, ultimately, permanent damage and disfigurement to the skin, nerves, limbs, eyes, and other body parts. It affects primarily the outer extremities such as the eyes, nose, earlobes, hands, testicles (in men), and feet.

Demographics

The **World Health Organization (WHO)** places the number of identified leprosy cases in the world at 192,246 as of 2012. According to **WHO**, the number of new cases globally decreased by about 16% from 2010 to 2011. Seventy percent of all cases are located in just three countries: India, Indonesia, and Myanamar (Burma). The infection can be acquired, however, in the Western Hemisphere as well. According to WHO, there were 169 reported cases in the United States in 2010, an increase of about 10 percent over the figure for 2005. Almost all of the U.S. cases involve immigrants from developing countries. Cases also occur in some areas of the Caribbean. Although it was thought for many years that only humans are affected by the disease, 15% of wild armadillos in southern Texas and Louisiana have been found to be infected with *M. leprae*.

Description

Leprosy is also known as Hansen's disease after Norwegian physician Gerhard Armauer Hansen (1841–1912), who in 1878 identified the bacillus (rod-shaped bacterium) *Mycobacterium leprae* (*M leprae*) that causes the disease.

The infection is characterized by abnormal changes of the skin. These changes, called lesions, are at first flat and red. Upon enlarging, they develop irregular shapes and a characteristic appearance. The lesions are typically darker in color around the edges with discolored pale centers. Because the organism grows best at lower body temperatures, the leprosy bacillus prefers the skin, the mucous membranes, and the nerves. Infection in the nerves and their eventual destruction leads to sensory loss. The loss of sensation in the fingers and toes increases the risk of injury. Inadequate care causes infection of open wounds. Gangrene may also follow, resulting in the deformation or death of body tissue.

Because of the disabling deformities associated with it, leprosy has been considered one of the most dreaded diseases since Biblical times (beginning at about 1500 B.C.), though much of what was called leprosy in the Old Testament most likely was not the same disease. Its victims were often shunned by the community, kept at arm's length, or sent to a leper colony. Many people still have misconceptions about the disease. Contrary to popular belief, it is not highly communicable and is extremely slow to develop. Household contacts of most cases and the medical personnel caring for Hansen's disease patients are not at particular risk. It is very curable, although the treatment is long-term, requiring multiple medications.

Causes and symptoms

The organism that causes leprosy is a rod-shaped bacterium called *Mycobacterium leprae*. This bacterium is related to *Mycobacterium tuberculosis*, the causative agent of **tuberculosis**. *M. leprae* is considered an obligate intracellular bacterium; that is, a bacterium that is able to grow only inside certain human and animal cells. Because special staining techniques involving acids are required to view these bacteria under the microscope, they are referred to as acid-fast bacilli (AFB).

When *Mycobacterium leprae* invades the body, one of two reactions can take place. In tuberculoid leprosy (TT), the milder form of the disease, the body's immune cells attempt to seal off the infection from the rest of the body by surrounding the offending pathogen. Because this response by the immune system occurs in the deeper layers of the skin, the hair follicles, sweat glands, and nerves can be destroyed. As a result, the skin becomes

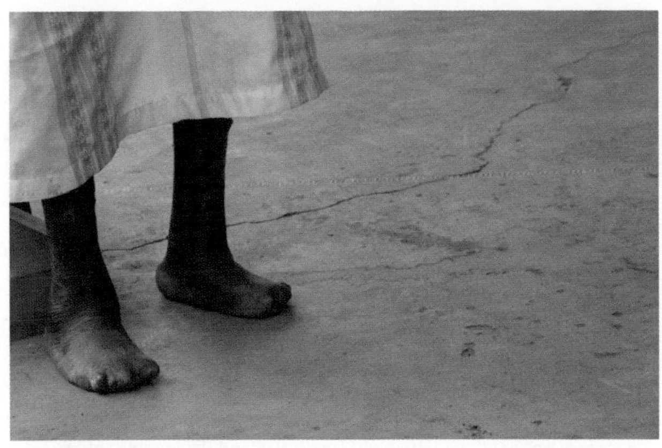

Dipiction of feet of a person with Leprosy. *(©iStockphoto .com/Shutterstitch)*

dry and discolored and loses its sensitivity. Involvement of nerves on the face, arms, or legs can cause them to enlarge and to become easily felt by the examining doctor. This finding is highly suggestive of TT. The scarcity of bacteria in this type of leprosy leads to its being referred to as paucibacillary (PB) leprosy. Approximately 70 to 80% of all leprosy cases are of the tuberculoid type.

In lepromatous (LL) leprosy, which is the second and more contagious form of the disease, the body's immune system is unable to mount a strong response to the invading organism. Hence, the organism multiplies freely in the skin. This type of leprosy is also called the multibacillary (MB) leprosy, because of the presence of large numbers of bacteria. The characteristic feature of this disease is the appearance of large nodules or lesions all over the body and face. Occasionally, the mucous membranes of the eyes, nose, and throat may be involved. Facial involvement can produce a lion-like appearance (leonine facies). This type of leprosy can lead to blindness, drastic change in voice, or mutilation of the nose. Leprosy can strike anyone; however, children seem to be more susceptible than adults.

The early symptoms of leprosy are not apparent, and they may very slowly develop over many years without much notice. Well-defined skin lesions that are numb are the first symptoms of tuberculoid leprosy. Numbness and a decreasing ability to sense hot and cold temperatures are two other early symptoms of leprosy. Lepromatous leprosy is characterized by a chronic stuffy nose due to invasion of the mucous membranes, and the presence of nodules and lesions all over the body and face. As the disease advances, the sense of touch, **pain**, and pressure are decreased and, eventually lost. Skin lesions of hypopigmented macules (flat and pale areas of the skin) also appear, as do nearly painless ulcers and increased dryness of the eyes. Eventually, large ulcerated areas are produced. Eventually facial disfiguration develops, along with loss of fingers and toes.

Although patients with leprosy are commonly thought not to suffer pain, neuroapthic pain caused by inflammation of peripheral nerve endings is increasingly recognized as a major complication of the disease in many patients. Corticosteroids may be given to reduce the inflammation.

The incubation period of the leprosy bacillus varies anywhere from six months to ten years. On an average, it takes four years for the symptoms of tuberculoid leprosy to develop. Probably because of the slow growth of the bacillus, lepromatous leprosy develops even more slowly, taking an average of eight years for the initial lesions to appear.

It is still not very clear how the leprosy bacillus is transmitted from person to person; about 50% of patients diagnosed with the disease have a history of close contact with an infected family member. Since untreated patients have a large number of *M. leprae* bacilli in their nasal secretions, it is thought that transmission may take place via nasal droplets. The milder tubercular form of leprosy may be transmitted by insect carriers or by contact with infected soil.

Some medical researchers contend that *M. leprae* is transmitted from one human to another through nasal secretions or droplets. However, other scientists think that the bacterium enters the body through breaks in the skin. As of 2012, the specific ways that the bacterium enters the body is being investigated by scientists.

The disease appears primarily in the poorest of the world's countries. In addition, environmental factors such as overpopulated areas, unhygienic living conditions, contaminated **water**, risk of other immune-compromising diseases, and insufficient diet/extreme malnutrition may also be contributing factors adding to the risk of leprosy.

Diagnosis

Leprosy is usually diagnosed through clinical investigations. One of the hallmarks of leprosy is the presence of AFB in smears taken from the skin lesions, nasal scrapings, or tissue secretions. In patients with LL leprosy, the bacilli are easily detected; however, in TT leprosy the bacteria are very few and almost impossible to find. In such cases, a diagnosis is made based on the clinical signs and symptoms, the type and distribution of skin lesions, and history of having lived in an endemic area. Generally, laboratory analysis is not used because such labs are rarely found in these very poor countries where leprosy is mostly found.

The signs and symptoms characteristic of leprosy can be easily identified by a health worker after a short training period. There is no need for a laboratory investigation to confirm a leprosy diagnosis, except in very rare circumstances.

In an endemic area, if smears from an individual show the presence of AFB, or if he/she has typical skin lesions, then that person should definitely be regarded as having leprosy. Usually, there is slight discoloration of the skin (sometimes called hypopigmented patches of skin) and loss of skin sensitivity along with redness of the area. Thickened nerves accompanied by weakness of muscles supplied by the affected nerve are very typical of the disease. One characteristic occurrence is a foot drop where the foot cannot be flexed upwards, affecting the ability to walk.

When laboratory tests are used, such tests usually include a CBC (complete blood count) test, liver function test, creatinine (clearance) test, and a nerve biopsy.

Public health response

The **World Health Organization** has declared that the way to eliminate leprosy is "to detect all patients and cure them with MDT," where "MDT" stands for "multidrug therapy." The first step in that process is for public health agencies to train representatives from villages in all areas where the disease is endemic. These trainees must learn how to recognize the symptoms of leprosy, get those diagnosed with the disease to a public health facility, and begin multidrug therapy as soon as possible. Trainees also need to learn how to educate members of a community about leprosy, explaining that it is generally not communicable and that it can be treated in much the same way as many other infectious disorders. Overcoming fears of the disease is a critical part of encouraging people to come forward and be tested for the disease. The cost of testing and treatment is now generally free almost anywhere in the world, so that an aggressive campaign against leprosy is not hindered by lack of resources by patients or their communities. Public health workers can also encourage members of a community to take responsibility for their own health practices by teaching them how to do self-examinations for leprosy and how to take MDT reliably during treatent of the disease.

Treatment

A vaccine for leprosy is still not available. The most widely used drug for leprosy is dapsone (DDS). However, the emergence of dapsone-resistant strains prompted the introduction of multidrug therapy, or MDT. MDT combines dapsone, rifampin (Rifadin; also known as rifampicin), and clofazimine (Lamprene), all of which are powerful antibacterial drugs. Patients with MB leprosy are usually treated with all three drugs, while patients with PB leprosy are given only rifampin and dapsone. Usually three months after starting treatment, a patient ceases being infectious, though not everyone with this disease is necessarily infectious before treatment. Depending on the type of leprosy, the time required for treatment may vary from six months to two years or more.

Each of the drugs has minor side effects. Dapsone can cause nausea, dizziness, palpitations, jaundice, and rash. A doctor should be contacted immediately if a rash develops. Dapsone also interacts with the second drug, rifampin. Rifampin increases the metabolizing of dapsone in the body, requiring an adjustment of the dapsone dosage. Rifampin may also cause muscle cramps, or nausea. If jaundice, flu-like symptoms or a rash appear, a doctor should be contacted immediately. The third drug, clofazimine may cause severe abdominal pain and diarrhea, as well as discoloration of the skin. Red to brownish black discoloration of the skin and bodily fluids, including sweat, may persist for months to years after use.

KEY TERMS

Endemic area—A geographical area where a particular disease is prevalent.

Gangrene—Death of tissue due to loss of blood supply followed by bacterial invasion and putrefaction.

Incubation period—The time it takes for symptoms to develop after initial exposure to a disease-causing organism.

Lesion—Any visible, local abnormality of the tissues of the skin, such as a wound, sore, rash, or boil.

Mucous membranes—The inner tissue that covers or lines body cavities or canals open to the outside, such as nose and mouth. These membranes secrete mucus and absorb water and salts.

Nasal scraping—Pathological material obtained for clinical study by scratching the inner surface of the nose with a clinical instrument.

Nodules—A small mass of tissue in the form of a protuberance or a knot that is solid and can be detected by touch.

Pathogen—Any disease-producing agent or microorganism.

Smear—A specimen prepared for microscopic study by spreading the material across a slide and treating it with a specific stain.

Thalidomide, the most famous agent of **birth defects** in the twentieth century, is now being used to treat complications of leprosy and similar diseases. Thalidomide regulates the immune response by suppressing a protein, tumor necrosis factor alpha.

Leprosy patients should be aware that treatment itself can cause a potentially serious immune system response called a lepra reaction. When **antibiotics** kill *M. leprae*, antigens (the proteins on the surface of the organism that initiate the body's immune system response) are released from the dying bacteria. In some people, when the antigens combine with the antibodies to *M. Leprae* in the bloodstream, a reaction called erythema nodosum leprosum may occur, resulting in new lesions and peripheral nerve damage. Cortisone-type medications and, increasingly, thalidomide are used to minimize the effects of lepra reactions.

Surgery may be performed in order to make cosmetic improvements to the patient. In some cases, severe ulcers caused by leprosy may be treated surgically with small skin grafts. In other cases, some movement of the limbs can be restored or, at least, some neural function improved.

Prognosis

Leprosy is curable; however, the deformities and nerve damage associated with leprosy are often irreversible. **Prevention** or rehabilitation of these defects is an integral part of management of the disease. Reconstructive surgery, aimed at preventing and correcting deformities, offers the greatest hope for disabled patients. Sometimes, the deformities are such that the patients will not benefit from this type of surgery.

Comprehensive care involves teaching patients to care for themselves. If the patients have significant nerve damage or are at high risk of developing deformities, they must be taught to take care of their insensitive limbs, similar to diabetics with lower leg nerve damage. Lacking the sensation of pain in many cases, the patients should constantly check themselves to identify cuts and bruises. If adequate care is not taken, these wounds become festering sores and a source of dangerous infection. Physiotherapy exercises are taught to the patients to maintain a range of movement in finger joints and prevent the deformities from worsening. Prefabricated standardized splints are available and are extremely effective in correcting and preventing certain common deformities in leprosy. Special kinds of footwear have been designed for patients with insensitive feet in order to prevent or minimize the progression of foot ulcers.

The genome of *M. leprae* has been sequenced as of 2010. The completion of this project has allowed much more research to be performed in the search for better treatments and a cure for leprosy. Scientists are currently working on how the bacterium infects humans, how the infection is transmitted within the body, what the period of incubation is for the disease, and many more avenues toward solving the problem.

QUESTIONS TO ASK YOUR DOCTOR

- If I have any reason to believe that I may have been exposed to leprosy, what signs and symptoms should I look for?
- What regions of the world are of special concern with respect to developing leprosy for the business or recreational traveler?
- How does one obtain information about leprosy, possible testing, and treatment programs in overseas countries?

Prevention

By early diagnosis and appropriate treatment of infected individuals, even a disease as ancient as leprosy can be controlled. People who are in immediate contact with the leprosy patient should be tested for leprosy. Annual examinations should also be conducted on these people for a period of five years following their last contact with an infectious patient. Some physicians have advocated dapsone treatment for people in close household contact with leprosy patients.

The WHO Action Program for the Elimination of Leprosy adopted a resolution calling for the elimination of leprosy around the world by the year 2005. This goal was not reached, however; a computer simulation performed for WHO by a team of Dutch researchers in 2004 indicates that leprosy is likely to persist in some parts of the world until 2020, although its incidence will continue to decline.

The WHO Action Program defined a strategy to eventually eliminate the disease as a public health problem. Members of the program hope to reach a rate of 1 or less leprosy case per 10,000 population. As of 2012, this "elimination" rate of 1 per 10,000 was reached in most countries with the highest rates of leprosy. The most recent country to achieve this distinction, Nepal, declared the elimination rate to have been reached in 2010 when only 2,331 new cases were reported, compared to more than 100,000 cases two decades earlier.

Resources

BOOKS

Brachman, Philip S., et al. eds. *Bacterial Infections of Humans: Epidemiology and Control.* New York: Springer Science and Business Media, 2009.

Dandel, Pieterson. *Understanding HIV/AIDS, Leprosy and TB-related Stigma among Health Care Workers*. Amsterdam: Royal Tropical Institute, 2011.

Makino, Jasanao, Masanori Matsuoka, Masamichi Goto, and Kentaro Hatano. *Leprosy: Science Working towards Dignity*. Hadano, Japan: Tokai University Press, 2011.

Nunzi, Enrico, and Cesare Massone, eds. *Leprosy: A Practical Guide*. Milan; New York: Springer, 2012.

Sehgal, Alfica. *Leprosy*. Philadelphia: Chelsea House, 2006.

WEBSITES

Leprosy. National Institutes of Health. http://health.nih.gov/topic/Leprosy (accessed August 20, 2012).

Leprosy (Hansen's Disease). MedicineNet.com. http://www.medicinenet.com/leprosy/article.htms (accessed August 20, 2012).

Leprosy Today. World Health Organization. http://www.who.int/lep/en/ (accessed August 20, 2012).

National Hansen's Disease (Leprosy) Program. Health Resources and Services Administration. http://www.hrsa.gov/hansens/ (accessed August 20, 2012).

ORGANIZATIONS

American Leprosy Missions, 1 ALM Way, Greenville, SC 29601. (864) 271-7040; (800) 543-135; Fax: (864) 271-7062. amlep@leprosy.org. http://www.leprosy.org/

International Federation of Anti-Leprosy Associations (ILEP), 234 Blythe Rd., London, United Kingdom, W14 0HJ. +44 (0) 20 7602 6925; +44 (0) 20 7371 1621; ilep@ilep.org.uk. http://www.ilep.org.uk.

LEPRA Health in Action, 28 Middleborough, Colchester, Essex, United Kingdom, CO1 1TG. +44 (0) 01206 216700; Fax: +44 (0) 01206 762151. http://www.lepra-healthinaction.org/.

Leprosy Mission International, 80 Windmill Rd. Brentford, Middlesex, United Kingdom, TW8 0QH. +44 (0) 20 8326 6767; Fax: +44 (0) 20 8326 6777. friends@timint.org. http://www.leprosymission.org/.

Lata Cherath, PhD
Rebecca J. Frey, PhD

Leptospirosis

Definition

Leptospirosis is a febrile (fever) disease caused primarily by infection with the bacterium *Leptospira interrogans*, but also by other bacteria within the genus *Leptospira*. It can be transmitted to humans by animals.

Description

The German physician Adolf Weil (1848–1916) first described the disease in 1886. It was later observed in 1907 from a slice of renal tissue during a post mortem procedure.

An infection by the bacterium *Leptospira interrogans* goes by different names in different regions. Alternate names for leptospirosis include mud fever, canefield fever, Rat Catcher's Yellows, seven–day fever, swamp fever, cane cutter's fever, rice field fever, Stuttgart disease, Swineherd's disease, and Fort Bragg fever. More severe cases of leptospirosis are called Weil's syndrome or icterohemorrhagic fever.

Leptospirosis is called a **zoonosis** because it is a disease of animals that can be transmitted to humans by various wild animals such as rats, opossums, raccoons, foxes, and skunks. It can be a very serious problem in the livestock industry. *Leptospira* bacteria have been found in dogs, rats, livestock, mice, voles, rabbits, hedgehogs, skunks, possums, frogs, fish, snakes, and certain birds and insects. Infected animals pass the bacteria in their urine for months, or even years. In the United States, rats and dogs are more commonly linked with human leptospirosis than other animals. Domesticated animals such as dogs and livestock can also carry and transmit the disease. Humans may also acquire the disease through soil or **water** infected by such animals. This rare disease and contagious infection can range from very mild and symptomless to a more serious, even life–threatening form, that may be associated with kidney (renal) failure.

Humans are considered accidental hosts and become infected with *Leptospira interrogans* by coming into contact with urine from infected animals. Transmission of the organism occurs through direct contact with urine, or through contact with soil, water, or plants that have been contaminated by animal urine. *Leptospira interrogans* can survive for as long as six months outdoors under favorable conditions. Leptospira bacteria can enter the body through cuts or other skin damage or through mucous membranes (such as the inside of the mouth and nose). Researchers believe that the bacteria may be able to pass through intact skin, although evidence for this hypothesis has not been obtained.

Once past the skin barrier, bacteria enter the blood stream and rapidly spread throughout the body. The infection causes damage to the inner lining of blood vessels. The liver, kidneys, heart, lungs, central nervous system, and eyes may be affected.

There are two stages in the disease process. The first stage is during the active Leptospira infection and is called the bacteremic or septicemic phase. The bacteremic phase lasts from three to seven days and presents as typical flu–like symptoms. During this phase, bacteria can be found in the patient's blood and cerebrospinal fluid. The second stage, or immune phase, takes place either immediately after the bacteremic stage or after a one to three day symptom-free period. The immune phase can last up to one month. During the immune phase, symptoms are milder but **meningitis** (inflammation of spinal cord and brain tissues) is common. Bacteria can be isolated only from the urine during this second phase.

Risk factors

Leptospirosis occurs all over the world, especially in temperate or tropical climates. It is considered an occupational hazard for many people who work outdoors or with animals, such as farmers, fish and meat processing workers, miners and sewer workers. Leptospirosis has also been associated with outdoor sports, such as swimming, wading, kayaking, and rafting in contaminated lakes and rivers. High–risk activities also include care of pets (especially dogs), raising of livestock, hunting and trapping.

Demographics

The disease is relatively rare in humans. Leptospirosis is usually found in tropical and subtropical areas, especially around stagnant or slow-moving waters, but can be present anywhere worldwide. It is also more likely to be a problem during the months of July through October and February through March. The infection is often transmitted to humans after drinking water contaminated with animal urine. It can also be contracted through such contamination of breaks in the skin and through mucous membranes such as the eyes.

Leptospirosis is rarely found in the continental part of the United States. However, when it is present in the United States, it is most often located in the state of Hawaii. According to the **Centers for Disease Control and Prevention (CDC)**, between 100 and 200 cases of leptospirosis are reported in the United States each year. In addition, nearly 75% of cases of leptospirosis in North America occur in males. Further, about 50% of cases happen in Hawaii, followed by the southern Atlantic, Gulf, and Pacific coastal states. However, because of the nonspecific symptoms of leptospirosis, it is believed that the occurrence in the United States is actually much higher. Leptospirosis occurs year–round in North America, but about half of the cases take place between July and October.

Causes and symptoms

Leptospirosis is caused primarily by an infection with the bacterium *Leptospira interrogans*. Bacteria are spread through contact with urine from infected animals.

Symptoms of *Leptospira* infection appear within two to 26 days following exposure to the bacteria, with 10 days being the average number of days. Because the symptoms can be nonspecific, most people who have antibodies to *Leptospira* do not remember having had an illness. Eighty five to 90% of the cases are not serious and clear up on their own. Symptoms of the first stage of leptospirosis last three to seven days and include:

- fever (with a temperature of 100–105°F [38–41°C])
- severe headache
- muscle pain
- stomach pain
- chills
- nausea
- vomiting
- diarrhea
- back pain
- joint pain
- neck stiffness
- extreme exhaustion

Dry cough, sore throat, and body rash sometimes also occur. Other symptoms, which are usually less frequently observed, are enlarged lymph glands, liver, and spleen, abnormal sounds from the lungs, skin rash, and muscle tenderness or rigidity.

Following the first stage of disease, a brief symptom-free period ensues for most patients. The symptoms of the second stage vary in each patient. Most patients have a low-grade fever, headache, vomiting, and rash. Aseptic meningitis is common in the second stage, symptoms of which include headache and photosensitivity (sensitivity of the eye to light). *Leptospira* can affect the eyes and make them cloudy and yellow to orange colored. Vision may be blurred.

Ten percent of the persons infected with *Leptospira* develop a serious disease called Weil's syndrome. The symptoms of Weil's syndrome are more severe than those described above and there is no distinction between the first and second stages of disease. The hallmark of Weil's syndrome is liver, kidney, and blood vessel disease. The signs of severe disease are apparent after 3–7 days of illness. In addition to those listed above, symptoms of Weil's syndrome include jaundice (yellow skin and eyes), decreased or no urine output, hypotension (low blood pressure), rash, anemia (decreased number of red blood cells), shock, and severe mental status changes.

Red spots on the skin, "blood shot" eyes, and bloody sputum signal that blood vessel damage and hemorrhage have occurred.

Diagnosis

Leptospirosis can be diagnosed and treated by doctors who specialize in infectious diseases. During the bacteremic phase of the disease, the symptoms are relatively nonspecific. This often causes an initial misdiagnosis because many diseases have similar symptoms to leptospirosis. The later symptoms of jaundice and kidney failure together with the bacteremic phase symptoms suggest leptospirosis. Blood samples will be tested to look for antibodies to *Leptospira interrogans*. Blood samples taken over a period of a few days would show an increase in the number of antibodies. Isolating *Leptospira* bacteria from blood, cerebrospinal fluid (performed by spinal tap), and urine samples is diagnostic of leptospirosis. Tests for white blood cell count and creatine kinase may also be performed. It may take six weeks for *Leptospira* to grow in laboratory media. Most insurance companies cover the diagnosis and treatment of this infection.

Several diagnostic tests for leptospirosis have been devised that are more accurate as well as faster than standard cultures. One test uses flow cytometry light scatter analysis; this method can evaluate a sample of infected serum in as little as 90 minutes. A second technique is an IgM-enzyme-linked immunosorbent assay (ELISA), which detects the presence of IgM antibodies to *L. interrogans* in blood serum samples.

Treatment

Leptospirosis is treated with **antibiotics** (such as tetracycline or chloramphenicol), penicillin (Bicillin, Wycillin), doxycycline (Monodox, Vibramycin), or erythromycin (E-mycin, Ery-Tab). However, many doctors prefer to treat patients with ceftriaxone, which is easier to use than intravenous penicillin. Ciprofloxacin may be combined with other drugs in caring for patients who develop uveitis. It is generally agreed that antibiotic treatment during the first few days of illness is helpful. However, leptospirosis is often not diagnosed until the later stages of illness. The benefit of antibiotic treatment in the later stages of disease, however, is controversial. A rare complication of antibiotic therapy for leptospirosis is the occurrence of the Jarisch–Herxheimer reaction, which is characterized by fever, chills, headache, and muscle **pain**.

Patients with severe illness require hospitalization for treatment and monitoring. Medication or other treatment for pain, fever, vomiting, fluid loss, bleeding, mental changes, and low blood pressure may be provided. Patients with kidney failure require hemodialysis to remove waste products from the blood.

KEY TERMS

Hemodialysis—The removal of waste products from the blood stream in patients with kidney failure. Blood is removed from a vein, passed through a dialysis machine, and then put back into a vein.

Jarisch–Herxheimer reaction—A rare reaction to the dead bacteria in the blood stream following antibiotic treatment.

Meningitis—Inflammation of tissues in the brain and spinal cord. Aseptic meningitis refers to meningitis with no bacteria present in the cerebral spinal fluid.

Spirochete—Any of a family of spiral- or coil-shaped bacteria known as Spirochetae. *L. interrogans* is a spirochete, as well as are the organisms that cause syphilis and relapsing fever.

Zoonosis (plural, zoonoses)—Any disease of animals that can be transmitted to humans. Leptospirosis is an example of a zoonosis.

Public health role and response

Leptospirosis is becoming an emerging **global public health** issue because of its increasing incidence in both developing and developed countries. A number of leptospirosis outbreaks have occurred in various regions such as Nicaragua, Brazil and India. Some outbreaks were due to natural calamities such as cyclone and floods that contaminated water supplies. Although most countries apply the basic principles of **prevention** such as source reduction, environmental **sanitation**, more hygienic work–related and personal practices, international monitoring efforts are being organized.

The Worls Health Organisation (**WHO**) has recommended standards and strategies for the surveillance, prevention and control of communicable diseases, developed by the WHO **Emerging Diseases** and **Pandemic** Response Department (EPR), in collaboration with the Department of **Food Safety** and Zoonoses (FOS), for major zoonoses involving livestock.

Prognosis

The majority of patients infected with *Leptospira interrogans* experience a complete recovery when treated promptly. Ten percent of patients develop eye

QUESTIONS TO ASK YOUR DOCTOR

- What is leptospirosis?
- How is it transmitted?
- What kinds of tests do I need to undergo?
- What is the best course of treatment?
- What are the best prevention measures?

inflammation (uveitis) up to one year after the illness. Other complications include excessive bleeding, meningitis, and Jarisch-Herxheimer reaction. In the United States, about one out of every 100 patients die from leptospirosis. Death is usually caused by kidney failure, but has also been caused by myocarditis (inflammation of heart tissue), septic shock (reduced blood flow to the organs because of the bacterial infection), organ failure, and/or poorly functioning lungs. Mortality is highest in patients over 60 years of age.

Prevention

Persons who are at an extremely high risk (such as soldiers training in wetlands) can be pretreated with 200 milligrams (mg) of doxycycline once a week. As of the early 2010s, no vaccine is available to prevent leptospirosis in humans, although similar vaccines have been formulated by veterinarians for dogs, swine, cattle, and other animals.

There are many ways to decrease the chances of being infected by *Leptospira*. These include:

- Avoid swimming or wading in freshwater ponds and slowly moving streams, especially those located near farms.
- Do not conduct canoe or kayak capsizing drills in freshwater ponds. Use a swimming pool instead.
- Boil or chemically treat pond or stream water before drinking it or cooking with it.
- Control rats and mice around the home.
- Have pets and farm animals vaccinated against *Leptospira*.
- Wear protective clothing (gloves, boots, long pants, and long-sleeved shirts) when working with wet soil or plants.

Resources

BOOKS

Russell, Jesse and Ronald Cohn. *Leptospirosis.* Great Malvern, UK: Book on Demand Ltd., 2012.

World Health Organization. *Human Leptospirosis: Guidance for Diagnosis, Surveillance and Control.* Geneva, Switzerland: WHO Press, 2003.

PERIODICALS

Del Carlo Bernardi, F., et al. "Immune receptors and adhesion molecules in human pulmonary leptospirosis."Human Pathology 43, no. 10 (October 2012): 1601–1610.

Dellagostin, O. A., et al. "Recombinant vaccines against leptospirosis."Human Vaccines 7, no. 11 (November 2011): 1215–1224.

Sarkar, J., et al. "Leptospirosis: a re–emerging infection."Asian Pacific Journal of Tropical Medicine 5, no. 6 (June 2012): 500–502.

Turhan, V. and O. Sezer. "Leptospirosis as a still unknown and underappreciated disease."International Journal of Preventive Medicine 3, no. 8 (August 2012): 591–592.

WEBSITES

Leptospirosis. Centers for Disease Control. January 13, 2012. http://www.cdc.gov/leptospirosis/

Leptospirosis. Medline Plus, 27 September 2012. http://www.nlm.nih.gov/medlineplus/ency/article/001376.htm

ORGANIZATIONS

American Veterinary Medical Association (AVMA), 1931 North Meacham Rd., Suite 100, Schaumburg, IL 60173–4360, (800) 248-2862, Fax: (847) 925-1329, http://www.avma.org

Centers for Disease Control and Prevention (CDC), 1600 Clifton Road, Atlanta, GA 30333, (800) 232-4636, cdcinfo@cdc.gov, http://www.cdc.gov

International Leptospirosis Society, Faculty of Medicine, Nursing and Health Sciences, Monash University, VictoriaAustralia 3800, +61 3 9905 4301, Fax: +61 3 9905 4302, enquiries@med.monash.edu.au, http://www.med.monash.edu.au/microbiology/staff/adler/ils.html.

Belinda Rowland, PhD
Rebecca J. Frey, PhD

Lesbian, gay, bisexual, and transgender (LGBT) health

Definition

Lesbian, gay, bisexual, and transgender (LGBT) individuals are as diverse as the general population in terms of race, ethnicity, age, religion, education, income, and family history. A number of health concerns, however, are unique to or shared by the LGBT community. These include an increased risk of certain cancers, infectious and **sexually transmitted diseases** (STDs), and mental health disorders. The LGBT community also has a higher incidence of issues relating to **nutrition** and weight, tobacco use, substance abuse, and may face discrimination from healthcare and insurance providers.

Description

The definitions of different sexual identities have shifted over the years, as have the perceptions and stereotypes encountered in the general population. The LGBT community encompasses a wide range of behaviors and identities. It includes:

- Gay men and lesbians, who are sexually attracted to or participate in sexual behaviors with individuals of the same gender.
- Bisexual men and women, who are sexually attracted to or participate in sexual behaviors with individuals of both genders.
- Transgender individuals, who live part-time or full-time in a gender role opposite to their genetic sex.

Important healthcare issues

Many LGBT individuals hesitate to reveal their sexual identity ("coming out") to their healthcare providers. They may fear discrimination from providers, may believe that their confidentiality might be breached, or simply may not see the need to provide that information. In some cases, healthcare workers have been poorly trained to address the needs of LGBT individuals, or have difficulty communicating with or feel uncomfortable providing care for patients with a non–traditional sexual orientation. In addition, many questions posed in questionnaires or examinations are heterosexually biased (e.g., asking a lesbian which birth-control methods she uses).

Other reasons why LGBT individuals are often cautious about sharing their sexual identity are more logistical. Many insurance companies deny benefits to long-term partners because they are not married and therefore do not meet the criteria for coverage. LGBT patients may have inadequate access to health care, either because they live in a remote rural area or in the crowded inner city. Some same-sex partners also find that they are denied the rights—visitation, input on medical decisions, and participation in consultations with physicians—usually provided to the spouses of patients who are in hospitals and clinics.

Some of the health concerns and risk factors that are relevant to LGBT individuals may be shared by the general population, while others are more specific to the LGBT community or to different subgroups of LGBT individuals. Areas of concern for the LGBT community include:

- Sexual behavior issues: STDs and sexually transmitted infections such as human immunodeficiency virus (HIV) and acquired immune deficiency syndrome (AIDS), hepatitis A virus, hepatitis B virus, bacterial vaginosis, gonorrhea, chlamydia, and genital warts (human papillomavirus or HPV); and anal, ovarian, and cervical cancer.
- Cultural issues: body image, nutrition, weight and eating disorders, drug and alcohol abuse, tobacco use, and parenting and family planning.
- Discrimination issues: inadequate medical care, harassment at work, school, or home; difficulty in obtaining housing, insurance coverage, or child custody; and violence.
- Sexual identity issues: conflicts with family members, friends, and fellow workers; psychological issues such as anxiety, depression, and suicide; and economic hardship.

CANCER. **Cancer** is the second leading cause of death (after **heart disease**) in the United States. In its *Cancer Facts & Figures* report, the U.S. **Centers for Disease Control and Prevention (CDC)** estimated that in 2012, about 1.64 million individuals would be diagnosed with cancer and about 577,190 would lose their lives as a result. LGBT individuals are at an increased risk for certain types of cancers.

Women who are lesbians have a higher risk of developing some cancers, including cervical and ovarian cancers. Compared to the heterosexual female population, lesbians are more likely to exhibit various risk factors for cancer. These include **obesity**, alcohol use, and tobacco use. Fewer lesbians give birth, and both pregnancy and breastfeeding are accompanied by a release of hormones that are believed to protect against ovarian, endometrial, and ovarian cervical cancers. Lesbians use oral contraceptives less frequently, and therefore do not receive any cancer-protective benefits from the hormones in the contraceptives. In addition, women who are lesbians are less likely than heterosexual women to visit a doctor for routine Pap screening that is used to detect cervical cancer. Lesbians also have a heightened danger of developing ovarian cancer due to inadequate access to health care.

Gay and bisexual men (or more generally, men who have sex with men [MSM]) are at higher risk of developing non-Hodgkin's lymphoma, Hodgkin's disease, and anal cancer. Kaposi's sarcoma, an AIDS-associated cancer, is also found in the gay community at rates higher than the general population. Anal cancer is associated with transmission of human papillomavirus, and the risk factors associated with MSM—such as

smoking, having many sexual partners, and receiving anal intercourse—are also associated with increased rates of anal cancer.

AIDS. According to the **CDC**, MSM make up about 49 percent of the approximately 1.2 million people in the United States who are living with **AIDS**, and MSM account for 61 percent of all new HIV infections in the country each year. The CDC report titled "HIV and AIDS Among Gay and Bisexual Men,", which was published in September 2011, noted a 48 percent increase in the number of new infections among young, black MSM aged 13–29 years old.

In the report, the CDC recognized several factors as contributing to the elevated rate of HIV infection in the overall MSM population:

- high risk of exposure during each sexual encounter, due to the already existing incidence of AIDS in the MSM population
- lack of knowledge of a sexual partner's HIV status
- lack of consistent use of safe-sex measures
- complacency driven in part by the belief that medical advancements have made HIV a less dangerous threat
- substance abuse, social discrimination, or other issues that may promote unwise decisions about risky sexual behaviors

PSYCHIATRIC DISORDERS. In 1973, the American Psychiatric Association removed homosexuality from their list of mental disorders. Nevertheless, American society has been slow to fully accept members of the LGBT community. As a result, members of this community often find themselves rejected by their families, socially stigmatized for their sexual orientation, treated unequally by laws and the justice system, and subject to physical and emotional abuse for their lifestyles. These pressures, plus the continuing **stress** caused by the need some LGBT individuals feel to conceal their sexual orientation from family, employers, and larger society lead to an increased occurrence of depressive illness, anxiety disorders, and drug and alcohol abuse. These, in turn, may manifest in risky sexual behaviors that can lead to sexually transmitted diseases, including AIDS.

NUTRITION AND BODY IMAGE. Diet and nutritional factors are associated with a number of medical issues, including cancer, **stroke**, diabetes, heart disease, and osteoporosis. Although lesbians are more likely than heterosexual women to be obese, to eat a nutritionally poorer diet, and have higher rates of smoking and alcohol use, they have a generally better body image. Compared to heterosexual men, on the other hand, gay men and adolescents have increased rates of eating-disorder behaviors, such as anorexia nervosa, bulimia, binge eating, and have a poorer body image.

KEY TERM

Nulliparity—The condition of being nulliparous, or not bearing offspring.

DEMOGRAPHICS. According to a 2011 study by the Williams Institute, 3.5 percent of U.S. adults identify as lesbian, gay or bisexual, and approximately 0.3 percent are transgender. The study notes that making such estimates is challenging, because they are based on self-reported information, and due to social stigmas or other reasons, individuals may not be forthcoming about their sexual orientation.

Certain issues arise when trying to define sexual orientation. Many gay men and lesbians have participated in or continue to participate in sexual activities with members of the opposite sex, but choose not to identify as heterosexuals or bisexuals. Others have never participated in sexual activities at all, yet still identify as gay, lesbian, or bisexual. Some men and women identifying as bisexuals are in long-term, monogamous relationships with individuals of the same or opposite sex. Male-to-female or female-to-male transgender individuals may or may not identify themselves as gay or lesbian.

The implications of these identity issues are far-reaching. Healthcare providers may mistakenly assume sexual behaviors or risks based on the patient's stated identity, and this may lead to misdiagnoses or improper medical recommendations. For example, a provider might incorrectly assume that a lesbian patient has never had sexual intercourse with a male and therefore would not have contracted STDs. These identity issues may also make it difficult to prepare accurate estimates of the numbers of LGBT individuals in the United States and elsewhere. Likewise, the statistics used in medical or social studies and surveys on LGBT issues may vary widely depending on what definitions were provided for the respondents. Because of this, many researchers have opted for the more inclusive terms of "men who have sex with men" and "women who have sex with women" (WSW) to categorize gay, lesbian, and bisexual respondents.

Effects on public health

Healthcare providers can take numerous measures to improve the access to and experience with healthcare services for LGBT individuals. These include:

- rewording questionnaires and examinations to be inclusive of LGBT patients

- providing referrals to social service agencies and counseling services that are LGBT-friendly
- taking educational courses that heighten sensitivity to the needs of LGBT patients
- treating the families of LGBT patients with the same respect and compassion as one would the families of heterosexual patients
- maintaining the strictest code of confidentiality
- developing and maintaining healthcare centers or clinics that address LGBT-specific needs
- asking non–threatening questions to determine if a person is at risk of an STD
- educating patients of risk factors associated with STDs, possible vaccines, and treatments available
- providing services to individuals in the process of disclosing their sexual identity and, if applicable, to their families

LGBT individuals can also take steps to protect their health. These include:

- finding and regularly visiting a doctor who is sensitive to LGBT individuals and knowledgeable about associated health risks
- engaging in all recommended and applicable health tests and exams, such as annual physicals, Pap tests, HPV tests, and AIDS screening
- maintaining a healthy lifestyle, including a good diet, regular exercise, proper weight, no smoking or illegal drug use, and moderate alcohol intake
- practicing safe sex

Resources

BOOKS

Committee on Lesbian, Gay, Bisexual, and Transgender Health Issues and Research Gaps and Opportunities, Board on the Health of Select Populations, Institute of Medicine. *The Health of Lesbian, Gay, Bisexual and Transgender People: Building a Foundation for Better Understanding*. Washington, DC: The National Academies Press, 2011.

WEBSITES

Cancer Facts & Figures 2012, American Cancer Society, http://www.cancer.org/acs/groups/content/@epidemiologysurveilance/documents/document/acspc-031941.pdf (accessed October 21, 2012).

Cancer Facts for Lesbians and Bisexual Women, American Cancer Society, http://www.cancer.org/Healthy/FindCancerEarly/WomensHealth/cancer-facts-for-lesbians-and-bisexual-women (accessed October 21, 2012).

Lesbians and Bisexual Health Fact Sheet, U.S. Department of Health and Human Services Office on Women's Health, http://womenshealth.gov/publications/our-publications/fact-sheet/lesbian-bisexual-health.cfm (accessed October 21, 2012).

CDC Report Finds Gay, Lesbian and Bisexual Students At Greater Risk for Unhealthy, Unsafe Behaviors, U.S. Centers for Disease Control Newsroom, http://www.cdc.gov/media/releases/2011/p0606_yrbsurvey.html (accessed October 21, 2012).

How Many People are Lesbian, Gay, Bisexual, and Transgender? The Williams Institute, http://williamsinstitute.law.ucla.edu/wp-content/uploads/Gates-How-Many-People-LGBT-Apr-2011.pdf (accessed October 21, 2012).

ORGANIZATIONS

Centers for Disease Control and Prevention (CDC), 1600 Clifton Road, Atlanta, GA 30333, (800) 232-4636, cdcinfo@cdc.gov, http://www.cdc.gov

Gay and Lesbian Medical Association, 1326 18th Street NW, Suite 22, Washington, DC 20036, (202) 600-8037, info@glma.org, http://www.glma.org

Parents, Families and Friends of Lesbians and Gays (PFLAG), 1828 L Street, NW, Suite 660, Washington, DC 20036, (202) 467-8180, info@pflag.org, http://community.pflag.org.

Stéphanie Dionne
Teresa G. Odle
Tish Davidson, AM
Leslie Mertz, PhD

Life expectancy

Definition

Life expectancy refers to the number of years a person can expect to live at any given age. For example, one can say that the life expectancy of a 60–year–old American in 2012 is 18.2 years. That is, he or she can expect to live to about age 78. A similar term is *life span*, the total number of years a person (or other animal or plant) can expect to live from birth to death. The expected life span for an American in 2012 is 78.2 years. In actual practice, the term *life expectancy* is often used as a synonym for *life span*, even if the two terms are not precisely comparable.

Description

Life expectancy and life span are mathematical concepts that represent average values. To determine either value for individuals in a country, one takes into consideration that ages at which everyone in the country has died. The average value of those numbers provides the expected life span for someone in the country at birth (age = 0). However, that expectation changes significantly over time, primarily because of the high fatality rate of young children in many cultures. The first year of life is generally the most dangerous because young children are susceptible to a host of diseases and other causes of death. For children surviving the first year, their chances of surviving increase significantly. Thus, newborns might have an anticipated life span at birth of 40 years, but, if they survive the first year of life, that expectation might increase to 50 years, 60 years, or older.

A number of factors affect the life expectancy of humans. Historically, the most important of these factors may have been disease. Before the mid-nineteenth century, very little was known about the causes of disease and medical practitioners could do little to prevent or cure diseases. As a consequence, many individuals died at a young age before their immune systems were well developed, and many more died at somewhat older ages because of infectious diseases. One consequence of this fact was that, even though life span was relatively short prior to the modern era, individuals who survived their childhood and youth often lived to a "ripe old age" comparable to what one might expect today. The effects of disease can be observed when infectious diseases strike in the modern world. For example, the average life span in most parts of the world has been increasing over the previous century. But in the United States in the 1980s, the average life span actually decreased for some subpopulations, such as African Americans. The reason for this decrease was the HIV/AIDS epidemic that caused the death of a disproportionate number of African Americans at an age younger than might otherwise have been expected. The same pattern is now playing out in parts of sub-Saharan Africa, where the HIV/AIDS epidemic continues to rage.

Any number of other factors have been shown to affect life expectancy, all of which influence a person's overall health and, hence, the ability to survive disease, injury, accidents, and other life-threatening events. Among those factors are:

- adverse geographic locations (the polar regions and deserts, for example)
- poor or inadequate nutrition
- access to adequate medical care
- adverse environmental conditions (such as crowded urban housing)
- type of employment (such as coal mining or other occupations that involve exposure to hazardous materials)
- genetic disorders
- lack of exercise
- obesity
- use of tobacco products
- use of illegal drugs
- excessive use of alcohol
- other employment factors (such as stress at work)
- marital status

Demographics

The interaction of these factors accounts for the fact that life expectancy has differed dramatically over the period of human existence and continues to differ significantly from country to country in the modern world. Adequate anthropological and archaeological evidence now exists to estimate the life expectancy of humans at various stages of evolution. According to that evidence, the life expectancy for certain evolutionary periods has been estimated:

- Late Paleolithic (30,000 - 9,000 BCE): male: 35.4; female: 30.0
- Early Neolithic (7,000 - 5,000 BCE): male: 33.6; female: 29.8
- Early Bronze (3,000 - 2,000 BCE): male: 33.6; female: 29.4
- Early Iron (1,150 - 650 BCE): male: 39.0; female: 30.9
- Classical Greek (650 - 300 BCE): male: 44.1; female: 36.8
- Roman (120 - 600 CE): male: 38.8; female: 34.2
- Late Middle Ages (1400 - 1800 CE): male: 33.9; female: 28.5
- Nineteenth century: male: 40.0; female: 38.4
- Modern American (1980): male: 71.0; female: 78.5

These data mask the considerable variations that exist among residents of various part of the world. As an example, the following data from the *CIA World Factbook* for 2011 show how life expectancy varies from country to country in the second decade of the twenty-first century (rank according to United Nations membership):

- Monaco: male: 85.77; female: 93.69; rank: 1
- San Marino: male: 80.5; female: 85.74; rank: 2
- Japan: male: 78.96; female: 85.72; rank: 4
- Australia: male: 79.4; female: 84.35; rank: 6
- Canada: male: 78.81; female: 84.1; rank: 9
- Israel: male: 78.79; female: 83.24; rank: 13
- South Korea: male: 75.84; female: 82.49; rank: 29
- United States: male: 75.92; female: 80.93; rank: 34
- Libya: male: 75.34; female: 80.08; rank: 41
- Mexico: male: 73.65; female: 79.43; rank: 51
- Hungary: male: 71.04; female: 78.76; rank: 65

- Thailand: male: 70.77; female: 75.55; rank: 82
- Russia: male: 64.3; female: 76.4; rank: 113
- Pakistan: male: 63.4; female: 65.64; rank: 136
- Haiti: male: 59.13; female: 62.48; rank: 149
- Ethiopia: male: 52.92; female: 57.97; rank: 160
- Mali: male: 48.38; female: 52.38; rank: 174
- Liberia: male: 40.71; female: 43; rank: 185
- Zambia: male: 38.53; female: 38.73; rank: 189
- Swaziland: male: 31.62; female: 32.15; rank: 191 (last)

Public health effects

Overall, increases in life expectancy throughout the developed world and in many parts of the developing world between 1900 and 2000 have been remarkable, with an improvement from roughly 50 years at the beginning of that period to well into the 70s at the end of the period. Almost everyone agrees that this change will have profound effects on nations around the world. But there is disagreement as to the precise nature of these changes and surprisingly little data to suggest the direction of future trends. The optimistic view of the future is that, as people tend to live longer lives, they will adopt more positive attitudes toward health issues and live healthier lives. Under this view, increasing life expectancies will produce stronger, healthier societies. The pessimistic view of the future is that, as people grow older, they will be more likely to develop diseases and disorders that were once relatively uncommon, such as **cancer** and cardiovascular disease. Under this view, societies will eventually be overwhelmed by the health costs associated with a new kind of crisis created by more and more unhealthy elderly. This new crisis has sometimes been called the *epidemiological transition*, in which the leading cause of death is no longer **infectious disease** and acute illness, but chronic disease and degenerative illness.

It appears to be too early to tell which of these scenarios is the more likely, although early data favor the optimistic view. For example, some studies have showed that the rates of certain types of chronic illness are declining overall among **aging** Americans. As people age, they appear to be getting better medical care and taking better care of themselves, providing them with not only longer lives, but better ones. Nonetheless, people who live longer still get sick and need medical care, and that medical care can often be more expensive than it is for younger patients. In a 2003 report, the **Centers for Disease Control and Prevention** noted that in the United States, medical care for individuals over the age of 65 averaged three times as much per person as it did for individuals under the age of 65. These higher costs result from a number of factors, such as surgeries that involve hip and knee replacements, heart bypasses, cataract and other eye procedures, and cancer treatments that younger patients do not require (because they often die of other causes before these procedures become necessary or desirable); more doctor and hospital visits; a greater number of an increased variety of medications, which may also be more expensive; and special provisions to deal with services that patients cannot provide for themselves, such as preparing their own meals and transporting themselves for medical appointments and other purposes.

These demands are a problem not only for the nation as a whole and for individual patients and their families, but also for the public health profession. New strategies and new programs have to be developed to help older men and women understand the nature of their health challenges, the resources that are available for dealing with them, and the changes in their lifestyles that may be necessary to cope with a new set of health and medical challenges. In fact, a whole new area of public health, generally known as geriatric public health or preventive geriatrics, has arisen to meet these needs. Some examples of geriatric public health programs that have been developed include the following:

- specialized activity programs that are designed for the elderly in their own homes or at easily accessible locations that take advantage of existing organizations wherever possible
- new types of provider/patient relationships that focus on specific health problems of the elderly on a more one-on-one basis and often occur in a home setting
- new and enhanced programs for meeting the special needs of elderly for obtaining meals, having access to alternative forms of transportation, and assisting with routine household tasks
- educational programs that provide the elderly with information about health issues, sources from which to get additional information, and suggested activities for maintaining their own health

KEY TERMS

Life expectancy—The number of years a person can expect to live at any given age.

Life span—The total number of years an organism can expect to live from birth to death.

Geriatrics—The field of medicine that deals with the health of elderly people.

QUESTIONS TO ASK YOUR DOCTOR

- Is there any way I can estimate how long I am going to live?
- What lifestyle changes can I make to increase the number of years I am likely to live?
- What kinds of health and medical problems would you anticipate that I should expect?
- What special facilities are available in our community to help my aged parents maintain a healthy lifestyle?

- improved data and information collecting in order to have a better understanding of the current status of the elderly population within a community

Resources

BOOKS

Crimmins, Eileen M., Samuel H. Preston, and Barney Cohen. *Explaining Divergent Levels of Longevity in High-income Countries*. Washington, DC: National Academies Press, 2011.

Global Health and Aging. [Washington, DC]: National Institute on Aging, 2011.

Kandel, Joseph, and Christine A. Adamec. *The Encyclopedia of Elder Care*. New York: Facts On File, 2009.

Taylor, David. *Active Ageing: Live Longer and Prosper: Realising the Benefits of Extended Healthy Life Expectancy*. London: University of London School of Pharmacy, 2012.

PERIODICALS

Griffin, B., B. Hesketh, and V. Loh. "The Influence of Subjective Life Expectancy on Retirement Transition and Planning: A Longitudinal Study." *Journal of Vocational Behavior* 81. 2. (2012): 129–37.

Le Bourg, E. "Forecasting Continuously Increasing Life Expectancy: What Implications?" *Ageing Research Reviews* 11. 2. (2012): 325–28.

Stoner, L., et al. "Preventing a Cardiovascular Disease Epidemic among Indigenous Populations through Lifestyle Changes." *International Journal of Preventive Medicine* 3. 4. (2012): 230–40.

Wirth, R., and C. C. Sieber. "Health Care Professionals Underestimate the Mean Life Expectancy of Older People." *Gerontology* 58. 1. (2012): 56–59.

WEBSITES

Aging and Community Care. American Medical Association. http://www.ama-assn.org/ama/pub/physician-resources/public-health/promoting-healthy-lifestyles/geriatric-health.page. Accessed on September 17, 2012.

Emerging Issues in Geriatric Care: Aging and Public Health Perspectives. Medscape Education. http://www.medscape.org/viewarticle/498939. Accessed on September 17, 2012.

The State of the Art of Geriatric Public Health Education and Training. ftp://ftp.hrsa.gov/migrated/bhpr/interdisciplinary/gecwhite/10publichealth.pdf. Accessed on September 17, 2012.

When It Comes to Public Health, Seniors Really Are Different. Long-term Living. http://www.ltlmagazine.com/article/when-it-comes-public-health-seniors-really-are-different. Accessed on September 17, 2012.

ORGANIZATIONS

National Institute on Aging (NAI), Bldg. 31, Rm. 5C27, 31 Center Dr., MSC 2292, Bethesda, MD USA 20892, (301) 496-1752, (800) 222-2225, Fax: (301) 496-1072, niaic@nia.nih.gov, http://www.nia.nih.gov/.

David E. Newton, Ed.D.

Listeriosis

Definition

Listeriosis, also called listeria infection, is an **infectious disease** caused by a bacterium, *Listeria monocytogenes*, which is most commonly acquired by eating contaminated food. The organism can spread to the blood stream and central nervous system. During pregnancy, listeriosis often causes miscarriage or stillbirth. It is also more likely to cause serious illness in the elderly, in newborns, or in people with weakened immune systems. Although listeriosis is infectious (caused by a disease organism), it is not contagious; that is, it is not spread by direct contact with other infected persons, with the exception of vaginal transmission during childbirth.

Demographics

Listeriosis is an uncommon disease in the general human population in North America and Western Europe. There are on average 9.7 cases per million persons per year in Canada and the United States, and five cases per million per year in Europe; however, European doctors reported in early 2012 that the rate of listeriosis in Europe had been rising since 2005. Listeriosis is far more common among domestic animals, farm animals (particularly cattle and sheep), game animals, poultry, and wild birds than among humans. Listeriosis outbreaks are sporadic (rare and scattered in occurrence) rather than epidemic; they are, however, more common in cold or temperate climates than in the tropics and more likely to occur in the summer in North America.

In 2011, there was a multistate outbreak of listeriosis linked to contaminated whole cantaloupes from Jensen Farms in Colorado. A total of 146 persons were infected with any of the four outbreak-associated strains of Listeria monocytogenes, and 30 deaths were reported. Seven of the illnesses were related to pregnancy; three were diagnosed in newborns and four were diagnosed in pregnant women. One miscarriage was reported.

About 800 laboratory-confirmed cases of Listeria infection are reported each year in the United States, and typically three or four outbreaks are identified. The foods that typically cause these outbreaks have been deli meats, hot dogs, and Mexican-style soft cheeses made with unpasteurized milk. Produce is not often identified as a source, but sprouts caused an outbreak in 2009, and celery caused an outbreak in 2010.

Before 2011, the largest outbreak occurred in 2002, when 54 illnesses, 8 deaths, and 3 fetal deaths in 9 states were found to be associated with consumption of contaminated turkey deli meat.

Description

Listeriosis is caused by an infection with the gram-positive bacterium *Listeria monocytogenes*. The bacterium was named for Joseph Lister (1827–1912), a British surgeon honored as the pioneer of antiseptic surgery. The bacterium is rod-shaped and moves about with the help of a small flagellum. It secretes a chemical that causes the destruction of red blood cells.

This bacterium is carried by at least 64 different species of animals, and it has also been found in soil, **water**, sewage, and animal feed. Five out of every 100 people carry *L. monocytogenes* in their intestines. The bacterium is hardy and can survive in a wide temperature range, from 39°F (3.9°C) to 111°F (43.9°C). It is found almost everywhere in the world in plants and soils.

Listeriosis is considered a foodborne disease because most people become infected after eating food contaminated with *L. monocytogenes*. However, a woman can pass the bacteria to her fetus during pregnancy. In addition, there have been a few cases in which veterinarians or farm workers have developed *Listeria* skin infections by touching infected calves or poultry.

There are five distinct clinical forms of listeriosis:

- Infection during pregnancy, most commonly in the third trimester.
- Neonatal (newborn) infection, which can take two forms: an early-onset inflammation of the entire body (sepsis), which usually results in premature birth, and a late-onset infection of the central nervous system, which the baby acquires during vaginal delivery.
- Central nervous system (CNS) infection. *L. monocytogenes* has a special predilection for the central nervous system of humans. The infection may take the form of inflammation of the membranes covering the brain (meningitis), paralysis of the cranial nerves, inflammation of the brain tissue itself (encephalitis), or abscesses. Patients may suffer from seizures and changes in mental status.
- Gastroenteritis (inflammation of the digestive tract). *L. monocytogenes* can cause diarrhea lasting one to three days.
- Cutaneous listeriosis. This infection of the skin is most likely to affect veterinarians and others who handle infected farm or wild animals.

Risk factors

Persons at particular risk for listeriosis include the elderly, pregnant women, newborns, those who take glucocorticosteroid medications (which suppress immune responses to infection), and those with a weakened immune system (immunocompromised). Risk is increased when a person suffers from diseases such as **AIDS**, **cancer**, kidney disease, **diabetes mellitus**, or by the use of certain medications. Infection is most common in babies younger than one month old and adults over 60 years of age. Pregnant women account for 27% of the cases, and immunocompromised persons account for almost 70%. Persons with AIDS are 280 times more likely to get listeriosis than others.

With the exception of pregnant women, sex is not a risk factor for listeriosis; neither is race nor ethnicity.

Causes and symptoms

Persons become infected with *L. monocytogenes* by eating contaminated food. *Listeria* has been found on raw vegetables, fish, poultry, raw (unpasteurized) milk, fresh meat, processed meat (such as deli meat, hot dogs, and canned meat), and certain soft cheeses, particularly Brie, Camembert, feta cheese, and bleu cheese. Listeriosis outbreaks in the United States between the 1980s and the early 2000s were linked to cole slaw, milk, Mexican-style cheese, undercooked hot dogs, undercooked chicken, and delicatessen or salad bar-type foods.

Unlike most other bacteria, *L. monocytogenes* does not stop growing when food is in the refrigerator; its growth is merely slowed. Although initial levels of the bacterium in contaminated foods are usually low, its ability to survive and multiply at low temperatures allows it to reach levels high enough to cause human disease, particularly if contaminated foods that allow for the growth of the organism are stored for prolonged times under refrigeration. Fortunately, typical cooking temperatures and the **pasteurization** process in milk kill this bacterium.

Listeria bacteria can pass through the wall of the intestines, and from there they can get into the blood stream. Once in the blood stream, they can be transported anywhere in the body but are commonly found the central nervous system (brain and spinal cord). In pregnant women they are often found in the placenta (the organ that connects the baby's umbilical cord to the uterus). *Listeria monocytogenes* live inside specific white blood cells called macrophages. Inside macrophages, the bacteria can hide from immune responses and become inaccessible to certain **antibiotics**. *Listeria* bacteria are capable of multiplying within macrophages, and then may spread to other macrophages.

Gastrointestinal listeriosis

After consuming food contaminated with this bacteria, symptoms of infection may appear anywhere from 11–70 days later. Most people do not get any noticeable symptoms. Scientists are unsure, but they believe that *L. monocytogenes* can cause upset stomach and intestinal problems just like other foodborne illnesses. Persons with listeriosis may develop such flu-like symptoms as fever, headache, nausea and vomiting, tiredness, and diarrhea.

Listeriosis in pregnancy

Pregnant women experience a mild, flu-like illness with fever, muscle aches, upset stomach, and intestinal problems. They recover, but the infection can cause miscarriage, premature labor, early rupture of the birth sac, and stillbirth. Unfortunately, half of the newborns infected with *Listeria* die from the illness.

Neonatal listeriosis

There are two types of listeriosis in the newborn baby: early-onset disease and late-onset disease. Early-onset disease refers to a serious illness that is present at birth and usually causes the baby to be born prematurely. Babies infected during pregnancy usually have a blood infection (sepsis) and may have a serious, whole body infection called granulomatosis infantisepticum. When a full-term baby becomes infected with *Listeria* during childbirth, that situation is called late-onset disease. Commonly, symptoms of late-onset listeriosis appear about two weeks after birth. Babies with this disease typically have **meningitis** (inflammation of the brain and spinal tissues), yet they have a better chance of surviving than those with early-onset disease.

Central nervous system involvement

Immunocompromised adults are at risk for a serious infection of the blood stream and central nervous system (brain and spinal cord). Meningitis occurs in about half of the cases of adult listeriosis. Symptoms of listerial meningitis occur about four days after flu-like symptoms and include fever, personality change, uncoordinated muscle movement, tremors, muscle contractions, seizures, and slipping in and out of consciousness.

L. monocytogenes causes endocarditis in about 7.5% of cases of listeriosis. Endocarditis is an inflammation of heart tissue due to bacterial infection. Listerial endocarditis causes death in about half of patients. Other diseases that have been caused by *Listeria monocytogenes* are brain abscess, eye infection, **hepatitis** (liver disease), peritonitis (abdominal infection), lung infection, joint infection, arthritis, **heart disease**, bone infection, and gallbladder infection.

Diagnosis

Listeriosis may be diagnosed and treated by infectious disease specialists and internal medicine specialists. The diagnosis and treatment of this infection should be covered by most insurance providers.

Examination

The doctor may or may not suspect listeriosis on the basis of an office examination, as the symptoms of a gastrointestinal listeria infection are not unique to *L. monocytogenes*. A patient with listerial meningitis or **encephalitis** may have seizures, problems with movement, or mental status changes. However, these can be caused by other disease organisms affecting the CNS. Laboratory tests are required to rule out other causes of the patient's symptoms.

Tests

The only way to confirm a diagnosis of listeriosis as of 2012 was to isolate *L. monocytogenes* from blood, cerebrospinal fluid (CSF), urine, or stool. A sample of cerebrospinal fluid is removed from the spinal cord using a needle and syringe. This procedure is commonly called a spinal tap. The amniotic fluid (the fluid that surrounds the unborn baby inside the uterus) may be tested in pregnant women with listeriosis. This sample is obtained by inserting a needle through the abdomen into the uterus and withdrawing fluid. *L. monocytogenes* grows well in laboratory media, and test results can be available within a few days. Blood cultures and CSF tests are more reliable for identifying *L. monocytogenes* than stool tests.

KEY TERMS

Abscess—An accumulation of pus caused by localized infection in tissues or organs. *L. monocytogenes* can cause abscesses in many organs, including the brain, spleen, and liver.

Brain stem—The posterior portion of the brain that connects directly to the spinal cord. It regulates breathing, heart function, and the sleep-wake cycle as well as maintaining consciousness.

Cutaneous—Pertaining to the skin.

Encephalitis—Acute inflammation of brain tissue.

Endocarditis—Inflammation of the endocardium, the inner layer of heart tissue.

Flagellum—A tail-like projection extending from the cell walls of certain bacteria. Its name is the Latin word for whip.

Glucocorticosteroids—Also called glucocorticoids, a class of steroid hormones that play important roles in metabolism and the immune system. Synthetic glucocorticosteroids are drugs given to control certain allergic and immune system disorders; they include cortisone, prednisone, aldosterone, and dexamethasone. These drugs suppress the immune response to infection; thus they can increase a person's risk of listeriosis.

Immunocompromised—To have a poor immune system due to disease or medication. Immunocompromised persons are at risk for developing infections because they cannot fight off microorganisms as can healthy persons.

Macrophages—White blood cells whose job is to destroy invading microorganisms. *Listeria monocytogenes* avoids being killed and can multiply within the macrophage.

Meningitis—Inflammation of the meninges, the layers of membranes that cover and protect the brain and spinal cord.

Sepsis—An inflammatory response of the whole body to an infection. Listeriosis in newborns may take the form of sepsis.

Sporadic—Rare and occasional in occurrence. Listeriosis in humans is a sporadic disease.

Imaging tests may be performed if endocarditis or involvement of the brain stem are suspect. Transesophageal echocardiographyis used to diagnose endocarditis. MRI is the most accurate form of imaging for identifying listeria infections in the brain stem.

Treatment

Traditional

Medications are the treatment of choice for listeriosis. Intravenous antibiotics must be started as soon as the diagnosis is suspected or confirmed.

Drugs

Listeriosis is treated with antibiotics, most often ampicillin (Omnipen), chloramphenicol (Chloromycetin), or sulfamethoxazole-trimethoprim (Bactrim, Septra). Because the bacteria live within macrophage cells, treatment may be difficult and the treatment periods may vary. Usually, pregnant women are treated for two weeks; newborns, two to three weeks; adults with mild disease, two to four weeks; persons with meningitis, three weeks; persons with brain abscesses, six weeks; and persons with endocarditis, four to six weeks.

Patients are often hospitalized for treatment and monitoring. However, it is not necessary to isolate them because listeriosis is not spread by human contact. Other drugs may be provided to relieve **pain** and fever and to treat other reactions to the infection.

Prognosis

Although listeriosis is a relatively uncommon infectious disease, it does cause significant mortality; the overall mortality rate for listeria infections in humans in 20%–30%. Listeriosis is the most virulent form of foodborne disease in North America, with fatality rates higher than those of botulism or **Salmonella** food **poisoning**. According to the **Centers for Disease Control and Prevention (CDC)**, there are on average 500 deaths from listeriosis each year in the United States.

Prevention

The **CDC** recommends the following precautions to prevent getting listeriosis:

- Cook all raw food thoroughly, and wash all raw vegetables carefully.
- Wash hands, knives, and cutting boards in hot soapy water after handling uncooked foods.

- Avoid drinking raw (unpasteurized) milk or consuming dairy products made from raw milk.
- Pregnant women or immunocompromised people should avoid Brie, Camembert, feta, Mexican queso blanco or queso fresco, and bleu cheese. Cream cheese, yogurt, and cottage cheese are safe to eat.
- Reheat leftovers or ready-to-eat foods such as hot dogs until they are steaming hot.
- Avoid delicatessen foods unless they can be thoroughly reheated.
- Cook all fish and meat to safe internal temperatures.

Resources

BOOKS

Baltimore, R. S. "Listeria Monocytogenes." In *Nelson Textbook of Pediatrics*, 19th ed. Philadelphia: Saunders Elsevier, 2011.

Bennett L. "Listeria Monocytogenes." In *Principles and Practice of Infectious Diseases*, 7th ed., edited by G. L. Mandell, J. E. Bennett, and R. Dolin, Chap. 207. Philadelphia: Elsevier Churchill Livingstone, 2009.

Lorber B. "Listerosis." In *Cecil Medicine*, 24th ed., edited by Lee Goldman and Andrew I. Schafer. Philadelphia: Saunders Elsevier, 2008.

Ryser, Elliott T., and Elmer H. Marth, eds. *Listeria, Listeriosis, and Food Safety*, 3rd ed. Boca Raton, FL: CRC Press, 2007.

Walker, W. Allan. *The Harvard Medical School Guide to Healthy Eating during Pregnancy*. New York: McGraw-Hill, 2006.

PERIODICALS

Allerberger, F., and M. Wagner. "Listeriosis: A Resurgent Foodborne Infection." *Clinical Microbiology and Infection* 16 (January 2010): 16–23.

Bortolussi R. "Listeriosis: A Primer." *Canadian Medical Association Journal* 179, no. 8 (2008):795–97.

Chan, Y. C., and M. Wiedmann. "Physiology and Genetics of *Listeria monocytogenes* Survival and Growth at Cold Temperatures." *Critical Reviews in Food Science and Nutrition* 49 (March 2009): 237–53.

Freitag, N. E., et al. "*Listeria monocytogenes*—From Saprophyte to Intracellular Pathogen." *Nature Reviews. Microbiology* 7 (September 2009): 623–28.

McClure, E. M., and R. L. Goldenberg. "Infection and Stillbirth." *Seminars in Fetal and Neonatal Medicine* 14 (August 2009): 182–89.

Posfay-Barbe, K. M., and E. R. Wald. "Listeriosis." *Seminars in Fetal and Neonatal Medicine* 14 (August 2009): 228–33.

Sleator, R. D., et al. "The Interaction between *Listeria monocytogenes* and the Host Gastrointestinal Tract." *Microbiology* 155 (August 2009): 2463–75.

Wilson, J., and J. S. Brownstein. "Early Detection of Disease Outbreaks Using the Internet." *Canadian Medical Association Journal* 180 (April 14, 2009): 829–31.

WEBSITES

Centers for Disease Control and Prevention (CDC). "Listeriosis." http://www.cdc.gov/nczved/divisions/dfbmd/diseases/listeriosis/ (accessed March 20, 2012).

Food and Drug Administration (FDA). "Listeria." http://www.fda.gov/ForConsumers/ByAudience/ForWomen/ucm118542.htm (accessed March 20, 2012).

Mayo Clinic. "Listeria Infection." http://www.mayoclinic.com/health/listeria–infection/DS00963 (accessed March 20, 2012).

Weinstein, Karen B., and Joanna Ortiz. "*Listeria monocytogenes*." eMedicine. (June 23, 2008). http://emedicine.medscape.com/article/220684–overview (accessed March 20, 2012).

ORGANIZATIONS

American College of Emergency Physicians (ACEP), 1125 Executive Cir., Irving, TX 75038-2522, (972) 550-0911, (800) 798-1822, Fax: (972) 580-2816, http://www.acep.org

American Veterinary Medical Association (AVMA), 1931 North Meacham Rd., Ste. 100, Schaumburg, IL 60173-4360, (847) 925-8070, Fax: (847) 925-1329, avmainfo@avma.org, http://www.avma.org

Centers for Disease Control and Prevention, 1600 Clifton Rd., Atlanta, GA 30333, (800) CDC-INFO (232-4636), cdcinfor@cdc.gov, http://www.cdc.gov

Food and Drug Administration, 10903 New Hampshire Ave., Silver Spring, MD USA 20993-0002, (888) INFO-FDA (463-6332), http://www.fda.gov

National Institute of Allergy and Infectious Diseases (NIAID), 6610 Rockledge Dr., MSC 6612, Bethesda, MD 20892-6612, (301) 496-5717, (866) 284-4107, Fax: (301) 402-3573, http://www3.niaid.nih.gov

World Health Organization (WHO), Avenue Appia 20, 1211 Geneva 27, Switzerland, + 41 22 791 21 11, Fax: + 41 22 791 31 11, info@who.int, http://www.who.int/en.

Belinda Rowland, PhD
Rebecca J. Frey, PhD
Karl Finley

Lyme disease

Definition

Lyme disease is an infection transmitted by the bite of ticks carrying the spiral-shaped bacterium *Borrelia burgdorferi*. The disease is characterized initially by a rash followed by flulike symptoms including fever, joint **pain**, and headache. The effects of this infection can be long-term and disabling and can include chronic arthritis and nerve and heart dysfunction, unless it is recognized and treated properly with **antibiotics**.

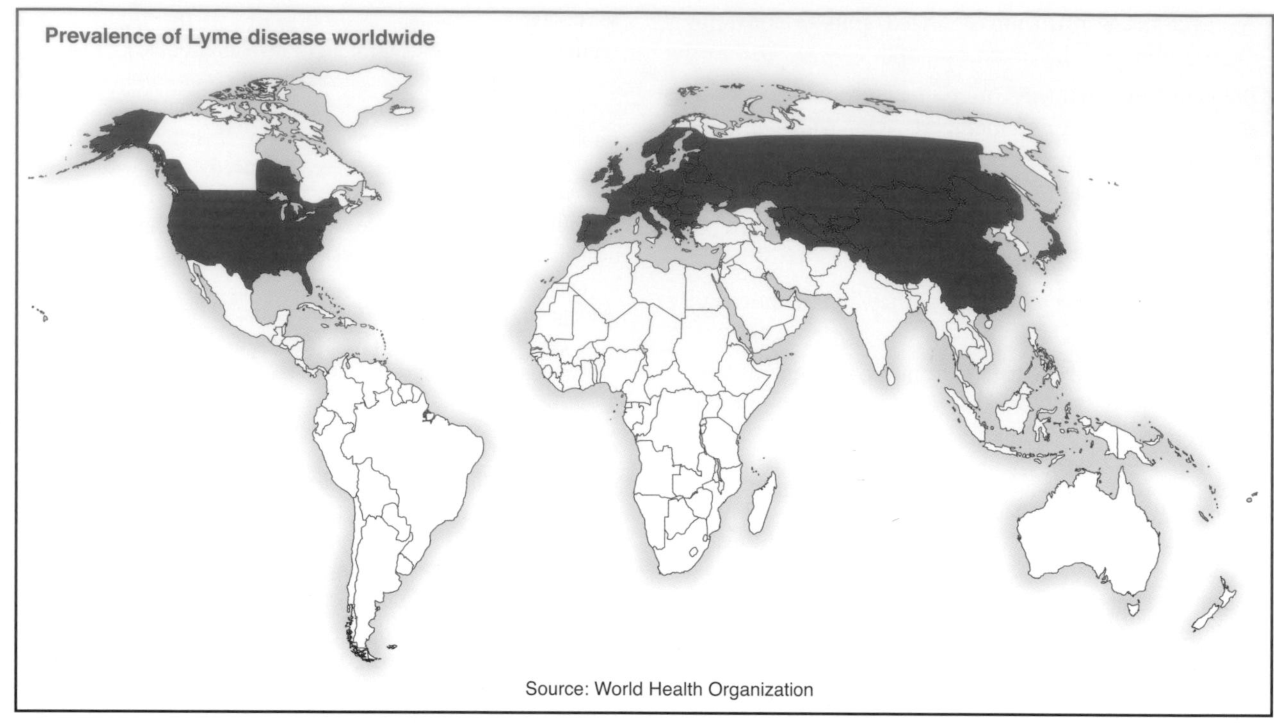

(Illustration by Electronic Illustrators Group. © 2013 Cengage Learning)

Demographics

The true incidence of Lyme disease is not known, because no test is 100% diagnostic for the disease, and many of its symptoms mimic those of many other diseases. Cases of Lyme disease have been reported in 49 of the 50 states (Montana has not reported cases); however, distribution is not uniform. The United States **Centers for Disease Control and Prevention (CDC)** report that 93% of cases come from 10 states: Connecticut, Delaware, Maryland, Massachusetts, Minnesota, New Jersey, New York, Pennsylvania, Rhode Island, and Wisconsin. Oregon and northern California also report a significant number of cases.

Prevalence estimates range for 4 in 100,000 **population** to 9.1 per 100,000 population. In states where Lyme disease is more common, the rate can be as high as 37.4 per 100,000 population. In 2011, 24,364 new cases were reported in the United States. Some epidemiologists believe that the actual incidence of Lyme disease in the United States may be 5–10 times greater than that reported by the **CDC**. The reasons for this difference include the narrowness of the CDC's case definition as well as frequent misdiagnoses of the disease.

Lyme disease has also been found in Canada, most countries in continental Europe, some countries of the former Soviet Union, Japan, China, and Australia. In Europe the disease has been found in Austria, Germany, Poland, Finland, and Norway, The highest rate reported as of mid-2010 was in Slovenia, where there were an estimated 206 cases per 100,000 population and in Austria where there were 135 cases per 100,000 population.

Lyme disease affects men and women equally. People ages 5–14 and 50–59 are most likely to contract Lyme disease because these groups are more likely to participate in outdoor activities where they are exposed to ticks. About one-quarter of cases occur in children under age 5, while the fewest cases are reported in the 20–24 year old age group.

Description

Lyme is named for Lyme, Connecticut, the town where it was first diagnosed in 1975 after a puzzling outbreak of arthritis. The organism causing the disease is named for its discoverer, Willy Burgdorfer. Lyme disease, which is also called Lyme borreliosis, is a vector-borne disease, which means that it is delivered from one host to another. It is also classified as a **zoonosis**, which is a disease of animals that can be transmitted to humans under natural conditions. In this case, a tick bearing the *B. burgdorferi* organism inserts it into a host's bloodstream when it bites the host to feed on its blood. It is important

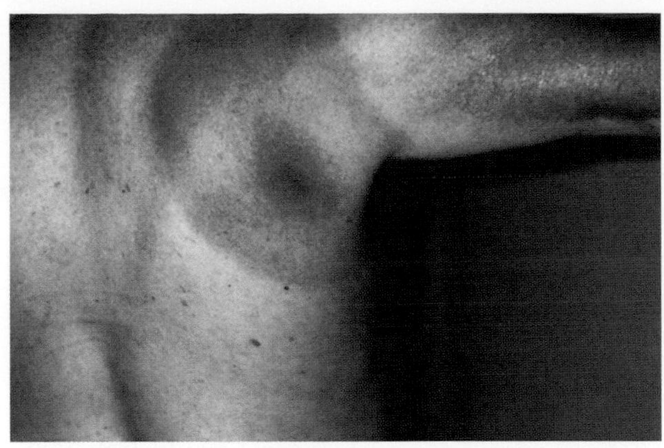

A patient presents with Lyme disease, displaying symptoms on his posterior right shoulder region. *(©CDC/ Anna Perez)*

to note that neither *B. burgdorferi* nor Lyme disease can be transmitted directly from one person to another or from pets to humans.

In the United States, Lyme disease accounts for more than 90% of all reported vector-borne illnesses. It is a significant public health problem and continues to be diagnosed in increasing numbers. The CDC attributes this increase to the growing size of the deer herd and the geographical spread of infected ticks rather than to improved diagnosis.

Risk factors

People who spend a lot of time outdoors in wooded areas are at greatest risk of encountering ticks and developing Lyme disease. The risk for acquiring Lyme disease also depends on what stage in its life cycle a tick has reached. A tick passes through three stages of development—larva, nymph, and adult—each of which is dependent on a live host for food. In the United States, *B. burgdorferi* is borne by ticks of several species in the genus *Ixodes*, which usually feed on the white-footed mouse and deer (and are often called deer ticks). In the summer, the larval ticks hatch from eggs laid in the ground and feed by attaching themselves to small animals and birds. At this stage they are not a problem for humans. It is the next stage—the nymph—that causes most cases of Lyme disease. Nymphs are very active from spring through early summer, at the height of outdoor activity for most people. Because they are still quite small (less than 2 mm), they are difficult to spot, giving them ample opportunity to transmit *B. burgdorferi* while feeding. Although far more adult ticks than nymphs carry *B. burgdorferi*, the adult ticks are much larger, more easily noticed, and more likely to be removed before the 24 hours or more of continuous feeding needed to transmit *B. burgdorferi*.

Causes and symptoms

Lyme disease is caused by *B. burgdorferi*. Once *B. burgdorferi* gains entry to the body through a tick bite, it can move through the bloodstream quickly. Only 12 hours after entering the bloodstream, *B. burgdorferi* can be found in cerebrospinal fluid (which means it can affect the nervous system). Treating Lyme disease early and thoroughly is important because Lyme disease can persist for long periods within the body in a clinically latent state. That persistence explains why symptoms can recur in cycles and can flare up after months or years, even over decades. It is important to note, however, that many people who are exposed to *B. burgdorferi* do not develop the disease.

Lyme disease usually is described in terms of length of infection (time since the person was bitten by a tick infected with Lyme disease) and whether *B. burgdorferi* is localized or disseminated (spread through the body by fluids and cells carrying *B. burgdorferi*). When and how symptoms of Lyme disease appear can vary widely from patient to patient. People who experience recurrent bouts of symptoms over time are said to have chronic Lyme disease.

Early localized Lyme disease

The most recognizable indicator of Lyme disease is a rash around the site of the tick bite. Often, the tick bite has not been noticed. The eruption might be warm or may itch. The rash—erythema migrans (EM)—generally develops within 3–30 days and usually begins as a round, red patch that expands outward. About 75% of patients with Lyme disease develop EM. Clearing may take place from the center out, leaving a bull's-eye effect; in some cases, the center gets redder instead of clearing. The rash may look like a bruise on people with dark skin. Of those who develop Lyme disease, about 50% notice flu-like symptoms, including fatigue, headache, chills and fever, muscle and joint pain, and lymph node swelling. However, a rash at the site can also be an allergic reaction to the tick saliva rather than an indicator of Lyme disease, particularly if the rash appears in less than three days and disappears only days later.

Late disseminated disease and chronic Lyme disease

Weeks, months, or even years after an untreated tick bite, symptoms can appear in several forms, including:

- Fatigue, forgetfulness, confusion, mood swings, irritability, numbness.

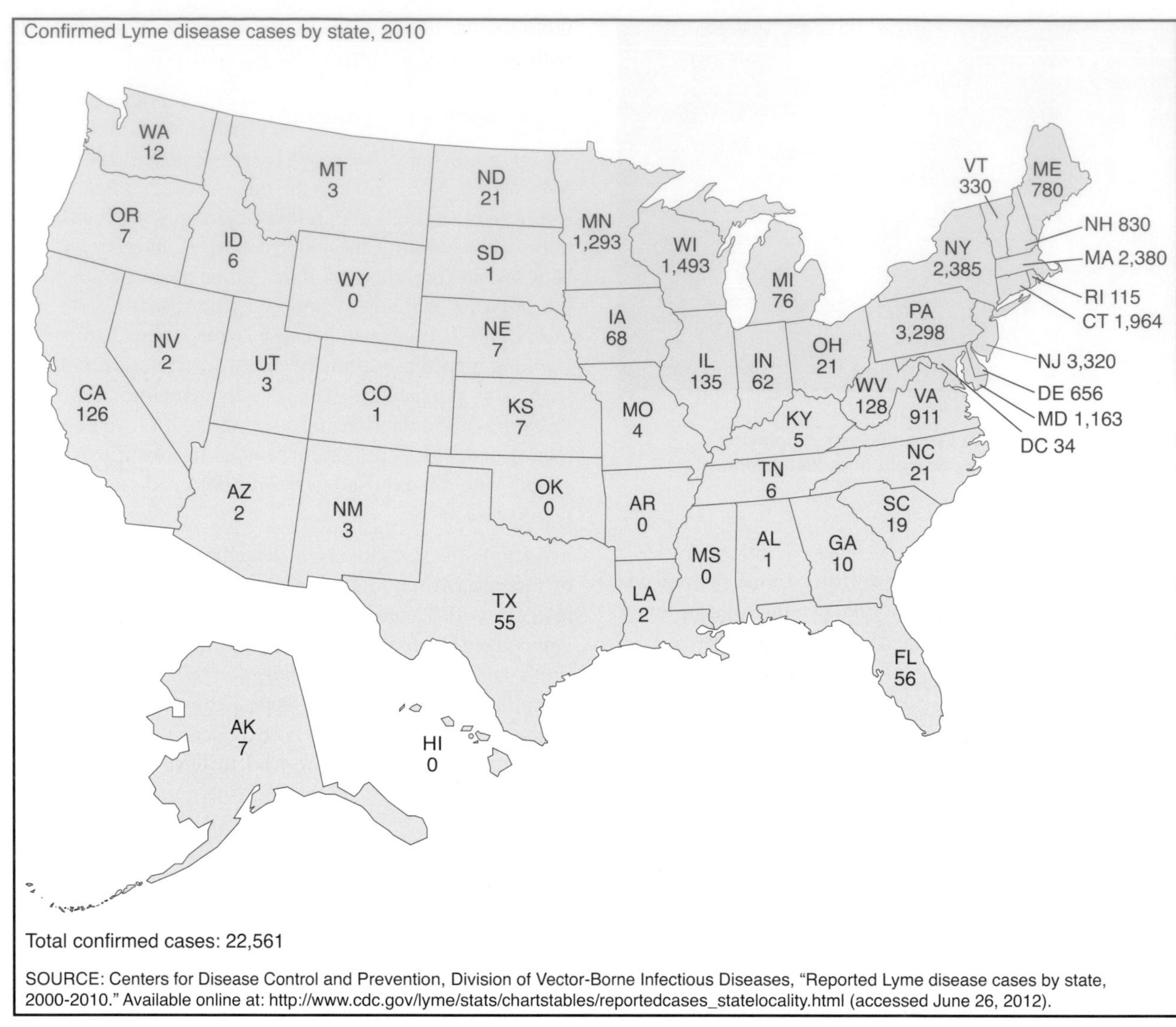

(Illustration by Electronic Illustrators Group. © 2013 Cengage Learning)

- Neurologic problems, such as pain (unexplained and not triggered by an injury), Bell's palsy (facial paralysis, usually one-sided but may be on both sides), and a mimicking of the inflammation of brain membranes known as meningitis; (fever, severe headache).
- Arthritis (short episodes of pain and swelling in joints) and other musculoskeletal complaints. Arthritis eventually develops in about 60% of patients with untreated Lyme disease.

Less common effects of Lyme disease are heart abnormalities such as irregular rhythm (arrhythmias) or cardiac block and eye abnormalities such as swelling of the cornea, tissue, or eye muscles and nerves.

A late-stage complication of Lyme disease that affects the skin is acrodermatitis chronica atrophicans, a disorder in which the skin on the person's lower legs or hands becomes inflamed and paper-thin. This disorder is seen more frequently in Europe than in the United States.

Diagnosis

Examination

A clear diagnosis of Lyme disease can be difficult and relies on information the patient provides and the doctor's clinical judgment, particularly through elimination of other possible causes of the symptoms. Lyme disease may mimic other conditions, including chronic fatigue syndrome (CFS), multiple sclerosis (MS), and other diseases with many symptoms involving multiple body systems. Differential diagnosis (distinguishing Lyme disease from other diseases) is based on clinical evaluation with laboratory tests used for clarification, when necessary.

Doctors generally know which disease-causing organisms are common in their geographic area. The most helpful piece of information is whether a tick bite or rash was noticed and whether it happened locally or while traveling. Doctors may not consider Lyme disease if it is rare locally, but will take it into account if a patient mentions vacationing in an area where the disease is commonly found.

Children may have difficulty effectively verbalizing their symptoms and as such, their symptoms may be misdiagnosed. Parents who suspect Lyme disease in their children should inform their doctor about the possibility of the disease and be proactive in requesting further medical evaluation and treatment.

Tests

As of 2010, the United States Food and Drug Administration (FDA) had approved two blood tests for Lyme disease. These tests look for antigens (substances that stimulate the production of antibodies) produced by *B. burgdorferi* rather than for the bacterium itself. Prevue B is a rapid test that can give results within one hour. The C6 Lyme Peptide ELISA (enzyme-linked immunosorbent assay) test takes longer to give results, but is more sensitive. A positive result from either test can be confirmed by a second blood test known as the Western blot test, which must be done in a laboratory.

Early diagnosis and prompt treatment are critical to preventing the neurologic complications of Lyme disease. Fewer than 50% of children realize that they have been bitten by a tick. Any child that develops a round, bull's-eye skin rash, joint pain, flu-like symptoms, and/or neurologic symptoms should see a doctor. Because the rash may not be readily visible (e.g., on the scalp under hair), children living in or visiting areas with a high incidence of Lyme disease and those participating in frequent outdoor activities during active tick months who develop joint pain and neurologic symptoms should see a doctor.

Treatment

Traditional

Immediate removal of an attached tick is the first step in treatment for people who know they have been bitten. Because black-legged ticks are slow feeders, it takes about 36 hours for *B. burgdorferi* to make its way into the body; infection is unlikely if the tick is removed within 24 hours of attachment. People who find ticks on themselves should *not* use a hot match, petroleum jelly, nail polish, or similar items to remove the tick. They should use fine-tipped tweezers, grasp the tick as close to the skin as possible, and pull the tick away from the skin with a steady motion. The area should then be cleansed with an antiseptic.

Because most children do not realize they have been in tick-infested areas or been bitten by a tick and because deer ticks can be the size of a poppy seed or smaller, parents should be diligent about checking children for ticks, especially if the family lives in or visits an area with a high incidence of Lyme disease or an area near tick habitats.

Drugs

For most patients, initial therapy consists of oral antibiotics such as doxycycline (Doryx, Vibramycin) or amoxicillin (Amoxil, Trimox) for 14–21 days. If the response is poor, alternative antibiotics such as Cefuroxime axetil (Ceftin), Clarithromycin (Biaxin), or azithromycin (Zithromax) are tried. When symptoms indicate nervous system involvement or a severe episode of Lyme disease, intravenous antibiotics such as ceftriaxone (Rocephin), cefotaxime (Claforan), or intravenous penicillin may be given for 14–30 days.

The physician may have to adjust the treatment regimen or change medications based on the patient's response. Treatment can be difficult because *B. burgdorferi* comes in several strains, some may react to different antibiotics than others. Also, *B. burgdorferi* can shut itself up in cell niches, allowing it to hide from antibiotics. Finally, antibiotics can kill *B. burgdorferi* only while it is active rather than dormant.

Lyme disease during pregnancy

Untreated Lyme disease during pregnancy may lead to infection of the placenta and possibly a stillbirth. However, no adverse effects on a fetus have been found in cases where the mother receives appropriate antibiotic treatment for her Lyme disease. In general, treatment for pregnant women with Lyme disease is similar to that of non-pregnant adults, although certain antibiotics, such as doxycycline, that can affect fetal development should not be used because they can affect fetal development. There have been no cases reported of Lyme disease being transmitted through breast milk.

Complementary and alternative treatments

Antibiotic therapy is essential in treating Lyme disease; however, complementary therapies may minimize symptoms of Lyme disease or improve the immune response. These include vitamin and nutritional supplements, mostly for chronic fatigue and increased susceptibility to infection. For example, yogurt and *Lactobacillus acidophilus* preparations help fight yeast infections, which are common in people on long-term antibiotic therapy. In

KEY TERMS

Antibody—A protein normally produced by the immune system to fight infection or rid the body of foreign material. The material that stimulates the production of antibodies is called an antigen. Specific antibodies are produced in response to each different antigen and can only inactivate that particular antigen.

Antigen—Any foreign substance, usually a protein, that stimulates the body's immune system to produce antibodies.

Babesiosis—A disease caused by protozoa of the genus *Babesia* characterized by a malaria-like fever, anemia, vomiting, muscle pain, and enlargement of the spleen. Babesiosis, like Lyme disease, is carried by a tick.

Bell's palsy—Facial paralysis or weakness with a sudden onset, caused by swelling or inflammation of the seventh cranial nerve, which controls the facial muscles. Disseminated Lyme disease sometimes causes Bell's palsy.

Blood-brain barrier—A specialized, semi-permeable layer of cells around the blood vessels in the brain that controls which substances can leave the circulatory system and enter the brain.

Cerebrospinal fluid—A clear fluid that fills the hollow cavity inside the brain and spinal cord. The cerebrospinal fluid has several functions, including providing a cushion for the brain against shock or impact, and removing waste products from the brain.

Disseminated—Scattered or distributed throughout the body. Lyme disease that has progressed beyond the stage of localized EM is said to be disseminated.

ELISA protocols—ELISA is an acronym for "enzyme-linked immunosorbent assay"; it is a highly sensitive technique for detecting and measuring antigens or antibodies in a solution.

Erythema migrans (EM)—A red skin rash that is one of the first signs of Lyme disease in about 75% of patients.

Lymph nodes—Small, bean-shaped masses of tissue scattered along the lymphatic system that act as filters and immune monitors, removing fluids, bacteria, or cancer cells that travel through the lymph system.

Opportunistic infection—An infection by organisms that usually do not cause infection in people whose immune systems are working normally.

Vector—An animal carrier that transfers an infectious organism from one host to another. The vector that transmits Lyme disease from wildlife to humans is the deer tick or black-legged tick.

Zoonosis (plural, zoonoses)—Any disease of animals that can be transmitted to humans under natural conditions. Lyme disease and babesiosis are examples of zoonoses.

addition, botanical medicine and homeopathy can be considered to help bring the body's systems back to a state of health and well being. A Western herb, spilanthes (*Spilanthes* spp.), may have an effect on diseases like Lyme disease that are caused by spirochetes (spiral-shaped bacteria), although this effect has not been proven to the satisfaction of practitioners of conventional medicine.

Other complementary and alternative therapies used in treating Lyme disease include:

- Chinese medicine. Formulae used to treat systemic bacterial infections include Wu Wei Xiao Du Yin (Five-Ingredient Decoction to Eliminate Toxin), Yin Hua Jie Du Tang (Honeysuckle Decoction to Relieve Toxicity), and Huang Lian Jie Du Tang (Coptis Decoction to Relieve Toxicity). Inflammation at the site of infection may be treated externally with Yu Lu San (Jade Dew Extract) or Jin Huang San (Golden Yellow Powder). Specific Chinese herbs and treatments can be used for specific symptoms. For examples, for systemic bacterial infection, one may use honeysuckle flower, forsythia, isatidis, scutellaria, and phellodendron. Acupuncture and ear acupuncture treatments are also used.
- Herbals. Botanical remedies include Echinacea (*Echinacea* species) to clear infection and boost the immune system, goldenseal (*Hydrastis canadensis*) to clear infection and boost the immune system, garlic to clear bacterial infection, and spilanthes (*Spilanthes* species) for spirochete infections.
- Hydrotherapy. The joint pain associated with Lyme disease can be treated with hydrotherapy. Dull, penetrating pain may be relieved by applying a warm compress to the affected area. Sharp, intense pain may be relieved by applying an ice pack to the affected area.
- Guided imagery. The patient may treat Lyme disease by visualizing Bb as looking like ticks swimming in the bloodstream being killed by the flame of a candle.

- Probiotics. Probiotics is treatment with beneficial microbes either by ingestion or through a suppository. Probiotics can restore a healthy balance of bacteria to the body in cases in which long-term antibiotic use has caused diarrhea or yeast infection. Yogurt or *Lactobacillus acidophilus* preparations may be ingested.

Public health role and response

Lyme disease is a reportable disease, with the requirements for reporting determined by state laws and regulations. In most states Lyme disease cases are reported by licensed health care providers, diagnostic laboratories, or hospitals. All personally identifiable information is removed from the reports before the information is provided to the CDC, which compiles and publishes the national surveillance data. The goal of Lyme disease surveillance is not to capture every case, but to systematically gather and analyze public health data in a way that enables public health officials to look for trends and take actions to reduce the disease and improve public health.

The United States CDC has developed a program of service, research, and education focusing on the **prevention** and control of Lyme disease. Activities of this program include:

- maintaining and analyzing national surveillance data for Lyme disease
- conducting epidemiologic investigations
- offering diagnostic and reference laboratory services
- developing and testing strategies for the control and prevention of this disease in humans
- supporting education of the public and health care providers.

Many states in the United States have also developed educational programs concerning Lyme disease for its citizens.

Prognosis

If aggressive antibiotic therapy is given early, and the patient cooperates fully and sticks to the medication regimen, recovery should be complete. Only a small percentage of Lyme disease patients fail to respond or relapse (have recurring episodes). Most long-term effects of the disease result when diagnosis and treatment is delayed or missed. Co-infection with other infectious organisms spread by ticks in the same areas as *B. burgdorferi* (babesiosis and ehrlichiosis, for instance) may be responsible for treatment failures or more severe symptoms. Most fatalities reported with Lyme disease involved patients co-infected with babesiosis.

QUESTIONS TO ASK YOUR DOCTOR

- I've been bitten by a tick. Do I have Lyme Disease?
- Can Lyme disease be transmitted sexually?
- Can Lyme disease be transmitted during a blood donation?
- Is it true that you can get Lyme disease anywhere in the United States?
- I have heard that the diagnostic tests that the CDC recommends for testing are not very accurate. Can I be treated based on my symptoms or do I need to use a different test?
- I am pregnant and just found out I have Lyme disease. What should I do?
- If I have been diagnosed with Lyme disease, do I need to get tested for other tickborne diseases (coinfections)?
- I have been sick for a few years with joint and muscle pain, fatigue, and difficulty thinking. I was tested for Lyme disease using a Western Blot test. The "IgM" Western Blot test was positive but the "IgG" Western Blot test was negative. Is Lyme disease the cause of my symptoms?
- Where can I get a test to make sure that I am cured?
- My serologic (blood) test for Lyme disease is still positive even though I finished three weeks of antibiotics. Does this mean I am still infected?
- I heard that if I get Lyme disease I will always have it. Is that true?

Prevention

Minimizing risk of exposure

Precautions to avoid contact with ticks include moving leaves and brush away from living quarters. Most important are personal protection techniques when outdoors, such as:

- spraying tick repellent on clothing and exposed skin
- wearing light-colored clothing to maximize ability to see ticks
- tucking pant legs into socks or boot top
- checking children and pets frequently for ticks
- inspecting each individual living in high-risk areas daily for ticks in the spring and summer

Minimizing risk of disease

The two most important factors are removing the tick quickly and carefully, and seeking a doctor's evaluation at the first sign of symptoms of Lyme disease. When in an area that may be tick-populated:

- Check for ticks, particularly in the area of the groin, underarm, behind ears, and on the scalp.
- Stay calm and grasp the tick as near to the skin as possible, using tweezers.
- To minimize the risk of squeezing more bacteria into the bite, pull straight back steadily and slowly to remove the tick.
- Do not try to remove the tick by using petroleum jelly, alcohol, or a lit match.
- Place the tick in a closed container (for species identification later, should symptoms develop) or dispose of it by flushing.
- See a physician immediately for any sort of rash or patchy discoloration that appears three to 30 days after a tick bite.

A vaccine for Lyme disease was available from 1998 to 2002, when it was removed from the United States market. Protection provided by the vaccine fades over time. Anyone who was vaccinated at the time the vaccine was available likely no longer has any protection against the disease. A vaccine still exists for dogs, although veterinarians have mixed ideas about its usefulness.

Resources

BOOKS

Singleton, Kenneth B. *The Lyme Disease Solution*. Charleston, SC: BookSurge Publishing, 2008.

Weintraub, Pamela. *Cure Unknown: Inside the Lyme Epidemic*. New York: St. Martin's Press, 2008.

WEBSITES

Learn About Lyme Disease. United States Centers for Disease Control and Prevention. http://www.cdc.gov/ncidod/dvbid/lyme

Lyme Disease. MedlinePlus. http://www.nlm.nih.gov/medlineplus/lymedisease.html

Meyerhoff, John O. Lyme Disease. eMedicine.com. http://emedicine.medscape.com/article/330178-overview

ORGANIZATIONS

American Lyme Disease Foundation, P. O. Box 466, Lyme, CT 06371, inquire@adlf.com, http://www.aldf.com

Lyme Disease Network of NJ., 43 Winton Road, East Brunswick, NJ 08816, http://www.lymenet.org

National Institute of Allergy and Infectious Diseases Office of Communications and Government Relations, 6610 Rockledge Drive, MSC 6612, Bethesda, MD 20892-6612, (301) 496-5717, (866) 284-4107 or TDD: (800)877-8339 (for hearing impaired), Fax: (301) 402-3573, http://www3.niaid.nih.gov

United States Centers for Disease Control and Prevention (CDC), 1600 Clifton Road, Atlanta, GA 30333, (404) 639-3534, 800-CDC-INFO (800-232-4636). TTY: (888) 232-6348, inquiry@cdc.gov, http://www.cdc.gov.

Rebecca J. Frey, Ph.D.
Jennifer E. Sisk, M.A.
Tish Davidson, A.M.
Judith L. Sims